Pediatric Radiation Oncology

Fourth Edition

Edward C. Halperin, M.D.

Vice Dean of the School of Medicine
Associate Vice Chancellor for Health Affairs
R.J. Reynolds Professor of Medical Education
Professor, Department of Radiation Oncology
Professor, Department of Pediatrics
Duke University Medical Center
Durham, North Carolina

Louis S. Constine, M.D.

Professor of Radiation Oncology and Pediatrics
Section Chief, Pediatric Radiation Oncology
Vice Chair, Department of Radiation Oncology
James P. Wilmot Cancer Center
University of Rochester Medical Center
Rochester, New York

Nancy J. Tarbell, M.D.

Professor of Radiation Oncology
Head, Pediatric Radiation Oncology Unit
Director, Office for Women's Careers
Massachusetts General Hospital
Harvard Medical School
Boston, Massachusetts

Larry E. Kun, M.D.

Chairman, Department of Radiological Sciences
St. Jude Children's Research Hospital
Professor, Departments of Radiology and Pediatrics
University of Tennessee College of Medicine
Memphis, Tennessee

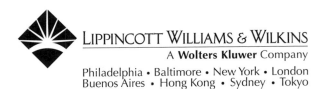

LIPPINCOTT WILLIAMS & WILKINS
A **Wolters Kluwer** Company

Philadelphia • Baltimore • New York • London
Buenos Aires • Hong Kong • Sydney • Tokyo

Acquisitions Editor: Jonathan Pine
Developmental Editor: Maureen Iannuzzi
Production Editor: Frank Aversa
Compositor: Graphic World
Printer: Edwards Brothers

© 2005 by LIPPINCOTT WILLIAMS & WILKINS
530 Walnut Street
Philadelphia, PA 19106 USA
LWW.com

Printed in the USA

Previous editions published: 1999, 1994, 1986

Library of Congress Cataloging-in-Publication Data

Care has been taken to confirm the accuracy of the information presented and to describe generally accepted practices. However, the editors, authors and publisher are not responsible for errors or omissions or for any consequences from application of the information in this book and make no warranty, expressed or implied, with respect to the currency, completeness, or accuracy of the contents of the publication. Application of this information in a particular situation remains the professional responsibility of the practitioner.

The editors, authors and publisher have exerted every effort to ensure that drug selection and dosage set forth in this text are in accordance with current recommendations and practice at the time of publication. However, in view of ongoing research, changes in government regulations, and the constant flow of information relating to drug therapy and drug reactions, the reader is urged to check the package insert for each drug for any change in indications and dosage and for added warnings and precautions. This is particularly important when the recommended agent is a new or infrequently employed drug.

Some drugs and medical devices presented in this publication have Food and Drug Administration (FDA) clearance for limited use in restricted research settings. It is the responsibility of the health care provider to ascertain the FDA status of each drug or device planned for use in their clinical practice.

10 9 8 7 6 5 4 3 2 1

For our children

Contents

Contributing Authors

Smita Bhatia, MD, MPH   *Director of Epidemiology and Outcomes Research, Division of Pediatric Hematology, Oncology and Bone Marrow Transplantation, City of Hope National Medical Center, Duarte, California*

Louis S. Constine, MD   *Department of Radiation Oncology, University of Rochester Medical Center, Rochester, New York*

Debra L. Friedman, MD   *Department of Pediatrics, Children's Hospital & Regional Medical Center, Division of Hematology/Oncology, Seattle, Washington*

Alison M. Friedmann, MD   *Pediatric Hematology/Oncology, Massachusetts General Hospital, Harvard Medical School, Boston, Massachusetts*

Daphne Haas-Kogan, MD   *Department of Radiation Oncology, University of California, San Francisco, San Francisco, California*

Edward C. Halperin, MD   *Department of Radiation Oncology, Duke University Medical Center, Durham, North Carolina*

Melissa M. Hudson, MD   *St. Jude Children's Research Hospital, Memphis, Tennessee*

John P. Kirkpatrick, MD, PhD   *Department of Radiation Oncology, Duke University Medical Center, Durham, North Carolina*

Larry E. Kun, MD   *Department of Radiological Sciences, Division of Radiation Oncology, St. Jude Children's Research Hospital, Memphis, Tennessee*

Kim Light, CMD   *Department of Radiation, Duke University; Duke University Medical Center, Durham, North Carolina*

Karen J. Marcus, MD   *Department of Radiation Oncology, Children's Hospital, Harvard Medical School, Boston, Massachusetts*

Katherine K. Matthay, MD   *Department of Pediatrics, University of California, San Francisco, San Francisco, California*

Scott R. Schulman, MD   *Departments of Anesthesiology and Pediatrics, Duke University Medical Center, Durham, North Carolina*

Nancy J. Tarbell, MD   *Department of Radiation Oncology and Office for Women's Careers, Massachusetts General Hospital, Harvard Medical School, Boston, Massachusetts*

Howard J. Weinstein, MD   *Pediatric Hematology/Oncology, Massachusetts General Hospital, Harvard Medical School, Boston, Massachusetts*

Preface

In 1986, we conceived the idea of a new textbook of pediatric radiation oncology. There was no shortage of general textbooks in radiation oncology at that time. There were, in fact, several in existence and many more to come. There was not, however, a textbook specifically devoted to the use of radiation therapy for the treatment of childhood cancer. The texts that were available in the marketplace of the mid-1980s were largely devoted to adult cancer. We believed that there was a need for a focused text in pediatric radiation oncology and we set out to write it.

Dr. Halperin contacted multiple medical publishing companies in the United States in an attempt to "sell the idea." The initial sample chapter, prepared with the proposal letter, eventually became chapter 17, "Langerhan's Cell Histiocytosis." Most publishing companies were impressed with the merit of the proposal but, paradoxically, most rejected the idea on the grounds that the market was too small to sustain a book of this type. Ultimately, Raven Press of New York agreed to publish the book. Dr. Halperin was joined in the project by Drs. Kun, Tarbell, and Constine, and the first edition of *Pediatric Radiation Oncology* went on sale in 1989.

Most clinical oncology textbooks are hefty tomes, edited by several physicians, with each chapter assigned to individual authors so that the book is written by one to three dozen experts. For the reader to do justice to any individual chapter, several hours of study are required. From its inception, our concept for *Pediatric Radiation Oncology* was at variance with this common textbook practice. We believed that a text was needed wherein each section, individually devoted to a specific tumor type, could be read at one sitting. We imagined the need of a house officer or practitioner, confronted with a case of childhood cancer at the end of a busy clinical day, and preparing to present the case the next day at morning rounds; time did not allow for a long trip to the library or hours at the computer, the downloading or copying of multiple articles from the primary literature, their synthesis, and the formulation of a case management plan by morning. We felt that we could and should write a book wherein this hypothetical clinician could find enough background information to understand the disease he or she faced, what was called for in diagnostic and staging studies, what the treatment strategy ought to be, and when and how to employ radiation therapy. By morning rounds the physician could not presume himself/herself to be an expert, but could present himself/herself as informed, competent, and ready to explore the topic in more depth.

As we conceived this book, we felt that it would be best written by a team. The chapters should reflect controversies in management and all major sides of an issue should be presented so that the reader may form their own opinion. We did not, and do not, shirk from offering our opinion on many topics of controversy, but we have striven to be fair to alternative views. This book is intentionally not a practice of pediatric radiation oncology book, i.e., a formulaic book that represents the treatment philosophy of one institution. We have tried to write all the chapters with a common voice, avoiding repetition and maintaining reasonable uniformity of style. We have included tables and illustrations that might be classified as historical. We believe that it is instructive and humbling to see how much was known about childhood cancer by our forebears in this discipline.

The response to our vision, as expressed in the first three editions of *Pediatric Radiation Oncology*, has been gratifying. We believe that the book has found a niche in the medical literature. We have been honored by supportive reviews and gracious praise and have benefitted from the many helpful suggestions we have received from readers over the past years. The selection of the book for the Association of Residents in Radiation Oncology (ARRO)'s "you should have" has been particularly appreciated. Buoyed by the medical community's support of the first three editions, and persuaded that new knowledge in the specialty warranted a thoroughly updated text, we undertook this fourth edition of *Pediatric Radiation Oncology.*

It is hard to believe that over eighteen years has passed since we began the first edition of this book. It is gratifying to have witnessed how far our discipline has come, and daunting to realize how far we have to go. We hope that the first three editions of this text have contributed to an improved understanding of the benefits and risks of radiotherapy for children. We trust that the dissemination of knowledge about pediatric radiation oncology will improve the quality and quantity of life for children affected with cancer.

Edward C. Halperin, M.D.
Louis S. Constine, M.D.
Nancy J. Tarbell, M.D.
Larry E. Kun, M.D.

Acknowledgments

For those children who have taught us about life, bravery, pain, and serenity; as well as for what they have taught us about clinical pediatric radiation oncology, we are grateful beyond words. We pray that the fourth edition of *Pediatric Radiation Oncology* will serve, in the ultimate measure of our days, as some small repayment of what our patients have given to us.

Much of the preparation and collation of this fourth edition of this book was done in Durham, North Carolina, by Ruth Aultman, Heidi Oehme, and Susan Kudler. Were it not for the skill and devoted work of these ladies, the book would never have been completed. Additional manuscript preparation was done by Ann G. Muhs (Rochester) and Rebecca Bunker (Memphis). Jonathan Pine, Maurene Iannuzzi, and the staff of Lippincott, Williams & Wilkins were, at all times, courteous and helpful.

We are indebted to our teachers: J. Robert Cassady, Juan A. del Regato, Sarah Donaldson, Samuel Hellman, Henry Kaplan, Rita M. Linngood, Leon Rosenberg, Philip Rubin, Herman D. Suit, Samuel O. Thier, and John Truman.

The love of our families who have been a source of constant strength to us.

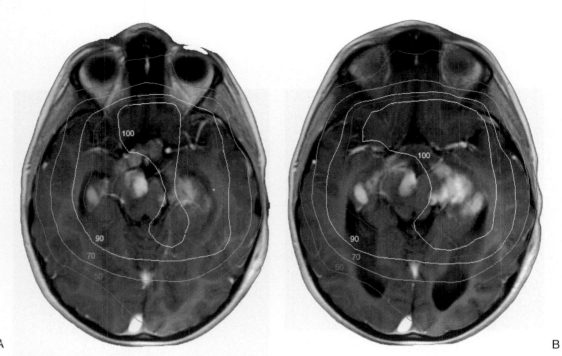

FIG. 3-4. 3D conformal radiation plan for a sizable optic pathway tumor in a 9-year-old boy. The disease involves the chiasm and the optic tracts bilaterally (to the geniculate bodies posteriorly) and the midbrain. The 95 percent volume (indicated on dosimetric plot) encompasses to planning target volume (PTV).

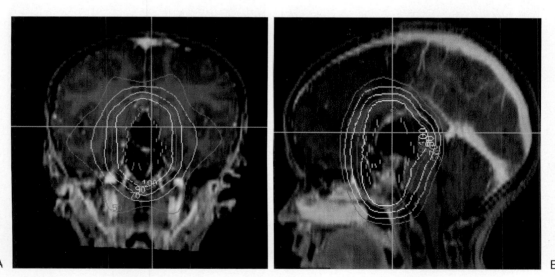

FIG. 3-10. Local irradiation for craniopharyngioma, including solid tumor and cyst extrusion into the third ventricle. The third ventricular cyst has been partially resected. The PTV (apparent as the outer hatch marks in the coronal and sagittal planes) represents the solid and residual cystic tumor (GTV) plus 5–10 mm expansion (CTV)—the inner hatch marks) and a 5 mm margin for the PTV. The 6-field 3D conformal 15 MeV plan achieve 100 percent coverage of the PTV.

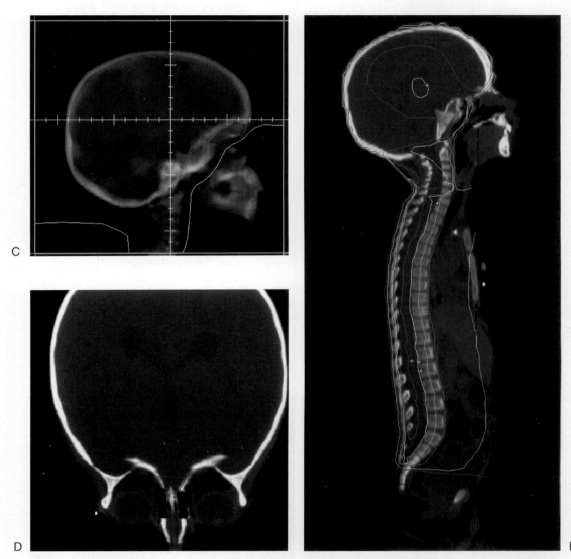

FIG. 4-4. Craniospinal irradiation (CSI) techniques, with two-dimensional fluoroscopic simulation outlining margins. **(C)** Computed tomography (CT) simulation technique for CSI: blocks derived from digital CT radiograph in treatment position, with the cribriform plate highlighted in blue derived from the axial dimension **(D). (E)** Dosage distribution through the neuraxis reflects a three-dimensional match at the craniocervical–spinal junction and use of two cranial and three spinal intensity-modulated radiation therapy components to homogenize the dosage in the subarachnoid space of the spine and calvaria.

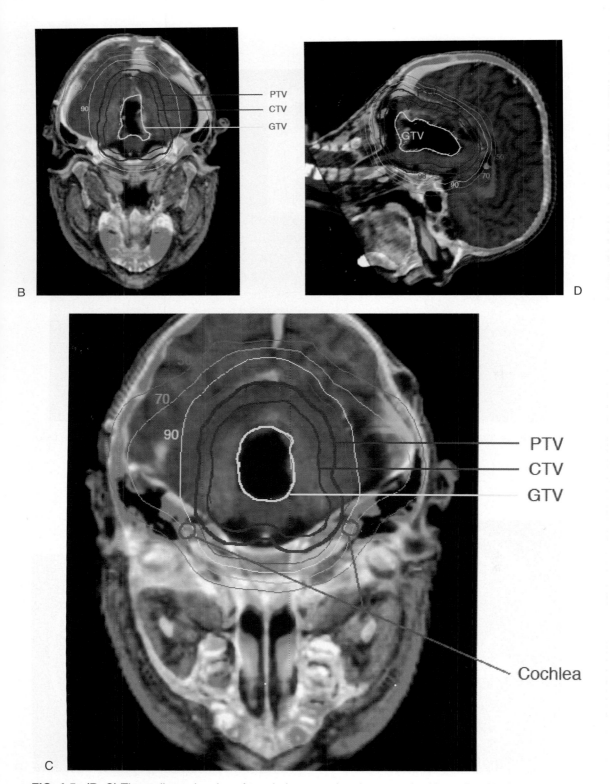

FIG. 4-5. (B, C) Three-dimensional conformal plan targeting the tumor bed is outlined in fused MRI and CT images showing the gross tumor volume as the tumor bed with a 1-cm expansion (protocol-defined) and CTV that has been anatomically corrected (to limit the CTV within the anatomic confines of the posterior fossa); a 5-mm geometric expansion defines the planning tumor volume (PTV). **(C)** The cochlea are shown on the upper axial view. Dosage distribution in axial and **(D)** sagittal projections indicates conformality of the 98–100% volume to the PTV, with lower-dose regions (50%, 30%) shown as appropriate.

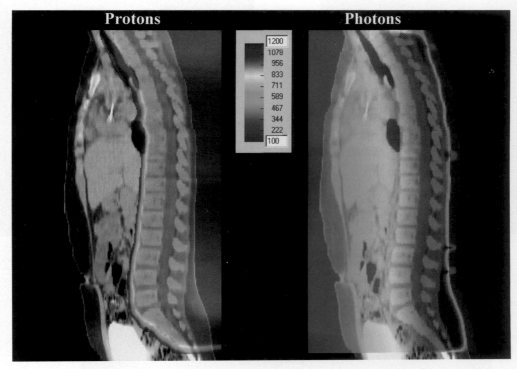

FIG. 4-6. A comparison of spinal irradiation with a posterior proton field and a posterior photon field.

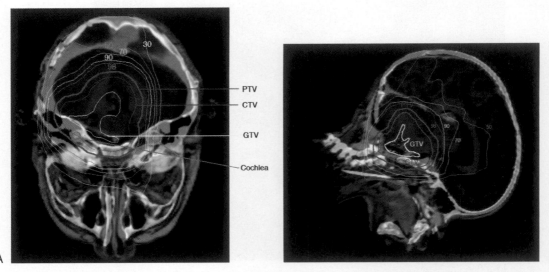

FIG. 4-12. Three-dimensional conformal radiation therapy for the fourth ventricular ependymoma following resection. The tumor bed (GTV) is here expanded by 1 cm to provide the clinical tumor volume (CTV); a 0.5 cm geometric expansion shows the planning tumor volume (PTV). Dose distributions depicted from 11-field 6 McV non-coplanar plan. Axial **(A)** and sagittal **(B)** dose distributions shown.

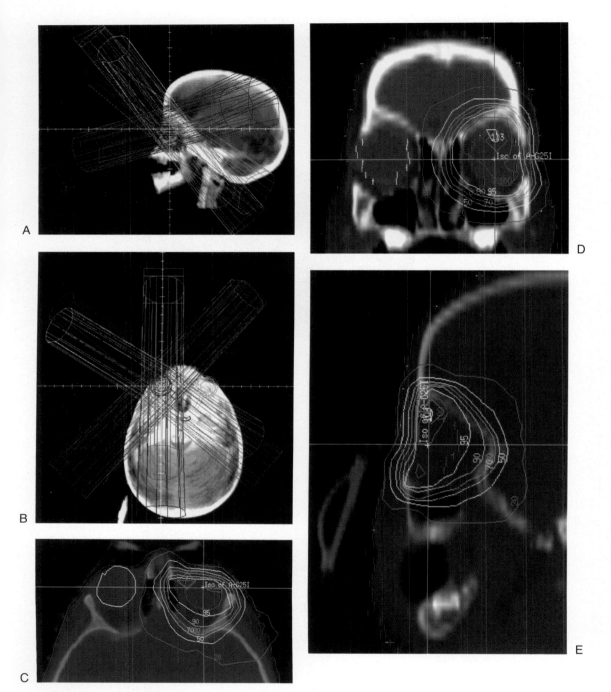

FIG. 5-20. Many centers now use conformal radiotherapy to treat retinoblastoma. Three-, five-, six-, and eight-field non-coplanar plans have been described using multileaf collimators. This plan is a six-field unilateral arrangement with non-coplanar fields. The left eye is being treated (image **B** is a view from above). **(A, B)** Reconstructed radiographs in the sagittal and axial views. **(C–E)** Dosage distributions in the axial, coronal, and sagittal views. The anesthesia mask is seen in image **E.**

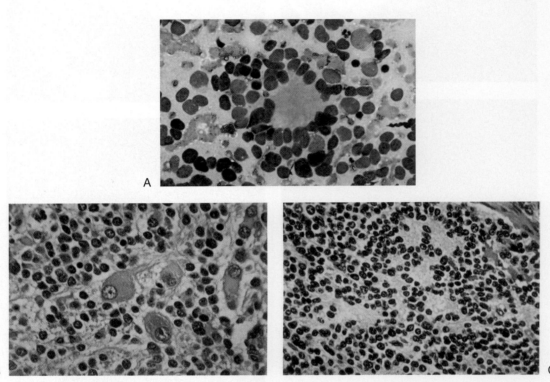

FIG. 6-4. (A) Fine-needle aspirate of neuroblastoma, showing typical Homer–Wright pseudorosettes with neurofibrillary material in the center. **(B)** Differentiating neuroblastoma, Schwannian stroma–poor. **(C)** Neuroblastoma (Schwannian stroma–poor), poorly differentiated subtype, composed of undifferentiated neuroblastic cells with clearly recognizable neuropil. (From Shimada H, Ambros IM, Dehner LP, et al. Terminology and morphologic criteria of neuroblastic tumors: recommendations by the International Neuroblastoma Pathology Committee. *Cancer* 1999;86(2):349–363, with permission.)

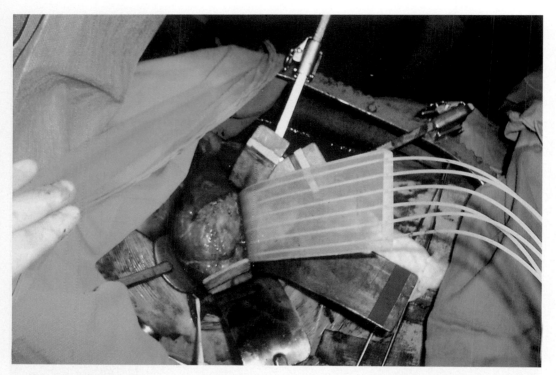

FIG. 13-11. Three weeks before birth, the patient was diagnosed with polyhydramnios. Ultrasound at birth, and periodically thereafter, showed bilateral renal enlargement. At 3 years of age bilateral solid renal masses were seen on abdominal computed tomography. Bilateral Wilms' tumors, favorable histology, were confirmed at exploratory laparotomy. She was treated with vincristine and actinomycin D and right nephrectomy. Biopsies of the left kidney were negative. She then received adriamycin. No radiotherapy was given.

Nine years later, the child, 12 years old, developed abdominal pain. She had a 16 $\times$ 9 $\times$ 16–cm left renal mass and multiple lung nodules consistent with metastases. Ultrasound-guided renal biopsy confirmed Wilms' tumor. After treatment with etoposide and carboplatin, the pulmonary nodules resolved, and the renal mass was smaller. She received 12 Gy of whole lung irradiation and 12 Gy to the left abdomen, followed by a 3-Gy boost, all at 1.5 Gy per fraction. The residual tumor was resected from the lower pole of the left kidney. Microscopic tumor was at the margin of resection. Intraoperative high–dose rate brachytherapy was administered with a 6-cm-wide applicator to the distal 5 cm of the tumor with ^{192}Ir. The dosage was 8 Gy at a depth of 0.5 cm in 403 seconds. Uninvolved tissue was shielded with lead sheets.

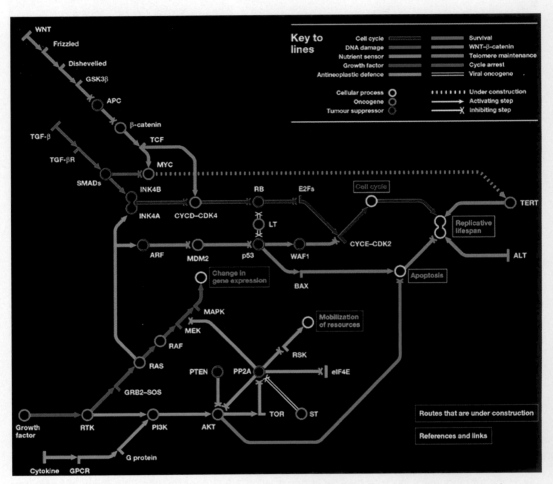

FIG. 20-1. A subway map of cancer pathways. (From Hahn W, Weinberg R. A subway map of cancer pathways. *Nat Rev Cancer* May 2002, with permission.)

1

The Cancer Problem in Children

Edward C. Halperin, M.D.

In 1900, cancer trailed typhoid fever, malaria, smallpox, measles, scarlet fever, whooping cough, diphtheria, croup, influenza, dysentery, erysipelas, tuberculosis, sexually transmitted disease, meningitis, acute bronchitis, pneumonia, accidents, birth injuries, and violence as a cause of death in children in the United States (1,2). Cancer mortality per 100,000 people in the United States and Canada from 1911 to 1916 was 3.7 for 1- to 4-year-olds, 1.4 for 5- to 9-year-olds, 1.3 for 10- to 14-year-olds, and 2.8 for 15- to 19-year-olds. Death from cancer constituted only 0.43% of mortality from all causes for these same age groups (1).

At the beginning of the twenty-first century in economically developed countries, more than 20,000 children die every year from preventable incidents such as traffic accidents, intentional injuries, drowning, falls, fire, and poisoning. The leading cause of death in children older than 1 year is murder by a close relative. The risk of a child's death from injury rises steeply with poverty. The likelihood of a child being injured and killed is also associated with single parenthood, low maternal education, young maternal age at birth, poor housing, and large family size (3).

Cancer in children has become a significant problem compared with other causes of childhood mortality (3,4). There were 8,600 new cases of cancer among children in the United States in 2001 and 1,500 to 1,700 cancer deaths (5). Cancer is the leading natural cause of death among children between the ages of 1 and 14 years in the United States (Table 1-1) (6). For the youngest children, however, cancer is not a major cause of mortality. Cancer does not even appear on the list of the ten leading causes of infant death in the United States (7). The leading causes of death in infants are congenital anomalies, disorders related to short gestation and low birth weight, and sudden infant death syndrome. In late adolescence, homicide surpasses cancer as a cause of death.

The mortality rate from cancer for children is approximately 3 deaths per 100,000 population per year (5). In the United States there are approximately 100 cancer deaths per year in 0- to 1-year-olds, 500 in 1- to 4-year-olds, and 1,100 in 5- to 14-year-olds (Figs. 1-1–1-3) (8,9).

Although cancer is a major cause of childhood death in developed countries, it continues to trail infections as a cause of mortality in developing countries (10–14). In many parts of the world, nutrition, housing, climate, and sanitation conditions create childhood mortality statistics similar to those reported for industrialized countries in the early twentieth century.

TABLE 1-1. *The five leading causes of death in 1- to 19-year-olds by sex, United States, 1999*

Male		Female	
Accidents	7,725	Accidents	3,952
Homicide	2,192	Cancer	945
Suicide	1,541	Homicide	709
Cancer	1,230	Congenital anomalies	535
Congenital anomalies	664	Heart disease	365

Data from Jemal A, Thomas A, Murray T, et al. Cancer statistics, 2002. *CA Cancer J Clin* 2002;52:23–47.

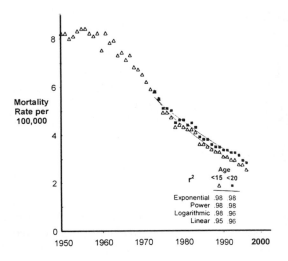

FIG. 1-1. Annual cancer mortality rates since 1944 among Americans younger than 15 years of age who were diagnosed between 1973 and 1996 *(lower curve)* and those less than 20 years of age when diagnosed in the same interval *(upper curve)* show a continuous downward trend. Changes in the mortality rate may be a function of improved diagnosis and treatment. Changes in incidence ultimately will have a direct effect on the mortality rate. For instance, a decrease in incidence lowers the mortality rate independently of any treatment advances. On the other hand, an increase in incidence raises mortality rates unless improvements in treatment overcome this effect. (From Bleyer WA. Reply: United States pediatric cancer mortality—an ominous trend? *Med Pediatr Oncol* 2001;36:337–338, with permission.)

While the incidence rate of cancers in people younger than 20 has increased since the 1970's, mortality rates are falling.

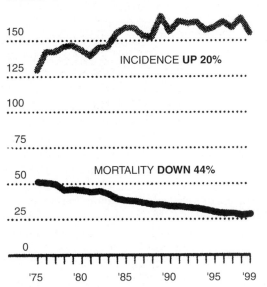

Source: National Cancer Institute

FIG. 1-2. The incidence of childhood cancer is rising in the United States while mortality rates are falling. (From Cushman JH Jr. U.S. reshaping cancer strategy as incidence in children rises. *New York Times* 1997 Sept. 29:1, with permission.)

SEER Incidence and U.S. Mortality
All Childhood Cancers, Under 20 Years of Age
Both Sexes, All Races, 1975-1999

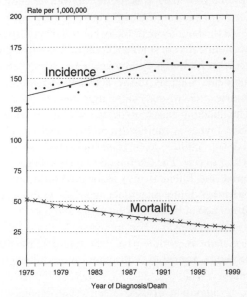

Source: SEER 9 areas and NCHS public use data file. Rates are age-adjusted to the 2000 U.S. standard million population by 5-year age groups. Regression lines are calculated using the Joinpoint Regression Program.

FIG. 1-3. A more detailed analysis of incidence and mortality rates from the Surveillance, Epidemiology, and End Results (SEER) program, using smoothed-out trend lines, confirms a rising incidence and a falling mortality rate. (SEER Cancer Statistics from http://seer.cancer.gov, http://seer.cancer.gov/iccol, and http://seer.cancer.gov/publications/childhood.)

However, it is likely that future improvements in the standard of living, the success of immunization programs, and dissemination of medical services will make inroads against infectious disease and thereby make childhood cancer a major cause of death in developing nations. Finally, there is almost certainly some variation in childhood cancer rates between countries because of differing abilities to diagnose and treat cases in different parts of the world.

THE RELATIVE FREQUENCY OF THE VARIOUS TYPES OF CHILDHOOD CANCER

The relative frequency of the various types of childhood cancer is influenced by whether we are examining incidence or mortality and by how we stratify by age, sex, or nation. Among the most commonly used data are those of the Surveillance, Epidemiology, and End Results (SEER) program. SEER is a continuing project of the Biometry Branch of the U.S. National Cancer Institute (NCI). The program draws data from several population-based cancer reporting systems covering approximately 10% of the total population of the United States (5,6,15). The adjusted relative frequency of the common forms of childhood cancer from SEER is shown in Table 1-2. Leukemias, brain and spinal tumors, lymphomas, sympathetic nervous system tumors (neuroblastoma), kidney (Wilms's) tumors, and soft tissue and bone sarcomas are the most common childhood cancers. The common epithelial tumors of adults are rare in children (Fig. 1-4).

Of the cancers that do afflict children, some are more common in specific age groups. For example, neuroblastomas are more common in infancy. The ratio of non-Hodgkin's lymphoma to Hodgkin's disease favors non-Hodgkin's lymphoma in younger children, but the reverse is true in adolescents. There is a steep rise in bone cancers among children ages 11 through 15, which coincides with the adolescent growth spurt.

Childhood cancer death rates for the United States are shown in Table 1-3. In general, approximately one-third of childhood cancer

deaths are caused by leukemia, and about one-fifth of these deaths are caused by brain tumors (5,6,15–17). The relative frequency of cancer types varies as a function of age. The most common tumors of neonates (younger than 28 days of age), for example, are teratomas, retinoblastoma, rhabdomyosarcoma, and neuroblastoma (18,19). In 15- to 20-year-olds, the list is headed by lymphoma (25%), epithelial tumors (18%), and bone malignancies (15%), followed by leukemia, central nervous system (CNS) tumors, and gonadal and germ cell tumors (10% each) (20).

Childhood cancer incidence varies throughout the world (Table 1-4). This may be related in part to fundamental issues of biology and demographics. It can also be related to the reporting system of a country and its level of economic development. For example, the distribution of childhood cancers in Uruguay is very similar to that of North America. Uruguay has a per capita

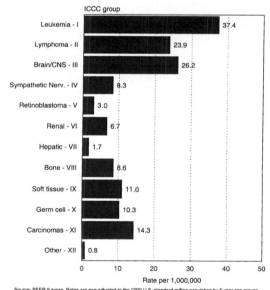

Childhood Cancer SEER Incidence Rates
1973-1999, by ICCC Group
Under 20 Years of Age, Both Sexes, All Races

Source: SEER 9 areas. Rates are age-adjusted to the 2000 U.S. standard million population by 5-year age groups.

FIG. 1-4. U.S. incidence rates for selected childhood cancers. (From Anonymous. US incidence rates for selected childhood cancer. *J Natl Cancer Inst* 2001;93:1201, with permission.)

TABLE 1-2. *SEER cancer incidence rates for 0- to 19-year-olds by ICCC group*

ICCC group	Incidence per 1,000,000	As a percentage of all childhood cancer
I. Leukemia	37.2	24%
a. Lymphoid leukemia	27.5	18%
ALL	27.2	18%
Lymphoid excluding ALL	0.4	—
b. Acute nonlymphoblastic leukemia	6.6	4%
c. Chronic myeloid leukemia	1.2	—
d. Other specified leukemias	0.2	—
e. Unspecified leukemias	1.6	1%
II. Lymphomas and reticuloendothelial neoplasms	24.1	16%
a. Hodgkin's disease	13.7	9%
b. Non-Hodgkin's lymphoma	6.9	4%
c. Burkitt's lymphoma	2.1	1%
d. Miscellaneous	0.4	—
e. Unspecified	1.0	—
III. Central nervous system and miscellaneous intracranial and intraspinal neoplasms (germ cells are found in category X)	26.6	17%
a. Ependymoma	2.2	1%
b. Astrocytoma	13.7	9%
c. Primitive neuroectodermal tumors	5.2	3%
d. Other gliomas	4.5	3%
e. Miscellaneous	0.4	—
f. Unspecified	0.5	—
IV. Sympathetic nervous system tumors	8.3	5%
a. Neuroblastoma and ganglioneuroblastoma	8.0	5%
b. Other	0.3	—
V. Retinoblastoma	3	2%
VI. Renal tumors	6.8	4%
a. Wilms's, rhabdoid, clear cell sarcoma	6.4	4%
b. Renal carcinoma	0.4	—
c. Unspecified	0	—
VII. Hepatic tumors	1.7	1%
a. Hepatoblastoma	1.1	1%
b. Hepatic carcinoma	0.5	—
c. Unspecified malignant	0	—
VIII. Malignant bone tumors	8.6	6%
a. Osteosarcoma	4.7	3%
b. Chondrosarcoma	0.5	—
c. Ewing's sarcoma	3	2%
d. Other specified malignant	0.3	—
e. Unspecified	0.1	—
IX. Soft tissue sarcomas	11	7%
a. Rhabdomyosarcoma and embryonal sarcoma	4.5	3%
b. Fibrosarcoma, neurofibrosarcoma, other fibromatous neoplasms	3.1	2%
c. Kaposi's	0.1	—
d. Other specified	2.3	1%
e. Unspecified	1.1	—
X. Germ cell, trophoblastic, and other gonadal neoplasms	10.5	7%
a. Intracranial and intrapial	1.3	1%
b. Other and unspecified nongonadal	1.6	1%
c. Gonadal germ cell tumor	6.3	4%
d. Gonadal carcinomas	1.0	1%
e. Other and unspecified malignant gonadal	0.2	—
XI. Carcinomas and other malignant epithelial neoplasms	14.4	9%
a. Adrenocortical carcinoma	0.2	—
b. Thyroid carcinoma	5.1	3%
c. Nasopharyngeal carcinoma	0.5	—
d. Malignant melanoma	4.6	3%
e. Skin carcinoma	0	—
f. Other and unspecified	3.9	3%
XII. Other and unspecified malignant neoplasms	0.8	—
Not classified by ICCC	0.3	—
All groups combined	153.4	100%

ALL, acute lymphoblastic leukemia; ICCC, International Classification of Childhood Cancer; SEER, Surveillance, Epidemiology, and End Results.

Data from SEER Cancer Statistics: http://seer.cancer.gov, http://seer.cancer.gov/iccol, and http://seer.cancer.gov/publications/childhood.

TABLE 1-3. *Reported cancer deaths for the five leading cancer sites in people younger than 20 years of age, by sex, United States, 1999*

	Males	Females
All sites	1,266	977
Leukemia	379	293
Brain and other nervous system	287	259
Bone and joint	117	92
Endocrine system	109	84
Soft tissue	92	60

Data from Jemal A, Thomas A, Murray T, et al. Cancer statistics, 2002. *CA Cancer J Clin* 2002;52:23–47.

income much higher than that of the rest of Latin America and the Caribbean (21). However, the frequency of malignant solid tumors in children in a report from Pakistan was distinctly different from that in the rest of the world. This may be related to artifacts of data collection and reporting (14,22–26). Although the absolute frequency of certain tumors is reported to be higher in developing countries than in industrialized states, there is likely to be variation in reporting standards, diagnostic techniques, and histopathologic review (25,27). In Cuba, the most common childhood tumor is leukemia (31%), followed by lymphoma (18%), CNS tumors (15%), sympathetic nervous system tumors (7%), soft tissue

TABLE 1-4. *The most common forms of childhood cancer, England and Wales, 1971–1990*

Diagnosis	Total cases
All leukemias	6,964
Brain and spinal cord[a]	4,404
Non-Hodgkin's lymphoma	1,195
Soft tissue sarcoma	1,259
Wilms's tumor	1,181
Hodgkin's disease	912
Osteosarcoma	559
Retinoblastoma	507
Germ and gonadal neoplasms	469
Ewing's tumor	413
Hepatoblastoma	116
Total	17,979

[a]It is likely that neuroblastoma cases have been included here.

From Coleman MP, Babb P, Damiecki P, et al. *Cancer survival trends in England and Wales, 1971–1995: deprivation and NHS region.* London: The Stationery Office, 1999, with permission.

sarcomas (6%), and renal tumors (5%) (11). In Thailand, leukemias are most common (40%), followed by CNS tumors (14%), lymphoma (12%), bone tumors (4%), and soft tissue sarcomas (4%) (28).

TRENDS IN CHILDHOOD CANCER MORTALITY RATES

Tables 1-5 and 1-6 demonstrate that the mortality rate from childhood cancer has fallen dramatically in the United States. Particularly impressive gains have been posted for acute lymphocytic leukemia, bone tumors (predominantly osteosarcoma and Ewing's sarcoma), Hodgkin's disease, non-Hodgkin's lymphoma, soft tissue sarcomas (including rhabdomyosarcoma and nonrhabdomyosarcoma soft tissue sarcomas), and Wilms's tumor. Although gains have also been achieved for acute myelocytic leukemia, neuroblastoma, and brain tumors, the improvements have been less dramatic or confined to certain subgroups or stages (Table 1-7). In general, however, the diagnosis and treatment of childhood cancer has been one of the success stories of modern medicine.

It is clear that when compared with adult cancer, childhood cancer is a vanishingly rare event. For example, in 2002 there were 154,900 reported deaths from lung cancer alone in the United States (5). The comparative infrequency of childhood cancer is highlighted by the fact that more people in the United States die of lung cancer in 1 week than children die of all forms of cancer in 1 year. Looking at the impact of cancer solely in this manner obscures the issue, however. If one looks at a death from cancer in terms of potential years of life lost, then one readily ap-

TABLE 1-5. *Trends in U.S. childhood cancer mortality rates*

Age group	1950	1975	1992
0–4 yr	11.0	5.1	2.9
5–14 yr	6.6	4.7	3.0

Age-adjusted to the 1970 U.S. population; rates per 100,000 population.

From SEER Cancer Statistics: http://seer.cancer.gov, http://seer.cancer.gov/iccol, and http://seer.cancer.gov/publications/childhood.

TABLE 1-6. *Trends in five-year relative cancer survival rates* (%) for children under age 15, US, 1974 to 1998*

	Five-year relative survival rates (%)						
	Year of diagnosis						
Cancer type	1974 to 1976	1977 to 1979	1980 to 1982	1983 to 1985	1986 to 1988	1989 to 1991	1992 to 1998
All Cancers	**56**	**62**	**65**	**68**	**70**	**73**	**77†**
Acute Lymphocytic Leukemia	53	67	71	69	78	80	85†
Acute Myeloid Leukemia	14	27‡	24‡	29‡	30‡	35‡	46†
Bones and Joints	55‡	52‡	55‡	57	63‡	62	73†
Brain and Other Nervous System	55	56	56	62	63	62	70†
Hodgkin Lymphoma	78	84	91	90	90	94	94†
Neuroblastoma	53	53	53	55	59	68	69†
Non-Hodgkin Lymphoma	44	50	62	71	70	75	81†
Soft Tissue	60	68	65	76	67	78	72†
Wilms Tumor	74	78	87	87	91	93	90†

*Survival rates are adjusted for normal life expectancy and are based on follow-up of patients through 1999.
†The difference in rates between 1974 to 1976 and 1992 to 1998 is statistically significant ($p < 0.05$).
‡The standard error of the survival rate is between 5 and 10 percentage points.
Note: "All Cancers" excludes basal and squamous cell skin cancers and in situ carcinomas, except urinary bladder.
Source: Surveillance, Epidemiology, and End Results program, 1973 to 1999, Division of Cancer Control and Population Sciences, National Cancer Institute, 2002.

preciates that the death of an 8-year-old from acute lymphocytic leukemia has greater statistical weight than the death of an 82-year-old from small cell carcinoma of the lung. Therefore, the success of medical treatment of childhood can-

cer has a significant public health impact when considered in terms of the person-years of potential life or lifetime earnings saved. A lifetime is saved for every child cured of cancer.

IS THE INCIDENCE OF CHILDHOOD CANCER INCREASING?

Some data suggest that the overall incidence of childhood cancer is rising in the United States. Experts disagree about what might account for this alleged increase. Some have asserted that new diagnostic techniques such as computed tomography, magnetic resonance imaging, needle biopsy, and serum chemical markers are increasing the rate of diagnosis of childhood cancer. Thus, the increase in childhood cancer is merely an artifact of improved diagnostic techniques. The counterargument is that the rise in the incidence of childhood cancer is real and may be linked to environmental toxins. So far, proposed links include pelvic radiography of mothers during pregnancy, the use of radioactive nucleotides during pregnancy, exposure to electromagnetic fields, radon, pesticides, solvents, parental occupational exposure, diet, environmental tobacco smoke, alcohol, and infec-

TABLE 1-7. *Difference in 5-year cancer survival between affluent and economically deprived children in England and Wales, 1986–1990*

	Affluent	Deprived
All leukemias	88.8%	84.1%
Hodgkin's disease	99.1%	98.6%
Non-Hodgkin's lymphoma	89.7%	80.9%
Brain and spinal cord	77.5%	74.0%
Retinoblastoma	Not available, $n = 104$	—
Wilms's tumor	95.4%	94.5%
Hepatoblastoma	Not available, $n = 32$	—
Osteosarcoma	92.6%	83.9%
Ewing's sarcoma	93.6%	84.8%
Soft tissue sarcoma	82.9%	75.8%
Germ cell and gonadal neoplasms	93.7%	88.9%

From Coleman MP, Bobb P, Damiecki P, et al. *Cancer survival trends in England and Wales, 1971–1995: deprivation and NHS region.* London: The Stationery Office, 1999, with permission.

tion. The alleged link to agricultural and home pesticide use is weak, and many studies find no correlation (29,30).

SEER, the Manchester Children's Tumor Registry in northwestern England, a registry for Queensland, Australia, the Greater Delaware Valley Pediatric Tumor Registry, and a study from Canada indicate an increase in cancer incidence in children of approximately 1% per year (31–33). Although a study in Denmark did not find a rising incidence, overall the evidence supports an increase in childhood cancer incidence (22).

The data concerning changes in the incidence of acute leukemia in childhood are somewhat conflicting. Some reports indicate that it is rising, and some show it to be stable. Improvements in diagnosis have decreased the number of children labeled as having "leukemia, not otherwise specified" and increased the number of children given a specific leukemia type as a diagnosis. However, most studies indicate an increase in the incidence of childhood brain tumors and lymphoma (31,32).

If we accept the premise that the overall incidence of childhood cancer is rising, then we must bear in mind three potential confounding factors. First, the frequency of childhood cancer is so low that it takes only a few cases, in registries covering a small population base, to suggest a change in incidence (34). Second, as the diagnostic tools of modern medicine improve, more children will be correctly diagnosed with cancer as opposed to another diagnosis. This may be particularly important for brain tumors (31). Third, it has been suggested that exposure to magnetic fields emanating from electric transmission and distribution lines and certain electrical household appliances may be associated with some childhood tumors. The available studies are contradictory (33). In summary, an explanation for the increase in childhood cancer incidence has not been established.

WHAT DOES *CURE* MEAN IN PEDIATRIC ONCOLOGY?

The English word *cure* is derived from the Latin term *cura* and the Old French term *cure,* both meaning "care." The generally accepted defini-

tion in medicine for *cure* is "successful medical treatment; the action or process of healing a wound, a disease, or a sick person; restoration to health" (35). There are several mathematical and statistical definitions of *cure*. In 1963 Easson and Russel suggested a definition for the cure of Hodgkin's disease that was a modification of an earlier definition proposed in 1929 by Greenwood (36,37): "We can speak of cure when in time—probably a decade or so after treatment—there remains a group of disease-free survivors whose progressive death rates from all causes is similar to that of a normal population of the same sex and age constitution." Frei and Gehan (38) suggested that survival should also be unassociated with continuing morbidity from the disease or its treatment.

Cure is not achieved when treatment stops or even after a 5-year disease-free period. For each child with cancer and his or her family, the meaning of *cure* is different. For some patients, it is the knowledge that the disease is gone and never coming back. To others it is the statement that they are well today and want to be so tomorrow. For all children with cancer, hope is the common denominator and getting on with life the goal (39).

One way of expressing this type of probability of survival is a relative survival rate. The relative survival rate is the ratio of the observed percentage of survival to the percentage expected on the basis of general population experience, adjusted for age, sex, race, and calendar year. Using this definition, a population of patients would be cured when a graph plotting relative survival rate showed a horizontal line (38).

Pinkel (40) summarizes the criteria of biologic cure as completion of all cancer treatment, continuous freedom from cancer relapse, and minimal or no risk of subsequent relapse. It is important to consider the continuous cancer-free survival (other commonly used terms are *relapse-free survival* and *event-free survival*) and the overall survival in constructing survival curves. Overall survival rates reflect factors other than biologic curability, including death caused by complications of treatment and subjective factors such as the patient's will to continue living with cancer or its repeated relapses, the physician's determination to keep the patient alive, and the technical and financial resources available to the physician and the patient.

Collins (41,42) provided a definition of *cure*, concerning Wilms's tumor, that is worth noting because it is of historical interest as well as practical use:

> If one accepts the prenatal origin of this tumor as occurring within a fixed period of embryonic development, then the time of recognition and diagnosis would depend upon the rate of growth. . . . If the rate of growth was characteristic of an individual tumor, then this would not only govern the time of first appearance of the primary tumor but would also place limits upon the length of time in which a recurrence might be expected to develop. A tumor present at birth had to develop to clinically recognizable size in a period of 9 months or less. If it were to recur following surgical removal, then this should require no longer than an additional 9 months. A tumor first recognized at the age of 5 years and incompletely removed should again reach the size of clinical recognition either as a recurrence at the primary site or as a distant metastasis in a period not to exceed 5 years plus 9 months.

Collins's argument was direct and vexingly simpleminded. It consisted of four parts:

- If a tumor is discovered shortly after birth, then it must arrive "within a fixed period of embryonic development."
- The "time of recognition and diagnosis" depends on the rate of tumor growth. By this line of argument, rapidly growing tumors would be identified at birth, average-growing tumors in third or fourth year of life, and slowly growing tumors in childhood or later in adult life.
- If the rate of growth is characteristic of a tumor, then this rate not only would "govern the time of first appearance" of that tumor "but would also place limits upon the length of time in which a recurrence might be expected."
- "A tumor present at birth had to develop . . . in a period of 9 months or less" (41–44).

Collins first reported his observations in children with Wilms's tumor. His work was later applied to CNS tumors. A recent comprehensive evaluation of the applicability of Collins's Law to brain tumors was conducted by Brown et al.

using the Childhood Brain Tumor Consortium database. Collins's Law was found to be a good predictor of survival for anaplastic astrocytoma, glioblastoma multiforme, pineoblastoma, medulloblastoma, primitive neuroectodermal tumor, teratoma, germinoma, ependymoma, and choroid plexus papilloma. It did not have predictive value in craniopharyngioma, oligodendroglioma, or fibrillary or pilocytic astrocytoma (43,44). In general, studies continue to confirm the value of Collins's Law in predicting cure rates in medulloblastoma (43–45). Exceptions to Collins's Law represent approximately 8–10% of all patients surviving past the period of risk of recurrence as defined by Collins (46).

The reported cure rates in pediatric cancer may be affected by artifacts of data acquisition and analysis. The zero time shift or lead time bias will extend the statistical length of survival without prolonging life. This phenomenon occurs when a new screening test or imaging study leads to the detection of a previously unknown tumor. Even if therapy is ineffectual, survival is increased by the interval provided by the earlier detection of the cancer. The "Will Rogers effect" occurs when there are improved techniques for detecting cancer metastases. These new data allow patients to migrate from lower stages of cancer to higher. Such migration improves survival in lower stages by eliminating those with metastatic disease. Survival also improves in higher stages because of the addition of people with minimal metastatic disease. Survival improves in each stage, but overall survival for the cancer is unaffected. This phenomenon is named after the American humorist Will Rogers, who is reputed to have remarked during the economic depression of the 1930s that "when the Okies left Oklahoma and moved to California, they raised the average intelligence in both states" (47).

With improving cure rates in childhood cancer, it is apparent that we must move beyond the statistical definition of *cure* (20,48). Cure is more than the absence of disease. It is important to provide the child with a functional cure, regaining or retaining the ability to function in society without major handicaps and minimizing the need for significant support. There are about

250,000 survivors of childhood cancer in the United States (49). The Childhood Cancer Survivor Study is a multicenter study funded by the NCI. This study of more than 14,000 survivors of childhood cancer shows that survivors are at a higher risk of impaired pulmonary function, growth abnormalities, endocrine dysfunction, obesity, physical limitations, infertility, cardiac problems, reduced quality of life, depression, special educational needs, and second malignant neoplasms. Pulmonary complications may develop years after treatment. They have higher rates of lung fibrosis, emphysema, pneumonia, pleurisy, and a need for oxygen compared with sibling control subjects. Survivors of childhood acute lymphoblastic leukemia treated with more than 20 Gy of cranial radiotherapy were significantly more likely to be overweight or obese than sibling control subjects (50).

Planning for adequate limb function, ambulation, and activities of daily living is crucial in planning a course of treatment. Rehabilitation including physical, occupational, and recreational therapy plays an important part in follow-up care. A comprehensive pediatric cancer rehabilitation program requires people with expertise in prosthetics, orthoses, ostomy care, gait training, and pain management (23,51–54).

Attention to the child's emotional status is also important. This includes preserving and nurturing a sense of well-being on the part of the child and his or her family. Childhood cancer survivors are more likely than their siblings to suffer symptoms of depression and somatic distress (55). The family should be given every measure of support in dealing with illness and restoring health. The diagnosis and treatment of cancer exert severe emotional and financial strains on a family.

Parental separation and divorce, sibling behavior problems, and the weight of family responsibilities during adversity complicate the treatment and rehabilitation of the child with cancer (56,57). The pediatric radiation oncologist should ensure an ongoing relationship with the child and family after treatment to contribute to rehabilitation. As the survival rates for pediatric cancers improve, we will have an increasing population of young adults who are cancer survivors. These people will pose new problems for medicine and society: What will be appropriate medical surveillance for late effects of treatment, including secondary malignancy? How shall these patients be counseled concerning reproduction? What special needs will such people have concerning employment, disability and health insurance, and psychological support (53)? The pediatric radiation oncologist will play an important role in understanding these issues and implementing solutions (58). Fortunately, an evolving body of literature is addressing these questions (59).

THE SITE OF CARE AND THE PEDIATRIC CANCER TEAM

The 1969 edition of *Nelson's Textbook of Pediatrics* reported that childhood "leukemia is a uniformly fatal malignant disease." The advances in the treatment of pediatric malignancies in the subsequent three decades have been remarkable. Success in the modern treatment of the child with cancer is the result of a complex, multidisciplinary process administered by a team of professionals (60).

Combined-modality therapy has been a rewarding approach. A coordinated group of medical and surgical specialists with expertise in the clinical care of children with cancer and in basic and clinical research best directs the child's care. The complete pediatric cancer center is staffed by a pediatric medical oncologist, specially trained nurses, a pediatric diagnostic radiologist, surgeons with expertise in pediatric oncology, anesthesiologists, psychiatrists, physiotherapists, physicians' assistants, and skilled social workers. The group must also include a radiation oncologist committed to pediatric care and with experience in radiotherapy for children (Table 1-8) (4,58,61).

Participation of the patient's parents and other significant family members is an integral part of the team approach. Parents will soon become extremely knowledgeable about their child's illness, its treatment, and the associated complications. They may be taught to become careful observers of physical signs and symptoms. Their report of changes in the child's

TABLE 1-8. *Requirements for a pediatric cancer center*

The **medical staff** should include a qualified pediatric hematologist or oncologist; a pediatric radiation oncologist; a pediatric general surgeon; surgeons with pediatric expertise in neurosurgery, urology, and orthopedic surgery; a pathologist with expertise in tumors of children and adolescents; and pediatric subspecialists in anesthesiology, diagnostic radiology, intensive care, infectious disease, cardiology, endocrinology, nephrology, and neurology.

The **allied health staff** should include pediatric nurses, social workers, pharmacists, psychologists, child life specialists, recreational therapists, physical and occupational therapists, and chaplains with expertise in childhood cancer.

The **physical plant** of the hospital or medical center should include an appropriate inpatient unit for the care of children with cancer, an ambulatory clinic for treatment and monitoring of children with cancer, a pediatric intensive care unit, a hematopathology laboratory capable of performing cell phenotype analysis, a clinical chemistry laboratory able to monitor antibiotic and antineoplastic drug levels, a blood bank, a pharmacy capable of preparing and dispensing antineoplastic agents and total parenteral nutrition, a diagnostic radiology suite, and a radiation oncology department.

The **institution** should conduct a regularly scheduled multidisciplinary pediatric tumor board and offer access to ongoing clinical protocols via one of the pediatric cancer treatment groups.

Based on American Academy of Pediatrics. Guidelines for the pediatric cancer center and role of such centers in diagnosis and treatment. *Pediatrics* 1986;77:916–917.

well-being will be invaluable to caregivers. Parents often develop important skills such as the care of indwelling venous access devices. Parents may be taught to administer medications, titrate their dosages, and oversee symptom management (61).

Going to school is the normal daytime activity for most children. The child with cancer should be encouraged to live as normally as possible. Participation in school is encouraged to whatever degree is reasonable. Many hospitals maintain a program for schooling children during their cancer care. In some states, the hospital itself is accredited as a public school and certified teachers are kept on staff. These teachers, working closely with the local school districts, can help children keep up with their studies and be more readily integrated back into their classrooms at home.

There is evidence that the diagnosis and treatment of some pediatric malignancies, particularly those dependent on complex radiotherapy, are better conducted at university-affiliated medical centers. In an analysis of children with brain tumors, survival was compared for children who received all or part of their treatment at university cancer centers and those who received all or part of their treatment at community hospitals (62). For children with medulloblastoma, the 5-year survival rate was 2.5 times greater for children treated at univer-

sity hospitals than for those treated at community hospitals. For brainstem gliomas there was also a greater probability of survival for children treated at university hospitals. The 5-year projected survival rates for cerebellar astrocytoma, grade I and II supratentorial astrocytoma, ependymoma, and glioblastoma multiforme (in which survival is arguably less dependent on irradiation) for university-treated patients were similar to those for community hospital–treated patients.

In another analysis, the survival rates of patients with Wilms's tumor were studied. Children treated in a coordinated university and cancer center treatment program in an upstate New York county were compared with those treated in smaller counties without large treatment centers (63). From 1950 to 1959, an era in which treatment for Wilms's tumor was poor, there was no significant difference in survival between these two groups. However, from 1967 to 1972 there was a significant improvement in survival for children treated in the county with the coordinated university and cancer center treatment program.

Another study addressed the influence of place of treatment on diagnosis, treatment, and survival in Wilms's tumor, rhabdomyosarcoma, and medulloblastoma in the Delaware Valley area (64). The probability of survival was higher for children treated for medulloblastoma and rhabdomyosarcoma at cancer centers than for children treated in noncancer centers. For Wilms's tumor, however, there were no major differences in management strategy or survival between cancer centers and noncancer centers. A study from the Children's Cancer Group indicated higher survival rates for children with acute leukemia treated at specialized pediatric institutions (20,48).

The available data suggest that there is a benefit to treatment at a university-based or regional cancer center when the treatment is rapidly evolving and when complex treatment approaches with technically difficult surgery or radiotherapy are needed. However, it appears that the site of treatment does not alter survival rates for patients in whom a cure may be achieved with surgical intervention alone, for tumors for which there is no significant curative treatment, and for tumors necessitating multimodality therapy when the most up-to-date protocol information and the services of a consulting expert are available in the community hospital (63–67).

POSTGRADUATE TRAINING IN PEDIATRIC RADIATION ONCOLOGY

There are serious gaps in residency training in pediatric radiation oncology in the United States. The incidence of childhood cancer is low. In addition, only a portion of childhood cancer cases are appropriate for radiotherapy. When one also considers the fact that pediatric cancer cases are not uniformly distributed among the radiation oncology training programs in the United States, one can readily understand why many residency programs see fewer than five pediatric cancer cases per year. In some residency programs the few pediatric radiation oncology cases that are seen are heavily weighted toward palliative cases, total body irradiation for bone marrow transplantation, or late adolescents with Hodgkin's disease. Therefore, it is very likely that a person could go through 4 years of postgraduate training in radiation oncology and never see a case of retinoblastoma, neuroblastoma, Wilms's tumor, or Langerhans cell histiocytosis.

There is an intrinsic problem with the way academic medical centers count the number of pediatric radiation oncology cases. In adult radiation oncology, guidelines exist for the appropriate number of lung, colorectal, breast, head and neck, and genitourinary malignancies necessary for training. In the case of pediatric cancer, however, all forms of cancer are lumped together to reach an acceptable number. Such a policy would never be acceptable in taking an inventory of the appropriate number of adult cases for training.

Some residency programs try to solve the problem by sending residents for away rotations. With a 1-month rotation at another center, residents are expected to acquire sufficient training to last them for the 4 years of the residency program. In 1 month, it is entirely likely that a resident would never see a patient taken from consultation through simulation and all the way through completion of a course of treatment. Long-term follow-up is also impossible.

Some have proposed eliminating pediatric radiation oncology training from general radiation oncology training. By this line of argument, pediatric radiation oncology would become a subspecialty, which would entail a separate fellowship at the end of a residency. Another proposed solution is to designate only certain residency programs as capable of providing pediatric radiation oncology training by virtue of the adequate number of cases and faculty with sufficient expertise. It is highly unlikely that there will be approved subspecialty training in pediatric radiation oncology in the near future. The designated accrediting boards in the United States have a series of requirements for subspecialty designation that are too formidable to be met in the case of pediatric radiation oncology. Therefore, it remains likely that for the foreseeable future pediatric radiation oncology residency training will continue to be inadequate (58).

THE PROBLEM OF EVIL AND CHILDHOOD CANCER

The philosophical problem of severe illness and death in children poses a tremendous challenge to the pediatric radiation oncologist. Why does premature death take the innocent? This question has troubled philosophers, theologians, and physicians.

Physicians use several defense mechanisms in dealing with adults with cancer. When faced with someone with advanced bronchogenic carcinoma, physicians may say to themselves, "The prognosis is grim. However, the patient has a long history of cigarette smoking." Faced with a patient with advanced carcinoma of the cervix, the physician may think, "The patient has a very bad malignancy, but this is almost certainly associated with significant risk factors associated with sexual behavior." When etiologic rational defenses do not come to mind in adult oncology, the physician may turn to the age defense: "The patient is 85 years old, and no one lives forever." Such rationalizations are not useful when a 40-year-old is faced with widespread metastatic breast cancer. In most cases, however, they do help the physician get through the day (68–70).

Rationalization defenses based on age or etiology break down when the pediatric radiation oncologist faces a child with a malignancy. We have nothing and no one to blame for a child dying of pontine glioma. There is no obvious rationalization.

The problem of evil is a long-standing one in the history of philosophy. For the physician who believes in a rational order to the universe, most often in the context of religious faith, there is a classic dilemma: Why is there evil? If there really is a God who permits cancer in children, is God omnipresent but not omnipotent? If so, then a logical contradiction exists in the concept of an omnipresent, omnipotent God. On the other hand, is the explanation for childhood cancer that God is all powerful but not all merciful? If so, again a contradiction exists in the general monotheistic view of the Supreme Being. One could also conclude that there is no God. If this is the case, then there is no rational order to the universe, everything is random, and evil is simply one more random event.

For some people, there is no response to the problem of evil. One Baptist minister wrote,

> Silence may be the most truly faithful response. This holds true at least in a Christian understanding that God is found not in the whirlwind, but in the silence. . . . The Old Testament tells

us that when Job cried out, "What does this all mean?" God responded, "Where were you when I created the heaven and the earth?" I think that this is a reminder that there are wisdom's beyond our wisdom (69).

In some philosophical schools, the greatest sin is the lack of knowledge. For others, however, the greatest sin is to be separated from one's conception of a Supreme Being.

The authors of this book clearly have no special knowledge concerning the problem of evil that enables us to counsel the pediatric radiation oncologist in training or to assuage the concerns of the long-standing practitioner. The child with cancer is discomforting to the physician. However, this discomfort should not paralyze the physician with indecision or doubt about a course of therapy. It is reasonable for the physician to be angry and distressed about the child with cancer. We should be more concerned about the physician who lacks rather than possesses such feelings.

> It is acceptable, in the context of the problem of evil, for physicians simply to accept the fact that they don't know the answer. In Medieval times, the population often went to cathedrals to seek the answers to the great questions of life. In the modern world, the grand complexes of medical centers supplanted cathedrals. We go into places like [a hospital] to seek our answers. [Physicians] are the new caste of priests. They are the persons to whom people come for the answers. You are asked to be without blame, faultless, and have absolute answers. Part of your training is the classic rationalization of an education which does not give you permission not to know. That is the issue for many [physicians]. You have to know that you cannot know all of the answers (69).

REFERENCES

References particularly recommended for further reading are indicated by an asterisk.

1. Dublin LI. *Mortality statistics of insured wage-earners and their families.* New York: Metropolitan Life Insurance Company, 1919.
2. North SND. *Special reports: mortality statistics 1900–1904.* Washington, DC: US Government Printing Office, 1906:76–89.

3. Anonymous. The dangers of childhood. *Lancet* 2002;360:811.

4. American Academy of Pediatrics. Guidelines for the pediatric cancer center and role of such centers in diagnosis and treatment. *Pediatrics* 1986;77: 916–917.

*5. SEER Cancer Statistics: http://seer.cancer.gov, http://seer.cancer.gov/iccol, and http://seer.cancer.gov/publications/childhood.

*6. Jemal A, Thomas A, Murray T, et al. Cancer statistics, 2002. *CA Cancer J Clin* 2002;52:23–47.

7. Ventura SJ, Peters KD, Martin JA, et al. Births and deaths: United States, 1996. *Mon Vital Stat Rep* 1997;46:29–34.

8. Dorgan CA, ed. *Statistical record of health & medicine.* New York: Gale Research Inc., 1995:49.

9. US Department of Commerce. *116th edition, statistical abstract of the United States 1996.* Washington, DC: US Department of Commerce, 1996:94–95.

10. *Canadian cancer incidence atlas,* volume 1: *Canadian cancer incidence.* Ottawa: Minister of National Health and Welfare, 1995:138–139.

11. Martin AA, Alpert JA, Reno JS, et al. Incidence of childhood cancer in Cuba (1986–1990). *Cancer* 1997;72:551–555.

12. Nkanza NK. Paediatric solid malignant tumors in Zimbabwe. *Cent Afr J Med* 1989;35:496–501.

13. Panda BK, Dandapat MC, Parida N. Patterns of paediatric solid malignant tumours in southern Orissa. *J Indian Med Assoc* 1989;87:136–137.

14. Shah SH, Pervez S, Hassan SH. Frequency of malignant solid tumors in children. *J Pakistan Med Assoc* 2000;50:86–88.

15. Anonymous. US incidence rates for selected childhood cancer. *J Natl Cancer Inst* 2001;93:1201.

16. Parkin DM, Stiller CA, Draper GJ, et al., eds. *International incidence of childhood cancer.* Lyon, France: World Health Organization, International Agency for Research on Cancer, 1988:101–107.

17. Gurney JG, Davis S, Severson RK, et al. Trends in cancer incidence among children in the US. *Cancer* 1996;78:532–541.

18. Plaschkes J. Epidemiology of neonatal tumours. In: Puri P, ed. *Neonatal tumours.* London: Springer-Verlag, 1996:1–1a.

19. Halperin EC. Neonatal neoplasms. *Int J Radiat Oncol Biol Phys* 2000;47:171–178.

20. Lewis IJ. Cancer in adolescence. *BMJ* 1996;52:887–897.

21. Costillo L, Fluchel M, Dabezies A, et al. Childhood cancer in Uruguay 1992–4. Incidence and mortality. *Med Pediatr Oncol* 2001;37:400–404.

22. DeNully Brown P, Hertz H, Olsen JH, et al. Incidence of childhood cancer in Denmark 1943–1984. *Int J Epidemiol* 1989;18:546–555.

23. Goodman MT, Yoshizawa CN, Kolonel LN. Ethnic patterns of childhood cancer in Hawaii between 1960 and 1984. *Cancer* 1989;64:1758–1763.

24. Groves FD, Craig JF, Chen VW, et al. Pediatric cancer in New Orleans. *J La State Med Soc* 1990;142:27–30.

25. McWhirter WR, Petroeschevsky AL. Childhood cancer incidence in Queensland, 1979–1988. *Int J Cancer* 1990;45:1002–1005.

26. Savitz DA, Zuckerman DL. Childhood cancer in the Denver metropolitan area 1976–1983. *Cancer* 1987;59:1539–1542.

27. Merrill RM, Feuer EJ. Risk-adjusted cancer incidence rates (United States). *Cancer Causes Control* 1996; 7:544–552.

28. Sriamporn S, Vatansapt V, Martin N, et al. Incidence of childhood cancer in Thailand 1988–1991. *Paediatr Perinat Epidemiol* 1996;10:73–85.

29. Massey-Stokes M, Lanning B. Childhood cancer and environmental toxins: the debate continues. *Fam Community Health* 2002;24:27–38.

30. Reynolds P, von Behren J, Gunier RB, et al. Childhood cancer and agricultural pesticide use: an ecologic study in California. *Environ Health Perspect* 2002; 110:319–324.

31. Bunin GR, Feurer EJ, Witman PA, et al. Increasing incidence of childhood cancer: report of 20 years experience from the Greater Delaware Valley Pediatric Tumor Registry. *Paediatr Perinat Epidemiol* 1996; 10:319–338.

32. Cushman JH Jr. U.S. reshaping cancer strategy as incidence in children rises. *New York Times* 1997 Sept 29:1.

33. Kraut A, Tate R, Tran N. Residential electric consumption and childhood cancer in Canada (1971–1986). *Arch Environ Health* 1994;3(49):156–159.

34. Walter SD. Letter to the editor. *Arch Environ Health* 1996;51(6):467.

35. *Compact edition of the Oxford English dictionary.* Oxford, UK: Oxford University Press, 1985.

36. Greenwood M. The errors of sampling of the survivorship table. In: *Reports on public health and medical subjects,* no. 33. Appendix I. London: His Majesty's Stationery Office, 1929.

37. Easson EC, Russel MH. The cure of Hodgkin's disease. *BMJ* 1963;1:1704–1707.

38. Frei E, Gehan EA. Definition of cure for Hodgkin's disease. *Cancer Res* 1971;31:1828–1833.

39. Podrasky PA. The family perspective of the cured patient. *Cancer* 1986;58:522–523.

40. Pinkel D. Cure of the child with cancer: definition and perspective. In: *American Cancer Society: proceedings of the national conference on the care of the child with cancer.* New York: American Cancer Society, Inc., 1979:191–200.

41. Collins VP. Wilms' tumor: its behavior and prognosis. *J La State Med Soc* 1955;107:474–480.

42. Collins VP. The treatment of Wilms' tumor. *Cancer* 1958;11:89–94.

43. Brown WD, Tavare CJ, Sobel EL, et al. The applicability of Collins' law to childhood brain tumors and its usefulness as a predictor of survival. *Neurosurgery* 1995;36:1093–1096.

44. Brown WD, Tavare CJ, Sobel EL, et al. Medulloblastoma and Collins' law: a critical review of the concept of a period of risk for tumor recurrence and patient survival. *Neurosurgery* 1995;36:691–697.

45. Sure U, Berghorn WJ, Bertalonfy H. Collins' law: prediction of recurrence or cure in childhood medulloblastoma? *Clin Neurol Neurosurg* 1997;99:113–116.

46. Friedberg MH, David O, Adelman LS, et al. Recurrence of medulloblastoma: violation of Collins' law after two decades. *Surg Neurol* 1997;47:571–574.

*47. Feinstein AR, Sasin DM, Wells CK. The Will Rogers

phenomenon: stage migration and new diagnostic techniques as a source of misleading statistics for survival in cancer. *N Engl J Med* 1985;312:1604–1608.

48. Nachman J, Sather HN, Buckley JD, et al. Young adults 16–21 years of age at diagnosis entered on Children's Cancer Group acute lymphoblastic leukaemia and acute myeloblastic leukaemia protocols. *Cancer* 1993;71:3377–3385.

49. Duenwald M, Grady M. Young survivors of cancer battle effects of treatment. *New York Times* 2002 Jan 8:1.

50. Boughton B. Childhood cancer treatment causes complications later in life. *Lancet Oncol* 2002;3:390.

51. Gerber LH, Binder H. Rehabilitation of the child with cancer. In: Pizzo PA, Poplack DG, eds. *Principles and practice of pediatric oncology.* Philadelphia: JB Lippincott, 1993:1079–1090.

52. Hammond D. Progress in the study, treatment and cure of the cancers of children. In: Burchenal JH, Oehgen HF, eds. *Cancer achievement, challenges, and prospects for the 1980s.* New York: Grune & Stratton, 1981:171–190.

53. Hays DM, Landsverk J, Ruccione K, et al. Employment problems and workplace experience of childhood cancer survivors. In: Green DM, D'Angio GJ, eds. *Late effects of treatment for childhood cancer.* New York: Wiley-Liss, 1992:171–178.

54. Meyer WH. Principles of total care: rehabilitation. In: Fernbach DJ, Vietti TJ, eds. *Clinical pediatric oncology.* St Louis: Mosby, 1991:285–294.

55. Zebrack BJ, Zeltzer LK, Whitten J, et al. Psychological outcomes in long-term survivors of childhood leukemia, Hodgkin's disease, and non-Hodgkin's lymphoma: a report from the childhood cancer survivor study. *Pediatrics* 2002;110:42–52.

56. Craft AW, Pearson ADJ. Three decades of chemotherapy for childhood cancer: from cure "at any cost" to "cure at least cost." *Cancer Surv* 1989;8:605–629.

57. Dickens M. *Miracles of courage.* New York: Dodd, Mead, 1985.

58. Constine LS, Donaldson SS. Pediatric radiation oncology: subspecialty training? *Int J Radiat Oncol Biol Phys* 1992;24:881–884.

59. Schwartz CL, Hobbie WL, Constine LS, et al. *Survivors of childhood cancer: assessment and management.* St Louis: Mosby, 1994.

60. Labotka RJ. Book review of *Principles and Practice of Pediatric Oncology. JAMA* 2002;288:894–895.

61. Meek RS. Pediatric oncology: the team approach of the medical center of Delaware. *Del Med J* 1988;60:169–172, 177–178.

62. Duffner PK, Cohen ME, Flannery JT. Referral patterns of childhood brain tumors in the state of Connecticut. *Cancer* 1982;50:1636–1640.

63. Griffel M. Wilms' tumor in New York State: epidemiology and survivorship. *Cancer* 1977;40:3140–3145.

64. Cohen ME, Duffner PK, Kun LE, et al. The argument for a combined cancer consortium research data base. *Cancer* 1985;56:1897–1901.

65. Lennox EL, Stiller CA, Morris-Jones P, et al. Nephroblastoma: treatment during 1970–1973 and the effect of inclusion in the first Medical Research Council trial. *BMJ* 1979;2:567–569.

66. Kramer S, Meadows AT, Pastore G, et al. Influence of place of treatment on diagnosis, treatment, and survival in 3 pediatric solid tumors. *J Clin Oncol* 1984; 2:917–923.

67. Stiller CA, Draper GJ. Treatment, centre size, trial entry and survival in acute lymphoblastic leukaemia. *Arch Dis Child* 1989;64:798–807.

68. Taylor EJ, Outlaw FH, Bernardo TR, et al. Spiritual conflicts associated with praying about cancer. *Psychooncology* 1999;8:386–394.

69. Halperin EC, Travis J, Browning IR III, et al. Children are not supposed to die: combined pediatric and radiation oncology grand rounds addresses severe illness and death. *NC Med J* 1997;58:445–448.

70. Halperin EC. Childhood cancers: overview. In: Gunderson LL, Tepper JE, eds. *Clinical radiation oncology.* New York: Churchill Livingstone, 2000:1044–1049.

2

Leukemias in Children

Larry E. Kun, M.D.

Leukemias are the most common cancer types in children, representing nearly 30% of all childhood cancers in North America. The most common leukemia is acute lymphoblastic leukemia (ALL), accounting for 80% of childhood leukemias and nearly 24% of all cancers in children. Approximately 3,000 children present with ALL annually in the United States (1). ALL was the prototype childhood cancer documenting response and, subsequently, cure with chemotherapy and the importance of combined modality therapy that incorporated irradiation for "sanctuary sites." The development of therapeutic approaches in ALL sets another precedent in oncology, demonstrating the value of serial, prospective clinical trials to introduce progressively more successful treatment regimens. It is no exaggeration to attribute the early success in leukemia control to the introduction of central nervous system (CNS) irradiation, a fundamental component of the earliest successful leukemia regimens developed in the late 1960s that is currently a selected part of therapy for "high-risk" ALL presentations (Fig. 2-1).

Approximately 20% of childhood leukemias are acute myeloblastic leukemia (AML), a disease that is more common in adults. Successful management of AML has lagged behind that of ALL historically, and the role of radiation therapy has been poorly defined. However, AML has been one of the more common indications for bone marrow transplantation in children, and the impact of total body irradiation (TBI) in this setting has been significant. Transplant regimens continue to evolve, with increasing indications for radiation immunosuppression as the host pool for allogeneic transplants expands beyond the usual "reservoir" of related, immuno-

logically matched siblings to matched, unrelated, and, more recently, haploidentical donors.

Biologic characterization of childhood leukemias indicates that up to 25% of children with ALL have some component of malignant myeloid features; although the presence of myeloid-associated antigen does not appear to have prognostic implications, it does represent a "marker" of value in genetically assessing disease response or potential "molecular residual" (2). Much less common are true mixed-lineage leukemias, wherein the cell lines express both lymphoid- and myeloid-associated antigens (3).

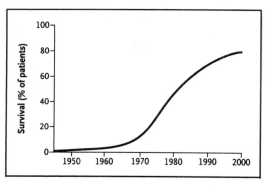

FIG. 2-1. There has been a progressive increase in long-term survival among children with acute lymphoblastic leukemia over the past five decades. The values shown in this curve are approximate. The results were obtained at major pediatric cancer centers and then in national cooperative groups. In medically underdeveloped countries, long-term survival rates are lower. Children who remain in first remission for the first 5 years after completion of therapy are generally cured. (From Simone JV. Childhood leukemia: successes and challenges for survivors. *N Engl J Med* 2003;349:627–628, with permission).

ACUTE LYMPHOBLASTIC LEUKEMIA

Biology

ALL results from a clonal expansion of dysregulated, immature lymphoid cells. The linkage of ALL subtypes to the major immunophenotypic lymphocyte lines provided the first biologic understanding of the disease types that correlate biologic characteristics with common clinical features. B-precursor leukemias account for 85% of ALL cases in children. Most cases of B-precursor ALL consist of leukemic clones from early pre–B cell lines (55%; cytoplasmic immunoglobulin [cIg] negative) or pre–B cell lines (25%; cIg positive); only 2–3% of B-progenitor ALL cases show mature B-cell differentiation with surface immunoglobulin that characterizes mature B cells. T-precursor ALL accounts for 15% of cases of childhood ALL (4). B cell–derived ALL classically occurs in young children, associated with a wide range of clinical manifestations and initial white blood cell (WBC) counts. Classically, T-cell ALL occurs in older children (more than 10 years old) and has been associated with extramedullary involvement (especially in the mediastinal lymph nodes) and high presenting WBC. Current immunophenotypic classifications rely on identification of clusters of differentiation (CDs), molecules found on white blood cells that characterize the leukocyte lineages. CD19 is a highly sensitive marker that is characteristic of B-precursor ALL; CD7, of T-cell ALL. Both so-called mature B-cell ALL and T-cell ALL, long associated with less favorable outcomes, now enjoy outcomes almost equal to those of "standard-risk" B-precursor ALL (5–7).

Enormous advances in the understanding of ALL have accompanied studies of the cytogenetics of this disease. More than 60% of ALL cell lines in children are identifiable as specific genetic abnormalities. The earliest distinct molecular characteristic included chromosomal translocations: The demonstration of Philadelphia chromosome (Ph+), associated with chronic myelogenous leukemia in adults, in up to 5% of children with B-precursor ALL, was recognized as an unfavorable biological characteristic in the 1980s. Ph+ cases have translocation of chromosomes 9 and 22 [t(9;22)] and often are associated with high WBC and a propensity for CNS involvement (8). Other translations have been described: More than 20% of children show t(12;21), and up to 6% of patients with B-precursor ALL show the t(1;19) defect, most often in boys, again with a high WBC (9). Less common genetic findings include t(4;11), noted predominantly in black children with high WBC, and t(8;14), noted in boys with mature B-cell ALL. The t(11;14) defect is found in 1% of cases, typically T-cell ALL with extramedullary involvement, and often in infants (10). The chromosomal gains and losses noted in leukemic cell lines result in hyperdiploid or hypodiploid ALL lines, respectively; the former finding is noted in almost one-fourth of childhood ALL presentations and is associated with a favorable outcome (3).

Translocations lead to the formation of transforming fusion genes or functional inactivation of tumor suppressor genes; the occurrence and relationships are outlined in Fig. 2-2. For example, t(12;21) is associated with the ETV6–CBRA2 gene rearrangement, defining a favorable genetic subset (11). Several chromosomal translocations [e.g., t(4;11), t(11;19), and t(1;11)] result in MLL gene rearrangements, a genetic factor associated with a significantly lower disease control rate (11). Infants younger than 1 year old typically show MLL gene rearrangements (3,10).

Clinical Presentation

The median age at presentation for ALL is 4 years, with a peak occurrence between ages 2 and 4 years. Boys are more commonly affected than girls; the sex distribution is particularly notable in T-cell ALL. ALL is less common in black children. Earlier studies demonstrated unfavorable outcome in adolescents and in black children; more recent results are similar to those in so-called standard-risk ALL (12).

The most common presenting symptoms include fever, bleeding, and bone pain. Findings at diagnosis include ecchymoses or petechiae, signs of lymph node enlargement, and hepatosplenomegaly. The diagnosis is suspected with a CBC demonstrating the presence of immature lymphoblasts in the peripheral blood or elevated

Genotypes in Childhood ALL

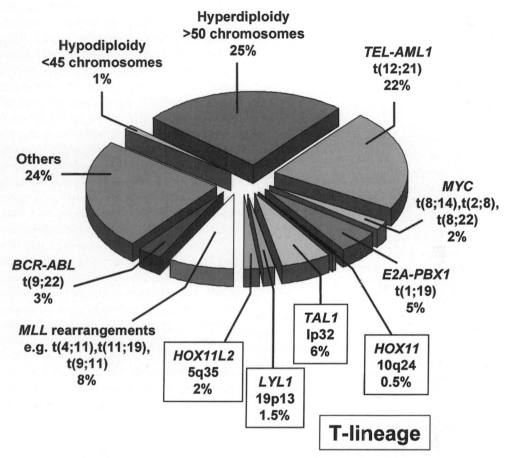

FIG. 2-2. Genetic findings in childhood acute lymphoblastic leukemia, illustrating the several genotypes identified in B-lineage and T-cell leukemias. (From Pui CH, Relling MV, Downing JR. Acute lymphoblastic leukemia. *N Engl J Med* [in press], with permission). (See color plate)

WBC (documented as within 10,000 WBC per cubic milliliter in 50% of presentations, 10–50,000 in 30%, and more than 50,000 in 15–20% at diagnosis). Less often, clinical symptoms or signs are associated with extramedullary involvement of the CNS, testis, or kidney.

ALL is a systemic disease by definition, usually involving the bone marrow diffusely and associated with lymphoblastic infiltration, either microscopic or overt, in a number of organ systems (e.g., lymph nodes, liver, and spleen).

Overt CNS leukemia is manifest clinically by irritability, headaches, sometimes vomiting or unanticipated weight gain, and, less often, cranial nerve palsies (especially VII; less often VI, III) or seizures. Advanced disease sometimes is manifest by papilledema and diffuse retinal infiltration. The pathophysiology was demonstrated in Price and Johnson's classic description of leukemic cells filling the subarachnoid space well into Virchow-Robin' spaces and throughout the basal cisterns (13).

Staging: Risk Categories for ALL

Although specified with somewhat different parameters in the major clinical trial groups addressing this disease in North America, Europe, and elsewhere, the "common risk assessment" criteria were agreed upon at a National Cancer Institute (NCI) consensus conference in 1995. ALL is classically considered "low risk" when presenting as B-precursor disease in children 1–9 years old with WBCs less than 50,000. Infants younger than 1 year of age and children older than 10 years are considered at "high risk," in addition to those with B-precursor disease and WBCs greater than 50,000 (14). The Berlin–Frankfurt–Munster (BFM) studies are the most commonly used worldwide; using an overall paradigm of "leukemic cell mass and response to therapy," cases are divided into standard, intermediate, and high risk. Additional high-risk features incorporated in BFM trials include T-cell immunophenotype, rearrangement BCR/ABL or translocation t(9;22), or CNS involvement (15).

Rapid or early response is increasingly recognized as a key correlate of ultimate disease control. Recent studies indicate a role for assessing "minimal residual disease" based on immunologic or molecular findings in bone marrow—beyond earlier identification of residual peripheral or marrow blasts—typically at 2–4 weeks of induction therapy (2,16–18).

By international convention, the definition of CNS leukemia is the presence of more than 5 WBC/μL and positive cerebrospinal fluid (CSF) cytology demonstrating blasts, or cranial nerve palsies. A generally accepted "staging" system defines CNS 1 as an absence of blasts on cytospin, CNS 2 as the presence of blasts but with CSF WBC less than 5/μL, and CNS 3 (overt CNS leukemia) as blasts with more than 5 WBC/μL (14,19).

Treatment: Chemotherapy

Current management incorporates three phases of therapy: remission induction, intensification (or consolidation), and continuation therapy. The "backbone" of induction is the combination of corticosteroids (prednisone or dexametha-

sone) and vincristine; current studies systematically also include asparaginase with or without the anthracycline daunorubicin. Remission induction is successful in 97–99% of children. The rationale for including a fourth agent is to increase the rapidity of response and the frequency of early biologic remission (20,21).

Intensification (or consolidation) follows remission induction and incorporates aggressive drugs and regimens to achieve maximal early cytoreduction. The most commonly used agents include methotrexate alone (at "high" dosages, typically 1–5 g/m^2 repeatedly during this phase) or with 6-mercaptopurine (6-MP), asparaginase (also at high dosages), an epipodophyllotoxin (VM-26 or VP-16) or cytosine arabinoside, or using a combination of vincristine, dexamethasone, asparaginase, doxorubicin, and thioguanine (6-TG) with or without cyclophosphamide.

Continuation therapy is a routine part of therapy for all ALL presentations, except the mature B-cell type; the latter is effectively treated with more intensive, less protracted chemotherapy. Continuation therapy is administered as chronic chemotherapy for 30–36 months (22). The classic continuation therapy is weekly methotrexate and 6-MP. Pulses of vincristine and prednisone (or dexamethasone) are a part of most current protocols; several also include reinduction, or repeating the induction regimen about 4 months into remission. The goal of continuation therapy is to eliminate any residual, slowly replicating leukemic blasts or to sufficiently suppress leukemic cell division to allow programmed cell death to intervene.

Long-term leukemia-free survival is now achieved in 80–90% of children with ALL (3,9,23–27). Standard-risk patients can anticipate disease-free survival rates greater than 80%, and children with high-risk features, 70–80% (Fig. 2-3) (23–25).

Treatment: CNS Preventive Therapy

Evolution of CNS Preventive Therapy in ALL

The initial concept for preventive CNS irradiation was derived from animal experiments with the mouse L1210 leukemia model, suggesting

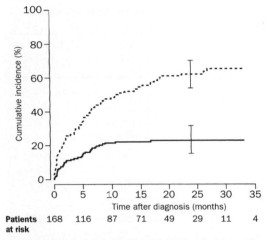

FIG. 2-3. In the economically advantaged world, childhood acute lymphoblastic leukemia (ALL) has become a generally curable disease. This is the result of complicated, intensive, and toxic therapy. For the 70% of the world's children who live in economically undeveloped countries, complex therapy for ALL often is nearly impossible to administer. Therefore, it is not surprising that the clinical results are much worse (159). In this study from Honduras, the cumulative incidence of treatment failure for children with ALL at 24 months was 62% *(upper line)* and specifically from therapy abandonment was 23% *(lower line),* both in striking contrast to the excellent survival rates described in clinical trials from economically developed countries. (From Metzger ML, Howard SC, Fu LC, et al. Outcome of childhood acute leukemia in resource poor countries. *Lancet* 2003;362:706–708, with permission).

that "leukemia control" was possible only when CNS irradiation was added to intraperitoneal chemotherapy. Investigators at St. Jude Children's Research Hospital (SJCRH) first applied the experimental model to children with ALL. Taking a "total" approach to the disease, they used induction chemotherapy (vincristine, prednisone) in sequence with prolonged, nonaggressive maintenance therapy (oral methotrexate and 6-MP) (28–30). The initial studies incorporated 5- to 12-Gy craniospinal irradiation (CSI) based on the mouse model cited earlier and the observation that CNS relapse was the dominant event terminating "remission" once chemotherapy was able to prolong hematologic remission beyond 6 months (28).

The evolution of CNS preventive therapy is highlighted by the serial studies at SJCRH (Table 2-1) and the early trials of Cancer and Leukemia Group B. The incidence of initial, isolated CNS relapse in SJCRH Total IV and VI (with no CNS preventive therapy) was 67%; for Total V, VI, and VII [with CSI or cranial irradiation to 24 Gy, the latter given with intrathecal methotrexate (IT-MTX)], the incidence was 8% (28,31). These investigators first noted the reduction in CNS relapse associated with preventive cranial irradiation (CrI) and IT-MTX and then compared preventive CSI with therapeutic CSI and CSI with CrI in conjunction with IT-MTX. The CSI and CrI dosage had been empirically derived and had been adopted as a "standard" for more than a decade (28).

Total VI randomly assigned children in hematologic remission to receive preventive CSI (24 Gy) or equivalent therapeutic CSI for overt CNS relapse. Event-free survival was strikingly higher with preventive therapy. For the 67% of patients who showed isolated CNS failure, treatment included prompt initiation of CSI (24 Gy) with continued maintenance chemotherapy. Although a surprising 23–35% of patients were cured by therapeutic CSI, the proportion of children ultimately free of leukemia was greater after early, preventive therapy (32). Subsequent studies showed that children who had sustained a CNS relapse had more significant functional deficits (e.g., seizure disorders and other neurologic sequelae, poorer cognitive function).

While demonstrating the efficacy of CSI, the SJCRH investigators noted hematologic and immune suppression that interfered with systemic therapy. IT-MTX was added to CrI based on apparently adequate distribution within the spinal subarachnoid space. Total VII showed that CrI (24 Gy) in conjunction with concurrent IT-MTX achieved results equivalent to those of CSI, and this remains a standard approach in selected presentations of ALL (28). Several subsequent trials have proved the relative equivalence of 18 Gy (at 1.5–1.8 Gy per fraction) and 24 Gy (similarly fractionated) (21,33–35).

Other approaches to preventive CNS therapy were developed in the 1970s, combining higher-dose systemic MTX with more prolonged inter-

TABLE 2-1. *Evolution of CNS therapy in acute lymphoblastic leukemia: St. Jude Children's Research Hospital total therapy studies IV–VIII*

Preventive CNS therapy	White blood cells	n	Initial (isolated) CNS relapse	Event-free survival at 5–10 years
Early Studies				
None (Total IV, VI)	<20,000	54	48–64%	
	>20,000	36	72–78%	
$CSI_{24 Gy/15 fx}$	<20,000	120	8%	
$CrI_{24 Gy/15 fx}$ + MTX_{IT} (Total V, VI, VII)	>20,000	50	12%	
Later Studies				
$CrI_{18 Gy/12 fx CNS 1,2}$ + MTX_{IT}				
$CrI_{24 Gy/16 fx CNS 3}$				
CrI 63% of cases (Total XI)	358	6%	70%	70%
$CrI_{18 Gy 12 fx CNS 1,2}$ + MTX/HC/$AraC_{IT}$				
$CrI_{24 Gy/16 fx CNS 3}$				
CrI 30% of cases (Total XII)	188	10%	62%	62%
CrI 17% of cases (Total XIIIA)	165	1%	77%	77%

$AraC_{IT}$, intrathecal cytosine arabinoside; CNS, central nervous system; CrI, cranial irradiation; CSI, craniospinal irradiation; fx, fractions; HC, hydrocortisone; MTX_{IT}, intrathecal methotrexate.

Modified from Schorin MA, Blattner S, Gelber RD, et al. Treatment of childhood acute lymphoblastic leukemia: results of Dana-Farber Cancer Institute/Children's Hospital Acute Lymphoblastic Leukemia Consortium Protocol 85-01. *J Clin Oncol* 1994;12(4):740–747; Hustu HO, Aur RJ. Extramedullary leukaemia. *Clin Haematol* 1978; 7(2):313–337.

mittent intrathecal (IT) therapy (33,34,36–39). Multiple trials have addressed serial reduction in the indications for CrI, balancing its proven efficacy with the potential toxicities (e.g., neurocognitive and neuroendocrine deficits; secondary cancers, especially brain tumors). Successful alternative regimens have relied on moderate- to high-dose intravenous methotrexate (HDMTX, varying from 0.5 to 8 g/m²) and prolonged exposure to repeated IT chemotherapy (either MTX alone or so-called triple IT therapy, also including hydrocortisone and cytosine arabinoside) throughout the 2–2.5 years of consolidation and continuation therapy (40). Comparative studies have shown that the combination of HDMTX and IT-MTX has been somewhat inferior to CrI in preventing overt CNS leukemia; however, overall disease control for all but the highest-risk subsets of ALL typically is equal or better with the chemotherapy approach because it significantly reduces systemic or extramedullary or extraneural failure (34,35, 37,40,41).

Yet to be fully evaluated is the balance of disease control and toxicities that might favor a chemotherapy or radiation therapy approach. The German BFM studies have explored risk-adapted proportional regimens that balance cranial irradiation (from 0 to 12 or 18 Gy for preventive therapy) and HDMTX (15,21,42).

Table 2-2 summarizes some of the major series reporting therapeutic approaches over the past 15 years. In sum, it is apparent that standard risk ALL may be treated without CrI (15,38,39, 41,43). The group for which CrI seems to be highly indicated is the cohort with T-cell ALL and a presenting WBC greater than 100,000 WBC/μL. Approximately 20% of children with T-cell ALL (or 2% of all children with ALL) present with high WBC and seem to benefit from preventive CrI (15,44). Because HDMTX and IT-MTX have been associated with neurologic sequelae, there is also interest in considering further dosage reduction (CrI = 12 Gy/8 fractions in the more recent BFM studies) (39).

Beyond the classic concerns regarding neurocognitive deficits (associated with both CrI and MTX) and neuroendocrine phenomena (especially growth hormone deficits and altered gonadotrophins), the major current concern limiting indications for CrI relates to secondary brain tumors (45–48). The incidence of secondary CNS tumors has ranged from 1–4% in several series to as high as 12% in a unique experience combining irradiation with high-dose antimetabolite therapy (23,49–51).

TABLE 2-2. *Major studies addressing CNS preventive therapy in acute lymphoblastic leukemia*

Study and risk category	CNS therapy	n	Event-free survival	CNS relapse
BFM 86: MR	$CrI_{18\ Gy}$	219	67%	2.3%
BFM 90: MR	$CrI_{12\ Gy}$	496	84%	1%
BFM 86: HR	$CrI_{18\ Gy}$	95	60%	7.4%
BFM 90: HR	$CrI_{12\ Gy}$	202	50%	2%
DFCC 87-01				
Standard risk	IT-MTX	142	77%	10%
High risk	$CrI_{18\ Gy}$	177	78%	1%
Very high risk	$CrI_{18\ Gy}$	50	62%	1%

BFM, Berlin–Frankfurt–Munster; CNS, central nervous system; CR, complete remission; CrI, cranial irradiation; DFCC, Dana–Farber Cancer Center; IT-MTX, intrathecal methotrexate; MR, CNS negative, medium risk with increased cell mass, non–T cell, age 2–9 years.
Standard risk = 2–8 yr, WBC < 20,000, CR ≤ 33 days; without CNS 2–3, mediastinal mass, T-cell, t(9;22).
High risk = not standard or very high risk.
Very high risk = WBC ≥ 100,000, <1 yr, t(9;22).
BFM data from Reiter A, Schrappe M, Ludwig WD, et al. Chemotherapy in 998 unselected childhood acute lymphoblastic leukemia patients. Results and conclusions of the multicenter trial ALL-BFM 86. *Blood* 1994;84(9):3122–3133; Gustafsson G, Schmiegelow K, Forestier E, et al. Improving outcome through two decades in childhood ALL in the Nordic countries: the impact of high-dose methotrexate in the reduction of CNS irradiation. Nordic Society of Pediatric Haematology and Oncology (NOPHO). *Leukemia* 2000;14(12):2267–2275.
DFCC data from Clarke M, Gaynon P, Hann I, et al. CNS-directed therapy for childhood acute lymphoblastic leukemia: Childhood ALL Collaborative Group overview of 43 randomized trials. *J Clin Oncol* 2003;21(9):1798–1809.

Current Recommendations for Preventive CNS Therapy

Current protocol-based CNS therapy reflects two different approaches. Most studies in the United States seek to minimize use of CrI, assessing radiation-related toxicities as substantially more concerning than chemotherapy-related toxicities (Fig. 2-4) (31,50–52). The BFM group has identified very high-risk patients as appropriately treated with CrI at lower dosages, feeling the balance of radiation- and chemotherapy-related toxicities has yet to be fully appreciated (21,25,31). Current "thresholds" for use of CrI and the dosages used are indicated in Table 2-3. To allow full-dose intensification and permit use of high-dose systemic MTX in the chemotherapy–irradiation sequence that is better tolerated, CrI typically is administered at the conclusion of intensification, 6–12 months after remission. Also to be considered is the role of CrI in patients treated for isolated mar-

TABLE 2-3. *Preventive CNS therapy: current protocol (recommendations)*

Study	Cohort	CrI
COG 0031 (very high risk, 5%)	Ph+, ≤ 44 chromosomes, M3 at end induction, M2 without CR at end extended induction and consolidation	18 Gy with CNS 3
		6 Gy if preceding TBI (TBI = 12 Gy/6 fractions/3 days)
POG 9906 (high risk)	CNS 3, testis (+), MLL gene rearrangement; no TEL-AML 1	86 Gy with CNS 3
	1 WBC > 100,000 or scaled with age for 20,000–80,000	
BFM 2000 (25% CrI)	Prednisone poor response, t(9;22), t(4;11), <CR end reduction, T cell, add high-level MRD week 12	12 Gy; 18 Gy with CNS 3
St. Jude Total XV	All cases (including high-risk, T cell, and CNS 3 at diagnosis)	0

AML, acute myeloblastic leukemia; BFM, Berlin–Frankfurt–Munster; CNS, central nervous system; COG, Children's Oncology Group; CR, complete remission; CrI, cranial irradiation; MRD, minimal residual disease; POG, Pediatric Oncology Group; TBI, total body irradiation; WBC, white blood cells.

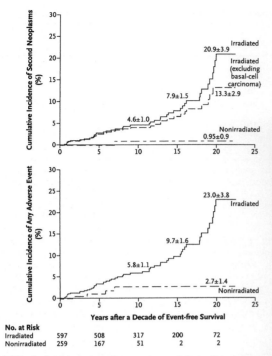

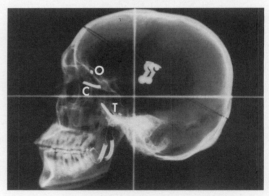

fossa anteriorly, located in the midline at a level that is typically below the orbital roof) and the lower limit of the temporal fossa at the skull base (Fig. 2-5). By convention, the lower border is at the inferior margin of the first or second

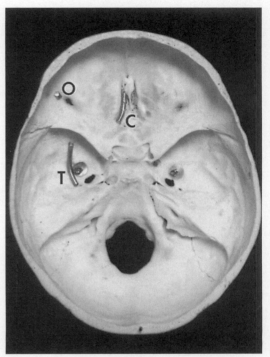

No. at Risk

Irradiated	597	508	317	200	72
Nonirradiated	259	167	51	2	2

FIG. 2-4. An extensive review of long-term survivors of childhood acute lymphoblastic leukemia (ALL) indicates that the cumulative incidence of second neoplasms or any significant adverse event among patients surviving 10 or more years free of relapsed leukemia is higher in those who were irradiated than in those who were not. This study also showed that children who underwent cranial irradiation had higher unemployment rates and lower marital rates as adults than age- and sex-matched members of the general population. Such results support current efforts to limit the use of cranial irradiation in initial therapy for ALL. (From Pui CH, Cheng C, Leung W, et al. Extended follow-up of long-term survivors of childhood acute lymphoblastic leukemia. *N Engl J Med* 2003;349:640–649, with permission).

row relapse; the threshold for CrI should be lower in children who relapse despite adequate initial systemic and IT therapy (53).

Radiotherapeutic Management

Volume

For preventive CNS therapy, the target volume includes the entire intracranial subarachnoid space. The key margins are at the skull base: the cribriform plate (the lowest point of the cranial

FIG. 2-5. Skull views outlining anatomic limits of the base of skull for inclusion of the intracranial subarachnoid space. **(A)** Lead markers have been placed in the subfrontal region at the level of the cribriform plate *(c)*, in contrast to the lateral subfrontal region representing the roof of the orbit *(o);* the inferior limits of the temporal fossa are outlined *(T)*. **(B)** The projection of the cribriform plate *(c)* and the temporal fossa *(T)* are indicated on the lateral radiograph of the skull.

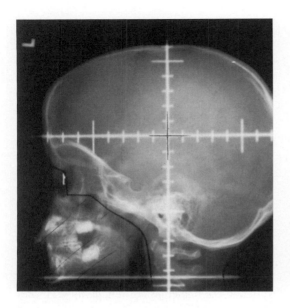

FIG. 2-6. Cranial irradiation field, outlining treatment that encompasses the entire cranial subarachnoid space, extending down to the second cervical vertebrae. Margins at the cribriform plate and temporal fossa are derived from anatomy, as demonstrated in Fig. 2-5. The lead markers outline the bony orbital rims, with inclusion of the posterior aspects of the orbit in the irradiated volume.

cervical vertebra (protocols differ). Familiarity with CrI in the setting of ALL and primary CNS tumors is important in achieving the desired coverage of the anatomic limits of the subarachnoid space (54).

Documentation of retinal involvement as a late manifestation of CNS leukemia has led to a standard requirement to include the posterior retina and orbital apex, subtending the extension of the subarachnoid space around the optic nerves (Fig. 2-6). Several techniques allow one to encompass the posterior orbit and globe while sparing the sensitive anterior aspect of the globe and lens. One approach uses inferior rotation of the gantry (i.e., angling the beam posteriorly for the supine patient) to achieve a parallel anterior margin at the bony orbital rim (Fig. 2-7) (55). The block or multileaf collimator margin for this

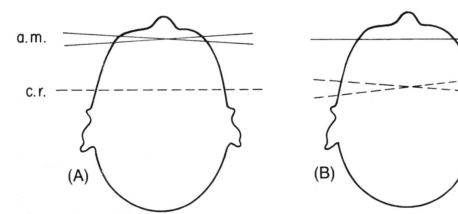

FIG. 2-7. Illustration of a simple means of achieving parallelism at the level of the anterior margin of the orbital rims for cranial irradiation. **(A)** Parallel opposed fields result in divergent beams at the orbital rims, resulting in irradiation of the anterior aspect of the contralateral eye. **(B)** A 4- to 5-degree gantry angle achieves a nonopposed field pair at the central ray *(c.r.)* while resulting in a parallel anterior margin *(a.m.)*. (From Li CK, Shing MMK, Chik KW, et al. Isolated testicular relapse after bone marrow transplantation with total body irradiation boost in acute lymphoblastic leukemia. *Bone Marrow Transplant* 1998;22:397–399, with permission.)

approach is identified by markers placed at the bony orbital rim during fluoroscopic simulation (Fig. 2-5). Alternatively, centers have used placement of the isocenter at the orbital rim to minimize divergence and allow one to use opposed lateral rather than gantry-angled field configurations. Detailed studies indicate that one needs to accept a dosage approximating 20% to the lens in order to adequately cover the cribriform plate (56). Dosimetric studies suggest that the use of custom beam blocking improves treatment when compared with a multileaf collimator alone (57).

Dosage

Dosages for preventive CrI range from 12 to 18 Gy in current protocols (Table 2-3). Fractionation typically is at 150–180 cGy once daily. A study at Dana–Farber Cancer Center (DFCC) in Boston has shown no difference in efficacy or apparent toxicity between conventional irradiation (180 cGy × 10) and hyperfractionated CrI (90 cGy twice daily to 18 Gy) (35).

Treatment of Established CNS Leukemia

CNS Leukemia at Diagnosis

CNS leukemia is present at diagnosis in 3–5% of children (19,58,59). Under the "staging" system proposed by Mahmoud, up to 20% of children show positive CSF cytology, but the incidence of true CNS leukemia (CNS 3: positive CSF cytology and WBC greater than 5/μL) is approximately 5% (19,59). Earlier trials found CNS leukemia at diagnosis associated with a negative outcome. More intensive systemic and IT chemotherapy has successfully eliminated CNS relapse in children with CNS 2 disease (positive CSF cytology and WBC less than 5/μL) (15,19–21,59). Therapeutic CrI or CSI has been used in most series for children with CNS 3 disease; the impact of CNS involvement on outcome has been diminished and, in some series, eliminated with such intervention (36,58–60).

Radiotherapeutic Management

Most current protocols include CrI after intensification therapy for children with CNS 3 disease

at diagnosis (Table 2-3). The recommended dosage of CrI is 18 Gy, based on 150- to 180-cGy fractions daily.

CNS Relapse

Despite CNS preventive therapy, 1–10% of children sustain an isolated CNS relapse (i.e., in the presence of continuous, maintained hematologic remission). More than 75% of children are diagnosed when asymptomatic based on surveillance lumbar puncture. Symptoms and signs related to CNS involvement include headaches with or without vomiting, papilledema, cranial nerve palsies (most often VI, VII; also V), and hyperphagia (61,62).

Therapy for isolated CNS relapse includes systemic chemotherapy for reinduction, IT chemotherapy (MTX alone or in combination with cytosine arabinoside and hydrocortisone) to clear the CSF, and irradiation. Several institutional reports documented the efficacy of CSI alone (28) or early after IT chemotherapy (63–66). Trials through the early 1990s showed moderate to high rates of CNS disease control but a rate of subsequent bone marrow relapse that exceeded 40% in every report (64,67,68). Reinduction chemotherapy without intensification similarly produced high rates of secondary CNS control while failing to cure more than 50% of children after CNS relapse (68–70). With the introduction of more intensive systemic chemotherapy, the secondary disease control rate increased to 70% (71).

Serial trials in Pediatric Oncology Group (POG) have shown the advantage of a more prolonged, intensive chemotherapy course before CSI: Ritchey et al. (61) documented 71% 4-year event-free survival (EFS) after systemic reinduction and intensification, delaying CSI (24-Gy CrI, 15-Gy spinal irradiation) until 6 months after second remission. Results also confirmed the impact of timing of CNS relapse: Children with initial remission exceeding 18 months had secondary EFS greater than 83%, compared with an EFS of 46% in those with early (less than 18 months) CNS relapse. A subsequent POG trial further delayed irradiation until 1 year after second remission to allow more intensive systemic therapy and selectively used just CrI (18 Gy) in those with initial remission duration of more than 18 months. Children with earlier CNS relapse (less than 18 months) received delayed CSI at dosages comparable to those of the earlier study. Preliminary data substantiate similar CNS and overall disease control: 65% overall EFS, with 76% EFS in those with later CNS relapse and 41% for those with earlier failure (72).

Volume

The standard therapy for CNS relapse is CSI. Evolving data seem to identify irradiation to the cranium only for children with onset of isolated CNS disease more than 18 months after first remission (72). Prospective studies in the setting of isolated CNS relapse use either technique, with no comparative data likely given the infrequency of isolated CNS failure in current protocols. The authors continue to recommend CSI, pending more mature data from the prospective POG trial reported earlier.

CrI techniques are as summarized earlier; CSI is described in detail in Chapter 4. The specific details of leptomeningeal leukemia management are outlined in Fig. 2-5, indicating slight modification of the cranial block at the skull base to account for the posterior retina and orbital apex, a standard for ALL therapy that differs from the type of cranial volumes indicated in primary CNS tumors.

Treatment of Other Extramedullary Sites

Testicular Leukemia

Treatment of ALL from 1985 to 1990 was associated with a significant risk of testicular relapse. Approximately 5–10% of boys showed clinical signs of testicular leukemia terminating remission; nearly 10–20% of all failures involved the testes (70,73,74). Testicular relapse typically is a late event. The median time from initial remission is 36 months in the Children's Cancer Group (CCG) experience (70,74). The occurrence is related to high-risk features (e.g., T-cell phenotype, high WBC at diagnosis) (70). Testicular relapse generally has been felt to rep-

resent a sign of inadequate systemic disease control rather than a true "sanctuary site" of inadequate chemotherapy penetrance analogous to the CNS. Enhanced systemic disease control, particularly the introduction of high-dose MTX into prolonged intensification regimens, has largely eliminated this occurrence in contemporary protocols (34,75). The Dutch Late Effects Study Group has recently reported successful management of testicular relapse without local irradiation, an approach without further documentation currently (76).

Radiotherapeutic Management

Treatment of testicular relapse involves systemic chemotherapy and consolidative irradiation. Although late failure may be associated with only unilateral involvement, most instances present with clinical or histologic evidence of bilateral infiltration (74,77). Irradiation is directed to both testes, often using an en face electron beam, calculating the energy to deliver 90% of the dose to the posterior aspect of the testes based on measurements in the treatment position or a superior oblique photon beam. Attention to daily positioning is important, ensuring the descent of the testes into the scrotum during therapy (Fig. 2-8). The recommended dosage is 20–24 Gy, usually given at 200 cGy per fraction (28,74). Because testicular irradiation is associated with both sterility and reduction in Leydig cell function, there is some interest in using chemotherapy alone, reserving orchiectomy for local disease control in boys who do not show prompt, histologically verified disease control after reinduction chemotherapy (3,43,78).

Other Sites of Extramedullary Disease

Other sites of extramedullary relapse are uncommon, representing only 2% of failures (70). An unusual pattern of involvement is disease confined to the anterior chamber of the eye. Unlike diffuse retinal disease that is associated with CNS leukemia, limited anterior chamber leukemia seems to be an isolated phenomenon, related more to lack of systemic disease control. Management with en face electrons superficially irradiating the

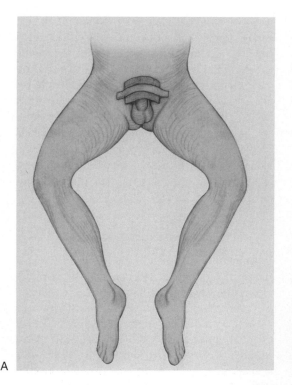

A

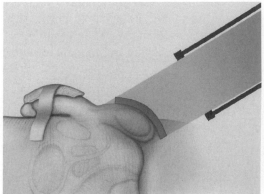

B

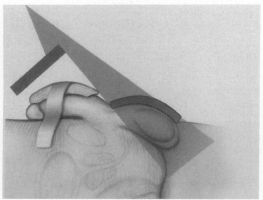

C

FIG. 2-8. Testicular irradiation for leukemia may be given with an en face electron field or a superior oblique photon field with a half beam block and bolus. The penile shaft is taped onto the abdominal wall with gauze to avoid irradiation.

eye has been successful at dosages of 12 Gy/6 fractions (79). Other sites of extramedullary involvement have included lymph nodes, ovaries or uterus, and bone (70). In the uncommon situation in which local extramedullary disease fails to respond to reinduction chemotherapy, or in the rare patient with massive local disease, it is appropriate to consider local consolidation either after intensification chemotherapy or in conjunction with bone marrow transplantation.

ACUTE MYELOGENOUS LEUKEMIA

Approximately 15–20% of children with leukemia present with AML, representing nearly 500 children per year in the United States. The disease occurs throughout the pediatric age range, with greater frequency in newborns and during adolescence. There is a high incidence of AML among young children with Down's syndrome (80). Presenting symptoms include pallor, fatigue, bleeding, and fever. Organomegaly at diagnosis is less common than in ALL. Localized extramedullary tumor deposits (chloromas or "granulocytic sarcomas") are rarely noted but can present as symptomatic masses involving the head and neck region, spinal cord, or brain. CNS disease is documented at presentation in 5–15% of cases (81). The initial WBC typically is below 50,000/mm^3; about 20% of cases present with hyperleukocytosis (WBC greater than 100,000/mm^3).

AML is classically categorized by cytomorphology, based on the French–American–British (FAB) classification (82). The common morphologic feature is the presence of Auer rods in cytoplasm of leukemic blasts. Cell types indicate primarily myeloblastic or monoblastic leukemia; less common are megakaryocytic types. Cytogenetic abnormalities have been documented in a majority of children with AML. One of the most common findings is translocation t(8;21), associated with AML1, a gene encoding AML1–CBFβ, a transcription factor that is essential for normal hematopoietic development (83,84). The t(8;21) often is combined with inversion of chromosome 16 [inv(16)] as "core binding factor" AML, commonly present in AML M2, the most common AML subtype (83,85). The t(8;21) translocation or inv(16) identifies patients with a comparably good prognosis. The t(9;22) translocation is associated with a poor outcome. Gene expression profiling has been used to match the chromosomal translocations in some cases. Children with CBF abnormalities appear to enjoy a favorable outcome (86). Changes in band q23 of chromosome 11 are common in secondary AML, especially after exposure to etoposides; outcome for secondary AML is particularly poor (83,87,88).

The mainstay of treatment for AML has been induction with daunorubicin (or idarubicin) in conjunction with cytarabine and thioguanine (89–92). Current regimens result in 30–40% disease-free survival rates in children. The subset of children with favorable prognostic features [t(15;17), t(8;21), and inv(16)] typically show long-term survival rates above 50% (81,83,86,89–91,93). Even more so than in ALL, the finding of minimal residual disease, by molecular or genetic analysis,

is associated with a poor outcome after induction in AML (94). Postinduction therapy is somewhat controversial, with recent data suggesting a role for either intensified consolidation chemotherapy or the use of allogeneic or autologous marrow transplant (91,93,95). Although earlier experience in pediatric AML had failed to prospectively identify a benefit with marrow transplant, trials in POG and CCG have demonstrated an apparent survival advantage for allogeneic transplant when compared with chemotherapy alone or autologous transplant (91,95).

Radiation therapy is occasionally needed for local manifestations of disease, typically chloromas in the spine or elsewhere in the CNS (Fig. 2-9). AML is radiosensitive, and dosages as low as 12 Gy often result in rapid local disease response. CNS involvement in AML is almost equivalent to that in ALL at diagnosis, more commonly associated with high initial WBC or children younger than 2 years old (96). CNS relapse is uncommon and is now most often treated with IT chemotherapy. Radiation therapy may be indicated for symptomatic or apparently resistant CNS involvement, treated in a manner comparable to that for ALL.

Bone Marrow Transplantation

Bone marrow transplantation (BMT) is a unique aspect of cancer therapy designed to allow higher dosages of cytolethal agents (chemotherapy, TBI), to "rescue" the attendant hematosuppression by engrafting new marrow stem cells to repopulate the bone marrow, and to take advantage of the immunotherapeutic effect of a donor graft in allogeneic BMT, combating otherwise aggressive or resistant neoplastic diseases. Developed initially by Donnell Thomas and colleagues at Fred Hutchinson Cancer Research Center, BMT has been used predominantly in leukemias, malignant lymphomas, and other hematologic disorders in both children and adults and increasingly in genetic diseases (e.g., aplastic anemia, Fanconi's syndrome, sickle cell disease, osteogenesis imperfecta) (97–101).

The principles of marrow transplantation include a conditioning regimen: "supralethal" dosages of chemotherapy (with TBI), and suc-

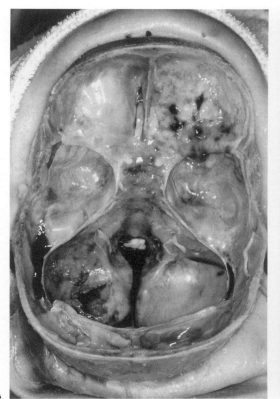

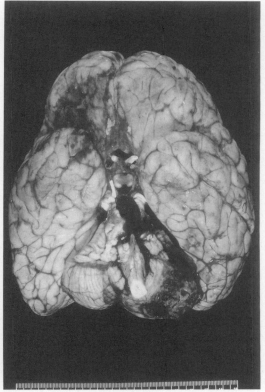

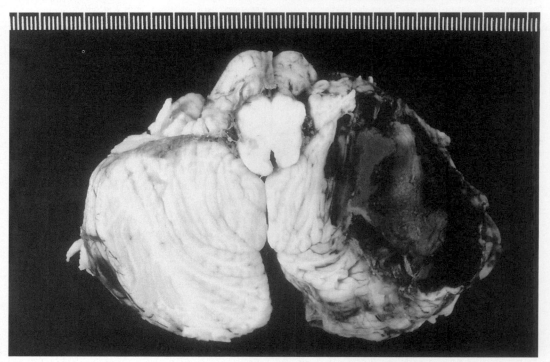

cessful engraftment of extrinsic hematopoietic stem cells. Initial work in BMT focused entirely on allogeneic transplantation, typically relying on a sibling or related donor found to be histocompatible based on human leukocyte antigen (HLA) typing. In the setting of malignant diseases, the cytolethal therapy is intended both to eliminate residual lymphoblasts or myeloblasts and to immunosuppress the host so that the donor marrow is accepted (97,102–104). More recently, the opportunity for BMT has been extended by the use of matched, unrelated donors, necessitating more significant immunosuppression but providing high-dose antineoplastic therapy to patients who lack a matched sibling donor (105–107). Unrelated donor transplants are more problematic in both the degree of immunosuppression needed to ensure engraftment and a higher rate of significant antihost immunoreactivity, called graft-versus-host disease (GVHD) (108). Syngeneic transplants (in which an identical twin is the donor) are technically similar to matched sibling donor transplants and are better tolerated immunologically.

In evaluating BMT, one looks at engraftment (implying both sufficient marrow depletion to allow the donor marrow access to "fertile ground" and immunosuppression to enable to graft to "take"); the rate of relapse or, conversely, leukemia- or cancer-free survival (i.e., disease control); and the rate of regimen-related (toxic) mortality, a significant proportion in most BMT data. Because of problems identifying suitable donors and regimen-related toxicities and mortalities often associated with GVHD, autologous transplants were developed to use the patient's own bone marrow stem cells (now often peripheral circulating stem cells), harvested and stored before the conditioning regimen, to repopulate the patient's bone marrow (with no immunocompatibility concerns). Autologous procedures are used in hematologic malignant diseases and "solid tumors" in both children and adults (95,109–111).

The first and current "standard" conditioning regimen is high-dose cyclophosphamide (CY) and TBI (27,97,103). The most commonly used non-TBI alternative is busulfan (BU) and cyclophosphamide (BU/CY) (112,113). Management of AML in remission and relapsed ALL are the most common indications for BMT in children and adolescents; data suggest that CY/TBI is superior to BU/CY in first or subsequent relapse of ALL (113–115).

Total Body Irradiation

The goals for TBI are similar to those outlined earlier (antineoplastic cell kill, bone marrow depletion to allow space for engraftment, and immunosuppression) (97,116–118). Initially, TBI was administered as a single fraction of approximately 10 Gy at 20–50 cGy per minute. Subsequent experience has demonstrated improved tolerance without sacrificing efficacy with lower dose rates (typically 5–10 cGy/minute) and with fractionated regimens (varying from the more common 2 Gy twice daily to

FIG. 2-9. The patient was a 3-year-old girl with a history of acute myelogenous leukemia diagnosed in January 2002. She developed cardiomyopathy and renal failure secondary to chemotherapy. In April 2002 she was hospitalized for chemotherapy and developed recurrent headaches. Computed tomography (CT) indicated the presence of left cerebral hemorrhage and a chloroma. A ventricular drain was placed. Radiotherapy was administered for increased intracranial pressure, but the patient's mental status declined. Review of her CT scan showed no significant change as result of radiation therapy. After a discussion with the child's family, a "do not resuscitate" order was issued, and the child died. These photographs, from the autopsy, show subdural hemorrhage most prominently in the left infratentorial region at the base of the skull. There was also tumor present in this area that measured 2 × 2 cm in diameter and 0.5 cm in thickness. Examination of the left interior cerebellum showed arachnoid hemorrhage and large viable tumor. There is also subarachnoid hemorrhage in the right frontal region. Microscopic evaluation showed tumor cells with pleomorphic nuclei of a myelomonocytic lineage. Myeloperoxide staining demonstrated numerous neoplastic cells in the hemorrhage.

12 Gy/6 fractions/3 days to a variety of regimens using 1–3 fractions per day to cumulative levels of 9–15.75 Gy) (116,119–123). For the increasingly used matched unrelated donor transplants, TBI-based regimens are standard to achieve sufficient immunosuppression (105–108).

BMT in Children and Adolescents

Acute Myeloblastic Leukemia

Consolidation of remission in childhood AML was one of the earlier successes in BMT (98). The overall disease-free survival rates of AML remain below 50%. There has been debate over the impact of postinduction intensification. More recent trials suggest a relationship between drug intensity and survival after remission (40,80,124). Improvements in supportive care have raised overall disease control rates after allogeneic BMT in childhood AML during first remission (112). Prospective studies comparing consolidation chemotherapy and BMT have shown improved disease control after allogeneic and autologous transplants in CCG and POG; regimen-related morbidities have limited the difference in overall survival with the allogeneic procedures (83,91, 95). Current trials independently emphasize rationally derived high-dose or drug-specific chemotherapy intensification or the use of allogeneic (or autologous) BMT. For children with relapse, the only curative approach is transplantation. Allogeneic transplants (at relapse or after reinduction) or autologous reinfusion (after second remission) result in survival rates of approximately 20–30% (83,119).

Conditioning regimens for allogeneic and autologous transplants in AML have ranged from variations of CY/TBI (with etoposide) to BU/CY or comparable chemotherapy combinations. Results suggest greater leukemia control with TBI in both children and adults, although overall survival rates usually are comparable, based on somewhat higher regimen-related mortality in the TBI-based transplants (111,114,116,119,125). Similarly, a prospective trial comparing TBI regimens (200 cGy daily to 12 Gy compared with 225 cGy daily to 15.75 Gy) showed equivalent outcome: Although relapse rates were much lower with the higher TBI dosage, the nonrelapse mortality was higher, resulting in similar event-free and overall survival rates (126). Current investigations also address low-dose TBI (2 Gy/fraction) in conjunction with fludarabine as "mini-transplants," purposefully inducing a chimeric state that relies on graft-versus-leukemia effect in a setting of postgraft immunosuppression (typically cyclosporine and mycophenolate mofetil) to maintain the chimerism (127).

Acute Lymphoblastic Leukemia

Indications for BMT in ALL differ from those in AML. Initial treatment regimens achieve overall disease-free survival rates of 80–90% (3). BMT typically is considered in children with early relapse (within 3 years of initial remission), poor initial response to induction therapy, or genetic signs of high-risk disease (Philadelphia chromosome (+) or BCR-ABL or MLL-AF4 fusion genes) (3,8,108). Both allogeneic and autologous transplants have been successful in ALL. Outcome depends on disease state: Several studies demonstrate long-term survival rates greater than 65% for ALL transplanted in first relapse (108,119–121,128–130). Comparative studies in relapsed ALL demonstrate an advantage for BMT, particularly in children with early relapse (131).

Allogeneic transplantation is the most common approach in relapsed ALL, using the standard matched sibling donor or, increasingly, matched unrelated or haploidentical (incompletely matched parent or sibling) donors (105,106,115,119,120). There has also been interest in using cord blood as a source of stem cells, less dependent on the degree of histocompatibility (104,107). It is unclear whether autologous transplants are superior to chemotherapy retrieval regimens (132).

The role of TBI has been addressed in children with ALL treated with allogeneic transplant using HLA-matched sibling donors. In a large retrospective comparison using data from the International Bone Marrow Transplant Registry, Davies et al. (115) found CY/TBI to be superior to BU/CY in preventing relapse, reducing treatment-related mortality, improving overall treatment failure, and reducing overall rate of mortality. Other series similarly suggest overall disease-free survival rates exceeding 55% (113, 115). The addition of etoposide to CY/TBI seems to further improve disease control and overall survival (119,130). For patients with extramedullary relapse (i.e., CNS, testis), the addition of local irradiation before (cranial) or during (testicular) the conditioning regimen results in excellent local disease control and outcomes equivalent to those with hematologic relapse alone (108,120).

Other Hematologic Diseases

Fanconi's anemia is an autosomal recessive disease characterized by progressive pancytopenia, thumb and radial abnormalities, growth retardation, abnormal skin pigmentation with café au lait spots, urinary tract abnormalities, microthalmia, small face, and cardiac malformations (100). The disease is associated with a number of chromosomal aberrations and is invariably fatal as a result of progressive marrow aplasia or the development of leukemia (133). BMT is potentially curative as "genetic therapy," reversing the underlying genetic clone and reintroducing normal hematopoiesis in approximately half of children without leukemic conversion (133,134). Transplant programs at some institutions rely on cyclophosphamide alone for those without overt leukemia based on greater radiation sensitivity in children with Fanconi's anemia. Other institutions use thoracoabdominal irradiation. Patients with leukemic conversion are treated with TBI at standard or reduced dosages similar to techniques used in other acute childhood leukemia settings.

Aplastic anemia is characterized by marrow hypoplasia and pancytopenia. The disease may be associated with chemical exposures or abnormal response to infectious or other agents; often, the origin is not apparent. Allogeneic BMT can be curative (101,135). Because it is a nonmalignant disorder, the conditioning regimen often is chemotherapy alone (cyclophosphamide with an additional alkylating agent). When additional immunosuppression is needed (e.g., initial failure at engraftment, incompletely matched donor), TBI or, preferably, total lymphoid irradiation is a part of the conditioning regimen (101,135). The latter has the advantage of sparing significant pulmonary irradiation while including sufficient volumes of the marrow and immune system to ensure engraftment (101,135).

Transplants have also been used successfully in sickle cell disease, although indications for the procedure and details of the conditioning regimen are evolving (136).

Abnormalities of the marrow stroma underlie the pathogenesis of bone development disorders (e.g., osteogenesis imperfecta, malignant osteopetrosis). BMT offers a potentially curative intervention, replacing the genetically abnormal stroma with stem cells capable of repopulating developing internal bone structure and reversing otherwise lethal aberrations in bone development (137). Preliminary investigations rely on TBI at lower dosages in these settings (138).

Radiotherapeutic Management

Volume

TBI is a fundamental component of BMT in most malignant and many genetic disease states. The target volume encompasses the entire body, key in any systemic disease (e.g., leukemia, disseminated malignant lymphomas). Techniques include a variety of physical configurations to achieve a field size adequate to subtend the entire body (Fig. 2-10). For infants and small children, an anterior–posterior (AP:PA) setup on the floor often allows sufficient field size and easy reproducibility. For larger children and adolescents, one of the extended distance techniques pictured in Fig. 2-10 is used to provide full coverage. AP:PA techniques (achieved with sitting or standing positions or with the supine or prone body rotated to be roughly perpendicular to the incident beam) offer the advantage of partial blocking for compensation or intentional diminution of dosages to critical structures (most often lungs, in some instances kidneys) (117,119,120,139–141).

Technical issues in TBI include identifying the desired dosage to the lungs. The incidence of inter-

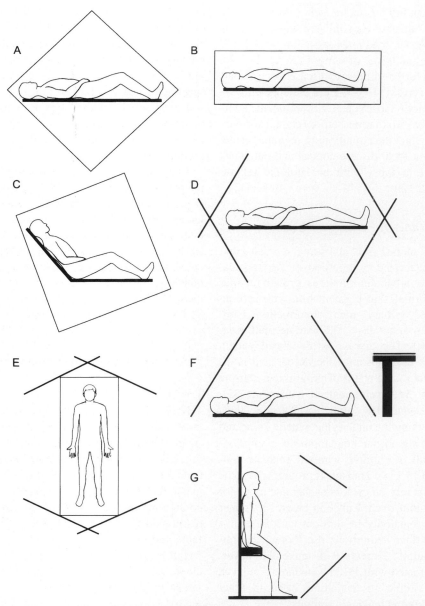

FIG. 2-10. A wide variety of techniques are available for administering total body irradiation (TBI). The techniques include **(A)** a lateral approach with the patient supine and the collimator of the treatment machine rotated to fit the patient in the beam; **(B)** a lateral approach with the patient supine and distant from the treatment machine so that a rectangular beam can be used; **(C)** a lateral approach with the patient in a semirecumbent position and the collimator of the treatment machine rotated to fit the patient in the beam; **(D)** a specially prepared TBI suite with one treatment machine mounted in the ceiling and one in the floor, with the patient placed on a treatment couch between the units; **(E)** a specially prepared TBI suite with two machines mounted at opposite ends of the room, with the patient irradiated in the lateral position while on a treatment couch between the units; **(F)** a conventional treatment unit used with the patient on the floor of the treatment room, rather than on the treatment couch, to obtain the necessary extended distance; and **(G)** the patient seated on a specially constructed seat to allow anterior and posterior treatment (some institutions use lung shielding during the photon treatment and then "boost" the ribs with electron beams).

stitial pneumonitis as one of the major regimen-related, often fatal acute toxicities is multifactorial. Factors include the transplant mode (syngeneic associated with the lowest incidence, allogeneic associated with an incidence that parallels the severity of acute GVHD), the combined conditioning regimen, and the radiation dosage, dose rate, and fractionation (121–123,126,140–143). Most current techniques compensate for added transmission through the measured lung volume and also deliver a dosage to the midplane of the lungs 10–15% lower than the dosage to the "total body" (119,120,126,140,142,143). Lung blocks should include the pulmonary volumes identified on AP:PA radiographs, typically excluding the upper mediastinum (i.e., thymus) from the lung shields. Ocular shields have also been explored, suggesting reduction in cataract formation and adequate disease control, perhaps excepting cases with overt CNS relapse before TBI (144). In lateral body techniques, the added width of the thorax in most children and adolescents compensates for the lung transmission.

Based on an initial testicular failure rate in 4 of 28 boys, Shank and colleagues at Memorial/Sloan–Kettering Cancer Center (117,145) recommended the addition of a testicular "boost" in TBI. Their use of a testicular boost almost completely eliminated testicular relapse. The use of testicular boosting has been similarly favored by other authors (146–152). However, not all institutions support the use of a testicular boost.

The recent French experience with TBI and high-dose cytosine arabinoside-busulphan used 12 Gy TBI in six fractions or 9–10 Gy as a single fraction with no testicular boost in two-thirds of the boys treated; no testicular failures were recorded (120).

Children with isolated CNS relapse may benefit from cranial irradiation given immediately before the start of the conditioning regimen (120). Studies at SJCRH typically use 9–10.8 Gy to the cranium (at 180 cGy once daily) timed to complete 1–3 days before TBI is initiated.

Dosage (Hematologic Malignancies)

The initial experience with TBI was based on a single fraction of 9–10 Gy (97,102,103,122).

Modifications in TBI delivery were stimulated by the occurrence of interstitial pneumonitis. Initial studies indicated a relative sparing by reducing the dosage below 10 cGy per minute (122,142). Parallel to the body of data regarding localized irradiation, a change to fractionated irradiation was suggested for TBI (123,153). Subsequent trials have generally indicated improvement in the therapeutic ratio with fractionated delivery based on one or two fractions per day (98,102,126,154). The most commonly used schedules include 2 Gy administered twice daily to 10–12 Gy; some centers have used an equal fraction size given once a day (98,102,120,126,154). Somewhat higher dosages have been used in study settings: 225 cGy once daily to 15.5 Gy or 1.7–1.75 Gy twice daily to 14 Gy (140,154). Alternative schedules deliver up to 12 Gy in 3- to 3.3-Gy fraction once daily (121,141,143). The range of fractionation regimens attests to the flexibility apparent at low total dosage levels for TBI. Suggestions that more fractionated regimens are better tolerated in terms of acute pulmonary and late somatic effects are difficult to prove across institutions and trials (117,123). Higher dosages typically are used in the setting of matched unrelated donor BMT (141). There is some suggestion that dosages beyond 14 Gy are associated with greater risks of TBI-related toxicities (116,154).

The use of a testicular boost is somewhat controversial, as noted earlier. The conventional approach in most current protocols uses 2 Gy on two consecutive days or 4 Gy in one fraction to the testes, most often via an en face electron field.

REFERENCES

1. Gurney JG, Davis S, Severson RK, et al. Trends in cancer incidence among children in the U.S. *Cancer* 1996;78(3):532–541.
2. Campana D, Pui CH. Detection of minimal residual disease in acute leukemia: methodologic advances and clinical significance. *Blood* 1995;85(6):1416–1434.
3. Pui CH, Evans WE. Acute lymphoblastic leukemia. *N Engl J Med* 1998;339(9):605–615.
4. Pui CH, Behm FG, Crist WM. Clinical and biologic relevance of immunologic marker studies in childhood acute lymphoblastic leukemia. *Blood* 1993;82(2):343–362.
5. Schorin MA, Blattner S, Gelber RD, et al. Treatment of childhood acute lymphoblastic leukemia: results of Dana-Farber Cancer Institute/Children's Hospital Acute

Lymphoblastic Leukemia Consortium Protocol 85-01. *J Clin Oncol* 1994;12(4):740–747.

6. Reiter A, Schrappe M, Ludwig WD, et al. Chemotherapy in 998 unselected childhood acute lymphoblastic leukemia patients. Results and conclusions of the multicenter trial ALL-BFM 86. *Blood* 1994;84(9):3122–3133.

7. Nachman J, Sather HN, Gaynon PS, et al. Augmented Berlin–Frankfurt–Munster therapy abrogates the adverse prognostic significance of slow early response to induction chemotherapy for children and adolescents with acute lymphoblastic leukemia and unfavorable presenting features: a report from the Children's Cancer Group. *J Clin Oncol* 1997;15(6):2222–2230.

8. Ribeiro RC, Abromowitch M, Raimondi SC, et al. Clinical and biologic hallmarks of the Philadelphia chromosome in childhood acute lymphoblastic leukemia. *Blood* 1987;70(4):948–953.

9. Pui CH, Crist WM. Biology and treatment of acute lymphoblastic leukemia. *J Pediatr* 1994;124(4):491–503.

10. Pui CH, Kane JR, Crist WM. Biology and treatment of infant leukemias. *Leukemia* 1995;9(5):762–769.

11. Look AT. Oncogenic transcription factors in the human acute leukemias. *Science* 1997;278(5340):1059–1064.

12. Pui CH, Boyett JM, Hancock ML, et al. Outcome of treatment for childhood cancer in black as compared with white children. The St. Jude Children's Research Hospital experience, 1962 through 1992. *JAMA* 1995;273(8):633–637.

13. Price RA, Johnson WW. The central nervous system in childhood leukemia. I. The arachnoid. *Cancer* 1973;31(3):520–533.

14. Smith M, Arthur D, Camitta B, et al. Uniform approach to risk classification and treatment assignment for children with acute lymphoblastic leukemia. *J Clin Oncol* 1996;14(1):18–24.

15. Schrappe M, Reiter A, Ludwig WD, et al. Improved outcome in childhood acute lymphoblastic leukemia despite reduced use of anthracyclines and cranial radiotherapy: results of trial ALL-BFM 90. German-Austrian-Swiss ALL-BFM Study Group. *Blood* 2000;95(11):3310–3322.

16. Gajjar A, Ribeiro R, Hancock ML, et al. Persistence of circulating blasts after 1 week of multiagent chemotherapy confers a poor prognosis in childhood acute lymphoblastic leukemia. *Blood* 1995;86(4):1292–1295.

17. Coustan-Smith E, Behm FG, Sanchez J, et al. Immunological detection of minimal residual disease in children with acute lymphoblastic leukaemia. *Lancet* 1998;351(9102):550–554.

18. Cave H, van der Werff ten Bosch J, Suciu S, et al. Clinical significance of minimal residual disease in childhood acute lymphoblastic leukemia. European Organization for Research and Treatment of Cancer: Childhood Leukemia Cooperative Group. *N Engl J Med* 1998;339(9):591–598.

19. Mahmoud HH, Rivera GK, Hancock ML, et al. Low leukocyte counts with blast cells in cerebrospinal fluid of children with newly diagnosed acute lymphoblastic leukemia. *N Engl J Med* 1993;329(5):314–319.

20. Pui CH, Mahmoud HH, Rivera GK, et al. Early intensification of intrathecal chemotherapy virtually eliminates central nervous system relapse in children with

acute lymphoblastic leukemia. *Blood* 1998;92(2):411–415.

21. Schrappe M, Reiter A, Henze G, et al. Prevention of CNS recurrence in childhood ALL: results with reduced radiotherapy combined with CNS-directed chemotherapy in four consecutive ALL-BFM trials. *Klin Padiatr* 1998;210(4):192–199.

22. Duration and intensity of maintenance chemotherapy in acute lymphoblastic leukaemia: overview of 42 trials involving 12,000 randomised children. Childhood ALL Collaborative Group. *Lancet* 1996;347(9018):1783–1788.

23. Pui CH, Cheng C, Leung W, et al. Extended follow-up of long-term survivors of childhood acute lymphoblastic leukemia. *N Engl J Med* 2003;349:640–649.

24. Pui CH. Childhood leukemias. *N Engl J Med* 1995;332(24):1618–1630.

25. Schrappe M, Reiter A, Zimmermann M, et al. Long-term results of four consecutive trials in childhood ALL performed by the ALL-BFM study group from 1981 to 1995. Berlin–Frankfurt–Munster. *Leukemia* 2000;14(12):2205–2222.

26. Brenner H, Kaatsch P, Burkhardt-Hammer T, et al. Long-term survival of children with leukemia achieved by the end of the second millennium. *Cancer* 2001;92(7):1977–1983.

27. Eden T. Translation of cure for acute lymphoblastic leukaemia to all children. *Br J Haematol* 2002;118(4):945–951.

28. Hustu HO, Aur RJ. Extramedullary leukaemia. *Clin Haematol* 1978;7(2):313–337.

29. Simone JV, Aur RJ, Hustu HO, et al. Three to ten years after cessation of therapy in children with leukemia. *Cancer* 1978;42(2 Suppl):839–844.

30. George P, Hernandez K, Hustu O, et al. A study of "total therapy" of acute lymphocytic leukemia in children. *J Pediatr* 1968;72(3):399–408.

31. Aur RJ, Simone JV, Hustu HO, et al. A comparative study of central nervous system irradiation and intensive chemotherapy early in remission of childhood acute lymphocytic leukemia. *Cancer* 1972;29(2):381–391.

32. George SL, Aur RJ, Mauer AM, et al. A reappraisal of the results of stopping therapy in childhood leukemia. *N Engl J Med* 1979;300(6):269–273.

33. Rivera GK, Raimondi SC, Hancock ML, et al. Improved outcome in childhood acute lymphoblastic leukaemia with reinforced early treatment and rotational combination chemotherapy. *Lancet* 1991;337(8733):61–66.

34. Abromowitch M, Ochs J, Pui CH, et al. Efficacy of high-dose methotrexate in childhood acute lymphocytic leukemia: analysis by contemporary risk classifications. *Blood* 1988;71(4):866–869.

35. LeClerc JM, Billett AL, Gelber RD, et al. Treatment of childhood acute lymphoblastic leukemia: results of Dana-Farber ALL Consortium Protocol 87-01. *J Clin Oncol* 2002;20(1):237–246.

36. Gaynon PS, Trigg ME, Heerema NA, et al. Children's Cancer Group trials in childhood acute lymphoblastic leukemia: 1983–1995. *Leukemia* 2000;14(12):2223–2233.

37. Freeman AI, Boyett JM, Glicksman AS, et al. Intermediate-dose methotrexate versus cranial irradiation in childhood acute lymphoblastic leukemia: a ten-year follow-up. *Med Pediatr Oncol* 1997;28(2):98–107.

38. Pullen J, Boyett J, Shuster J, et al. Extended triple intrathecal chemotherapy trial for prevention of CNS relapse in good-risk and poor-risk patients with B-progenitor acute lymphoblastic leukemia: a Pediatric Oncology Group study. *J Clin Oncol* 1993;11(5): 839–849.

39. Mahoney DH Jr, Shuster JJ, Nitschke R, et al. Intensification with intermediate-dose intravenous methotrexate is effective therapy for children with lower-risk B-precursor acute lymphoblastic leukemia: a Pediatric Oncology Group study. *J Clin Oncol* 2000;18(6):1285–1294.

40. Clarke M, Gaynon P, Hann I, et al. CNS-directed therapy for childhood acute lymphoblastic leukemia: Childhood ALL Collaborative Group overview of 43 randomized trials. *J Clin Oncol* 2003;21(9):1798–1809.

41. Laver JH, Barredo JC, Amylon M, et al. Effects of cranial radiation in children with high risk T cell acute lymphoblastic leukemia: a Pediatric Oncology Group report. *Leukemia* 2000;14(3):369–373.

42. Pui CH. Toward optimal central nervous system–directed treatment in childhood acute lymphoblastic leukemia. *J Clin Oncol* 2003;21(2):179–181.

43. Gustafsson G, Schmiegelow K, Forestier E, et al. Improving outcome through two decades in childhood ALL in the Nordic countries: the impact of high-dose methotrexate in the reduction of CNS irradiation. Nordic Society of Pediatric Haematology and Oncology (NOPHO). *Leukemia* 2000;14(12):2267–2275.

44. Conter V, Schrappe M, Arico M, et al. Role of cranial radiotherapy for childhood T-cell acute lymphoblastic leukemia with high WBC count and good response to prednisone. Associazione Italiana Ematologia Oncologia Pediatrica and the Berlin–Frankfurt–Munster groups. *J Clin Oncol* 1997;15(8):2786–2791.

45. Waber DP, Shapiro BL, Carpentieri SC, et al. Excellent therapeutic efficacy and minimal late neurotoxicity in children treated with 18 grays of cranial radiation therapy for high-risk acute lymphoblastic leukemia: a 7-year follow-up study of the Dana-Farber Cancer Institute Consortium Protocol 87-01. *Cancer* 2001; 92(1):15–22.

46. Mulhern RK, Fairclough D, Ochs J. A prospective comparison of neuropsychologic performance of children surviving leukemia who received 18-Gy, 24-Gy, or no cranial irradiation. *J Clin Oncol* 1991;9(8):1348–1356.

47. Jankovic M, Brouwers P, Valsecchi MG, et al. Association of 1800 cGy cranial irradiation with intellectual function in children with acute lymphoblastic leukaemia. ISPACC. International Study Group on Psychosocial Aspects of Childhood Cancer. *Lancet* 1994;344(8917):224–227.

48. Ochs J, Mulhern R, Fairclough D, et al. Comparison of neuropsychologic functioning and clinical indicators of neurotoxicity in long-term survivors of childhood leukemia given cranial radiation or parenteral methotrexate: a prospective study. *J Clin Oncol* 1991;9(1): 145–151.

49. Loning L, Zimmermann M, Reiter A, et al. Secondary neoplasms subsequent to Berlin–Frankfurt–Munster therapy of acute lymphoblastic leukemia in childhood: significantly lower risk without cranial radiotherapy. *Blood* 2000;95(9):2770–2775.

50. Walter AW, Hancock ML, Pui CH, et al. Secondary brain tumors in children treated for acute lymphoblastic leukemia at St. Jude Children's Research Hospital. *J Clin Oncol* 1998;16(12):3761–3767.

51. Relling MV, Rubnitz JE, Rivera GK, et al. High incidence of secondary brain tumours after radiotherapy and antimetabolites. *Lancet* 1999;354(9172):34–39.

52. Pui CH, Boyett JM, Rivera GK, et al. Long-term results of Total Therapy studies 11, 12 and 13A for childhood acute lymphoblastic leukemia at St. Jude Children's Research Hospital. *Leukemia* 2000;14(12):2286–2294.

53. Buhrer C, Hartmann R, Fengler R, et al. Importance of effective central nervous system therapy in isolated bone marrow relapse of childhood acute lymphoblastic leukemia. BFM (Berlin–Frankfurt–Munster) Relapse Study Group. *Blood* 1994;83(12):3468–3472.

54. Halperin EC, Laurie F, Fitzgerald TJ. An evaluation of the relationship between the quality of prophylactic cranial radiotherapy in childhood acute leukemia and institutional experience: a Quality Assurance Review Center–Pediatric Oncology Group study. *Int J Radiat Oncol Biol Phys* 2002;53(4):1001–1004.

55. Kline RW, Gillin MT, Kun LE. Cranial irradiation in acute leukemia: dose estimate in the lens. *Int J Radiat Oncol Biol Phys* 1979;5(1):117–121.

56. Weiss E, Krebeck M, Kohler B, et al. Does the standardized helmet technique lead to adequate coverage of the cribriform plate? An analysis of current practice with respect to the ICRU 50 report. *Int J Radiat Oncol Biol Phys* 2001;49(5):1475–1480.

57. Kalapurakal JA, Sathiaseelan V, Bista T, et al. Adverse impact of multileaf collimator field shaping on lens dose in children with acute leukemia receiving cranial irradiation. *Int J Radiat Oncol Biol Phys* 2000;48(4):1227–1231.

58. Cherlow JM, Sather H, Steinherz P, et al. Craniospinal irradiation for acute lymphoblastic leukemia with central nervous system disease at diagnosis: a report from the Children's Cancer Group. *Int J Radiat Oncol Biol Phys* 1996;36(1):19–27.

59. Burger B, Zimmermann M, Mann G, et al. Diagnostic cerebrospinal fluid examination in children with acute lymphoblastic leukemia: significance of low leukocyte counts with blasts or traumatic lumbar puncture. *J Clin Oncol* 2003;21(2):184–188.

60. Kun LE. CNS disease at diagnosis: a continuing challenge in childhood lymphoblastic leukemia. *Int J Radiat Oncol Biol Phys* 1996;36(1):257–259.

61. Ritchey AK, Pollock BH, Lauer SJ, et al. Improved survival of children with isolated CNS relapse of acute lymphoblastic leukemia: a pediatric oncology group study. *J Clin Oncol* 1999;17(12):3745–3752.

62. Ha CS, Woong-ki C, Koller CA, et al. Role of radiation therapy to the brain in leukemic patients with cranial nerve palsies in the absence of radiological findings. *Leuk Lymphoma* 1999;32(5–6):497–503.

63. Wells RJ, Weetman RM, Baehner RL. The impact of isolated central nervous system relapse following initial complete remission in childhood acute lymphocytic leukemia. *J Pediatr* 1980;97(3):429–432.

64. Kun LE, Camitta BM, Mulhern RK, et al. Treatment of meningeal relapse in childhood acute lymphoblastic leukemia. I. Results of craniospinal irradiation. *J Clin Oncol* 1984;2(5):359–364.

65. Behrendt H, van Leeuwen EF, Schuwirth C, et al. The

significance of an isolated central nervous system relapse, occurring as first relapse in children with acute lymphoblastic leukemia. *Cancer* 1989;63(10):2066–2072.

66. Willoughby MCN. Treatment of CNS leukemia. In: Mastrangelio A, Poplak DG, Riccardi R, eds. *Central nervous system leukemia: prevention and treatment.* Boston: Martinus Nijhoff, 2003:113.

67. Land VJ, Thomas PR, Boyett JM, et al. Comparison of maintenance treatment regimens for first central nervous system relapse in children with acute lymphocytic leukemia. A Pediatric Oncology Group study. *Cancer* 1985;56(1):81–87.

68. Winick NJ, Smith SD, Shuster J, et al. Treatment of CNS relapse in children with acute lymphoblastic leukemia: a Pediatric Oncology Group study. *J Clin Oncol* 1993;11(2):271–278.

69. Kumar P, Kun LE, Hustu HO, et al. Survival outcome following isolated central nervous system relapse treated with additional chemotherapy and craniospinal irradiation in childhood acute lymphoblastic leukemia. *Int J Radiat Oncol Biol Phys* 1995;31(3): 477–483.

70. Gaynon PS, Qu RP, Chappell RJ, et al. Survival after relapse in childhood acute lymphoblastic leukemia: impact of site and time to first relapse—the Children's Cancer Group Experience. *Cancer* 1998;82(7):1387–1395.

71. Ribeiro RC, Rivera GK, Hudson M, et al. An intensive re-treatment protocol for children with an isolated CNS relapse of acute lymphoblastic leukemia. *J Clin Oncol* 1995;13(2):333–338.

72. Barredo JC, Lauer S, Billet A, et al. Isolated CNS relapse of acute lymphoblastic leukemia (ALL) treated with intensive systemic chemotherapy and delayed CNS radiation: A Pediatric Oncology Group study. Proceedings of ASCO 2003;22:796.

73. Nesbit ME Jr, Robison LL, Ortega JA, et al. Testicular relapse in childhood acute lymphoblastic leukemia: association with pretreatment patient characteristics and treatment. A report for Childrens Cancer Study Group. *Cancer* 1980;45(8):2009–2016.

74. Bowman WP, Aur RJ, Hustu HO, et al. Isolated testicular relapse in acute lymphocytic leukemia of childhood: categories and influence on survival. *J Clin Oncol* 1984;2(8):924–929.

75. Rivera GK, Pinkel D, Simone JV, et al. Treatment of acute lymphoblastic leukemia. 30 years' experience at St. Jude Children's Research Hospital. *N Engl J Med* 1993;329(18):1289–1295.

76. van den BH, Langeveld NE, Veenhof CH, et al. Treatment of isolated testicular recurrence of acute lymphoblastic leukemia without radiotherapy. Report from the Dutch Late Effects Study Group. *Cancer* 1997;79(11):2257–2262.

77. Testicular disease in acute lymphoblastic leukaemia in childhood. Report on behalf of the Medical Research Council's Working Party on leukaemia in childhood. *BMJ* 1978;1(6109):334–338.

78. Jahnukainen K, Salmi TT, Kristinsson J, et al. The clinical indications for identical pathogenesis of isolated and non-isolated testicular relapses in acute lymphoblastic leukaemia. *Acta Paediatr* 1998;87(6): 638–643.

79. Bunin N, Rivera G, Goode F, et al. Ocular relapse in the anterior chamber in childhood acute lymphoblastic leukemia. *J Clin Oncol* 1987;5(2):299–303.

80. Vormoor J, Boos J, Stahnke K, et al. Therapy of childhood acute myelogenous leukemias. *Ann Hematol* 1996;73(1):11–24.

81. Boulad F, Kernan NA. Treatment of childhood acute nonlymphoblastic leukemia: a review. *Cancer Invest* 1993;11(5):534–553.

82. Ebb DH, Weinstein HJ. Diagnosis and treatment of childhood acute myelogenous leukemia. *Pediatr Clin North Am* 1997;44(4):847–862.

83. Lowenberg B, Downing JR, Burnett A. Acute myeloid leukemia. *N Engl J Med* 1999;341(14):1051–1062.

84. Miyoshi H, Shimizu K, Kozu T, et al. t(8;21) Breakpoints on chromosome 21 in acute myeloid leukemia are clustered within a limited region of a single gene, AML 1. *Proc Natl Acad Sci U S A* 1991;88:10431–10434.

85. Downing JR. The AML1-ETO chimaeric transcription factor in acute myeloid leukaemia: biology and clinical significance. *Br J Haematol* 1999;106(2):296–308.

86. Raimondi SC, Chang MN, Ravindranath Y, et al. Chromosomal abnormalities in 478 children with acute myeloid leukemia: clinical characteristics and treatment outcome in a cooperative pediatric oncology group study-POG 8821. *Blood* 1999;94(11):3707–3716.

87. Hale GA, Heslop HE, Bowman LC, et al. Bone marrow transplantation for therapy-induced acute myeloid leukemia in children with previous lymphoid malignancies. *Bone Marrow Transplant* 1999;24(7): 735–739.

88. Pui CH, Relling MV. Topoisomerase II inhibitor-related acute myeloid leukaemia. *Br J Haematol* 2000;109(1):13–23.

89. Creutzig U, Ritter J, Zimmermann M, et al. Idarubicin improves blast cell clearance during induction therapy in children with AML: results of study AML-BFM 93. AML-BFM Study Group. *Leukemia* 2001; 15(3):348–354.

90. Krance RA, Hurwitz CA, Head DR, et al. Experience with 2-chlorodeoxyadenosine in previously untreated children with newly diagnosed acute myeloid leukemia and myelodysplastic diseases. *J Clin Oncol* 2001; 19(11):2804–2811.

91. Woods WG, Neudorf S, Gold S, et al. A comparison of allogeneic bone marrow transplantation, autologous bone marrow transplantation, and aggressive chemotherapy in children with acute myeloid leukemia in remission. *Blood* 2001;97(1):56–62.

92. Stevens RF, Hann IM, Wheatley K, et al. Marked improvements in outcome with chemotherapy alone in paediatric acute myeloid leukemia: results of the United Kingdom Medical Research Council's 10th AML trial. MRC Childhood Leukaemia Working Party. *Br J Haematol* 1998;101(1):130–140.

93. Bloomfield CD, Shuma C, Regal L, et al. Long-term survival of patients with acute myeloid leukemia: a third follow-up of the Fourth International Workshop on Chromosomes in Leukemia. *Cancer* 1997;80(11 Suppl):2191–2198.

94. Sievers EL, Lange BJ, Buckley JD, et al. Prediction of relapse of pediatric acute myeloid leukemia by use of multidimensional flow cytometry. *J Natl Cancer Inst* 1996;88(20):1483–1488.

95. Ravindranath Y, Yeager AM, Chang MN, et al. Autologous bone marrow transplantation versus intensive consolidation chemotherapy for acute myeloid leukemia in childhood. Pediatric Oncology Group. *N Engl J Med* 1996;334(22):1428–1434.

96. Pui CH, Dahl GV, Kalwinsky DK, et al. Central nervous system leukemia in children with acute nonlymphoblastic leukemia. *Blood* 1985;66(5):1062–1067.

97. Thomas E, Storb R, Clift RA, et al. Bone-marrow transplantation. *N Engl J Med* 1975;292(16):832–843.

98. Thomas ED, Clift RA, Hersman J, et al. Marrow transplantation for acute nonlymphoblastic leukemic in first remission using fractionated or single-dose irradiation. *Int J Radiat Oncol Biol Phys* 1982;8(5):817–821.

99. Thomas ED. ALL and beyond: implications for other hematologic malignancies. *Leukemia* 1997;11(Suppl 4):S43–S45.

100. Alter BP. Fanconi's anemia. Current concepts. *Am J Pediatr Hematol Oncol* 1992;14(2):170–176.

101. McGlave PB, Haake R, Miller W, et al. Therapy of severe aplastic anemia in young adults and children with allogeneic bone marrow transplantation. *Blood* 1987;70(5):1325–1330.

102. Altschuler C, Resbeut M, Blaise D, et al. Fractionated total body irradiation and bone marrow transplantation in acute lymphoblastic leukemia. *Int J Radiat Oncol Biol Phys* 1990;19(5):1151–1154.

103. Gale RP, Butturini A, Bortin MM. What does total body irradiation do in bone marrow transplants for leukemia? *Int J Radiat Oncol Biol Phys* 1991;20(3):631–634.

104. Kurtzberg J, Laughlin M, Graham ML, et al. Placental blood as a source of hematopoietic stem cells for transplantation into unrelated recipients. *N Engl J Med* 1996;335(3):157–166.

105. Sierra J, Radich J, Hansen JA, et al. Marrow transplants from unrelated donors for treatment of Philadelphia chromosome–positive acute lymphoblastic leukemia. *Blood* 1997;90(4):1410–1414.

106. Hongeng S, Krance RA, Bowman LC, et al. Outcomes of transplantation with matched-sibling and unrelated-donor bone marrow in children with leukaemia. *Lancet* 1997;350(9080):767–771.

107. Gluckman E, Rocha V, Boyer-Chammard A, et al. Outcome of cord-blood transplantation from related and unrelated donors. Eurocord Transplant Group and the European Blood and Marrow Transplantation Group. *N Engl J Med* 1997;337(6):373–381.

108. Woolfrey AE, Anasetti C, Storer B, et al. Factors associated with outcome after unrelated marrow transplantation for treatment of acute lymphoblastic leukemia in children. *Blood* 2002;99(6):2002–2008.

109. Vaidya SJ, Atra A, Bahl S, et al. Autologous bone marrow transplantation for childhood acute lymphoblastic leukaemia in second remission: long-term follow-up. *Bone Marrow Transplant* 2000;25(6):599–603.

110. Dusenbery KE, Daniels KA, McClure JS, et al. Randomized comparison of cyclophosphamide–total body irradiation versus busulphan–cyclophosphamide conditioning in autologous bone marrow transplantation for acute myeloid leukemia. *Int J Radiat Oncol Biol Phys* 1995;31(1):119–128.

111. Biagi E, Rovelli A, De Lorenzo P, et al. Autologous hematopoietic stem cell transplantation (AHSCT) as consolidation therapy for childhood acute myelogenous leukemia in 1st complete remission. *Pediatr Hematol Oncol* 2001;18(5):359–362.

112. Michel G, Gluckman E, Esperou-Bourdeau H, et al. Allogeneic bone marrow transplantation for children with acute myeloblastic leukemia in first complete remission: impact of conditioning regimen without total-body irradiation—a report from the Société Francaise de Greffe de Moelle. *J Clin Oncol* 1994;12(6):1217–1222.

113. Ringden O, Ruutu T, Remberger M, et al. A randomized trial comparing busulfan with total body irradiation as conditioning in allogeneic marrow transplant recipients with leukemia: a report from the Nordic Bone Marrow Transplantation Group. *Blood* 1994;83(9):2723–2730.

114. Litzow MR, Perez WS, Klein JP, et al. Comparison of outcome following allogeneic bone marrow transplantation with cyclophosphamide–total body irradiation versus busulphan–cyclophosphamide conditioning regimens for acute myelogenous leukaemia in first remission. *Br J Haematol* 2002;119(4):1115–1124.

115. Davies SM, Ramsay NK, Klein JP, et al. Comparison of preparative regimens in transplants for children with acute lymphoblastic leukemia. *J Clin Oncol* 2000;18(2):340–347.

116. Bieri S, Helg C, Chapuis B, et al. Total body irradiation before allogeneic bone marrow transplantation: is more dose better? *Int J Radiat Oncol Biol Phys* 2001;49(4):1071–1077.

117. Shank B, Chu FC, Dinsmore R, et al. Hyperfractionated total body irradiation for bone marrow transplantation. Results in seventy leukemia patients with allogeneic transplants. *Int J Radiat Oncol Biol Phys* 1983;9(11):1607–1611.

118. Down JD, Tarbell NJ, Thames HD, et al. Syngeneic and allogeneic bone marrow engraftment after total body irradiation: dependence on dose, dose rate, and fractionation. *Blood* 1991;77(3):661–669.

119. Duerst RE, Horan JT, Liesveld JL, et al. Allogeneic bone marrow transplantation for children with acute leukemia: cytoreduction with fractionated total body irradiation, high-dose etoposide and cyclophosphamide. *Bone Marrow Transplant* 2000;25(5):489–494.

120. Bordigoni P, Esperou H, Souillet G, et al. Total body irradiation–high-dose cytosine arabinoside and melphalan followed by allogeneic bone marrow transplantation from HLA-identical siblings in the treatment of children with acute lymphoblastic leukaemia after relapse while receiving chemotherapy: a Societe Francaise de Greffe de Moelle study. *Br J Haematol* 1998;102(3):656–665.

121. Corvo R, Paoli G, Barra S, et al. Total body irradiation correlates with chronic graft versus host disease and affects prognosis of patients with acute lymphoblastic leukemia receiving an HLA identical allogeneic bone marrow transplant. *Int J Radiat Oncol Biol Phys* 1999;43(3):497–503.

122. Kim TH, Rybka WB, Lehnert S, et al. Interstitial pneumonitis following total body irradiation for bone marrow transplantation using two different dose rates. *Int J Radiat Oncol Biol Phys* 1985;11(7):1285–1291.

123. Cosset JM, Girinsky T, Malaise E, et al. Clinical basis for TBI fractionation. *Radiother Oncol* 1990;18(Suppl 1):60–67.

124. Ravindranath Y, Steuber CP, Krischer J, et al. High-dose cytarabine for intensification of early therapy of

childhood acute myeloid leukemia: a Pediatric Oncology Group study. *J Clin Oncol* 1991;9(4):572–580.

125. Robin M, Guardiola P, Dombret H, et al. Allogeneic bone marrow transplantation for acute myeloblastic leukaemia in remission: risk factors for long-term morbidity and mortality. *Bone Marrow Transplant* 2003;31(10):877–887.

126. Clift RA, Buckner CD, Appelbaum FR, et al. Allogeneic marrow transplantation in patients with acute myeloid leukemia in first remission: a randomized trial of two irradiation regimens. *Blood* 1990;76(9):1867–1871.

127. Niederwieser D, Maris M, Shizuru JA, et al. Low-dose total body irradiation (TBI) and fludarabine followed by hematopoietic cell transplantation (HCT) from HLA-matched or mismatched unrelated donors and postgrafting immunosuppression with cyclosporine and mycophenolate mofetil (MMF) can induce durable complete chimerism and sustained remissions in patients with hematological diseases. *Blood* 2003;101(4):1620–1629.

128. Zecca M, Pession A, Messina C, et al. Total body irradiation, thiotepa, and cyclophosphamide as a conditioning regimen for children with acute lymphoblastic leukemia in first or second remission undergoing bone marrow transplantation with HLA-identical siblings. *J Clin Oncol* 1999;17(6):1838–1846.

129. Brochstein JA, Kernan NA, Groshen S, et al. Allogeneic bone marrow transplantation after hyperfractionated total-body irradiation and cyclophosphamide in children with acute leukemia. *N Engl J Med* 1987;317(26):1618–1624.

130. Biagi E, Rovelli A, Balduzzi A, et al. TBI, etoposide and cyclophosphamide as a promising conditioning regimen for BMT in childhood ALL in second remission. *Bone Marrow Transplant* 2000;26(11):1260–1262.

131. Barrett AJ, Horowitz MM, Pollock BH, et al. Bone marrow transplants from HLA-identical siblings as compared with chemotherapy for children with acute lymphoblastic leukemia in a second remission. *N Engl J Med* 1994;331(19):1253–1258.

132. Borgmann A, Schmid H, Hartmann R, et al. Autologous bone-marrow transplants compared with chemotherapy for children with acute lymphoblastic leukaemia in a second remission: a matched-pair analysis. The Berlin–Frankfurt–Munster Study Group. *Lancet* 1995;346(8979):873–876.

133. Flowers ME, Doney KC, Storb R, et al. Marrow transplantation for Fanconi anemia with or without leukemic transformation: an update of the Seattle experience. *Bone Marrow Transplant* 1992;9(3):167–173.

134. MacMillan ML, Auerbach AD, Davies SM, et al. Haematopoietic cell transplantation in patients with Fanconi anaemia using alternate donors: results of a total body irradiation dose escalation trial. *Br J Haematol* 2000;109(1):121–129.

135. Castro-Malaspina H, Childs B, Laver J, et al. Hyperfractionated total lymphoid irradiation and cyclophosphamide for preparation of previously transfused patients undergoing HLA-identical marrow transplantation for severe aplastic anemia. *Int J Radiat Oncol Biol Phys* 1994;29(4):847–854.

136. Walters MC, Storb R, Patience M, et al. Impact of bone marrow transplantation for symptomatic sickle cell disease: an interim report. Multicenter investigation of bone marrow transplantation for sickle cell disease. *Blood* 2000;95(6):1918–1924.

137. Eapen M, Davies SM, Ramsay NK, et al. Hematopoietic stem cell transplantation for infantile osteopetrosis. *Bone Marrow Transplant* 1998;22(10):941–946.

138. Horwitz EM, Gordon PL, Koo WKK, et al. Isolated allogeneic bone marrow-derived mesenchymal cells engraft and stimulate growth in children with osteogenesis imperfecta: implications for cell therapy of bone. *Proc Natl Acad Sci U S A* 2003;99:8932–8937.

139. Broerse JJ, Dutriex A, Noordijk EM. Physical, biological and clinical aspects of TBI. *Radiother Oncol* 1990;18(Suppl 1):11–162.

140. Harden SV, Routsis DS, Geater AR, et al. Total body irradiation using a modified standing technique: a single institution 7 year experience. *Br J Radiol* 2001; 74(887):1041–1047.

141. Corvo R, Lamparelli T, Bruno B, et al. Low-dose fractionated total body irradiation (TBI) adversely affects prognosis of patients with leukemia receiving an HLA-matched allogeneic bone marrow transplant from an unrelated donor (UD-BMT). *Bone Marrow Transplant* 2002;30(11):717–723.

142. Barrett A, Depledge MH, Powles RL. Interstitial pneumonitis following bone marrow transplantation after low dose rate total body irradiation. *Int J Radiat Oncol Biol Phys* 1983;9(7):1029–1033.

143. Gopal R, Ha CS, Tucker SL, et al. Comparison of two total body irradiation fractionation regimens with respect to acute and late pulmonary toxicity. *Cancer* 2001;92(7):1949–1958.

144. van Kempen-Harteveld ML, van Weel-Sipman MH, Emmens C, et al. Eye shielding during total body irradiation for bone marrow transplantation in children transplanted for a hematological disorder: risks and benefits. *Bone Marrow Transplant* 2003;31:1151–1156.

145. Shank B, O'Reilly RJ, Cunningham I, et al. Total body irradiation for bone marrow transplantation: the Memorial Sloan–Kettering Cancer Center experience. *Radiother Oncol* 1990;18(Suppl 1):68–81.

146. Koike M, Hino K, Onizuka T, et al. Testicular relapse with Ph-positive chromosome after bone marrow transplantation for acute lymphocytic leukemia. *Rinsho Ketsueki* 1993;34(1):63–67.

147. Matsue K, Tohi T, Massauji N, et al. Second bone marrow transplantation following high dose busulfan, etoposide, and Ara-C after testicular relapse in a patient with AML. *Rinsho Ketsueki* 1992;33(3):338–342.

148. Godinho C, Trindale AJ, Vale L, et al. Testicular relapse in acute lymphoblastic leukemia. *Acta Med Port* 1995;8(11):613–618.

149. Li CK, Shing MMK, Chik KW, et al. Isolated testicular relapse after bone marrow transplantation with total body irradiation boost in acute lymphoblastic leukemia. *Bone Marrow Transplant* 1998;22: 397–399.

150. Forrest DL, Dalal BI, Naiman SC, et al. Testicular relapse of acute promyelocytic leukemia after allogeneic BMT. *Bone Marrow Transplant* 1997;20:689–690.

151. Lehmann LE, Guinan EC, Halpern SL, et al. Isolated testicular relapse in an adolescent 5 years following allogeneic bone marrow transplantation for acute myelogenous leukemia. *Bone Marrow Transplant* 1997; 19:849–851.

152. Locatelli F, Gambarana D, Zecca M, et al. Prophylactic orchiectomy after bone marrow transplantation for boys with acute lymphoblastic leukaemia and previous testicular relapse. *Bone Marrow Transplant* 1991; 8(Suppl 1):57–59.

153. Peters LJ, Withers HR, Cundiff JH, et al. Radiobiological considerations in the use of total-body irradiation for bone-marrow transplantation. *Radiology* 1979; 131(1):243–247.

154. Clift RA, Buckner CD, Appelbaum FR, et al. Long-term follow-up of a randomized trial of two irradiation regimens for patients receiving allogeneic marrow transplants during first remission of acute myeloid leukemia. *Blood* 1998;92(4):1455–1456.

3

Supratentorial Brain Tumors Except Ependymomas; Brain Tumors in Babies and Very Young Children

Larry E. Kun, M.D.

Nearly 20% of all neoplasms in children arise in the central nervous system (CNS). The incidence of CNS tumors in children has increased over the past three decades (1). The frequency of brain tumors by site and histology is indicated in Table 3-1. The current World Health Organization (WHO) classification of CNS neoplasms is summarized in Table 3-2 (2,3).

Nearly one-half of pediatric CNS tumors are supratentorial tumors. Anatomically, the supratentorial cranial compartment (Fig. 3-1) includes the cerebral hemispheres (i.e., the frontal, parietal, temporal, and occipital lobes), the diencephalon (i.e., the hypothalamus, the optic chiasm, and the thalamic, caudate nucleus, putamen, and basal ganglion structures, the latter generally considered together as the thalamic region), and the pineal region (i.e., the pineal gland and posterior third ventricular region). Tumors are commonly categorized by regions that correlate with specific clinical findings and histologic types: suprasellar lesions (including glial tumors of the optic chiasm and adjacent hypothalamic area, craniopharyngiomas, and germ cell tumors of the anterior third ventricular region), central or deep-seated lesions (gliomas of the thalamic region and pineal region tumors including germ cell, embryonal, and glial neoplasms), and peripheral lesions (gliomas, ependymomas, and embryonal tumors of the cerebral hemispheres).

Advances in neuroimaging have greatly improved the accuracy of diagnosis and staging of CNS tumors. Magnetic resonance imaging (MRI) often is the only imaging tool sensitive enough to identify small hemispheric tumors presenting with seizures. Although MRI provides unique and often diagnostic information in suprasellar and pineal region lesions, computed tomography (CT) better delineates calcification (typically seen in craniopharyngiomas and malignant germ cell tumors). Positron emission tomography, single photon emission tomography, and magnetic resonance spectroscopy are of potential value in assessing tumor type or grade, particularly in evaluating tissue viability to differentiate tumor progression from radiation-related changes (e.g., intralesional necrosis) (4–7).

Modern neurosurgical techniques have largely eliminated the need to consider radiation therapy or chemotherapy without a histologic diagnosis in supratentorial tumors (8). There is no apparent advantage to the patient or radiation oncologist in considering therapy based on imaging alone. Exceptions include malignant germ cell tumors diagnosed by elevated levels of α-fetoprotein or β-human chorionic gonadotropin (β-HCG) and optic pathway tumors that involve the optic nerve alone or the chiasm in conjunction with adjacent optic pathway structures, particularly in the setting of neurofibromatosis (9). For craniopharyngiomas, the imaging diagnosis often can be confirmed by simple cyst aspiration, documenting the presence of diagnostic squamous cells or cholesterol crystals in the cyst fluid (10).

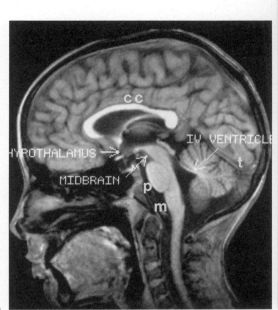
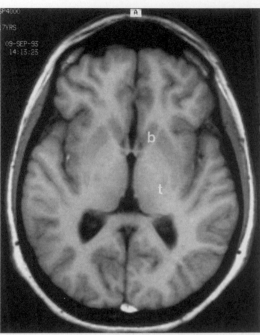

A   B

FIG. 3-1. (A) Sagittal and **(B)** axial MRI of the normal brain. Note tentorium *(t)* separating supraten-torial volume from infratentorial or posterior fossa region **(A).** The supratentorial compartment in-cludes the cerebral hemispheres, basal ganglia *(b),* and thalamic nuclei *(t),* and the lateral ventricles **(B)** contain the hypothalamus and corpus callosum *(cc)* **(A).** The posterior fossa **(A)** includes the cerebellum and the brainstem (midbrain, pons *[P],* medulla *[M]*); the fourth ventricle is central in the posterior fossa **(A).**

ETIOLOGY

Although brain tumors are mostly sporadic, a number of pediatric brain tumor presentations are associated with recognized neurocutaneous or other genetic syndromes (11).

Neurofibromatosis is a common congenital disorder associated with CNS tumors (12). Clini-cal criteria for type I neurofibromatosis (NF1) in-clude six or more café au lait spots and peripheral neurofibromas. NF1 is an autosomal dominant syndrome linked to a 17q chromosomal defect. Fully 15–20% of children with neurofibromatosis ultimately present with CNS neoplasms, usually gliomas of the visual pathways or low-grade tu-

TABLE 3-1. *Relative incidence of common brain tumors in children*

Supratentorial tumors	(45–50%)	Infratentorial tumors	(50–55%)
Astrocytoma	23%	Medulloblastoma	20%
Malignant gliomas (anaplastic	6%	Astrocytoma	15%
astrocytoma, glioblastoma multiforme)		Brainstem glioma	10%
Craniopharyngioma	6%	Ependymoma	6%
Embryonal tumors (PNET and others)	4%		
Pineal region tumors/intracranial germ			
cell tumors	4%		
Ependymoma	3%		
Oligodendroglioma	2%		
Other (meningioma, ganglioma, choroids			
plexus tumors, others)	2%		

From references 2, 146, and 150, with permission.

TABLE 3-2. *Histopathologic classification of CNS tumors—WHO classification 1994*

1. Tumors of neuroepithelial tissue
   astrocytic tumors (astrocytoma, anaplastic
      astrocytoma, glioblastoma, pilocytic
      astrocytoma, pleomorphic xanthoastrocytoma,
      subependymal giant cell astrocytoma)
   oligodendroglial tumors (oligodendroglioma,
      anaplastic oligodendroglioma)
   ependymal tumors (ependymoma, anaplastic
      ependymoma, myxopapillary ependymoma)
   mixed gliomas (oligodendroglioma, others)
   choroids plexus tumors
   neuronal tumors (gangliocytoma, gnaglioglioma,
      desmoplastic infantile neuroepithelioma,
      dysembryoplastic neuroepithelial tumor)
   pineal tumors (pineocytoma, pineoblastoma)
2. Embryonal tumors
   medulloepithelioma
   neuroblastoma
   ependymoblastoma
   primitive neuroectodermal tumors (PNETs)
      medulloblastoma (posterior fossa, cerebellar)
      cerebral or spinal PNETs
3. Tumors of meningothelial cells
   meningioma
   malignant meningioma
4. Tumors of the uncertain histogenesis
   hemangioblastoma
5. Germ cell tumors
   germinoma
   embryonal carcinoma
   endodermal sinus tumor
   choriocarcinoma
   teratoma
   mixed germ cell tumors
   ependymoblastoma
6. Tumors of the sellar region
   pituitary adenoma
   craniopharyngioma

From references 3 and 188, with permission.

mors of the diencephalon, cerebral hemispheres, or posterior fossa (13). Low-grade gliomas associated with NF1 may be biologically less aggressive than similar gliomas in the general population (14,15).

The indolent subependymal giant cell astrocytoma occurs in children with tuberosclerosis, a hereditary disorder signified also by cutaneous acneiform lesions and angiofibromas, mental retardation, and renal insufficiency; CNS findings include hamartomatous periventricular lesions known as tubers.

The Li-Fraumeni familial tumor syndrome includes brain tumors and sarcomas in children in association with breast cancer, sarcomas, and brain tumors in related young adults (16). The syndrome is associated with p53 deletion abnormalities and a high incidence of secondary, treatment-related neoplasms (17).

Radiation-induced meningiomas have long been recognized. Reports indicate a disturbing incidence of secondary gliomas, most often malignant or high grade, in long-term survivors of childhood acute lymphoblastic leukemia (18, 19). The estimated risk is 1–3% after routine preventive cranial irradiation (CrI); a dose–response relationship has been suggested, with minimal incidence after dosages less than 20 Gy and a risk of approximately 10% after cumulative dosages greater than 30 Gy (generally in children with repeated courses of cranial irradiation in association with CNS relapse) (19). A unique experience at St. Jude Children's Research Hospital found a 12% incidence in a particular study associated with 18-Gy CrI and high-dose, concurrent antimetabolite therapy (6-mercaptopurine); the incidence is now approximately 19% in the latter trial (20) (L. Kun, personal communication, 2003).

CLINICAL PRESENTATION

Supratentorial tumors generally present with localizing neurologic symptoms. Seizures are the most common symptom in cerebral hemispheric lesions, especially in those arising in the temporal lobe. Lateralizing neurologic signs (motor or sensory) occur in thalamic region tumors, often associated with symptoms of increased intracranial pressure. Suprasellar tumors typically occlude the foramen of Monro, resulting in symptoms of elevated intracranial pressure. Visual signs (e.g., visual field cuts or decreased acuity) and endocrine abnormalities (e.g., diminished growth hormone, cortisol, or thyroid-stimulating hormone or signs of delayed or precocious puberty) often are apparent with the midline suprasellar lesions. Youngsters with suprasellar tumors may show features of the diencephalic syndrome, signified by hyperactivity and asthenia, the latter despite normal or high food intake (21). Pineal region tumors produce hydrocephalus by compressing the aqueduct of Sylvius; specific ocular signs (i.e., Parinaud's syndrome) are classically noted (22).

LOW-GRADE HEMISPHERIC AND DIENCEPHALIC ASTROCYTOMAS

Low-grade supratentorial astrocytomas of childhood occur predominantly in the central regions of the diencephalon, including the hypothalamic–optic chiasmatic region and the thalamus. Cerebral hemispheric astrocytomas account for 40% of the supratentorial lesions, occurring primarily in the temporal and frontal lobes (23–25).

The astrocytic neoplasms are classified histologically by the dominant cell type (3,26–28).

Fibrillary astrocytomas consist of long, thin cells highlighted by a crisscrossing background matrix of neuroglial fibrils. The tumors often are circumscribed in the diencephalon but may be diffuse or poorly marginated in the cerebral hemispheres. Gemistocytic astrocytomas are an uncommon variant that present as benign-appearing, often circumscribed lesions with a high rate of recurrence; these tumors often demonstrate malignant degeneration within several years after initial presentation (29). Protoplasmic astrocytomas are characterized by large, rounded astrocytes with abundant cytoplasm and a background largely devoid of fibrils (30).

The fibrillary, gemistocytic, and protoplasmic astrocytomas may be grouped together with "astrocytomas, not otherwise specified (NOS)" as ordinary astrocytomas to distinguish them from the common juvenile pilocytic astrocytoma (JPA) (26,28). Ordinary astrocytomas may show malignant degeneration, accruing successive genetic abnormalities that result in a more malignant phenotype in up to 40% of recurrent, uncontrolled lesions (24,31,32). Whether the genotypical progression documented in adult malignant gliomas occurs in children is unclear (33–37).

The classic Kernohan system for grading ordinary astrocytomas (cytologically identifying astrocytomas as grades I, II, III, or IV) has largely been replaced by a histologic system advanced by Burger et al. (26,38), the WHO (3), and others (27). The WHO system categorizes JPA as grade 1, other differentiated astrocytoma as grade 2, anaplastic (malignant) astrocytoma as grade 3, and glioblastoma multiforme (GBM) as grade 4 (3).

JPAs are low-grade neoplasms histologically signified by elongated bipolar astrocytes organized in a parallel array of glial fibers, giving a hairlike or piloid appearance (27). The sparsely cellular tumors are signified by microcysts and Rosenthal's fibers (amorphous eosinophilic material formed by plump, degenerating astrocytes). Macroscopically, visible cystic components often are present, sometimes with much less prominent solid tumor components. The tumors may be circumscribed or may extend along white matter tracks, depending on location (Fig. 3-2) (27). JPA is the most common tumor in the diencephalic region and makes up 25% of hemispheric astrocytomas (8,23). JPA is unique in retaining low-grade characteristics even when uncontrolled or recurrent. The tumor typically is nonaggressive, although rapid progression and dissemination (or multifocal presentations) certainly occur (39–42). The incidence of leptomeningeal dissemination among low-grade gliomas ranges from 1% to 20%; a recent review of more than 500 children and adolescents with low-grade neuroepithelial tumors indicated a 3% incidence (43). As in prior reports, such involvement typically is present at diagnosis (in contradistinction to metastatic tumors) and associated with JPA or grade II astrocytomas, most often arising in the diencephalon (39,43).

Pilomyxoid astrocytomas were recently identified as a more aggressive subset of lesions previously classified as JPAs (44). Occurring primarily in the hypothalamic region in young children (median age, 10 months), they appear to have a higher rate of early recurrence and may necessitate a more aggressive approach than classic JPAs.

Less common astrocytic tumors include pleomorphic xanthoastrocytomas and subependymal giant cell astrocytomas.

Pleomorphic xanthoastrocytomas are benign astrocytic tumors presenting in children as large, peripherally located hemispheric lesions, often involving the leptomeninges (45). The tumor appears aggressive histologically, with cellular pleomorphism and numerous mitoses, but is biologically benign. A small percentage of

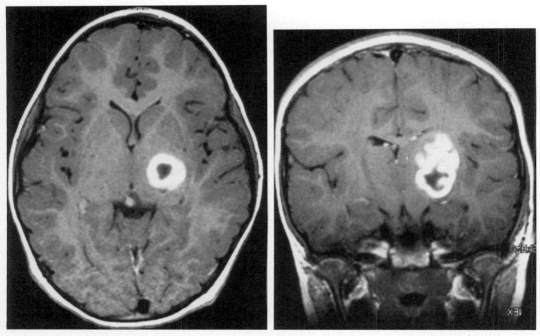

A   B

FIG. 3-2. Juvenile pilocytic astrocytoma of left thalamus, a localized, well-circumscribed lesion occurring in a 7-year-old boy. This type of lesion can be approached surgically but is also an excellent target for three-dimensional conformal irradiation (Fig. 3-4) or stereotactic radiotherapy (fractionated radiosurgery).

these lesions show mitotic activity or areas of necrosis; designated as pleomorphic xanthoastrocytoma with anaplastic features, tumors with high proliferative indices (with or without necrosis) appear to be somewhat more aggressive clinically (46,47). Long-term disease control usually is obtained through surgery alone; a proportion of cases do recur late and may show malignant degeneration (48,49).

Subependymal giant cell astrocytomas are sharply marginated tumors that occur along the linings of the lateral ventricles (3). The lesions occur in the setting of tuberous sclerosis, a congenital disease complex associated with hamartomas and benign neoplasms of the brain (cortical hamartomas known as tubers and the subependymal lesions here noted most often) in conjunction with cutaneous angiofibromas and angiomyolipomas of the kidney; children often show significant developmental delays (50). CNS manifestations of tuberosclerosis are most often related to the tuber sclerosis complex gene

1 (*TSC1*), identified as a 9q34 mutation (51). The tumors are benign, nearly hamartomatous lesions necessitating therapy (most often surgery alone) only if progressive or symptomatic.

Uncommonly, low-grade gliomas present as diffusely infiltrating tumors involving two or more cerebral lobes. The latter tumors often are nonenhancing on CT and MRI, and in children they may show little mass effect (52). A subset of patients with gliomatosis cerebri present with an obvious mass lesion in addition to the diffuse pattern of involvement (53). These diffuse lesions appear to represent an uncommon entity, usually called gliomatosis cerebri (3,26,54). Surgery is limited to biopsy; early response to irradiation is almost always followed by recurrence within 2 years (55,56). Low-grade gliomas involving both right and left thalamic regions (i.e., bithalamic tumors) are noted in up to 25% of pediatric thalamic region astrocytomas and seem to have an aggressive course similar to that of the more diffuse gliomatosis cerebri (57).

Therapy

Surgery

Management of low-grade gliomas generally is determined by the site of origin. Tumors arising in the cerebral hemispheres often are resectable. Pediatric reports indicate total removal in up to 90% of cerebral hemispheric astrocytomas and mixed oligoastrocytomas (23,24,58). Low recurrence rates are reported for both JPA and ordinary astrocytomas after total resection (23,24, 58–60). Early data from the Children's Cancer Group (CCG) and Pediatric Oncology Group (POG) study of primary surgery in low-grade gliomas indicate 5-year progression-free survival in 92% of children after gross total resection (GTR), ranging from 95–100% for juvenile pilocytic astrocytomas and gangliogliomas to 80% for grade II diffuse astrocytomas in this age group (61,62). Tumors involving the dominant medial temporal lobe, motor strip region, or Broca's speech cortex may be unresectable because of the neurologic deficits attendant to surgery.

Resection has been increasingly reported in the central thalamic and hypothalamic astrocytomas (63–65). The surgical series are selected by tumor size and anatomic location; resection is feasible in fewer than one-third of children with diencephalic gliomas. Reports indicate safety in resecting selected tumors, with serious morbidity limited to fewer than 10% of cases (63, 66–69). Short-term follow-up indicates freedom from recurrence in a majority of children after resection, although long-term results are pending (68,69). The CCG and POG study, available in preliminary abstract form, indicates progression-free survival after surgery alone of 50–60% for diencephalic tumors and 80–90% for lesions originating in the cerebellar or cerebral hemispheres (61,62,70). For most diencephalic presentations, surgery is limited to stereotactic biopsy, cyst decompression, and ventriculoperitoneal shunt as needed.

Radiation Therapy

Radiation therapy is effective in low-grade gliomas, achieving tumor response measured by serial imaging studies and durable disease control in a significant proportion of pediatric cases (Fig. 3-3) (24,59,71–73). An analysis from Pollack et al. (24) showed improved disease control at 10 years after irradiation following incomplete resection of cerebral hemispheric astrocytomas: 82% progression-free survival with irradiation versus 42% after surgery alone. The same study showed no significant benefit in overall survival (24). There are no contemporary data suggesting a benefit to postoperative irradiation for completely resected low-grade astrocytomas. For incompletely resected astrocytomas, the current indications for radiation therapy include postsurgical progression in a location not amenable to safe, definitive second resection; symptomatic disease, as with tumor-related neurologic signs that might be diminished after radiation response (e.g., long tract signs in thalamic tumors); or evolving identification of disease factors including the size of residual disease (61) or aggressive subtypes of astrocytomas based on histology (e.g., pilomyxoid tumors) or biology (JPAs that are associated with markers of increased proliferative activity, e.g., high MIB-1 labeling index) (44,60). For incompletely resected tumors that are asymptomatic and limited in volume, it is prudent to follow up with children until progression is documented by neurologic findings or imaging.

Preliminary reports from the large CCG and POG low-grade trial mentioned earlier in this chapter confirm previous institutional reports suggesting that a significant proportion of incompletely resected astrocytomas remain indolent over 3–5 years: progression-free survival at 5 years is 53–60% after near total or subtotal resection (14,61). A decision to observe children with residual astrocytomas should involve the radiation oncologist and the neurosurgeon, indicating the importance of regular imaging follow-up that allows one to comfortably follow a child with the anticipation that irradiation can be initiated upon documented tumor progression (58). Such an approach balances the recognized efficacy of radiation therapy with potential toxicities related, in part, to the anatomic location and volume of the tumor and the age of the patient (14,25). Inherent in such an approach is the commitment to intervene appropriately

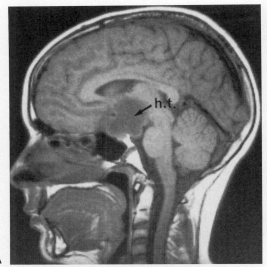

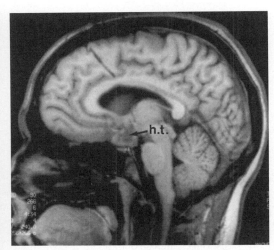

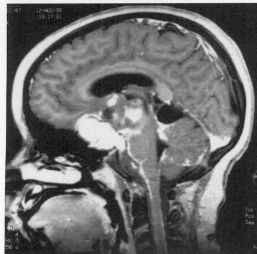

FIG. 3-3. Tumors of the optic chiasm and hypothalamic region: **(A)** a well-delineated lesion involving the posterior aspect of the chiasm and adjacent hypothalamus; **(B)** appearance 5 years after local irradiation. Current treatment approach is highlighted in Fig. 3-4. **(C)** Approximately 10–20% of these lesions demonstrate multifocal or metastatic tumor at diagnosis, a presentation that may be compatible with long-term response or stabilization.

with documented disease progression, including use of primary radiation therapy or additional surgery, as indicated.

JPAs predominate in diencephalic childhood gliomas. Prolonged progression-free survival after irradiation alone for hypothalamic and chiasmatic tumors reflects both the indolent nature of tumors in this site and the efficacy of irradiation. Survival rates greater than 70% at 10 years after irradiation are common for these tumors (10,72). In thalamic astrocytomas, pilocytic histology is less prevalent; 10-year survival results range from 33% to 60% after therapy (10,57, 72). For central diencephalic gliomas, precision

volume radiation techniques, including three-dimensional (3D) conformal and intensity-modulated radiation therapy (IMRT), proton beam therapy, and highly selected use of single-fraction radiosurgery, may offer advantages that alter the risk–benefit ratio in favor of earlier radiation therapy (74–78).

Diffuse low-grade gliomas are uncommon outside the brainstem in children. Gliomatosis cerebri or bithalamic astrocytomas may represent supratentorial counterparts of the more common infiltrating brainstem astrocytomas (56,57). These tumors respond to radiation therapy both symptomatically and by imaging, although recurrence and progression often are apparent within 2 years (similar to the radiation response noted in diffuse brainstem gliomas) (56,57).

Chemotherapy

The use of initial chemotherapy for low-grade gliomas has been studied primarily in hypothalamic and chiasmatic tumors. Follow-up studies suggest similar response and disease control rates for astrocytomas at other sites, primarily using the now-standard carboplatin and vincristine regimen (79–81). Although chemotherapy has been associated with only a modest objective response rate, data indicate a prolonged disease stabilization interval in progressive low-grade gliomas of approximately 3 years (79). The goal of delayed irradiation for such an interval may be worthwhile, especially in young children. Use of carboplatin, alone or with vincristine, has been the standard, associated with few serious late toxicities to date (79,80,82). The five-drug University of California at San Francisco regimen (6-thioguanine, procarbazine, dibromodulcitol, lomustine, and vincristine) has been reported to be similarly efficacious; a randomized comparison with carboplatin and vincristine is ongoing in the COG (83). Temozolomide appeared to be effective in a phase II trial including both children and adults (84).

Radiotherapeutic Management

Volume

The target volume for low-grade astrocytomas usually is localized to the imaging-defined tumor with limited margin. JPAs usually are well-circumscribed lesions; with image-guided therapy, the typically enhancing or circumscribed lesion is defined as the gross tumor volume (GTV), most often using the T1 sequence on MRI with gadolinium enhancement (for nonenhancing tumors, T1, T2, or flair sequence may best identify the lesion). The clinical tumor volume (CTV) may be defined as a 1-cm margin; early data in a prospective study at St. Jude indicated a dearth of marginal recurrences with tight targeting (73). Similar guidelines appear to be appropriate for grade II (fibrillary) astrocytomas, recognizing that most such tumors in children have readily identifiable margins on imaging; expansion of the GTV by 1 cm apparently has resulted in few marginal failures (73,85). Shrinking fields typically are not used in JPAs; when target volumes for infiltrating fibrillary astrocytomas are broader than typically needed because of difficulty identifying tumor margins, fields may be reduced to more narrowly encompass the obvious tumor on T1 or T2 at 45–50.4 Gy.

Diffuse low-grade gliomas outside the brainstem are most often identified as gliomatosis cerebri or bithalamic astrocytomas; both necessitate wide-field irradiation (56,57). Such lesions are best identified on T2 or flair sequences; a margin of 2 to 3 cm is recommended. For gliomatosis cerebri that is bilateral and involving much of the cerebral hemispheres, corpus callosum, and, sometimes, thalamic nuclei, it is appropriate to include the whole brain, at least to a dosage level of 45 Gy, before using a more imaging-defined "boost" volume (56,86).

Astrocytomas with multifocal presentations or subarachnoid seeding generally are treated with craniospinal irradiation (CSI), although the need to cover the entire neuraxis is unproven (39–41).

Dosage

There are few direct dose-response data specific for pediatric astrocytomas in the literature. Shaw et al. (86) showed an advantage with radiation therapy in JPA and other low-grade astrocytomas only at dosages greater than 53 Gy. It seems ironic that the adult low-grade glioma trials have established no clear benefit for dosage levels greater than 45 Gy (the European Organization for Research and Treatment of Cancer study showed no difference between 45 and 59.4 Gy; the North Central Cancer Treatment Group, Radiation Therapy Oncology Group, and Eastern Cooperative Oncology Group study showed no difference between 50.4 and 64.8 Gy) (87,88), yet planned national trials in children continue to focus on dosage levels approaching tolerance (i.e., 50–54 Gy). The primary justification is the long-term disease control rates documented in studies of pediatric JPA and, to a lesser extent, other low-grade astrocytomas. For children 2 to 5 years old, we recommend 50 to 54 Gy using 150 to 180 cGy per fraction. For children younger than 2 years of age, one generally tries to delay irradiation, particularly with increasing data indicating the efficacy of chemotherapy in delaying irradiation for an average of 3 years. When radiation therapy is needed, a dosage of 45 to 50 Gy to small volumes is appropriate. In children at least 5 years old, the traditional dosage of 54 to 55 Gy is recommended at 150 to 180 cGy per fraction (73).

Technique

Ideal techniques achieve close conformation of the high-dose region to a well-defined local target volume. Both 3D conformal and IMRT achieve such conformality, with potential differences in sparing adjacent dose-limiting structures (e.g., optic chiasm, eye, and pituitary–hypothalamic region) and in intralesional homogeneity. Given the nature of low-grade gliomas and recognized dose-related toxicities, attention to intralesional dosage maps is critical in designing treatment techniques. Multiple fields, based on single-plane or noncoplanar techniques as available, are used to a dosage distribution maximally conformed to the target volume (Fig. 3-4). The impact of low-dose irradiation on broader regions of the developing brain has not yet been fully explored; early results suggest that 3D conformal techniques achieve greater sparing of neuropsychologic function, for example, than past experience has shown for conventional therapies (89). Experience with stereotactic radiotherapy or fractionated radiosurgery seems to have been succeeded by the greater conformality of 3D conformal radiation therapy (CRT) or IMRT (74). The potential advantage of proton therapy is being explored (76,90).

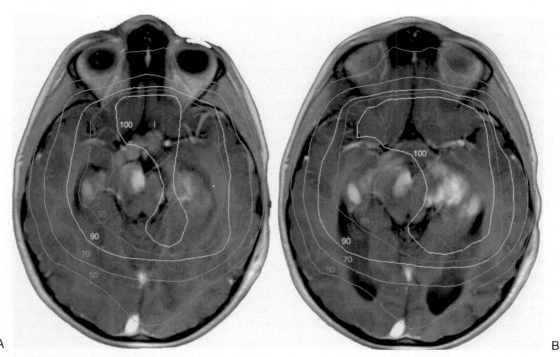

A · · B

FIG. 3-4. Three-dimensional conformal radiation plan for a sizable optic pathway tumor in a 9-year-old boy. The disease involves the chiasm and the optic tracts bilaterally (to the geniculate bodies posteriorly) and the midbrain. The 95 percent volume (indicated on dosimetric plot) encompasses the planning target volume (PTV). (See color plate)

The use of single-fraction radiosurgery for primary management of pediatric low-grade gliomas has been reported in several small institutional series (77,78). In selected instances where truly focal lesions can be targeted while key normal neurologic structures are spared, the early data suggest reasonable efficacy and intermediate-term tolerance (75,77,78).

Results

Long-term disease-free survival has been reported in 90% of children after complete resection of cerebral hemispheric tumors; for similarly managed thalamic tumors, smaller series report 60–90% disease control (24,58,61,62,68, 70,91). Incomplete resection alone results in approximately 50% progression-free survival at 5 years (61,62). The addition of therapeutic irradiation has been shown to achieve progression-free survival in hemispheric astrocytomas in approximately 80% of children measured at 10 years (24); indications for therapeutic (rather than routine adjuvant) irradiation are discussed earlier in this chapter. For thalamic tumors treated primarily with irradiation, 40–50% survive free of progression (8,10,57,67). Hypothalamic tumors have a more favorable outcome after primary irradiation, with 10-year progression-free survival rates of approximately 70%; current literature typically groups these tumors with chiasmatic lesions as "hypothalamic/chiasmatic gliomas" (8, 10,92). Particularly when one is treating central (diencephalic or midbrain) JPAs, it is noteworthy that tumor size may appear to increase within 6 months after irradiation, often by apparent intralesional necrosis or cyst formation; such changes typically remit over several months, and the majority of lesions respond by imaging criteria after radiation therapy (both in size and in gradual loss of enhancement), but the median time to objective response often is greater than 15 months (Fig. 3-3) (93).

Long-term follow-up of children treated with carboplatin and vincristine indicates age-related differences in disease control: for children younger than 5 years old, 3-year progression-free survival is reported at 74%, compared with 39% for children older than 5 years similarly treated

(79,81). Similar results have been reported with the UCSF regimen described earlier (83).

OPTIC PATHWAY TUMORS

Optic pathway tumors (OPTs) represent 5% of childhood brain tumors. OPTs may involve the optic nerves alone (20–25% of cases) or the optic chiasm (alone or in combination with optic nerve infiltration) in 20–40% of children; in 30–60% of cases, tumors involve both the chiasm and the hypothalamus, often with additional extension to the optic tracts (Fig. 3-5) (14,71,94,95). OPTs occur predominantly in young children; 25% present before 18 months of age, and 50% present before 5 years (71,92, 94,95).

Between 25% and 40% of childhood OPTs occur in children with NF1 (64,71,81). Conversely, of children with neurofibromatosis, up to 10% are found to have tumors of the optic pathways either on screening evaluation or during follow-up (64,96). Children with NF1 may have a more indolent disease course (71,81, 92,96).

Clinical presentation is most often with diminished vision. In young children, increased intracranial pressure endocrinopathies and diencephalic syndrome (hyperactivity and low weight) may predominate. Histologically, more than 90% of OPTs are low-grade astrocytomas, most often JPAs (more than 65% of all cases) and grade II astrocytomas (25%), with infrequent gangliogliomas or hamartomas; malignant gliomas are uncommon (14,66,72,92,97).

The nature of OPTs has been debated. Hoyt and Baghdassarian (98) and Imes and Hoyt (99) argued that OPTs are hamartomatous lesions associated with clinical progression or death in fewer than 25% of cases. The pediatric neuro-oncology literature over the past two decades differs with this view (9,64,94,95). While acknowledging the sometimes indolent nature of OPTs, serial observations in major pediatric neuro-oncology clinics indicate progression in 75–85% of children, typically within 2 years of initial presentation (14,92). Children with NF1 have a lower rate of progression and a longer latency interval (92,96). Other signs of the neo-

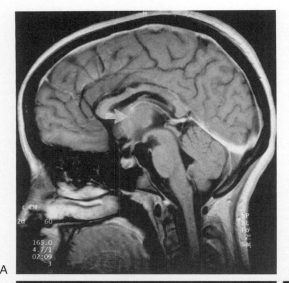

A

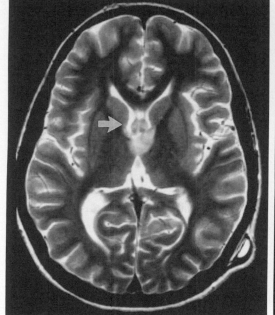

B

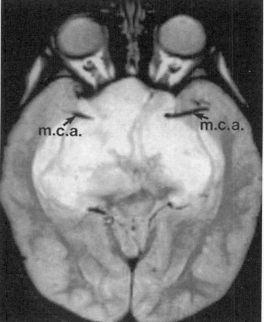

C

FIG. 3-5. Optic chiasm gliomas present as **(A, B)** localized lesions or as **(C)** tumors that extend along the optic tracts; tumors may extend to involve the optic nerves and may extend posteriorly to the lateral geniculate body. Notice the tracking of the middle cerebral arteries *(m.c.a.)* through the tumor.

plastic behavior of OPTs include frequent extension to (or invasion of) the adjacent hypothalamus and posterior extension to the optic tracts (and, uncommonly, the optic radiation). Infrequently, optic chiasmatic and hypothalamic tumors demonstrate extension into the subarachnoid space or diffuse leptomeningeal disease (39–43). Mortality within 10 years of diagnosis is uncommon, although ultimate disease-related mortality has been documented in up to 40% of cases (10,14,71,94,100). Also to be noted is the rare but documented occurrence of spontaneous regression of OPTs (101).

Several series identify chiasmatic OPTs as optic pathway/hypothalamic gliomas, acknowledging the difficulty in identifying the origin of tumors that intimately involve both the chiasm and the hypothalamus (81,102). Although lesions extending to or originating in the hypothalamus may be somewhat more aggressive than lesions confined to the visual pathways, up to 50% of selected, asymptomatic children have been free of progression for 5 years or longer without therapeutic intervention. Preliminary data suggest adequate retrieval with secondary therapy at the time of progression during observation (14,92).

Therapy

Surgery

Surgery has been the preferred treatment for unilateral tumors of the optic nerve (94,95,97). Observation may be selected, especially if there is residual vision associated with a lesion confined to the intraorbital optic nerve. Alvord and Lofton (94) reported progression in 70% of children with untreated lesions within 6 years of diagnosis, although it was rarely associated with tumor-related mortality. Most series indicate more indolent, perhaps truly hamartomatous behavior in children with neurofibromatosis (14,97).

For lesions involving the optic chiasm, there are limited data suggesting a role for surgical resection. Decompression or limited resection may be successful in restoring vision (65,66, 103). Series from the Hospital for Sick Children, Toronto, and New York University suggest a somewhat broader role for local excision in selected presentations. The latter authors indicate removal of lesions of partially infiltrating low-grade optic pathway astrocytomas with surprisingly little added visual compromise; approximately 50% of such cases have remained stable without further intervention for 3 to 5 years. (63, 66,97,103). Whether less aggressive surgery or observation would have achieved similar results relates to the selection of cases for surgery, a debate in the surgical community (9).

Typical chiasmatic lesions that involve components of the visual pathways beyond the optic chiasm and hypothalamic region (i.e., with imaging extension to the optic nerves, optic tracts, or optic radiation) may be managed without biopsy confirmation. Most of these tumors are low-grade astrocytomas and most often can be managed based on the clinical and imaging diagnosis. Globular tumors that involve the chiasm and hypothalamus are best biopsied; a small percentage of these lesions may be germ cell tumors, unusual types of low-grade neoplasms, or more aggressive malignant gliomas (65,72).

Radiation Therapy

Treatment is indicated for significant visual or neurologic deficits at presentation or documented progression by clinical evaluation or neuroimaging (14,64,79,81,82,94). Radiation therapy is highly effective for chiasmal gliomas: 10-year progression-free survival rates (i.e., disease control) exceed 80% (14,71,72,104). Although overall survival at 10 years is unaffected by the initial therapeutic approach (i.e., observation, resection, chemotherapy, or irradiation), progression-free survival rates at 5 and 10 years are substantially higher after radiation therapy (10,14,58). Serial imaging studies document significant tumor response in more than 50% of children after irradiation (72,92). Transient postirradiation tumor enlargement, often in the setting of central cystic degeneration, has been well documented, indicating a role for close observation and medical management for lesions that may appear to progress within 6 months of therapy (71). Visual improvement has been reported in 25–35% of children after irradiation (71,92,104). Visual deterioration is reported in 10–20% of children after irradiation, largely related to cystic degeneration (and consequent increased mass effect at the chiasm) or unrecognized elevated intracranial pressure (14,71,92, 104).

Balancing the indications for radiation therapy and the timing requires judgment and, often, serial evaluations to determine the nature of the disease process. OPTs are associated with unique late radiation-related sequelae. The young age at diagnosis, central location, and often extensive optic anatomic involvement challenge the ability to deliver adequate radiation therapy while preserving neurocognitive function most associated with the adjacent temporal lobe; the problem is further accentuated in children with NF1, itself associated with cognitive delays (72,81,92,96). Furthermore, there is concern about late vascular events: the incidence of occlusive vasculopathy at the circle of Willis in children with brain tumors is highest among those with OPTs, especially in children presenting before 3 years of age (72,81,105,106). Moyamoya syndrome is signified by total obliteration of the major vessels at the circle of Willis; incomplete brain perfusion is provided by peripheral meningeal vessels. The syndrome has been noted after irradiation, perhaps related to cicatricial constriction of vessels tracking through chiasmal and hypothalamic gliomas. An incidence approaching 18% has been reported, especially noted among young children (less than 2 years old) with NF1 (72,105).

The Toronto group has uniquely reported a 10% incidence of second malignant neoplasms after irradiation for OPTs; of interest, a series from Children's Hospital of Los Angeles showed the same rate of anaplastic degeneration in JPA after surgery alone (14,31,91).

Chemotherapy

Mostly because of the radiation-associated toxicities in young children, Packer et al. (107) explored primary chemotherapy in children younger than 5 years old with primary optic pathway gliomas. Initial experience with actinomycin D and vincristine resulted in stabilization in a majority of children and objective tumor reduction in approximately 25%. Although more than 60% of children needed irradiation by 5 years after diagnosis, the approach resulted in a substantial delay in radiation therapy, with a median time to progression of 3 years (107). Subsequent experience with an 18-month regimen of carboplatin and vincristine has shown a significant rate of objective tumor reduction (reporting greater than 50% tumor reduction in one-third of patients), early progression in only 10%, and 3-year progression-free survival that ranges from 75% for children younger than 5 years old to 39% for those older than 5 years

(79,81). Similar results have been reported with the UCSF five-drug regimen (83).

Early experience suggests favorable outcome with secondary irradiation after progression during or after chemotherapy; recent observations related to the timing of initiating radiation therapy question whether ultimate disease control and function may be diminished with prolonged preirradiation intervals (14,79,92,108). Toxicity with carboplatin and vincristine has been limited, and early data suggest continued intellectual development during chemotherapy (9,81). There is a balance between duration of disease control (clearly superior with radiation therapy) and moderate-term control, apparently without some of the toxicities associated with irradiation in the younger age group (14,92). Current therapeutic approaches address initial chemotherapy in a variably defined set of eligible age groups (2–3, 5, 10, or 15 years or until completion of puberty). Additional experience and follow-up will determine the appropriate age thresholds for initial chemotherapy or irradiation in those needing treatment.

Radiotherapeutic Management

Volume and Technique

Local volumes are used, often confined to the suprasellar region for lesions that are limited to the chiasm with or without hypothalamic involvement. Central lesions necessitate multifield, often noncoplanar arrangements to optimize 3D conformal approaches, limiting the dosage to the surrounding cerebral hemispheres (73,74). The use of proton beam therapy will be prospectively explored in the next several years (76). The target volume includes only the involved aspects of the optic pathway, often confined to the chiasm. Optic nerve involvement, most often in NF1, necessitates inclusion of the nerve to the posterior aspect of the globe in defining the target volume. For lesions extending along the optic tracts or beyond (occasionally to involve the optic radiation, toward or to the occipital lobes), it is key to discern where apparent neoplastic changes differ from the extensive T2 changes often visualized in NF1 (71,81,96).

Dosage

The extensive literature on radiation therapy for OPTs typically calls for dosage levels of 50 to 54 Gy, most often at 180 cGy per fraction (14,71,73,95,104). Reduction to 45 Gy at 150 cGy daily may be appropriate in children younger than 3 years old (10,104).

OLIGODENDROGLIOMA

Oligodendrogliomas represent 2% of supratentorial tumors in children. The generally circumscribed tumors occur most often in the cerebral hemispheres. In adults, loss of chromosome 1p or 19q is noted in 50–80% of cases. Data specific for pediatric oligodendrogliomas are limited but suggest that similar molecular findings are uncommon in adolescents and not apparent in children younger than 10 years old (54,109). Treatment recommendations are based largely on adult experience with surgery and irradiation (110). Adults show excellent response to procarbazine, lomustine, and vincristine (PCV) chemotherapy, particularly in anaplastic oligodendrogliomas with isochromosome 1p or p53 mutations (28,111,112). Given differences in biology, it is unclear whether chemosensitivity to PCV can be extrapolated to children.

Total surgical resection is the treatment of choice for accessible lesions. GTR has been documented in 20–25% of all cases, apparently more often in children and adolescents (110, 113). The survival rate at 10 years after total excision is reported to be 60% in the Mayo Clinic series; of six children, five survived (86,113).

For incompletely resected oligodendrogliomas, a short-term benefit for radiation therapy has been documented. Shaw et al. (86) reported 5-year survival of 25% after subtotal resection, compared with 62% with the addition of radiation dosages greater than 50 Gy; by 10 years, the survival rates were similar with (31%) and without (25%) irradiation. Adjuvant irradiation typically is withheld for differentiated oligodendrogliomas in children, even with incomplete resection. Histologic grade has been cited as a prognostic indicator in oligodendrogliomas (86, 114). Anaplastic oligodendrogliomas are managed similarly to other malignant supratentorial gliomas in children, although the outcome tends to be superior to those of anaplastic astrocytoma and glioblastoma (115,116).

Combined radiation therapy and PCV has been associated with excellent disease control in adults, specifically with anaplastic oligodendroglioma (112). Limited chemotherapy has been associated with sufficient tumor reduction to permit delayed GTR in tumors initially felt to be unresectable (117).

The "benign" nature of oligodendrogliomas is open to some question, with few reports documenting survival rates greater than 25% beyond 15 years (86). Long-term results after contemporary surgery and irradiation are limited in the literature; given the added facility of stereotactic neurosurgery, one might anticipate improved outcome in the larger proportion of children with grossly resected lesions (86).

RARE LOW-GRADE NEOPLASMS

Gangliogliomas are biologically benign neoplasms containing neuronal (ganglion cells) and glial (astrocytes) elements (118). The tumors occur primarily in children. Gangliogliomas arise throughout the CNS, most often in the cerebral hemispheres, especially in the temporal lobes (3,119,120). The tumors usually are well circumscribed and often resectable; recurrence is uncommon (118,120). Malignant transformation is rare in these tumors; when documented, it is generally the glial elements that are identified as anaplastic or malignant (27). There are few indications for radiation therapy in children. Progressive, unresectable lesions may respond to irradiation with treatment factors similar to those used for low-grade astrocytomas (120).

Neurocytomas are clinically indolent tumors that present as intraventricular lesions, usually in the third ventricle; most are diagnosed in adolescents and young adults. Neurocytomas are composed of small neuronal cells thought to represent a benign neoplasm derived from cells midway in the maturation process of neuronal differentiation (27,121,122). These tumors are genetically distinct from the oligodendrogliomas and dysembryoplastic neuroepithelial tumors (DNETs), with which they can be confused both clinically and histologically (123). The lesion generally is resectable (124). Some consider hemispheric neurocytomas more likely to be DNETs; the lesions seem to necessitate only local excision (122). Prognosis seems to relate to the rate of proliferation (gauged by MIB-1) (125). These tumors respond to irradiation; small series have suggested improved outcome for cases with less than total resection when followed by radiation therapy (dosage levels of 54 Gy in 30 fractions) (125–127).

DNETs are biologically indolent, often large cerebral cortical tumors typically presenting with a long-standing seizure history (128,129). Symptoms typically arise in children younger than 12 years of age; the mean age at diagnosis is 14 years (130). The tumors may be considered quasi-hamartomatous, classically well demarcated, and without contrast on MRI (130). These tumors may be followed, but surgery often is needed for seizure control; although they are anecdotally responsive to irradiation, there is no documented role for postoperative therapy (128,129,131).

MALIGNANT GLIOMAS

Supratentorial malignant gliomas represent approximately 6% of brain tumors in children. Children seem to present a continuation of the adult data, suggesting that more favorable histology and outcome are inversely related to age. Histologic grading divides high-grade (or malignant) gliomas into anaplastic astrocytoma and GBM (38). Children have a higher proportion of anaplastic astrocytomas among the malignant gliomas and have arguably longer survival intervals (132,133). The tumors are biologically separate from the more common adult malignant gliomas. Adult primary malignant gliomas appear to arise *de novo* and are as-

sociated with amplification of the epidermal growth factor receptor (*EGFR*) gene; less common secondary malignant gliomas evolve from low-grade tumors and typically have *TP53* mutations (3,28,134). Overexpression of p53 and mutations in *TP53* have been noted in pediatric malignant glial tumors; *EGFR* is less commonly expressed (34–36).

Supratentorial malignant gliomas arise primarily as cerebral hemispheric tumors; 20–30% present primarily in the thalamus or basal ganglia (116,132). Imaging characteristics are similar to those in adults, with often poorly marginated, peripherally enhancing lesions on MRI or CT associated with surrounding white matter changes ("edema") and often central necrosis. Adult studies have shown infiltration of the small, round anaplastic cells well into the perilesional low-density areas on CT or areas of abnormal signal on T2 MRI (3,26,38,135). The infiltrative characteristics of high-grade gliomas necessitate some caution in aggressive surgery and high-dose local radiation techniques; the histologic studies are at odds with clinical data substantiating a direct relationship between tumor control and degree of resection and the incidence of primarily local failure even after high-dose focal radiation therapy (116,132,133,135, 136). There is only limited evidence that more aggressive surgery or local irradiation might be associated with a higher rate of failure beyond the primary site (137). Leptomeningeal dissemination had been reported in up to 15% of children at diagnosis; however, the large prospective CCG trial (CCG-945) showed disease beyond the primary site only anecdotally (133,135).

The diagnosis of high-grade glioma in children has been fraught with uncertainties. Central review of pathology in the CCG-945 trial showed that fully 36% of cases entered based on an institutional diagnosis of anaplastic astrocytomas or GBM were felt to have a discordant diagnosis, primarily a low-grade glioma, based on a single or panel reviewer's interpretation, respectively (133,138). As might be anticipated, the favorable results of that combined-modality study (surgery, radiation therapy, chemotherapy) are reported to be significantly less impressive when corrected for reviewed histopathology (133,138).

Therapy

Surgery

Surgical resection often has been limited in extent by the poorly circumscribed nature of the tumor and the attendant lack of aggressive neurosurgical intent. The large CCG series indicated that more than 90% resection (gross total and near total, by definition) was achieved in 37% of cases: 49% of lesions arising in the superficial cerebral hemispheres, 45% of lesions arising in the cerebellum, and only 8% of those arising in the central structures (diencephalons, midbrain) (139). GTR has been less common (approximately 25% of supratentorial cases in children) (116,132,133,139). There is a significant relationship between degree of resection and outcome. Five-year progression-free survival in the initially reported CCG-945 experience was 44% and 26% for anaplastic astrocytomas and GBM, respectively, after more than 90% removal, compared with 22% and 4%, respectively, after less aggressive resection (139).

Radiation Therapy

Radiation therapy is a primary component of initial management of pediatric malignant gliomas. Adult studies have documented the impact of adequate radiation therapy on survival, although survival beyond 2 years occurs almost entirely among those with anaplastic astrocytoma rather than GBM. Treatment has evolved to local irradiation, with margins reflecting the known pattern of microscopic extension, and a series of dose-escalating trials that have yet to demonstrate a convincing impact on disease control (135–137,140).

Pediatric experience with interstitial brain implants suggested improved outcome in highly selected children eligible for stereotactic brachytherapy, similar to that earlier apparent in adults (141,142). Lack of sustained disease control in most such cases and the frequency of symptomatic treatment-related intralesional necrosis have dampened enthusiasm for this intervention (Fig. 3-6) (115,143).

Stereotactic radiosurgery for pediatric high-grade tumors paralleled the broader experience in adults (74,144). Current trials use 3D conformal radiation therapy or IMRT to dosage levels similar to those used in adults.

Chemotherapy

Chemotherapy for adult malignant gliomas has shown a statistically significant, if clinically marginal, gain in time to progression and survival (145). The greater benefit in adults younger than 40 years old and with anaplastic astrocytomas (compared with GBM) leads one to anticipate greater benefit in children. The first significant prospective trial addressing chemotherapy (vincristine, lomustine, and prednisone) and irradiation showed an apparently significant benefit in the cohort treated with combined modality therapy: Sposto et al. (146) reported 5-year event-free survival approaching 45%, compared with 17% for those who received radiation therapy alone postoperatively. Later follow-up of this study showed a significant number of cases misinterpreted as malignant gliomas (133). The subsequent CCG-945 trial showed overall survival at 5 years in 21% of children with reviewed malignant gliomas treated on the same regimen (133,138). Interest in overcoming the theoretical blood–brain barrier and the potential advantage of dosage intensification have stimulated investigation of high-dose chemotherapy with autologous bone marrow rescue in childhood malignant gliomas (147). Trials using variations of two- and three-drug regimens (based largely on thiotepa and busulfan, carboplatin and thiotepa, thiotepa and cyclophosphamide, or thiotepa and etoposide) with autologous bone marrow or, more commonly, peripheral stem cell rescue have shown response rates of 10–30% but no apparent improvement in survival (115,147–150). Some of the more commonly used high-dose regimens have been associated with fatal acute toxicities in 15% of children (148).

Current trials in COG address the addition of temozolomide to irradiation in pediatric high-

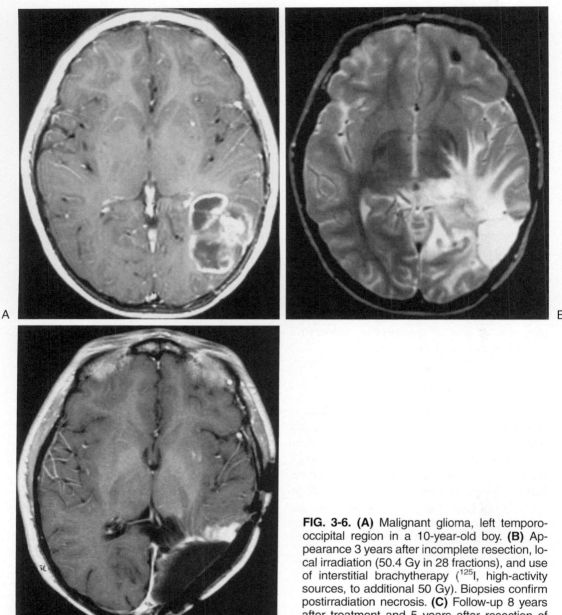

FIG. 3-6. (A) Malignant glioma, left temporo-occipital region in a 10-year-old boy. **(B)** Appearance 3 years after incomplete resection, local irradiation (50.4 Gy in 28 fractions), and use of interstitial brachytherapy (^{125}I, high-activity sources, to additional 50 Gy). Biopsies confirm postirradiation necrosis. **(C)** Follow-up 8 years after treatment and 5 years after resection of necrotic site.

grade gliomas (151). In the Pediatric Brain Tumor Consortium (PBTC), the addition of biologic agents targeting growth factors (STI 571, or Gleevec®, which targets platelet-derived growth factor receptors, and ZD 1839, or Iressa®, which targets the epidermal growth factor receptor) is being tested both concurrently and sequentially with irradiation (152,153).

Radiotherapeutic Management

Volume and Technique

The target volume is best defined by the enhancing lesion and surrounding low-density change (on CT) or signal abnormality (on T2 MRI). A detailed review of imaging and histologic extent in untreated patients with malignant gliomas suggests that a 2–3-cm margin around the target volume as defined provides adequate coverage, avoiding full-brain irradiation in most patients (135). Detailed correlations of imaging and histology indicate that the "surrounding edema" in most supratentorial malignant glioma cases contains tumor cells (135). The lack of local disease control, even after irradiation dosages as high as 90 Gy, eliminates the opportunity to test whether more limited target definitions will ultimately result in a change in the pattern of failure away from the more commonly, if not uniformly, identified local, in-field pattern of recurrence (135–137). The use of image-guided radiation planning in pediatric malignant gliomas is important in sparing the normal brain. Although survival rates remain poor, a cohort of survivors in childhood malignant glioma are at risk for treatment-related sequelae, favoring the introduction of volume-defined targeting and planning now a part of prospective cooperative group studies in the COG and the PBTC.

Dosage

The conventional dose–volume relationships in children have favored levels of 45 to 54 Gy to the wide local volume (3 cm beyond tumor extent, as described previously), with subsequent boost, often defined as a 1-cm margin around the enhancing lesion, to a cumulative dosage of 55 to 60 Gy (116,133). Use of interstitial brain implants has recently been evaluated for recurrent GBM, with apparent efficacy using low-activity ^{125}I in a single-institution experience (154).

Results

Median survival times for pediatric malignant gliomas are 18 to 24 months in all recent series (116,132,133). Event-free survival at 3–5 years is as high as 45% among the minority of patients in whom GTR is apparent, confirmed by postoperative neuroimaging and treated subsequently with both irradiation and chemotherapy (116, 132,133,139). For the 65–75% of childhood malignant gliomas with residual disease identifiable after surgery, the progression-free survival rate at 3 to 5 years is only 5–20%, slightly

higher among the anaplastic astrocytomas than the GBMs (116,133,138,139).

BRAIN TUMORS IN INFANTS AND YOUNG CHILDREN

Children younger than 2 years old account for 10–15% of pediatric CNS neoplasms (10,155, 156). Symptoms in this age group usually include enlarged head, lethargy, and vomiting. Tumors are predominantly supratentorial; in comparison to older children, lesions are more often histologically malignant and overtly metastatic within the neuraxis (10,155,157). The most common tumor types include the embryonal neoplasms (medulloblastoma and the supratentorial embryonal tumors, including primitive neuroectodermal tumors [PNETs] and pineoblastomas), astrocytomas (particularly optic chiasmatic and hypothalamic lesions), ependymomas, and malignant gliomas. Unique to this age group are the atypical teratoid/rhabdoid tumors (AT/RTs), often confused with medulloblastomas in the very young. Intracranial teratomas and choroid plexus tumors occur most often in this age group; the median age for choroid plexus carcinomas is 18 months (158). The latter tumors include papillomas and carcinomas, typically arising in the lateral ventricles but occurring in third and fourth ventricles as well. Histology can be uncertain in predicting benign or malignant behavior; outcome correlates with the degree of brain invasiveness as a sign of malignant biology (26,27,158,159).

The infantile desmoplastic neuroepithelial tumors (desmoplastic infantile gangliogliomas and astrocytomas) also arise predominantly in the very young. These lesions often are quite large, are peripherally located, and appear aggressive at first histologic inspection but typically represent low-grade neoplasms rarely recurring after primary resection (26,27,160).

Most pediatric series indicate lower survival rates for brain tumors presenting in children younger than 4 years old (100,156,161). In addition to the unfavorable tumor characteristics noted, the therapeutic ratio for surgery and radiation therapy is less favorable (139,162,163). Operative morbidity and mortality rates are higher in infants than in older children, in part because of the incomplete myelinization and diminished plasticity of the infant brain; mortality rates approaching 10% have been documented (162). After radiation therapy, cognitive dysfunction, somatic alterations, endocrine deficits, and neurotoxicity are more pronounced than in older children (155,164).

Conventional surgery and irradiation have resulted in 5-year survival rates of 50% or less in infants with brain tumors (10,160,165). Outcome in medulloblastoma is significantly poorer in young children: 22–48% compared with 50–80% for those older than 2 years old in major institutional and cooperative group studies (157,166–170). A similar difference is apparent in ependymomas; younger children have experienced survival rates of 22–30%, compared with rates approaching 80% in children older than 2 years old (73,166,171,172). In malignant gliomas, there has been little age-related difference in outcome among children (133,157,173). Overall, survival rates in infants with malignant brain tumors have been recorded at 25–30% (155,174). Survival rates for low-grade or benign tumors approach 85% in this age group (79,100,155).

Therapy

For low-grade neoplasms, the approach in infants and younger children is similar to that in older children but with greater reliance on surgery or initial chemotherapy for central lesions because it is better to delay irradiation. It is important for the radiation oncologist to be involved in the initial decision process; despite favorable initial disease control rates with chemotherapy in these tumors, there is preliminary evidence that prolonged delay to initiating irradiation may result in less favorable functional results (79,82,107,108).

For malignant lesions, cooperative group studies in North America and Europe between 1985 and 2000 explored the use of prolonged primary postoperative chemotherapy using delayed, diminished, or no irradiation depending on the goals and philosophy of the respective group or institution (Table 3-3) (155,157,166, 167,174–178). The experience allowed unparal-

leled assessment of the frequency and durability of response in malignant CNS tumors using prolonged or high-dose, multiagent chemotherapy. Several large series have documented a high rate of chemoresponsiveness; durable disease control without irradiation in only a small minority of cases, primarily those with localized disease amenable to complete resection at diagnosis; disease control rates disappointingly similar to those achieved with surgery and irradiation in older series, still well below 50% at 3 to 5 years; and small amounts of data suggesting a role for additional exploration of altered radiation parameters (i.e., limited dosage and volume) in selected protocol settings (155,157,166,167,171, 174–179). The overall rate of disease control for malignant histiotypes in this age group, only 20–40% in studies between 1985 and 2000, has stimulated interest in sophisticated radiation techniques, the use of intrathecal chemotherapy, and dose-intensive cytotoxic regimens in attempts to improve local and overall disease control while preserving functional integrity (73,89, 167,174,180,181).

Surgery

Contemporary neurosurgical techniques increasingly allow primary resection of low-grade gliomas, including selected hypothalamic and thalamic and basal ganglia lesions in addition to the more traditionally approachable cerebral hemispheric tumors (61–63,66,97,155). Long-term outcome after radical resection of diencephalic tumors is unavailable with reference to ultimate pituitary–hypothalamic function and intellectual development (63,66,97).

For malignant tumors, GTR often is feasible for posterior fossa tumors (primarily medulloblastomas and ependymomas); supratentorial lesions (primarily malignant gliomas and embryonal tumors) tend to be more extensive and less often amenable to complete resection (9,163,176,182). Complete resection often is the primary predictor of disease control (155,157, 158,174,177,183). For infant medulloblastoma and ependymoma, the differences in outcome strongly favor attempted GTR: in the Baby POG study, overall survival for medulloblastoma was

TABLE 3-3. *Malignant infant CNS tumors—outcome of prominent series*

Histiotype	Series	Interval	n (age)	Surgery	Chemotherapy	RT	EFS @ 5 yr	OS @ 5 yr
medulloblastoma	POG 8633 [157, 174]	1986–1990	198 (<3 y.o.)	all	vcr-cyclo-CDDP-VP-16[a]	PD>18 mo (CSI 30–36Gy + PF 50–54 Gy) consolidation (CSI 24 Gy + PF 45–50 Gy)	32%	40%
	MSKCC + collaborators [167]	1991–1995	13 (<6 y.o.)	GTR, M₀ all	same vcr-CDDP-cyclo-CDDP thio-topa-etoposide (ABMR)[b]	same PD only	38% @ 2 yr	69% 62% @ 2 yr
	Institut Gustav Roussy + collaborators [315]	1988–1994	13 (<4 y.o.)	all, s/p PD (33% 2nd GTR) on infant chemotherapy	cyclo-melphalan (ABMR)	PF (50–55 Gy)	70%	
ependymoma	POG 8633 [157, 171, 174]	1986–1990	48 (<3 y.o.)	48% GTR	as in [a] above	PD>18 mos. (local-50–54 Gy) consol-idation (45–50 Gy)	38%	45%
	SFOP [41]	1990–1998	73 (<5 y.o.)	60% GTR	CBCDA-procarbazine CDDP-VP-16; vcr-cyclo[c]	PD (local 50 Gy)	23% @ 4 yr	52% @ 5 yr
	St. Jude RT-1 [73]	1997–2003	48 (<3 y.o.)	84% GTR	0	local (54–59.4 Gy)	77% @ 3 yr	

[a]vcr (vincristine)-cyclo (cyclophosphamide); VP-16, etoposide; CDDP, cisplatinum.
[b]ABMR, autologous bone marrow rescue.
[c]CBCDA, carboplatin.

40%, compared with 60% for the one-third of children who had undergone GTR and 69% for those with GTR and localized disease (174). Similar differences were seen in ependymomas, where 5-year survival rates were 66% and 25%, respectively, after complete and incomplete resection (171,174).

Delayed definitive surgery has been an effective approach for selected malignant tumors in this age group. After initial chemotherapy, tumors may be reduced in size and vascularity, resulting in more successful tumor resection (120, 157,158).

Radiation Therapy

Radiation therapy is an option for low-grade gliomas in this age group, generally reserved for tumors that have documented progression after surgery and chemotherapy. It is important to recognize the indications for radiation therapy and to intervene promptly and definitively when imaging or clinical signs indicate tumor progression (14,92,100,108).

The majority of children with malignant tumors treated in studies with initial chemotherapy ultimately need irradiation (79,81,155,157). Even in trials that have avoided planned consolidative irradiation, management of incomplete chemotherapy responders and children selected for salvage irradiation has made radiation therapy an ultimate component of therapy for up to one-half of the children in this age group (158,167,174,180,184). The earlier data from the POG infant study were based on systematic irradiation at planned completion of 12 to 24 months of chemotherapy (157). Subsequent studies used a primary chemotherapy approach, typically using irradiation for disease that progressed during or after chemotherapy or for instances in which residual tumor was apparent at completion of planned chemotherapy (167,177, 181). The data from Kalifa's program in Paris showed the value of local posterior fossa irradiation for recurrent or progressive M_0 medulloblastoma in infants also treated with high-dose systemic chemotherapy (Table 3-3) (180). Irradiation seems to add significantly to disease control upon completion of chemotherapy in

ependymomas and is effective in achieving secondary disease control among children with medulloblastoma treated at the time of disease progression or residual disease (171,178,179).

The percentage of cases of medulloblastoma and ependymoma that are ultimately controlled without irradiation is estimated at 10–30% in several large, protocol-based reports (157,166, 167,174). Progression typically has been documented within 6 to 12 months of surgery, during initial chemotherapy (166,174,178). Incorporating consolidative, local irradiation within 4 months of surgery seems to be an attractive alternative to using irradiation for secondary disease control after progression (174,178). It is important to note that the first Baby POG trial and the German HIT studies reported impressive results in resected, localized medulloblastoma even without irradiation, suggesting that one might identify a cohort of children who can be treated with postoperative chemotherapy alone (157,174,177).

Even among the more aggressive AT/RTs, current recommendations incorporate aggressive but localized irradiation to the primary site after just 2 or 3 months of chemotherapy (185,186).

Although salvage CSI (at therapeutic dosage levels of 30 to 36 Gy equivalent using 180-cGy daily fractions) was successful in controlling more than 40% of recurrent medulloblastomas (in fact, it was equally effective in M_0 and $M+$ cases) in the St. Jude data, the ultimate 40–60% disease control was balanced by a median IQ of only 62 at 7 years (Fig. 3-7) (178). The latter finding has dampened enthusiasm for salvage CSI, at least at dosage levels greater than 24 Gy, in this age group.

Chemotherapy

The initial study of primary mechlorethamine, vincristine, procarbazine, and prednisone chemotherapy at M.D. Anderson Cancer Center showed long-term survival in eight of 11 infants with medulloblastoma; six of eight survivors had not received radiation therapy (175).

Duffner et al. (157) reported the first POG trial with initial postoperative chemotherapy in 1993. The regimen included cycles of cy-

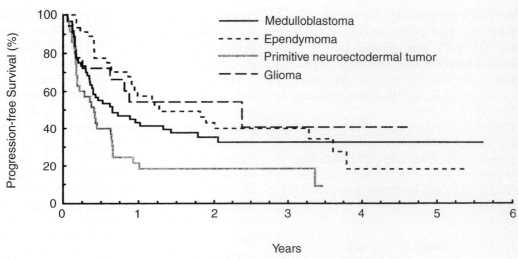

A

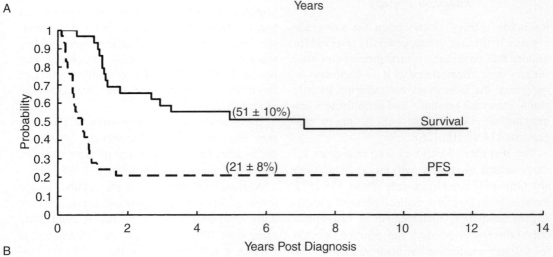

B

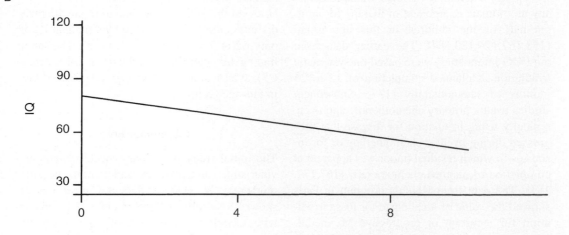

C

clophosphamide with vincristine and cisplatin with etoposide; response rates varied between medulloblastoma (48% partial and complete response rate among those with imaging disease residual), ependymoma (48%), and malignant gliomas (60%) (157,174). Progression-free survival and overall survival rates have been updated to provide 5-year data: 32% and 40% for medulloblastoma, 38% and 45% for ependymomas, 43% and 50% for malignant gliomas, and 0% and 0% for pineoblastomas, respectively (Fig. 3-7). Overall 5-year survival among children with supratentorial PNETs was 27% (174). As in other infant trials, failures beyond 2 years have been uncommon with the "malignant" histiotypes (i.e., medulloblastoma, malignant gliomas and brainstem gliomas, supratentorial PNETs); notably, ependymomas have continued to fail at and beyond 5 years after therapy (155, 159,166,171,173–175,178).

A CCG trial in medulloblastoma and PNETs used postoperative multi-agent chemotherapy alone. There was little adherence to the suggested use of local or neuraxis irradiation. Geyer et al. (166) reported 3-year disease control in only 22% of children. A similar regimen in malignant gliomas showed disease control in 44% with anaplastic astrocytoma and 0% with GBM (176).

The Headstart program initiated by Finlay and reported by Mason et al. (167) used induction chemotherapy followed by a high-dose regimen (busulphan, etoposide, and thiotepa) and autologous marrow rescue. Long-term disease control is not significantly different from the experience reported by Geyer; only among the cohort successfully proceeding through the high-

dose regimen did a subset analysis show disease control approaching 50% (167).

Although limited in number, the series reported by Dupuis-Girod and colleagues (180) showed a 75% objective response rate to high-dose busulfan and thiotepa in medulloblastoma progressing after a traditional infant chemotherapy regimen. Among 13 patients with only local tumor progression treated with consolidative posterior fossa irradiation, 70% were progression free at 3 years; by comparison, none of the nine patients with metastatic disease achieved durable disease control despite CSI (180).

Radiotherapeutic Management

Volume and Technique

For low-grade gliomas, the target volume should include the primary tumor as the GTV with a 1-cm margin to define the CTV for the majority of lesions that are discrete and circumscribed on imaging; for infiltrating low-grade tumors that extend along white matter tracts, the target volume should include all areas of known extension (being careful to differentiate tumor involvement from imaging changes more typically associated with NF1 in such patients). Similar targeting has been suggested for ependymomas, most often in the posterior fossa in this age group (73,187). Limiting the CTV to a 5-mm expansion of the GTV for well-circumscribed lesions has been considered; there are no data substantiating this change. Those with malignant gliomas

FIG. 3-7. (A) Outcome in infants with malignant brain tumors after initial postoperative chemotherapy and delayed postoperative consolidative irradiation: progression-free survival (PFS) by histiotype from original report of Baby POG 8633 (1986–1990, $n = 198$). Late update of results indicates 5-year PFS and overall survival (OS): 32% and 40% in medulloblastoma, 38% and 45% in ependymoma, 43% and 50% in malignant glioma, and 27% OS in supratentorial primitive neuroectodermal tumor (157,174). **(B)** OS and PFS in medulloblastoma after initial postoperative chemotherapy and delayed consolidative ($n = 6$) or therapeutic (i.e., for progressive disease on chemotherapy, $n = 23$) irradiation, St. Jude Children's Research Hospital (1984–1995, $n = 29$ consecutive children younger than 4 years old) (178). **(C)** Serial full-scale IQ in survivors of infant medulloblastoma, St. Jude experience ($n = 19$ surviving more than 2 years after diagnosis; 17 received therapeutic craniospinal irradiation at median 35.2 Gy cranial irradiation, two received 24 Gy consolidative irradiation); median follow-up IQ is 62 at 4.8 years (178).

typically are treated with 2- to 3-cm margins, as described for older children.

For the embryonal tumors (medulloblastoma and supratentorial PNETs, pineoblastomas, and choroid plexus carcinomas), traditional therapy has included CSI. CSI has been used at reduced dosage levels for consolidation after initial postoperative chemotherapy, with outcome among localized, resected children approaching 70% long-term survival (174). More recent trials have emphasized the potential role of local irradiation, initially defined as targeting the entire posterior fossa for medulloblastomas in infants and children younger than 4 years old (180). Ongoing studies in COG and the PBTC have investigationally identified the posterior fossa as the primary target volume, including a boost to the tumor bed that uses the initial tumor volume as modified by resection to identify the GTV and includes a 1.5- to 2-cm expansion to define the CTV for planning. Results of this approach are premature, but regular monitoring of the ongoing trials ensures one that the number of marginal failures must be at or below the level one would expect based on prior cooperative group infant studies.

The use of CSI in this age group has been discouraged based on the functional outcomes of earlier primary therapeutic approaches and more recent retrieval studies; it seems clear that conventional dosages to the neuraxis (30–36 Gy) result in unacceptable functional consequences in children younger than 3 years of age (155,178). Even in conjunction with intensive chemotherapy, more moderate dosage levels to the neuraxis have not achieved secondary disease control in children who had failed earlier, conventional chemotherapy (180). Use of lower dosages (18 Gy CSI) in conjunction with chemotherapy for primary postoperative therapy has been only anecdotally reported (188).

Three-dimensional conformal or intensity-modulated irradiation offer a potential advantage in targeting and delivering the intended dosage with greater sparing of the critical, adjacent normal brain for supratentorial tumors, posterior fossa boost volumes, and localized infratentorial lesions (e.g., dorsally exophytic brainstem gliomas and, investigationally, ependymomas) (73). Whether one is planning the full posterior fossa or a tumor region in the posterior fossa or supratentorial brain, the advantage to image-guided planning and delivery seems axiomatic in sparing the normal brain. Such target definition is key to achieving disease control with acceptable morbidity in this age group (89). For centrally located tumors with spherical configuration, earlier trials of fractionated stereotactic radiosurgery (or stereotactic radiotherapy) showed favorable outcome, preceding the more sophisticated image-guided techniques available with 3D CRT or, in selected settings, IMRT (73,74,189).

Dosage

For embryonal CNS tumors, response-adjusted irradiation is a component of most open trials in North America. Most regimens use 23.4 to 24 Gy (using 180- or 150-cGy daily fractions, respectively) to the initial planning target volume (PTV, e.g., the entire posterior fossa or supratentorial residual tumor volume or operative bed with wider margins) while targeting the reduced PTV (i.e., the tumor bed with 1.5- to 2-cm margins for infratentorial or supratentorial lesions) at dosages of 45 Gy (for children younger than 2 years old with no imaging residual upon commencing irradiation), 50.4 Gy (for children younger than 2 years old with residual tumor or children 2 to 3 years old with no residual), or 54 Gy (for children older than 2 years old with imaging residual). The French series that combined high-dose chemotherapy and local posterior fossa consolidation for progressive medulloblastoma used only 36 Gy total dosage to the posterior fossa (180).

Reduced-dose neuraxis irradiation has been successful, if not always indicated, in children with localized disease (the initial POG study used only 24 Gy for children in "complete response" in that setting, and Goldwein et al. [188] reported disease control of 70% in a small series of similar children who received 18 Gy to the neuraxis in conjunction with conventional chemotherapy for initial postoperative therapy) (157,174).

Dosages for low-grade gliomas are 45 to 50 Gy for those younger than 1 year old, 50 Gy for those 1 to 2 years old, and 50 to 54 Gy in children older than 2 years old. Data reported for malignant gliomas have been based on dosage levels of 50 to 54 Gy in this age group (73,173).

Results

Overall results in children with malignant histiotypes are 20–35% disease control at 5 years. (10,157,166,167,174,176). Pineoblastomas and AT/RTs in this age group have done poorly, with few survivors beyond 1 year (157,166,174,190, 191). Outcome in young children with low-grade gliomas is more favorable, with disease control rates approaching 80% after surgery, initial chemotherapy, or initial or delayed use of irradiation (8,10,14,24,39,92,100,155).

EMBRYONAL CNS TUMORS (PRIMITIVE NEUROECTODERMAL TUMORS OR PNETS AND AT/RTS)

The WHO classification of embryonal CNS tumors clarifies the controversies regarding PNETs (3,192). Hart and Earle (193) initially reported the supratentorial primitive neuroectodermal tumor (S-PNET) in 1973 as an aggressive cerebral tumor occurring predominantly in young children. The tumor consists of undifferentiated neuroepithelial cells with focal areas of divergent differentiation toward glial, neuronal, and mesenchymal lines and unique molecular markings (192–195). In 1983, Rorke (196) introduced the PNET as a unifying concept grouping together the cellular "small blue cell" CNS tumors with or without focal or uniform differentiation. Included among PNETs were several "primitive" supratentorial tumors (cerebral neuroblastomas, ependymoblastomas, pineoblastomas, medulloepitheliomas, and undifferentiated "PNETs" as identified by Hart and Earle) in addition to medulloblastomas (included as "posterior fossa PNET") (196). The tumors share similar histologic appearances, a tendency to seed along the cerebrospinal fluid (CSF) pathways, and relative responsiveness to irradiation and chemotherapy. Those skeptical of the broad PNET designation had argued that malignant transformation could occur not only at the level of the primitive multipotential neuroepithelial

cell precursor, as suggested by the PNET concept, but also in the committed neuronal and glial cell lines at later stages of differentiation (3,26,197). Recent biologic studies have demonstrated that the finding of isochromosome 17p in medulloblastoma is absent in supratentorial PNETs, loss of chromosome 14q or 19q is noted in S-PNETs but not in medulloblastoma, and gene profiling convincingly demonstrates medulloblastoma to be similar to normal cerebellar granular cells but molecularly distinct from S-PNETs, suggesting a unique cerebellar origin for medulloblastoma (198,199).

The clinical outcomes of medulloblastoma and the supratentorial embryonal tumors continue to differ; even the several different supratentorial entities show varying survival rates in reported series (3,166,182,192,200–203).

Table 3-2 shows the WHO classification of embryonal CNS tumors, maintaining the distinct clinical entities (i.e., the primitive medulloepithelioma, pineoblastoma, ependymoblastoma, cerebral neuroblastoma, and supratentorial PNETs). The category of "primitive neuroectodermal tumors" is specifically distinguished for medulloblastoma ("posterior fossa PNET") (3).

Embryonal tumors occur predominantly in young children. In the POG infant malignant CNS tumor study, 18% of cases were grouped as embryonal supratentorial tumors; one-half of these can be classified as PNETs, lacking a recognizable dominant line of differentiation, and the other half can be classified as one of the specific embryonal tumor types (157).

Medulloepithelioma is the most primitive embryonal tumor, histologically showing features of primitive medullary epithelium and primitive tubular structures. Focal differentiation toward glial, neuronal, or mesenchymal lines is often present (202). Primitive polar spongioblastoma is a rare cerebral tumor thought to be derived from migrating glial precursor cells and characterized by immature unipolar glial cells with or without focal differentiation toward astrocytic or oligodendroglial elements (197).

Ependymoblastoma is a poorly differentiated embryonal tumor including ependymal differentiation signified by multilayered rosettes similar to those seen in retinoblastoma (Flexner-Wintersteiner rosettes) (27). The tumor is felt to be a specific embryonal neoplasm, different from the differentiated and anaplastic ependymomas (discussed in Chapter 4) that occur both in the posterior fossa and supratentorially (3,197).

The cerebral neuroblastoma ranges histologically from an undifferentiated tumor similar to the extra-CNS childhood neuroblastoma, often including unilayered Homer–Wright rosettes, to lesions demonstrating ganglionic differentiation (197,204).

The tumor most often confused with medulloblastoma histologically and by contiguous anatomic location is the pineoblastoma (Fig. 3-8). The tumor is believed to arise from pineal parenchymal cells, histologically signified by undifferentiated small round cells, usually including scattered Homer–Wright rosettes. The tumor may mimic retinoblastoma, including fleurettes and Flexner–Wintersteiner rosettes (190,205).

The embryonal tumors present as solid or partially cystic lesions (Fig. 3-8). Although the undifferentiated classic PNET and cerebral neuroblastoma may present as well-demarcated lesions, the embryonal tumors are generally invasive (165, 192,193,197). Leptomeningeal dissemination is apparent at the time of diagnosis or at the time of initial tumor recurrence or progression in approximately one-third of children with pineoblastoma, ependymoblastoma, and undifferentiated supratentorial PNET (157,165,182,206). Although questions have been raised regarding the frequency of CSF failure in localized cerebral neuroblastoma, most reports indicate a frequency of CNS dissemination similar to that noted previously (201,204,207). Also controversial is the frequency of extra-CNS and peritoneal metastases associated with ventricular peritoneal shunts (208,209). Occasionally children develop peritoneal seeding of tumor concentrated around the shunt tip after a ventriculoperitoneal shunt. In the

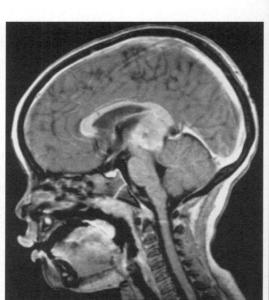
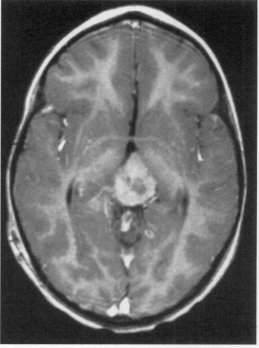

A   B

FIG. 3-8. Pineoblastoma in a 2-year-old girl, a sizable central lesion that often responds promptly to chemotherapy or irradiation; experience in this age group shows few long-term survivals despite aggressive intervention.

absence of any other tumor relapse, these nodules are considered shuntborne metastases. However, it is not clear whether there is a statistically significant elevated risk of systemic dissemination of CNS tumors in shunted children.

Separate from the PNETs are the immature, highly aggressive tumors identified as AT/RTs (210,211). The tumors are of uncertain histogenesis and occur almost exclusively in young children as posterior fossa or supratentorial lesions (210). Rorke et al. (210) reported that on review, up to 25% of presumed infant medulloblastomas are actually AT/RTs. The lesions are associated with monosomy of chromosome 22, a finding in common with extraneural primary rhabdoid tumors (212). Mutations of *INI1* are almost always noted in AT/RTs; the hSNF5/*INI1* appears to function as a tumor suppressor gene (213). Approximately 25% of cases are associated with leptomeningeal dissemination at diagnosis (186,213,214). Although AT/RTs often respond to chemotherapy (especially carboplatin-containing regimens) and irradiation, the disease course typically has been marked by rapid recurrence and neuraxis dissemination (210). The outcome in this disease appears to have improved over the past decade; initially, survival beyond 2 years had been reported only anecdotally. A recent National Cancer Institute consensus conference identified the degree of resection and the use of focal irradiation early in disease management as the primary factors associated with survival (185).

Therapy

The basic principle of surgical resection is limited by disease extent and site. Undifferentiated supratentorial PNET, cerebral neuroblastoma, and ependymoblastoma may be resectable in up to 50% of cases, more often in tumors that are grossly cystic (157,166,182,192,193,201). Pineoblastomas are generally approached by stereotactic biopsy or limited resection (165,190, 215).

Postoperative irradiation is indicated for the embryonal CNS tumors. Classic studies indicate disease control in fewer than 25% of cases with supratentorial PNET and pineoblastoma (192, 215–217). The addition of chemotherapy to of-

ten limited surgery and CSI has been associated with a 60% survival rate in pineoblastomas in children older than 18 months old (190). Similar rates are preliminarily reported after similar chemotherapy (vincristine, lomustine, prednisone, or the "8-in-1" regimen) (200). In small series, outcome after surgery and irradiation for cerebral neuroblastoma has approached 60% survival beyond 2 years (201,204).

Radiotherapeutic Management

Volume and Technique

Most series documenting more favorable outcome in the literature have included full neuraxis irradiation for embryonal CNS tumors (182,190,200,206,216). The exception is a single report documenting disease control in six children with localized cystic cerebral neuroblastoma after surgery and limited-volume irradiation (201). The technique for CSI is discussed in Chapter 4. The local boost is confined to the preoperative tumor volume, corrected for tissue shifts that occur during resection of often sizable lesions; in practice, the preoperative volume is diminished to the tumor bed and residual neoplasm. Margins of 2 to 3 cm are indicated for all but the most circumscribed tumors, often followed by a more limited field with 1-cm dosimetric margins for a final boost. As in other supratentorial lesions, the use of 3D conformal irradiation offers a potential advantage in coverage and limits the dosage to adjacent normal brain volumes.

Dosage

The dosage of CSI is comparable to that used in medulloblastoma, with full neuraxis dosages of 35 to 36 Gy in children older than 3 years of age (182,190). There has been little experience documenting outcomes after reduced neuraxis irradiation (similar to the 23.4-Gy level used in favorable or low-stage medulloblastoma; see Chapter 4) in conjunction with chemotherapy (170). Ongoing trials will address this issue as a potentially valid alternative. Treatment to the primary tumor volume generally is to a cumulative dosage of 54 to 55 Gy, often incorporating an additional reduction in target volume after 50 Gy.

CRANIOPHARYNGIOMA

Craniopharyngiomas are benign tumors of epithelial origin believed to arise from remnants of Rathke's pouch in the suprasellar region. The typical adamantinous craniopharyngioma is a calcified, cystic tumor derived from embryonic cell rests of enamel organs located adjacent to the tuber cinereum along the pituitary stalk (26,218). The less common squamous cell craniopharyngioma occurs almost exclusively in adults; the latter type is rarely calcified and often presents as a solid lesion without cyst formation. The adamantinous craniopharyngioma seen in children and adolescents includes solid components and often large, complex cysts filled with fluid containing high lipid content and cholesterol granules, typically described as "crankcase oil."

Craniopharyngiomas are well-circumscribed, encapsulated extra-axial lesions. The argument for surgical resection is based on the marginated nature of the tumor. It is confounded by the interdigitating pattern of adhesion to adjacent neurologic structures and the location of the tumor, often found adherent to the optic nerves or chiasm, the major vessels at the circle of Willis, the tuber cinereum, and the hypothalamus (219). Infiltration into the tuber cinereum and the presence of small tumor islets in the adjacent hypothalamus have been noted, indicating locally invasive potential (218,220).

Anatomically, 70% of childhood craniopharyngiomas are retrochiasmatic in location, usually extending superiorly into the third ventricle and along the hypothalamus (Fig. 3-9) (221). The multicystic lesion may include cystic extension into the basal cisterns and even into the posterior fossa. In 30% of cases, the tumor is prechiasmatic, occurring between the optic nerves and pushing the chiasm posteriorly (220,222,223). The latter tumors are more accessible and less adherent to vital suprasellar structures.

Children present with visual disturbances (visual field deficits or impaired acuity) and symptoms of elevated intracranial pressure (headaches, nausea, vomiting). Endocrine deficits at diagnosis are apparent in 50–90% of children studied, most often including diminished growth hormone, diabetes insipidus (noted in only 10–15% of cases preoperatively), and decreased gonadotropin, thyroid-stimulating hormone, or adrenocorticotropic hormone (224–226). Noteworthy is the low incidence of diabetes insipidus and hypothalamic obesity at diagnosis (224,226–228). Changes in personality and altered cognitive function have been noted in up to 50% of children at presentation (218,229–232).

Therapy

The treatment of craniopharyngiomas is one of the most controversial issues in pediatric neuro-oncology (219,233). Total resection often is curative in this technically "benign" neoplasm. Matson's classic 1969 neurosurgical text (234) described complete resection in 44 of 57 children preceding the modern era of the operating microscope; 10 of the 44 had needed more than one surgical procedure to effect gross total removal. Numerous contemporary series reporting primary surgical intent in children note attempted total resection in 50–80% of cases (220,222, 227,232-235). A review of treatment strategies in academic pediatric neurosurgical centers in North America indicated that most programs are oriented toward surgical resection in most childhood craniopharyngiomas (233). Postoperative imaging indicates residual calcification, consistent with residual tumor, in 15–50% of "totally resected" cases (222,232,236,237). The rate of clinical recurrence after total resection is 10–30%, linked to tumor volume and location and the presence of residual tumor (including small "calcified flecks" that may alone signal residual tumor) (222,223,232,233,236–240).

Balanced against the low failure rate after aggressive surgery are risks of mortality (1–3%) and major postoperative morbidity (defined as significant visual loss or neurologic dysfunction, 10–20%) (220,222,232,233,237). The skill and experience of the surgeon are important; tumor control and morbidity rates correlate with the number of cases performed annually in neurosur-

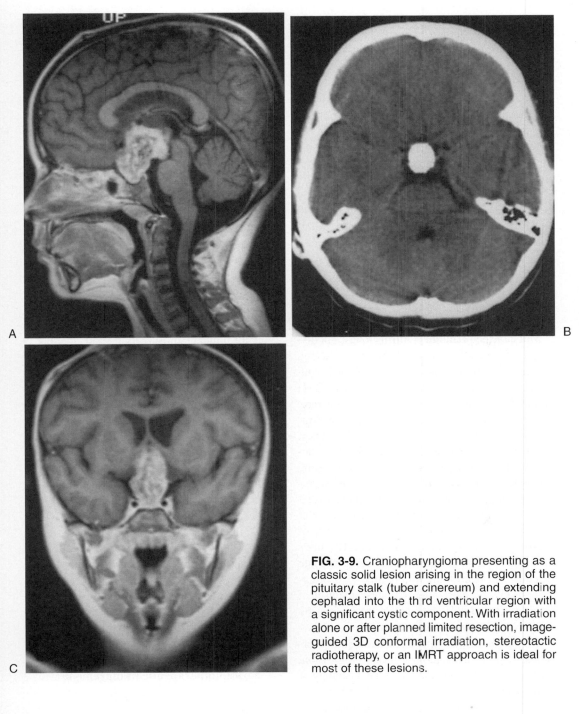

FIG. 3-9. Craniopharyngioma presenting as a classic solid lesion arising in the region of the pituitary stalk (tuber cinereum) and extending cephalad into the third ventricular region with a significant cystic component. With irradiation alone or after planned limited resection, image-guided 3D conformal irradiation, stereotactic radiotherapy, or an IMRT approach is ideal for most of these lesions.

gical centers (233,239). One of the most common operative sequelae is an 80–90% incidence of diabetes insipidus, one of the most difficult endocrinopathies to manage in long-term survivors, and an incidence of morbid hypothalamic obesity as high as 50% (220,222,224,227,228,237,238, 240,241). Dissection can also be associated with fusiform dilation of the internal carotid artery in up to 15% of cases (242). Personality changes also attend extensive surgery.

Kramer and colleagues (243) first reported the efficacy of limited surgical decompression and primary irradiation for craniopharyngiomas from London's Royal Marsden Hospital in 1961. An update indicated 15-year progression-free survival in all six children (244). Subsequent experience at the Royal Marsden Hospital has documented survival rates at 10 and 15 years of 84% and 79%, respectively, in patients treated between 1950 and 1981 by simple cyst aspiration or limited decompression followed by irradiation (10). Among 27 children treated by modern supervoltage techniques between 1970 and 1981, survival at 5, 10, and 15 years are reported at 100%, 96%, and 96%, respectively; these results are equal to or better than those of the best radical resection series (10,230). Kramer's (245) additional experience at Jefferson also demonstrated 80% 20-year disease control after limited surgery and irradiation.

Much of the literature confirms long-term disease control in 80–95% of children with varying degrees of nonradical surgery combined with irradiation (226,230,233,235,236,238,245–251) (Table 3-4). Although acute reactions are rare, one anticipates late endocrine changes after irradiation (including growth hormone deficiency, less frequent accelerated or delayed sexual development, and diminished thyroid-stimulating hormone or adrenocorticotropic hormone secretion). Radiation-related diabetes insipidus is distinctly uncommon (228,238,247). Late vascular events are reported, if infrequently, as a cause of neurologic toxicity after irradiation; Kramer's (245) later Jefferson experience documented late vascular and neurologic events in 10% of long-term survivors, most often amongst a subset of children treated at dosage levels (more than 61 Gy) beyond those used in current practice.

The option of incomplete resection and observation, delaying irradiation until later progression, is unattractive. Despite the low-grade histology of craniopharyngiomas, clinically detectable progression is apparent in 70% of incompletely removed tumors within 3 years (220,222,231). Second surgery is associated with lower efficacy and much higher surgical morbidity (222,232,233, 241). Results of delayed irradiation at the time of recurrent disease are inferior to those achieved with planned postoperative irradiation: 25% versus 78% (245). Experience at Children's Memorial Hospital in Chicago demonstrated secondary disease-free survival after irradiation at 100% after irradiation and 0% after surgery alone; late follow-up showed 88% relapse-free survival after irradiation administered at the first or second recurrence (240,241). It should be noted that some patients who have cyst enlargement in the first few months after radiotherapy may not have truly progressive tumor. A majority of children ultimately have stabilization and later regression of the cyst or need simple cyst aspiration for associated neurologic symptoms (244,252). It appears that craniopharyngioma cells may continue, for a period of time, to secrete fluid despite having sustained a lethal radiation injury (252). In some instances, progressive but isolated cystic enlargement may be treated with intracystic irradiation using ^{32}P or other pure beta emitters (253–256). There may be a role for limited radiosurgery if residual tumor is limited in size and anatomically positioned to allow one to avoid the chiasm and hypothalamus (254,257–259).

Primary total resection and limited surgery with planned primary irradiation achieve excellent disease control. The controversy regarding primary treatment includes the balance of high rates of immediate postsurgical sequelae (endocrinopathies including diabetes insipidus, visual deterioration in up to 25% of cases, and major neurologic complications) and recognized rates of late postirradiation sequelae (growth hormone and other endocrinopathies, late vascular events, secondary carcinogenesis) (233,235,240,249). Comparative reports of neurocognitive and overall functional levels favor children treated by limited surgery and irradiation (230,235,238,246,247,260).

Radiotherapeutic Management

Volume and Technique

The volume of irradiation is limited to the well-marginated tumor, including its cystic components. It is important to accurately map out the cystic areas; cystic extensions posteriorly or inferiorly may be obscured by the basal cisterns.

TABLE 3-4. *Craniopharyngioma—outcome in children*

Primary therapy/series	Interval	n	% Complete resection	RT	PFS @ 5 yrs	PFS @ 10 yrs	PFS @ 20 yrs
Surgery							
JCRT, Boston [238][b]	1970–1990	15	66% (op), 4/6 (NI)	0[a]	52%	31%	
Hospital Sick Children, Toronto [222]	1975–1989	50	90% (op)	0	66%		
Great Ormond St. Hosp, London [237]	1973–1994	29 (GTR)	66% (op), 49% (NI)	0[a] (GTR only)	89%	78%	
U. Virginia [227]	1974–1999	32	57% (op, NI)[c]	0[a]	77%[a]		
Child Memorial Hosp, Chicago [240]	1983–1996	25	76% (op + NI)	0[a]	55%		
St. Jude [226][b]	1984–1997	15	53% (NI)	0[a]	73%		
Limited Surgery + Primary RT							
Royal Marsden, London [230]	1950–1986	77 (all)	<27%	56 Gy median (median 1.5 Gy/fx)		83%	79%
Thomas Jefferson Univ [245]	1961–1981	12	8%	55.8 Gy mean (1.8–2 Gy/fx)	83%	81%	
JCRT, Boston [238][b]	1970–1990	38		54.6 Gy median (1.8–2 Gy/fx)	92%	89%	
U. Pittsburgh [249]	1971–1992	24	4%	≥54 Gy (1.2–3.1 Gy/fx)	95%	89%	54%
St. Jude [226][b]	1984–1997	15	0	55.8 Gy (1.8 Gy/fx)[d]	93%		

GTR, gross total resection; op, neurosurgical assessment of degree of resection; NI, postoperative neuro-imaging assessment.

[a] Without RT by primary intention; RT used for recurrent disease only.

[b] Comparative results of primary S and primary RT presented in Table for JCRT (Joint Center for Radiation Therapy) and St. Jude (Children's Research Hospital, Memphis).

[c] Degree of operability and 77% overall PFS in adults *and* children; 50% of children listed as "good outcome" (i.e., PFS without major operative or neurologic/quality of life sequelae beyond anticipated endocrine changes).

[d] 13/15 → external beam RT; 2 → ^{32}P (including the 1 failure within 5 yrs).

With close margins and image-guided radiation planning and delivery, it is often fruitful to surgically decompress, or resect, cystic extensions to minimize the radiation volume. Craniopharyngiomas often interdigitate or invade at the hypothalamic and chiasmatic regions; it is unusual to see invasion at other sites. Accordingly, one can define the GTV as the residual solid tumor and diminished cyst volume after surgical intervention. Definition should include both MRI (for soft tissue and cyst extent) and CT (for calcified residual tumor). The CTV has been defined as narrowly as the GTV itself in an experience from Heidelberg reporting preliminary results with fractionated stereotactic radiotherapy using CTV as GTV and an additional margin of just 2 mm to identify the PTV (250). The recent protocol-based experience at St. Jude has been based on a GTV defined as the minimal postoperative residual, a CTV derived from a 1-cm 3D expansion of the GTV, and a PTV 3 to 5 mm beyond the CTV (Fig. 3-10). Caution is warranted in documenting the sometimes significant reexpansion of cystic components during the 6-week course of irradiation, leading us to repeatedly aspirate cysts through indwelling Ommaya reservoirs or stereotactic access as necessary to maintain a limited target volume.

Conventional external beam techniques had included coronal arcs using head position to avoid exit through the thyroid, three-field coronal or four-field axial obliqued configurations (avoiding exit through the eyes and, preferably, the neck and torso), or opposed lateral high-energy beams when necessitated by disease extent (226). Stereotactic or 3D conformal techniques based on image-guided planning should replace other approaches in almost all instances (250,261). These techniques decrease the volume of normal tissue irradiated and offer the promise of reduced neuropsychological sequelae of irradiation (189,250,262).

Experience with single-fraction radiosurgery has been reported largely in the context of minimal residual solid tumor components (i.e., after attempted complete resection with minimal residual in the sella or in areas of tumor not adherent to the chiasm or hypothalamus) or limited, localized recurrence (257–259). The target volume for such interventions is limited to residual solid tumor in most instances, typically smaller than 2 cm in diameter (254,258).

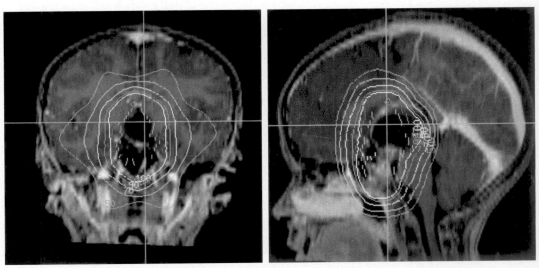

A   B

FIG. 3-10. Local irradiation for craniopharyngioma, including solid tumor and cyst extrusion into the third ventricle. The third ventricular cyst has been partially resected. The PTV (apparent as the outer hatch marks in the coronal and sagittal planes) represents the solid and residual cystic tumor (GTV) plus 5–10 mm expansion (CTV)—the inner hatch marks) and a 5 mm margin for the PTV. The 6-field 3D conformal 15 MeV plan achieve 100 percent coverage of the PTV. (See color plate)

Intracavitary radionuclide insertion, in an effort to delay primary surgery or external irradiation (e.g., in children younger than 4 years of age) or to treat residual or recurrent cyst formation after definitive surgery or radiation therapy, is a valid approach for tumors that are largely cystic. A catheter is passed into the cyst at craniotomy or by stereotactic guidance. Based on the cyst volume, an appropriate dosage of isotope in diluent is instilled into the cavity. Most contemporary experience is with beta emitters such as ^{32}P and ^{90}Yt, delivering a high dosage (i.e., 200 Gy) to the cyst wall (253,263,264). Centers selectively using intracystic brachytherapy as primary management report high rates of uncomplicated disease control in a majority of tumor presentations (253,264).

Dosage

An external beam dosage response has been documented at 54 to 55 Gy using 180-cGy fractions daily (10,230,245). A review from Institut Gustave Roussy (Paris) suggested improved 10-year event-free survival with dosages of 55 Gy or more (251). A report from Pittsburgh also suggested superior disease control with dosages above 60 Gy (12 of 12 patients progression free) compared with dosages of 54 to 57 Gy (seven of 12 patients disease free) (249). Other data, from Paris, indicate excellent intermediate-term disease control with dosage levels of 52.2 Gy (at the isocenter; periphery of narrowly targeted tumor = 90% level) (226). There is insufficient evidence that dosages greater than 55 Gy add to disease control in pediatric craniopharyngioma; late complications, including chiasmal injury, are increased with dosages greater than 60 Gy (10,230,245,249).

Results

Long-term disease control rates for craniopharyngioma should be 80–90%, with a plateau on both disease-free and overall survival beyond 5 years. Such results are achievable among those selected for surgery who have successfully undergone GTR (222,223,232,233,236–238). Most data suggest that postoperative irradiation is indicated with imaging evidence of residual disease (233,240,241,245). Control rates after limited surgery and irradiation are equivalent to those of radical resection (10,226,230,235,245,248–251, 260,265). Quality of life is particularly important in a tumor setting marked by significant potential neurologic deficits (vision, integrity of major cerebral vasculature), hypothalamic dysfunction, and neurocognitive compromise (219,226,237, 249,251).

INTRACRANIAL GERM CELL TUMORS

Intracranial germ cell tumors (GCTs) are rare in North America and Europe, representing fewer than 2% of pediatric CNS neoplasms; in Japan and Taiwan they are reported to represent up to 9% of childhood brain tumors (22,266). The full range of germ cell histiotypes present as primary CNS tumors: germinomas (accounting for 60–70% of intracranial GCT), "malignant" germ cell types (i.e., embryonal carcinomas, endodermal sinus tumors and choriocarcinomas, collectively 15–20% of CNS GCTs), and teratomas (benign, immature, and malignant types, 15–20%) (22,266–268). Malignant teratomas are admixtures of benign teratomatous lesions with one or more malignant germ cell lines such as embryonal carcinoma, endodermal sinus tumor, or choriocarcinoma or with malignant elements of rhabdomyosarcoma, neuroblastoma, or epithelial carcinoma (26,27,267,269).

CNS GCTs usually occur in the diencephalic structures, almost exclusively as midline third ventricular lesions. The tumors are located most often in the pineal region (50–60% of presentations) or in the anterior third ventricular (suprasellar) region (30–35% of cases). Uncommonly, primary intracranial germ cell tumors originate in the basal ganglia or thalamic nuclei (22,266,269–272). It is not uncommon to see germinomas, in particular, presenting with multiple tumor sites around the third ventricle, most often the pineal and suprasellar (pituitary stalk) region concurrently; such tumors are called multiple midline germinomas and appear to represent multicentric tumor development or subependymal laminar infiltration around the third ventricle rather than subarachnoid or CSF pathway metastasis (22,209,269,273–275). Up to 20% of intracranial germinomas present as multiple midline tumors.

Pineal germinomas occur with a unique predilection in adolescent boys. Suprasellar germinomas occur throughout the first two decades; there is no gender predilection (22,269,276). Teratomas tend to occur in younger children, and other malignant histiotypes (e.g., embryonal carcinoma, endodermal sinus tumor) present in older children, adolescents, and young adults.

GCTs are the most common tumors arising in the pineal region. A unique spectrum of neoplasms presents a broad differential diagnosis for tumors arising in the posterior third ventricular region (Table 3-5). Approximately 80% of the pineal region tumors in children and adolescents are GCTs (representing 60–70%) or pineal parenchymal tumors (i.e., pineoblastomas and less common pineocytomas, representing 10–20%). In very young children, the most common tumor type is the pineoblastoma. Less common histiotypes include glial tumors (astrocytomas, ependymomas) and arachnoid cysts. Low-grade and malignant astrocytomas have been reported as pineal region tumors (215,277). Pineoblastomas are embryonal CNS tumors believed to originate from pineal parenchymal cells. Pineocytomas are "mature" parenchymal cell neoplasms, which are rare lesions in children, clinically benign in adolescents, and potentially malignant in young children (278–280). The differential diagnosis for suprasellar tumors is also rather broad, including astrocytomas and craniopharyngiomas (together, more than 80% of lesions in this location in children and adolescents) as well as GCTs.

Pineal GCTs present most often with elevated intracranial pressure caused by compression of the adjacent Sylvian aqueduct. Ocular signs are classically noted as Parinaud's syndrome: decreased upward gaze, abnormal pupillary responses described as near-light dissociation (i.e., limited constriction to light but retained pupillary response to accommodation), and diminished convergence (22,281).

In suprasellar GCTs, the classic triad of presenting symptoms is diabetes insipidus, precocious or delayed sexual development, and visual deficits (271,282). In adolescent boys, one may find symptoms of suprasellar involvement associated with primary pineal tumors, occasionally in the absence of imaging evidence of suprasellar involvement. Diabetes insipidus or other suprasellar signs in conjunction with apparently isolated pineal tumors is virtually diagnostic of the multiple midline germinoma.

Alpha-fetoprotein may be present in serum or CSF in embryonal carcinoma, endodermal sinus tumor, or malignant teratoma; elevated levels are diagnostic of a malignant germ cell histiotype and exclude the diagnosis of a pure germinoma (267,268). β-HCG is elevated in a subset of germinomas (10–20% of pure germinomas show levels above 10 IU, up to 70 IU; higher levels are found in germinomas with syncytiotrophoblastic

TABLE 3-5. *Pineal region tumors—relative incidence*

Tumor type	Relative frequency (%)	Characteristics
Germinoma	40–60%	Predominately adolescent males, (−) AFP; may have isolated (+) BHCG (typically to <15–75 units)

Malignant germ cell tumors
  endodermal sinus tumor
  choriocarcinoma
  malignant teratoma
  immature teratoma
	20–25%	(+++) AFP
		(+++) HCG; frequent intralesional hemorrhage

Pineal parenchymal tumor
  pineoblastoma
  pineocytoma
	14%	Predominately in young children
		Uncommon in children/adolescent

Glioma
  astrocytoma
  ependymoma
	15%	

giant cells); significant elevation (typically more than 1,000 IU) is diagnostic of choriocarcinoma (22,267,268,283–286).

Therapy

Treatment of CNS GCTs is controversial, from the decision to establish histology to the role of surgery, radiation parameters, and the appropriate role of chemotherapy. Although excellent disease control has been reported in series based on clinical and imaging diagnosis (i.e., without histologic confirmation), specific radiation, chemotherapy, and surgical interventions are best guided by a histologic diagnosis. Most North American clinicians routinely recommend histologic confirmation for pineal region tumors. In the suprasellar region, the surgical approach is simpler and the differential diagnosis often more difficult to establish on clinical and imaging grounds; biopsy has always been considered essential in these tumors. When there is significant elevation of tumor markers in serum or CSF (any clear elevation of α-fetoprotein or marked elevation of β-HCG, typically more than 100 IU), some clinicians consider the diagnosis of a "malignant" GCT (i.e., a tumor with embryonal or endodermal sinus tumor components or choriocarcinoma) without biopsy adequate.

Historically, the nonoperative approach for pineal region tumors had been to assume the relative dominance of germinoma cell type, especially among adolescent boys, and initiate local irradiation as a "histologic test." Prompt tumor reduction (after 20 to 25 Gy) was interpreted to be diagnostic of germinoma, and subsequent therapy used modified radiation parameters based on institutional use of local, cranial, or craniospinal fields (276,287,288). If a tumor showed limited early response to the "test" dosage, then surgical intervention was entertained, or subsequent therapy (modified radiation parameters with chemotherapy) was based on the presumption of a benign (e.g., teratoma, glioma) or malignant (i.e., malignant germ cell histiotype) tumor (10,288). In modern practice the "radiation test dosage" is not a standard approach.

Radiation therapy has been the standard treatment for germinomas; it is a significant compo-

nent of therapy for the malignant germ cell types (287,289–292). Intracranial germinomas are quite chemoresponsive; the use of combined chemotherapy and limited-volume and limited-dose irradiation has been an alternative approach in treating these tumors (289,293–297) (Table 3-6). The use of chemotherapy alone has been associated with unacceptable recurrence and mortality rates (283,284). For the more malignant histiotypes, irradiation alone has achieved disease control in only 20–35% of tumors, and combined-modality therapy, including chemotherapy and potential surgical resection, is standard (22,295,298,299).

Surgery

Contemporary surgical techniques permit stereotactic or open biopsy for pineal region tumors with low rates of mortality (1–3%) and morbidity (293,300,301). A prior suggestion that biopsy predisposed the patient to a higher risk of subarachnoid dissemination has not been confirmed (288,300,302).

There is no advantage to attempting a GTR in intracranial germinomas (303,304). The more aggressive germ cell histiotypes, known to experience higher failure rates after irradiation and chemotherapy, have been operated on at diagnosis or, sometimes more safely, after initial chemotherapy and before irradiation (293,295,298,305). Choriocarcinomas tend to be markedly vascular tumors; there may be an advantage to resection, often simpler after chemotherapy-induced reduction in tumor size and vascularity (295). Significant deterioration in functional status can be noted at presentation or after shunt insertion or biopsy in malignant pineal region GCTs. Patients with dramatic neurologic impairment often respond to radiotherapeutic intervention, warranting intensive supportive care early in the course of urgent irradiation.

Radiation Therapy

Radiation therapy has been the major curative modality for pineal and suprasellar germinomas. Long-term disease control rates range from 75% to more than 90% (209,271,285,288,

TABLE 3-6. *Intracranial germinoma—outcome[a]*

Primary therapy/series	n	RT volume/dose	Chemotherapy timing	Drugs	PFS @ 5 yrs	OS @ 5 yrs
Radiation Therapy						
JCRT, Boston [321]	40	CrI (15–44 Gy, median 32 Gy) local (median 52 Gy) Spl (n = 30, median = 25 Gy)	n = 4	CDDP-based	97%	100%
Mayo Clinic [275]	32	CrI or CSI (median = 30 Gy), local (median = 48.5 Gy)[b]	n = 5	CDDP/VP-16	70%	91%
Kyoto Univ [303]	38	local (n = 13)/36–50 Gy[b] CSI (n = 25) M+ or selected/21–24Gy CSI (primary as above)	0		95%	97%
MAKEI 83/86/89[c] [319]	11	CSI (36 Gy), local (50 Gy)	0		100%	100%
	49	CSI (30 Gy), local (45 Gy)			89%	92%
St. Jude [313]	12	CSI (median = 25.5 Gy), local (median = 50.4 Gy)	0		100%	100%
Chemotherapy → Reduced RT						
NYU [293]	11	local/30 Gy, CSI (M+)	pre-RT	cyclo		91%
Hokkaido Univ [310]	15	local (n = 11), (pre-RT volume)/24 Gy CSI (n = 2 M+)/24 Gy	pre-RT x 4	CDDP/VP-16 (n = 6, localized) ifos/CDDP/VP-16 (n = 9, ↑ HCG, multifocal, or M+)	83% @ 4 yrs	100%
SFOP[d] [311, 324]	57	local (n = 51, pre-RT volume)/40 Gy local/30 Gy, CSI (M+)	pre-RT x 2	CBCDA/VP-16/ifos	96% @ 3 yrs	98% @ 3 yrs

CSI, craniospinal irradiation; CrI, cranial irradiation; CDDP, cisplatin; ifos, ifosfamide; VP-16, etoposide; CBCDA, carboplatin; cyclo, cyclophosphamide.
[a]Outcome in series of children and, in several, adults to 30–40 years old.
[b]Local tumor RT dose size-dependent.
[c]German Society Pediatric Oncology & Hematology studies.
[d]French Society of Pediatric Oncology.

291,292,300,302,306). Areas of current controversy include the appropriate radiation volume (local tumor with or without wider volumes that have included third ventricular, full ventricular, full cranial, or craniospinal) and dosage (40 to 50 Gy for primary irradiation). Whether primary radiation therapy is the best option is often a complex decision based on tumor site and extent, the child's age, and the child's functional status at presentation, necessitating a choice between irradiation alone or a combination of chemotherapy and reduced-dose, limited-volume irradiation (300,307).

For malignant teratomas and more aggressive germ cell histiotypes, combined chemotherapy and irradiation is the standard, again with some uncertainty regarding appropriate radiation volume (local to craniospinal) (22,295,298). The use of stereotactic radiosurgery to boost local disease visible on imaging after fractionated radiation therapy is rational but investigational in children with malignant intracranial germ cell types that are not locally resected (308,309).

Chemotherapy

Intracranial GCTs are chemosensitive, with excellent objective response rates documented for cyclophosphamide; carboplatin; cisplatin and etoposide; ifosfamide, carboplatin, and etoposide; and cisplatin, etoposide, and bleomycin (284,293–296). Objective response rates approach 100% for germinomas (284,293,296,310,311).

Several series using preirradiation chemotherapy and limited-volume, "response-adjusted" radiation therapy have shown excellent disease control rates. Initially explored in the United States by Allen, use of cyclophosphamide and, more recently, platinating agents has resulted in a large proportion of complete or substantial response, with long-term disease control after local irradiation to dosage levels of 24 to 36 Gy (293–296,310,311). Carboplatin, most often now in combination with etoposide, has been an effective regimen that has largely replaced cisplatin for germinomas because the drug is associated with fewer long-term sequelae (294,296,311). The major short-term morbidity has related to difficulties handling fluid and electrolyte balance

in children with suprasellar tumors, often associated with diabetes insipidus or salt-wasting syndromes. In some settings, this has been associated with early mortality during chemotherapy (284). The relative advantage of primary irradiation or combined chemotherapy and irradiation has been not in disease control but in the potential difference in long-term functional outcome based on lower radiation dosages and, often, lower radiation volumes in combined-modality approaches (276,294,307,312). The COG is planning a prospective comparative trial, the design parameters of which assume equivalent disease control and seek to determine differences in quality of life after radiation therapy alone or in combination with chemotherapy.

The use of chemotherapy alone for intracranial germinomas has been tested in the international protocols coordinated by Balmaceda and colleagues (284). The first drug regimen tested in this context (cisplatin, etoposide, and bleomycin) achieved high initial response rates, but disease progression or recurrence occurred in 50% of patients; also, unacceptable chemotherapy-related mortality was approximately 15% (284). Disease control was particularly inferior among children with germinomas and elevated β-HCG (284). Although Merchant et al. (313) reported systematic salvage after high-dose cyclophosphamide and CSI, the use of the more aggressive combined-therapy regimen is excessive in a significant cohort of children treated initially with chemotherapy alone (276).

For the malignant GCT histiotypes, cisplatin and etoposide, typically with an alkylating agent (cyclophosphamide in North American studies, ifosfamide in European trials), has been effective in combination with local or, more commonly, neuraxis irradiation (295,298,311).

Radiotherapy Management

Volume and Technique

There has been continuing debate regarding the need for large-volume irradiation (full cranial or CSI or inclusion of the entire ventricular system) in pineal region and suprasellar germinomas. The concept originated in the pre-CT era when Sung and colleagues (282) showed a more than 10% risk of subarachnoid dissemination in pineal region tumors; among biopsied suprasellar germinomas, neuraxis dissemination occurred in 43%. Several more recent studies have proposed limiting the radiation volume to the primary tumor alone, a portion of the third ventricle and the pineal, the whole ventricles and the pineal, or the whole brain followed by the whole ventricles followed by the pineal (300, 302,303,314,315).

Evidence of disease beyond the primary site is apparent in 10–20% of intracranial germinomas at diagnosis. Third ventricular disease occurs as multiple midline presentations, classically involving the pineal and suprasellar recess areas but sometimes showing multiple nodules along the linings of the ventricle (209,276,287, 302,306,316). CSF involvement has been documented in fewer than 15% of cases in North American series (275,282,288). However, overt spinal seeding is rarely demonstrable by imaging (287,306). A higher rate of positive CSF cytology has been reported in Japanese series, where Shibamoto et al. (317) described disease-free survival in six of six children with positive CSF cytology after irradiation limited to the third ventricular volume (291).

A large proportion of clinical series reporting disease control rates higher than 90% in the past 15 years have been based on low-dose CSI as a component of therapy (206,270,287,288,295, 300,312,318). Other series report favorable results with local radiation volumes (286,287,300, 302,303,314,319). The incidence of spinal failure, specifically, has been reported to be 0–10% after irradiation to volumes not including the spinal axis (286,287,291,292,302,303,314,319). Radiation volumes limited to the local tumor bed without irradiating the ventricles have been associated with significant rates of intracranial recurrence in several series (275,300,306,319).

In light of these data, there is recognition that CSI has a marginal benefit for intracranial germinomas treated solely by radiation therapy (276,300,307). The potential 10–15% gain is not uniformly recognized and must be weighed against the potential added toxicities of 24 to 25 Gy to the neuraxis. In considering the debate on

therapeutic volume, studies reporting functional outcome or quality of life among long-term survivors of CSI in childhood and adolescence have shown remarkably normal achievement in this disease setting (312,318). For older teenagers, the use of CSI is considered appropriate therapy by many. Perhaps the conventional approach has migrated toward treatment of the full ventricular system as the large field component, the standard arm to be tested against combined-modality therapy in the upcoming COG trial. For prepubertal children, one might argue that the putative gain from CSI may not exceed even the low likelihood of significant functional toxicities.

Local radiation volumes have included the primary tumor only, using a 1- to 2-cm dosimetric margin, or broader fields encompassing the third ventricle. Image-guided therapy using multiple, often noncoplanar fields or stereotactic radiotherapy techniques is superior in treating midline GCTs (309,310,316). When initial wide-field irradiation is used, local fields are determined by the initial tumor extent; dosages beyond 30 Gy may be defined as boost volumes restricted to the reduced tumor or the pineal region as reconfigured after tumor reduction. For tumors with multiple midline involvement, the initial radiation volume should include the neuraxis or, with intent to avoid spinal irradiation, either the entire ventricular system or the full cranium (303,314,316). Although sizable, a 3D approach to the ventricular volume can spare significant cortical tissue when compared with full cranial irradiation (320). A treatment policy of local irradiation restricts indications for CSI to those with overt imaging evidence of dissemination, often beyond those with multiple midline involvement (i.e., with signs of subependymal extension beyond the third ventricle or less common subarachnoid disease outside the ventricular system) (271,275,280,287,300,302,306, 309,317).

Guidelines for radiation therapy after initial chemotherapy most often target the prechemotherapy extent of the local tumor (294,310,311). It is unknown whether full CSI or therapy targeted to the ventricular system is appropriate for multiple midline tumors in combined-modality therapy. Tumors with clear subarachnoid dissemination receive CSI at low dosage levels after chemotherapy (294,310,311). Experience from German and Italian studies suggests that local volumes might include at least the full ventricular system for a component of therapy (319). The planned COG trial will use wide local fields after partial or complete response to chemotherapy in the experimental combined-modality arm.

For malignant germ cell histiotypes, data suggest that CSI is an important component of combined-modality therapy (295,298). Incorporation of a final stereotactic radiosurgical "boost" to the local tumor site may be appropriate for unresected malignant GCTs (308,309).

Dosage

Dose–response data for intracranial germinomas classically identified the 50-Gy level, despite the known radioresponsiveness of extracranial seminomas and germinomas (209,271,288,300,306). More recent analyses suggest that a dosage of 45 Gy is appropriate (275,291,303,317,321).

The elective dosage to the neuraxis (i.e., for M_0 disease) is 24 to 25 Gy; in patients with positive cytology, neuraxis levels of 24 to 30 Gy have been used successfully. Similarly, in patients receiving full cranial or ventricular volumes, the dosage to the initial volume typically is 24 to 30 Gy (276,316,318,319).

In conjunction with chemotherapy, radiation dosages of 24 to 30 Gy typically are administered after complete or near complete response, with dosages of 30 to 36 Gy for patients with partial or incomplete response (294,310,311). Patients with less than partial response usually receive full-dose irradiation (45 Gy). Successful salvage (for patients with progressive or recurrent disease during or after primary chemotherapy) has been reported with 30 Gy to the neuraxis and 45 to 50 Gy to the local tumor region (313).

The malignant GCT histiotypes necessitate consolidative irradiation with CSI to 30 to 36 Gy and local tumor boost to 35 to 45 Gy (295,298).

Results

Five-year disease-free survival is documented at 80–90% in intracranial germinomas treated with primary radiation therapy. Comparable control rates are now reported for suprasellar germinomas (271,288,290,291,300,303,306,316–319,321). Comparable results are reported with induction chemotherapy and more limited irradiation (293,294,296,310,311). It is important to recognize a 10% incidence of late failure (between 5 and 15 years) (209,275,306,316). Disease control with primary chemotherapy has been only about 50% (284). It is of interest that results with chemotherapy are diminished with β-HCG levels above 50 IU; series based on primary radiation therapy have shown little relationship of β-HCG to outcome within the range associated with pure germinomas (typically less than 100 IU) (283,285,286).

A comparison of primary radiation therapy with combined chemotherapy and reduced-dose, limited-volume irradiation is planned by the COG; the outcome comparison is to be based on relative quality of life measures, anticipating disease control to be at least 90% in both arms.

For the aggressive malignant GCTs (i.e., other than germinomas), survival rates at 5 years are 0–33% after radiation therapy alone (22,206, 288,293). The use of combined-modality therapy has been associated with disease control rates of 50–65%, potentially improved with the addition of surgical resection or selected use of radiosurgical boost to the primary residual tumor (295,298,308,309,322,323).

REFERENCES

References particularly recommended for further reading are indicated by an asterisk.

1. Gurney JG, Davis S, Severson RK, et al. Trends in cancer incidence among children in the U.S. *Cancer* 1996;78(3):532–541.
2. Childhood Brain Tumor Consortium. A study of childhood brain tumors based on surgical biopsies from ten North American institutions: sample description. *J Neurooncol* 1988;6(1):9–23.
3. Kleihues P, Cavenee WK. *Pathology and genetics of tumours of the nervous system.* Lyon, France: IARC Press, 2000.
4. Broniscer A, Gajjar A, Bhargava R, et al. Brain stem involvement in children with neurofibromatosis type 1: role of magnetic resonance imaging and spectroscopy in the distinction from diffuse pontine glioma. *Neurosurgery* 1997;40(2):331–337.

5. Sutton LN, Wang ZJ, Wehrli SL, et al. Proton spectroscopy of suprasellar tumors in pediatric patients. *Neurosurgery* 1997;41(2):388–394.

6. Tzika AA, Vigneron DB, Ball WS Jr, et al. Localized proton MR spectroscopy of the brain in children. *J Magn Reson Imaging* 1993;3(5):719–729.

7. Poussaint TY. Magnetic resonance imaging of pediatric brain tumors: state of the art. *Top Magn Resonance Imaging* 2001;12:411–433.

8. Albright AL, Price RA, Guthkelch AN. Diencephalic gliomas of children. A clinicopathologic study. *Cancer* 1985;55(12):2789–2793.

9. Sutton LN, Molloy PT, Sernyak H, et al. Long-term outcome of hypothalamic/chiasmatic astrocytomas in children treated with conservative surgery. *J Neurosurg* 1995;83(4):583–589.

*10. Bloom HJ, Glees J, Bell J, et al. The treatment and long-term prognosis of children with intracranial tumors: a study of 610 cases, 1950–1981. *Int J Radiat Oncol Biol Phys* 1990;18(4):723–745.

11. Mulvihill JJ. Clinical ecogenetics: cancer in families. *N Engl J Med* 1985;312(24):1569–1570.

12. Riccardi VM. Neurofibromatosis: past, present, and future. *N Engl J Med* 1991;324(18):1283–1285.

13. Lewis RA, Gerson LP, Axelson KA, et al. von Recklinghausen neurofibromatosis. II. Incidence of optic gliomata. *Ophthalmology* 1984;91(8):929–935.

14. Jenkin D, Angyalfi S, Becker L, et al. Optic glioma in children: surveillance, resection, or irradiation? *Int J Radiat Oncol Biol Phys* 1993;25(2):215–225.

15. Listernick R, Darling C, Greenwald M, et al. Optic pathway tumors in children: the effect of neurofibromatosis type 1 on clinical manifestations and natural history. *J Pediatr* 1995;127(5):718–722.

16. Li FP, Fraumeni JF Jr. Soft-tissue sarcomas, breast cancer, and other neoplasms. A familial syndrome? *Ann Intern Med* 1969;71(4):747–752.

17. Birch JM, Hartley AL, Tricker KJ, et al. Prevalence and diversity of constitutional mutations in the p53 gene among 21 Li-Fraumeni families. *Cancer Res* 1994;54(5):1298–1304.

18. Neglia JP, Meadows AT, Robison LL, et al. Second neoplasms after acute lymphoblastic leukemia in childhood. *N Engl J Med* 1991;325(19):1330–1336.

19. Walter AW, Hancock ML, Pui CH, et al. Secondary brain tumors in children treated for acute lymphoblastic leukemia at St Jude Children's Research Hospital. *J Clin Oncol* 1998;16(12):3761–3767.

20. Relling MV, Rubnitz JE, Rivera GK, et al. High incidence of secondary brain tumours after radiotherapy and antimetabolites. *Lancet* 1999;354(9172):34–39.

21. Poussaint TY, Barnes PD, Nichols K, et al. Diencephalic syndrome: clinical features and imaging findings. *Am J Neuroradiol* 1997;18:1499–1505.

22. Jennings MT, Gelman R, Hochberg F. Intracranial germ-cell tumors: natural history and pathogenesis. *J Neurosurg* 1985;63(2):155–167.

23. Hirsch JF, Sainte RC, Pierre-Kahn A, et al. Benign astrocytic and oligodendrocytic tumors of the cerebral hemispheres in children. *J Neurosurg* 1989;70(4):568–572.

24. Pollack IF, Claassen D, al Shboul Q, et al. Low-grade gliomas of the cerebral hemispheres in children: an analysis of 71 cases. *J Neurosurg* 1995;82(4):536–547.

25. Watson GA, Kadota RP, Wisoff JH. Multidisciplinary management of pediatric low-grade gliomas. *Semin Radiat Oncol* 2001;11(2):152–162.

*26. Burger PC, Scheithauer BW, Vogel FS. *Surgical pathology of the nervous system and its coverings,* 4th ed. New York: Churchill Livingstone, 2002.

*27. Bigner DD, McLendon RE, Bruner JM. *Russell & Rubinstein's pathology of tumors of the nervous system,* 6th ed. London: Arnold, 1998.

28. Louis DN, Holland EC, Cairncross JG. Glioma classification: a molecular reappraisal. *Am J Pathol* 2001;159(3):779–786.

29. Krouwer HG, Davis RL, Silver P, et al. Gemistocytic astrocytomas: a reappraisal. *J Neurosurg* 1991;74(3):399–406.

30. Prayson RA, Estes ML. Protoplasmic astrocytoma. A clinicopathologic study of 16 tumors. *Am J Clin Pathol* 1995;103(6):705–709.

31. Dirks PB, Jay V, Becker LE, et al. Development of anaplastic changes in low-grade astrocytomas of childhood. *Neurosurgery* 1994;34(1):68–78.

32. Linskey ME, Gilbert MR. Glial differentiation: a review with implications for new directions in neuro-oncology. *Neurosurgery* 1995;36(1):1–21.

33. Cheng Y, Ng HK, Zhang SF, et al. Genetic alterations in pediatric high-grade astrocytomas. *Hum Pathol* 1999;30(11):1284–1290.

34. Pollack IF, Hamilton RL, Finkelstein SD, et al. The relationship between TP53 mutations and overexpression of p53 and prognosis in malignant gliomas of childhood. *Cancer Res* 1997;57(2):304–309.

35. Pollack IF, Finkelstein SD, Burnham J, et al. Age and TP53 mutation frequency in childhood malignant gliomas: results in a multi-institutional cohort. *Cancer Res* 2001;61(20):7404–7407.

36. Pollack IF, Finkelstein SD, Woods J, et al. Expression of p53 and prognosis in children with malignant gliomas. *N Engl J Med* 2002;346(6):420–427.

37. Rickert CH, Strater R, Kaatsch P, et al. Pediatric high-grade astrocytomas show chromosomal imbalances distinct from adult cases. *Am J Pathol* 2001;158(4):1525–1532.

38. Burger PC, Vogel FS, Green SB, et al. Glioblastoma multiforme and anaplastic astrocytoma. Pathologic criteria and prognostic implications. *Cancer* 1985;56(5):1106–1111.

39. Gajjar A, Bhargava R, Jenkins JJ, et al. Low-grade astrocytoma with neuraxis dissemination at diagnosis. *J Neurosurg* 1995;83(1):67–71.

40. Mamelak AN, Prados MD, Obana WG, et al. Treatment options and prognosis for multicentric juvenile pilocytic astrocytoma. *J Neurosurg* 1994;81(1):24–30.

41. Pollack IF, Hurtt M, Pang D, et al. Dissemination of low grade intracranial astrocytomas in children. *Cancer* 1994;73(11):2869–2878.

42. Prados M, Mamelak AN. Metastasizing low grade gliomas in children. Redefining an old disease. *Cancer* 1994;73(11):2671–2673.

43. Hukin J, Siffert J, Cohen H, et al. Leptomeningeal dissemination at diagnosis of pediatric low-grade neuroepithelial tumors. *Neuro-oncology* 2003;5(3):188–196.

44. Tihan T, Fisher PG, Kepner JL, et al. Pediatric astrocytomas with monomorphous pilomyxoid features and a less favorable outcome. *J Neuropathol Exp Neurol* 1999;58(10):1061–1068.

45. Kepes JJ, Rubinstein LJ, Eng LF. Pleomorphic xanthoastrocytoma: a distinctive meningocerebral glioma of young subjects with relatively favorable prognosis. A study of 12 cases. *Cancer* 1979;44(5): 1839–1852.

46. Giannini C, Scheithauer BW, Burger PC, et al. Pleomorphic xanthoastrocytoma: what do we really know about it? *Cancer* 1999;85(9):2033–2045.

47. Pahapill PA, Ramsay DA, Del Maestro RF. Pleomorphic xanthoastrocytoma: case report and analysis of the literature concerning the efficacy of resection and the significance of necrosis. *Neurosurgery* 1996; 38(4):822–828.

48. Fouladi M, Jenkins J, Burger P, et al. Pleomorphic xanthoastrocytoma: favorable outcome after complete surgical resection. *Neuro-oncology* 2001;3(3):184–192.

49. Fuller CE, Perry A. Pathology of low- and intermediate-grade gliomas. *Semin Radiat Oncol* 2001;11(2): 95–102.

50. Shepherd CW, Scheithauer BW, Gomez MR, et al. Subependymal giant cell astrocytoma: a clinical, pathological, and flow cytometric study. *Neurosurgery* 1991;28(6):864–868.

51. van Slegtenhorst M, Verhoef S, Tempelaars A, et al. Mutational spectrum of the TSC1 gene in a cohort of 225 tuberous sclerosis complex patients: no evidence for genotype-phenotype correlation. *J Med Genet* 1999;36(4):285–289.

52. Carpio-O'Donovan R, Korah I, Salazar A, et al. Gliomatosis cerebri. *Radiology* 1996;198(3):831–835.

53. Pyhtinen J, Paakko E. A difficult diagnosis of gliomatosis cerebri. *Neuroradiology* 1996;38(5):444–448.

54. Perry A. Pathology of low-grade gliomas: an update of emerging concepts. *Neuro-oncology* 2003;5(3): 168–178.

55. Jennings MT, Frenchman M, Shehab T, et al. Gliomatosis cerebri presenting as intractable epilepsy during early childhood. *J Child Neurol* 1995;10(1): 37–45.

56. Perkins GH, Schomer DF, Fuller GN, et al. Gliomatosis cerebri: improved outcome with radiotherapy. *Int J Radiat Oncol Biol Phys* 2003;56(4): 1137–1146.

57. Reardon D, Gajjar A, Walter A, et al. Pediatric thalamic gliomas: 10 year St. Jude Children's Research Hospital experience. *J Neurooncol* 1997;33:285.

58. Gajjar A, Sanford RA, Heideman R, et al. Low-grade astrocytoma: a decade of experience at St. Jude Children's Research Hospital. *J Clin Oncol* 1997;15(8): 2792–2799.

59. Shibamoto Y, Kitakabu Y, Takahashi M, et al. Supratentorial low-grade astrocytoma. Correlation of computed tomography findings with effect of radiation therapy and prognostic variables. *Cancer* 1993;72(1): 190–195.

60. Bowers DC, Gargan L, Kapur P, et al. Study of the MIB-1 labeling index as a predictor of tumor progression in pilocytic astrocytomas in children and adolescents. *J Clin Oncol* 2003;21(15):2968–2973.

61. Wisoff JH, Sanford R, Holmes E, et al. Impact of surgical resection on low grade gliomas of childhood: a report from the CCG9891/POG 9130 low grade astrocytoma study. Presented at the International Society for Pediatric Neuro-oncology, Porto, Portugal, 2002.

62. Sanford A, Kun L, Sposto R, et al. Low-grade gliomas of childhood: impact of surgical resection. *J Neurosurg* 2002;96:427–428.

63. Hoffman HJ, Soloniuk DS, Humphreys RP, et al. Management and outcome of low-grade astrocytomas of the midline in children: a retrospective review. *Neurosurgery* 1993;33(6):964–971.

64. Listernick R, Louis DN, Packer RJ, et al. Optic pathway gliomas in children with neurofibromatosis 1: consensus statement from the NF1 Optic Pathway Glioma Task Force. *Ann Neurol* 1997;41(2):143–149.

65. Medlock MD, Scott RM. Optic chiasm astrocytomas of childhood. 2. Surgical management. *Pediatr Neurosurg* 1997;27(3):129–136.

66. Wisoff JH, Abbott R, Epstein F. Surgical management of exophytic chiasmatic-hypothalamic tumors of childhood. *J Neurosurg* 1990;73(5):661–667.

67. Krouwer HG, Prados MD. Infiltrative astrocytomas of the thalamus. *J Neurosurg* 1995;82(4):548–557.

68. Bernstein M, Hoffman HJ, Halliday WC, et al. Thalamic tumors in children. Long-term follow-up and treatment guidelines. *J Neurosurg* 1984;61(4):649–656.

69. Kelly PJ. Stereotactic biopsy and resection of thalamic astrocytomas. *Neurosurgery* 1989;25(2):185–194.

*70. Shaw EG, Wisoff JH. Prospective clinical trials of intracranial low-grade glioma in adults and children. *Neuro-oncology* 2003;5(3):153–160.

71. Tao ML, Barnes PD, Billett AL, et al. Childhood optic chiasm gliomas: radiographic response following radiotherapy and long-term clinical outcome. *Int J Radiat Oncol Biol Phys* 1997;39(3):579–587.

72. Cappelli C, Grill J, Raquin M, et al. Long-term follow up of 69 patients treated for optic pathway tumours before the chemotherapy era. *Arch Dis Child* 1998;79(4):334–338.

73. Merchant TE, Zhu Y, Thompson SJ, et al. Preliminary results from a Phase II trail of conformal radiation therapy for pediatric patients with localised low-grade astrocytoma and ependymoma. *Int J Radiat Oncol Biol Phys* 2002;52(2):325–332.

74. Dunbar SF, Tarbell NJ, Kooy HM, et al. Stereotactic radiotherapy for pediatric and adult brain tumors: preliminary report. *Int J Radiat Oncol Biol Phys* 1994;30(3):531–539.

75. Grabb PA, Lunsford LD, Albright AL, et al. Stereotactic radiosurgery for glial neoplasms of childhood. *Neurosurgery* 1996;38(4):696–701.

76. Loeffler JS, Smith AR, Suit HD. The potential role of proton beams in radiation oncology. *Semin Oncol* 1997;24(6):686–695.

77. Somaza SC, Kondziolka D, Lunsford LD, et al. Early outcomes after stereotactic radiosurgery for growing pilocytic astrocytomas in children. *Pediatr Neurosurg* 1996;25(3):109–115.

78. Kida Y, Kobayashi T, Mori Y. Gamma knife radiosurgery for low-grade astrocytomas: results of long-term follow up. *J Neurosurg* 2000;93[Suppl 3]:42–46.

79. Packer RJ, Ater J, Allen J, et al. Carboplatin and vincristine chemotherapy for children with newly diagnosed progressive low-grade gliomas. *J Neurosurg* 1997;86(5):747–754.

80. Friedman HS, Krischer JP, Burger P, et al. Treatment of children with progressive or recurrent brain tumors with carboplatin or iproplatin: a Pediatric Oncology Group randomized phase II study. *J Clin Oncol* 1992;10(2):249–256.

81. Packer RJ. Chemotherapy: low-grade gliomas of the

hypothalamus and thalamus. *Pediatr Neurosurg* 2000;32(5):259–263.

82. Packer RJ, Lange B, Ater J, et al. Carboplatin and vincristine for recurrent and newly diagnosed low-grade gliomas of childhood. *J Clin Oncol* 1993; 11(5):850–856.

83. Prados MD, Edwards MS, Rabbitt J, et al. Treatment of pediatric low-grade gliomas with a nitrosourea-based multiagent chemotherapy regimen. *J Neurooncol* 1997;32(3):235–241.

84. Quinn JA, Reardon DA, Friedman AH, et al. Phase II trial of temozolomide in patients with progressive low-grade glioma. *J Clin Oncol* 2003;21(4):646–651.

85. Pu AT, Sandler HM, Radany EH, et al. Low grade gliomas: preliminary analysis of failure patterns among patients treated using 3D conformal external beam irradiation. *Int J Radiat Oncol Biol Phys* 1995;31(3):461–466.

86. Shaw EG, Scheithauer BW, O'Fallon JR. Management of supratentorial low-grade gliomas. *Oncology (Huntingt)* 1993;7(7):97–104, 107.

*87. Karim AB, Maat B, Hatlevoll R, et al. A randomized trial on dose-response in radiation therapy of low-grade cerebral glioma: European Organization for Research and Treatment of Cancer (EORTC) Study 22844. *Int J Radiat Oncol Biol Phys* 1996;36(3): 549–556.

*88. Shaw E, Arusell R, Scheithauer B, et al. Prospective randomized trial of low- versus high-dose radiation therapy in adults with supratentorial low-grade glioma: initial report of a North Central Cancer Treatment Group/Radiation Therapy Oncology Group/Eastern Cooperative Oncology Group study. *J Clin Oncol* 2002;20(9):2267–2276.

*89. Merchant TE, Kiehna EN, Miles MA, et al. Acute effects of irradiation on cognition: changes in attention on a computerized continuous performance test during radiotherapy in pediatric patients with localized primary brain tumors. *Int J Radiat Oncol Biol Phys* 2002;53(5):1271–1278.

90. Miralbell R, Lomax A, Cella L, et al. Potential reduction of the incidence of radiation-induced second cancers by using proton beams in the treatment of pediatric tumors. *Int J Radiat Oncol Biol Phys* 2002;54(3):824–829.

91. Krieger MD, Gonzalez-Gomez I, Levy ML, et al. Recurrence patterns and anaplastic change in a long-term study of pilocytic astrocytomas. *Pediatr Neurosurg* 1997;27(1):1–11.

92. Janss AJ, Grundy R, Cnaan A, et al. Optic pathway and hypothalamic/chiasmatic gliomas in children younger than age 5 years with a 6-year follow-up. *Cancer* 1995;75(4):1051–1059.

93. Fisher BJ, Bauman GS, Leighton CE, et al. Low-grade gliomas in children: tumor volume response to radiation. *J Neurosurg* 1998;88(6):969–974.

94. Alvord EC Jr, Lofton S. Gliomas of the optic nerve or chiasm. Outcome by patients' age, tumor site, and treatment. *J Neurosurg* 1988;68(1):85–98.

95. Wong JY, Uhl V, Wara WM, et al. Optic gliomas. A reanalysis of the University of California, San Francisco experience. *Cancer* 1987;60(8):1847–1855.

96. Grill J, Laithier V, Rodriguez D, et al. When do children with optic pathway tumours need treatment? An oncological perspective in 106 patients treated in a single centre. *Eur J Pediatr* 2000;159(9): 692–696.

97. Hoffman HJ, Humphreys RP, Drake JM, et al. Optic pathway/hypothalamic gliomas: a dilemma in management. *Pediatr Neurosurg* 1993;19(4):186–195.

98. Hoyt WF, Baghdassarian SA. Optic glioma of childhood. Natural history and rationale for conservative management. *Br J Ophthalmol* 1969;53(12):793–798.

99. Imes RK, Hoyt WF. Childhood chiasmal gliomas: update on the fate of patients in the 1969 San Francisco Study. *Br J Ophthalmol* 1986;70(3):179–182.

100. Jenkin D, Greenberg M, Hoffman H, et al. Brain tumors in children: long-term survival after radiation treatment. *Int J Radiat Oncol Biol Phys* 1995;31(3): 445–451.

101. Schmandt SM, Packer RJ, Vezina LG, et al. Spontaneous regression of low-grade astrocytomas in childhood. *Pediatr Neurosurg* 2000;32(3):132–136.

102. Fouladi M, Wallace D, Langston JW, et al. Survival and functional outcome of children with hypothalamic/chiasmatic tumors. *Cancer* 2003;97(4):1084–1092.

103. Garvey M, Packer RJ. An integrated approach to the treatment of chiasmatic-hypothalamic gliomas. *J Neurooncol* 1996;28(2–3):167–183.

104. Bataini JP, Delanian S, Ponvert D. Chiasmal gliomas: results of irradiation management in 57 patients and review of literature. *Int J Radiat Oncol Biol Phys* 1991;21(3):615–623.

105. Kestle JR, Hoffman HJ, Mock AR. Moyamoya phenomenon after radiation for optic glioma. *J Neurosurg* 1993;79(1):32–35.

106. Rudoltz MS, Regine WF, Langston JW, et al. Multiple causes of cerebrovascular events in children with tumors of the parasellar region. *J Neurooncol* 1998; 37(3):251–261.

107. Packer RJ, Sutton LN, Bilaniuk LT, et al. Treatment of chiasmatic/hypothalamic gliomas of childhood with chemotherapy: an update. *Ann Neurol* 1988;23(1): 79–85.

108. Awdeh RM, Drewry RD, Kerr NC, et al. Visual outcome after conformal radiation therapy in children with optic pathway gliomas. The Association for Research in Vision and Ophthalmology Annual Meeting, Ft. Lauderdale, FL; May 4–9, 2003.

109. Raghavan R, Balani J, Perry A, et al. Pediatric oligodendrogliomas: a study of molecular alterations on 1p and 19q using fluorescence in situ hybridization. *J Neuropathol Exp Neurol* 2003;62(5):530–537.

110. Razack N, Baumgartner J, Bruner J. Pediatric oligodendrogliomas. *Pediatr Neurosurg* 1998;28(3): 121–129.

111. Ino Y, Betensky RA, Zlatescu MC, et al. Molecular subtypes of anaplastic oligodendroglioma: implications for patient management at diagnosis. *Clin Cancer Res* 2001;7(4):839–845.

*112. Allison RR, Schulsinger A, Vongtama V, et al. Radiation and chemotherapy improve outcome in oligodendroglioma. *Int J Radiat Oncol Biol Phys* 1997; 37(2):399–403.

*113. Shaw EG, Scheithauer BW, O'Fallon JR, et al. Oligodendrogliomas: the Mayo Clinic experience. *J Neurosurg* 1992;76(3):428–434.

114. Burger PC, Rawlings CE, Cox EB, et al. Clinicopathologic correlations in the oligodendroglioma. *Cancer* 1987;59(7):1345–1352.

115. Heideman RL, Douglass EC, Krance RA, et al. High-dose chemotherapy and autologous bone marrow rescue followed by interstitial and external-beam radiotherapy in newly diagnosed pediatric malignant gliomas. *J Clin Oncol* 1993;11(8):1458–1465.

116. Heideman RL, Kuttesch J Jr, Gajjar AJ, et al. Supratentorial malignant gliomas in childhood: a single institution perspective. *Cancer* 1997;80(3):497–504.

117. Gajjar A, Heideman RL, Kovnar EH, et al. Response of pediatric low grade gliomas to chemotherapy. *Pediatr Neurosurg* 1993;19(3):113–118.

118. Johnson JH Jr, Hariharan S, Berman J, et al. Clinical outcome of pediatric gangliogliomas: ninety-nine cases over 20 years. *Pediatr Neurosurg* 1997;27(4):203–207.

119. Garrido E, Becker LF, Hoffman HJ, et al. Gangliogliomas in children. A clinicopathological study. *Childs Brain* 1978;4(6):339–346.

120. Mickle JP. Ganglioglioma in children. A review of 32 cases at the University of Florida. *Pediatr Neurosurg* 1992;18(5–6):310–314.

121. Burger PC, Fuller GN. Pathology: trends and pitfalls in histologic diagnosis, immunopathology, and applications of oncogene research. *Neurol Clin* 1991; 9(2):249–271.

122. Nishio S, Takeshita K, Fujii K, et al. Supratentorial astrocytic tumours of childhood: a clinicopathologic study of 41 cases. *Acta Neurochir* 1989;101:3–8.

123. Fujisawa H, Marukawa K, Hasegawa M, et al. Genetic differences between neurocytoma and dysembryoplastic neuroepithelial tumor and oligodendroglial tumors. *J Neurosurg* 2002;97(6):1350–1355.

124. Yasargil MG, von Ammon K, von Deimling A, et al. Central neurocytoma: histopathological variants and therapeutic approaches. *J Neurosurg* 1992;76(1): 32–37.

125. Brown DM, Karlovits S, Lee LH, et al. Management of neurocytomas: case report and review of the literature. *Am J Clin Oncol* 2001;24(3):272–278.

126. Kim DG, Paek SH, Kim IH, et al. Central neurocytoma: the role of radiation therapy and long term outcome. *Cancer* 1997;79(10):1995–2002.

127. Schild SE, Scheithauer BW, Haddock MG, et al. Central neurocytomas. *Cancer* 1997;79(4):790–795.

128. Daumas-Duport C, Scheithauer BW, Chodkiewicz JP, et al. Dysembryoplastic neuroepithelial tumor: a surgically curable tumor of young patients with intractable partial seizures. Report of thirty-nine cases. *Neurosurgery* 1988;23(5):545–556.

129. VandenBerg SR, May EE, Rubinstein LJ, et al. Desmoplastic supratentorial neuroepithelial tumors of infancy with divergent differentiation potential ("desmoplastic infantile gangliogliomas"). Report on 11 cases of a distinctive embryonal tumor with favorable prognosis. *J Neurosurg* 1987;66(1):58–71.

130. Daumas-Duport C. Dysembryoplastic neuroepithelial tumours. *Brain Pathol* 1993;3:283–295.

131. Cervera-Pierot P, Varlet P, Chodkiewicz JP, et al. Dysembryoplastic neuroepithelial tumors located in the caudate nucleus area: report of four cases. *Neurosurgery* 1997;40(5):1065–1069.

132. Campbell JW, Pollack IF, Martinez AJ, et al. High-grade astrocytomas in children: radiologically complete resection is associated with an excellent long-term prognosis. *Neurosurgery* 1996;38(2):258–264.

*133. Finlay JL, Boyett JM, Yates AJ, et al. Randomized phase III trial in childhood high-grade astrocytoma comparing vincristine, lomustine, and prednisone with the eight-drugs-in-1-day regimen. *J Clin Oncol* 1995;13(1):112–123.

134. Collins VP. Progression as exemplified by human astrocytic tumors. *Semin Cancer Biol* 1999;9(4):267–276.

135. Halperin EC, Bentel G, Heinz ER, et al. Radiation therapy treatment planning in supratentorial glioblastoma multiforme: an analysis based on post mortem topographic anatomy with CT correlations. *Int J Radiat Oncol Biol Phys* 1989;17(6):1347–1350.

136. Chan JL, Lee SW, Fraass BA, et al. Survival and failure patterns of high-grade gliomas after three-dimensional conformal radiotherapy. *J Clin Oncol* 2002;20(6):1635–1642.

137. Nakagawa K, Aoki Y, Fujimaki T, et al. High-dose conformal radiotherapy influenced the pattern of failure but did not improve survival in glioblastoma multiforme. *Int J Radiat Oncol Biol Phys* 1998;40(5):1141–1149.

138. Pollack IF, Boyett JM, Yates AJ, et al. The influence of central review on outcome associations in childhood malignant gliomas: results from the CCG-945 experience. *Neuro-oncology* 2003;5(3):197–207.

139. Wisoff JH, Boyett JM, Berger MS, et al. Current neurosurgical management and the impact of the extent of resection in the treatment of malignant gliomas of childhood: a report of the Children's Cancer Group trial no. CCG-945 *J Neurosurg* 1998;89(1):52–59.

*140. Walker MD, Strike TA, Sheline GE. An analysis of dose-effect relationship in the radiotherapy of malignant gliomas. *Int J Radiat Oncol Biol Phys* 1979;5(10):1725–1731.

141. Florell RC, Macdonald DR, Irish WD, et al. Selection bias, survival, and brachytherapy for glioma. *J Neurosurg* 1992;76(2):179–183.

142. Fontanesi J, Heideman RL, Muhlbauer M, et al. High-activity ^{125}I interstitial irradiation in the treatment of pediatric central nervous system tumors: a pilot study. *Pediatr Neurosurg* 1995;22(6):289–297.

143. Taylor JS, Langston JW, Reddick WE, et al. Clinical value of proton magnetic resonance spectroscopy for differentiating recurrent or residual brain tumor from delayed cerebral necrosis. *Int J Radiat Oncol Biol Phys* 1996;36(5):1251–1261.

144. Loeffler JS, Alexander E III, Shea WM, et al. Radiosurgery as part of the initial management of patients with malignant gliomas. *J Clin Oncol* 1992;10(9): 1379–1385.

*145. Fine HA, Dear KB, Loeffler JS, et al. Meta-analysis of radiation therapy with and without adjuvant chemotherapy for malignant gliomas in adults. *Cancer* 1993;71(8):2585–2597.

146. Sposto R, Ertel IJ, Jenkin RD, et al. The effectiveness of chemotherapy for treatment of high grade astrocytoma in children: results of a randomized trial. *J Neurooncol* 1989;7(2):165–177.

147. Kalifa C, Valteau D, Pizer B, et al. High-dose chemotherapy in childhood brain tumours. *Childs Nerv Syst* 1999;15:498–505.

148. Papadakis V, Dunkel IJ, Cramer LD, et al. High-dose carmustine, thiotepa and etoposide followed by autologous bone marrow rescue for the treatment of high risk central nervous system tumors. *Bone Marrow Transplant* 2000;26(2):153–160.

149. Finlay JL, Goldman S, Wong MC, et al. Pilot study of

high-dose thiotepa and etoposide with autologous bone marrow rescue in children and young adults with recurrent CNS tumors. *J Clin Oncol* 1996;14(9): 2495–2503.

150. Bouffet E, Mottolese C, Jouvet A, et al. Etoposide and thiotepa followed by ABMT (autologous bone marrow transplantation) in children and young adults with high-grade gliomas. *Eur J Cancer* 1997;33(1): 91–95.

151. Lashford LS, Thiesse P, Jouvet A, et al. Temozolomide in malignant gliomas of childhood: a United Kingdom Children's Cancer Study Group and French Society for Pediatric Oncology Intergroup Study. *J Clin Oncol* 2002;20(24):4684–4691.

152. Jones HA, Hahn SM, Bernhard E, et al. Ras inhibitors and radiation therapy. *Semin Radiat Oncol* 2001;11(4):328–337.

153. Valerie K, Dritschilo A, McKenna G, et al. Novel molecular targets for tumor radiosensitization: Molecular Radiation Biology and Oncology Workshop: translation of molecular mechanisms into clinical radiotherapy. *Int J Cancer* 2000;90(1):51–58.

154. Rostomily RC, Halligan J, Geyer R, et al. Permanent low-activity ^{125}I seed placement for the treatment of pediatric brain tumors: preliminary experience. *Pediatr Neurosurg* 2001;34(4):198–205.

155. Cohen BH, Packer RJ, Siegel KR, et al. Brain tumors in children under 2 years: treatment, survival and long-term prognosis. *Pediatr Neurosurg* 1993;19(4): 171–179.

156. Duffner PK, Cohen ME, Myers MH, et al. Survival of children with brain tumors: SEER Program, 1973–1980. *Neurology* 1986;36(5):597–601.

157. Duffner PK, Horowitz ME, Krischer JP, et al. Postoperative chemotherapy and delayed radiation in children less than three years of age with malignant brain tumors. *N Engl J Med* 1993;328:1725–1731.

158. Fitzpatrick LK, Aronson LJ, Cohen KJ. Is there a requirement for adjuvant therapy for choroid plexus carcinoma that has been completely resected? *J Neurooncol* 2002;57(2):123–126.

159. Duffner PK, Kun LE, Burger PC, et al. Postoperative chemotherapy and delayed radiation in infants and very young children with choroid plexus carcinomas. *Pediatr Neurosurg* 1995;22(4):189–196.

160. Taratuto AL, Monges J, Lylyk P, et al. Superficial cerebral astrocytoma attached to dura. Report of six cases in infants. *Cancer* 1984;54(11):2505–2512.

161. Saran FH, Driever PH, Thilmann C, et al. Survival of very young children with medulloblastoma (primitive neuroectodermal tumor of the posterior fossa) treated with craniospinal irradiation. *Int J Radiat Oncol Biol Phys* 1998;42(5):959–967.

162. Albright AL, Wisoff JH, Zeltzer PM, et al. Current neurosurgical treatment of medulloblastoma in children. *Pediatr Neurosurg* 1989;177:633–641.

163. Albright AL, Wisoff JH, Zeltzer PM, et al. Effects of medulloblastoma resections on outcome in children: a report from the Children's Cancer Group. *Neurosurgery* 1996;38(2):265–271.

164. Johnson DL, McCabe MA, Nicholson HS, et al. Quality of long-term survival in young children with medulloblastoma. *J Neurosurg* 1994;80(6):1004–1010.

165. Jooma R, Hayward RD, Grant DN. Intracranial neo-

plasms during the first year of life: analysis of one hundred consecutive cases. *Neurosurgery* 1984;14(1): 31–41.

166. Geyer J, Zelter P, Boyett J, et al. Survival of infants with primitive neuroectodermal tumors or malignant ependymomas of the CNS treated with eight drugs in 1 day: a report from the Children's Cancer Group. *J Clin Oncol* 1994;12:1607–1615.

167. Mason WP, Grovas A, Halpern S, et al. Intensive chemotherapy and bone marrow rescue for young children with newly diagnosed malignant brain tumors. *J Clin Oncol* 1998;16(1):210–221.

168. Evans AE, Jenkin RD, Sposto R, et al. The treatment of medulloblastoma. Results of a prospective randomized trial of radiation therapy with and without CCNU, vincristine, and prednisone. *J Neurosurg* 1990;72(4):572–582.

169. Tait DM, Thornton-Jones H, Bloom HJ, et al. Adjuvant chemotherapy for medulloblastoma: the first multi-centre control trial of the International Society of Paediatric Oncology (SIOP I). *Eur J Cancer* 1990;26(4):464–469.

170. Goldwein JW, Radcliffe J, Johnson J, et al. Updated results of a pilot study of low dose craniospinal irradiation plus chemotherapy for children under five with cerebellar primitive neuroectodermal tumors (medulloblastoma). *Int J Radiat Oncol Biol Phys* 1996; 34(4):899–904.

171. Duffner PK, Krischer JP, Sanford RA, et al. Prognostic factors in infants and very young children with intracranial ependymomas. *Pediatr Neurosurg* 1998;28(4): 215–222.

172. Kellie SJ, Wong CK, Pozza LD, et al. Activity of postoperative carboplatin, etoposide, and high-dose methotrexate in pediatric CNS embryonal tumors: results of a phase II study in newly diagnosed children. *Med Pediatr Oncol* 2002;39(3):168–174.

*173. Duffner PK, Krischer JP, Burger PC, et al. Treatment of infants with malignant gliomas: the Pediatric Oncology Group experience. *J Neurooncol* 1996; 28(2–3):245–256.

*174. Duffner PK, Horowitz ME, Krischer JP, et al. The treatment of malignant brain tumors in infants and very young children: an update of the Pediatric Oncology Group experience. *Neuro-oncology* 1999; 1(2):152–161.

*175. Ater JL, van Eys J, Woo SY, et al. MOPP chemotherapy without irradiation as primary postsurgical therapy for brain tumors in infants and young children. *J Neurooncol* 1997;32(3):243–252.

176. Geyer JR, Finlay JL, Boyett JM, et al. Survival of infants with malignant astrocytomas. *Cancer* 1995; 75(4):1045–1050.

177. Kuhl J, Beck J, Bode U, et al. Delayed radiation therapy after postoperative chemotherapy in children less than 3 years of age with medulloblastoma. Results of the trial HIT-SKK '87, and preliminary results of the pilot trial HIT-SKK '92. *Med Pediatr Oncol* 1995;25:250.

178. Walter AW, Mulhern RK, Gajjar A, et al. Survival and neurodevelopmental outcome of young children with medulloblastoma at St Jude Children's Research Hospital. *J Clin Oncol* 1999;17(12):3720–3728.

179. Gajjar A, Mulhern RK, Heideman RL, et al. Medulloblastoma in very young children: outcome of defin-

itive craniospinal irradiation following incomplete response to chemotherapy. *J Clin Oncol* 1994;12(6): 1212–1216.

180. Dupuis-Girod S, Hartmann O, Benhamou E, et al. Will high dose chemotherapy followed by autologous bone marrow transplantation supplant cranio-spinal irradiation in young children treated for medulloblastoma? *J Neurooncol* 1996;27(1):87–98.

181. Strother D, Kepner J, Aronin P, et al. Dose-intensive chemotherapy prolongs event-free survival for very young children with ependymoma. Results of Pediatric Oncology Group study 9233. *Proc ASCO* 2000;19:2302.

182. Albright AL, Wisoff JH, Zeltzer P, et al. Prognostic factors in children with supratentorial (nonpineal) primitive neuroectodermal tumors. A neurosurgical perspective from the Children's Cancer Group. *Pediatr Neurosurg* 1995;22(1):1–7.

183. Cohen BH, Zeltzer PM, Boyett JM, et al. Prognostic factors and treatment results for supratentorial primitive neuroectodermal tumors in children using radiation and chemotherapy: a Children's Cancer Group randomized trial. *J Clin Oncol* 1995;13(7):1687–1696.

184. Fisher PG, Needle MN, Cnaan A, et al. Salvage therapy after postoperative chemotherapy for primary brain tumors in infants and very young children. *Cancer* 1998;83(3):566–574.

185. Packer RJ, Biegel JA, Blaney S, et al. Atypical teratoid/rhabdoid tumor of the central nervous system: report on workshop. *J Pediatr Hematol Oncol* 2002; 24(5):337–342.

186. Hilden JM, Watterson J, Longee DC, et al. Central nervous system atypical teratoid tumor/rhabdoid tumor: response to intensive therapy and review of the literature. *J Neurooncol* 1998;40(3):265–275.

*187. Merchant TE, Jenkins JJ, Burger PC, et al. Influence of tumor grade on time to progression after irradiation for localized ependymoma in children. *Int J Radiat Oncol Biol Phys* 2002;53(1):52–57.

188. Goldwein JW, Radcliffe J, Packer RJ, et al. Results of a pilot study of low-dose craniospinal radiation therapy plus chemotherapy for children younger than 5 years with primitive neuroectodermal tumors. *Cancer* 1993;71(8):2647–2652.

189. Shrieve DC, Tarbell NJ, Alexander E, et al. Stereotactic radiotherapy: a technique for dose optimization and escalation for intracranial tumors. *Acta Neurochir* 1994;62:118–123.

190. Jakacki RI, Zeltzer PM, Boyett JM, et al. Survival and prognostic factors following radiation and/or chemotherapy for primitive neuroectodermal tumors of the pineal region in infants and children: a report of the Children's Cancer Group. *J Clin Oncol* 1995;13(6):1377–1383.

191. Duffner PK, Cohen ME, Sanford RA, et al. Lack of efficacy of postoperative chemotherapy and delayed radiation in very young children with pineoblastoma. *Med Pediatr Oncol* 1995;25(1):38–44.

192. Pigott TJ, Punt JA, Lowe JS, et al. The clinical, radiological and histopathological features of cerebral primitive neuroectodermal tumours. *Br J Neurosurg* 1990;4(4):287–297.

193. Hart MN, Earle KM. Primitive neuroectodermal tumors of the brain in children. *Cancer* 1973;32(4): 890–897.

194. Cruz-Sanchez FF, Rossi ML, Hughes JT, et al. Differentiation in embryonal neuroepithelial tumors of the central nervous system. *Cancer* 1991;67(4):965–976.

195. Raffel C, Gilles FE, Weinberg KI. Reduction to homozygosity and gene amplification in central nervous system primitive neuroectodermal tumors of childhood. *Cancer Res* 1990;50(3):587–591.

196. Rorke LB. The cerebellar medulloblastoma and its relationship to primitive neuroectodermal tumors. *J Neuropathol Exp Neurol* 1983;42(1):1–15.

197. Rubinstein LJ. Embryonal central neuroepithelial tumors and their differentiating potential. A cytogenetic view of a complex neuro-oncological problem. *J Neurosurg* 1985;62(6):795–805.

198. Pomeroy SL, Tamayo P, Gaasenbeek M, et al. Prediction of central nervous system embryonal tumour outcome based on gene expression. *Nature* 2002; 415(6870):436–442.

199. Burnett ME, White EC, Sih S, et al. Chromosome arm 17p deletion analysis reveals molecular genetic heterogeneity in supratentorial and infratentorial primitive neuroectodermal tumors of the central nervous system. *Cancer Genet Cytogenet* 1997;97(1):25–31.

200. Zeltzer P, Boyett J, Finlay J, et al. Prognostic factors for survival in high risk primitive neuroectodermal tumors (PNET)s in children: report from the Children's Cancer Group CCG-921. *Proc ASCO* 2003; 12:415.

201. Berger MS, Edwards MS, Wara WM, et al. Primary cerebral neuroblastoma. Long-term follow-up review and therapeutic guidelines. *J Neurosurg* 1983;59(3): 418–423.

202. Molloy PT, Yachnis AT, Rorke LB, et al. Central nervous system medulloepithelioma: a series of eight cases including two arising in the pons. *J Neurosurg* 1996;84(3):430–436.

203. Reddy AT, Janss AJ, Phillips PC, et al. Outcome for children with supratentorial primitive neuroectodermal tumors treated with surgery, radiation, and chemotherapy. *Cancer* 2000;88(9):2189–2193.

204. Bennett JP Jr, Rubinstein LJ. The biological behavior of primary cerebral neuroblastoma: a reappraisal of the clinical course in a series of 70 cases. *Ann Neurol* 1984;16(1):21–27.

205. Herrick MK, Rubinstein LJ. The cytological differentiating potential of pineal parenchymal neoplasms (true pinealomas) a clinicopathological study of 28 tumours. *Brain* 1979;102:280–320.

206. Linggood RM, Chapman PH. Pineal tumors. *J Neurooncol* 1992;12(1):85–91.

207. Horten BC, Rubinstein LJ. Primary cerebral neuroblastoma: a clinicopathological study of 35 cases. *Brain* 1976;99:735.

208. Gururangan S, Heideman RL, Kovnar EH, et al. Peritoneal metastases in two patients with pineoblastoma and ventriculo-peritoneal shunts. *Med Pediatr Oncol* 1994;22(6):417–420.

209. Rich TA, Cassady JR, Strand RD, et al. Radiation therapy for pineal and suprasellar germ cell tumors. *Cancer* 1985;55(5):932–940.

210. Rorke LB, Packer RJ, Biegel JA. Central nervous system atypical teratoid/rhabdoid tumors of infancy and childhood: definition of an entity. *J Neurosurg* 1996;85(1):56–65.

211. Hanna SL, Langston JW, Parham DM, et al. Primary

malignant rhabdoid tumor of the brain: clinical, imaging, and pathologic findings. *Am J Neuroradiol* 1993;14:107–115.

212. Biegel JA, Fogelgren B, Zhou JY, et al. Mutations of the INI1 rhabdoid tumor suppressor gene in medulloblastomas and primitive neuroectodermal tumors of the central nervous system. *Clin Cancer Res* 2000; 6(7):2759–2763.

213. Biegel JA, Kalpana G, Knudsen ES, et al. The role of INI1 and the SWI/SNF complex in the development of rhabdoid tumors: meeting summary from the workshop on childhood atypical teratoid/rhabdoid tumors. *Cancer Res* 2002;62(1):323–328.

214. Burger PC, Yu IT, Tihan T, et al. Atypical teratoid/rhabdoid tumor of the central nervous system: a highly malignant tumor of infancy and childhood frequently mistaken for medulloblastoma: a Pediatric Oncology Group study. *Am J Surg Pathol* 1998; 22(9):1083–1092.

215. Edwards MS, Hudgins RJ, Wilson CB, et al. Pineal region tumors in children. *J Neurosurg* 1988;68(5): 689–697.

216. Gaffney CC, Sloane JP, Bradley NJ, et al. Primitive neuroectodermal tumours of the cerebrum. Pathology and treatment. *J Neurooncol* 1985;3(1):23–33.

217. Kosnik EJ, Boesel CP, Bay J, et al. Primitive neuroectodermal tumors of the central nervous system in children. *J Neurosurg* 1978;48(5):741–746.

218. Adamson TE, Wiestler OD, Kleihues P, et al. Correlation of clinical and pathological features in surgically treated craniopharyngiomas. *J Neurosurg* 1990; 73(1):12–17.

219. Rutka JT. Craniopharyngioma. *J Neurosurg* 2002; 97(1):1–2.

220. Tomita T, McLone DG. Radical resections of childhood craniopharyngiomas. *Pediatr Neurosurg* 1993; 19(1):6–14.

*221. Van Effenterre R, Boch AL. Craniopharyngioma in adults and children: a study of 122 surgical cases. *J Neurosurg* 2002;97(1):3–11.

222. Hoffman HJ, De Silva M, Humphreys RP, et al. Aggressive surgical management of craniopharyngiomas in children. *J Neurosurg* 1992;76(1): 47–52.

223. Hoffman HJ. Surgical management of craniopharyngioma. *Pediatr Neurosurg* 1994;21[Suppl 1]:44–49.

224. Curtis J, Daneman D, Hoffman HJ, et al. The endocrine outcome after surgical removal of craniopharyngiomas. *Pediatr Neurosurg* 1994;21[Suppl 1]:24–27.

225. Merchant TE, Williams T, Smith JM, et al. Preirradiation endocrinopathies in pediatric brain tumor patients determined by dynamic tests of endocrine function. *Int J Radiat Oncol Biol Phys* 2002;54(1):45–50.

*226. Merchant TE, Kiehna EN, Sanford RA, et al. Craniopharyngioma: the St. Jude Children's Research Hospital experience 1984–2001. *Int J Radiat Oncol Biol Phys* 2002;53(3):533–542.

227. Duff JM, Meyer FB, Ilstrup DM, et al. Long-term outcomes for surgically resected craniopharyngiomas. *Neurosurgery* 2000;46(2):291–302.

228. Sklar CA. Craniopharyngioma: endocrine sequelae of treatment. *Pediatr Neurosurg* 1994;21[Suppl 1]: 120–123.

229. Anderson CA, Wilkening GN, Filley CM, et al. Neurobehavioral outcome in pediatric craniopharyngioma. *Pediatr Neurosurg* 1997;26(5):255–260.

*230. Rajan B, Ashley S, Gorman C, et al. Craniopharyngioma: long-term results following limited surgery and radiotherapy. *Radiother Oncol* 1993;26(1): 1–10.

*231. Weiss M, Sutton L, Marcial V, et al. The role of radiation therapy in the management of childhood craniopharyngioma. *Int J Radiat Oncol Biol Phys* 1989;17(6):1313–1321.

232. Yasargil MG, Curcic M, Kis M, et al. Total removal of craniopharyngiomas. Approaches and long-term results in 144 patients. *J Neurosurg* 1990;73(1):3–11.

233. Sanford RA. Craniopharyngioma: results of survey of the American Society of Pediatric Neurosurgery. *Pediatr Neurosurg* 1994;21[Suppl 1]:39–43.

234. Matson DD. Neurosurgery of infancy and childhood. *Craniopharyngiomas*. Springfield, IL: Charles C. Thomas, 1969:544–574.

*235. Scott RM, Hetelekidis S, Barnes PD, et al. Surgery, radiation, and combination therapy in the treatment of childhood craniopharyngioma: a 20-year experience. *Pediatr Neurosurg* 1994;21[Suppl 1]:75–81.

236. Wen BC, Hussey DH, Staples J, et al. A comparison of the roles of surgery and radiation therapy in the management of craniopharyngiomas. *Int J Radiat Oncol Biol Phys* 1989;16(1):17–24.

237. De Vile CJ, Grant DB, Kendall BE, et al. Management of childhood craniopharyngioma: can the morbidity of radical surgery be predicted? *J Neurosurg* 1996;85(1):73–81.

*238. Hetelekidis S, Barnes PD, Tao ML, et al. 20-year experience in childhood craniopharyngioma. *Int J Radiat Oncol Biol Phys* 1993;27(2):189–195.

239. Sweet WH. History of surgery for craniopharyngiomas. *Pediatr Neurosurg* 1994;21[Suppl 1]:28–38.

240. Kalapurakal JA, Goldman S, Hsieh YC, et al. Clinical outcome in children with craniopharyngioma treated with primary surgery and radiotherapy deferred until relapse. *Med Pediatr Oncol* 2003;40(4):214–218.

241. Kalapurakal JA, Goldman S, Hsieh YC, et al. Clinical outcome in children with recurrent craniopharyngioma after primary surgery. *Cancer J* 2000;6(6):388–393.

242. Sutton LN. Vascular complications of surgery for craniopharyngioma and hypothalamic glioma. *Pediatr Neurosurg* 1994;21[Suppl 1]:124–128.

243. Kramer S, McKissock W, Concannon JP. Craniopharyngiomas: treatment by combined surgery and radiation therapy. *J Neurosurg* 1961;18:217–226.

244. Kramer S, Southard M, Mansfield CM. Radiotherapy in the management of craniopharyngiomas: further experiences and late results. *Am J Roentgenol Radium Ther Nucl Med* 1968;103(1):44–52.

245. Regine WF, Kramer S. Pediatric craniopharyngiomas: long term results of combined treatment with surgery and radiation. *Int J Radiat Oncol Biol Phys* 1992;24(4):611–617.

246. Brada M, Thomas DG. Craniopharyngioma revisited. *Int J Radiat Oncol Biol Phys* 1993;27(2):471–475.

247. Fischer EG, Welch K, Shillito J Jr, et al. Craniopharyngiomas in children. Long-term effects of conservative surgical procedures combined with radiation therapy. *J Neurosurg* 1990;73(4):534–540.

248. Laws ER Jr. Conservative surgery and radiation for childhood craniopharyngiomas. *J Neurosurg* 1991; 74(6):1025–1026.

249. Varlotto JM, Flickinger JC, Kondziolka D, et al. External beam irradiation of craniopharyngiomas: long-

term analysis of tumor control and morbidity. *Int J Radiat Oncol Biol Phys* 2002;54(2):492–499.

250. Schulz-Ertner D, Frank C, Herfarth KK, et al. Fractionated stereotactic radiotherapy for craniopharyngiomas. *Int J Radiat Oncol Biol Phys* 2002;54(4):1114–1120.

251. Habrand JL, Ganry O, Couanet D, et al. The role of radiation therapy in the management of craniopharyngioma: a 25-year experience and review of the literature. *Int J Radiat Oncol Biol Phys* 1999;44(2): 255–263.

*252. Constine LS, Randall SH, Rubin P, et al. Craniopharyngiomas: fluctuation in cyst size following surgery and radiation therapy. *Neurosurgery* 1989;24(1):53–59.

253. Backlund EO, Axelsson B, Bergstrand CG, et al. Treatment of craniopharyngiomas: the stereotactic approach in a ten to twenty-three years' perspective. I. Surgical, radiological and ophthalmological aspects. *Acta Neurochir* 1989;99:11–19.

254. Mokry M. Craniopharyngiomas: a six year experience with gamma knife radiosurgery. *Stereotact Funct Neurosurg* 1999;72[Suppl 1]:140–149.

255. Hader WJ, Steinbok P, Hukin J, et al. Intratumoral therapy with bleomycin for cystic craniopharyngiomas in children. *Pediatr Neurosurg* 2000;33(4):211–218.

256. Mottolese C, Stan H, Hermier H, et al. Intracystic chemotherapy with bleomycin in the treatment of craniopharyngiomas. *Childs Nerv Syst* 2001;17:724–730.

257. Lunsford LD, Pollock BE, Kondziolka DS, et al. Stereotactic options in the management of craniopharyngioma. *Pediatr Neurosurg* 1994; 21[Suppl 1]:90–97.

258. Plowman PN, Wraith C, Royle N, et al. Stereotactic radiosurgery. IX. Craniopharyngioma: durable complete imaging responses and indications for treatment. *Br J Neurosurg* 1999;13(4):352–358.

259. Chiou SM, Lunsford LD, Niranjan A, et al. Stereotactic radiosurgery of residual or recurrent craniopharyngioma, after surgery, with or without radiation therapy. *Neuro-oncology* 2001;3(3):159–166.

260. Vernet O, Montes JL, Farmer JP, et al. Long term results of multimodality treatment of craniopharyngioma in children. *J Clin Neurosci* 1999;6(3):199–203.

261. Kooy HM, van Herk M, Barnes PD, et al. Image fusion for stereotactic radiotherapy and radiosurgery treatment planning. *Int J Radiat Oncol Biol Phys* 1994;28(5):1229–1234.

262. Stephanian E, Lunsford LD, Coffey RJ, et al. Gamma knife surgery for sellar and suprasellar tumors. *Neurosurg Clin N Am* 1992;3(1):207–218.

263. Pollack IF, Lunsford LD, Slamovits TL, et al. Stereotaxic intracavitary irradiation for cystic craniopharyngiomas. *J Neurosurg* 1988;68(2):227–233.

264. Van den Berge JH, Blaauw G, Breeman WA, et al. Intracavitary brachytherapy of cystic craniopharyngiomas. *J Neurosurg* 1992;77(4):545–550.

265. Flickinger JC, Lunsford LD, Singer J, et al. Megavoltage external beam irradiation of craniopharyngiomas: analysis of tumor control and morbidity. *Int J Radiat Oncol Biol Phys* 1990;19(1):117–122.

266. Ho DM, Liu HC. Primary intracranial germ cell tumor. Pathologic study of 51 patients. *Cancer* 1992; 70(6):1577–1584.

267. Bjornsson J, Scheithauer BW, Okazaki H, et al. Intracranial germ cell tumors: pathobiological and immunohistochemical aspects of 70 cases. *J Neuropathol Exp Neurol* 1985;44(1):32–46.

268. Felix I, Becker LE. Intracranial germ cell tumors in children: an immunohistochemical and electron microscopic study. *Pediatr Neurosurg* 1990;16(3):156–162.

269. Glenn OA, Barkovich AJ. Intracranial germ cell tumors: a comprehensive review of proposed embryologic derivation. *Pediatr Neurosurg* 1996;24(5): 242–251.

270. Huh SJ, Shin KH, Kim IH, et al. Radiotherapy of intracranial germinomas. *Radiother Oncol* 1996;38(1): 19–23.

271. Legido A, Packer RJ, Sutton LN, et al. Suprasellar germinomas in childhood. A reappraisal. *Cancer* 1989;63(2):340–344.

272. Yasue M, Tanaka H, Nakajima M, et al. Germ cell tumors of the basal ganglia and thalamus. *Pediatr Neurosurg* 1993;19(3):121–126.

273. Kollias SS, Barkovich AJ, Edwards MS. Magnetic resonance analysis of suprasellar tumors of childhood. *Pediatr Neurosurg* 1991;17(6):284–303.

274. Dayan AD, Marshall AH, Miller AA, et al. Atypical teratomas of the pineal and hypothalamus. *J Pathol Bacteriol* 1966;92( ):1–28.

*275. Haddock MG, Schild SE, Scheithauer BW, et al. Radiation therapy for histologically confirmed primary central nervous system germinoma. *Int J Radiat Oncol Biol Phys* 1997;38(5):915–923.

276. Paulino AC, Wen BC, Mohideen MN. Controversies in the management of intracranial germinomas. *Oncology (Huntingt)* 1999;13(4):513–521.

277. Herrick MK. Pathology of pineal tumors. In: Neuwelt EA, ed. *Diagnosis and treatment of pineal region tumors.* Baltimore: Williams & Wilkins, 1984:31–60.

*278. Borit A, Blackwood W, Mair WG. The separation of pineocytoma from pineoblastoma. *Cancer* 1980; 45(6):1408–1418.

279. Disclafani A, Hudgins RJ, Edwards MS, et al. Pineocytomas. *Cancer* 1989;63(2):302–304.

280. Schild SE, Scheithauer BW, Schomberg PJ, et al. Pineal parenchymal tumors. Clinical, pathologic, and therapeutic aspects. *Cancer* 1993;72(3):870–880.

281. Erlich SS, Apuzzo ML. The pineal gland: anatomy, physiology, and clinical significance. *J Neurosurg* 1985;63(3):321–341.

*282. Sung DI, Harisliadis L, Chang CH. Midline pineal tumors and suprasellar germinomas: highly curable by irradiation. *Radiology* 1978;128(3):745–751.

283. Balmaceda C, Diez B, Villablanca J, et al. Chemotherapy only strategy in primary central nervous system germ cell tumors (CNS GCT): results of an international study. *J Neurooncol* 1993;15:S3.

284. Balmaceda C, Heller G, Rosenblum M, et al. Chemotherapy without irradiation—a novel approach for newly diagnosed CNS germ cell tumors: results of an international cooperative trial. *J Clin Oncol* 1996;14(11):2908–2915.

285. Shibamoto Y, Takahashi M, Sasai K. Prognosis of intracranial germinoma with syncytiotrophoblastic giant cells treated by radiation therapy. *Int J Radiat Oncol Biol Phys* 1997;37(3):505–510.

286. Sawamura Y, Ikeda J, Shirato H, et al. Germ cell tumours of the central nervous system: treatment consideration based on 111 cases and their long-term clinical outcomes. *Eur J Cancer* 1998;34(1): 104–110.

*287. Shibamoto Y, Abe M, Yamashita J, et al. Treatment results of intracranial germinoma as a function of the irradiated volume. *Int J Radiat Oncol Biol Phys* 1988;15(2):285–290.

288. Dearnaley DP, A'Hern RP, Whittaker S, et al. Pineal and CNS germ cell tumors: Royal Marsden Hospital experience 1962–1987. *Int J Radiat Oncol Biol Phys* 1990;18(4):773–781.

289. Allen JC. Controversies in the management of intracranial germ cell tumors. *Neurol Clin* 1991;9(2):441–452.

290. Shibamoto Y, Takahashi M, Abe M. Reduction of the radiation dose for intracranial germinoma: a prospective study. *Br J Cancer* 1994;70(5):984–989.

*291. Shirato H, Nishio M, Sawamura Y, et al. Analysis of long-term treatment of intracranial germinoma. *Int J Radiat Oncol Biol Phys* 1997;37(3):511–515.

*292. Wolden SL, Wara WM, Larson DA, et al. Radiation therapy for primary intracranial germ-cell tumors. *Int J Radiat Oncol Biol Phys* 1995;32(4):943–949.

293. Allen JC, Kim JH, Packer RJ. Neoadjuvant chemotherapy for newly diagnosed germ-cell tumors of the central nervous system. *J Neurosurg* 1987; 67(1):65–70.

294. Allen JC, DaRosso RC, Donahue B, et al. A phase II trial of preirradiation carboplatin in newly diagnosed germinoma of the central nervous system. *Cancer* 1994;74(3):940–944.

295. Calaminus G, Bamberg M, Baranzelli MC, et al. Intracranial germ cell tumors: a comprehensive update of the European data. *Neuropediatrics* 1994;25(1):26–32.

296. Sawamura Y, Shirato H, Ikeda J, et al. Induction chemotherapy followed by reduced-volume radiation therapy for newly diagnosed central nervous system germinoma. *J Neurosurg* 1998;88(1):66–72.

297. Yoshida J, Sugita K, Kobayashi T, et al. Prognosis of intracranial germ cell tumours: effectiveness of chemotherapy with cisplatin and etoposide (CDDP and VP16). *Acta Neurochir* 1993;120:111–117.

298. Robertson PL, DaRosso RC, Allen JC. Improved prognosis of intracranial non-germinoma germ cell tumors with multimodality therapy. *J Neurooncol* 1997;32(1):71–80.

299. Schild SE, Haddock MG, Scheithauer BW, et al. Nongerminomatous germ cell tumors of the brain. *Int J Radiat Oncol Biol Phys* 1996;36(3):557–563.

300. Jenkin D, Berry M, Chan H, et al. Pineal region germinomas in childhood treatment considerations. *Int J Radiat Oncol Biol Phys* 1990;18(3):541–545.

301. Regis J, Bouillot P, Rouby-Volot F, et al. Pineal region tumors and the role of stereotactic biopsy: review of the mortality, morbidity, and diagnostic rates in 370 cases. *Neurosurgery* 1996;39(5):907–912.

*302. Linstadt D, Wara WM, Edwards MS, et al. Radiotherapy of primary intracranial germinomas: the case against routine craniospinal irradiation. *Int J Radiat Oncol Biol Phys* 1988;15(2):291–297.

*303. Shibamoto Y, Sasai K, Oya N, et al. Intracranial germinoma: radiation therapy with tumor volume-based dose selection. *Radiology* 2001;218(2):452–456.

304. Sawamura Y, de Tribolet N, Ishii N, et al. Management of primary intracranial germinomas: diagnostic surgery or radical resection? *J Neurosurg* 1997;87(2):262–266.

305. Stein BM. Surgical therapy of benign pineal tumors. In: Neuwelt EA, ed. *Diagnosis and treatment of pineal region tumors.* Baltimore: Williams & Wilkins, 1984:254–272.

306. Glanzmann C, Seelentag W. Radiotherapy for tu-

mours of the pineal region and suprasellar germinomas. *Radiother Oncol* 1989;16(1):31–40.

307. Paulino AC. Induction chemotherapy and involved-field radiotherapy for intracranial germinoma. *J Clin Oncol* 2002;20(12):2911–2912.

308. Kondziolka D, Hadjipanayis CG, Flickinger JC, et al. The role of radiosurgery for the treatment of pineal parenchymal tumors. *Neurosurgery* 2002; 51(4):880–889.

309. Dempsey PK, Lunsford LD. Stereotactic radiosurgery for pineal region tumors. *Neurosurg Clin N Am* 1992;3(1):245–253.

310. Kitamura K, Shirato H, Sawamura Y, et al. Preirradiation evaluation and technical assessment of involved-field radiotherapy using computed tomographic (CT) simulation and neoadjuvant chemotherapy for intracranial germinoma. *Int J Radiat Oncol Biol Phys* 1999;43(4):783–788.

311. Baranzelli MC, Patte C, Bouffet E, et al. Nonmetastatic intracranial germinoma: the experience of the French Society of Pediatric Oncology. *Cancer* 1997;80(9):1792–1797.

312. Sutton LN, Radcliffe J, Goldwein JW, et al. Quality of life of adult survivors of germinomas treated with craniospinal irradiation. *Neurosurgery* 1999;45(6): 1292–1297.

313. Merchant TE, Davis BJ, Sheldon JM, et al. Radiation therapy for relapsed CNS germinoma after primary chemotherapy. *J Clin Oncol* 1998;16(1):204–209.

314. Dattoli MJ, Newall J. Radiation therapy for intracranial germinoma: the case for limited volume treatment. *Int J Radiat Oncol Biol Phys* 1990;19(2):429–433.

315. Aoyama H, Shirato H, Kakuto Y, et al. Pathologically proven intracranial germinoma treated with radiation therapy. *Radiother Oncol* 1998;47(2):201–205.

316. Zissiadis Y, Dutton S, Kieran M, et al. Stereotactic radiotherapy for pediatric intracranial germ cell tumors. *Int J Radiat Oncol Biol Phys* 2001;51(1):108–112.

317. Shibamoto Y, Oda Y, Yamashita J, et al. The role of cerebrospinal fluid cytology in radiotherapy planning for intracranial germinoma. *Int J Radiat Oncol Biol Phys* 1994;29(5):1089–1094.

*318. Merchant TE, Sherwood SH, Mulhern RK, et al. CNS germinoma: disease control and long-term functional outcome for 12 children treated with craniospinal irradiation. *Int J Radiat Oncol Biol Phys* 2000;46(5):1171–1176.

319. Bamberg M, Kortmann RD, Calaminus G, et al. Radiation therapy for intracranial germinoma: results of the German cooperative prospective trials MAKEI 83/86/89. *J Clin Oncol* 1999;17(8):2585–2592.

320. Roberge D, Sontag M, Merchant T, et al. Intracranial germinoma: dosimetric issues of whole-ventricular irradiation. *Int J Radiat Oncol Biol Phys* 2003;[Suppl 1].

*321. Hardenbergh PH, Golden J, Billet A, et al. Intracranial germinoma: the case for lower dose radiation therapy. *Int J Radiat Oncol Biol Phys* 1997;39(2):419–426.

322. Kobayashi T, Yoshida J, Ishiyama J, et al. Combination chemotherapy with cisplatin and etoposide for malignant intracranial germ-cell tumors. An experimental and clinical study. *J Neurosurg* 1989;70(5):676–681.

323. Patel SR, Buckner JC, Smithson WA, et al. Cisplatin-based chemotherapy in primary central nervous system germ cell tumors. *J Neurooncol* 1992;12(1):47–52.

4

Tumors of the Posterior Fossa and the Spinal Canal

Larry E. Kun, M.D.

The posterior fossa occupies the lower half of the posterior aspect of the cranium, bounded anteriorly by the clivus and posterior clinoid and posteriorly by the calvaria, at and below the level of the inion (the midline bony prominence at the confluence of the straight and sagittal sinuses). Inferiorly, the posterior fossa is bordered by the occipital bone (to the foramen magnum); laterally, it is bordered by portions of the temporal, occipital, and parietal bones. Superiorly, the margin is defined by the tentorium cerebellae, that is, the portion of the dura mater extending from the basisphenoid adjacent to the posterior clinoid, rising to cover the cerebellum, and extending posteriorly and inferiorly to insert at the level of the inion. The cerebellum and brainstem are contained in the posterior fossa.

More than one-half of all childhood brain tumors arise in the posterior fossa. The most common types are medulloblastoma, low-grade astrocytomas of the cerebellum, brainstem tumors, and ependymomas (see Table 3-1, Chapter 3) (1-4).

MEDULLOBLASTOMA

Medulloblastoma is a primitive cerebellar tumor of neuroectodermal origin. The tumor is the most common malignant tumor in children and adolescents, accounting for 20% of pediatric brain tumors, or approximately 540 cases per year in the United States (1,4). Medulloblastoma was first identified in Bailey and Cushing's 1925 classification of central nervous system (CNS) tumors (5,6). The classic description defined medulloblastoma as a primitive or embryonal tumor of the cerebellum, theoretically derived from the progenitor medulloblasts located in the external granular layer of the cerebellum.

The World Health Organization (WHO) classification of CNS neoplasms identifies embryonal tumors as a component of neuroepithelial neoplasms that are particularly prominent among pediatric brain tumors (7,8). There has been much progress in rationalizing the histopathology and emerging molecular biology of the more common undifferentiated, small round cell tumors that have been generically classified as primitive neuroectodermal tumors (PNETs) or embryonal neoplasms. The umbrella concept of primitive neuroectodermal tumors proposed by Rorke (9) in 1983 grouped a number of previously recognized, related "small, round, blue cell" tumors occurring throughout the CNS based on similar morphology, a common tendency to seed through cerebrospinal fluid (CSF) pathways, and relative sensitivity to both irradiation and chemotherapy. The current WHO classification is included in Table 3-2 of Chapter 3, separately categorizing three tumor types often considered generically as PNETs: ependymoblastoma, medulloblastoma, and supratentorial PNETs. Also listed as embryonal tumors are medulloepithelioma and atypical teratoid/rhabdoid tumors (AT/RTs), with notably distinct pathology and apparent lines of genetic evolution (8). Pineoblastomas, clinically and histologically similar to the medulloblastomas and supratentorial PNETs, are classified among the pineal parenchymal tumors in the WHO classification.

The most common of the embryonal tumors is medulloblastoma, by definition a malignant, invasive embryonal tumor arising in the cerebellum, with predominantly neuronal differentiation

(8). The supratentorial PNETs, initially identified by Hart and Earle (10), are tumors typically of the cerebrum or suprasellar region that are composed of undifferentiated or poorly differentiated neuroepithelial cells that often display divergent differentiation along neuronal, astrocytic, or ependymal lines (8). Previously distinct cerebral neuroblastomas and cerebral ganglioneuroblastomas often are included in the category of supratentorial PNETs (8).

A recent study by Pomeroy et al. (11) adds credence to the WHO classification. Using DNA microarray gene expression patterns, they confirmed the apparent derivation of medulloblastoma from the molecularly similar cerebellar granule cells while showing medulloblastoma to be molecularly distinct from supratentorial PNETs.

Histologically, medulloblastoma is a densely cellular neoplasm composed predominantly of undifferentiated small, round, blue cells. Differentiation may be apparent toward neuronal or glial (astrocytic, oligodendroglial, and, less commonly, ependymal) lines (8,12). Differentiation along mesenchymal lines (striated muscle) may be present as a variant called medullomyoblastoma (8,12). Approximately 10–20% of medulloblastomas can be identified as desmoplastic medulloblastoma, marked histologically by hypoplastic nodules and dense reticulin-rick perinodular zones; the tumor is of interest because it is linked to the mutations of the *PTCH* gene, related to the sonic hedgehog pathway responsible for cerebellar granular cell proliferation and associated with activation of *GLI* (13–15).

The histologic grade of medulloblastoma has been more recently appreciated as of prognostic importance. Extensive nodularity has been correlated with favorable outcome, and the degree of anaplasia (and, particularly, the subset of large call anaplastic tumors) has been associated with inferior survival rates (3,8,16). Tumors with metastatic disease, either at diagnosis or as a pattern of failure, are more often associated with markedly anaplastic histology (17).

The most common genetic abnormality found in medulloblastomas is 17p deletion or isochromosome 17q (18,19). Amplification of *MYC* is apparent in tumors with double minutes and appears to be related to anaplastic large cell tumors (16).

Other molecular correlations important in understanding current directions in medulloblastoma include TrkC expression (directly proportional to survival in one major study) and ErbB2 expression (elevated levels of this factor, biologically related to cerebellar granular cell proliferation, migration, and invasion, are associated with poor outcome) (13,19,20).

The median age at diagnosis is 5 to 6 years. Approximately 20% of medulloblastomas present in infants younger than 2 years old; the tumor is uncommon in adults. Boys are affected more often than girls. Presenting symptoms are those classically associated with posterior fossa lesions in children: symptoms related to elevated intracranial pressure (headaches and vomiting, especially in the morning) and ataxia. Elevated intracranial pressure results from the tumor obstructing CSF flow through the sylvian aqueduct and fourth ventricle.

Medulloblastomas arise most often in the midline cerebellar vermis. The tumor characteristically grows into and fills the fourth ventricle. Infiltration around the fourth ventricle is common, often involving the brachium pontis and extending onto the ventricular floor (i.e., the brainstem). On magnetic resonance imaging (MRI), medulloblastomas are well-defined, typically solid lesions with uniform or, less often, nonhomogeneous contrast enhancement. By computed tomography (CT) scan, the tumor often is hyperdense, reflecting high cellularity.

Medulloblastoma is the classic CNS tumor associated with CSF seeding or metastasis. Subarachnoid dissemination is reported at diagnosis in 20–35% of children (21–23). A review of 106 consecutive cases staged at diagnosis showed leptomeningeal disease in 32%, noted on both spinal MRI and CSF cytology in 12%, positive CSF alone in 8%, and MRI alone in 11% (23). Neuraxis disease typically involves the spinal subarachnoid space; intracranial metastasis is less common, noted as isolated disease in the basal or suprasellar cisterns (Fig. 4-1) or diffusely in the subarachnoid space (24).

The standard of care requires postoperative staging, typically based on imaging of the brain to assess degree of resection and potential subarachnoid metastasis (ideally within 24 hours,

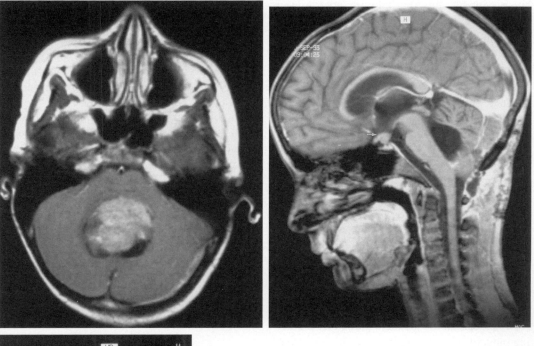

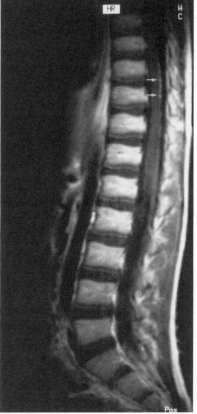

FIG. 4-1. Medulloblastoma, originating classically in the cerebellar vermis **(A, B),** with signs of subarachnoid spread in the hypothalamic region **(B)** and along the spine **(C).**

but acceptable up to 72 hours postsurgery), spinal MRI (gadolinium-enhanced study approximately 10 to 14 days after surgery to assess potential overt metastasis), and lumbar CSF cytology (best obtained immediately after spinal imaging).

Since publication by a radiation oncologist, the Chang (25) staging system has been used for clinical staging in medulloblastoma. The system was developed in the pre-CT era and is based on the size and invasiveness of the primary tumor at surgery ("T stage") and evidence of spread outside the posterior fossa ("M stage") (Table 4-1). Progressive tumor size and invasion of the brainstem defined increasing local tumor burden and aggressive behavior, classified as T_{1-4}. With the advent of CT and MRI, it became apparent that imaging identification of brainstem invasion is not as reliable as surgical observation. There is no modern data to substantiate a role for T stage as an independent parameter predicting outcome or defining therapy (26–30). Comparisons in otherwise early medulloblastoma (defined as M_0 with complete or near total resection) and in series addressing advanced medulloblastoma have shown equivalent outcome among those with brainstem invasion (T_{3b}) and those without such (T_{1-3a}) (26,31).

M stage is based on subarachnoid metastasis, progressively coding abnormal CSF cytology (M_1) or imaging evidence of noncontiguous tumor in the cranium (M_2) or spine (M_3). Extra-neural disease (most often confined to the bone marrow) is present in fewer than 2% of cases at presentation, coded as M_4. M stage remains a highly significant prognostic factor; intensity of therapy in current protocols and outcome are strongly related to the presence or absence of metastatic disease (26,28,30,32).

Current clinical trials and standard management in North America define risk categories for medulloblastoma as average risk (children older than 3 years with no metastatic disease after near total or total resection, with less than 1.5 cm^2 residual on early postoperative imaging) or high risk (overt metastatic disease based on CSF cytology or neuroimaging, or the presence of more than 1.5 cm^2 residual on early postoperative imaging; more recently, all children younger than 3 years of age typically have been classified as high risk based on outcome studies) (33).

Therapy

Surgery

Harvey Cushing's (5) classic 1930 report of his experience with medulloblastoma demonstrated the inability of surgery alone to cure this tumor; only one of 61 patients survived 3 years after surgery with or without limited irradiation.

The importance of maximal, judicious surgical resection is apparent in most contemporary

---

TABLE 4-1. *Chang staging for medulloblastoma[a]*

T_1	Tumor <3 cm in diameter	M_0	No evidence of subarachnoid or hematogenous metastasis
T_2	Tumor ≥3 cm in diameter	M_1	Tumor cells found in cerebrospinal fluid
T_{3a}	Tumor >3 cm in diameter with extension	M_2	Intracranial tumor beyond primary site (e.g., into the aqueduct of Sylvius and/or into the subarachnoid space or in the third or foramen of Luschka or lateral ventricles
T_{3b}[b]	Tumor >3 cm in diameter with unequivocal extension into the brain stem	M_3	Gross nodular seeding in spinal subarachnoid space
T_4	Tumor >3 cm in diameter with extension up past the aqueduct of Sylvius and/or down past the foramen magnum (i.e., beyond the posterior fossa)	M_4	Metastasis outside the cerebrospinal axis (esp. bone marrow, bone)

[a]A pre-CT era system described by Chang (25), modified by J. Langston (*personal communication*, 1988).
[b]T_{3b} is generally defined by *intraoperative* demonstration of tumor extension into the brainstem.

series (26,34–37). Gross total resection (i.e., no evidence of residual tumor seen at surgery and negative postoperative imaging) and near total resection (best defined as minimal residual: more than 90% resection estimated by the surgeon and less than 1.5 cm^2 residual on postoperative imaging) are associated with superior outcome in comparison to subtotal (51–90% resection) or partial (11–50% removal) resection and biopsy only (less than 10% removal) (28).

Table 4-2 summarizes data from series documenting the influence of degree of surgical resection on survival. A correlation between degree of resection and local tumor extent (i.e., infiltration into the brainstem or cerebellopontine peduncle, limiting complete removal) can be inferred. Data from the Children's Cancer Group (CCG) indicate gross total or near total resection in approximately 90% of children (26,28). Survival appears to correlate more significantly with amount of tumor residual (i.e., the surgical result as documented on immediate postoperative imaging) than with the surgeon's impression of degree of resection; data confirming the value of minimal residual disease are most apparent among children with M_0 disease (28,38). In one earlier CCG trial, 5-year event-free survival (EFS) was 78% for children with M_0 disease and less than 1.5 cm^2 residual, compared with 54% for those with larger residual volumes (26). For tumors adherent to or invading the brainstem, a report from St. Jude Children's Research Hospital showed no advantage to pursuing gross total resection compared with near total removal, with none of the cases exhibiting more than 1.5 cm^2 residual; morbidity appeared to be greater with the more aggressive surgical approach (39).

Operative mortality has been reduced to 2% or less in pediatric neurosurgical centers. However, aggressive surgery may be associated with significant morbidity (28,40,41). The posterior fossa syndrome has been described in up to 15% of children after posterior fossa craniotomy. The syndrome is signified by difficulty swallowing, truncal ataxia, mutism, and, less often, respiratory failure. Symptoms and signs typically are noted after a 12- to 24-hour period of initially uneventful postoperative recovery (27,40,41). Disabling neurologic signs often improve dramatically, sometimes over many months after surgery. It is important to maintain an aggressive, curative approach (including radiation therapy) in children with this syndrome, anticipating significant neurologic recovery, which may not be apparent early in the course of irradiation.

The routine use of ventriculoperitoneal shunts to reduce intracranial pressure before posterior fossa craniotomy resulted in significant improvement in operative morbidity and mortality when introduced 40 years ago. The risk of shuntborne metastases is minimal (42). Several earlier reports implicated shunts in the dissemi-

TABLE 4-2. *Medulloblastoma—results of radiation therapy*

Series	Interval	No. patients	Post-op therapy	5-yr DFS	5-yr OS	10-yr OS
Royal Marsden [44]	1950–1964	71	Crl (30-40r), Spl (25–30r), PF (45–50r)		40%	30%
Toronto [36]	1977–1987	72	CSI (35 Gy), PF (50–52.5 Gy)	64%	71%	63%
SIOP II [32]	1984–1989	40	CSI (35 Gy), PF (50 Gy)	60%		
POG/CCG [31]	1986–1990	126	CSI (23.4 Gy), PF (54 Gy) CSI (36 Gy), PF (54 Gy)	52% 67% $\Big\rangle p = .08$	63% 80% $\Big\rangle$n.s.	

CSI, Craniospinal irradiation; Crl, cranial irradiation; Spl, spinal irradiation; r, converted to rad; Gy, Gray; DFS, disease- or event-free survival; OS, overall survival.

nation of medulloblastoma (36). More recent studies find no increased incidence of medulloblastoma dissemination in the presence of a shunt (42). We may conclude that although shuntborne metastases do occur, they are not common enough to warrant a change in tumor management policy. Children with ventriculoperitoneal shunts typically become shunt dependent. Shunt failure or infection may complicate long-term survival, necessitating revision or replacement in nearly 25% of children measured 5 years after insertion. In many academic pediatric neurosurgical centers, it is standard procedure to place a ventricular drain (ventriculostomy), as needed, at the time of surgery. The surgeon often can document reestablishment of CSF flow after fourth ventricular tumor resection. Later shunt insertion may be needed in up to 25% of children (27). A delayed shunt insertion approach provides physiologic CSF dynamics for the majority of children, avoiding potential late events related to an indwelling ventriculoperitoneal shunt.

Radiation Therapy

The efficacy of radiation therapy in medulloblastoma was reported within a decade of Cushing's initial description of the tumor. Cutler et al. (43) reported the radiation responsiveness of medulloblastoma and the value of preventive irradiation of the entire neuraxis based on Cushing's clinical series. The seminal report documenting cure of medulloblastoma with craniospinal irradiation (CSI) was published by Bloom et al. in 1969 (44), documenting 32% survival at 5 years and 25% disease-free survival at 10 years. Numerous subsequent reports confirm increasing rates of disease control with modern radiation techniques (Table 4-2) (27,31,32,36,37,45–47). Modifications of radiation volume, dosage, and fractionation have been explored. Data confirm the value of standard full neuraxis irradiation rather than more limited treatment volumes (with the possible exception of very young children); established neuraxis dosage levels are superior to reduced-dose CSI when postoperative therapy is limited to radiation therapy (31,45). However, reduction in CSI dosage is effective

when given in conjunction with contemporary, cis-platinum–based chemotherapy (48).

Chemotherapy

Phase II trials have documented the chemoresponsiveness of medulloblastoma to alkylating agents (especially cyclophosphamide), platinum compounds (cisplatin, carboplatin), etoposide (administered orally or intravenously), and camptothecins (topotecan) (49–52).

Randomized trials in both CCG and International Society for Pediatric Oncology (SIOP) between 1978 and 1981 documented the impact of adjuvant chemotherapy (lomustine and vincristine, with prednisone added in the CCG study). The early, preplatinum regimens had no overall benefit but did show a significant improvement in disease control and survival among patients with locally advanced, incompletely resected, and metastatic disease (i.e., cases now identified as high risk) and in children younger than 2 years old (Table 4-3) (29,53). A parallel Pediatric Oncology Group (POG) study suggested an overall survival benefit in children receiving adjuvant mechlorethamine, vincristine, procarbazine, and prednisone chemotherapy (54).

The addition of platinating agents appears to have further enhanced the efficacy of chemotherapy. Packer et al.'s (30) earlier studies of postoperative irradiation and concurrent vincristine, followed by adjuvant lomustine, cisplatin, and vincristine in high-risk patients (defined as T_{3b} or brainstem invasion, significant local residual tumor, or metastatic disease) reported disease-free and overall survival at 5 years of 85% and 83%, respectively. Although one would no longer identify $T_{3b}M_0$, resected patients as high risk, the outcome in the M_0 cohort (related as 90% EPS at 5 years) stimulated further study of platinum-based chemotherapy (30). A subsequent trial by CCG tested the same chemotherapy regimen after reduced neuraxis dosage irradiation (23.4 Gy CSI) in average-risk children between 3 and 10 years old. The results, with 79% progression-free survival at 5 years, seem to be superior in a cross-study comparison to similarly staged patients treated in the earlier CCG and POG low-stage

TABLE 4-3. *Medulloblastoma-combined postoperative radiation therapy and chemotherapy*

Series	Interval	Cohort	n	RT	Chemotherapy	EFS @ 5 yrs	OS @ 5 yrs
CCG-9892 [48]	1990–1994	std risk, 3–10 y.o.	65[a]	CSI (23.4 Gy/13 fx), PF (55.2 Gy)	(vcr-CDDP-CCNU) x 8 post-RT[b]	78%	
SIOP/UKCCSG PNET-3 [47]	1992–2000	std risk, M_0, 3–16 y.o.	179[c]	CSI (35 Gy/21 fx), PF (55 Gy)	0 (n = 89) (vcr-VP-16-CBCOA-cyclo) x 4 pre-RT[d]	60% / 74% p = 0.04	65% / 77% p = .09
GPOH HIT '91 [21]	1991–1997	std risk, M_{0-11}, 3–18 y.o.	118[e]	CSI (35.2 Gy/16 fx), PF (55.2 Gy)	(ifos-VP-16-MTX-CDDP-AM-C) x 2 pre-RT[f] / (vcr-CDDP-CCNV) x 8 post-RT[b]	65% / 78% p < .03 (@ 3 yrs)	
POG 9031 [58]	1990–1996	hi-risk, 3–21 y.o. (T_{3-4}, > 1.5 cm^3 residual, M_{1-3})	224[g]	CSI (35.2 Gy/22 fx to 40 Gy/25 fx), PF (53.2–54.4 Gy)	(CDDP-VP-16) x 3 pre-RT plus (vcr-cyclo) x 8 post-RT[h] / (CDDP-VP-16) x 3 post-RT plus (vcr-cyclo) x 8 post-RT[h]	66% / 70% n.s.	73% / 76%

[a]65 assessable of 85 registered

[b]vcr, vincristine, *during RT*; vcr, CDDP (cisplatinum), CCNU

[c]179 eligible of 217 randomized

[d]vcr, VP16 (= etoposide), CBCDA (carboplatin); vcr, VP-16, cyclo (= cyclophosphamide)

[e]118 randomized without M_{2-3} disease of total 137 randomized and 184 analyzed; NOTE EFS is at *3 years*

[f]ifos (= ifosfamide), VP-16, MTX (hi-dose methotrexate); CDDP–ara-c (= cytosine arabinoside)

[g]224 of 229 registered

[h](CDDP-VP-16) x 3 given pre-irradiation, with sequential (vcr-cyclo) administered post-RT or post- (CDDP-VP-16), respectively

study (with 67% 5-year EFS after 36-Gy CSI without the addition of chemotherapy) (31,48). Taken together, and without the benefit of a prospective randomized trial further assessing neuraxis radiation dosage and postirradiation chemotherapy, the standard of care for children with average-risk medulloblastoma throughout North America has been accepted as reduced-dose CSI (23.4 Gy) in conjunction with a platinum-based chemotherapy regimen. In Europe, the recent SIOP PNET-3 study seems to confirm this conclusion for average-risk disease, showing 5-year EFS of 74% after combined chemotherapy and irradiation (vincristine, etoposide, carboplatin, and cyclophosphamide; note CSI at 35 Gy) compared with 60% with irradiation alone (47).

For high-risk medulloblastoma, an intervening CCG trial confirmed the earlier studies demonstrating disease control rates of about 60% when lomustine, vincristine, and prednisone were added to standard-dose (36-Gy) CSI (26). The earlier Packer et al. (30) study showed 67% 5-year disease-free survival for children with M_{1-3} disease, the cohort that remains most challenging in achieving disease control.

Trials of up-front, often phase II chemotherapy for patients with measurable residual disease (incomplete resection or neuraxis dissemination) have shown excellent response rates to cisplatin and etoposide; carboplatin; carboplatin and etoposide; high-dose methotrexate; and cyclophosphamide, cisplatin, and vincristine (50, 51,55). Problematic is a low but recognized rate of disease progression, even during a 12- to 16-week course of preirradiation chemotherapy (50,56,57).

POG completed a randomized trial comparing preirradiation and postirradiation CDDP and etoposide for high-risk disease in 1996; results indicate no difference in disease control related to sequence of chemotherapy and irradiation (58). It is of interest that the overall EFS of 65% among M_{1-3} cases is nearly identical to results quoted earlier; among patients with measurable disease receiving preirradiation chemotherapy, outcome is highly dependent on the degree of response to chemotherapy (58). Earlier SIOP data suggested a negative impact of preirradiation chemotherapy

in favorable-stage disease when combined with lower neuraxis dosage irradiation (32). A more recent trial from the German Pediatric Oncology Group indicated superior results with irradiation followed by CDDP, lomustine, and vincristine when compared with a cohort receiving postoperative ifosfamide, etoposide, high-dose methotrexate, CDDP, and ara-C before the same irradiation–chemotherapy combination (21). Pending additional data, postoperative irradiation followed by chemotherapy appears to be the preferable sequence in most settings.

For disease recurrent after radiation therapy (with or without chemotherapy), demonstration of chemotherapy responsiveness and subsequent high-dose chemotherapy with autologous bone marrow or peripheral stem cell rescue has resulted in a small proportion of durable secondary disease control (59).

Radiotherapeutic Management

Volume

Medulloblastoma is the seminal tumor identified with subarachnoid dissemination. The need for full CSI has been recognized for more than five decades. In reviewing serial treatment regimens in Sweden, Landberg et al. (60) noted serial improvements in survival rates with increasing radiation volume: 5% 10-year survival after limited posterior fossa irradiation, 15% after irradiation to the posterior fossa and spinal canal, and 53% after CSI. Reported failures in the subfrontal region additionally indicate the need to completely encompass the cranial and spinal subarachnoid space; such failures clearly represent inadequate dosage to the subfrontal area, a potential site of geographic miss or underdosage that necessitates particular attention in CSI planning and delivery (61,62).

A French cooperative trial of limited-volume irradiation (including the posterior fossa and spinal axis only but not the supratentorial brain) in conjunction with aggressive chemotherapy confirmed the importance of comprehensive CSI in children older than 3 years old. The notably poor outcome with early neuraxis failures (both supratentorial and spinal in location) asso-

ciated with limited-volume therapy led to early closure of the study (63).

All prospective trials reported from the North American and European pediatric cooperative groups have been based on the standard use of boost irradiation to the entire posterior fossa. Early experience with three-dimensional conformal irradiation (3D CRT) to the tumor bed only, replacing the posterior fossa as the local or "boost" volume, was reported by Merchant et al. (64) from Memorial Sloan–Kettering in 1999. A pattern of failure analysis detailing the relative infrequency of posterior fossa failures outside the tumor bed supported further study of this approach (65). A subsequent update of the Memorial Sloan–Kettering experience documented only one posterior fossa failure among 32 consecutive patients who received 3D CRT to the local tumor bed (45). A preliminary report of the more recent St. Jude collaborative experience, similarly targeting only the local tumor bed beyond 36 Gy, confirmed a low rate of posterior fossa failures with only two isolated and one combined posterior fossa recurrence among 73 consecutive patients; eight of 11 failures involved the leptomeninges (Table 4-4) (46). The French M-SFOP 98 trial also incorporated tumor bed boost volumes, with pre-

liminary reports suggesting a low rate of posterior fossa recurrences despite more limited volume irradiation (66).

Although the earlier literature suggested a predominance of posterior fossa failures in medulloblastoma despite surgery and higher-dose irradiation to the primary tumor region, more recent studies consistently indicate a shift in the pattern of failure to diffuse leptomeningeal recurrences (31,45,46,48,65–68). Together with the several trials reporting outcome after local boost to the tumor bed, recent experience supports a major prospective trial of image-guided irradiation to limited tumor bed boost volumes, as planned for 2004 in COG.

Dosage

Medulloblastoma is a radiosensitive tumor. *In vitro* studies by Fertil and Malaise (69) demonstrated a favorable surviving fraction at 2 Gy (28%), comparable to most other embryonal pediatric tumors and notably different from the clinically less responsive malignant gliomas. There is much data indicating a correlation between dosage to the posterior fossa primary site and outcome; local disease control and survival

TABLE 4-4. *Medulloblastoma—radiation therapy (preliminary data reporting reduced tumor/target volume techniques)*

Series	Interval	n	RT	Chemotherapy	EFS	OS
MSKCC [45,64]	1994–2002	32[a]	CSI (23.4–36 Gy) TBed (CTV = GTV + 1–2 cm; PTV = CTV + 0.5 cm; 55.8–59.4 Gy)	CDDP; vcr; CCNU or cyclo	84% @ 5 yrs	85% @ 5 yrs
SJCRH + collaborators [46]	1996–2002	73[b]	CSI (23.4 Gy) PF (36 Gy) TBed (CTV = GTV + 2 cm; PTV = CTV + 0.5 cm, 55.8 Gy)	CDDP; cyclo; vcr	92% @ 4 yrs	
M-SFOP 98 [66]	1998–2001	55[b]	CSI (36 Gy @ 100 cGy bid) TBed (68 Gy @ 100 cGy bid)	no	83% @ 2.5 yrs	94% @ 2.5 yrs

[a]Standard risk = 27, hi-risk = 5
[b]Standard risk
CSI, craniospinal irradiation; TBed, Tumor Bed; PF, posterior fossa; GTV, gross tumor volume; CTV, clinical target volume; PTV, planning target volume; CDDP, cisplatinum; vcr, vincristine; cyclo, cyclophosphamide.

have been related to posterior fossa dosages of 50 to 55 Gy using conventional fractionation at 160 to 180 cGy per fraction (36,70). The use of limited volume boost to 59.4 Gy for patients with imaging evidence of residual disease at the primary site has been reported, with no clear evidence that further dosage escalation is fruitful (45,64).

Recent trials support the use of 23.4 Gy (at 180 cGy/fraction) to the neuraxis for average-risk presentations when combined irradiation and chemotherapy is planned (48). Although the overwhelming percentage of failures now occur in the neuraxis and a limited comparative analysis suggests superior outcome after the previously standard 36 Gy compared with the 23.4 Gy dosage level in the Memorial Sloan–Kettering report, the current standard approach is to use the lower (23.4-Gy) CSI dosage (31,45,48,65). The recommendation is based upon apparent confirmation that 80% long-term disease control is achievable with 23.4-Gy CSI and platinum-based chemotherapy, now undergoing further analysis in the COG and POG trial that ended in 2001; agreement across several major radiation-alone studies showing long-term disease control in 60–65% of cases after 36-Gy CSI (31,47); and documentation that the reduced neuraxis dosage has been associated with significantly less neurocognitive decline than the higher-dose (36-Gy) CSI regimen when compared in the first POG and CCG trial of postoperative irradiation alone (31,45,46,48,52,71).

Largely in response to age-related concerns regarding neurocognitive changes, a small pilot study of 10 children younger than 10 years old was undertaken at Children's Hospital of Philadelphia and the University of Pennsylvania. Late follow-up showed disease control in seven of ten children who received only 18 Gy to the neuraxis, with reportedly minor neuropsychologic deficits (72). The COG average-risk medulloblastoma protocol, scheduled to open in 2004, will compare 23.4-Gy CSI with 18-Gy CSI for children younger than 8 years old, prospectively addressing the potential adequacy and related toxicities for further reduction in CSI dosage.

For patients with high-risk disease, particularly those with overt metastasis (including M_1

in most studies in addition to M_{2-3}), 36 Gy to the neuraxis remains the standard. Several studies have used 39.6 to 40 Gy for cases with significant bulk disease through the intracranial and spinal meninges.

Trials of hyperfractionated CSI include neuraxis dosages of 30 to 48.4 Gy at 100 to 110 cGy per fraction twice daily, with an interfraction interval greater than 6 hours; cumulative dosages for the posterior fossa have been 66 to 72 Gy with similar fractionation (73–75). None of the North American trials showed a significant benefit in disease control or reduction in toxicities supportive of further study. A recent report of hyperfractionated CSI (36 Gy in 36 fractions) with tumor bed boost (cumulative dosage, 68 Gy in 68 fractions) from the M-SFOP 98 study showed disease control rates greater than 80% with limited (less than 3-year) follow-up (66). The current SIOP (PNET 4) and UK-CCSG (CNS 2001) are addressing hyperfractionated and accelerated hyperfractionated delivery, respectively, in standard-risk (36 Gy at 100 cGy twice daily, boosting the posterior fossa and tumor bed to 60 Gy and 68 Gy, respectively) and metastatic (39.68 Gy at 1.24 Gy twice daily CSI, boosting the posterior fossa to 62 Gy at 50 fractions for 5 weeks). The potential value of altered fractionation has yet to be demonstrated.

Technique

The goal of achieving uniform dosage throughout the subarachnoid space, encompassing the entire intracranial vault and spinal canal, is one of the most technically demanding aspects of radiation oncology. Several techniques are appropriate for CSI administration (76). Fundamental is the use of opposed lateral fields including the cranium and upper cervical spinal canal, matching a posterior spinal field including the full spinal subarachnoid space or, in larger children, the upper one-half of the spinal canal (with a separate, matched lower posterior spinal field) (67,77).

It is important to establish immobilization and reproducibility of setup. Prone positioning is generally preferable because it allows greater immobilization and better extension of the chin

(minimizing potential bone growth changes caused by the exit of the posterior spinal field) and simplifies technical maneuvers at the critical junction between the lateral craniocervical fields and the posterior spinal field. Immobilization can be achieved through a customized plaster cast, use of the Alpha Cradle system, or a vacuum bag (discussed in Chapter 22) (78). Contemporary techniques and use of CT simulation for planning CSI are discussed in Mah et al.'s 1998 report (79). Supine techniques may be appropriate for very young children needing sedation or anesthesia; detailed attention to the junction area is needed when one adapts the more familiar prone geometry to supine CSI use.

In planning CSI, it is simpler to first simulate the spinal fields: establishing the length of the spinal field defines the collimator angle necessary for homogeneity with the craniocervical fields. The lower border of the spinal field is set to encompass the lowest level of the thecal sac as determined by MRI, typically at or below S2 (80,81). The upper portion of the spinal field is set in the area of C4 to C7. In small children the entire spine can be encompassed in one field; in children older than 5 years, extended distance or use of two adjacent spinal fields often is needed. If conventional fluoroscopic simulation is used and two spinal fields are necessary, lateral radiographs are taken to include the isocenter and junctional margin of each spinal field to establish the spinal cord depth for dosage prescription and calculation of the gap at the surface to provide uniformity at the spinal depth. Whenever two spinal fields are needed, it is important to change the level of the junction concurrently when feathering the craniocervical junction. The width of the spinal field should be sufficient to dosimetrically encompass the full width of the spinal canal. There has been debate whether a spade configuration is necessary to allow adequate lateral coverage at the lower sacral margin. Halperin's (81) anatomic study documents the importance of covering the sacral foramina, often necessitating some blocking of the superior component of the spinal volume (Fig. 4-2).

The brain and upper cervical spine are treated with lateral fields. The collimators for the lateral fields are angled to match the divergence of the posterior spinal field (Fig. 4-3). The cranial fields must accommodate serial decreases in length to feather the junction zone; if asymmetric collimators are not available to allow diminution of the caudal portion of the lateral fields while maintaining the isocenter, the length of the craniocervical fields must be sufficient to permit ultimate symmetric shrinkage by 6 to 10 cm. A table angle generally is used to correct for caudal divergence of the craniocervical fields (Fig. 4-3). Although detailed analysis shows only minimal inhomogeneity if a correcting table angle is not used (76), full 3D attention at the junction zone permits more confident abutting of the lateral craniocervical and posterior spinal fields. Eliminating a gap typically simplifies daily setup; with proper attention to technique and feathering to anatomically distribute any potential inhomogeneity, a 3D junction with abutting fields provides maximal homogeneity in the spinal canal. As an alternative, asymmetric jaws can be used to avoid divergence at this junction; the technique creates somewhat greater divergence in blocking the eyes at the critical cribriform plate region and limits the spinal length, necessitating a spinal junction even with younger children. Even with the ideal craniocervical match using asymmetric jaws, it is important to feather all junctional zones, shifting the anatomic junction site by at least 5 mm every 8 to 9 Gy, effectively once a week.

The cranial fields must be planned carefully to include the entire intracranial subarachnoid space. The most difficult area is at the level of the cribriform plate, where there is often little margin to allow one to block the eyes and dosimetrically encompass the critical subfrontal cribriform site. Reports of subfrontal recurrences have been noted even by highly respected institutions, documenting the particular technical difficulty in achieving adequate coverage at this site (61,62,82,83). For older children, the pneumatized frontal sinuses allow sufficient margin to obviate concern for the cribriform anatomy (Fig. 4-4). In younger children, the margin above the eye may be extremely close but should permit coverage of the subfrontal area as a first priority, minimizing dosage to the eye and, in particular, the optic lens. The literature supports the use of customized blocking rather

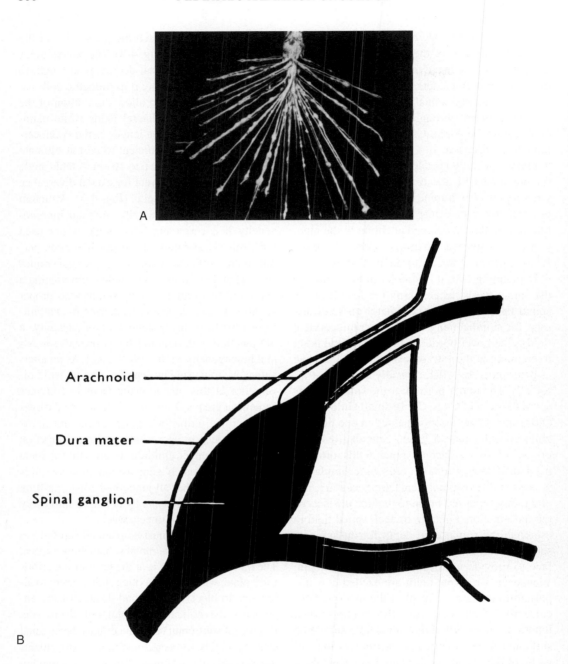

FIG. 4-2. Consideration of spinal volume for craniospinal irradiation. **(A)** Nerve root seeding in medulloblastoma; this figure first appeared in the *Bulletin of the Los Angeles Neurological Society* (8:1–10, 1943), representing advanced, diffuse leptomeningeal seeding. **(B)** Typical anatomy of the nerve roots, demonstrating the extension of the subarachnoid space laterally along the nerve root to a location in the neural foramen. (From Romanes GJ, ed. *Cunningham's textbook of anatomy,* 12th ed. Oxford: Oxford University Press, 1981:732–733, with permission.)

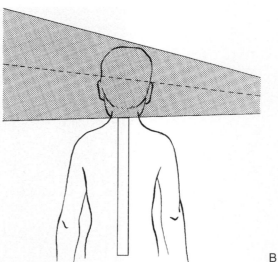

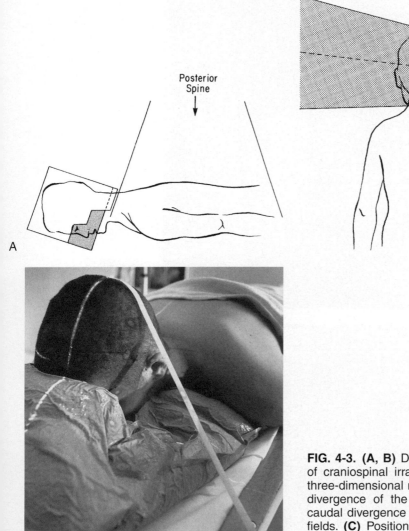

FIG. 4-3. (A, B) Diagrammatic representation of craniospinal irradiation technique, using a three-dimensional match that corrects for both divergence of the posterior spinal field and caudal divergence of the lateral craniocervical fields. **(C)** Positioning and immobilization device for the patient for CSI.

than the multileaf collimator to ensure adequate subfrontal coverage while minimizing dosage to the eye (84).

The classic posterior fossa boost was delivered by parallel opposed lateral fields. From a historical perspective, the anterior border of the posterior fossa was set at the posterior clinoid on a lateral simulation radiograph. The superior border of the tentorium was identified on postoperative sagittal MRI scans; anatomically, one could estimate the superior margin as 1 cm

higher than the midpoint between the foramen magnum and the vertex. To cover the inferior and posterior borders, field edge margins were set beyond the calvaria, with a lower border typically at the lower border of C1.

Current techniques typically include 3D CRT or intensity-modulated radiation therapy (IMRT) to encompass the posterior fossa, measured on CT or fused CT and MRI. The accuracy of identifying the tentorium and the anterior margins of the posterior fossa structures is facilitated by im-

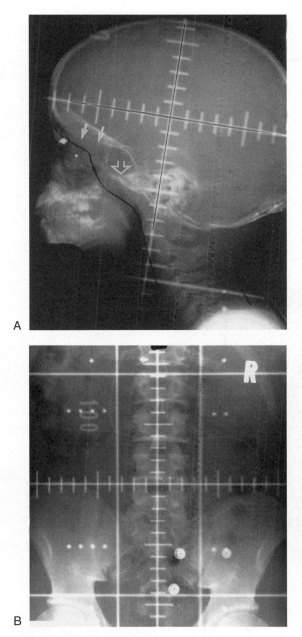

FIG. 4-4. Craniospinal irradiation (CSI) techniques, with two-dimensional fluoroscopic simulation out-lining margins for **(A)** cranial irradiation and **(B)** lower border of spinal fields. Computed tomography (CT) simulation technique for CSI: blocks derived from digital CT radiograph in treatment position **(C)**, with the cribriform plate highlighted in blue derived from the axial dimension **(D).** Dosage distribution through the neuraxis **(E)** reflects a three-dimensional match at the craniocervical–spinal junction and use of two cranial and three spinal intensity-modulated radiation therapy components to homogenize the dosage in the subarachnoid space of the spine and calvaria. (See color plate)

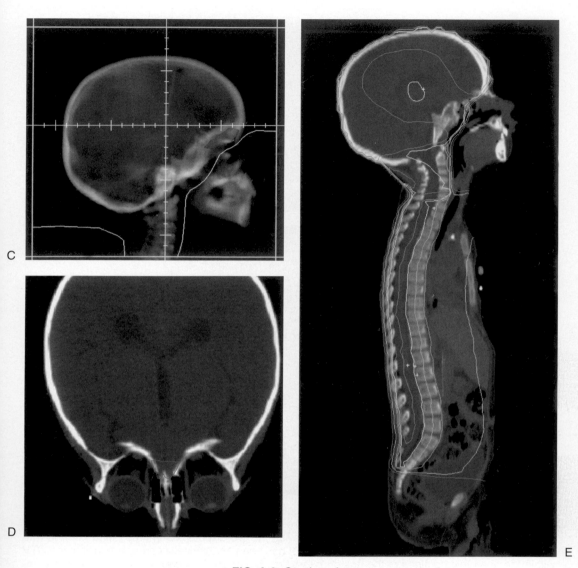

C

D

E

FIG. 4-4. *Continued.*

age-guided methods and by CT simulation (79). In protocol settings, there is now sufficient information to suggest the adequacy of boost volumes confined to the tumor bed. This sophisticated approach entails analyzing the initial tumor extent and identifying on CT images through the posterior fossa (with further guidance by MRI) the tumor bed based on postoperative imaging (Fig. 4-5). The gross tumor volume (GTV) is defined as the tumor bed; studies to date have used a 2-cm, anatomically corrected expansion to create the clinical tumor volume (CTV); depending on immobilization available, a further geometric margin of 5 to 7 mm is used to define the planning tumor volume (PTV) (64,79,85). The goal of image-guided irradiation and narrow margins in targeting the tumor bed is to diminish the dosage to the cochlea (especially important with combined irradiation and cisplatin), the temporal lobes, and the hypothalamic–pituitary region (Fig. 4-5).

The proposed COG trial for average-risk medulloblastoma will prospectively compare targeting the full posterior fossa with targeting only the tumor bed, based on 3D CRT or IMRT planning and delivery.

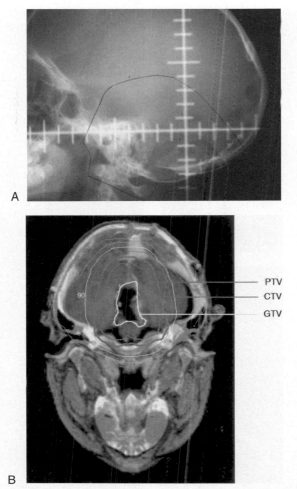

FIG. 4-5. (A) Posterior fossa irradiation, shown in two-dimensional fluoroscopic simulation for prior standard full posterior fossa coverage. **(B, C)** Three-dimensional conformal plan targeting the tumor bed is outlined in fused MRI and CT images showing the gross tumor volume as the tumor bed with a 1-cm expansion (protocol-defined) and CTV that has been anatomically corrected (to limit the CTV within the anatomic confines of the posterior fossa); a 5-mm geometric expansion defines the planning tumor volume (PTV). **(C)** The cochlea are shown on the upper axial view. Dosage distribution in axial and **(D)** sagittal projections indicates conformality of the 98–100% volume to the PTV, with lower-dose regions (50%, 30%) shown as appropriate. (See color plate)

The use of spinal electron irradiation has been explored to minimize the exit dosage through the length of the body (86). Theoretically, one can reduce potential late effects on the lungs and heart and the absorbed dosage in the childhood thyroid. Detailed dosimetry has been performed in phantoms for the use of electron fields in CSI (86,87). Whether inhomogeneity across the vertebral bodies will result in accentuated kyphoscoliosis is yet unclear. The clinical outcome of this technique has been summarized by Gaspar et al. (87), who noted no apparent difference in late complications between electron and photon spinal irradiation. There has been little recent interest in exploring electrons in this capacity, although there is now interest in exploring proton beam irradiation for CSI, based on greater homogeneity across the target volume than electrons and limited fall-off into the anterior structures (Fig. 4-6) (88).

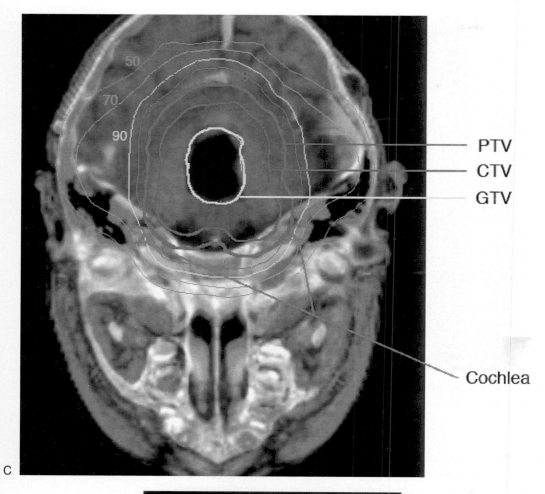

PTV

CTV

GTV

Cochlea

C

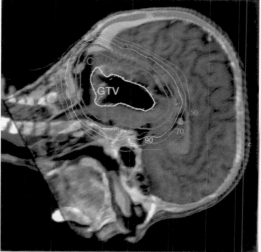

D

FIG. 4-5. *Continued.*

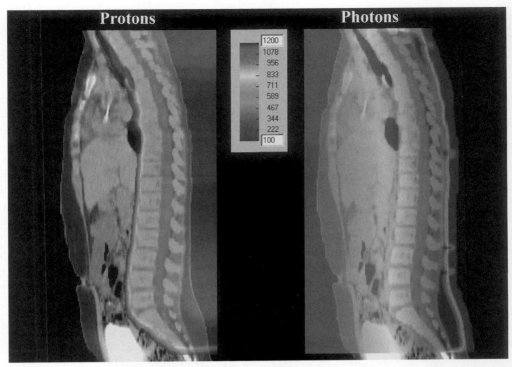

FIG. 4-6. A comparison of spinal irradiation with a posterior proton field and a posterior photon field. (See color plate)

The quality of radiation therapy has been correlated with improved outcome, based on both volume adequacy (in several but not all prospective cooperative group reviews) and duration of therapy (with several reports indicating inferior disease control when the interval to complete irradiation exceeds 45 days (67,89–91).

Delivery

CSI results in predictable, if quantitatively variable, acute changes in the peripheral blood counts. Monitoring for neutropenia or thrombocytopenia, most often noted during or after the third week of CSI without preceding chemotherapy, is critically important. Traditionally, CSI is interrupted if the neutrophil count falls below 1,000 cells per milliliter, especially if the child is febrile. When necessary to permit completion of neuraxis irradiation, granulocyte colony-stimulating factor may be used to correct neutropenia; thrombocytopenia may necessitate platelet transfusion (92). In most settings, radiation therapy for medulloblastoma

begins with CSI. If blood counts necessitate interrupting CSI for more than 2 consecutive days, initiation of posterior fossa irradiation will provide continuity and limit unnecessary interruption in irradiation at the primary site. One should return to CSI as soon as hematologic status permits. When CSI follows chemotherapy, extended hematosuppression delaying initiation of CSI may favor beginning with posterior fossa irradiation to allow earlier radiation therapy and delay neuraxis therapy until hematologically feasible.

Nausea and vomiting are generally more pronounced in older children. Use of antiemetics is important in preventing "anticipatory" vomiting, which may be more difficult to control. Ondansetron usually is successful. Rarely, corticosteroids may be necessary at low dosage levels, particularly early in the postoperative period.

Results

Long-term disease-free survival after surgery and irradiation is 60–70% (Fig. 4-6, Table 4-4).

Factors associated with more favorable outcome include age greater than 3 years, localized presentations (i.e., M_0), and tumors amenable to near total or total resection. Biologic factors may be even more important, particularly with reference to histologic subtype, ErbB2, c-myc, and TrkC expression, as well as specific genetic findings (11,13,17,19,20,93). Investigations to additionally improve outcome seek improvement in disease control and reduction in functional limitations attendant to therapy.

BRAINSTEM GLIOMA

The brainstem is the connecting structure that joins the long tracts from the cerebral hemispheres and midline diencephalic nuclei with the cerebellar tracks, forming the spinal cord as the tracts exit through foramen magnum. Within the brainstem are the nuclei of the cranial

nerves, the reticular activating system, and vital functional centers (e.g., respiratory). The brainstem includes three anatomic segments: the midbrain rostrally, the pons, and the medulla caudally. Brainstem tumors are a heterogeneous group of tumors that share common astrocytic histologies but evidence divergent clinical behavior related to the anatomic region of involvement and the pattern of growth. The tumor types are identified by their apparent anatomic segment of origin and the macroscopic appearance, defined as diffuse or focal lesions. Focal lesions are tumors that are limited in size (typically identified as involving less than 50% of the anatomic structure of origin, or less than 2 cm in maximal diameter), well circumscribed on imaging (with no evidence of infiltration or edema beyond the primary lesion), and often showing juvenile pilocytic histology if biopsied (Fig. 4-7) (94,95). The classically quoted incidence of brainstem tumors in children identifies 70–80%

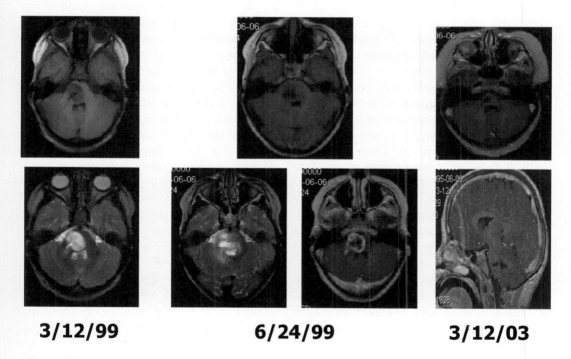

3/12/99   **6/24/99**   **3/12/03**

FIG. 4-7. Focal, intrinsic pontomedullary juvenile pilocytic astrocytoma after biopsy (3/12/99). Appearance 6 weeks after radiation therapy (54 Gy in 30 fractions): symptoms progressed from isolated right sixth nerve palsy with subtle left hyperreflexia to complete right seventh nerve palsy and dense left hemiparesis, associated with intralesional necrosis and expansion of the lesion (6/24/99). Patient treated supportively, with gradual improvement of left hemiparesis but persistent right seventh and sixth nerve palsies, associated with virtual resolution of lesion showing residual area of focal encephalomalacia on late imaging follow-up (3/12/03).

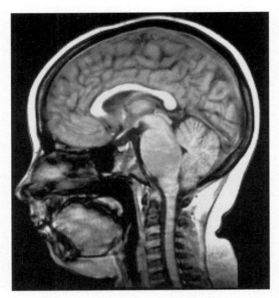

FIG. 4-8. Brainstem gliomas: classic and most common diffusely infiltrating pontine glioma.

as diffusely infiltrating lesions (primarily arising in the pons) (Fig. 4-8), with the remainder identified as one of the focal or benign tumor types discussed later in this chapter.

As a group, brainstem tumors constitute more than 10% of intracranial tumors in children. The peak incidence occurs between the ages of 5 and 9 years; boys are affected more commonly than girls. The most common presenting symptoms for the diffusely infiltrating pontine gliomas (the usual interpretation of "brainstem gliomas") include diplopia, motor weakness, and difficulty with speech, swallowing, and walking. Neurologic signs include ataxia, cranial nerve palsies (most common are the pontine nerves, VI and VII, followed by the medullary nerves, IX, X, XI, and XII, and, less often, the midbrain nerves, III, IV, and V), and long tract signs (motor weakness, most often hemiparesis) (34,95, 96). A review of the anatomy of the brainstem readily demonstrates why this constellation of signs occurs (Fig. 4-9).

Tumors of the midbrain and medulla may be diffuse or focal; even diffuse tumors typically show much less infiltration and expansion of the brainstem than seen with the pontine gliomas. Focal intrinsic tumors do occur in the pons, as do

dorsally exophytic tumors; both types enjoy much more favorable outcome than the more typical diffusely infiltrating pontine tumors (34,94–99).

The duration of symptoms correlates with the type of brainstem glioma. Children with diffusely infiltrating pontine gliomas relate a brief history of neurologic symptoms, almost uniformly measured in weeks and certainly less than 6 months. Neurologic signs necessary for pontine glioma protocols include at least two of three major categories of neurologic signs (i.e., cranial nerve deficits, long tract signs, ataxia) (95,100,101). Elevated intracranial pressure (secondary to obstructive hydrocephalus) is present in fewer than 15% of children with pontine gliomas. Midbrain tumors and dorsally exophytic tumors of the pons or pontomedullary junction typically present with elevated intracranial pressure caused by obstruction at the aqueduct of Sylvius or the fourth ventricle, respectively. The more focal, less aggressive brainstem tumors often are associated with prolonged symptoms, typically confined to deficits in one or two cranial nerves alone, ataxia, or gradual onset of elevated intracranial pressure (102–104).

MRI is the definitive test for diagnosis and delineation of tumor extent and type (Figs. 4.7 and 4.8). The typical diffusely infiltrating pontine glioma is homogeneous or hypodense on T1 imaging but readily appreciated on T2 sequence. The tumor expands the pons, often showing exophytic growth in the ventral, dorsal,

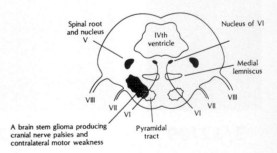

FIG. 4-9. A lower pontine glioma interferes with motor function on one side of the body and with contralateral function of the sixth and seventh cranial nerves. These two cranial nerves are most commonly affected by brainstem tumors. Ataxia can result from involvement of the fibers of the middle cerebellar peduncle.

or lateral projections (Fig. 4-8). The disease infiltrates into the other brainstem segments, sometimes as far rostrally as into the thalamus, and often extends into the cerebellopontine peduncle (brachium pontis) toward or into the cerebellum. There is often little enhancement, although inhomogeneous areas of focal enhancement or signs of intralesional hemorrhage or necrosis may be noted (94).

Biopsy of the classic, diffusely infiltrating pontine glioma is generally unnecessary (34,95, 96,105,106). Histologic series show roughly equal proportions of low-grade (fibrillary astrocytoma or WHO grade II astrocytoma) and malignant (anaplastic astrocytoma or glioblastoma multiforme) types (34,96,105,107,108). There is no consistent correlation between histology and outcome; all diffusely infiltrating pontine tumors show extremely poor duration of response to irradiation and median survival of less than 1 year (95,98,109–111). It is of interest that most such tumors show malignant astrocytoma at autopsy; even tumors showing low-grade histology at biopsy often are malignant when analyzed at autopsy less than 2 years after diagnosis (107,112). Lacking evidence that low-grade tumors warrant a less aggressive approach or demonstrate superior outcome, there is no apparent benefit derived from a biopsy procedure when the imaging and clinical picture indicate a typical diffusely infiltrating, expansile pontine glioma (34,106). Brainstem tumors have recently been shown to express *ERBB1*, with the degree of overexpression or less common amplification proportional to increasing histologic grade (113). The finding suggests that ErbB or EGFR inhibitors may be worth studying in these tumors, as is being done in the Pediatric Brain Tumor Consortium's study of ZD1839 in conjunction with irradiation.

Hoffman et al. (103) identified a less common, highly specific brainstem tumor now recognized as a dorsally exophytic "benign" brainstem tumor. This tumor type represents 15–20% of brainstem lesions (104,106,114). The lesion characteristically fills the fourth ventricle, presenting with symptoms and signs of elevated intracranial pressure. In most cases, the tumor enhances briskly with gadolinium (Fig. 4-10). The origin from the floor of the fourth ventricle (the dorsal surface of the pons or medulla, with the tumor often arising at the pontomedullary junction) may be suggested by MRI but is usually apparent only at the time of surgery. These tumors are almost always juvenile pilocytic astrocytomas (JPAs); the prognosis has been quite favorable (104,106,114).

Focal tumors of the pons are uncommon. One specific presentation includes isolated facial nerve palsy or similar, limited neurologic dysfunction associated with a small, enhancing intrapontine lesion (102). Such tumors are low grade (often JPA or WHO grade I) and enjoy a favorable prognosis (Fig. 4-7) (95,105).

Tumors of the midbrain may involve the tegmentum or the tectal plate. Tegmental tumors usually are fibrillary astrocytomas (WHO grade II). The tumors may involve the tegmentum focally or may infiltrate through much of the midbrain. Lesions may show uniform enhancement or little contrast enhancement. Presenting signs include extraocular muscle palsy or long track involvement. Biopsy is preferred, especially for lesions contiguous with the pineal region. Tectal plate tumors usually are quite small and well demarcated, confined to the tectal plate, and best visualized on MRI. Many such tumors probably accounted for the former diagnosis of "idiopathic obstructive hydrocephalus," small mass lesions obstructing the aqueduct often not demonstrable on CT scan (95,105). Ventriculoperitoneal shunt usually is needed. MRI shows the focal nature of tectal lesions, most often signified by brisk enhancement; biopsy generally confirms juvenile pilocytic histology (WHO grade I). These tumors typically are indolent; observation alone usually is the treatment of choice (95,105,115). If the tumor is anatomically confined to the tectum and stable over an initial 3- to 6-month period of observation, biopsy may be deferred unless there is evidence of tumor progression necessitating therapy (95,105). When lesions are atypical (e.g., cystic) or when there is some question whether the lesion originated in the adjacent pineal region, biopsy may be needed at diagnosis. If it is confirmed as a low-grade astrocytoma, observation is appropriate.

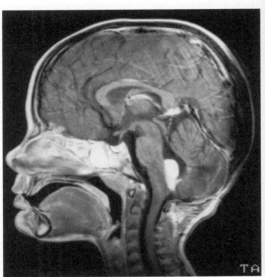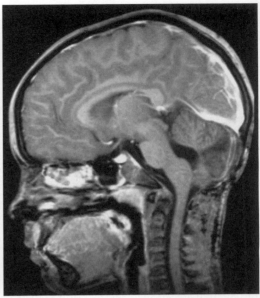

A   B

FIG. 4-10. Brainstem astrocytomas. **(A)** Dorsally exophytic brainstem juvenile pilocytic astrocytoma presents as a sizable lesion filling the fourth ventricle but is attached only along the floor at the level of the pontomedullary junction (**B**, postoperative); appearance 4 years after irradiation for documented postsurgical progression shows decreased mass effect and lack of enhancement.

Therapy

Surgery

The role of surgery in classic pontine gliomas is limited. Routine biopsy is not recommended. A small proportion of tumors that are otherwise characteristic of diffusely infiltrating gliomas present with large cysts or focal areas of hemorrhage or necrosis in the pons. When such components are peripheral in location and can be approached safely, an initial surgical procedure to "decompress" the lesion may be helpful (34,96,106,116).

For dorsally exophytic tumors, judicious incomplete resection will establish the diagnosis (by surgical observation of the origin from the brainstem and histology) and reduce the obstructing mass in the fourth ventricular region. Although there is no documented advantage to aggressive surgery, it may be advantageous to remove the bulk of the lesion posteriorly, establishing CSF flow and reducing the bulk of tumor

when it can be reasonably separated from the underlying margin of normal, functioning brainstem. Aggressive resection as a primary intervention often is associated with unnecessary morbidity. (104;114) Partial resection alone is associated with 60–70% freedom from progression at 5 to 10 years (103,104,108,114).

Small focal lesions intrinsic to the pons may be biopsied if safely approachable; one cannot insist on biopsy if the differential diagnosis is limited and the biopsy-associated morbidity is high (95,102,105).

Lesions in the tegmentum should be biopsied, although the potential morbidity of stereotactic biopsy is recognized because of the proximity of the central veins. Occasional resection has been reported for midbrain tumors (99,105). Tumors of the lower medulla or cervicomedullary region are similar to low-grade astrocytomas of the spinal cord. Biopsy and attempted gross total resection have been reported; results after surgery alone have been impressive but limited to a small number of neurosurgical centers (99,116,117). Histology usually is low-grade astrocytoma (WHO grade II). Malignant gliomas have been reported (34,116).

Radiation Therapy

Children with diffusely infiltrating pontine gliomas often respond impressively to irradiation initially. Approximately 70% show improvement in neurologic symptoms and signs over the several weeks during and after irradiation. Improvement in MRI has been reported in 30–70% of children. However, objective response is almost always followed by signs of progressive disease within 8 to 12 months (95, 97,98,100,105,110).

Clinical response has also been noted in tegmental midbrain lesions and tumors of the medulla, where radiation therapy is more likely to achieve long-term disease control (97,98, 105). For tectal plate or dorsally exophytic pontomedullary astrocytomas, irradiation is safely deferred until signs of disease progression are apparent on imaging (104,105,108,114). Once progression has been documented on serial imaging (noted in up to 25% of dorsally exophytic tumors), there has been almost uniform disease control measured out to more than 5 years after local irradiation (104,105,108,114). Intrinsic focal pontine lesions often must be irradiated at diagnosis because of the attendant neurologic signs (102,105). With the availability of precision volume techniques (i.e., 3D CRT or fractionated radiosurgery), the risk:benefit ratio may favor earlier radiation intervention in localized, low-grade brainstem lesions.

Chemotherapy

Despite many studies, there is little evidence of efficacy for chemotherapy in brainstem tumors. An earlier prospective, randomized trial of lomustine, vincristine, and prednisone showed no benefit in these tumors despite purported efficacy in supratentorial high-grade gliomas (118). For the classic pontine gliomas, preirradiation chemotherapy has shown some responsiveness. A small series testing high-dose cyclophosphamide demonstrated objec-

tive response in four children with brainstem gliomas; a POG study revealed objective response (by imaging criteria) in three of 32 patients (119). It is difficult to measure objective response in this tumor system; for example, the POG series showed few imaging measurable responders, and the majority of patients needed radiotherapeutic intervention before the planned completion of four cycles of cisplatin and cyclophosphamide (119). Cross-study analyses of the serial POG brainstem glioma trials actually suggested a detrimental effect when cis-platinum was added to high-dose hyperfractionated irradiation (70.2 Gy in 60 fractions) (120). Although anecdotal responses to oral etoposide in pontine gliomas have been documented, there have been no durable responders reported in the several phase II studies that have included children with brainstem gliomas (121).

Demonstration that large molecules can be perfused directly through the brainstem via intra-axial catheter placement raises the possibility of direct infusion of biologic agents for brainstem gliomas, a concept now being addressed in a phase I trial at the U.S. National Institutes of Health (122).

For focal, low-grade gliomas, the use of chemotherapy before irradiation is an extrapolation from diencephalic low-grade tumors, which may be rational in selected settings (121). For the majority of children, even those younger than 4 years old, symptomatic or progressive dorsally exophytic or focal pontine lesions can be treated effectively with focal radiation techniques. It is difficult to anticipate any significant advantage in delaying definitive therapy with intervening chemotherapy.

Radiotherapeutic Management

Volume

MRI and autopsy studies document contiguous extension of pontine gliomas linearly through the adjacent medulla or midbrain and axially into the brachium pontis, the cerebellopontine angle, and adjacent portions of the cerebellar hemispheres (94,123). Leptomeningeal involvement has been noted in up to 15% of children with diffusely infiltrating pontine lesions, most often involving the subarachnoid space about the brainstem, the basal cistern, or the upper cervical cord; spinal canal involvement has also been documented (95,107,124,125). A small proportion of focal, low-grade brainstem lesions (often JPAs) are associated with neuraxis dissemination, most often noted at diagnosis (102,126).

The pattern of failure for pontine gliomas generally is one of local recurrence. Local irradiation is indicated, with target volumes subtending both the pons and the adjacent regions both linearly (the adjacent midbrain and medulla) and axially (the adjacent anterior cerebellum). Diffusely infiltrating pontine gliomas often are incompletely or nonenhancing lesions; the greatest tumor extent on T1 or T2 images should define the GTV. For infiltrating tumors of the midbrain and medulla, margins of 1 to 2 cm beyond the imaging evident lesion are appropriate.

Focal lesions of the tectum can be treated with limited target volumes; treatment of discrete lesions generally entails treating only the identifiable tumor with a 1-cm or less CTV (95). Fractionated stereotactic radiosurgery (also called stereotactic radiotherapy) has been used for the latter tumor types (127); more recent experience may favor 3D CRT or IMRT in this setting.

For dorsally exophytic tumors, the volume can conform to the disease process based on MRI; the anterior margin at the brainstem should encompass at least 5 mm of apparently normal brainstem ventral to the tumor as documented on MRI. A 3D CRT or IMRT approach can spare radiation dosage to the temporal lobes, especially important in this young age group.

Dosage

A decade-long series of trials explored the impact of high-dose, hyperfractionated irradiation for brainstem gliomas. Despite dosage escalation from 66 to 70–72 to 75.6–78 Gy using twice-daily fractions of 100 to 126 cGy, no durable improvement was documented in disease control of survival based on dosage escalation with altered fractionation. Outcome after conventionally fractionated irradiation to 54 Gy or hyperfractionated irradiation to between 70 and 78 Gy has been consistently documented at median times to pro-

gression of only 8 months and 2-year survival rates of only 10% (95,97,98,100,109–111,120, 128). The use of conventionally fractionated irradiation (typically 180 cGy once daily) has been shown to be equivalent to the best of the hyperfractionated regimens (70.2 Gy in 60 fractions using 117 cGy twice daily with a 6-hour interfraction interval) in a prospective randomized trial in POG (129). A trial of accelerated fractionation in Europe, using 180 cGy twice daily with interfraction intervals of 8 hours to 48.6 and 50.4 Gy showed similar results, with 32% survival at 1 year and 11% at 2 years (130).

The experience with hyperfractionated irradiation may have been most important because it encouraged neurosurgeons, pediatric neurologists, and pediatric oncologists to focus on brain tumor trials and develop some understanding of radiation parameters (131,132). The number of long-term survivors with diffusely infiltrating pontine gliomas remains small; a late update of the POG study, including all three serially escalating dose arms studied between 1984 and 1990, shows only nine survivors of 130 enrolled (109). The standard for management of diffusely infiltrating brainstem gliomas is to use conventional fractionation (typically 180 cGy once daily) to 54 to 55.8 Gy, often in a protocol addressing radiosensitization or biologically targeted therapy. For focal or dorsally exophytic brainstem tumors, similar dosage and fractionation are incorporated in a cohort in which one anticipates a higher likelihood of longer-term survival, avoiding the potential risks of higher radiation dosages, accelerated fractionation regimens, or concurrent chemotherapeutic or molecularly targeted therapies.

Attempts to identify radiosensitization by concurrent chemotherapy (using cisplatin or etoposide), biologic response modifiers (with concurrent interferon or tamoxifen), and hypoxic cell sensitizers (testing estramustine) have been uniformly disappointing (129,133).

Technique

Diffusely infiltrating pontine gliomas typically were irradiated with parallel opposed lateral fields intended to encompass the tumor volume with a margin of 2 to 3 cm (100). Current approaches more often include 3D CRT or, less often, IMRT, approaches that enable one to spare the temporal lobes, although very few patients are long-term survivors and subject to late ill effects of therapy. Radiation delivery often is facilitated by prone positioning. The lower border of the radiation volume typically extends to C1 or C2 to allow a 2-cm axial margin beyond the GTV in defining the CTV, with an additional 5-mm expansion to identify the PTV. Because of narrower separation at the C2 level, one should assess off-axis dosimetry to avoid dosages to the upper cervical cord greater than the PTV. With high-dose regimens, it may be appropriate to block the C1–C2 volume as it approaches the intended cumulative dosage level.

For focal brainstem gliomas (including tectal plate lesions, dorsally exophytic pontomedullary tumors, and focal intrinsic lesions of the midbrain, pons, or medulla), tumor size, margination, and location demand 3D CRT or IMRT approaches to minimize dosage beyond the primary target volume while maintaining intralesional homogeneity in the CTV within 5%.

Children with diffusely infiltrating brainstem gliomas usually need corticosteroids at diagnosis to control neurologic symptoms. For those not receiving corticosteroids at the initiation of radiation therapy, one should consider initiating a low-dose regimen (e.g., dexamethasone at 2 to 4 mg twice daily) only for children with large intrinsic tumors or early development of additional or progressive neurologic signs. Children with rapidly deteriorating neurologic signs may need high-dose corticosteroids and use of mannitol to control local edema and mass effect before irradiation.

Irradiation generally is well tolerated. Acute reactions include radioepidermitis, most pronounced in the external auditory canal and the retroauricular region; such reactions may be more pronounced with hyperfractionated delivery (100,110,111).

A significant proportion of patients with brainstem tumors demonstrate clinical and imaging evidence of apparent progressive tumor within 1 to 4 months of completing radiation therapy (100,105,111,124). After high-dose hyperfractionated irradiation, 10–40% of patients may need reinstitution of corticosteroids or remain corticosteroid dependent for several months after therapy (100,110,111,124). Patients should not be considered therapeutic failures immediately; a majority of children stabilize or improve after 3 to 12 weeks. Imaging changes during this interval include focal enhancement (often in a previously nonenhancing lesion), cyst formation (or cystic cegeneration), or intralesional hemorrhage and necrosis (124,130). Differentiating such subacute phenomena from tumor progression may be extremely difficult, often apparent only with time to observe the clinical course. Positron emission tomography using fluorodeoxyglucose and magnetic resonance spectroscopy have been of some value in differentiating tumor progression from postirradiation changes in this interval (134,135). Similar changes, with apparent tumor progression and worsening of neurologic signs, can occur 1 to 4 months after irradiation for focal intrinsic JPAs (Fig. 4-7). Medical support, including corticosteroids, may be necessary until the lesion regresses over several months.

Results

Approximately 60–70% of patients with classic pontine gliomas have a stabilization or improvement of their functional status after irradiation. Time to progression may be difficult to document in this tumor system; cooperative group studies report median time to progression of 6 to 8 months. Median survival is 8 to 12 months in patients selected for high-risk pontine glioma studies, and the proportion surviving at 2 years is less than 20% (95,97,98,100, 109–111,120,129).

Children with focal, intrinsic tumors of the midbrain or medulla show long-term survival after irradiation of 50–70%. (34,94,95,97,105). Survival at 10 years after surgery with or without necessary irradiation for dorsally exophytic brainstem gliomas approaches 75% (95,103–105,114). Similar rates are quoted for the focal pontine lesions of limited size after localized irradiation (102,105).

EPENDYMOMAS

Intracranial ependymomas represent 3–6% of intracranial neoplasms in children. More than 95% of pediatric ependymomas occur as intracranial tumors; primary spinal cord ependymomas are uncommon. Two-thirds of the tumors in children present as infratentorial lesions, arising along the linings of the fourth ventricle. Tumors originate from the ventricular floor as midline neoplasms, where attachment is commonly noted at the level of the obex (the caudalmost aspect of the fourth ventricle along the posterior surface of the medulla, where the fourth ventricle ends and the central spinal canal begins). It is quite common for the tumors to grow into the foramina of Lushka (on either side of the brainstem) toward the cerebellopontine (CP) angle (136–138). Presentation in the CP angle is noted less commonly, occurring particularly in very young children (139). Tumor extension caudally along the upper cervical spine occurs classically in nearly 50% of fourth ventricular lesions, resulting from direct downward extension of the CP angle component of the tu-

mor (Fig. 4-11) (136–138). Some writers have called this the tongue of tumor. Supratentorial ependymomas account for one-third of childhood presentations, occurring predominantly as cerebral hemispheric tumors, often adjacent to the third or lateral ventricular regions. Ependymomas can arise in the suprasellar (lower third ventricular) or pineal (posterior third ventricular) regions (137,140,141).

Ependymomas consist histologically of polygonal cells with large vesicular nuclei and cytoplasmic granules. Characteristic are ependymal rosettes, formed by tumor cells oriented radially around a central lumen; cells also have a tendency to orient themselves around blood vessels, forming perivascular pseudorosettes (142–145). The origin is from the ependymal central neuroepithelial cells during embryogenesis or as malignant degeneration of mature ependymal cells in the ventricular linings or the subependymal zones of cellular proliferation. Supratentorial ependymomas may be remote from the ventricular system; such tumors theoretically arise from ependymal cell rests (8,146).

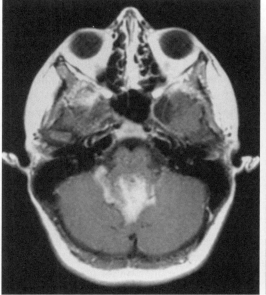
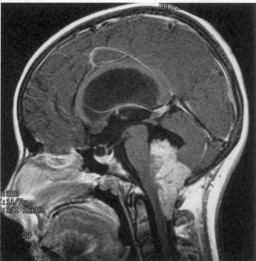

A   B

FIG. 4-11. Posterior fossa ependymoma, typically extending from the region of the fourth ventricle, through the right foramen of Luschka **(A)** and caudally beyond the cerebellopontine angle along the cervicomedullary junction to a level below the foramen magnum **(B)**. (See color plate)

There has been much debate over the clinical significance of the histologic classification or grading of ependymomas (8,136–138,143–146). The major tumor types in current histopathologic classifications include the following:

- Differentiated, or ordinary, ependymomas.
- Anaplastic ependymomas (identified by focal or diffuse areas of increased cellular density or cytologic evidence of cellular anaplasia); anaplastic characteristics are more common in supratentorial than in fourth ventricular lesions.
- Clear cell ependymomas, an uncommon cell type occurring in somewhat older children, typically in the supratentorial region; the tumor is associated with an aggressive course and a noted frequency of extracranial extension or metastasis (23).
- Myxopapillary ependymomas: well-differentiated, papillary-like tumors occurring most often as primary spinal cord lesions, typically at the level of the cauda equina.
- Ependymoblastoma: an extremely rare, highly malignant form of primitive embryonal supratentorial tumor occurring in infants with undifferentiated embryonal cells but definite, predominant features of an ependymal neoplasm. Ependymoblastomas are not considered in the classification of ependymomas and are not discussed further here. Their biology and management are considered in Chapter 3 (146).

There have been conflicting reports with respect to the correlation between tumor grade (i.e., ependymoma versus anaplastic ependymoma) and survival. Three of the most prominent neuropathologists in the 1980s specifically indicated a lack of apparent correlation between anaplasia or grade and clinical behavior (143–145). However, more recent series identify histology as one of the dominant features related to disease control after aggressive surgery and irradiation (138,146–149). Merchant et al. (148) recently reviewed the St. Jude historical experience, noting 3-year progression-free survival of 84% among the 70% of children with differentiated ependymomas and 28% for the remainder with anaplastic features. A multi-institutional review reflecting the experience at 11 major U.S. centers between 1987 and 1991 noted 5-year EFS of 54% for the 60% of children with WHO grade II tumors and 14% for the WHO grade III lesions (149). Earlier data suggesting a correlation between the presence of anaplasia and the frequency of neuraxis dissemination, particularly among fourth ventricular lesions (150), have been superseded by recent experience demonstrating a higher risk of local failure with inconsistent trends toward more frequent recurrences also involving intracranial or, uncommonly, spinal seeding (85,137,141,148, 149).

The biology of ependymomas has not been as well explored as that of medulloblastoma. Chromosomal abnormalities are present in approximately 50% of tumors, most commonly loss of the long arm of chromosome 22 or 6 or gain in chromosome 1q (151). The tumors show expression of the ErbB receptors (19).

The tumor is somewhat more common in boys, although young children show equal sex distribution or even a slight female predominance. The median age at diagnosis is 3 to 4 years; younger children have less favorable outcome, particularly in posterior fossa ependymomas (136,137,141,147,149,152).

Symptoms usually are nonspecific and related to fourth ventricular obstruction with attendant headaches, vomiting, and ataxia. Children with disease involving the CP angle, with or without tumor growing into the upper cervical spine, often show torticollis or CP angle cranial nerve signs (including unilateral hearing loss and facial weakness) (139,153). MRI often shows a nonhomogeneously enhancing lesion, diagnostic when there is characteristic involvement through the foramen of Lushka. The tumor characteristically grows toward or into the CP angle, may extend circumferentially around the brainstem (at the level of the medulla or the pontomedullary junction), and commonly grows caudally from there to extend along the upper cervical spine. Approximately 50% of children show contiguous tumor involving the upper cervical spinal canal; tumor often extends to the C2 area and has been documented to the C5 level (136,154).

Therapy

Surgery

Extent of resection is the dominant factor influencing outcome (136–138,141,147–149,153). Fourth ventricular lesions usually are adherent along the brainstem, especially at the level of the obex, where surgical damage can result in significant cardiorespiratory compromise. Total or near total resection is feasible with current neurosurgical techniques in 50–75% of cases (136,137,141,147,148,153). Aggressive resection is consistently associated with higher rates of disease control. Recent reports confirm earlier series in documenting disease control rates of 50–75% after gross total resection with no evident tumor on postoperative imaging, compared with 30–45% with incomplete removal (Table 4-5) (137,141,147–149,152–155).

Total resection is associated with a low but acknowledged rate of operative mortality (2.5% or less in the 1990s). Postoperative cranial nerve deficits are common, including components of the posterior fossa syndrome (e.g., significant difficulties with speech, swallowing, and balance) (41,136–138,153). The nature of the fourth ventricular lesions is particularly challenging, with tumors extending through the foramen of Lushka to the anterior aspect of the medulla, onto the brainstem, and intertwined with cranial nerves in the CP angle. Total resection of supratentorial ependymomas is more readily achieved.

Radiation Therapy

Radiation therapy has been a routine component of therapy for ependymomas since the 1950s (Fig. 4-3). The favorable results summarized previously after surgical resection are based on the addition of postoperative irradiation (85, 136,137,147,154,155). Two classic series earlier confirmed the contribution of radiation therapy: Pollack et al. (147) recorded overall 5-year survival of 45% with surgery and irradiation, compared with 13% with surgery alone; Rousseau et al. (154) noted similar results: 63% survival at 5 years after irradiation and 23% without irradiation. The report from Hôpital Necker–Enfants Malades, Paris, documented EFS rates of 65% after postoperative irradiation, compared with 25% with primary postoperative chemotherapy, specifically in patients younger than 5 years old (137,141). Among those with gross total resection, the difference between irradiated children (5-year EFS 75%) and those treated on an infant SIOP chemotherapy-alone protocol (EFS 21%) was highly significant (137). The impact of irradiation on disease control in young children has also been suggested in the first POG infant brain tumor study: children 2 to 3 years old received irradiation after 1 year of chemotherapy, and those younger than 2 years old were scheduled to receive irradiation after 2 years of chemotherapy. Long-term disease control has been significantly higher in the older cohort, interpreted as likely to be related to earlier irradiation (156).

The current impetus to study surgery alone comes from the young age at presentation (half the children present before age 4 years) and limited data from New York (New York University and Beth Israel) suggesting the apparent ability of surgery alone to achieve disease control after confirmed gross total resection of supratentorial tumors in young children (157). The latter group showed complete resection in 14 of 15 supratentorial lesions; six of eight followed without irradiation were free of disease at a median time exceeding 4 years (157). The same group achieved gross removal in ten of 17 fourth ventricular ependymomas; only two were followed without irradiation, one of whom recurred locally (157).

The excellent results with complete resection and postoperative irradiation continue to support early, systematic use of radiation therapy, especially for posterior fossa lesions.

Chemotherapy

Ependymomas are chemosensitive tumors, with objective responses demonstrated after cisplatin or carboplatin and alkylating agents in phase II trials (50,51,137,156). The only prospective, randomized trial tested adjuvant chemotherapy (lomustine, vincristine, prednisone) after surgery and irradiation. The trial was small, but there was no suggestion of improved disease control with chemotherapy (158).

TABLE 4-5. *Ependymoma—outcome following surgery and irradiation*

Series	Interval	n	Site	Surgery	RT	EFS @ 5 yrs	OS @ 5 yrs
Institut Gustave Roussy, Paris [154]	1975–1989, < 16 y.o.	65 65	all all	48% GTR	local (n = 28) with Crl or CSI (n = 37) 0	45%⟩p < .001 0	63%⟩⟩p < .003 23%
Children's Hospital, Pittsburgh [147]	1975–1993	10 27	all all	62% GTR	local (n = 11) with CSI (n = 16) 0	59%⟩p = .03 13%	67%⟩n.s. 38%
Hopital Necker-Enfants Malades, Paris [137]	1980–1998, < 15 y.o.	44 25	all all	73% GTR 84% GTR	local (n = 25) with CSI or SPI (n = 19) 0 (received BBSFOP[a] chemotherapy)	64%⟩⟩p < .002 26%	80%⟩⟩p < .04 69%
St. Jude RT-1 [162]	1997–2003, 1–22 y.o.	88	all	84% GTR	T Bed (CTV = GTV+1 cm, 54–59.4 Gy)	81% (3 yrs)	

GTR, gross total resection
[a]BBSFOP, carboplatin-procarbazine; etoposide-cisplatin; vincristine-cyclophosphamide.

The infant studies may be interpreted positively in documenting that approximately 20–25% of children with ependymomas can be controlled with surgery and chemotherapy, absent radiation therapy (141,156). The multidrug regimens have included the traditional four-drug combination (CDDP, etoposide, vincristine, and cyclophosphamide) or the BBSFOP regimen used by the French Society of Pediatric Oncology (SFOP), which also includes carboplatin and procarbazine. Part of the rationale for continuing primary chemotherapy in this age group is the potential ability for postchemotherapy (including postprogression) surgery and irradiation to achieve ultimate disease control: the overall 5-year survival in the SFOP series was 59% despite the 22% rate of progression-free survival (141). Still unclear is the longer-term ability to achieve durable disease control after postchemotherapy progression compared with more definitive postoperative irradiation in infants or older children (141,149,159).

Radiotherapeutic Management

Volume

The selection of treatment volume for ependymomas has been an issue of ongoing controversy, from before 1990, when debate focused on use of craniospinal irradiation for a significant subset of childhood ependymomas, to the current era, in which treatment is evolving from full posterior fossa therapy to local tumor bed volumes and consideration of high-dose volumes restricted to residual tumor sites (136,137, 142,148,150,154,160,161). Posterior fossa ependymomas tend to adhere to the floor of the fourth ventricle and to cranial nerves and vessels rather than invading the normal brain, suggesting that more limited margins may be appropriate for this tumor. Recurrence patterns for fourth ventricular tumors identify sites of attachment, typically areas of potential residual tumor after aggressive resection, as the most common area of disease recurrence (i.e., areas of initial involvement, often contiguous to the brainstem or at the CP angle) (85,136,142,148, 152,154,159). Data since the mid-1980s have highlighted the use of local radiation volumes

rather than full cranial or CSI previously used (136,150,154). More recent experience highlights comparable or superior results after maximal surgery with irradiation limited to the tumor bed (142,148,162). The experience at St. Jude, with 80% disease-free survival at 4 years in a series of 80 children with ependymomas, reflects narrow target volumes (defined as a 1 cm CTV beyond the tumor bed and any residual defined as the GTV) often diminished to spare the cervical spinal cord beyond 54 Gy (148,162).

Ependymomas have the ability to seed the craniospinal axis via the CSF. The incidence of neuraxis dissemination varies in the literature; several review articles summarize the frequency at approximately 12% (137,163–165). Bloom et al. (150) initially reported a high frequency of seeding among high-grade posterior fossa ependymomas, recommending CSI for such presentations (165). Late follow-up of Bloom's Royal Marsden experience reported neuraxis dissemination in only two of 33 children with local posterior fossa tumor control, also noting no difference between children who had received CSI and those treated with only local volumes (165). More recent experience indicates a higher rate of disease recurrence with anaplastic histology but defines an infrequent pattern of neuraxis dissemination (136,137,148,154,166). Superior outcome was recently reported in the Hôpital Necker–Enfants Malades after CSI: 74% 5-year EFS compared with 54% with local volumes (137). The broad body of recent experience and reviews supports use of more limited radiation volumes (136,142,148,154,160,166).

Local irradiation traditionally has implied incorporation of the full posterior fossa, the primary target including the anatomic limits of the posterior fossa extending inferiorly to the C2 level (or lower to allow 2 to 3 cm below disease when there is extension below the foramen magnum). Reduction of the target volume to cover only the initial tumor bed rather than the entire posterior fossa appears to be adequate and is the basis for the current prospective trial of 3D CRT in patients 1 to 21 years old in the COG protocol. Use of a limited-volume boost to encompass areas of attachment or residual has been explored, both as a smaller volume to a higher fractionated dosage (59.4 Gy focally) or as a stereotactic radiosurgical boost as a single fraction of 8 to 12 Gy (148,161).

152,154,163,166). Recent experience has focused on dosage levels of 54 Gy as a standard, with investigational trials incorporating limited-volume irradiation to 59.4 Gy (138,148).

Dosage

Dose–response data for ependymoma are incomplete. Most series confirm improved disease control with dosage levels above 45 Gy (142,

Technique

The standard of practice now entails use of 3D CRT or IMRT to target the tumor bed (rather

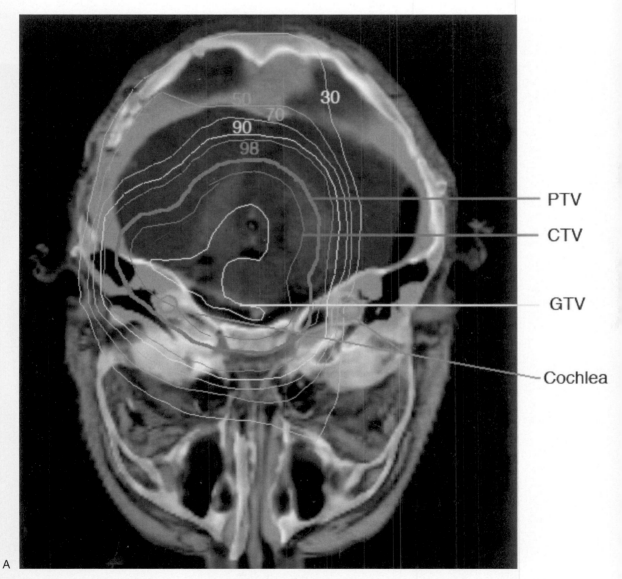

A

FIG. 4-12. Three-dimensional conformal radiation therapy for the fourth ventricular ependymoma following resection. The tumor bed (GTV) is here expanded by 1 cm to provide the clinical tumor volume (CTV); a 0.5 cm geometric expansion shows the planning tumor volume (PTV). Dose distributions depicted from 11-field 6 McV non-coplanar plan. Axial **(A)** and sagittal **(B)** dose distributions shown. *Continued.* (See color plate)

than the entire posterior fossa), with a CTV defined as 1 to 1.5 cm and a PTV expanded by an additional 5 to 7 mm, depending on the immobilization techniques and experience of the treating institution (Fig. 4-12). Dosage distributions should show good conformality to the target volume, with dosages limited to the temporal lobes and hypothalamic–pituitary regions (for fourth ventricular lesions) and the surrounding cerebrum plus the chiasmatic region (for supratentorial lesions). Immobilization in the prone position is most effective for fourth ventricular

tumors; most often, supratentorial tumors are treated in the supine position.

Significant acute treatment-related toxicities are largely limited to cutaneous reactions. For most children treated after complete or near total resection, it is unnecessary to use corticosteroids during irradiation.

Results

Overall results in various series indicate 5-year survival rates of 45–65% for children older than 2

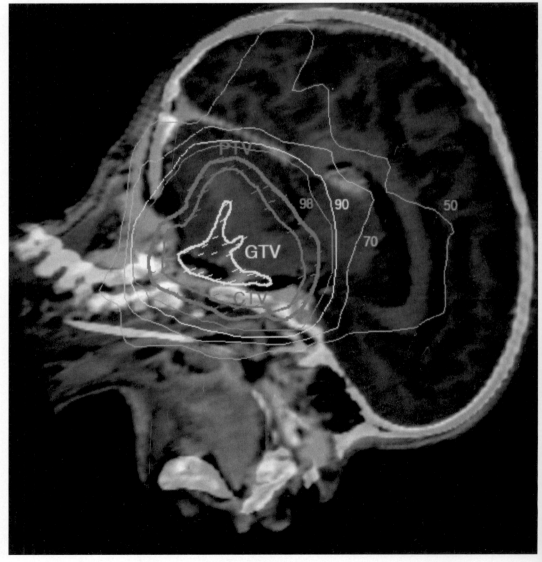

B

FIG. 4-12. *Continued.*

years old (Table 4-5). Progression-free survival rates approach 50% (136,137,147,149,152,154, 163,165). For children with gross total resection followed by irradiation, disease-free survival at 5 years ranges from 60% to more than 80% in the most recent series (137,148,162). After incomplete resection and irradiation, or with anaplastic histology, progression-free survival rates have averaged only 20–40% at 5 years (85,137,147, 149,152,154,163,165).

CEREBELLAR ASTROCYTOMAS

Cerebellar astrocytomas make up 10–15% of childhood brain tumors and 25% of posterior fossa neoplasms. The tumors typically are well-circumscribed, slowly growing lesions with prominent cyst formation (167,168). The classic cystic cerebellar astrocytoma presents as a unilocular cyst with a prominent mural nodule (Fig. 4-11). Cushing (169) was the first to describe the entity in 1931, commenting on the "benign" nature of cerebellar astrocytomas, associated with low morbidity and mortality. Initially, Cushing failed to recognize that the mural nodule represented the active neoplastic portion of cystic cerebellar astrocytomas. Without removal of the nodule, the cyst was likely to recur. Once the neoplastic nature of the nodule was recognized and the nodule was removed at surgery, results improved dramatically (170).

Cerebellar astrocytomas are divided histologically into JPAs (noted in up to 80–95% of cases) and nonpilocytic or diffuse low-grade astrocytomas (5–15%) (146,171–173). The classic JPA consists of bipolar (piloid) astrocytes intermixed with Rosenthal fibers and areas of microcystic, loose-textured astrocytes (146). The other low-grade astrocytomas, sometimes called diffuse astrocytomas in this location, are identified as fibrillary astrocytomas or astrocytomas not otherwise specified; uncommonly, such tumors are oligoastrocytomas (146,170,171,174). Malignant gliomas are quite uncommon in the childhood cerebellum. A recent review found only 26 documented malignant gliomas (14 glioblastoma multiforme, 12 anaplastic astrocytomas) in children (175). The tumors do not appear to have unique imaging or gross characteristics but are associated with aggressive behavior based on time to recurrence, almost uniformly fatal outcome, and potential neuraxis dissemination (175,176). Although some of the standard neuropathology texts have debated whether true malignant astrocytomas arise in the cerebellum in this age group, there does appear to be documentation for up to 5% of cerebellar astrocytomas occurring as malignant histiotypes (175,176).

The median age at diagnosis is 5 to 6 years. Although 20% occur in young children (younger than 3 years old), it is rarely found in infants in the first year of life (167,172,177). Presenting symptoms often are confined to those associated with elevated intracranial pressure (headaches, vomiting, less often diplopia), with less frequent altered cerebellar function (primarily ataxia, less often poor coordination or dyspraxic speech); cranial nerve deficits are uncommon.

The majority of tumors arise in the cerebellar hemispheres; approximately one-third are primary vermis lesions. More than two-thirds of the lesions are confined to the cerebellum; one-third extend to the cerebellopontine peduncle or the posterior aspect of the brainstem, sometimes called transitional cerebellar lesions (167,168, 172,177,178). The most characteristic appearance on CT or MRI is a large, well-circumscribed tumor with prominent cysts (unilocular or multilocular). The nodular or solid portion of the tumor characteristically enhances briskly. The cyst wall may or may not demonstrate contrast enhancement. The classic interpretation that a nonenhancing cyst wall is not truly a component of the neoplasm has been questioned in the more recent literature, and contemporary approaches usually involve resection or biopsy of the cyst wall to determine its potential neoplastic character (172,176,177). Cerebellar JPAs have uncommonly been associated with multifocal CNS involvement, representing either neuraxis dissemination or multifocal tumorigenesis (179,180).

Therapy

Surgery

Surgical resection is the treatment of choice for cerebellar astrocytomas. Long-term disease control, even in the presence of known postoperative residual, has been well documented since Cushing's operative series (169). For classic cystic cerebellar astrocytomas, gross total resection has been reported in 70–90% of cases (170–172,181). The clinical behavior of these tumors remains indolent, often with long-term disease stabilization despite documented tumor residual. After surgery- and imaging-confirmed gross total resection, recurrence is uncommon, noted at 5–10% in major series (170,172,174,177,178,181,182). After incomplete resection, disease progression (or recurrence) has been reported in 30–60% of cases at 5 years or more. Importantly, long-term survival remains above 65% (168,170, 172,181). Tumors that extend into the peduncle or onto the brainstem are less likely to be totally resected and are associated with a higher rate of disease progression and recurrence (172,175). Despite the "indolent" nature of these tumors, the median time to recurrence is about 2 years (168,170,172,178).

Radiation Therapy

There is no established role for radiation therapy in the primary management of cerebellar astrocytomas. The primary issue revolves around prognostic factors that may predict recurrence after surgery alone. Most series indicate greater risk of recurrence in solid (rather than cystic) tumors, in tumors that extend into the peduncle or onto the brainstem, and in nonpilocytic or "diffuse" histologic types (167,168,171,172,177,181).

Indications for radiation therapy have included incompletely resected tumors or those with diffuse or unfavorable histologies. (172; 174) There are no data substantiating improvement in disease control with postoperative irradiation (177,181,183). Infrequent malignant gliomas seem to benefit from immediate postoperative irradiation (175).

Chemotherapy

There are no substantial data addressing the impact of chemotherapy in cerebellar astrocytomas to date.

Radiotherapeutic Management

Indications for radiation therapy are generally limited to documented progressive or recurrent disease that has undergone a second incomplete resection or is felt to be unresectable at the time of progression or recurrence (172,183). Some centers withhold irradiation even after multiple recurrences when further surgery seems to be an option (178). Judicious use of local radiation therapy seems appropriate for patients who have shown a second or subsequent recurrence, particularly when the lesion has extended into or onto the peduncle or brainstem. Such lesions are targeted with minimal expansion of the CTV to 1 cm or less beyond the tumor bed and residual lesion, at 50 to 54 Gy (85).

The treatment of high-grade cerebellar astrocytomas is controversial. Postoperative irradiation to the local tumor is recognized as the standard of care (172,183). CSF dissemination was a pattern of failure in two of the four cases recently reviewed from Toronto, raising the unanswered question of CSI for this uncommon tumor presentation in children (172). Current recognized indications for CSI are generally limited to children with documented subarachnoid metastasis or multifocal disease, regardless of histology (179,180,183).

Results

Overall survival rates in childhood cerebellar astrocytomas are more than 80% at 10 to 20 years (167,168,172,177). Survival rates are highest among those with tumor confined to the cerebellar hemispheres or vermis, JPA histology, and gross total resection. For incompletely resected diffuse astrocytomas, long-term survival rates of 50–80% have been reported (167,170–172,178).

SPINAL CORD NEOPLASMS

Spinal cord neoplasms are uncommon in children. Tumors involving the spinal canal are classified as intradural when confined to the spinal canal (called intramedullary) or arising from the cauda equina or intradural components of the nerve

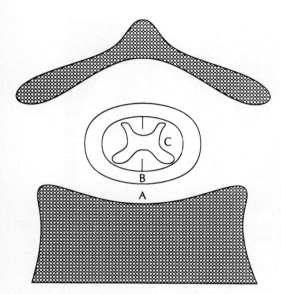

FIG. 4-13. Classification of spinal tumors. **(A)** Extramedullary, extradural. **(B)** Extramedullary, intradural. **(C)** Intramedullary, intradural.

roots (extramedullary). Extradural tumors are extraneural neoplasms that arise outside the nervous system (Fig. 4-13). The extradural lesions extend into the canal by direct growth (from osseous tumors of the vertebrae or adjacent soft tissue lesions) or by insinuation through the spinal foramina. Tumors that grow through a spinal foramen (or adjacent foramina) extend linearly beyond the cord segment of entry, accounting for the "dumbbell" description; such presentations are most common in neuroblastomas, paravertebral soft tissue tumors of the Ewing type (i.e., peripheral PNET), or neurofibromas (184). Management of extradural presentations is discussed in chapters related to the primary tumor type. Nervous system tumors arising in the spinal cord and cauda equina are discussed in this section.

Primary spinal cord neoplasms account for 5% of CNS neoplasms in children. It is difficult to extrapolate adult data regarding spinal cord tumors to children; spinal cord tumors represent a greater proportion of CNS neoplasms in adults, and the relative histologic and anatomic frequencies are almost mirror image presentations of those in children (185–188). Astrocytomas account for 60% of primary spinal cord tumors in children. Ependymomas account for 30%; other

gliomas (gangliogliomas, oligodendrogliomas) and neurilemomas (neurofibromas usually associated with neurofibromatosis type I) make up the remaining 10% (185,186,189–191).

More than 80% of pediatric spinal cord astrocytomas are low-grade neoplasms, most often fibrillary and less commonly pilocytic in type. Astrocytomas occur primarily in the cervical and thoracic regions of the cord, presenting as circumscribed or more infiltrating lesions (Fig. 4-14). The tumors diffusely widen the involved cord; tumor length averages six spinal cord segments (186). More than 30% are associated with sizable intraspinal cysts (185,189,191). The cysts typically extend in cephalad and caudal directions from the solid tumor, representing fluid-filled components that may more than double the overall length of the lesion. The cyst wall usually is not a part of the tumor process (185,189,192). Malignant gliomas (high-grade astrocytomas: anaplastic astrocytoma and glioblastoma multiforme) account for fewer than 20% of astrocytic lesions of the cord. The spinal malignant gliomas are clinically aggressive lesions. The literature suggests that such tumors are more common in infants (185,188,189,191).

Holocord astrocytomas extend over much of the length of the cervicothoracic cord. The majority of these tumors appear to represent lengthy cystic extensions of more localized neoplasms; the solid tumor components may involve a significant length of the spinal cord (187,192,193).

The less common glial tumors include oligodendrogliomas and gangliogliomas. These tumors usually are discrete, well-circumscribed intraspinal lesions that occur in the cervical, thoracic, or cervicomedullary junction regions. Presenting characteristics are similar to those of the astrocytomas (187,194,195).

Spinal cord ependymomas represent no more than 5% of all ependymomas in children (185,196). The majority arise in the low thoracic–lumbar region, involving the conus medullaris or the cauda equina. Ependymomas tend to be discrete, focal tumors when presenting as intramedullary lesions of the cervical or thoracic cord (190,197). Most such ependymal lesions are histologically differentiated ependy-

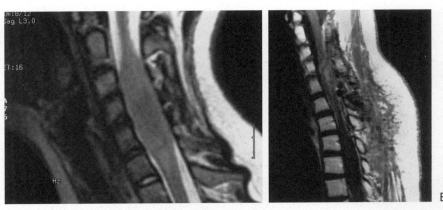

FIG. 4-14. Intramedullary spinal cord astrocytoma. **(A)** Lesion involving the cervicothoracic cord. **(B)** The child is free of disease after subtotal resection and irradiation.

momas. The more common pediatric tumor is the myxopapillary ependymoma (187,196). The latter tumors are low-grade, indolent lesions signified histologically by papillary growth and mucin formation (198). Two-thirds occur in the cauda equina, presumably arising from the filum; 30% present as tumors of the conus medullaris and 5% as atypical myxopapillary tumors of the cervical or thoracic cord (198).

Spinal cord tumors usually present with slowly progressive symptoms. The average duration of symptoms in children was 2 years in a review from the Mayo Clinic (185). The most common symptoms include long tract signs, most apparent as subtle, gradually progressive changes in gait. Spinal pain is common, usually limited to the thoracic or cervical region of origin. Pain is classically greater at night, when the child is recumbent (193,194). It is not rare to see lower thoracic cord pain evaluated as an intra-abdominal symptom, including by laparotomy for suspected appendicitis. Numbness or sphincter dysfunction occurs in 10% of cases (185, 187,192). Symptoms and signs of elevated intracranial pressure may be noted at diagnosis of a primary, localized spinal cord tumor (199).

MRI provides ideal evaluation of spinal cord neoplasms. One can usually distinguish intramedullary from extramedullary lesions. Tumor extent is generally well appreciated on MRI (Fig. 4-15). It is sometimes difficult to discern subtle cystic changes from solid tumor exten-

sion; intraoperative ultrasound can be a more sensitive tool in this regard. Low-grade astrocytomas and gangliogliomas usually are nonenhancing tumors, best delineated on T2 or proton spin density sequences. Pilocytic astrocytomas enhance uniformly. Ependymomas typically are enhancing lesions. In evaluating spinal cord tumors, it is important to image the entire length of the spinal canal; one can see "skip" intramedullary involvement uncommonly in astrocytomas. In ependymomas, it is standard to image the entire neuraxis. Rarely, intracranial ependymomas can masquerade as a primary intraspinal or cauda equina tumor, with an occult intracranial primary and symptoms caused by spinal metastasis. Subarachnoid dissemination can occur in malignant gliomas and ependymomas; staging is appropriate before postoperative management is considered (189,197).

Therapy

Surgery

The primary management for most intradural spinal tumors is surgery. Current technology and experience with intramedullary lesions have greatly facilitated the radical or gross total resection of a large percentage of pediatric intraspinal neoplasms. The use of midline myelotomy and ultrasonic dissection has allowed discrete dissection of intraspinal gliomas. Pediatric neurosurgeons

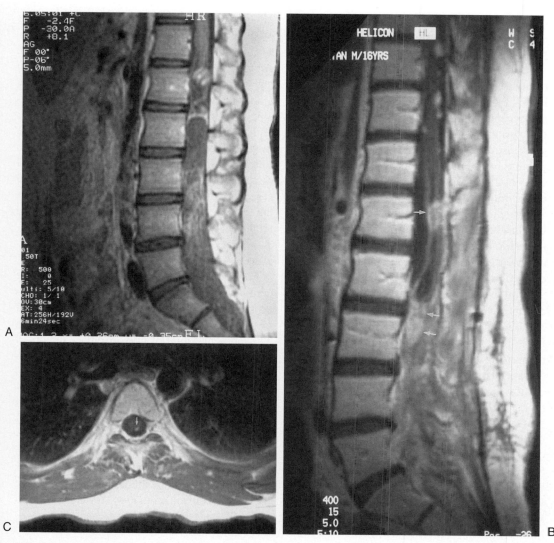

FIG. 4-15. Myxopapillary ependymoma of the cauda equina, documenting extensive disease that involves the cauda and nerve roots **(A)**; postoperative imaging shows residual and subarachnoid deposits **(B)** and **(C)**. Disease controlled at 5 years following surgery and CSI.

relate less long-term morbidity after judicious complete resection, often technically approached from just outside the tumor margin, than after biopsy with attendant intralesional swelling or potential hemorrhage (187,188,190,192,195,196, 200). Spinal evoked potentials guide the surgical procedure, allowing intraoperative monitoring for preservation of long track function (192,195). Postoperative morbidity, defined as increased neurologic deficit, is reported to be limited and often transient for tumors above the T9 level; intraspinal astrocytomas at the T9–T12 level

are reported to have the most significant operative-related morbidity (187,188,190,192).

Summary data from ten earlier series combining pediatric and adult experience indicated total excision in 16% of low-grade spinal gliomas (primarily astrocytoma) (189,192,193,200) and serially presented experience with radical resection of spinal cord astrocytomas, relating excellent functional outcome and nearly uniform disease control among children with low-grade astrocytomas managed by aggressive resection. For low-grade histologies, the New York experience indicates progression-free survival after surgery alone exceeding 90% at more than 5 years in spinal cord and cervicomedullary junction tumors, data that have been confirmed in smaller series (117,185,191,192,196). The high rates of disease control after radical resection and acceptable morbidity for spinal surgery suggest primary surgical management for low-grade astrocytomas. Outcome among malignant gliomas has been systematically poor, with only anecdotal survival beyond 3 years for anaplastic astrocytomas or glioblastomas (185,189–191).

For spinal ependymomas, gross total resection has been documented in 25–100% of cases in series often combining pediatric and adult experience (187,190,197,198,201). The more common myxopapillary ependymomas in children often are amenable to gross total resection, especially when they involve the cauda equina. Although detailed dissection often is necessary for lesions that adhere to numerous nerve roots comprising the cauda, data from the Royal Marsden Hospital (1950–1987) indicate total resection in 42% of 24 cases of cauda equina tumors, with 92% progression-free survival at 5 years (197). For lesions of the conus medullaris, the latter series indicated resection in only two of 14 cases (197). By contrast, McCormick et al. (201) indicated resection in all 23 children and adults with intramedullary tumors, only one of whom experienced recurrence. Surgery alone has been associated with survival rates at 5 years of 86–100% (117,187,195–197).

gliomas (especially pilocytic histologies and for prepubertal children in whom the risk:benefit ratio may favor delaying radiation intervention). Although long-term freedom from progression has been documented after incomplete surgery alone, postoperative radiation therapy is generally indicated for sizable residual tumors that are unlikely to be amenable to later, more complete resection (185,188,196,202,204). If one elects to follow a child with suspected or definite residual disease, it is important to commit to later second surgery (when feasible) and irradiation (unless the second surgery results in imaging-confirmed total resection) with evidence of progressive disease (based on imaging or on changes in symptoms or neurologic signs).

For spinal cord ependymomas, there is more certain evidence supporting surgery alone for intramedullary tumors and for initial management of cauda equina tumors (187,190,195,201,203). The indolent nature of myxopapillary tumors of the cauda equina favors observations in the settings of total resection or minimal residual disease (189,196,197,204). Recurrence after complete resection of intramedullary tumors is less than 10% in large series (189,190,197). Although the impact of histologic grade in ependymomas is apparent in adult series, anaplastic lesions of the spine are uncommon in children; extrapolation from the adult data suggests a role for postoperative irradiation for such lesions (190,197,202).

Radiation Therapy

The use of postoperative irradiation for spinal cord tumors has been controversial and largely inconsistent. With improved neurosurgical methods, there appears to be no clear benefit from systematic postoperative radiation therapy in spinal gliomas or ependymomas in this age group (187–189,196).

The literature readily documents 50–60% survival rates at 5 years after surgery and irradiation for largely incompletely resected spinal astrocytomas (185,189,196,202,203). Lacking comparative data, a rational approach includes maximal surgical resection. For incompletely resected tumors, one can support observation for low-grade

Radiotherapeutic Management

Volume

Neuraxis staging is an important component of preirradiation assessment for extensive intramedullary tumors and for myxopapillary ependymomas. Local irradiation is used for most spinal cord tumors. Localized intramedullary astrocytomas and ependymomas are generally treated to the tumor bed, based on preoperative and postoperative MRI; a margin of 2 to 3 cm cord length is indicated for low-grade, focal lesions. For astrocytomas, one typically sees decompression or obliteration of the rostral and caudal cystic components after resection of the solid tumor. In such instances, it appears that radiation therapy can be limited to the bed of the solid component (189,191,192,196,197,200). For spinal ependymomas, local volumes are also indicated (189, 196,197). For cauda equina tumors, there is some debate regarding the use of local or craniospinal volumes; most recent series suggest local irradiation that includes a 5-cm margin above imaging documentation of the initial tumor volume and caudal coverage to include the proximal sacral nerve roots to the bottom of the thecal sac (with a lateral margin to encompass the sacral dorsal roots) (196–198).

Dosage

The local radiation dosage for spinal cord gliomas has been fairly consistently reported as 50 Gy. The dosage is based at least as much on estimated cord tolerance as on documentation of tumoricidal dosages. Single-institution and collected series indicate no apparent dose–response relationship beyond 50 Gy (at 200 cGy per fraction) or 50 to 54 Gy (at 180 cGy per fraction) for astrocytomas (189,203). For ependymomas, similar analyses indicate a response at the 45- to 50-Gy level, with most authors favoring a dosage of 50 Gy (typically at 180 cGy per fraction) (189,203,204). With current localization techniques, the use of 54 Gy at 180 cGy per fraction is considered acceptable to volumes of gross residual disease, typically defined as the GTV with a 1-cm CTV expansion linearly along the cord for focal or discrete lesions (196).

Technique

Current techniques for spinal cord tumors use image-guided definition of the target volume, with 3D CRT or IMRT approaches to avoid excessive irradiation of the underlying viscera, especially the kidneys, lung, or heart. Electrons have also been used. Among the planning parameters should be reasonably homogeneous irradiation of the vertebral bodies.

Results

Overall survival in spinal cord astrocytomas is estimated at 80% at 5 years and 55% at 10 years (185,187–191,195). Prognosis is af-

fected by histologic grade and the extent of surgical resection. For ependymomas, overall survival is comparable, with recent figures indicating 70% 5-year survival and more than 60% 10-year survival. Outcome depends on the site of origin (with long-term survival rates greater than 90% for cauda equina tumors and 60% for intramedullary tumors or those arising in the conus medullaris) (187,188,190, 197,204). Patients with radical or complete resection appear to enjoy a favorable outcome (188–190,197).

REFERENCES

References particularly recommended for further reading are indicated by an asterisk.

1. Gurney JG, Davis S, Severson RK, et al. Trends in cancer incidence among children in the U.S. *Cancer* 1996;78(3):532–541.
2. Barnholtz-Sloan JS, Sloan AE, Schwartz AG. Relative survival rates and patterns of diagnosis analyzed by time period for individuals with primary malignant brain tumor, 1973–1997. *J Neurosurg* 2003; 99(3):458–466.
3. Eberhart CG, Kepner JL, Goldthwaite PT, et al. Histopathologic grading of medulloblastomas: a Pediatric Oncology Group study. *Cancer* 2002;94(2): 552–560.
4. McNeil DE, Cote TR, Clegg L, et al. Incidence and trends in pediatric malignancies medulloblastoma/ primitive neuroectodermal tumor: a SEER update. *Med Pediatr Oncol* 2002;39(3):190–194.
5. Cushing H. Experiences with the cerebellar medulloblastomas: a critical review. *Acta Pathol Microbiol Scand* 1930;1:1–86.
6. Bailey J, Cushing H. Medulloblastoma cerebelli, common type of mid-cerebellar glioma of childhood. *Arch Neurol Psychiatry* 1925;14:192–224.
*7. Kleihues P, Burger PC, Scheithauer BW. The new WHO classification of brain tumours. *Brain Pathol* 1993;3(3):255–268
8. Kleihues P, Cavenee WK. *Pathology & genetics of tumours of the nervous system.* Lyon, France: IARC Press, 2000.
9. Rorke LB. The cerebellar medulloblastoma and its relationship to primitive neuroectodermal tumors. *J Neuropathol Exp Neurol* 1983;42(1):1–15.
*10. Hart MN, Earle KM. Primitive neuroectodermal tumors of the brain in children. *Cancer* 1973;32(4): 890–897.
11. Pomeroy SL, Tamayo P, Gaasenbeek M, et al. Prediction of central nervous system embryonal tumour outcome based on gene expression. *Nature* 2002; 415(6870):436–442.
12. Burger PC, Grahmann FC, Bliestle A, et al. Differentiation in the medulloblastoma. A histological and immunohistochemical study. *Acta Neuropathol (Berl)* 1987;73(2):115–123.
13. Louis DN, Pomeroy SL, Cairncross JG. Focus on

central nervous system neoplasia. *Cancer Cell* 2002; 1(2):125–128.

14. Taylor MD, Liu L, Raffel C, et al. Mutations in SUFU predispose to medulloblastoma. *Nat Genet* 2002;31(3):306–310.

15. Wechsler-Reya R, Scott MP. The developmental biology of brain tumors. *Annu Rev Neurosci* 2001;24: 385–428.

16. Brown HG, Kepner JL, Perlman EJ, et al. "Large cell/anaplastic" medulloblastomas: a Pediatric Oncology Group Study. *J Neuropathol Exp Neurol* 2000;59(10):857–865.

17. Eberhart CG, Cohen KJ, Tihan T, et al. Medulloblastomas with systemic metastases: evaluation of tumor histopathology and clinical behavior in 23 patients. *J Pediatr Hematol Oncol* 2003;25(3):198–203.

18. Bigner SH, Mark J, Friedman HS, et al. Structural chromosomal abnormalities in human medulloblastoma. *Cancer Genet Cytogenet* 1988;30(1):91–101.

19. Gilbertson R. Paediatric embryonic brain tumours. Biological and clinical relevance of molecular genetic abnormalities. *Eur J Cancer* 2002;38(5):675–685.

20. Gilbertson R, Wickramasinghe C, Hernan R, et al. Clinical and molecular stratification of disease risk in medulloblastoma. *Br J Cancer* 2001;85(5):705–712.

*21. Kortmann RD, Kuhl J, Timmermann B, et al. Postoperative neoadjuvant chemotherapy before radiotherapy as compared to immediate radiotherapy followed by maintenance chemotherapy in the treatment of medulloblastoma in childhood: results of the German prospective randomized trial HIT '91. *Int J Radiat Oncol Biol Phys* 2000;46(2):269–279.

22. Kuhl J, Muller HL, Berthold F, et al. Preradiation chemotherapy of children and young adults with malignant brain tumors: results of the German pilot trial HIT '88/'89. *Klin Padiatr* 1998;210(4):227–233.

23. Fouladi M, Gajjar A, Boyett JM, et al. Comparison of CSF cytology and spinal magnetic resonance imaging in the detection of leptomeningeal disease in pediatric medulloblastoma or primitive neuroectodermal tumor. *J Clin Oncol* 1999;17(10):3234–3237.

24. Helton KJ, Gajjar A, Hill DA, et al. Medulloblastoma metastatic to the suprasellar region at diagnosis: a report of six cases with clinicopathologic correlation. *Pediatr Neurosurg* 2002;37(3):111–117.

25. Chang CH, Housepian EM, Herbert C Jr. An operative staging system and a megavoltage radiotherapeutic technic for cerebellar medulloblastomas. *Radiology* 1969;93(6):1351–1359.

*26. Zeltzer PM, Boyett JM, Finlay JL, et al. Metastasis stage, adjuvant treatment, and residual tumor are prognostic factors for medulloblastoma in children: conclusions from the Children's Cancer Group 921 randomized phase III study. *J Clin Oncol* 1999; 17(3):832–845.

27. David KM, Casey AT, Hayward RD, et al. Medulloblastoma: is the 5-year survival rate improving? A review of 80 cases from a single institution. *J Neurosurg* 1997;86(1):13–21.

28. Albright AL, Wisoff JH, Zeltzer PM, et al. Effects of medulloblastoma resections on outcome in children: a report from the Children's Cancer Group. *Neurosurgery* 1996;38(2):265–271.

29. Evans AE, Jenkin RD, Sposto R, et al. The treatment of medulloblastoma. Results of a prospective randomized trial of radiation therapy with and without CCNU, vincristine, and prednisone. *J Neurosurg* 1990;72(4):572–582.

30. Packer RJ, Sutton LN, Elterman R, et al. Outcome for children with medulloblastoma treated with radiation and cisplatin, CCNU, and vincristine chemotherapy. *J Neurosurg* 1994;81(5):690–698.

*31. Thomas PR, Deutsch M, Kepner JL, et al. Low-stage medulloblastoma: final analysis of trial comparing standard-dose with reduced-dose neuraxis irradiation. *J Clin Oncol* 2000;18(16):3004–3011.

*32. Bailey CC, Gnekow A, Wellek S, et al. Prospective randomised trial of chemotherapy given before radiotherapy in childhood medulloblastoma. International Society of Paediatric Oncology (SIOP) and the (German) Society of Paediatric Oncology (GPO): SIOP II. *Med Pediatr Oncol* 1995;25(3):166–178.

33. Packer RJ, Rood BR, MacDonald TJ. Medulloblastoma: present concepts of stratification into risk groups. *Pediatr Neurosurg* 2003;39(2):60–67.

34. Albright AL, Guthkelch AN, Packer RJ, et al. Prognostic factors in pediatric brain-stem gliomas. *J Neurosurg* 1986;65(6):751–755.

35. Gentet JC, Bouffet E, Doz F, et al. Preirradiation chemotherapy including "eight drugs in 1 day" regimen and high-dose methotrexate in childhood medulloblastoma: results of the M7 French Cooperative Study. *J Neurosurg* 1995;82(4):608–614.

36. Jenkin D, Goddard K, Armstrong D, et al. Posterior fossa medulloblastoma in childhood: treatment results and a proposal for a new staging system. *Int J Radiat Oncol Biol Phys* 1990;19(2):265–274.

37. Jenkin D, Greenberg M, Hoffman H, et al. Brain tumors in children: long-term survival after radiation treatment. *Int J Radiat Oncol Biol Phys* 1995;31(3): 445–451.

38. Bourne JP, Geyer R, Berger M, et al. The prognostic significance of postoperative residual contrast enhancement on CT scan in pediatric patients with medulloblastoma. *J Neurooncol* 1992;14(3):263–270.

39. Gajjar A, Sanford RA, Bhargava R, et al. Medulloblastoma with brain stem involvement: the impact of gross total resection on outcome. *Pediatr Neurosurg* 1996;25(4):182–187.

40. Aguiar PH, Plese JP, Ciquini O, et al. Transient mutism following a posterior fossa approach to cerebellar tumors in children: a critical review of the literature. *Childs Nerv Syst* 1995;11(5):306–310.

41. Cochrane DD, Gustavsson B, Poskitt KP, et al. The surgical and natural morbidity of aggressive resection for posterior fossa tumors in childhood. *Pediatr Neurosurg* 1994;20(1):19–29.

42. Berger MS, Baumeister B, Geyer JR, et al. The risks of metastases from shunting in children with primary central nervous system tumors. *J Neurosurg* 1991; 74(6):872–877.

43. Cutler EC, Sosman MC, Vaughan WW. Place of radiation in treatment of cerebellar medulloblastoma: report of 20 cases. *Am J Roentgenol Radium Ther Nucl Med* 1936;35:429–453.

44. Bloom HJG, Glees J, Bell J. The treatment and prognosis of medulloblastoma in children. *AJR Am J Roentgenol* 1969;105:43–62.

45. Wolden SL, Dunkel IJ, Souweidane MM, et al. Patterns of failure using a conformal radiation therapy

tumor bed boost for medulloblastoma. *J Clin Oncol* 2003;21(16):3079–3083.

*46. Merchant TE, Kun LE, Krasin MJ, et al. Multi-institution prospective trial of reduced-dose craniospinal irradiation (23.4 Gy) followed by conformal posterior fossa (36 Gy) and primary site irradiation (55.8 Gy) and dose-intensive chemotherapy for average-risk medulloblastoma. *Proceedings of the 45th Annual ASTRO Meeting* 2003;57:S194–S195.

*47. Taylor RE, Bailey CC, Robinson K, et al. Results of a randomized study of preradiation chemotherapy versus radiotherapy alone for nonmetastatic medulloblastoma: the International Society of Paediatric Oncology/United Kingdom Children's Cancer Study Group PNET-3 Study. *J Clin Oncol* 2003;21(8):1581–1591.

*48. Packer RJ, Goldwein J, Nicholson HS, et al. Treatment of children with medulloblastomas with reduced-dose craniospinal radiation therapy and adjuvant chemotherapy: a Children's Cancer Group Study. *J Clin Oncol* 1999;17(7):2127–2136.

49. Ashley DM, Meier L, Kerby T, et al. Response of recurrent medulloblastoma to low-dose oral etoposide. *J Clin Oncol* 1996;14(6):1922–1927.

50. Heideman RL, Kovnar EH, Kellie SJ, et al. Preirradiation chemotherapy with carboplatin and etoposide in newly diagnosed embryonal pediatric CNS tumors. *J Clin Oncol* 1995;13(9):2247–2254.

51. Kovnar EH, Kellie SJ, Horowitz ME, et al. Preirradiation cisplatin and etoposide in the treatment of high-risk medulloblastoma and other malignant embryonal tumors of the central nervous system: a phase II study. *J Clin Oncol* 1990;8(2):330–336.

52. Strother D, Ashley D, Kellie SJ, et al. Feasibility of four consecutive high-dose chemotherapy cycles with stem-cell rescue for patients with newly diagnosed medulloblastoma or supratentorial primitive neuroectodermal tumor after craniospinal radiotherapy: results of a collaborative study. *J Clin Oncol* 2001;19(10):2696–2704.

53. Tait DM, Thornton-Jones H, Bloom HJ, et al. Adjuvant chemotherapy for medulloblastoma: the first multi-centre control trial of the International Society of Paediatric Oncology (SIOP I). *Eur J Cancer* 1990;26(4):464–469.

54. Krischer JP, Ragab AH, Kun L, et al. Nitrogen mustard, vincristine, procarbazine, and prednisone as adjuvant chemotherapy in the treatment of medulloblastoma. *J Neurosurg* 1991;74(6):905–909.

55. Mastrangelo R, Lasorella A, Riccardi R, et al. Carboplatin in childhood medulloblastoma/PNET: feasibility of an in vivo sensitivity test in an "up-front" study. *Med Pediatr Oncol* 1995;24(3):188–196.

56. Hartsell WF, Gajjar A, Heideman RL, et al. Patterns of failure in children with medulloblastoma: effects of preirradiation chemotherapy. *Int J Radiat Oncol Biol Phys* 1997;39(1):15–24.

57. Mosijczuk AD, Nigro MA, Thomas PR, et al. Preradiation chemotherapy in advanced medulloblastoma. *Cancer* 1993;72(9):2755–2762.

*58. Tarbell NJ, Friedman H, Kepner J, et al. High-risk medulloblastoma: a Pediatric Oncology Group (POG 9031) randomized trial of chemotherapy before or after radiation therapy. *J Clin Oncol* 2003.

59. Mahoney DH Jr, Strother D, Camitta B, et al. High-dose melphalan and cyclophosphamide with autologous bone marrow rescue for recurrent/progressive malignant brain tumors in children: a pilot Pediatric Oncology Group study. *J Clin Oncol* 1996;14(2):382–388.

60. Landberg TG, Lindgren ML, Cavallin-Stahl EK, et al. Improvements in the radiotherapy of medulloblastoma, 1946–1975. *Cancer* 1980;45(4):670–678.

61. Wara WM, Le QT, Sneed PK, et al. Pattern of recurrence of medulloblastoma after low-dose craniospinal radiotherapy. *Int J Radiat Oncol Biol Phys* 1994;30(3):551–556.

62. Sun LM, Yeh SA, Wang CJ, et al. Postoperative radiation therapy for medulloblastoma: high recurrence rate in the subfrontal region. *J Neurooncol* 2002;58(1):77–85.

63. Bouffet E, Bernard JL. Frappaz D, et al. M4 protocol for cerebellar medulloblastoma: supratentorial radiotherapy may not be avoided. *Int J Radiat Oncol Biol Phys* 1992;24(1):79–85.

64. Merchant TE, Happersett L, Finlay JL, et al. Preliminary results of conformal radiation therapy for medulloblastoma. *Neuro-oncology* 1999;1(3):177–187.

65. Fukunaga-Johnson N. Lee JH, Sandler HM, et al. Patterns of failure following treatment for medulloblastoma: is it necessary to treat the entire posterior fossa? *Int J Radiat Oncol Biol Phys* 1998;42(1):143–146.

*66. Carrie C, Muracciole X, Gomez F, et al. Conformal radiotherapy, reduced boost volume, hyperfractionated radiotherapy and on-line quality control in standard risk medulloblastoma without chemotherapy, results of the French M-SFOP 98. *Proceedings of the 45th Annual ASTRO Meeting* 2003;57:S195.

67. Miralbell R, Bleher A, Huguenin P, et al. Pediatric medulloblastoma: radiation treatment technique and patterns of failure. *Int J Radiat Oncol Biol Phys* 1997;37(3):523–529.

68. Merchant TE, Wang MH, Haida T, et al. Medulloblastoma: long-term results for patients treated with definitive radiation therapy during the computed tomography era. *Int J Radiat Oncol Biol Phys* 1996;36(1):29–35.

69. Fertil B, Malaise EP. Intrinsic radiosensitivity of human cell lines is correlated with radioresponsiveness of human tumors: analysis of 101 published survival curves. *Int J Radiat Oncol Biol Phys* 1985;11(9):1699–1707.

70. Pratt D, Mansur DB, Michalski JM, et al. Patterns of failure in medulloblastoma after optimal radiation therapy. *Proceedings of the 45th Annual ASTRO Meeting* 2003;57:S373.

71. Mulhern RK, Kepner JL, Thomas PR, et al. Neuropsychologic functioning of survivors of childhood medulloblastoma randomized to receive conventional or reduced-dose craniospinal irradiation: a Pediatric Oncology Group study. *J Clin Oncol* 1998;16(5):1723–1728.

*72. Goldwein JW, Radcliffe J, Johnson J, et al. Updated results of a pilot study of low dose craniospinal irradiation plus chemotherapy for children under five with cerebellar primitive neuroectodermal tumors (medulloblastoma). *Int J Radiat Oncol Biol Phys* 1996;34(4):899–904.

73. Allen JC, Nirenberg A, Donahue B. Hyperfraction-

ated radiotherapy and adjuvant chemotherapy for high risk PNET. *J Neurooncol* 1992;12:262.

74. Hudes RS, Gajjar A, Heideman RL, et al. High dose hyperfractionated craniospinal irradiation (HF-CSI): feasibility, acute toxicity, outcome and late sequelae. *Proceedings of the 40th Annual ASTRO Meeting* 1999;185.

75. Prados MD, Wara WM, Edwards MS, et al. Hyperfractionated craniospinal radiation therapy for primitive neuroectodermal tumors: early results of a pilot study. *Int J Radiat Oncol Biol Phys* 1994;28(2):431–438.

*76. Tatcher M, Glicksman AS. Field matching considerations in craniospinal irradiation. *Int J Radiat Oncol Biol Phys* 1989;17(4):865–869.

*77. Holupka EJ, Humm JL, Tarbell NJ, et al. Effect of set-up error on the dose across the junction of matching cranial-spinal fields in the treatment of medulloblastoma. *Int J Radiat Oncol Biol Phys* 1993;27(2):345–352.

78. Goldschmidt EJ Jr, Holst RJ. Second place Alpha Cradle Award winner. Medulloblastoma immobilization and treatment considerations. *Med Dosim* 1990;15(1):7–11.

79. Mah K, Danjoux CE, Manship S, et al. Computed tomographic simulation of craniospinal fields in pediatric patients: improved treatment accuracy and patient comfort. *Int J Radiat Oncol Biol Phys* 1998;41(5):997–1003.

80. Dunbar SF, Barnes PD, Tarbell NJ. Radiologic determination of the caudal border of the spinal field in cranial spinal irradiation. *Int J Radiat Oncol Biol Phys* 1993;26(4):669–673.

*81. Halperin EC. Concerning the inferior portion of the spinal radiotherapy field for malignancies that disseminate via the cerebrospinal fluid. *Int J Radiat Oncol Biol Phys* 1993;26(2):357–362.

*82. Halperin EC. Impact of radiation technique upon the outcome of treatment for medulloblastoma. *Int J Radiat Oncol Biol Phys* 1996;36(1):233–239.

*83. Donnal J, Halperin EC, Friedman HS, et al. Subfrontal recurrence of medulloblastoma. *Am J Neuroradiol* 1992;13:1617–1618.

84. Liu M, Carrie C, Parker W, et al. Comparison of manual and computer-generated customized blocks for whole brain fields used in the treatment of medulloblastoma. *Med Pediatr Oncol* 2002;38(1):55–57.

*85. Merchant TE, Zhu Y, Thompson SJ, et al. Preliminary results from a phase II trail of conformal radiation therapy for pediatric patients with localised low-grade astrocytoma and ependymoma. *Int J Radiat Oncol Biol Phys* 2002;52(2):325–332.

86. Maor MH, Fields RS, Hogstrom KR, et al. Improving the therapeutic ratio of craniospinal irradiation in medulloblastoma. *Int J Radiat Oncol Biol Phys* 1985;11(4):687–697.

*87. Gaspar LE, Dawson DJ, Tilley-Gulliford SA, et al. Medulloblastoma: long-term follow-up of patients treated with electron irradiation of the spinal field. *Radiology* 1991;180(3):867–870.

*88. Miralbell R, Lomax A, Russo M. Potential role of proton therapy in the treatment of pediatric medulloblastoma/primitive neuro-ectodermal tumors: spinal theca

irradiation. *Int J Radiat Oncol Biol Phys* 1997;38(4):805–811.

89. Paulino AC, Wen BC, Mayr NA, et al. Protracted radiotherapy treatment duration in medulloblastoma. *Am J Clin Oncol* 2003;26(1):55–59.

90. del Charco JO, Bolek TW, McCollough WM, et al. Medulloblastoma: time-dose relationship based on a 30-year review. *Int J Radiat Oncol Biol Phys* 1998;42(1):147–154.

91. Carrie C, Alapetite C, Mere P, et al. Quality control of radiotherapeutic treatment of medulloblastoma in a multicentric study: the contribution of radiotherapy technique to tumour relapse. *Radiother Oncol* 1992;24(2):77–81.

92. Marks LB, Halperin EC. The use of G-CSF during craniospinal irradiation. *Int J Radiat Oncol Biol Phys* 1993;26(5):905–906.

93. Rubin JB, Rowitch DH. Medulloblastoma: a problem of developmental biology. *Cancer Cell* 2002;2(1):7–8.

94. Barkovich AJ, Krischer J, Kun LE, et al. Brain stem gliomas: a classification system based on magnetic resonance imaging. *Pediatr Neurosurg* 1990;16(2):73–83.

*95. Freeman CR, Farmer JP. Pediatric brain stem gliomas: a review. *Int J Radiat Oncol Biol Phys* 1998;40(2):265–271.

96. Albright AL, Price RA, Guthkelch AN. Brain stem gliomas of children. A clinicopathological study. *Cancer* 1983;52(12):2313–2319.

97. Prados MD, Wara WM, Edwards MS, et al. The treatment of brain stem and thalamic gliomas with 78 Gy of hyperfractionated radiation therapy. *Int J Radiat Oncol Biol Phys* 1995;32(1):85–91.

98. Shrieve DC, Wara WM, Edwards MS, et al. Hyperfractionated radiation therapy for gliomas of the brainstem in children and in adults. *Int J Radiat Oncol Biol Phys* 1992;24(4):599–610.

99. Vandertop WP, Hoffman HJ, Drake JM, et al. Focal midbrain tumors in children. *Neurosurgery* 1992;31(2):186–194.

*100. Freeman CR, Krischer JP, Sanford RA, et al. Final results of a study of escalating doses of hyperfractionated radiotherapy in brain stem tumors in children: a Pediatric Oncology Group study. *Int J Radiat Oncol Biol Phys* 1993;27(2):197–206.

101. Freeman CR. Hyperfractionated radiotherapy for diffuse intrinsic brain stem tumors in children. *Pediatr Neurosurg* 1996;24(2):103–110.

102. Edwards MS, Wara WM, Ciricillo SF, et al. Focal brain-stem astrocytomas causing symptoms of involvement of the facial nerve nucleus: long-term survival in six pediatric cases. *J Neurosurg* 1994;80(1):20–25.

103. Hoffman HJ, Becker L, Craven MA. A clinically and pathologically distinct group of benign brain stem gliomas. *Neurosurgery* 1980;7(3):243–248.

104. Pollack IF, Hoffman HJ, Humphreys RP, et al. The long-term outcome after surgical treatment of dorsally exophytic brain-stem gliomas. *J Neurosurg* 1993;78(6):859–863.

105. Farmer JP, Montes JL, Freeman CR, et al. Brainstem gliomas. A 10-year institutional review. *Pediatr Neurosurg* 2001;34(4):206–214.

106. Pierre-Kahn A, Hirsch JF, Vinchon M, et al. Surgical management of brain-stem tumors in children: results

and statistical analysis of 75 cases. *J Neurosurg* 1993;79(6):845–852.

107. Yoshimura J, Onda K, Tanaka R, et al. Clinicopathological study of diffuse type brainstem gliomas: analysis of 40 autopsy cases. *Neurol Med Chir (Tokyo)* 2003;43(8):375–382.

108. Stroink AR, Hoffman HJ, Hendrick EB, et al. Diagnosis and management of pediatric brain-stem gliomas. *J Neurosurg* 1986;65(6):745–750.

109. Freeman CR, Bourgouin PM, Sanford RA, et al. Long term survivors of childhood brain stem gliomas treated with hyperfractionated radiotherapy. Clinical characteristics and treatment related toxicities. *Cancer* 1996;77(3):555–562.

110. Packer RJ, Boyett JM, Zimmerman RA, et al. Hyperfractionated radiation therapy (72 Gy) for children with brain stem gliomas. A Children's Cancer Group phase I/II trial. *Cancer* 1993;72(4):1414–1421.

111. Packer RJ, Boyett JM, Zimmerman RA, et al. Outcome of children with brain stem gliomas after treatment with 7800 cGy of hyperfractionated radiotherapy. A Children's Cancer Group phase I/II trial. *Cancer* 1994;74(6):1827–1834.

*112. Mantravadi RV, Phatak R, Bellur S, et al. Brain stem gliomas: an autopsy study of 25 cases. *Cancer* 1982;49(6):1294–1296.

113. Gilbertson RJ, Hill DA, Hernan R, et al. ERBB1 is amplified and overexpressed in high-grade diffusely infiltrative pediatric brain stem glioma. *Clin Cancer Res* 2003;9(10 Pt 1):3620–3624.

114. Khatib ZA, Heideman RL, Kovnar EH, et al. Predominance of pilocytic histology in dorsally exophytic brain stem tumors. *Pediatr Neurosurg* 1994; 20(1):2–10.

115. Boydston WR, Sanford RA, Muhlbauer MS, et al. Gliomas of the tectum and periaqueductal region of the mesencephalon. *Pediatr Neurosurg* 1991;17(5): 234–238.

116. Epstein F, McCleary EL. Intrinsic brain-stem tumors of childhood: surgical indications. *J Neurosurg* 1986;64(1):11–15.

117. Epstein F, Wisoff J. Intra-axial tumors of the cervicomedullary junction. *J Neurosurg* 1987;67(4): 483–487.

118. Jenkin RD, Boesel C, Ertel I, et al. Brain-stem tumors in childhood: a prospective randomized trial of irradiation with and without adjuvant CCNU, VCR, and prednisone. *J Neurosurg* 1987;66(2):227–233.

119. Kretschmar CS, Tarbell NJ, Barnes PD, et al. Preirradiation chemotherapy and hyperfractionated radiation therapy 66 Gy for children with brain stem tumors. A phase II study of the Pediatric Oncology Group, Protocol 8833. *Cancer* 1993;72(4):1404–1413.

*120. Freeman CR, Kepner J, Kun LE, et al. A detrimental effect of a combined chemotherapy-radiotherapy approach in children with diffuse intrinsic brain stem gliomas? *Int J Radiat Oncol Biol Phys* 2000;47(3): 561–564.

121. Allen JC, Siffert J. Contemporary chemotherapy issues for children with brainstem gliomas. *Pediatr Neurosurg* 1996;24(2):98–102.

122. Lonser RR, Walbridge S, Garmestani K, et al. Successful and safe perfusion of the primate brainstem: in vivo magnetic resonance imaging of macromolecular distribution during infusion. *J Neurosurg* 2002; 97(4):905–913.

123. Halperin EC. Pediatric brain stem tumors: patterns of treatment failure and their implications for radiotherapy. *Int J Radiat Oncol Biol Phys* 1985;11(7): 1293–1298.

124. Packer RJ, Zimmerman RA, Kaplan A, et al. Early cystic/necrotic changes after hyperfractionated radiation therapy in children with brain stem gliomas. *Cancer* 1993;71(8):2666–2674.

125. Donahue B, Allen J, Siffert J, et al. Patterns of recurrence in brain stem gliomas: evidence for craniospinal dissemination. *Int J Radiat Oncol Biol Phys* 1998;40(3):677–680.

126. Gajjar A, Sanford RA, Heideman R, et al. Low-grade astrocytoma: a decade of experience at St. Jude Children's Research Hospital. *J Clin Oncol* 1997;15(8): 2792–2799.

127. Dunbar SF, Tarbell NJ, Kooy HM, et al. Stereotactic radiotherapy for pediatric and adult brain tumors: preliminary report. *Int J Radiat Oncol Biol Phys* 1994;30(3):531–539.

*128. Mandell L, Kadota R, Douglass EC, et al. It is time to rethink the role of hyperfractionated radiotherapy in the management of children with newly diagnosed brainstem? Results of a Pediatric Oncology Group Phase III trial comparing conventional versus hyperfractionated radiotherapy. *Int J Radiat Oncol Biol Phys* 1997;39:143.

129. Packer RJ, Prados M, Phillips P, et al. Treatment of children with newly diagnosed brain stem gliomas with intravenous recombinant beta-interferon and hyperfractionated radiation therapy: a Children's Cancer Group phase I/II study. *Cancer* 1996;77(10): 2150–2156.

130. Lewis J, Lucraft H, Gholkar A. UKCCSG study of accelerated radiotherapy for pediatric brain stem gliomas. *Int J Radiat Oncol Biol Phys* 1997;38(5): 925–929.

131. Hebert ME, Halperin EC, Oakes WJ, et al. Multiple fraction-per-day radiotherapy for patients with brain stem tumors. *J Neurooncol* 1993;17(2):131–138.

132. Fisher PG, Donaldson SS. Hyperfractionated radiotherapy in the management of diffuse intrinsic brainstem tumors: when is enough enough? *Int J Radiat Oncol Biol Phys* 1999 43(5):947–949.

133. Walter AW, Gajjar A, Ochs JS, et al. Carboplatin and etoposide with hyperfractionated radiotherapy in children with newly diagnosed diffuse pontine gliomas: a phase I/II study. *Med Pediatr Oncol* 1998;30(1):28–33.

134. Griebel M, Friedman HS, Halperin EC, et al. Reversible neurotoxicity following hyperfractionated radiation therapy of brain stem glioma. *Med Pediatr Oncol* 1991;19(3):182–186.

135. Taylor JS, Langston JW, Reddick WE, et al. Clinical value of proton magnetic resonance spectroscopy for differentiating recurrent or residual brain tumor from delayed cerebral necrosis. *Int J Radiat Oncol Biol Phys* 1996;36(5):1251–1261.

136. Nazar GB, Hoffman HJ, Becker LE, et al. Infratentorial ependymomas in childhood: prognostic factors and treatment. *J Neurosurg* 1990;72(3):408–417.

137. Veelen-Vincent ML, Pierre-Kahn A, Kalifa C, et al. Ependymoma in childhood: prognostic factors, extent of surgery, and adjuvant therapy. *J Neurosurg* 2002;97(4):827–835.

138. Merchant TE. Current management of childhood ependymoma. *Oncology (Huntingt)* 2002;16(5):629–642, 644.

139. Sanford RA, Kun LE, Heideman RL, et al. Cerebellar pontine angle ependymoma in infants. *Pediatr Neurosurg* 1997;27(2):84–91.

140. Centeno RS, Lee AA, Winter J, et al. Supratentorial ependymomas. Neuroimaging and clinicopathological correlation. *J Neurosurg* 1986;64(2):209–215.

141. Grill J, Le Deley MC, Gambarelli D, et al. Postoperative chemotherapy without irradiation for ependymoma in children under 5 years of age: a multicenter trial of the French Society of Pediatric Oncology. *J Clin Oncol* 2001;19(5):1288–1296.

*142. Paulino AC. The local field in infratentorial ependymoma: does the entire posterior fossa need to be treated? *Int J Radiat Oncol Biol Phys* 2001;49(3):757–761.

143. Rawlings CE III, Giangaspero F, Burger PC, et al. Ependymomas: a clinicopathologic study. *Surg Neurol* 1988;29(4):271–281.

144. Rorke LB. Relationship of morphology of ependymoma in children to prognosis. *Prog Exp Tumor Res* 1987;30:170–174.

145. Ross GW, Rubinstein LJ. Lack of histopathological correlation of malignant ependymomas with postoperative survival. *J Neurosurg* 1989;70(1):31–36.

146. Bigner DD, McLendon RE, Bruner JM. *Russell & Rubinstein's pathology of tumors of the nervous system,* 6th ed. London: Arnold, 1998.

147. Pollack IF, Gerszten PC, Martinez AJ, et al. Intracranial ependymomas of childhood: long-term outcome and prognostic factors. *Neurosurgery* 1995;37(4):655–666.

*148. Merchant TE, Jenkins JJ, Burger PC, et al. Influence of tumor grade on time to progression after irradiation for localized ependymoma in children. *Int J Radiat Oncol Biol Phys* 2002;53(1):52–57.

149. Horn B, Heideman R, Geyer R, et al. A multi-institutional retrospective study of intracranial ependymoma in children: identification of risk factors. *J Pediatr Hematol Oncol* 1999;21(3):203–211.

150. Bloom HJ, Glees J, Bell J, et al. The treatment and long-term prognosis of children with intracranial tumors: a study of 610 cases, 1950–1981. *Int J Radiat Oncol Biol Phys* 1990;18(4):723–745.

151. Grill J, Avet-Loiseau H, Lellouch-Tubiana A, et al. Comparative genomic hybridization detects specific cytogenetic abnormalities in pediatric ependymomas and choroid plexus papillomas. *Cancer Genet Cytogenet* 2002;136:121–125.

*152. Goldwein JW, Leahy JM, Packer RJ, et al. Intracranial ependymomas in children. *Int J Radiat Oncol Biol Phys* 1990;19(6):1497–1502.

153. Kim BS, Roonprapunt C, LaMarca V, et al. The current management of intracranial ependymomas in children. *Ann Neurosurg* 2002;2:1–10.

154. Rousseau P, Habrand JL, Sarrazin D, et al. Treatment of intracranial ependymomas of children: review of a 15-year experience. *Int J Radiat Oncol Biol Phys* 1994;28(2):381–386.

155. Healey EA, Barnes PD, Kupsky WJ, et al. The prognostic significance of postoperative residual tumor in ependymoma. *Neurosurgery* 1991;28(5):666–671.

156. Duffner PK, Krischer JP, Sanford RA, et al. Prognostic factors in infants and very young children with intracranial ependymomas. *Pediatr Neurosurg* 1998;28(4):215–222.

*157. Hukin J, Epstein F, Lefton D, et al. Treatment of intracranial ependymoma by surgery alone. *Pediatr Neurosurg* 1998;29(1):40–45.

158. Evans AE, Anderson JR, Lefkowitz-Boudreaux IB, et al. Adjuvant chemotherapy of childhood posterior fossa ependymoma: cranio-spinal irradiation with or without adjuvant CCNU, vincristine, and prednisone: a Children's Cancer Group study. *Med Pediatr Oncol* 1996;27(1):8–14.

159. Goldwein JW, Glauser TA, Packer RJ, et al. Recurrent intracranial ependymomas in children. Survival, patterns of failure, and prognostic factors. *Cancer* 1990;66(3):557–563.

160. Goldwein JW, Corn BW, Finlay JL, et al. Is craniospinal irradiation required to cure children with malignant (anaplastic) intracranial ependymomas? *Cancer* 1991;67(11):2766–2771.

161. Aggarwal R, Yeung D, Kumar P, et al. Efficacy and feasibility of stereotactic radiosurgery in the primary management of unfavorable pediatric ependymoma. *Radiother Oncol* 1997;43(3):269–273.

*162. Merchant TE, Mulhern RK, Krasin MJ, et al. A phase II trial of conformal radiation therapy and evaluation of radiation-related CNS effects for pediatric patients with localized ependymoma. *J Clin Oncol* 2003.

163. Kovalic JJ, Flaris N, Grigsby PW, et al. Intracranial ependymoma long term outcome, patterns of failure. *J Neurooncol* 1993;15(2):125–131.

164. Rezai AR, Woo HH, Lee M, et al. Disseminated ependymomas of the central nervous system. *J Neurosurg* 1996;85(4):618–624.

*165. Vanuytsel LJ, Bessell EM, Ashley SE, et al. Intracranial ependymoma: long-term results of a policy of surgery and radiotherapy. *Int J Radiat Oncol Biol Phys* 1992;23(2):313–319.

166. Merchant TE, Haida T, Wang MH, et al. Anaplastic ependymoma: treatment of pediatric patients with or without craniospinal radiation therapy. *J Neurosurg* 1997;86(6):943–949.

167. Ilgren EB, Stiller CA. Cerebellar astrocytomas. Clinical characteristics and prognostic indices. *J Neurooncol* 1987;4(3):293–308.

168. Schneider JH Jr, Raffel C, McComb JG. Benign cerebellar astrocytomas of childhood. *Neurosurgery* 1992;30(1):58–62.

169. Cushing H. Experiences with the cerebellar astrocytomas: a critical review of 76 cases. *Surg Gynecol Obstet* 1931;52:129–191.

170. Ilgren EB, Stiller CA. Cerebellar astrocytomas: therapeutic management. *Acta Neurochir (Wien)* 1986;81(1–2):11–26.

171. Hayostek CJ, Shaw EG, Scheithauer B, et al. Astrocytomas of the cerebellum. A comparative clinicopathologic study of pilocytic and diffuse astrocytomas. *Cancer* 1993;72(3):856–869.

172. Pencalet P, Maixner W, Sainte-Rose C, et al. Benign cerebellar astrocytomas in children. *J Neurosurg* 1999;90(2):265–273.

173. Desai KI, Nadkarni TD, Muzumdar DP, et al. Prognostic factors for cerebellar astrocytomas in children: a study of 102 cases. *Pediatr Neurosurg* 2001;35(6): 311–317.

174. Gjerris F, Klinken L. Long-term prognosis in children with benign cerebellar astrocytoma. *J Neurosurg* 1978;49(2):179–184.

175. Kulkarni AV, Becker LE, Jay V, et al. Primary cerebellar glioblastomas multiforme in children. Report of four cases. *J Neurosurg* 1999;90(3):546–550.

176. Campbell JW, Pollack IF. Cerebellar astrocytomas in children. *J Neurooncol* 1996;28(2–3):223–231.

177. Sgouros S, Fineron PW, Hockley AD. Cerebellar astrocytoma of childhood: long-term follow-up. *Childs Nerv Syst* 1995;11(2):89–96.

178. Tomita T, McLone DG. Medulloblastoma in childhood: results of radical resection and low-dose neuraxis radiation therapy. *J Neurosurg* 1986;64(2): 238–242.

179. Pollack IF, Hurtt M, Pang D, et al. Dissemination of low grade intracranial astrocytomas in children. *Cancer* 1994;73(11):2869–2878.

180. Prados M, Mamelak AN. Metastasizing low grade gliomas in children. Redefining an old disease. *Cancer* 1994;73(11):2671–2673.

181. Garcia DM, Marks JE, Latifi HR, et al. Childhood cerebellar astrocytomas: is there a role for postoperative irradiation? *Int J Radiat Oncol Biol Phys* 1990;18(4):815–818.

182. Sutton LN, Cnaan A, Klatt L, et al. Postoperative surveillance imaging in children with cerebellar astrocytomas. *J Neurosurg* 1996;84(5):721–725.

183. Larson DA, Wara WM, Edwards MS. Management of childhood cerebellar astrocytoma. *Int J Radiat Oncol Biol Phys* 1990;18(4):971–973.

184. Schick U, Marquardt G. Pediatric spinal tumors. *Pediatr Neurosurg* 2001;35(3):120–127.

185. Reimer R, Onofrio BM. Astrocytomas of the spinal cord in children and adolescents. *J Neurosurg* 1985;63(5):669–675.

186. DeSousa AL, Kalsbeck JE, Mealey J Jr, et al. Intraspinal tumors in children. A review of 81 cases. *J Neurosurg* 1979;51(4):437–445.

187. Nadkarni TD, Rekate HL. Pediatric intramedullary spinal cord tumors. Critical review of the literature. *Childs Nerv Syst* 1999;15(1):17–28.

188. Albright AL. Pediatric intramedullary spinal cord tumors. *Childs Nerv Syst* 1999;15(9):436–438.

189. Curran WJ Jr, D'Angio GJ. Nonsurgical management of spinal tumors. In: Ashley DG, Curran WJ Jr, D'Angio GJ, et al., eds. *Spinal tumors in children and adolescents: the international review of child neurology.* New York: Raven Press, 1990:71–84.

190. Innocenzi G, Raco A, Cantore G, et al. Intramedullary astrocytomas and ependymomas in the pediatric age group: a retrospective study. *Childs Nerv Syst* 1996;12(12):776–780.

191. Rossitch E Jr, Zeidman SM, Burger PC, et al. Clinical and pathological analysis of spinal cord astrocytomas in children. *Neurosurgery* 1990;27(2):193–196.

192. Epstein F. Spinal cord astrocytomas of childhood. *Prog Exp Tumor Res* 1987;30:135–153.

193. Epstein F, Epstein N. Surgical management of holocord intramedullary spinal cord astrocytomas in children. *J Neurosurg* 1981;54(6):829–832.

194. Pascual-Castroviejo I. *Spinal cord tumors in children and adolescents.* New York: Raven Press, 1990.

195. Houten JK, Weiner HL. Pediatric intramedullary spinal cord tumors: special considerations. *J Neurooncol* 2000;47(3):225–230.

196. Merchant TE, Kiehna EN, Thompson SJ, et al. Pediatric low-grade and ependymal spinal cord tumors. *Pediatr Neurosurg* 2000;32(1):30–36.

197. Whitaker SJ, Bessell EM, Ashley SE, et al. Postoperative radiotherapy in the management of spinal cord ependymoma. *J Neurosurg* 1991;74(5):720–728.

198. Sonneland PR, Scheithauer BW, Onofrio BM. Myxopapillary ependymoma. A clinicopathologic and immunocytochemical study of 77 cases. *Cancer* 1985; 56(4):883–893.

199. Rifkinson-Mann S, Wisoff JH, Epstein F. The association of hydrocephalus with intramedullary spinal cord tumors: a series of 25 patients. *Neurosurgery* 1990;27(5):749–754.

200. Epstein F, Epstein N. Surgical treatment of spinal cord astrocytomas of childhood. A series of 19 patients. *J Neurosurg* 1982;57(5):685–689.

201. McCormick PC, Torres R, Post KD, et al. Intramedullary ependymoma of the spinal cord. *J Neurosurg* 1990;72(4):523–532.

*202. Linstadt DE, Wara WM, Leibel SA, et al. Postoperative radiotherapy of primary spinal cord tumors. *Int J Radiat Oncol Biol Phys* 1989;16(6):1397–1403.

203. O'Sullivan C, Jenkin RD, Doherty MA, et al. Spinal cord tumors in children: long-term results of combined surgical and radiation treatment. *J Neurosurg* 1994;81(4):507–512.

204. Chun HC, Schmidt-Ullrich RK, Wolfson A, et al. External beam radiotherapy for primary spinal cord tumors. *J Neurooncol* 1990;9(3):211–217.

5

Retinoblastoma

Edward C. Halperin, M.D., and John P. Kirkpatrick, M.D., Ph.D.

HISTOLOGY AND PATTERNS OF GROWTH

Retinoblastoma (RB) is the most common malignant intraocular tumor of childhood. The tumor is of neuroepithelial origin and arises from the nucleated layers of one or both eyes (1). RB consists of undifferentiated small anaplastic cells, which may be round or polygonal. Scant cytoplasm surrounds the large nuclei, which characteristically stain deeply with hematoxylin. Calcification commonly occurs in necrotic areas (2,3). Both Flexner and Wintersteiner described the arrangement of the more differentiated malignant cells of RB in neuroepithelial rosettes. These Flexner–Wintersteiner rosettes appear to represent an attempt to differentiate into photoreceptor cells (Figs. 5-1–5-3) (4).

As RB grows, it may cause a retinal detachment secondary to a solid or multifocal mass (endophytic type of growth). Endophytic tumors may break through the inner layers of the retina to the vitreous. The tumor may also form a pedunculated mass (exophytic type of growth). Both patterns of growth may occur in the same eye, and neither one is of prognostic significance (5). It is not unusual for RB to seed the vitreous. These vitreous seeds may grow even though they lack a blood supply (2).

INCIDENCE

The reported incidence of RB ranges from 1 in 14,000 live births to 1 in 34,000 (4,6). There are approximately 200 to 350 new cases per year in the United States and 50 in the United Kingdom (2,4–8). The tumor may be more common in Latin America (9).

RB shows no predilection for sex, race, or the right or left eye. Between 65% and 80% of cases are unilateral (2,4,10–14). The frequency of bilateral tumors is higher at institutions serving as referral centers for more complicated cases. Bilaterality may be ascertained concurrently or sequentially.

The diagnosis may be made from shortly after birth until 7 years of age. The mean age of detection is 2 to 4 months, and most cases are discovered before 3 years of age (2,4,15,16). In general,

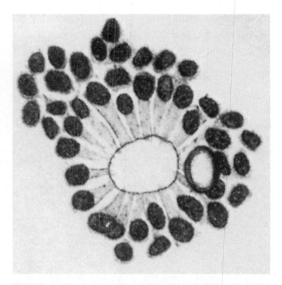

FIG. 5-1. A rosette characteristic of differentiated retinoblastoma, after a drawing by Wintersteiner. Note the cylindrical nuclei and fine protoplasm extensions toward the lumen. (From Dudgeon J. Retinoblastoma: trends in conservative management. *Br J Ophthalmol* 1995;79:104, with permission.)

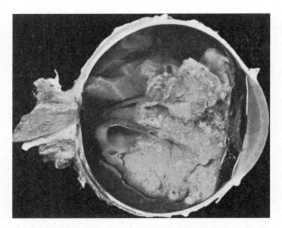

FIG. 5-2. Renowned pathologist James Ewing, in the 1919 edition of his textbook of tumor pathology, recognized the "glioma of the retina" as being composed of "small round-cells . . . arranged in small alveoli or rosettes after the manner of neuro-epithelial rosettes . . . [occurring] almost exclusively in infants. . . . The congenital character is most remarkable." (From Ewing J. *Neoplastic diseases: a text-book on tumors.* Philadelphia: WB Saunders, 1919, with permission.)

unilateral RB is diagnosed at a later age than is bilateral disease. In the Mayo Clinic series the median ages at diagnosis were 4.5 months for bilateral disease and 22 months for unilateral disease, an observation supported by others (5,8,17).

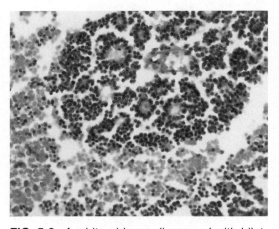

FIG. 5-3. A white girl was diagnosed with bilateral retinoblastoma at 7 weeks of age. OD enucleation was performed. Note the characteristic Flexner–Wintersteiner rosettes in the enucleated eye.

THE GENETICS AND MOLECULAR BIOLOGY OF RB*

The infectious nature of some cancers was demonstrated by Francis Peyton Rous (1879–1970). In a 1910 experiment he showed that submicroscopic, filterable agents (viruses) isolated from a chicken sarcoma could induce new sarcomas in healthy chickens. Rous's work languished in obscurity before it was rediscovered and recognized with the Nobel Prize in Physiology or Medicine in 1966. In his Nobel lecture, "The Challenge to Man of the Neoplastic Cell," Rous (18) considered the possible existence of growth-promoting genes. He called them *oncogens;* today they are called *oncogenes.*

> The chemical and physical initiators [of cancer] are ordinarily called *carcinogens;* but it is a misleading term because they not only induce the malignant epithelial growths known as carcinomas but other neoplasms of widely various kinds. In the present paper the less used term *oncogens* will be employed, meaning thereby capable of producing a tumor. It hews precisely to the fact. . . .
>
> What can be the nature of the generality of neoplastic changes, the reason for their persistence, their irreversibility, and for the discontinuous, steplike alterations that they frequently undergo? A favorite explanation has been that oncogens cause alterations in the genes of the body, somatic mutations as these are termed. But numerous facts, when taken together, decisively exclude this supposition.

Rous was wrong about oncogenes. Theodor Boveri (19), on the other hand, was right. In 1914 he used studies of normal mitosis in sea urchins and worms as a platform for suggesting that cancer might be caused by the abnormal gain or loss of chromosomes and their function. In a 1929 English translation of his 1926 book *The Origin of Malignant Tumors,* Boveri wrote,

> Most cancers have many chromosomal abnormalities, both in number and in structure, whereas some show only a single aberration. In the era before molecular biology, cancer researchers, study-

*Some of this material originally appeared in Chapter 1 of Perez C, Brady L, Halperin EC, et al. *Principles and practice of radiation oncology,* 4th ed. Philadelphia: JB Lippincott, 2003.

ing both human and animal cancers, proposed that a small number of events was needed for carcinogenesis. Evidence from the recent molecular era indicate that cancers can arise from small numbers of events that affect common cell birth and death processes. . . . The unlimited tendency to rapid proliferation in malignant tumor cells [could result] from a permanent predominance of the chromosomes that promote division. . . . Another possibility [to explain cancer] is the presence of definite chromosomes which inhibit division. . . . Cells of tumors with unlimited growth would arise if those "inhibiting chromosomes" were eliminated. . . . [Because] each kind of chromosome is represented twice in the normal cell, the depression of only one of these two might pass unnoticed (19).

Boveri predicted that the genetic abnormalities leading to the development of cancer are of two sorts: growth-promoting genes and growth-suppressing genes. If the growth-promoting genes are excessive in number or activity, they lead to cell proliferation. If the growth-suppressing genes are defective in amount or activity, they fail to halt cell proliferation and lead to unbridled cell replication. These growth promoting genes are called *oncogenes*. The growth-suppressing genes are called *tumor suppressor genes*.

We may think of oncogenes and tumor suppressor genes as analogous to the accelerator and brake pedals of an automobile. When it is idling with the transmission in drive, one can move the car forward by pushing on the accelerator pedal, by taking pressure off the brake pedal, or by doing both simultaneously. Similarly, cell growth and proliferation, leading to cancer, can occur by the activity of the oncogenes or inactivity of the suppressor genes (20–23).

A wide variety of physiologic conditions call for the effective use of growth-promoting and growth-suppressing genes. There must be a mechanism to cause the fetus to grow and then, at the appropriate time, to restrain growth. There must be a way of causing fibroblasts to proliferate to heal a wound and then, at the appropriate time, halting the fibroblasts (except in the case of keloid formation). Uncontrolled cell growth, or cancer, may be thought of as a set of physiologic controls of cell growth gone awry.

In 1972, Alfred G. Knudson Jr. proposed a simple genetic model to explain the origins of RB. Almost 30 years after the original article was published, Knudson described the origins of his discovery.

I was interested in the fact that the germ-line mutation, which is a *de novo* mutation in 80% of the germ-line mutants, is not a sufficient condition for tumorigenesis—some children with an affected parent do not develop a tumour, but later produce an affected child, indicating that they carried the germ-line mutation. Most affected children with an affected parent develop tumors bilaterally but some do so unilaterally. Approximately 60% of all cases are unilateral in the United States and do not carry a predisposing germ-line mutation. I calculated that the numbers of tumors per heritable case fall in a Poisson distribution with a mean of 3. From this, in can be inferred that 5% ($e^{-3} = 0.05$) of carriers of the germ-line mutation developed no tumor which fits approximately with observation. The distribution of bilateral cases that have not yet been diagnosed (S) at different ages showed a linear decline on a semi log plot. That is, $\ln S = -kt$ (where k is a constant that incorporates the mutation rate and t is time), as expected for a one hit phenomenon. From this, I predicted that hereditary retinoblastoma involves two mutations and, knowing that one of these had to be a germ-line mutation, I hypothesized that the other one would be somatic. The unilateral cases with no positive family history, only a minority of whom carry a germ-line mutation, showed a distribution consistent with two mutations, so both of these ought to be somatic. The hereditary and non-hereditary forms of the tumor seem to entail the same number of events—a hypothesis that became known as the "two-hit hypothesis" [Fig. 5-4] (24).

Knudson (20,21) sought to understand how the disease might have a familial (i.e., hereditary) form and a sporadic (i.e., nonhereditary) form. In a retrospective statistical analysis, he plotted the logarithm of the proportion of cases not yet diagnosed against the age for bilateral (i.e., hereditary) and unilateral (largely nonhereditary) forms of RB. The graph for the bilateral type generated a straight line, whereas the unilateral type created a curved line with second-order kinetics. Knudson in-

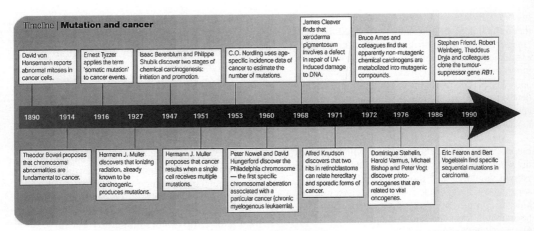

FIG. 5-4. The idea that cancer is a genetic disease of somatic cells involved in the work of multiple investigators. The term *somatic mutation* was first applied to cancer by Tyzzer, who observed that tumors sequentially transplanted in mice developed an increasingly broad host specificity among recipients from different inbred strains. Firm support for the genetic concept of mutations came from Muller's discovery that ionizing radiation, which was already known to be carcinogenic, was also mutagenic. (From Knudson AG. Two genetic hits [more or less] to cancer. *Nat Rev Cancer* 2001; 1:157–162, with permission.)

ferred that the bilateral type was explicable by a single random somatic event acting in the presence of an existing germ line mutation, whereas the unilateral form resulted from two somatic events. He also analyzed the number of tumors in patients with bilateral RB. He found that the mean number was three and that the distribution of the number of tumors followed the Poisson equation. He concluded that the tumor events were random and independent (20,21).

In its simplest statement, Knudson's model suggests that children with sporadic RB are genetically normal at conception. During embryonic development, two somatic mutations (also called two genetic "hits") occur in the cell line leading to the retinal photoreceptors. The resulting doubly mutated primordial retinal cell proliferates into RB tumors. In familial RB, the fertilized egg already carries one copy of the mutant gene (one hit). All descendants of this cell carry the mutation. If any cell sustains a somatic mutation (a second hit) to reach the doubly mutated state needed for tumor induction, RB develops. The two-hit hypothesis had the potential to explain both forms of RB (Figs. 5-5 and 5-6) (14,20,21,25,26).

Knudson's hypothesis explained neither the precise gene affected nor the nature of the mutation or gene product that caused the malignancy. Evidence concerning the gene product came from the work of Cavenee and colleagues. They used DNA restriction fragment length polymorphisms (RFLPs) in the study of cancer. The cytogenic analysis was vital in uncovering the mechanism behind the two hits of RB. Investigators found that a few cases were associated with deletion of chromosomal band 13q14. Heterozygosities for linked but external markers of chromosome 13 were lost with the deletion but not with intragenic mutations. RFLPs supported the conclusion that either of these mechanisms can occur as a second event in RB. This work provided direct evidence for the identification of RB1 as a tumor suppressor gene (25,27–30).

What protein is normally produced by the deleted 13q14 RB gene? How does it regulate cell growth? Why does its absence lead to malignancy? The search for the answers to these questions is at the heart of molecular cancer biology (150). In general, we may think of tumor formation as the possible result of mutations in two classes of genes: proto-oncogenes and tumor suppressor genes. When mutations occur in proto-

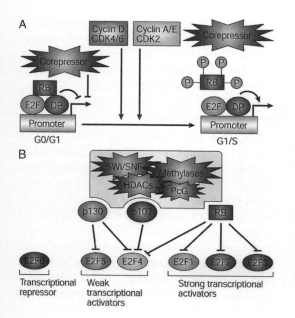

FIG. 5-5. It has recently been shown that the growth-repressive action of retinoblastoma (RB) occurs, in part, via the recruitment of chromatin-remodeling complexes to promote a region. These complexes mediate chromatin condensation and the subsequent inhibition of transcription. In addition to its role in self cycle control, RB has been implicated in regulating a wide variety of cellular processes, including DNA replication, differentiation, and apoptosis. RB potentially interacts with more than 100 different cellular proteins. The functional relevance of most of these interactions has not been elucidated. (From Classon M, Harlow E. The retinoblastoma tumor suppressor in development and cancer. *Nat Rev Cancer* 2002;2:910–917, with permission.)

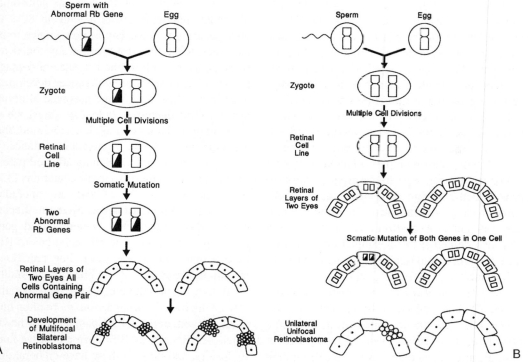

FIG. 5-6. (A) In heritable bilateral retinoblastoma, a gamete carrying a defective Rb gene (the first hit) forms a zygote heterozygous at the Rb locus. A later somatic mutation inactivates the other Rb gene (the second hit), allowing bilateral multifocal tumors. **(B)** In nonheritable retinoblastoma, inactivation of both genes in a retinal cell (two hits) by somatic mutations leads to the development of unilateral unifocal disease. (Modified from Toma NMG, Hungerford JL, Plowman PN, et al. External beam radiotherapy for retinoblastoma: II: lens sparing technique. *Br J Ophthalmol* 1995;79:112–117 with permission.)

oncogenes, which result in a gain of function and unbridled cell growth, they are called oncogenes. Proto-oncogenes participate in cell growth and proliferation via several mechanisms: the elaboration of cellular growth factors; the production and deployment of membrane growth factor receptors; intracellular signal transducers, which conduct growth-promoting signals from the membrane deep into the interior of the cell; and transcription factors that promote the ultimate production of proteins, which lead to cell proliferation. It is clear that proto-oncogenes have desirable physiologic functions in fetal development, normal childhood growth, wound healing, and desirable cell proliferation, as occurs in the aerodigestive tract, gut, and bone marrow. However, when proto-oncogenes go awry and become oncogenes, the persistent cell growth that results, without appropriate restraints of time and space, leads to cancer.

In contrast, tumor suppressor genes provide signals that constrain cell proliferation. Mutations in the tumor suppressor genes behave in a recessive manner at the molecular level. Consistent with Knudson's hypothesis, when mutations occur in both alleles (two hits), the suppressive behavior of the gene is fully lost (i.e., only when both copies of the gene are inactivated by mutations does an abnormal phenotype, a malignant transformation, occur in a cell). A child born with one defective copy of a tumor suppressor gene has a predisposition to cancer. If the second copy of the gene is rendered inactive by a mutation, then the carcinogenic potential is realized. However, a child with two defective tumor suppressor genes has fully lost a constraint on cell growth, and cancer will ensue.

The RB protein (pRB) is intimately involved in control of the cell cycle. A transcription factor called *E2F* (the name comes from its initial identification as being involved in the adenovirus E2 promoter) helps drive the cell through the cell cycle to mitosis. When pRB binds E2F, E2F is not free to activate promoters of DNA synthesis. In addition, the pRB–E2F complex downregulates the expression of many G_1 exit-promoting genes such as c-*myc* and c-*myb*. In this way, pRB inhibits the cell from duplicating itself. If pRB is phosphorylated, the phosphorus groups displace the E2F from its binding site. Then the E2F launches into action and promotes cell division. If the pRB is absent or defective, then the factors leading to cell proliferation have no countervailing force.

The growth repressive action of RB occurs, in part, via the recruitment of chromatin-remodeling complexes to promote a region. These complexes mediate chromatin condensation and the subsequent inhibition of transcription. In addition to its role in self cycle control, RB has been implicated in regulating a wide variety of cellular processes. These include DNA replication, differentiation, and apoptosis. RB potentially interacts with more than 100 different cellular proteins. The functional relevance of most of these interactions has not been elucidated (31).

A generation of pediatric radiation oncologists were taught that RB has an autosomal dominant inheritance pattern with an 80% to 90% penetrance (1,8). This is now known to be incorrect. RB is the result of an autosomal recessive pattern; only in the presence of damage to two alleles (two hits) will cancer develop. It must be the case that, in the presence of an inherited single defective allele, the occurrence of a mutation in the second allele is common; this gives the impression of dominant inheritance.

RB may be inherited from an affected parent or may be the result of sporadic mutations (32). Although most cases of RB are sporadic, 25–40% are familial (inherited from an affected parent who survived RB, a nonaffected gene carrier parent who has no clinical signs of RB, or a parent with a new germ line mutation). Hereditary cases usually are bilateral and multifocal; they occur at a younger age than sporadic cases, which are, in comparison, more often unifocal and unilateral. Of all patients with newly diagnosed RB, about 10% have a positive family history, and most of these have bilateral disease. Of the 90% with no family history, 20–30% have hereditary, bilateral disease. The remaining 65% to 80% are unilateral. Of these unilateral cases, about 10% are hereditary and 90% nonhereditary (Fig. 5-7) (14).

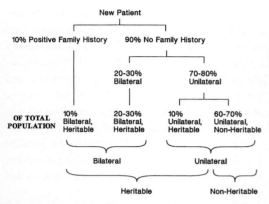

FIG. 5-7. The distribution of unilateral, bilateral, heritable, and nonheritable cases of retinoblastoma.

WORKUP

RB commonly presents with a white pupillary light reflex (called *leukocoria*) (5,11,33). The parents may notice this abnormal appearance in a flash photograph (Figs. 5-8 and 5-9) because a photographic flash bounces light through the pupil and conjunctiva to produce a red appearance in a color snapshot. However, large RB, or an RB producing retinal detachment, produces the white reflex when the flash bounces off it. This effect can also be seen with a handheld ophthalmoscope. RB may also be discovered by

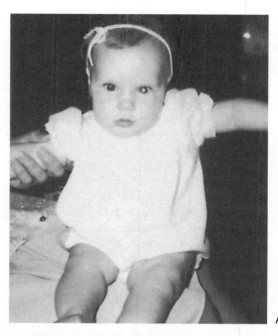

A

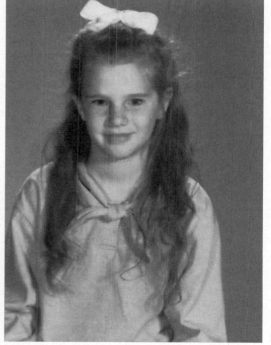

B

FIG. 5-9. Leukocoria in a flash photograph of a 6-month-old girl with retinoblastoma. Over time, the eye improved, and irradiated with 43.6 Gy, she retained excellent vision at 20-year follow-up. (Reproduced with permission of the patient's parents.)

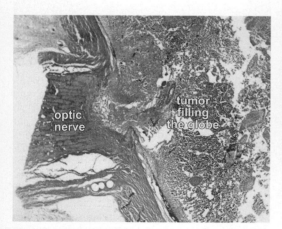

FIG. 5-8. OD enucleation of the child shown in Fig. 5-3. Tumor fills the globe but does not involve the optic nerve.

a pediatrician or ophthalmologist doing a surveillance examination of a child with a positive family history or during the course of a routine examination.

On physical examination one notes a raised white, white-yellow, or white-pink mass (2). Tortuous vessels may be seen feeding the tumor. Cells may break off from the main tumor mass and grow as small vitreous seeds (5). Because RB may be multifocal, it is necessary to examine the entire retinal surface, generally with the patient under anesthesia.

When RB presents as a mass, the differential diagnosis includes astrocytic hamartoma, *Toxo-*

cara canis granuloma, the infected emboli of subacute bacterial endocarditis or toxoplasmosis, and other types of severe uveitis. When RB causes retinal detachment, the differential diagnosis includes Coats's disease, retrolental fibroplasia, and persistent hyperplastic vitreous (2,4–6,8). Biopsy of a suspected RB or vitreous aspiration for enzyme studies is generally felt to be contraindicated because of the risk of choroidal seeding (5). The consequences of intraocular procedures in patients with RB are discussed later in this chapter.

Retinal drawings and photographs, along with a written description, are used to record whether single or multifocal tumors are present (Fig. 5-10). Ultrasound is also useful for documenting tumor location and size (Fig. 5-11). The distance from the cornea to the back of the lens can also be measured with ultrasound to aid in lateral field radiotherapy planning. Computed tomography (CT) scan is effective in demonstrating tu-

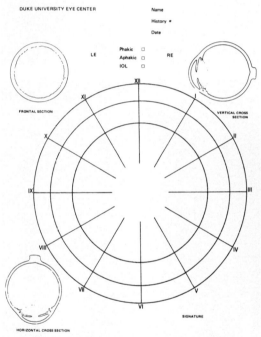

FIG. 5-10. A standard retinal drawing used to localize intraocular tumors. The drawing represents the inner curved surface of the eye. The space between the outermost circle and the middle circle represents the pars plana. The middle circle is the ora serrata, the anterior termination of the retina. The most inner circle is the geometric equator of the globe. The macula, the yellow spot in the center of the retina, is indicated by the central area of the drawing. The macula contains a pit, the fovea centralis, where closely packed cones function as the area of most acute vision. The optic nerve's exit (the optic nerve head or disk) is 2-mm medial to the macula. The disk is approximately 1.5 mm in diameter and is often used as a measure of tumor dimensions.

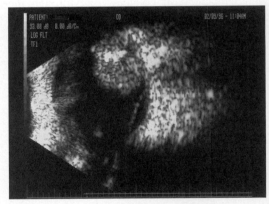

FIG. 5-11. Ultrasonography may aid the pediatric radiation oncologist in the diagnosis and treatment of retinoblastoma. This 18-month-old child had unilateral retinoblastoma. The circular globe is clearly seen in the image with the lens on the left. The tumor mass with internal calcification is seen in the upper right portion of the image of the globe. (The tumor was located superior–temporal in the patient.) Adjacent to the tumor, an area of retinal detachment is clearly seen. Preservation and restoration of vision depended on the ability to control the tumor and on reattachment of the detached retina. The ultrasound was also used to determine the distance between the front of the cornea and the back of the lens to direct the use of the Schipper device (see also Fig. 5-19).

mor calcification. A cranial CT scan may accompany the orbital study to assess the presence of intracranial extension of the primary tumor and the possibility of a synchronous pineal tumor.

Among the tests used to detect metastatic disease are a lumbar puncture with cerebrospinal fluid (CSF) cytology and a bone marrow biopsy and aspirate (34). Pratt et al. (35) reported no positive CSF cytologies or bone marrow aspirates in 109 children with RB confined to the globe. The only positive studies were in patients with extraocular tumor extension (i.e., through the sclera or beyond the cut end of the optic nerve) or with bone, distant soft tissue, or brain metastases. Pratt et al.'s data are supported by a 1997 study from Riyadh, Saudi Arabia. In children with disease confined to the eye who were treated with external beam irradiation, 0 of 49 had a positive CSF, 0 of 50 had a positive bone marrow biopsy and aspirate, and 0 of 54 had a positive bone scan. In children with more advanced disease necessitating enucleation and orbital irradiation, the frequency of positive staging studies was 0 in 27 for CSF cytology, 0 in 28 for bone marrow examination, and 0 in 26 for bone scan. In the patients presenting with locally advanced or metastatic disease there were some positive staging studies: CSF cytology positive in 7 of 31 (23%) and bone scan positive in 5 of 27 (19%) (36). In review from the Mayo Clinic, Mohney and Robertson (37) identified 100 patients seen between 1939 and 1952. Of this group, 35 had undergone bone marrow aspiration, lumbar puncture, or both within 1 month of diagnosis. In all cases, the bone marrow aspiration and lumbar puncture were negative for metastatic disease. A second review by Karcioglu (38) of patients from Riyadh, Saudi Arabia, was published in 1997. In this study, there was only 1 positive lumbar puncture among 176 tests done in patients with stages 1 and 2 disease. There were 1 positive lumbar puncture and 1 positive bone marrow aspirate among 38 patients with stage 3 disease. In patients with stage 4 disease, there were 2 positive lumbar punctures and 9 positive bone marrow aspirates among 31 patients. All of the positive diagnostic tests were in patients with choroidal RB undergoing lumbar puncture and bone marrow aspirate. None of the 11 patients with disease stages 1 through 3 had positive studies. There

was one suspicious bone marrow aspirate among 49 patients with disease stages 4 and 5. This patient had extensive orbital inflammation with adhesions of the globe to the adjacent soft tissue. None of the staging lumbar punctures, performed at the time of diagnosis, showed evidence of RB. There have been reports of positive lumbar punctures at the time of relapse, all in symptomatic patients (39). In modern practice, routine lumbar puncture and bone marrow aspiration are not justified for RB confined to the retina without optic nerve involvement or other suggestion of extraocular extension. In the presence of symptoms suggestive of metastatic disease, a bone scan and plain bone films are indicated.

PROGNOSTIC FACTORS AND STAGING

The staging system for RB must fulfill at least two requirements. First, it must predict the likelihood of cure, a requirement of all malignancy staging systems. However, an important goal of RB treatment is preservation of sight in the affected eye. To this end, some eyes are treated with chemotherapy, cryotherapy, laser photocoagulation, hyperthermia, radioactive plaque, and external beam radiotherapy as an alternative to enucleation. Therefore, the second requirement for staging is to predict the likelihood of visual preservation.

The most widely used grouping system for RB was proposed by Algernon Reese (6) and Robert Ellsworth (Table 5-1) (40). This system does not predict survival probability well. However, it does predict the chance of visual preservation with conservative therapy. At least two staging systems have attempted to predict prognosis for survival and include information on disease extension beyond the globe (9,35). Of these systems, the St. Jude Children's Research Hospital (SJCRH) system has been used somewhat more frequently (Table 5-2). The most recent clinical protocols for combined-modality RB therapy use a new system based on the work of the Children's Oncology Group and Murphee et al. of Children's Hospital of Los Angeles. This staging system is gaining increasing popularity. There is also a system that addresses intraocular and extraocular RB described by Grabowski and Abramson (Tables 5-3 and 5-4).

TABLE 5-1. *The Reese–Ellsworth system of classifying retinoblastoma*

Group I: Very favorable
  A. Solitary tumor, less than 4 DD[a] in diameter, at or behind the equator
  B. Multiple tumors, none larger than 4 DD in diameter, all at or behind the equator
Group II: Favorable
  A. Solitary tumor, 4–10 DD in diameter, at or behind the equator
  B. Multiple tumors, 4–10 DD in diameter, all at or behind the equator
Group III: Doubtful
  A. Any lesion anterior to the equator
  B. Solitary tumors, larger than 10 DD in diameter, behind the equator
Group IV: Unfavorable
  A. Multiple tumors, some larger than 10 DD
  B. Any lesion extending anterior to the ora serrata
Group V: Very unfavorable
  A. Massive tumors involving more than half of the retina
  B. Vitreous seeding

[a]The optic nerve's exit (the optic nerve head or disk) is approximately 1.5 mm in diameter. The disk diameter (DD) often is used as a measure of tumor dimensions.
Based on references 2, 6, 15, and 40.

TABLE 5-2. *The St. Jude Children's Research Hospital staging system of retinoblastoma*

  I. Intraocular diseases
    Ia. Retinal tumor, single or multiple
    Ib. Extension to lamina cribrosa
    Ic. Uveal extension
  II. Orbital disease
    IIa. Orbital tumor
      IIa1. Scattered episcleral cells
      IIa2. Orbital invasion
    IIb. Optic nerve
      IIb1. Invasion of optic nerve to cut end
      IIb2. Invasion of optic nerve beyond cut end
  III. Intracranial metastases
    IIa. Positive cerebrospinal fluid
    IIb. Mass lesion in the central nervous system
  IV. Hematogenous metastasis
  IVa. Positive bone marrow
  IVb. Facial bone lesions with or without positive marrow
  IVc. Other organ involvement

From Schvartzman E, Chantado G, Fandino A, et al. Results of a stage-based protocol for the treatment of retinoblastoma. *J Clin Oncol* 1996;14:1532–1536 and Chan HSL, DeBaer G, Thiessen JJ, et al. Combining cyclosporin with chemotherapy controls intraocular retinoblastoma without requiring radiation. *Clin Cancer Res* 1996;2:1499–1508.

TABLE 5-3. *Staging retinoblastoma with separate classifications for intraocular and extraocular advanced disease: Grabowski and Abramson staging for intraocular and extraocular retinoblastoma*

Stage	Tumor localization
I	Intraocular disease
	a. Retinal disease
	b. Extension to lamina cribrosa
	c. Uveal extension
II	Orbital disease
	a. Orbital tumor
	a1. Scattered episcleral cells
	a2. Orbital invasion
	b. Optic nerve
	b1. Invasion up to cut end
	b2. Invasion beyond cut end
III	Intracranial metastasis
	a. Positive cerebrospinal fluid alone
	b. Mass lesion in the central nervous system
IV	Hematogenous metastasis
	a. Positive bone marrow alone
	b. Focal bone lesions with or without bone marrow disease

From Grabowski EF, and Abramson DH. Intraocular and extraocular retinoblastoma. *Hematol Oncol Clin North Am* 1987;1:721–735, with permission.

TABLE 5-4. *ABC Classification for Intraocular Retinoblastoma*

Group A
  Small tumors confined to the retina
  No tumor greater than 3 mm in diameter
  No tumor less than 2 DD (3 mm) from fovea or 1 DD (1.5 mm) from optic nerve
  No vitreous seeding
  No RD
Group B
  Tumors confined to the retina; any location
  No vitreous seeding
  No retinal detachment more than 5 mm from tumor base
Group C
  Fine diffuse or localized vitreous or subretinal seeding
  No tumor masses, clumps, or snowballs in the vitreous or the subretinal space
  More than 5 mm RD to total RD
Group D
  Massive vitreous or subretinal seeding
  Snowballs or tumor masses in the vitreous or subretinal space
  More than 5 mm RD to total RD
Group E
  No visual potential or presence of one or more of the following:
    Tumor in the anterior segment
    Tumor in or on the ciliary body
    Neovascular glaucoma
    Vitreous hemorrhage obscuring the tumor or significant hyphema
    Phthisical or prephthisical eye
    Orbital cellulitis-like presentation

DD, disk diameter; RD, retinal detachment.

HISTOLOGIC EVALUATION OF RB

RB is a poorly differentiated malignant neuro-ectodermal tumor. There are often significant necrotic and apoptotic changes. Although the cytologic details of the tumor may vary from case to case, the cell type, the degree of differentiation, and necrosis have not been defined in themselves as risk factors for local recurrence or metastasis (41). Some have asserted that poorly differentiated tumors are more likely to respond to radiation, but this information is not available at the time of radiation treatment. Some investigators believe that there is an association between vascular density and prognosis in RB. This may merit further investigation (42).

Classically, four growth patterns are recognized in RB:

- Endophytic RB, which grows from the retina toward the vitreous, appears to be a mass protruding into the vitreous chamber. These often friable and necrotic tumors may produce small clusters of tumor cells that are detached from the main mass and form satellite tumor nodules. These can range from localized tumor nodules within the vitreous, known as vitreous seeding, up to diffuse involvement, which some call the *snowstorm effect*.
- Exophytic RB typically grows from the outer retinal layers and extends beneath the detached retina toward the choroid. Dislodged masses may implant on the retinal pigment epithelium and erode through Bruch's membrane into the choroid.
- Diffuse plaquelike RB defies common morphologic patterns. It grows diffusely and insidiously in the retina without forming a detectable mass. Such a growth pattern can present a confusing clinical picture.
- A mixed endophytic and exophytic pattern may also occur (42).

RISK FACTORS FOR METASTASES IN RB THAT CAN BE IDENTIFIED AT THE TIME OF ENUCLEATION

The ocular pathologist plays a crucial role in determining whether RB has a risk of dissemination because it has broken out of its ocular confines. Reported risk factors include the following:

- Optic nerve invasion: The presence of tumor beyond the lamina cribrosa is a risk factor for metastatic disease because access to the subarachnoid space allows RB cells to spread to the spinal fluid and central nervous system. Optic nerve invasion is present in approximately one-third of nucleated globes and often correlates the presence of choroidal or scleral extension. Optic nerve invasion is categorized as preliminary, laminar, postlaminar, and up to the line of transection. The latter occurrence is quite rare. In a study of 261 cases, the multivariate risk of metastasis was 9 when the optic nerve was involved up to the resection line, compared with 4 when the RB extended retrolaminar but not up to the resection line. A study of 172 patients found that the disease-free survival rate was 97% when the optic nerve was not involved and 55% when it was involved up to the line of resection. The prognosis was intermediate with retrolaminar involvement. When patients with extrascleral extension and optic nerve involvement up to the resection line were excluded, retrolaminar involvement still was a significant prognostic factor for metastasis (43,156).
- Uveal invasion: Choroidal invasion has long been considered an important risk factor for metastatic disease because it allows the tumor access the scleral and emissary veins. However, choroidal invasion is difficult to quantify. In a study from Wills Eye Hospital, it appeared that patients with choroidal invasion were more likely to develop distant metastasis than those without. However, when patients with optic nerve invasion were excluded, there was no longer a significant risk, although there was still a trend toward the metastasis with choroidal invasion ($p = 0.1$) (43).
- Orbital invasion: When tumor extends to the sclera, it gains access to the vascular and lymphatic channels outside the eye. This creates a significant risk for metastatic disease and is generally considered an indication for more aggressive local and systemic treatment. Microscopic orbital extension often is impossi-

ble to diagnose by clinical examination. Preoperatively, larger extensions may be imaged by ultrasound, CT, or magnetic resonance imaging (MRI).

- Choroidal involvement: Invasion of the choroid usually is considered a poor prognostic sign. It is almost certainly true that hematogenous spread of RB occurs via choroidal vessels. However, choroidal invasion is not rare; it occurs in up to 62% of cases. Distant metastases are rare. It seems that the prognostic correlation is less with choroidal invasion alone than with the *volume* of choroidal invasion and its correlation with other risk factors.

Involvement of the optic nerve beyond the lamina cribrosa is a risk factor for orbital recurrence and central nervous system (CNS) dissemination. Even worse is the involvement of the distal cut end of the optic nerve with tumor (3). Tumor involvement of the scleral emisseric veins and episcleral tissues also forebodes a poor prognosis. Multivariate analysis of data from 330 children at St. Bartholomew's Hospital and Moorfield's Eye Hospital showed that the deleterious effect of extensive choroidal invasion as a prognostic factor was lost in the absence of retrolaminar invasion or invasion of the cut end of the optic nerve. Two patient groups had a particularly poor prognosis: retrolaminar extension and extensive choroidal invasion (5-year survival 31%) and extensive choroidal invasion and invasion of the cut end of the optic nerve (5-year survival 25%) (5). In 62 children only one death was attributable to metastatic disease from choroidal invasion alone (44,45).

SELECTION OF THERAPY

The primary goal of RB therapy is cure. Because RB infrequently metastasizes, the chance of cure is excellent. The actuarial overall 5-year survival rate for 731 children with RB seen at St. Bartholomew's Hospital and Moorfield's Eye Hospital from 1960 to 1988 was 87% (5). The 50-month actuarial overall survival of 52 SJCRH patients with initial intraocular disease was 97% (9). Therefore, it is ap-

propriate to assert that a secondary goal of treatment is preservation of vision in the affected eye. Enucleation is recommended only in a blind eye or an eye for which there is no reasonable expectation of sight after cryotherapy, phototherapy, or radiotherapy. Every effort should be made to preserve vision in a sighted eye. This rule pertains to both bilateral and unilateral disease. Often, however, children with unilateral disease have locally advanced tumors with little hope of vision, so many of these patients undergo enucleation. In bilateral disease, enucleation of the more severely affected eye is indicated only if this eye is blind. If both eyes are sighted, then an effort should be made to preserve both eyes.

Enucleation

In an enucleation for RB, anterior traction is placed on the globe after the rectus muscles are severed. The optic nerve is then cut near its exit from the socket. Obtaining a long segment of nerve is important if the tumor is within the nerve. In young children, orbital growth slows after enucleation. As the child grows, the orbit appears small. This may be ameliorated by a properly fitting orbital prosthesis.

A review of the New York Hospital experience showed that primary enucleation was performed in 97% of eyes in unilateral cases seen from 1951 to 1965 and 87% from 1966 to 1980. Enucleation was used in 67% of eyes in bilateral cases treated from 1951 to 1965 and 58% in 1966 to 1980 (46). Similarly, Shields et al. reported a reduction in the proportion of children having an eye removed for RB from 96% in 1974 to 1978 to 75% for 1984 to 1988 (38,39, 47,48).

Enucleation is indicated in unilateral RB, where the eye is blind. In bilateral RB when both eyes are blind, a bilateral enucleation is done. If one eye is blind, a unilateral enucleation is done. Enucleation is also indicated in unilateral or bilateral tumor when glaucoma follows rubeosis iridis with visual loss. It is also recommended when local recurrence of tumor can no longer be controlled with more conservative measures (15,49) (Fig. 5-12).

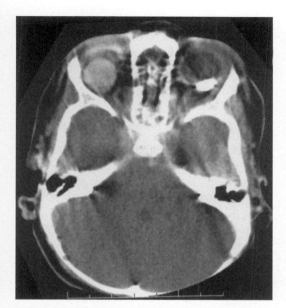

FIG. 5-12. Bilateral retinoblastoma treated with enucleation on one side with a prosthesis in place. A calcified macular lesion is seen in the remaining eye.

Exenteration

An exenteration is the removal of the globe, extraocular muscles, lids, nerves, and orbital fat. Blood loss may be significant. In the opinion of some ophthalmologists, the indications for exenteration in RB include extensive local tumor breaching the globe (exenteration in this situation generally is followed by postoperative radiotherapy and chemotherapy) and recurrence of tumor in the socket after enucleation. However, some cases of local recurrence may be locally managed with external beam radiotherapy, a radioactive implant or a radioactive mold, and chemotherapy.

Local Therapy

The four local therapies for RB are cryotherapy, photocoagulation, laser hyperthermia, and radioactive plaque applications.

Until the early 1990s, in children at high risk for multicentric disease, local therapy was thought to be appropriate only when there could be serial follow-up with repeated local therapy or with external beam radiotherapy when neces-

sary. In children with bilateral disease, an average of five tumor foci are randomly distributed (2,50). These foci may not appear simultaneously but may occur months after successful local treatment of the sentinel lesion. In children with multifocal disease or in those at high risk of developing multifocal disease, as well as in children with large tumors, it was believed that local therapy generally should not be used.

Modern thinking concerning local therapy is very different. With the increase in use of systemic chemotherapy, local therapy is now used in multifocal disease. Local therapy may be interspersed with chemotherapy or follow it. Programs using focal therapy in this way are reviewed later in this chapter.

Photocoagulation

The technique of photocoagulation is based on obliteration of the retinal vessels. With the child under anesthesia, a white retinal burn, surrounding the tumor by 1 mm, is painted with the laser beam. Special attention is directed to closing feeding vessels (57). The tumor is encircled by the burn, and regression depends on interruption of blood supply. Direct photocoagulation of RB should be avoided because small explosions can release viable tumor cells into the vitreous and lead to tumor recurrence (5). In primary therapy, photocoagulation may be used for tumors up to 4.5 mm at the base and up to 2.5 mm thick if they are not close to the macula or disk, where retinal damage would generate a large scotoma. Vitreous seeding is a contraindication (12,49). Photocoagulation may be used for small tumor recurrences after irradiation to avoid the risks of reirradiation. With proper case selection, photocoagulation has a local tumor control probability of about 70% (51).

Laser Hyperthermia

Laser hyperthermia is generated by a diode laser (810 nm) on continuous mode. A single spot, 0.8 to 2.0 mm in diameter, is placed on the center of the tumor using the aiming beam. An output of 300 to 700 mW is selected based on the tumor size. Tumors are heated for 10 to 30 minutes per session. It is estimated that a central tumor temperature of about 46°C is reached. As the heat disperses through the tumor, the temperature decreases about 2°C for each millimeter beyond the treatment spot. In this technique the heat is used principally to enhance the binding and cytotoxicity of platinum drugs, a method supported by experiments using rabbit ocular melanoma (52,153,154). Whole eye hyperthermia in combination with external beam irradiation has been shown to be effective in controlling murine transgenic RB but to our knowledge has not been used in humans (53).

Cryotherapy

With cryotherapy a tumor is localized and indented, transsclerally, with a nitrous oxide cryoprobe. The freeze (−80°C) is then applied until the tumor is completely covered with a frozen vitreous. The freeze–thaw cycle is repeated at least three times (54,55). Cryotherapy is indicated for the primary therapy of RB in small tumors anterior to the equator, without vitreous seeding, which can be reached with the cryoprobe (posterior tumors are difficult to reach, and the risks of freezing the macula or nerve increase); in local recurrence or tumor persistence after irradiation; and in conjunction with chemotherapy (46).

Cryotherapy can induce acute retinal edema and accumulation of subretinal fluid. To avoid retinal detachment, some ophthalmologists use the laser to create a retinal barrier to fluid leakage. Disruption of the retina by cryotherapy may increase intravitreal penetration of systemic carboplatin (55).

Radioactive Plaque Application

Plaques are used for solitary 2- to 16-mm basal diameter unilateral lesions located more than 3 mm from the optic disk or fovea, generally less than 10 mm thick, for two lesions that are small enough or close enough to be covered by one plaque, and for local failure after other therapy (Fig. 5-13). Plaques can be used if there is a small amount of vitreous seeding over the tumor apex (11,33,56–59).

Before the operative procedure, the tumor's maximum basal diameter and maximum height are ascertained by physical examination and ultrasonography. In treatment planning, it is customary to allow 1 mm for scleral thickness, although there is some normal variation in this measurement (60,61). The operative procedure begins with a careful eye examination using magnifying lenses. After confirming the tumor anatomy, the surgeon opens the conjunctiva around the periphery of the limbus (a peritomy). Muscle hooks are used to snare rectus muscles and rotate the eye. Traction sutures sometimes are used. It may be necessary to disinsert a muscle in order to visualize the tumor. With the

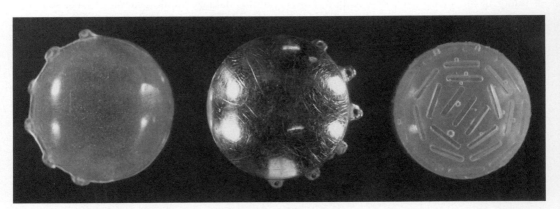

FIG. 5-13. Equipment for ^{125}I ocular plaque construction and placement includes a dummy plaque to aid in the placement of the necessary retention sutures *(left)*, a gold backing with lug holes for sutures *(center)*, and a plastic insert to hold the radioactive ^{125}I seeds *(right)*.

room darkened, a transilluminator is placed over the pupil. The shadow cast by the tumor is marked on the sclera with a marking pen or with electrocautery. Tumors that cannot be transilluminated are located by ultrasound. A clear dummy plaque is then brought into the operative field. We allow 2 mm of margin on either side of the basal diameter; that is, an 8-mm tumor is plaqued with a 12-mm device. The dummy is used to place the two sutures through the lug holes and into the sclera. The dummy is then replaced with the radioactive plaque. The retention sutures are tied, and the eye is rotated back into place. The conjunctiva is then closed. The patient generally remains hospitalized for the duration of the application. The plaque is then removed (62).

Several plaque types are available. The ^{60}Co plaque (1.17 and 1.33 MeV, half-life 5.2 years) may be purchased in a circular or crescentic configuration to fit around the optic nerve (63). The ^{60}Co ball applicator is a platinum-coated 6-mm sphere attached to a ring (16). The ^{125}I plaque (27 to 35 keV, half-life 60 days) with lip consists of ^{125}I seeds glued in a carrier within a gold shield. These plaques are available in a circular or notched configuration. ^{192}Ir (295 to 612 keV, half-life 74.5 days) and ^{109}Ru (beta emitter) plaques are also available (64,65).

Each of the four available plaques (^{60}Co, ^{125}I, ^{192}Ir, and ^{109}Ru) has advantages and disadvantages. ^{60}Co plaques may be purchased and assembled in standard sizes. The long half-life means that the plaque may be used for several years before the treatment times become unacceptably long. The high-energy ^{60}Co and the breadth of the high-dose isodose curves mean that thick and infiltrative tumors can be treated. However, shielding of periocular normal tissues behind the plaque is impossible. Effective shielding on the back of the plaque is achievable with ^{125}I and ^{109}Ru. Shielding from the gold lip on the ^{125}I plaque necessitates expert placement lest tumor be missed. ^{125}I plaques must be assembled for each case; although this involves extra work, it allows individualization of the plaque. Hospital personnel exposure is minimal with ^{125}I or ^{109}Ru. A shielded ^{125}I plaque with a lead eye patch allows the nursing staff and the

child's parents to provide care while observing appropriate radiation safety precautions (11,33,56–59).

Using ^{60}Co plaques, Stallard (66) administered 40 Gy to the tumor apex in 1 week. Sixty-three of 69 children with tumor involving one-fourth of the retinal area or less were successfully treated with a plaque. When the tumor involved one-fourth to one-half of the retinal area, success was achieved in eight of ten instances. Among the best-characterized clinical series of plaque brachytherapy for RB is that of the Wills Eye Hospital of Philadelphia (11,33, 57–59,68). This series describes the outcome for more than 140 children with RB treated between 1976 and 1999. In these children, 148 tumors were treated with radioactive plaques for recurrent or residual RB after other therapies failed, and 60 tumors were treated primarily with plaques. The median tumor dosage at the tumor apex was 40 Gy, with ^{125}I used in almost 90% of all plaques. During a median follow-up of 34 months, recurrences developed in 17% and 20% of cases at 1 and 4 years, respectively. In tumors treated with a radioactive plaque as primary therapy, recurrences were observed in 12%, and 20% of tumors for which other treatments failed exhibited recurrence after plaque radiotherapy. Metastases developed in only four patients, all with Reese–Ellsworth group Vb tumors. On multivariate analysis, the risk of recurrence was increased significantly by the presence of vitreous or retinal seeds and by increasing age at diagnosis (68). In earlier studies, visual acuity of 20/400 or better was obtained in 62% (57–59).

In the past, it was reported that for large tumors with vitreous seeds, multiple sequential plaques (rotating plaques) could be used. In this technique, two plaques are applied in one operation to opposite quadrants of the eye. In a second operation these two plaques are rotated to the remaining quadrants. In a third operation the plaques are removed. This technique delivers about 40 Gy to the midvitreous and 160 Gy to the sclera. Initial reports indicated that useful vision was retained in 14 of 16 patients treated with plaques as the single irradiation modality. Useful vision was retained in 22 of 36 patients plaqued after failure of some other treatment (11,33,58). Later reports showed a significant incidence of radiation retinopathy with this technique, and it has been largely abandoned (62).

In carefully selected patients with small primary RB or for recurrent tumors after other treatment, a radioactive single-plaque application of 30 to 40 Gy to the tumor apex is reasonable therapy. With growth in the use of chemotherapy as primary treatment for RB, plaque therapy has joined photocoagulation, laser treatment, and cryotherapy as an adjuvant focal treatment after or interspersed with chemotherapy. When a plaque is used in a child who has also received chemotherapy, many ophthalmologists believe that 40 Gy as an apical dosage is too high. The occurrence of a few cases of postbrachytherapy retinitis has led to a dosage reduction to 25 to 30 Gy to the tumor apex (52). Plaques have little chance of producing orbital bone hypoplasia and should not contribute to the risk of orbital bone sarcoma. Long-term complications of plaque radiotherapy include retinopathy, cataracts, maculopathy, papillopathy, and glaucoma (33,58,68). In the Wills Eye Hospital series of more than 140 children treated with plaque radiotherapy, only one second cancer was observed in the field of plaque irradiation over a mean follow-up of 49 months (68).

External Beam Radiotherapy

When RB is multifocal or close to the macula or optic nerve with preservation of vision, it has been found that cryotherapy, photocoagulation, or plaque therapy by itself is not adequate and that enucleation is too drastic. In such situations, which are quite common, external beam irradiation or chemotherapy with focal therapy is used. These types of therapy are also indicated for large tumors and vitreous seeding. Hilgartner (69) reported treatment of a case of bilateral RB with X-rays in 1910. Verhoeff cured a case of RB with X-ray treatment in 1918. The patient died in 1972 with tumor controlled (70). Historically, the Reese–Ellsworth grouping system has been used to predict the probability of success for external beam irradiation (Tables 5-1, 5-5, and 5-6). Large lesions tend to fail after teletherapy. Some say that anterior lesions are also more likely to fail after teletherapy, but the risk of failure of anterior lesions probably was related to the practice, by some radiotherapists, of treating with a lateral beam with the anterior field edge at the rim of the bony orbit. This technique underdoses the anterior globe (8,12, 71–74). Technical factors play a large role in the probability of success of external beam therapy and the frequency of complications.

Technique

The goals of conventional external beam radiotherapy are to provide a homogeneous and tumoricidal dose to the retinal anlage and vitreous and to respect tolerance of normal tissue structures. At least five arguments have been put forward in support of this expansive view of treatment volume. First, in many cases RB represents a field change in which all retinal cells have a genetic neoplastic potential; therefore, the entire retina must be treated. Second, vitreous seeding can occur. Third, multiple tumors may arise from a primary RB. Fourth, the tumor may spread via the subretinal space. Finally, retinal differentiation progresses from posterior to anterior and from superior to inferior. Subclinical disease may exist in the immature retina and must be included in the treatment (17). The argument in favor of a more restrictive tumor volume is that selected cases will be unilateral and unifocal and therefore amenable to more focal irradiation, as might be delivered to a fixed target with protons.

The dimensions of the eye of young children have been well characterized. The outer sagittal diameter of the eye varies from 16 to 17 mm at birth and increases rapidly to an average of 22.5 to 23 mm at 3 years of age (60,61). In any individual patient the axial intraocular dimensions may be measured by ultrasonic biometry and ocular CT (Fig. 5-14).

One of the earliest techniques for the external beam irradiation of RB was developed by Algernon Reese in the 1930s. Using an orthovoltage unit, treatment was delivered through temporal and nasal portals. The technique attempted to

TABLE 5-5. *Visual preservation in retinoblastoma with external beam irradiation as a function of initial Reese–Ellsworth group[a]*

Study (reference number)	Reese–Ellsworth group				
	I	II	III	IV	V
Columbia 1969 (12)[a]	84%(43)[b]	67% (45)	69% (33)	30% (37)	15% (66)
Stanford 1987 (13)[a]	88% (8)	60% (5)	67% (8)	0% (2)	33% (15)
Cornell 1983, children < 6 months old (64)[c,d]	89%	82%	80%	56%	10%
Utrecht 1985 (83)	100% (14)	100% (9)	83% (10)	79% (14)	0% (5)
Norwegian Radium Hospital 1986 (153)[a]	100% (5)	100% (5)	100% (1)	100% (1)	—
Curie Institute 1987 (152)[e]	0% (1)	100% (2)	0% (1)	50% (2)	38% (13)
Cornell 1988 (72,73)[a,d,f]	—	—	100% (31)	—	60% (14)
Mayo 1989[a] (17)	100% (1)	100% (1)	85% (13)	50% (14)	83% (6)
Arhus 1989 (151)[c]	—	—	61% (46)	—	—
Wills Eye Hospital 1990 (11)[g]	100% (2)	83%	100% (6)	67% (3)	50% (5)
Duke 1992 (80)[a,h]	—	—	100% (8)	100% (8)	100% (4)s
University of Washington and South Florida 1994 (92a)[e,h,i]	—	83%/100% (6)	71%/71% (7)	—	—
St. Jude Children's Research Hospital 1995, >1 yr old (77)[j]	100% (1)	67%/67% (6)	67%/100% (3)	100% (1)	57%/100% (7)
St. Bartholomew's Hospital 1995 (75), whole eye technique[j]	88%/100% (16)	56%/84% (55)	59%/82% (68)	14%/43% (7)	45%/66% (29)
St. Bartholomew's Hospital 1995 (84), lens-sparing technique[j]	78%/100% (18)	67%/88% (33)	64%/91% (11)	100% (5)	—
St. Jude Children's Research Hospital 1996, <1 yr old (90)[j]	75%/100% (20)	100% (6)	50%/100% (6)	100% (2)	43%/57% (7)
Memorial Sloan–Kettering and the New York Hospital–Cornell 1996 (71)[j]	67%/88% (96)	67%/88% (96)	67%/88% (96)	44%/60%	44%/60%
Duke 1996 (81)	86% (15)	86% (15)	86% (15)	86% (15)	—
Hahneman University and Wills Eye Hospital 1996 (93)	79% (4)	79% (10)	20% (7)	20% (2)	20% (11)
King Faisal Specialist Hospital and Research Center 1997 (36)[a,e]	86% (7)	100% (6)	50% (3)	67% (15)	54% (28)
University of Miami and University of California at San Francisco 1999 (166)	—	—	—	—	83% (24)
St. Jude Children's Research Hospital 2002 (167)[d,e]	—	95% (24)	—	66% (20)	—

[a]Patients were treated with external beam radiotherapy, but cryotherapy, plaques, or laser therapy may have been used for salvage. In some series, the need for additional treatment after radiotherapy approaches 50%.
[b]The numbers in parentheses in the body of the table are the number of eyes per group.
[c]Patients were treated with a variety of primary therapies.
[d]These series probably share some patients.
[e]These patients also received chemotherapy.
[f]Modified lateral beam technique was used.
[g]Primary therapy included external beam treatment or plaque.
[h]These series principally contained macular tumors.
[i]Lateral field only.
[j]The first number is control with radiotherapy alone; the second number is eye preservation including focal salvage therapy.

avoid the lens by having the nasal portal angled 24 to 30 degrees (Fig. 5-15). A high bone dosage was given by the orthovoltage apparatus. A "saddle nose" deformity developed in long-term survivors along with depression of the temporal bone (7).

In modern pediatric radiation oncology, patient immobilization is recognized as crucial to delivering the designated treatment volume precisely while minimizing radiation to normal tissue. In RB treatment, anesthesia is generally needed.

TABLE 5-6. *Reported eye preservation rates after lens-sparing external beam radiation therapy (RT)*

Author (reference)	Year of report	Number of eyes irradiated	Groups I–V		Groups I–III	
			RT	RT and salvage	RT	RT and salvage
Cassady (12)	1969	223	49%	69%	—	73%
Egbert (13)	1978	38	—	58%	—	80%
Schipper (83)	1985	54	41%	81%	54%	94%
Foote (17)	1989	25	29%	79%	40%	80%
Fontanesi (77,90)	1995, 1996	7[a]	71%	71%	67%	67%
		13[b]	67%	76%	60%	100%
Toma (84)	1995	67	72%	93%	69%	92%
Blach (71)	1996	67[c]	38%	71%	37%	81%
Scott (166)	1999	113[d]	65%	78%	84%	94%

[a]>1 yr of age.
[b]<1 yr of age.
[c]Anterior lens-sparing technique or modified lateral beam technique.
[d]Modified lateral beam technique.

Immobilization and anesthesia for pediatric radiotherapy are fully discussed in Chapters 21 and 22. Two special points are warranted in this discussion. When a plaster or thermoplastic head holder is prepared for treatment and the anesthesia gas mask is placed, care must be taken to allow an unobstructed view of the eye so that the fields may be correctly set. Second, ketamine anesthesia produces lateral nystagmus. If a blocking technique is used that relies on the eye being a stable target, then ketamine generally is unacceptable as the anesthetic agent.

The contemporary radiotherapist may consider a large number of techniques. However, several have passed from favor as conformal radiotherapy has gained popularity.

- A lateral-beam megavoltage technique with the anterior field border set at the lateral bony orbit has been used. A direct lateral field is

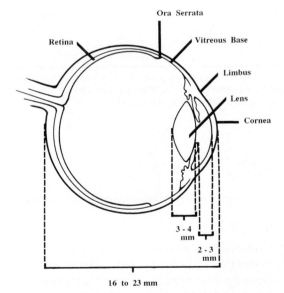

FIG. 5-14. The range of measurements of relevant dimensions of a young child's eye. Measurements may be made by ultrasound.

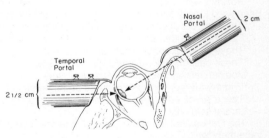

FIG. 5-15. In the 1930s, Reese used orthovoltage beams to externally irradiate retinoblastoma while attempting to spare the lens. The high bone dosage produced cosmetic deformities. (From Abramson DH. Treatment of retinoblastoma. In: Blodi FC, ed. *Contemporary issues in ophthalmology,* vol 2: *Retinoblastoma.* New York: Churchill Livingstone, 1985:63–93, with permission.)

used after enucleation in the contralateral side. When the contralateral globe is in place, the beam is slightly angled posteriorly in an attempt to avoid exit radiation into the lens of the other eye (Fig. 5-16) (74). The distance from the back of the lens to the ora serrata is 1 to 1.5 mm, making techniques that endeavor to treat the entire retina from a lateral approach but miss the posterior part of the lens highly impractical (64). Use of only a lateral beam may result in tumor recurrence at or near the ora serrata (7,12,74). However, small anterior failures can be treated with cryother-

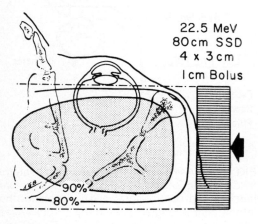

22.5 MeV
80cm SSD
4 x 3cm
1cm Bolus

90%
80%

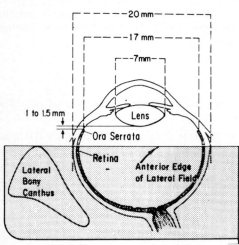

20 mm
17 mm
7mm
1 to 1.5mm
Lens
Ora Serrata
Retina
Lateral Bony Canthus
Anterior Edge of Lateral Field

FIG. 5-16. A direct lateral supervoltage field with anterior border set at the bony orbit. (From Cassady JR, Sagerman RH, Tretter P, et al. Radiation therapy in retinoblastoma. *Radiology* 1969; 93:405–409, with permission.)

apy, so if there is no gross disease near the ora serrata, this technique may be adequate (7). The lateral field is shaped to spare the pituitary and some of the tooth buds. This produces a *D*-shaped field.

- A direct anterior ^{60}Co or linear accelerator field treats the entire eye and spares the opposite eye. There is no sparing of the lens, cataract formation is almost certain, the lacrimal gland is fully irradiated (thereby potentially impairing tear production), and radiation exits through the brain. However, the single anterior field is easy to set up, is reproducible, and homogeneously irradiates the entire vitreous and retina (7,15,40,71–73,75). Because the cataract takes time to develop, mitigating the problem of disuse amblyopia, and may be treated surgically, advocates of the anterior field are assuaged (76–78).

- A half-beam blocked lateral field has been used to sharpen the beam edge. Field sizes ranging from 3 × 6 cm to 5 × 10 cm typically are used for a 3 × 3-cm to 5 × 5-cm treatment area. The field edge may be set at the bony orbit or between the bone and the limbus. A field anterior edge about halfway between the limbus and the edge of the bony orbit will cover the ora serrata. Treatment may be given with a lateral beam with photons alone or with mixed photon and electron straight lateral and lateral oblique beams (7, 40,71–73,79) For children with unilateral disease, many clinicians replace straight lateral fields with oblique fields. Superior and inferior oblique fields miss the uninvolved eye. The price of an inferior oblique field is exit radiation into the frontal lobe of the brain. A superior oblique field exits into the maxillary sinus and mouth (Fig. 5-17).

- A two-field technique using a lateral field and an anterior field with a hanging lens block is an attempt to achieve a homogeneous retinal dosage yet spare the lens (Fig. 5-18) (7,8, 23,77,78,80,81). The fields are weighted 75–80% from the lateral and 20–25% from the anterior. There are two alternative techniques. One continues to use the lateral field but uses an anterior electron field with a contact lens–mounted lead block for the lens.

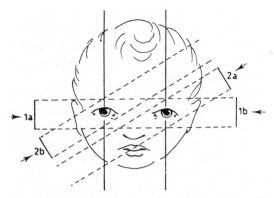

FIG. 5-17. In this schematic, fields 1a and 1b demonstrate simultaneous irradiation of bilateral disease with opposed fields. Fields 2a and 2b illustrate the use of oblique fields in unilateral disease intended to spare the opposite eye. (From Dr. Jan Schipper, *Thesis retinoblastoma,* 1980, illustrated in *Ophthalmology* 1996;103:263–268, with permission.)

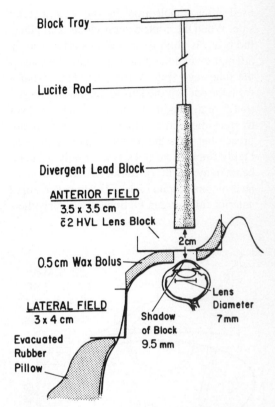

FIG. 5-18. A two-field technique using a lateral field with an anterior field and a hanging eye block. If the contralateral eye is in place, the lateral field is angled posteriorly. (From Weiss DR, Cassady JR, Peterson R. Retinoblastoma: a modification in radiation therapy technique. *Radiology* 1975;114:705–708, with permission.)

Small displacements of the contact lens will significantly affect the dosage from the anterior field (7,40,71–73). A second modification uses anterior photons without the hanging eye block when it is feared that the hanging block will shield a posterior pole tumor (81).

• Schipper (82,83) has described a precision lateral technique that calls for a specially devised machine-mounted device that, by way of a scale, sets the anterior field edge just behind the lens (Fig. 5-19). Measurement of the lens depth in each patient is necessary for proper beam alignment (79,82, 83). This elegant technique is particularly appropriate for posterior pole lesions (5). Schipper's technique uses a linear accelerator, modified with a beam splitter and extended collimation system, to produce a nondivergent and almost penumbra-free anterior beam edge. The depth of the posterior margin of the lens is measured by ultrasound. A contact lens or plumb bob with an attached rod and scale measuring system allows placement of the beam behind the lens. A straight or angled lateral beam is used, depending on whether the clinician wants to avoid exit radiation to the other eye (84).

• A superior dosage distribution for RB treatment might be achieved with a proton beam. With a lateral approach, the patient with unilateral RB would benefit from sparing of the other eye because of the stopping characteristics of the protons related to deposition of energy via the Bragg peak. Even in bilateral cases the possibility of sparing some normal tissue is held out as a benefit to reduce the risks of radiation-induced malignancy. Several institutions worldwide are treating RB with proton therapy. The conformal dosage

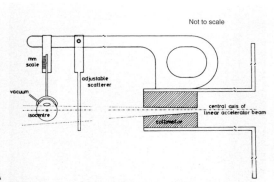
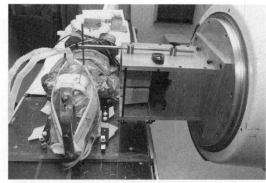

A   B

FIG. 5-19. (A) A special retinoblastoma treatment applicator designed to set the treatment beam just at the posterior pole of the lens. The position is adjusted with the scale and contact lens assembly. (From Harnett AN, Hungerford J, Lambert G, et al. Modern lateral external beam [lens sparing] radiotherapy for retinoblastoma. *Ophthalmic Paediatr Genet* 1987;8:53–61, with permission.) **(B)** A modification of such a device in operation. Such devices eventually may be replaced by intensity-modulated radiation therapy.

distribution related to the spread-out Bragg peak of proton beams makes it attractive in the external beam treatment of RB. One would hope to reduce late effects by using protons insofar as one can minimize the dosage to surrounding bone and soft tissue. This is intended to reduce the risk of treatment-related second malignant neoplasms (37–39). Proton irradiation conformal techniques in a fractionated schema are also available (85–87).

• Intensity-modulated radiation therapy (IMRT) is used to externally irradiate RB at many centers. It can be used to treat the entire globe or to spare the lens while irradiating all or part of the retina. IMRT may deliver substantially less radiation to surrounding periocular bone or soft tissues than conventional photon or electron beams do. Six to eight lateral or oblique fields may be used (Fig. 5-20).

Which is the best technique for external beam treatment of RB? In a retrospective review from Riyadh, Saudi Arabia, Pradhan et al. (36) compared eye survival in 26 children treated with external beam radiotherapy with lateral fields to 38 children in whom anterior fields were used for part or all of the treatment. Forty-four of the total population of 64 children (84%) had group IV or V disease. No difference in eye survival

was found between the two groups. However, Foote et al. (17) at the Mayo Clinic reported a benefit to whole eye irradiation using anterior fields rather than a lateral lens-sparing technique. The tumor control rate with the former (7 of 11, 64%) was stated to be superior to the latter (29%), but the overall ocular survival was comparable between the two techniques (whole eye 82%, lens sparing 79%). An excellent retrospective comparison of lens-sparing and whole eye irradiation for disease groups I to III from St. Bartholomew's Hospital, London, included 201 children. The eye preservation rate was 85% after whole eye and 92% after lens-sparing radiotherapy (*p* = 0.55) (75,84).

Blach et al. (71) updated a series by McCormick et al. (72,73) that indicated, in a retrospective review, that a lateral beam technique with the beam edge set 2 to 3 mm behind the limbus is preferred to a technique using a more posteriorly set lateral beam and an anterior electron field with lens-sparing block. The more posterior field arrangement was associated with anterior failures. Many other series confirm anterior failures when anterior segment–sparing techniques are used (Fig. 5-19) (71–73). Twenty patients with large macular RB were treated at Duke with a lateral 4-MV photon half-blocked beam set halfway between the limbus and bony orbit and an anterior field (sometimes using a

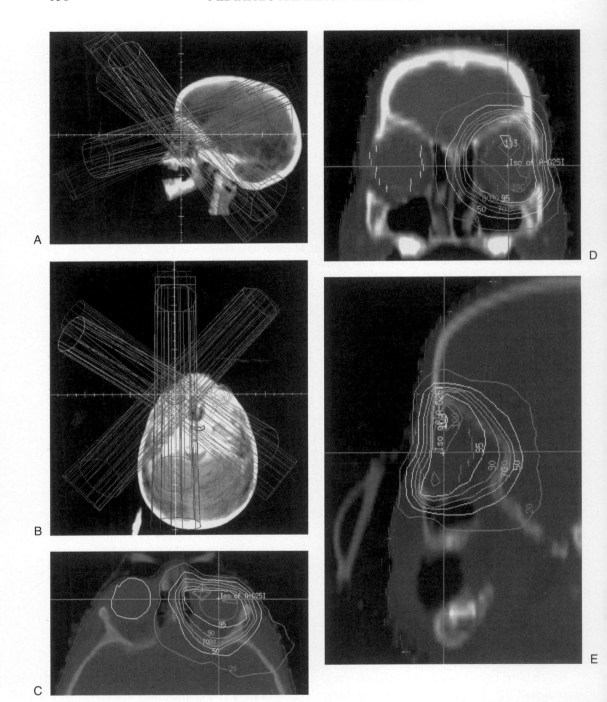

FIG. 5-20. Many centers now use conformal radiotherapy to treat retinoblastoma. Three-, five-, six-, and eight-field non-coplanar plans have been described using multileaf collimators. This plan is a six-field unilateral arrangement with non-coplanar fields. The left eye is being treated (image **B** is a view from above). **(A, B)** Reconstructed radiographs in the sagittal and axial views. **(C–E)** Dosage distributions in the axial, coronal, and sagittal views. The anesthesia mask is seen in image **E**. (See color plate)

hanging eye block, weighted lateral to anterior 4:1 or 5:1). With 1 to 8 years' follow-up, there have been no local failures and four clinically significant cataracts (80).

Scott et al. (166) reviewed children irradiated at the University of Miami and the University of California at San Francisco and retrospectively compared a lateral beam technique (the anterior field border is 2–3 mm behind the limbus) with a relative lens-sparing technique that treats the entire globe and the optic nerve to the conus. A total of 42 patients were described. Eye conservation rates were equivalent, but local control with radiotherapy was superior with the lateral beam technique. Cataract rates were similar.

Inspection of Table 5-5 shows that, in general, control of disease groups I to III with lens-sparing external beam irradiation alone is fairly good in contemporary series (i.e., 40–80%). The addition of photocoagulation, cryotherapy, and plaque therapy results in an ultimate eye preservation rate of 67–100% for disease groups I–III. When new tumors develop in patients treated with lens-sparing external beam techniques, the majority of the recurrences are located anterior in the eye (84). Clearly, failure to irradiate the anterior retina in a tumor in which the entire retinal surface is at risk for tumor will lead to recurrence. Even when careful placement of the anterior beam edge is done with a half-beam blocked lateral field or a Schipper device, it is almost impossible to perfectly irradiate the most anterior retina and reproducibly miss the lens. It is for this reason that many radiation oncologists supplement a lateral beam with some radiation from an anterior field (with an 80:20 lateral-to-anterior weighting) or use three-dimensional (3D) conformal therapy or IMRT to raise the dosage anteriorly. The overall eye preservation rate in patients with anterior failures after lateral beam alone treatment remains quite good. This is because of the frequent success of focal salvage therapies such as cryotherapy, laser therapy, or plaque therapy (84).

Lateral techniques that use a sufficiently anterior field border (with or without a lightly weighted anterior beam), a single anterior field, or 3D conformal therapy or IMRT are the best techniques to avoid anterior failures. Defenders

of the former technique cite the possibility of reducing the risk of injury to anterior structures and brain, whereas supporters of the second invoke ease of setup and the manageability of complications (5,8,17,71–73).

There will undoubtedly be a move toward IMRT techniques for RB. Such techniques allow highly conformal fields around the globe with lower dosages to the surrounding tissue. IMRT may prolong treatment and pose some problems for the anesthesiologist. There is also the theoretical risk that a higher integral dosage may increase the risk of second malignant neoplasms.

Any external beam RB technique should encompass the entire retinal anlage, avoid the other eye if uninvolved, and limit the dosage to normal tissue. Radiotherapists must adopt a technique that fulfills the aforementioned criteria within the context of their own equipment and expertise and the patient's needs.

DOSAGE

Two recent studies have evaluated the radiosensitivity for RB grown in culture. Zhang et al. (157) found that the clonogenic survival rates after 2 Gy of two RB cell lines were 14% and 6%—highly radiosensitive (Fig. 5-21). Hayden et al. (158) found that murine transgenic RB was locally controlled at a significantly lower dose by 1.2 Gy twice daily than 2 Gy once daily (Fig. 5-21).

Is there a clinical radiation dose–response relationship for external beam therapy for RB? Stallard (66) performed serial sections of RB treated with brachytherapy and concluded that 35 Gy was the appropriate dosage delivered in 7 days. A large number of dosage and fraction schemes have been proposed for external beam treatment, ranging from 2 to 3.8 Gy per fraction to a total dosage of 30 to 60 Gy (2,40,71–73, 77,79,82–84,89–92a). Objective data that speak to the establishment of an optimum tumor dosage include a 1969 report by Cassady et al. (12) that 32 to 35 Gy was no less effective than 40 to 45 Gy and the observation that late ill effects of irradiation on the retina (i.e., chorioretinitis) are uncommon at dosages of <50 Gy or less (12,72,73). In 1972, Thompson et al. (92)

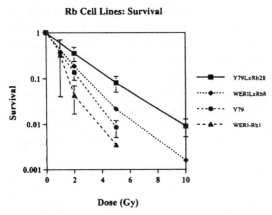

Rb Cell Lines: Survival

FIG. 5-21. Clonogenic survival curves were obtained using a linear quadratic model for human RB cells grown in culture. All cell lines are extremely sensitive, with a small B component and no shoulder region. (From Zhang M, Stevens G, Madigan MC. In vitro effects of radiation on human retinoblastoma cells. *Int J Cancer* 2001; 96[Suppl]:7–14, with permission.).

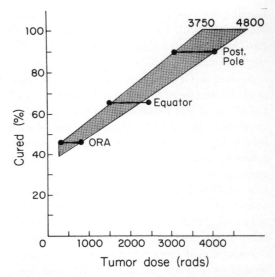

FIG. 5-22. With a single lateral photon technique for the treatment of retinoblastoma, particularly if the beam is not half-beam blocked, the dosage across the retinal anlage is quite heterogeneous. Abramson has observed that if the beam's anterior edge is not set sufficiently close to the limbus, then the ora serrata may receive only 10–30% of the prescribed dosage, the equator 50%, and the posterior pole 90–100%. He plotted the local tumor control of tumors as a function of their ocular location. The more posterior the tumor, the higher the rate of local control. By relating the dosage that was probably administered to the eye at the ora, equator, and posterior pole and plotting it against the local control rate, one can generate a dose–response curve. Although the observation is interesting, it only argues in favor of a dosage of at least 37.5 Gy. This analysis does not provide guidance as to the best dosage in the 37.5- to 50-Gy range that can be administered homogeneously with a multiple-field technique. (From Abramson DH. Treatment of retinoblastoma. In: Blodi FC, ed. *Contemporary issues in ophthalmology*, vol 2: *Retinoblastoma*. New York: Churchill Livingstone, 1985:63–93, with permission.)

published an analysis of treatment time and total dosage suggesting improved local control at higher dosages. These authors recommend 2.5 Gy per fraction, four fractions per week, to 50 Gy.

In 1985, Abramson (7), reviewing the Cornell and Columbia experience, reported no influence of tumor size on the control rate with radiotherapy. Tumors less than 3 disk diameters (DD) in diameter were cured as often as those 3 DD in diameter or larger. However, Abramson did observe a dose–response relationship as a result of dosage inhomogeneities from lateral beam treatment. This is shown in Fig. 5-22. A review of the Mayo Clinic experience by Foote et al. (17) in 1989 found no dose–response relationship over the 45- to 50-Gy dose range in 4 to 5.5 weeks for tumors less than 4 DD in diameter, tumors 4 to 10 DD in diameter, or Reese–Ellsworth group III disease. Based on a small number of patients, local control was thought to be associated with higher dosages in group V cases and in tumors more than 10 DD in diameter. However, in 1996 a group from Wills Eye Hospital in Philadelphia found an inverse relationship between tumor control and tumor size after external beam irradiation. Tumor control with radiation alone as a function of maximum

basal tumor diameter was 88% (less than 5 mm), 93% (5.1 to 10 mm), 72% (10.2 to 15 mm), and 50% (more than 15 mm) (93).

A review of the St. Bartholomew's Hospital, London, data described the using of varying dosage and fraction schemes over the period 1970 to 1985. Tumor control was minimally better with 40 to 44 Gy in 20 fractions than 35 to 36 Gy in 9 to 12 fractions, but little can be concluded from this retrospective review with multiple uncontrolled variables (65). Messmer et al. (94) from Germany reported a higher tumor recurrence rate with a mean dosage of 40 Gy versus 50 Gy (49% vs. 22%). However, Fontanesi et al. (77,90) found the reverse in a small number of patients: Control with less than 36 Gy (71%) was superior to that obtained with more than 36 Gy (50%).

What can we conclude? First, a high dosage per fraction is associated with an increasing risk of late effects. Data from Lausanne, Switzerland, demonstrate an increase in retinopathy at 2.5 Gy or more per fraction (36). Second, with improvements in anesthesia technique, it is not plausible to argue in favor of high-dosage irradiation with three fractions per week because the anesthesia is too difficult. Patients with RB should be treated 5 days per week at 2 Gy or less per fraction. Third, in view of the somewhat contradictory data, most clinicians choose a dosage based on the tolerance of normal tissue rather than on an unfounded belief in unassailable dose–response information. Daily dosages of 1.8 to 2.0 Gy, 5 days per week, are used. Finally, the most controversial aspect of external beam dosage selection is the appropriate total dosage. Let us consider this matter in some detail.

As described earlier, the traditional dosage for treating intraocular RB with external beam radiotherapy is 40 to 45 Gy. When radiation therapy is used after cytoreduction with chemotherapy and intensive focal therapy, however, one must consider modifying the dosage. The arguments in favor of reducing the dosage, in this setting, are as follows:

- In pediatric radiation oncology there is precedent for using a reduced dosage for "consolidation" after surgery and chemotherapy. For example, in Wilms' tumor, Hodgkin's disease, and neuroblastoma, radiation oncologists have reduced conventional dosages of radiation for the purpose of "boosting" or "consolidating" treatment after chemotherapy.
- There may be a higher risk of toxicity with the use of 40 to 45 Gy of irradiation after chemotherapy. This would further argue for a dosage reduction in an attempt to minimize ill effects.

- There is some evidence that institutions using dosages on the order of 36 Gy have reasonable control of RB when radiotherapy is used alone (155).

Based on these arguments, protocols in development for treating locally advanced RB call for chemotherapy and focal therapy (cryotherapy, laser therapy, or laser hyperthermia). Then, after completion of chemotherapy and focal therapy, 26 Gy of irradiation in 2.5 weeks is administered with conformal fields. It is hoped that protocols of this sort ultimately will maintain a high rate of local control of RB with a lower risk of second malignant neoplasms and bone growth abnormalities.

Clearly, if dosage reduction is used in external beam treatment of RB, careful attention must be paid to defining which patients are being "consolidated" and which patients have relapsed. For example, a child whose tumors regressed on chemotherapy and focal therapy and who is promptly referred for radiotherapy, to begin within 4 weeks after the chemotherapy, would be considered "consolidated." But what are we to make of a child whose tumors start to grow immediately after chemotherapy or during chemotherapy? If this latter patient is judged to have relapsed, then one cannot justify using 26 Gy of irradiation. Rather, one should treat with 40 to 45 Gy. Clearly, as the role of chemotherapy in RB management evolves, radiation oncologists will have to use careful judgment to choose the correct dosage. Careful studies of patterns of failure and late effects over the coming years may better define appropriate treatment guidelines.

POSTENUCLEATION CHEMOTHERAPY

A multi-institutional study conducted under the auspices of the Pediatric Oncology Group (POG) and the Children's Cancer Study Group (CCSG) and reported in 1981 evaluated chemotherapy (cyclophosphamide 30 mg/kg and vincristine 0.05 mg/kg) every 3 weeks for 37 weeks in 88 children with group V disease after enucleation. No overall survival or disease-free survival advantage was shown over enucleation alone (5,7,8,95). In 1969, Cassady et al. (12) found no advantage to intracarotid triethylene-mamine in conjunction with radiotherapy when compared with radiotherapy alone in terms of local control or survival for advanced intraocular disease.

Initially, cyclophosphamide was said to be the most active agent in treating metastatic RB (5,8). However, many clinicians favor carboplatin combined with vincristine and etoposide in the setting of extraocular extension, trilateral RB, or distant metastases. In addition, adjuvant chemotherapy may be effective in reducing the frequency of postenucleation metastases in patients at high risk for metastatic disease (i.e., tumor in the cut end of the optic nerve, massive choroidal invasion, and retrolaminar optic nerve invasion) (9). In a retrospective review of patients at high risk for postenucleation RB treated at Wills Eye Hospital, Honavar et al. (96) reported metastases in 2 of 46 (4%) patients treated with adjuvant chemotherapy and 8 of 34 (24%, $p = 0.02$) patients not receiving adjuvant chemotherapy. Chemotherapy consisted of vincristine, adriamycin, and cyclophosphamide in 21 patients and vincristine, etoposide, and carboplatin in 26. The addition of chemotherapy significantly reduced the incidence of metastases in patients with massive choroidal infiltration or retrolaminar optic nerve invasion.

Mustafa et al. (96a) described the results of treatment with vincristine, adriamycin, and cyclophosphamide in a group of 26 patients at high risk for postenucleation RB. With a median follow-up of 5.6 years, five of 36 patients developed distant metastases and subsequently died. All of these patients had massive tumors. Six other patients developed recurrent disease in the intact eye. On multivariate analysis, only optic nerve involvement was a significant factor in predicting poor outcome. Uusitalo et al. (97) analyzed the histopathology and outcome in 129 patients with high-risk, unilateral RB treated by enucleation with and without chemotherapy followed for a median of 54 months. Patients with prelaminar optic nerve disease or isolated choroidal involvement did not receive chemotherapy, and none of these patients developed metastatic disease. Of the 11 patients receiving adjuvant multiagent chemotherapy for positive surgical margin of the optic nerve or tumor extending more than 1 cm beyond the posterior extent of the lamina cribrosa, only one patient developed metastases.

CHEMOTHERAPY FOR INTRAOCULAR DISEASE

Beginning in 1996, a series of publications in refereed journals, as well as platform presentations, described attempts to treat intraocular RB primarily with chemotherapy (98). Because the control of advanced RB is poor with external beam irradiation alone and because external beam irradiation is associated with orbital and midfacial bone deformity, lacrimal gland dysfunction, and an increased risk of second malignant neoplasms, it is not unreasonable to seek alternatives. Primary chemotherapy is seldom used as the sole treatment modality. Instead, chemotherapy typically is combined with one or more focal therapies (cryotherapy, laser photocoagulation, laser hyperthermia, or plaque radiotherapy) (152a,153a).

More than 400 patients with RB treated with primary chemotherapy have been described in detail (Table 5-7). These cases include a mix of Reese–Ellsworth groups, focal therapies, classification of responses and failures, and reporting of results by the number of patients, eyes, and, in some series, tumors. Although chemotherapy most often consists of carboplatin, etoposide, and vincristine, the number of cycles, dosage, and sequencing of these drugs and the optimum regimen have not been established (165). Although the acute effects of chemotherapy appear minimal, long-term follow-up is limited.

Nevertheless, multiagent chemotherapy combined with vigorous focal therapy appears to permit some patients to avoid, or at least delay, enucleation and external beam radiotherapy or allow the dosage of radiotherapy to be reduced. This strategy appears most effective in patients with Reese–Ellsworth group I to III disease. Conversely, the presence of vitreous seeding (i.e., Reese–Ellsworth group Vb disease) or subretinal seeds is associated with a worse outcome. For example, Shields et al. reported a respective study of 103 patients with RB treated primarily with carboplatin, etoposide, and vincristine plus focal therapies at the Wills Eye Hospital. At 5-year follow-up, external beam radiation therapy (EBRT) or enucleation was needed in 10% and 15%, respectively, of Reese–Ellsworth group I to IV patients. In contrast, EBRT or enucleation was needed in 47% and 53% of Reese–Ellsworth groups IV to V. On multivariate analysis, only the presence of subretinal seeds predicted tumor recurrence (99–102). Similar observations were made in retrospective studies of multiagent chemotherapy in intraocular RB at other institutions (52,103–109).

The use of cyclosporine A in the Toronto series is based on the notion that the activity of the multidrug resistance gene (MDR) correlates with chemotherapy resistance in RB. The MDR gene product is a transmembrane pump that promotes the efflux of many drugs from cells (110,111). Cyclosporine A blocks the MDR pump and might increase tumor cell kill by increasing the intracellular drug levels. However, the importance of MDR in human tumors and the efficacy of cyclosporine A are both matters of debate. MDR has been shown to be of questionable importance in neuroblastoma, and the clinical data for RB are conflicting.

Cooperative group trials are in preparation to optimize chemotherapy regimens. Several protocols have been drafted to test the benefits of carboplatin, etoposide, and vincristine regimens. These protocols generally address more advanced cases of disease and combine the chemotherapy with vigorous local therapies such as cryotherapy, laser therapy, and thermotherapy. Some of the more interesting studies, in group V disease, will involve the use of 26 Gy of "consolidation" irradiation. This is justified by the high rate of relapse when these tumors are treated with chemotherapy alone. It is hoped that chemotherapy will allow a reduction from previous dosages of 40 to 45 Gy and be accompanied by a lower risk of long-term ill effects with treatment. Such studies are analogous to the radiotherapy dosage reduction programs that have been attempted in neuroblastoma and Wilms' tumor. Given the absence of mature trials, it will be critical to monitor the long-term side effects of mul-

tiagent chemotherapy, especially as regards the development of secondary malignancies.

SPECIAL SITUATIONS

Trilateral Disease

Trilateral RB is a rare but well-recognized entity consisting of bilateral RB associated with ectopic RB of the pineal or suprasellar region. A forme fruste of trilateral RB has been described in which unilateral RB is associated with intracranial tumor (112). The intracranial lesion can cause signs of raised intracranial pressure (anorexia, ataxia, lethargy, vomiting) or, when the lesion is suprasellar, diabetes insipidus (113,114).

Since the publication of earlier editions of this book, several estimates of the incidence of trilateral RB have appeared in the literature from the United Kingdom and the United States (Table 5-8). Most cases appear in children with bilateral RB. The frequency of trilateral RB has led some authorities to argue in favor of screening cranial CT or MRI to make the diagnosis. Those at prime risk are children with bilateral RB within the first 3 to 4 years after diagnosis (112–114). Some patients develop intracranial diseases as late as 7 years after the diagnosis of RB (114). A meta-analysis of 106 patients with trilateral RB demonstrated that trilateral RB was detected earlier and the child survived longer (16 vs. 8 months after diagnosis) when screening neuroimaging was performed (162). Although median age at death was similar whether or not screening neuroimaging was performed, cumulative 5-year survival was higher in the screened group (27% vs. 0%).

A Wills Eye Hospital study compared the frequency of trilateral RB in patients treated with carboplatin, etoposide, and vincristine chemotherapy with those receiving no chemotherapy (115,163). During the mean follow-up of 47 months, no associated intracranial neuroblastic tumor was observed in 99 patients at risk for trilateral RB (162) receiving multiagent chemotherapy. Based on the results of the meta-analysis of trilateral RB, five to 15 cases were anticipated. In contrast, one of 18 at-risk pa-

TABLE 5-7. *Selected published reports of chemotherapy as primary treatment for intraocular retinoblastoma, 1996–2002*

Institution	Number of patients	Number of eyes	Reese–Ellsworth group	Primary treatment plan	Median follow-up (mo)	Success rate	Comments
Centre Hospitalier Universitaire Vausdois (104)	24	33	I 5 II 10 III 3 IV 1 V 14	2–5 cycles CBP + E ± CrT ± ThT + plaque RT (33 eyes) Enucleation (9 eyes)	31	R–E I–III: 71% R–E IV–V: 0%	Salvage by EBRT or enucleation needed in 0/18 R–E group I–III and 13/15 R–E group IV–V eyes ($p < 0.0001$).
Children's Hospital Los Angeles (52)	73		I 18 II 16 II 4 IV 4 V 31	CBP + ThT (38 eyes) CBP + E + V ± ThT ± CrT ± plaque (35 eyes)	NS	24/38 (63%) of eyes 11/35 (31%) of eyes	In CBP + E + V group at 30 mo follow-up, 100% of R–E I–IV had avoided enucleation or EBRT, compared with ~35% and 11% of patients with subretinal and vitreous seeding, respectively ($p < 0.002$).
Children's Hospital of Philadelphia (105)	47	75	I 6 II 12 III 21 IV 6 V 30	6 cycles CBP + V + E	13	Overall 74% RE I–III: 100% RE V: 39%	No dissemination outside eyes, treatment-related mortality or second neoplasms ($p < 0.001$ for EFS of R–E I–III vs. V).
Children's Memorial Hospital, Chicago (54)	6	11	II 1 III 3 IV 1 V 6	CBP + E ± CrT ± ThT + plaque	23	6/11 (55%) of eyes	8/11 eyes salvaged.
Hospital for Sick Children, Toronto (29,110)	21	26	I 5 II 5 III 4 IV 1 V 11	V + TEN + CBP + CSA ± CrT ± ThT	53	89% overall (7/8 in R–EVb)	1 therapy-related death. 1 remission sustained with ^{125}I plaque.
Institut Curie (164)	51	65 (103 tumors)	I 23 II 18 III 54 IV 4 V 4	Previous 2 cycles CBP + E in 78 tumors. All: 1–6 cycles of CBP + laser ThT	30	92% at 1 yr 90% at 2 yr	Salvage needed in 11 patients.
Institute Rotary Cancer Hospital (108)	19	22	NS	2–12 cycles CBP + V E + CYP + ADR ± ThT ± CrT + EBRT	13 (mean)	3/19 (16%)	CR in 35% of tumors at 6 mo.
King Faisal Specialist Hospital (36)	28	31	I–III 9 IV–V 22	V + ADR + CYP + EBRT	49 (mean)	R–E I–III: 78% R–E IV–V: 28%	Nonrandomized study; no benefit from addition of chemotherapy.

Institution	No.	No.	Reese–Ellsworth stage	Chemotherapy	Age (mo)		Outcome	Comments
St. Bartholomew's Hospital (107)	36	42	I 4 / II 19 / III 9 / IV 2 / V 8	6–8 cycles CBP + V + E	33 (for tumors that did not recur)	57%		On bivariate analysis, odds ratio for successful response to chemotherapy significant for age <2 mo, macular location.
St. Jude Children's Research Hospital (103)	20	36	0 2 / I 5 / II 11 / III 2 / IV 2 / V 14	8 cycles CBP + V	19		R–E I–III: 8% R–E IV–V: 0%	In all patients with multifocal retinoblastoma, 15 eyes (42%) needed EBRT; 81% of eyes were salvaged.
Wills Eye Hospital (100,101)	103	158	I 9 / II 26 / III 16 / IV 32 / V 75	2–6 cycles CBP + V + E	28	Retinal tumor recurrence 51% at 3 and 5 yr		On multivariate analysis, only presence of subretinal seeds predicted tumor recurrence. Treatment failure necessitated EBRT or enucleation at 5 yr in 10% and 15%, respectively, of R–E I–IV and 47% and 53%, respectively, of R–E V ($p < 0.001$). Factors predicting enucleation: age < 12 mo at diagnosis, single tumor, tumor <2 mm from foveola. Factors predicting need for EBRT: male sex, nonwhite race, R–E V.
Wills Eye Hospital (102)	30	30 (all unilateral)	II 9 / III 4 / IV 5 / V 12	2–6 cycles CBP + V + F + CrT or ThT	29		68% at 5 yr	Treatment failure necessitated EBRT or enucleation at 5 yr in 11% and 27%, respectively, of R–E II–IV and 50% and 67%, respectively, of R–E V ($p = 0.001$).
Université Catholique de Louvain (109)	21	33	I–IV 12 / V 21	2–6 cycles CBP + V + E ± ThT ± CrT (24 eyes) Enucleation (9 eyes)	21	NS		Tumor control in 12/12 (100%) R–E I–IV eyes. 8/21 (38%) of R–E V eyes salvaged.

ADR, adriamycin; CBP, carboplatin; CR, complete response; CrT, cryotherapy; CSA, cyclosporine; CYP, cyclophosphamide; E, etoposide; EBRT, external beam radiotherapy; EFS, event-free survival; NS, not stated; R–E, Reese–Ellsworth group; RT, radiotherapy; TEN, teniposide; ThT, thermotherapy; V, vincristine.

TABLE 5-8. *Incidence of midline intracranial tumors (trilateral disease) in RB*

	Overall	Bilateral familial RB	Bilateral sporadic RB
West Midlands Regional Children's Tumour Research Group (112)	3%	5%	12.5%
Wills Eye Hospital (150)	4%	8%	5%
New York Hospital/Memorial Sloan–Kettering Cancer Center (113)	5%	10%	6%
St. Bartholomew's Hospital (149)	2%	—	—

RB, retinoblastoma.

tients treated without chemotherapy developed an associated intracranial tumor (163). Thus, it seems reasonable to perform intracranial imaging at the diagnosis of all cases of RB (when many clinicians do CT of the orbits) and every 3 to 6 months thereafter for 3 to 4 years in bilateral RB. If a pineal or suprasellar mass is found, a decision must be made concerning biopsy.

For some clinicians the presence of a calcified, discrete midline mass of the pineal or suprasellar regions in the setting of heritable bilateral RB is sufficient to make the diagnosis of trilateral disease (5). However, other oncologists feel more comfortable with a biopsy of the intracranial lesion. The authors of this chapter recently saw a 10-month-old with heritable RB and a pineal mass who, on pineal biopsy, was shown to have a benign pineal cyst.

The treatment of trilateral disease with surgery alone or in combination with radiotherapy resulted in no long-term survivors (112,113, 116–118). Six cases of trilateral RB were reported in 1994 from Memorial Sloan–Kettering Cancer Center. Three were treated with craniospinal irradiation (CSI) and chemotherapy, two with chemotherapy alone, and one with no treatment. All patients died of the tumor in 2 to 12 months (113). Five patients with trilateral RB seen in the West Midlands Health Authority, United Kingdom, reported in 1996, died at 1–31 months after diagnosis (112). In 1986, the pediatric neuro-oncology group at Duke reported that cyclophosphamide and vincristine were active in patients with recurrent trilateral RB (116). Subsequently, the same group has described three children with newly diagnosed trilateral RB treated with systemic (cyclophosphamide, vincristine) and intrathecal (methotrexate, hydro-cortisone, cytarabine) chemotherapy along with orbital irradiation and, in two cases, CSI. Two patients are alive without evidence of disease 3 and 8 years after diagnosis. One is alive with persistent disease 2 years after diagnosis (118).

Paulino (114) performed a Medline search of all English-language articles pertaining to trilateral RB published between 1977 and 1997. Of the 94 different cases identified, the median age at the time of diagnosis of RB was 6 months. In 78 patients (83%) the intracranial tumor was in the pineal region, and in 16 patients (17%) it was in the suprasellar region. The location of the tumor had no impact on survival. For patients who received no treatment the median survival was 1 month, whereas it was 8 months for those who received treatment. Therapy in 25 of the patients was craniospinal radiotherapy with chemotherapy, 20 patients received CSI, 10 received chemotherapy alone, and a variety of other treatment combinations were used in the remainder of the patients. The median survival was 8 months. Of the six children who survived more than 2 years after diagnosis of intracranial primitive neuroectodermal tumor, all received chemotherapy and four received craniospinal radiotherapy. For the 75 children for whom patterns of failure were reported, 55% had disseminated neuroaxis disease.

The use of radiotherapy in trilateral RB poses an interesting challenge to the radiotherapist. The orbital disease usually is irradiated first, accompanied and followed by chemotherapy, with CSI given last in the sequence. Knowing this, the radiotherapist must set up the orbital fields with the understanding that they will be called on to partially overlap and then match the CSI fields. Particular attention is paid to the optic chiasm dosage in this situation. Using rigid patient immobilization and 3D treatment planning, it is possible to administer CSI and a boost to the intracranial tumor with reasonable safety even apart from ocular irradiation (117).

Ocular Retreatment

Among the most difficult problems confronting the pediatric radiation oncologist is therapy selection in a child who has suffered recurrent RB in an eye previously externally irradiated to full dosage. If the recurrent lesion is small and favorably located, it may be treated with photocoagulation, cryotherapy, or a radioactive plaque, often with success. Amendola and coworkers (11,33,57) plaqued 29 eyes, 28 with group V disease, for recurrent tumor. Tumor progression in 14 eyes ultimately necessitated enucleation. The remaining 15 eyes (52%) have preservation of vision.

In some situations, the clinician faces the choice of enucleation or reirradiation with external beam. Abramson reported retreatment of 15 eyes that, at the time of tumor recurrence, could be classified as groups I to III. Twelve (80%) of these eyes survived. Of the 89 eyes that were group IV or V at the time of tumor recurrence, only 2 (2.2%) survived. Nine of the 14 salvaged eyes had useful vision. The overwhelming cause of enucleation was progressive tumor, not radiation damage. There appears to be no increase in secondary nonocular tumors in children receiving two courses of radiotherapy (119).

MANAGEMENT OF EXTRAOCULAR EXTENSION, ORBITAL RECURRENCE, AND METASTATIC DISEASE

In developed countries, cases of extraocular extension or orbital recurrence after initial treatment of RB are rare. At academic centers, such cases often are referred from institutions where the initial treatment was given by physicians who thought, at first, that they were dealing with another diagnosis. By making the best possible use of the available data and by relying on sound clinical reasoning, the pediatric radiation oncologist can make the best of these vexing cases.

Earlier in this chapter, we pointed out that histologic evaluation of the enucleated eye can predict prognosis to some extent (44,120–123). Extensive involvement of the choroid along with retrolaminar extension of tumor or, even worse, involvement of the cut end of the optic nerve predicts a poor outcome. Patients with these problems are subject to either local recurrence of tumor in the orbit, CNS disease, or systemic tumor. It is reasonable to consider more aggressive adjuvant treatment in these cases in an attempt to improve the outcome.

Another important prognostic factor is the performance of a prior intraocular procedure in patients with RB. RB may be initially misdiagnosed. As an unforeseen consequence, the increase in the availability of technology in vitreous surgery has resulted in more children undergoing intraocular surgery in an attempt to confirm an inflammatory cause of visual loss or in an attempt to improve vision (124). The surgeon will be surprised and dismayed to find that RB is the true diagnosis. By such procedures, RB may be seeded by breach of the scleral or corneal barrier. One of the authors has seen a patient with tumor growing directly through the previous incision. Children who have undergone an intraocular operative procedure before definitive enucleation are at risk for orbital recurrence of tumor and nodal and hematogenous dissemination.

Historically, recurrence of RB in the orbit after enucleation has carried an extremely poor prognosis for survival. Only one of 16 children with orbital recurrence was a long-term survivor in the St. Bartholomew's and Moorefield Eye Hospital's 1987 report (90). Children succumbed to CNS tumor, systemic disease, and uncontrolled orbital tumor.

Fortunately, clinical results are now better. We will now consider the appropriate treatment for children found to have one or more identified risk factors.

Optic Nerve Involvement

Tumor may extend beyond the lamina cribrosa or to the end of the transected optic nerve. The mortality rate when the optic nerve is involved up to the line of transection is 40–45% (125,126) Retrolaminar involvement also markedly affects survival, although not as severely. This argues strongly for the use of adjuvant therapy, but there are no prospective, randomized data proving the value of adjuvant therapy in this situation.

Contemporary practice generally includes adjuvant chemotherapy for optic nerve involvement (carboplatin and etoposide or vincristine, carboplatin, and etoposide). Orbital external beam irradiation to 40 to 50 Gy in 4 to 5 weeks is commonly used for tumor up to the line of transection. The posterior aspect of the irradiated volume should encompass the pathway of the optic nerve back to the optic chiasm. Some radiation oncologists advocate whole brain and orbital irradiation in this situation, but this approach is less popular. Retrolaminar tumor, without extension to the line of transection, is treated by adjuvant chemotherapy and orbital irradiation by some and by chemotherapy alone by others (127). Some clinicians are guided by the extent of the margin (i.e., they will not irradiate minimal extralaminar extension as long as there is a 4- to 5-mm negative margin) (128).

When postoperative radiotherapy is used for the orbit, external beam treatment is most commonly used. Popular field arrangements include an anterior wedge pair, a single anterior field, or a three-dimensionally planned set of fields, usually four to six. Coralline hydroxyapatite prostheses do not significantly affect the radiation dosage distribution (129).

Some institutions prefer to treat the postenucleation socket with brachytherapy. There are at least three techniques. The Groote Schuur Hospital of Cape Town, South Africa, has described a technique using six rows of ^{125}I arrayed around the periphery of the orbit, one central row, and seeds on a metal disc sutured beneath the eyelids. The median dosage is 34–40 Gy in about 3 days. The benefits of this procedure compared with external beam treatment are felt to be a lower risk of bone growth abnormality, less failure of tooth eruption, a reduced risk of neuroendocrine injury, and a possible reduction in second malignant neoplasms. Local tumor control in the South African series has been excellent, al-

though there have been some deaths from distant metastases (128,130).

Another technique for postenucleation orbital brachytherapy is the creation of a mold. This technique is similar to that used at some institutions for brachytherapy for cervical or vaginal carcinoma. In an anesthetized child, the walls of the socket are lined with petroleum jelly gauze or plastic wrap. The socket is filled with modeling compound that, when it hardens, creates an impression of the cavity. The mold is then removed. A permanent mold is created in the hospital prosthetics shop with impregnated catheters to carry ^{125}I or ^{192}Ir afterloading seeds. A dosimetry plan is prepared. At the time of the actual implant the mold, if skillfully prepared, should pop readily into place, the seeds are loaded, and a covering lead eye patch placed. A dosage of 35 to 45 Gy is given to the orbital wall in 3 to 4 days. The mold usually is prepared so that there is room for some petroleum jelly gauze between the mold and the orbital wall for a better depth dosage.

A third brachytherapy technique uses a spherical orbital prosthesis. The prosthesis is drilled and ^{192}Ir or ^{125}I is placed in the center of the sphere. This creates an applicator with a uniform dosage on the sphere's surface (131).

Orbital Extension and Orbital Recurrence

As previously described in this chapter, orbital extension of intraocular RB or orbital relapse after enucleation is associated with a high mortality rate. Small series have been reported showing long-term survival with postoperative chemotherapy and radiotherapy (36,96,131,132). As regards chemotherapy, there is some debate concerning whether systemic treatment is adequate or intrathecal chemotherapy should also be used. Concerning radiotherapy, there is some debate concerning whether orbital or whole brain radiotherapy is appropriate (5). It would be best if we had detailed patterns of failure analyses that made it clear what predicted for orbital only, brain only, systemic only, or some combination of sites relapses. This would guide us in selecting radiotherapy treatment volumes. Because most clinical series are small and describe a mixture of patients with orbital involvement at presentation, at relapse, and of varying sizes and extent, it is impossible to make unequivocal pronouncements on this topic. For the radiation oncologist, a sound policy is to irradiate the orbit alone unless there is extension into the brain or there are brain metastases. If the orbital disease is bulky, some treat with a combination of external beam and brachytherapy (5,7,16,73,124,131–132).

Metastases

Radiotherapy has been used in the curative and palliative treatment of metastatic RB. Whole brain irradiation or CSI is used for brain metastases or leptomeningeal dissemination. Bone or nodal metastases often respond to involved field irradiation. When bone marrow transplantation is attempted for advanced disease, total body irradiation (TBI) has been included in the preparative program, albeit infrequently (133–135).

High-dose chemotherapy (HDC) with autologous stem cell rescue may also be an option in treating advanced disease (136,137). In a study of 25 patients with RB receiving HDC with autologous stem cell rescue for relapsed or high-risk disease, Namouni et al. (136) reported a 67% disease-free survival at 3 years. Of the eight patients who relapsed, seven of the relapses were in the CNS. Seven patients died with disease at a median of 13 months after HDC. Hertzberg et al. (137) described the use of HDC with peripheral hematopoietic stem cell transplantation in five children with RB metastatic to bone marrow and one child with extraorbital disease. One child was salvaged with surgery and conventional therapy after suffering a meningeal relapse and is alive at 105 months after treatment. The other four did not relapse and are in complete remission 8, 9, 57, and 107 months after HDC.

Results in the Management of Extraocular RB

Patients with extraocular RB limited to the orbit or preauricular nodes, treated with postoperative radiotherapy and chemotherapy, have a widely variable reported progression-free survival. With 1 to 5 years of follow-up, in small series, it ranges from 30% to 80% (9,36,45,130,132,135,138). Widespread metastatic disease outside the CNS, treated with HDC, local irradiation or TBI, and stem cell rescue, may be curable in about one-fourth to one-half of cases (135). The prognosis of CNS metastases, treated with cranial or craniospinal irradiation and systemic and intrathecal chemotherapy, is grim.

PALLIATION OF METASTASES

For bony metastases causing pain, palliative radiotherapy is appropriate. A dosage of 20 to 40 Gy, similar to that for neuroblastoma, is used (8). (See Chapter 6.)

LATE EFFECTS

Secondary Nonocular Tumors

The evidence is persuasive that the 13q–14q deletion of heritable RB produces a malignant diathesis. The relative risk (RR) for death from a second tumor is much higher among patients with bilateral RB (RR = 60) than among those with unilateral disease (RR = 3.8). This first manifests itself in the development of the index case of RB. In long-term survivors of heritable RB, there is an extremely high incidence of secondary nonocular tumors. The most common secondary malignant neoplasms (SMNs) occurring in the radiation field in survivors of heritable RB are osteosarcoma, fibrosarcoma, and other spindle cell sarcomas. SMNs developing out of the radiotherapy field also include osteosarcoma and the soft tissue sarcomas. However, this list must be broadened to include malignant melanoma and thyroid carcinoma. In addition, there is a long list of less common SMNs that have developed in long-term survivors of heritable RB (22,139,140).

In children treated with hereditary RB, the incidence of SMNs increases with time. The median latency period is 15 years (141,142). At 10 years, the incidence of SMNs is about 10%, at 20 years it is about 20%, at 30 years it is estimated to be about 25%, and at 50 years, 51% (44,111,142). Initially, Abramson et al. (7,10), described even higher risks: 20% at 10 years,

50% at 20 years, and 90% at 30 years. A comprehensive evaluation of SMNs in RB by Eng et al. (139) is based on a large number of patients with RB, including patients from New York and Boston. In a 1993 report, at 40 years of follow-up, the cumulative mortality for all second tumors was 26% for bilateral RB and 1.5% for unilateral RB. The Eng study includes those previously reported by Abramson and therefore supersedes those reports (Figs. 5-23–5-25).

In a 1997 report, the cumulative incidence of second cancer at 50 years after diagnosis was 51% (142). All the major studies agree that the risk of SMN is greater in survivors of heritable RB who received radiotherapy than in those who did not. For example, Roarty et al. (140) found a 30-year SMN incidence rate of 29% in the radiation field for 137 patients who received radiotherapy. The incidence of 8% outside the radiation field was similar to the 6% rate for the 78 patients who did not receive radiation. Abramson et al. (7,10) also found a significant reduction in the incidence of SMN outside the field of radiation or in patients never irradiated. Among patients with bilateral RB, Eng et al. (139) found that cumulative mortality from second neoplasms at 40-year follow-up was 30% for irradiated patients and 6% for those who did not receive irradiation. Wong et al. (142) found that, at 50 years, the cumulative incidence of

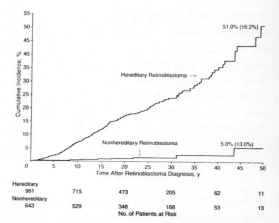

FIG. 5-24. Cumulative incidence (± standard error) of second cancers after the diagnosis of retinoblastoma in 961 patients with hereditary disease and 643 patients with nonhereditary disease. (From Wong FL, Boice JD Jr, Abramson DH, et al. Cancer incidence after retinoblastoma: radiation dose and sarcoma risk. *JAMA* 1997; 278:1262–1267, with permission.)

second cancers was 58% in irradiated heritable RB patients and 27% in nonirradiated patients. Dosimetry data, collected for patients with secondary bone and soft tissue sarcoma, showed a stepwise increase in secondary tumor relative

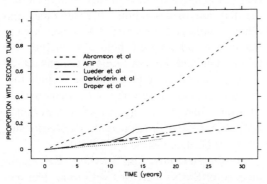

FIG. 5-23. The risk of secondary nonocular tumors for children with bilateral retinoblastoma from several published studies described in the text. (From Roarty JD, McLean IW, Zimmerman LE. Incidence of second neoplasms in patients with bilateral retinoblastoma. *Ophthalmology* 1988;95: 1583–1587, with permission.)

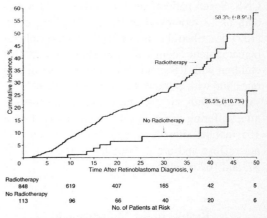

FIG. 5-25. Cumulative incidence (± standard error) of second cancers after diagnosis of retinoblastoma in patients with hereditary disease, by presence or absence of radiation treatment. (From Wong FL, Boice JD Jr, Abramson DH, et al. Cancer incidence after retinoblastoma: radiation dose and sarcoma risk. *JAMA* 1997; 278:1262–1267, with permission.)

risk with increasing dosage (142). In an analysis confined to bilateral cases the incidence of second tumors at 30 years was 34% for children irradiated at less than 12 months of age, 22% for children irradiated at more than 12 months of age, and 18% for those not irradiated (141).

Cavenee et al. (143) have developed some evidence to implicate cyclophosphamide as a risk factor for SMN in heritable RB. In an extensive review of heritable RB, they found that the estimated incidence rate 12 years after diagnosis for tumors in the field of radiation was 4.2% for patients given chemotherapy and 2.9% for patients not given chemotherapy. The rates for tumors outside the radiation field (including patients not irradiated) was 4.6% for those receiving chemotherapy and 1% for those not receiving it.

Children with heritable RB have a field change rendering them subject to malignant transformation. Radiotherapy and perhaps chemotherapy are an additional insult. Radiotherapy shortens the latent period for SMN, increases the incidence of SMN, and affects the distribution of SMN (141). In summary, for heritable RB radiotherapy compounds the risk of SMN on a background of high risk.

CATARACTS

Fontanesi et al. (90) noted that clinically significant posterior pole cataracts developed in 23 of 27 eyes (85%) treated with anterior fields. The Mayo Clinic reported four of 14 (28%) posterior cataracts using a lens-sparing technique (17). In seven eyes followed for more than 36 months, Hernandez et al. (93), generally using lateral and anterior fields, observed lens changes in all cases, with three necessitating lens extraction. Radiation-induced cataracts after radiotherapy of RB can be removed successfully and vision can be corrected. Brooks et al. (76) removed cataracts in 38 patients with RB (42 eyes) from 1973 to 1989. Nineteen eyes (45%) had final visual acuities of 20/20 to 20/50. Twelve eyes (29%) had macular tumors with postoperative visual acuities of 20/80 to counting fingers. Buckley and Heath (80) extracted cataracts from three eyes with macular tumors and observed near vision acuities of 20/60, 10/200, and local-

izing 2-mm beads at 13 inches. The risks of cataract removal after RB treatment include amblyopia, retinal detachment, and the risk of tumor dissemination if RB was not controlled by irradiation (76).

ORBITAL DEVELOPMENT

Children treated with radiotherapy or enucleation for RB are at significant risk for orbital and midfacial growth retardation insofar as their orbital bones are growing during treatment. In long-term survivors of RB, these orbital growth injuries may be apparent. In recent years, investigators have sought to quantify the changes in orbital development wrought by treatment.

Imhof et al. (144,145) examined children treated at Utrecht University Hospital in the Netherlands and followed for a mean of approximately 8 years. Direct measurements were made of the orbital width and height and the orbital–tragus distance. In general, high-dose-per-fraction external beam irradiation had been used (3 Gy per fraction × 15 = 45 Gy, 8-MV photons). The mean orbital width, height, and distance between the tragus and the outer orbital edge were significantly shorter in irradiated orbits compared with nonirradiated orbits in patients with unilateral RB and compared with control eyes. EBRT given to children younger than 6 months old was more injurious than when it was used in older children. Enucleation with EBRT was not worse than EBRT alone.

Findings by Imhof et al. are supported by a slightly less detailed study from Essen, Germany, by Messmer et al. (146). The German researchers evaluated 99 patients, diagnosed at the median age of 10 months, and at a median age at last follow-up of 16 years. In children and adolescents with anophthalmic sockets, there was a significantly less satisfactory cosmetic and functional outcome in patients who received EBRT before or after enucleation (Fig. 5-26). Midfacial hypoplasia was also clearly related to the use of enucleation or irradiation (Figs. 5-27 and 5-28).

Kaste et al. (63) at SJCRH evaluated the orbital development in long-term survivors of RB using a CT scan obtained at a median age of 13 years. Because the orbital interior is roughly

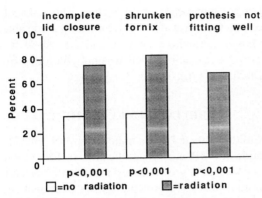

FIG. 5-26. Radiation with enucleation can produce significant orbital problems. In anophthalmic children, deformities were heightened by the addition of radiation. (From Messmer EP, Frize H, Mohr C, et al. Long-term treatment effects in patients with bilateral retinoblastoma: ocular and mid-facial findings. *Graefes Arch Clin Exp Ophthalmol* 1991;229:309–314, with permission.)

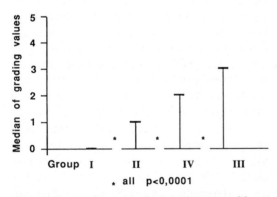

FIG. 5-27. Using a clinical grading system, Messmer et al. did subjective grading of deformity of midfacial structures after treatment for retinoblastoma. Midfacial hypoplasia correlated with therapy. Group 1 consists of patients treated with photocoagulation or cryotherapy only, group 2 comprises patients treated with enucleation without irradiation, group 3 comprises patients treated with enucleation with radiation, and group 4 includes children treated with radiation without enucleation. (From Messmer EP, Frize H, Mohr C, et al. Long-term treatment effects in patients with bilateral retinoblastoma: ocular and mid-facial findings. *Graefes Arch Clin Exp Ophthalmol* 1991;229: 309–314, with permission.)

conical, the orbital volume was assessed with a scan slice at the level of the optic nerve using the equation for the volume of a cone ($v = \frac{1}{3}\pi r^2 h$).

In patients with unilateral RB, the orbit on the enucleated side was smaller in 20 of 24 cases and larger in 4 cases. The median orbital volume difference was 1.5 cm^3. This small difference may be the result of the use of orbital prostheses that stimulate bony orbital growth. In 18 children with bilateral disease treated with enucleation on one side and irradiation on the other, the enucleated side had the smaller volume in six cases, the irradiated side was smaller in ten, and there was no difference in two.

Nahum et al. (168) from Haifa, Israel, using CT volume reconstruction, showed that enucleation and postoperative irradiation produced significant orbital volume loss. The available literature confirms the impression of senior clinicians caring for children with RB that radiation and, to some extent, enucleation without a properly fitting prosthesis can lead to retardation of bony and soft tissue growth of the midface (orbits, ethmoid bones, nasal bridge). Hypotelorism, enophthalmos, depressed temporal bones, atrophy of the temporalis muscle, narrow and deep orbits, and a depressed nasion can be the result (147). These effects are accentuated if radiotherapy is used in the very young (younger than 6 months of age) and at dosages greater than 35 Gy (63,145).

LACRIMAL GLAND

In 1955 Cogan et al. (148), of the Massachusetts Eye and Ear Infirmary, did a series of experiments concerning the irradiation of the orbital glands of rabbits. Rabbits have two orbital glands opening onto the conjunctiva; one is a sebaceous gland, called a Harderian gland, and the other is a true lacrimal gland. They irradiated rabbit orbits to varying dosages and excised and weighed the glands at 45 days or later. The results, shown in Fig. 5-29, demonstrate a definite decrease in gland size with increasing dosage.

Imhof et al. (145) studied lacrimal function in 45 eyes of 34 irradiated patients who underwent tear function tests a mean of 86 months after irradiation. Irradiated eyes had significantly less tear production and significantly less tear

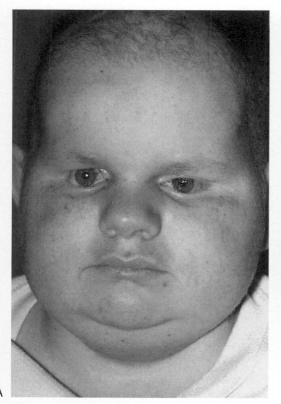
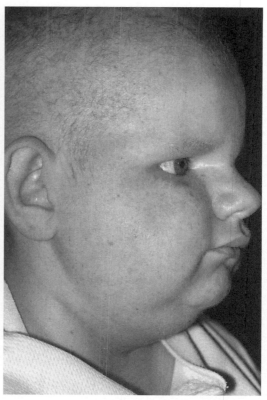

A

B

FIG. 5-28. A 10-month-old Caucasian boy presented with bilateral leukocoria. Cranial computed tomography scan showed bilateral orbital masses and suggested extraglobal extension of the right orbital mass and a calcified pineal. The left eye was enucleated, and histologic examination demonstrated retinoblastoma. The right eye was treated with external beam irradiation. A total dosage of 45 Gy was administered at 1.8 Gy per fraction with an anterior and right lateral field. The pineal mass was not biopsied but was presumed to represent trilateral retinoblastoma. The child was treated with systemic and intrathecal chemotherapy. Craniospinal irradiation was administered to the patient when he was 2 years old. Careful blocking was used to avoid overdose to the previously irradiated volume used for the treatment of the right eye. The whole brain, with partial overlap of the previously irradiated volume, received 13.5 Gy. Then the treatment volume was reduced with blocking of the previously irradiated fields for an additional 10.5 Gy. The pineal region was treated to an additional 30.6 Gy. Thus, the pineal lesion received a cumulative dosage of 54.6 Gy. The spine was irradiated to 24 Gy. When the child was 14 years old he developed distal right ulnar tenderness. Magnetic resonance imaging showed a permeative lesion in the right ulna associated with periosteal reaction and a pathologic nondisplaced fracture. Biopsy demonstrated a small blue cell malignancy most consistent with recurrent, metastatic retinoblastoma. Additional chemotherapy and local palliative irradiation were administered. These photographs, taken when the child was 14 years old, demonstrate the long-term consequences on bone development of enucleation, irradiation administered at 10 months of age, and craniospinal irradiation administered at 2 years of age. In modern practice, biopsy of the pineal lesion at the time of original presentation would be more likely. (Photographs are reproduced with the permission of the patient's father.)

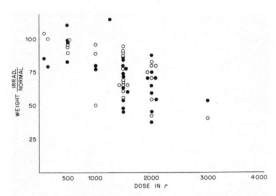

FIG. 5-29. In a study by Cogan et al., the two or-bital glands of the rabbit were weighed after irradi-ation. The Harderian gland is the sebaceous gland. Rabbits also have a true lacrimal gland. The relative weights of the irradiated and normal Harderian glands *(open circles)* are compared with the weights of the irradiated and normal lacrimal glands *(closed circles)*. Although there is great individual variation, there is clearly a de-crease in gland size with increasing dosages of ir-radiation. (From Cogan DG, Fink R, Donaldson DD. X-ray irradiation of orbital glands of the rabbit. *Radiology* 1955;64:731–737, with permission.)

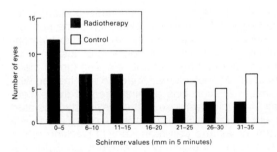

FIG. 5-30. The Schirmer test may be used to quantify the effects of retinoblastoma irradiation on lacrimal function. A small piece of filter paper is inserted into the lower conjunctival fornix, folded at right angles over the ciliary body of the lid, where it is left in position. Normal secretion ought to moisten at least 1.5 cm of the strip, as measured from the fold in 5 minutes. Though crude, the test provides an indication of exces-sive lacrimation or marked hyposecretion. In this study, from researchers in Amsterdam and Utrecht, children irradiated with a lateral beam for retinoblastoma are shown, on average, to have less tear production than nonirradiated controls. (From Imhof SM, Hofman P, Tan KEWP. Quantifi-cation of lacrimal function after D-shaped field ir-radiation for retinoblastoma. *Br J Ophthalmol* 1993;77:482–484, with permission.)

protein production than a control group (Fig. 5-30). Although many radiation oncologists at-tempt to shield the lacrimal gland, some long-term survivors of RB have diminished tears and diminished stability of the tear film. Such chil-dren may be prone to keratopathies. Keratitis as a side effect of irradiation for RB has been re-ported with varying frequency: 28% by Imhof et al., 3 of 30 (10%) of patients treated at less than 1 year of age, and 2 of 15 patients (13%) treated after 1 year of age by Fontanesi et al. (77,90,145).

REFERENCES

References particularly recommended for fur-ther reading are indicated by an asterisk.

1. Cowell JK, Hungerford J, Jay M, et al. Retinoblas-toma—clinical and genetic aspects: a review. *J R Soc Med* 1987;81:220–223.
2. Abramson DH. Retinoblastoma: diagnosis and man-agement. *CA Cancer J Clin* 1982;32:130–140.
3. Redler LD, Ellsworth RM. Prognostic importance of choroidal invasion in retinoblastoma. *Arch Ophthal-mol* 1973;90:294–296.
4. Duke-Elder S, Darbree JH, eds. Diseases of the retina. In: *System of ophthalmology,* vol 10. St. Louis: Mosby, 1957:671–727.
5. Kingston JE, Hungerford JL. Retinoblastoma. In: Plowman PN, Pinkerton CR, eds. *Paediatric oncol-ogy: clinical practice and controversies.* London: Chapman & Hall, 1992:268–290.
6. Reese AB. *Tumors of the eye,* 3rd ed. Hagerstown, MD: Harper & Row, 1976:90–122.
7. Abramson DH. Treatment of retinoblastoma. In: Blodi FC, ed. *Contemporary issues in ophthalmol-ogy,* vol 2: *Retinoblastoma.* New York: Churchill Liv-ingstone, 1985:63–93.
8. Donaldson SS, Egbert PR, Lee WH. Retinoblastoma. In: Pizzo PA, Poplack DG, eds. *Principles and prac-tice of pediatric oncology.* Philadelphia: JB Lippin-cott, 1993:683–696.
9. Schvartzman E, Chantado G, Fandino A, et al. Re-sults of a stage-based protocol for the treatment of retinoblastoma. *J Clin Oncol* 1996;14:1532–1536.
10. Abramson DH, Ellsworth RM, Kitchin FD, et al. Sec-ond nonocular tumors in the retinoblastoma sur-vivors: are they radiation-induced? *Ophthalmology* 1984;91:1351–1355.
11. Amendola BE, Lamm FR, Markae AM, et al. Radio-therapy of retinoblastoma: a review of 63 children treated with different irradiation techniques. *Cancer* 1990;66:21–26.
*12. Cassady JR, Sagerman RH, Tretter P, et al. Radia-tion therapy in retinoblastoma. *Radiology* 1969;93: 405–409.
13. Egbert PR, Donaldson SS, Moazed K, et al. Visual re-sults and ocular complications following radiother-

apy for retinoblastoma. *Arch Ophthalmol* 1978;96: 1826–1830.

13a. Stannard C, Sealy R, Hering E, et al. Localized whole eye radiotherapy for retinoblastoma using a ^{125}I applicator, "claws." *Int J Radiat Oncol Biol Phys* 2001; 51:399–409.

14. Brantley MA Jr, Harbour JW. The molecular biology of retinoblastoma. *Ocul Immun Inflamm* 2001;11: 59–76.

15. Bedford MA, Bedotta C, MacFaul PA. Retinoblastoma: a study of 139 cases. *Br J Ophthalmol* 1971; 55:19–27.

16. Gaitan-Yanguas M. Retinoblastoma: analysis of 235 cases. *Int J Radiat Oncol Biol Phys* 1978;4:359–365.

*17. Foote RL, Garretson BR, Schamberg PJ, et al. External beam irradiation for retinoblastoma: patterns of failure and dose-response analysis. *Int J Radiat Oncol Biol Phys* 1989;116:823–830.

18. Rous P. Nobel Prize lecture, "The Challenge to Man of the Neoplastic Cell," 1966, at http://www.nobel.se/medicine/laureates/1966/rous-lecture.html.

19. Boveri T. *Frage der Entstehung maligner Tumoren.* Jena: Gustav Fischer, 1926. Translated as *The origin of malignant tumors.* Baltimore: Williams & Wilkins, 1929. M Boveri, translator.

20. Knudson AG. Hereditary cancer, oncogenes, and antioncogenes. *Cancer Res* 1985;45:1437–1443.

*21. Knudson AG, Strong LC. Mutation and cancer: a model for Wilms' tumor of the kidney. *J Natl Cancer Inst* 1972;48:313–324.

22. Druja TP, Cavanee W, White R, et al. Homozygosity of chromosome 13 in retinoblastoma. *N Engl J Med* 1984;310:550–553.

23. Leis JF, Livingston DM. Tumor suppressor genes and their mechanism of action. In: Bishop JM, Weinberg RA, eds. *Scientific American: molecular oncology.* New York: Scientific American, 1996: 111–142.

24. Knudson AG. Two genetic hits (more or less) to cancer. *Nat Rev Cancer* 2001;1:157–162.

25. Weinberg RA. The retinoblastoma gene and gene product. *Cancer Surv* 1992;12:43–57.

26. Varmus H, Weinberg RA. *Genes and the biology of cancer.* New York: Scientific American Library, 1993.

27. Gallie BL. Gene carrier detection in retinoblastoma. *Ophthalmology* 1980;87:591–595.

*28. Gallie BL, Budning A, DeBoer G, et al. Chemotherapy with focal therapy can cure intraocular retinoblastoma without radiotherapy. *Arch Ophthalmol* 1996; 114:1321–1328.

29. Gallie BL, Dunn JM, Chan HSL, et al. The genetics of retinoblastoma: relevance to the patient. *Pediatr Clin North Am* 1991;38:299–315.

30. Stiegler P, Glordano A. The family of retinoblastoma proteins. *Crit Rev Eukaryot Gene Expr* 2001;11:59–76.

31. Classon M, Harlow E. The retinoblastoma tumor suppressor in development and cancer. *Nat Rev Cancer* 2002;2:910–917.

32. Cavenee WK, Hansen MF, Nordenskjold M, et al. Genetic origin of mutations predisposing to retinoblastoma. *Science* 1985;228:501–503.

33. Amendola BE, Markoe AM, Augsburger JJ, et al. Analysis of treatment results in 36 children with retinoblastoma treated by scleral plaque irradiation. *Int J Radiat Oncol Biol Phys* 1989;17:63–70.

34. MacKay CJ, Abramson DH, Ellsworth RM. Metastatic patterns of retinoblastoma. *Arch Ophthalmol* 1984; 102:391–396.

*35. Pratt CB, Meyer D, Chenaille P, et al. The use of bone marrow aspirations and lumbar punctures at the time of diagnosis of retinoblastoma. *J Clin Oncol* 1989; 7:140–143.

36. Pradhan DG, Sandridge AL, Mullaney P, et al. Radiation therapy for retinoblastoma: a retrospective review of 120 patients. *Int J Radiat Oncol Biol Phys* 1997;39:3–13.

37. Mohney BG, Robertson DM. Ancillary testing for metastasis patients with newly diagnosed retinoblastoma. *Am J Ophthalmol* 1994;118:707–711.

38. Karcioglu ZA, Al-Mesfer SA, Abboud E, et al. Workup for metastatic retinoblastoma: a review of 261 patients. *Ophthalmology* 1997;104:307–312.

39. Moscinski LC, Pendergrass TW, Weiss A, et al. Recommendations for the use of routine bone marrow aspiration and lumbar punctures in the follow-up of patients with retinoblastoma. *J Pediatr Hematol Oncol* 1996;18(2):130–134.

40. Abramson DH, Jereb B, Ellsworth RM. External beam radiation for retinoblastoma. *Bull N Y Acad Med* 1981;57:787–803.

41. Stannard C, Lipper S, Sealy R, et al. Retinoblastoma: correlation of invasion of the optic nerve and choroid with prognosis and metastases. *Br J Ophthalmol* 1979; 63:560–570.

*42. Finger P, Harbour JW, Karacioglu ZA. Risk factors for metastasis in retinoblastoma. *Surv Ophthalmol* 2002;47:1–16.

43. Singh AD, Shields CL, Shields JA. Prognostic factors in retinoblastoma. *J Pediatr Ophthalmol Strabismus* 2000;37:134–141.

44. Hungerford J. Factors influencing metastasis in retinoblastoma. *Br J Ophthalmol* 1993;77:541.

45. Hungerford J, Kingston J, Plowman N. Orbital recurrence of retinoblastoma. *Ophthalmic Paediatr Genet* 1987;8:63–68.

46. Abramson DH, Niksarli K, Ellsworth RM, et al. Changing trends in the management of retinoblastoma: 1951–1965 vs. 1966–1980. *J Pediatr Ophthalmol Strabismus* 1994;31:32–37.

47. Dudgeon J. Retinoblastoma: trends in conservative management. *Br J Ophthalmol* 1995;79:104.

48. Shields JA, Shields CL, Sivalingam V. Decreasing frequency of enucleation in patients with retinoblastoma. *Am J Ophthalmol* 1989;108:185–188.

49. Abramson DH, Ellsworth RM. The surgical management of retinoblastoma. *Ophthalmic Surg Lasers* 1980; 11:596–598.

50. Abramson DH, Ellsworth RM, Rozakis GW. Cryotherapy for retinoblastoma. *Arch Ophthalmol* 1982;100:1253–1256.

51. Shields CL, Shields JA, Kiratli H, et al. Treatment of retinoblastoma with indirect ophthalmoscope laser photocoagulation. *J Pediatr Ophthalmol Strabismus* 1995;32:317–322.

*52. Murphree AL, Villablanca JG, Deegan WF, et al. Chemotherapy plus local treatment in the management of intraocular retinoblastoma. *Arch Ophthalmol* 1996;114:1348–1356.

53. Murray TG, Roth DB, O'Brien JM, et al. Local carboplatin and radiation therapy in the treatment of

murine transgenic retinoblastoma. *Arch Ophthalmol* 1996;114:1385–1389.

54. Greenwald MJ, Strauss LC. Treatment of intraocular retinoblastoma with carboplatin and etoposide chemotherapy. *Ophthalmology* 1996;103:1989–1997.

55. Wilson AH, Karr DJ, Kalina RE, et al. Visual outcomes of macular retinoblastoma after external beam radiation therapy. *Ophthalmology* 1994;101:1244–1249.

56. Kock E, Rosengren B, Tengrath B, et al. Retinoblastoma treated with a ^{60}Co applicator. *Radiother Oncol* 1986;7:19–26.

57. Shields JA, Giblin ME, Shields CL, et al. Episcleral plaque radiotherapy for retinoblastoma. *Ophthalmology* 1989;96:530–537.

58. Shields CL, Shields JA, DePotter P, et al. Plaque radiotherapy for retinoblastoma. *Int Ophthalmol Clin* 1993;33:107–118.

59. Shields JA, Shields CL, DePotter P, et al. Plaque radiotherapy for residual or recurrent retinoblastoma in 91 cases. *J Pediatr Ophthalmol Strabismus* 1994;31:242–245.

60. Charles MW, Brown N. Dimensions of the human eye relevant to radiation protection. *Phys Med Biol* 1975;20:202–218.

61. Duke-Elder S, ed. The anatomy of the visual system. In: *System of ophthalmology*, vols. 2 and 10. London: Henry Kimpton, 1961;2:78–82, 1961;10:672–678.

62. Freire JE, DePotter P, Brady LW, et al. Brachytherapy in primary ocular tumors. *Semin Surg Oncol* 1997;13:167–176.

63. Kaste SC, Chen G, Fontanesi J, et al. Orbital development in long-term survivors of retinoblastoma. *J Clin Oncol* 1997;15(3):1183–1189.

64. Abramson DH, Notterman RB, Ellsworth RM, et al. Retinoblastoma treated in infants in the first six months of life. *Arch Ophthalmol* 1983;101:1362–1366.

65. Abramson DH, Servodidio CA, DeLillo AR, et al. Recurrence of unilateral retinoblastoma following radiation therapy. *Ophthalmic Genet* 1994;15:107–113.

66. Stallard HB. The treatment of retinoblastoma. *Ophthalmologica* 1966;151:214–230.

67. Hernandez JC, Brady LW, Shields CL, et al. Conservative treatment of retinoblastoma. The use of plaque brachytherapy. *Am J Clin Oncol* 1993;16(5):397–401.

*68. Shields CL, Shields JA, Cater J, et al. Plaque radiotherapy for retinoblastoma: long-term tumor control and treatment complications in 208 tumors. *Ophthalmology* 2001;108:2116–2121.

69. Hilgartner HL. Report of a case of double glioma treated by x-rays. *Tex Med J* 1910;18:322.

70. Marcus DM, Craft JL, Albert DM. Histopathologic verification of Verhoeff's 1918 irradiation cure of retinoblastoma. *Ophthalmology* 1990;97:221–224.

*71. Blach LE, McCormick B, Abramson DH. External beam radiation therapy and retinoblastoma: long-term results in the comparison of two techniques. *Int J Radiat Oncol Biol Phys* 1996;35:45–51.

72. McCormick B, Ellsworth R, Abramson D, et al. Radiation therapy for retinoblastoma: comparison of results with lens-sparing versus lateral beam techniques. *Int J Radiat Oncol Biol Phys* 1988;15:567–574.

73. McCormick B, Ellsworth R, Abramson D, et al. Results of external beam radiation for children with retinoblastoma: a comparison of two techniques. *J Pediatr Ophthalmol Strabismus* 1989;26:239–243.

74. Weiss DR, Cassady JR, Peterson R. Retinoblastoma: a modification in radiation therapy technique. *Radiology* 1975;114:705–708.

*75. Hungerford JL, Toma NMG, Plowman PN, et al. External beam radiotherapy for retinoblastoma: I: whole eye technique. *Br J Ophthalmol* 1995;79:109–111.

76. Brooks HL Jr, Meyer D, Shields JA, et al. Removal of radiation-induced cataracts in patients treated for retinoblastoma. *Arch Ophthalmol* 1990;108:1701–1708.

77. Fontanesi J, Pratt CB, Hustu HO, et al. Use of irradiation for therapy of retinoblastoma in children more than 1 year old: the St. Jude Children's Research Hospital experience and review of literature. *Med Pediatr Oncol* 1995;24:321–326.

78. Fontanesi J, Pratt C, Meyer D, et al. Asynchronous bilateral retinoblastoma: the St. Jude Children's Research Hospital experience. *Ophthalmic Genet* 1995;16:109–112.

79. Harnett AN, Hungerford J, Lambert G, et al. Modern lateral external beam (lens sparing) radiotherapy for retinoblastoma. *Ophthalmic Paediatr Genet* 1987;8:53–61.

80. Buckley EG, Heath H. Visual acuity after successful treatment of large macular retinoblastoma. *J Pediatr Ophthalmol Strabismus* 1992;29:103–106.

81. Merrill PT, Buckley EG, Halperin EC. New and recurrent tumors in germinal retinoblastoma: is there a treatment effect? *Ophthalmol Genet* 1996;17:115–118.

82. Schipper J. An accurate and simple method for megavoltage radiation therapy of retinoblastoma. *Radiother Oncol* 1983;1:31–41.

83. Schipper J, Tan KEWP, Van Peperzeel HA. Treatment of retinoblastoma by precision megavoltage radiation therapy. *Radiother Oncol* 1985;3:117–132.

*84. Toma NMG, Hungerford JL, Plowman PN, et al. External beam radiotherapy for retinoblastoma: II: lens sparing technique. *Br J Ophthalmol* 1995;79:112–117.

85. Croughs P, Deman C, Richard F, et al. Treatment of retinoblastoma using accelerated protons. *Bull Soc Belge Ophtalmol* 1992;243:81–85.

86. Smith EV, Gragoudas ES, Kolodny NH, et al. Magnetic resonance imaging: an emerging technique for the diagnosis of ocular disorders. *Int Ophthalmol* 1990;14(2):119–124.

87. Fitzek MN, Dahlberg WK, Nagasawa H, et al. Unexpected sensitivity to radiation of fibroblasts from unaffected parents of children with hereditary retinoblastoma. *Int J Cancer* 2002;99(5):764–768.

88. Loeffler JS, Alexander E III, Kooy HM, et al. Stereotactic radiotherapy: rationale, techniques, and early results. In: DeSalles AAF, Goetsch SJ, eds. *Stereotactic surgery and radiosurgery*. Madison, WI: Medical Physics Publishing, 1993:307–320.

89. Chatterjee B, Dulta TK, Ayyagari S, et al. Radiation schedules for advanced retinoblastoma in children. *Int J Radiol* 1977;31:100–103.

90. Fontanesi J, Pratt CB, Kun LE, et al. Treatment outcome and dose–response relationship in infants younger than 1 year treated for retinoblastoma with primary irradiation. *Med Pediatr Oncol* 1996;26:297–304.

91. Shidnia H, Hornback NB, Helveston EM, et al. Treatment results of retinoblastoma at Indiana University Hospitals. *Cancer* 1977;40:2917–2922.

92. Thompson RW, Small RC, Stein JJ. Treatment of retinoblastoma. *AJR Am J Roentgenol* 1972;114: 16–23.

92a. Weiss AH, Karr DJ, Kalina RE, et al. Visual outcomes of macular retinoblastoma after external beam radiation therapy. *Ophthalmology* 1994;101(7):1244–1249.

*93. Hernandez JC, Brady LW, Shields JA, et al. External beam radiation for retinoblastoma: results, patterns of failure, and a proposal for treatment guidelines. *Int J Radiat Oncol Biol Phys* 1996;35:125–132.

94. Messmer EP, Saverwin W, Heinrich T, et al. New and recurrent tumor foci follow local treatment as well as external beam retinoblastoma in eyes of patients with hereditary retinoblastoma. *Graefes Arch Clin Exp Ophthalmol* 1990;228:426–431.

95. Wolff JA, Baesel CP, Dyment PG. Treatment of retinoblastoma: a preliminary report. *Int Congress Ser* 1981;570:364–368.

96. Honavar SG, Singh AD, Shields CL, et al. Postenucleation adjuvant therapy in high risk retinoblastoma. *Arch Ophthalmol* 2002;120:923–931.

96a. Mustafa MM, Jamshed A, Khafaga Y, et al. Adjuvant chemotherapy with vincristine, doxorubicin, and cyclophosphamide in the treatment of post enucleation high risk retinoblastoma. *J Pediatr Hematol Oncol* 1999;21(5):364–369.

97. Uusitalo MS, Van Quill KR, Scott IU, et al. Evaluation of chemoprophylaxis in patients with unilateral retinoblastoma with high-risk features on histopathologic examination. *Arch Ophthalmol* 2001;119(1): 41–48.

*98. Ferris FL, Chew EY. A new era for the treatment of retinoblastoma. *Arch Ophthalmol* 1996;114:1412.

99. Shields CL, Shields JA, Needle M, et al. Combined chemoreduction and adjuvant treatment for intraocular retinoblastoma. *Ophthalmology* 1997;104:2101–2111.

*100. Shields CL, Honavar SG, Meadows AT. Chemoreduction plus focal therapy for retinoblastoma: factors predictive of need for treatment with external beam radiotherapy or enucleation. *Am J Ophthalmol* 2002; 133:657–664.

*101. Shields CL, Honavar SG, Shields JA, et al. Factors predictive of recurrence of retinal tumors, vitreous seeds, and subretinal seeds following chemoreduction for retinoblastoma. *Am J Ophthalmol* 2002;120: 460–464.

*102. Shields CL, Honavar SG, Meadows AT, et al. Chemoreduction for unilateral retinoblastoma. *Arch Ophthalmol* 2002;120:1653–1658.

103. Wilson MW, Rodriguez-Galindo C, Haik BG, et al. Multiagent chemotherapy as neoadjuvant treatment for multifocal intraocular retinoblastoma. *Ophthalmology* 2001;108:2106–2114.

104. Beck MN, Balmer A, Dessing C, et al. First-line chemotherapy with local treatment can prevent external-beam irradiation and enucleation in low-stage intraocular retinoblastoma. *J Clin Oncol* 2000;18: 2881–2887.

105. Friedman DL, Himelstein B, Shields CL, et al. Chemoreduction and local ophthalmic therapy for intraocular retinoblastoma. *J Clin Oncol* 2000;18:12–17.

*106. De Potter P. Current treatment for retinoblastoma. *Curr Opin Ophthalmol* 2002:13:331–336.

107. Gombos DS, Kelly A, Coen PG, et al. Retinoblastoma treated with primary chemotherapy alone: the significance of tumor size, location, and age. *Br J Ophthalmol* 2002;86:80–83.

108. Ghose S, Niziamuddin SH, Sethi A, et al. Efficacy of induction chemotherapy in retinoblastoma, alone or combined with other adjuvant modalities. *J Pediatr Ophthalmol Strabismus* 2002;39:143–150.

109. Brichard B, DeBruycker JJ, De Potter P, et al. Combined chemotherapy and local treatment in the management of intraocular retinoblastoma. *Med Pediatr Oncol* 2002;38:411–415.

110. Chan HSL, DeBaer G, Thiessen JJ, et al. Combining cyclosporin with chemotherapy controls intraocular retinoblastoma without requiring radiation. *Clin Cancer Res* 1996;2:1499–1508.

111. Chan HSL, deBaer G, Thorner PS, et al. Multidrug resistance: clinical opportunities in diagnosis and circumvention. *Hematol Oncol Clin North Am* 1994; 8:383–410.

112. Amoaku WMK, Willishaw HE, Parkes SE, et al. Trilateral retinoblastoma: a report of five patients. *Cancer* 1996;78:858–863.

113. Blach LE, McCormick B, Abramson DH, et al. Trilateral retinoblastoma incidence and outcome: a decade of experience. *Int J Radiat Oncol Biol Phys* 1994;29:729–733.

114. Paulino AC. Trilateral retinoblastoma: is the location of the intracranial tumor important? *Cancer* 1999;86: 135–141.

115. Shields CL, Shields JA, Meadows AT. Chemoreduction for retinoblastoma may prevent trilateral retinoblastoma. *J Clin Oncol* 2000;18:236–237.

116. Malik RK, Friedman HS, Djang W, et al. Treatment of trilateral retinoblastoma with vincristine and cyclophosphamide. *Am J Ophthalmol* 1986;102:650–656.

117. Marks LB, Bentel G, Sherouse GW, et al. Craniospinal irradiation for trilateral retinoblastoma following ocular irradiation. *Med Dosim* 1993;18:125–128.

118. Nelson SC, Friedman HS, Oakes WJ, et al. Successful therapy for trilateral retinoblastoma. *Am J Ophthalmol* 1992;114:23–29.

119. Abramson DH, Ellsworth RM, Rosenblatt M, et al. Retreatment of retinoblastoma with external beam irradiation. *Arch Ophthalmol* 1982;100:1257–1260.

120. Taktikas A. Investigation of retinoblastoma with special reference to histology and prognosis. *Br J Ophthalmol* 1966;50:225–234.

121. Kopelman JE, McLean IW, Rosenberg SH. Multivariate analysis of risk factors for metastasis in retinoblastoma treated by enucleation. *Ophthalmology* 1987;94:371–377.

122. Khelfaou F, Validire P, Auprin A, et al. Histologic risk factors for retinoblastoma: a retrospective study of 172 patients treated in a single institution. *Cancer* 1996;77:1206–1213.

123. Shields CL, Shields JA, Viaz EK, et al. Choroidal invasion of retinoblastoma: metastatic potential and clinical risk factors. *Br J Ophthalmol* 1993;77:544–548.

124. Stevenson KE, Hungerford J, Garner A. Local extraocular extension of retinoblastoma following in-

traocular surgery. *Br J Ophthalmol* 1989;73:739–742.

125. Khelfaoui F, Validire P, Auperin A, et al. Histopathologic risk factors in retinoblastoma: a retrospective study of 172 patients treated in a single institution. *Cancer* 1996;77:1206–1213.

126. Kopelman JE, McLean IW, Rosenberg SH. Multivariate analysis of risk factors for metastasis in retinoblastoma treated by enucleation. *Ophthalmology* 1987;94:371–377.

127. Schvartzman E, Chantada G, Fandino A, et al. Results of a stage-based protocol for the treatment of retinoblastoma. *J Clin Oncol* 1996;14:1532–1536.

128. Stannard C, Sealy R, Hering E, et al. Postenucleation orbits in retinoblastoma: treatment with ^{125}I brachytherapy. *Int J Radiat Oncol Biol Phys* 2002;54:1446–1454.

129. Arora V, Weeks K, Halperin EC, et al. Influence of coralline hydroxyapatite used as a ocular implant on the dose distribution of external bean photon radiation therapy. *Ophthalmology* 1992;99(3):380–382.

130. Dunkel IJ, Aledo A, Kernan NA, et al. Successful treatment of metastatic retinoblastoma. *Cancer* 2000; 89:2117–2121.

131. Bentel G, Halperin EC, Buckley EG. Iodine-125 embedded in an orbital prosthesis for re-treatment of recurrent retinoblastoma. *Med Dosim* 1993:18:1–5.

132. Goble RR, McKenzie J, Kingston JE, et al. Orbital recurrence of retinoblastoma successfully treated by combined therapy. *Br J Ophthalmol* 1990;74:97–98.

133. Ekert H, Tiedeman K, Waters KD, et al. Experience with high dose multiagent chemotherapy and autologous bone marrow rescue in the treatment of twenty-two children with advanced tumours. *Aust Paediatr J* 1984;20:195–201.

134. Saarinen UM, Sariola H, Hovi L. Recurrent disseminated retinoblastoma treated by high-dose chemotherapy, total body irradiation, and autologous bone marrow rescue. *Am J Pediatr Hematol Oncol* 1991; 13:315–319.

135. Yue NC, Benson ML. The hourglass facial deformity as a consequence of orbital irradiation for bilateral retinoblastoma. *Pediatr Radiol* 1996;26:421–423.

136. Namouni F, Doz F, Tanguy ML, et al. High-dose chemotherapy with carboplatin, etoposide and cyclophosphamide followed by a haematopoietic stem cell rescue in patients with high-risk retinoblastoma: a SFOP and SFGM study. *Eur J Cancer* 1997;33: 2368–2375.

137. Hertzberg H, Kremens B, Velten I, et al. Recurrent disseminated retinoblastoma in a 7-year-old girl treated successfully by high-dose chemotherapy and CD34-selected autologous peripheral blood stem cell transplantation. *Bone Marrow Transplant* 2001;27(6): 653–655.

138. Chantada G, Fandino A, Casak S, et al. Treatment of overt extraocular retinoblastoma. *Med Pediatr Oncol* 2003;40:158–161.

139. Eng C, Li FP, Abramson DH, et al. Mortality from second tumors among long-term survivors of retinoblastoma. *J Natl Cancer Inst* 1993;85:1121–1128.

140. Roarty JD, McLean IW, Zimmerman LE. Incidence of second neoplasms in patients with bilateral retinoblastoma. *Ophthalmology* 1988;95:1583–1587.

141. Frank CM, Abramson DH. Second non-ocular tumors

in retinoblastoma survivors: something new you need to know. *Int Symp Ocul Tumors* 1997:23(abst).

142. Wong FL, Boice JD Jr, Abramson DH, et al. Cancer incidence after retinoblastoma: radiation dose and sarcoma risk. *JAMA* 1997;278:1262–1267.

143. Cavenee WK, Murphree AL, Shull MM, et al. Prediction of familial predisposition to retinoblastoma. *N Engl J Med* 1986;314:1201–1207.

144. Imhof SM, Hofman P, Tan KEWP. Quantification of lacrimal function after D-shaped field irradiation for retinoblastoma. *Br J Ophthalmol* 1993;77:482–484.

145. Imhof SM, Mourits MP, Hofman P, et al. Quantification of orbital and mid-facial growth retardation after megavoltage external beam irradiation in children with retinoblastoma. *Ophthalmology* 1996;103:263–268.

146. Messmer EP, Frize H, Mohr C, et al. Long-term treatment effects in patients with bilateral retinoblastoma: ocular and mid-facial findings. *Graefes Arch Clin Exp Ophthalmol* 1991;229:309–314.

147. Chantada G, Fandino A, Casak S, et al. Treatment of overt extraocular retinoblastoma. *Med Pediatr Oncol* 2003;40:158–161.

148. Cogan DG, Fink R, Donaldson DD. X-ray irradiation of orbital glands of the rabbit. *Radiology* 1955;64: 731–737.

149. Kingston JE, Plowman PN, Hungerford JL. Ectopic intracranial retinoblastoma in childhood. *Br J Ophthalmol* 1985;69(10):742–748.

150. DePotter P, Shields CL, Shields JA. Clinical variations of trilateral retinoblastoma: a report of 13 cases. *J Pediatr Ophthalmol Strabismus* 1994; 31:26–31.

151. Holbek S, Ehlers N. Long-term visual results in eyes cured for retinoblastoma by radiation. *Acta Ophthalmol* 1989;67:560–566.

152. Haye C, Desjardins L, Schlienger P, et al. Treatment of bilateral retinoblastoma stage V at the Curie Foundation. *Ophthalmol Paediatr Genet* 1987;8:73–76.

152a. DePotter P. Current treatment of retinoblastoma. *Curr Opin Ophthalmol* 2002;13:331–336.

153. Monge OR, Flage T, Hatlevoli R, et al. Sightsaving therapy in retinoblastoma experience with external megavoltage radiotherapy. *Acta Ophthalmol* 1986; 64:414–420.

153a. Levy C, Doz F, Quintana E, et al. Role of chemotherapy alone or in combination with hyperthermia in the primary treatment of intraocular retinoblastoma: preliminary results. *Br J Ophthalmol* 1998;82:1154–1158.

154. Shields CL, Santos MC, Dini W, et al. Thermotherapy for retinoblastoma. *Arch Ophthalmol* 1999;117: 885–893.

155. Schouten-Van Meeteren AYN, Moll AC, Imhof SM, et al. Chemotherapy for retinoblastoma: an expanding area of clinical research. *Med Pediatr Oncol* 2002;38:428–438.

156. Magramm I, Abramson DH, Ellsworth RM. Optic nerve involvement in retinoblastoma. *Ophthalmology* 1989;96:217–222.

157. Zhang M, Stevens G, Madigan MC. In vitro effects of radiation on human retinoblastoma cells. *Int J Cancer* 2001;96(Suppl):7–14.

158. Hayden BC, Murray TG, Cicciarelli N, et al. Hyperfractionated external beam radiation therapy in the treatment of murine transgenic retinoblastoma. *Arch Ophthalmol* 2002;120:353–359.

159. Lal P, Biswal BM, Mohanti BK, et al. Management of retinoblastoma with radiation. *Indian Pediatr* 2001;38:15–23.

160. Kao LY, Tsang NM. Advanced bilateral retinoblastoma treated conservatively with lens sparing external beam radiation therapy: report of three cases. *Changgeng Yi Xue Za Zhi* 1999;22:100–105.

161. Hall LS, Ceisler E, Abramson DH. Visual outcomes in children with bilateral retinoblastoma. *J AAPOS: Am Assoc Pediatr Ophthalmol Strabismus* 1999;3: 138–142.

162. Kivela T. Trilateral retinoblastoma: a meta-analysis of hereditary retinoblastoma associated with primary ectopic intracranial retinoblastoma. *J Clin Oncol* 1999; 17:1829–1837.

163. Shields CL, Meadows AT, Shields JA, et al. Chemoreduction for retinoblastoma may prevent intracranial neuroblastic malignancy (trilateral retinoblastoma). *Arch Ophthalmol* 2001;119:1269–1272.

164. Lumbroso L, Doz F, Urbieta M, et al. Chemotherapy in the management of retinoblastoma. *Ophthalmology* 2002;109:1130–1136.

*165. Finger, Czechonska G, Demirci H, et al. Chemotherapy for retinoblastoma: a current topic. *Drugs* 1999;58:983–996.

166. Scott IU, Murray TG, Feuer WJ. et al. External beam radiotherapy in retinoblastoma: tumor control and comparison of 2 techniques. *Arch Ophthalmol* 1999; 117:766–770.

167. Merchant TE, Gould CJ, Hilton NE, et al. Ocular preservation after 36 Gy external beam radiation therapy for retinoblastoma. *J Pediatr Hematol Oncol* 2002;24:246–249.

168. Nahum MP, Gdal-On M, Kuten A, et al. Long-term follow-up of children with retinoblastoma. *J Pediatr Hematol Oncol* 2001;13:173–179.

6

Neuroblastoma

Katherine K. Matthay, M.D., Daphne Haas-Kogan, M.D.,
and Louis S. Constine, M.D.

Neuroblastoma (NB) is a malignancy derived from embryonic neural crest cells of the peripheral sympathetic nervous system. It is the most common extracranial solid tumor of childhood, accounting for 15% of cancer-related deaths. The behavior of NB is marked by clinical heterogeneity, which leads to differences in behavior ranging from spontaneous maturation in some patients to inexorable rapid metastatic progression in others. It was noted as early as 1927 to be a tumor in which spontaneous maturation could occur, when Cushing and Wolbach (1) reported the case of a 2-year-old boy whose thoracic paravertebral sympathetic NB, over the course of 10 years, transformed into a completely differentiated ganglioneuroma. However, advanced NB is the most lethal of childhood solid tumors, often resistant to all attempts at disease eradication (2). The enigmatic behavior of this tumor is beginning to be elucidated by new research into the genetic and biologic diversity, but the treatment of advanced disease is a continuing challenge. This chapter discusses the biologic features of NB associated with differing behavior, the evaluation and staging, and a risk-based approach to therapy, with an emphasis on local control issues.

EPIDEMIOLOGY AND SCREENING

There are approximately 650 cases of NB annually in the United States, with an overall incidence of 10.3 per million per year from birth to age 15. NB accounts for nearly 10% of pediatric cancer in children younger than 15 years old, making it the fourth most common malignancy in children after leukemias, brain tumors, and lymphomas. However, it is the most common malignancy of children younger than 18 months old, with an incidence of 29.1 per million per year in children younger than 5 years old (3). Ninety percent of patients with NB are diagnosed by 10 years, 79% before 4 years, and 36% are infants less than 1 year old. The incidence is slightly higher in boys than girls. The median age at diagnosis is 22 months (4). NB is responsible for 15% of childhood cancer mortality, with an annual mortality rate of 5 per million for all children and 9 per million for the 0- to 4-year-old subgroup (5).

NB arises from primitive (fetal) adrenergic neuroblasts of neural crest tissue, which may explain its high incidence in infancy. In the embryo, continuous columns of neural crest tissue form dorsolateral to the developing neural tissue. These columns are the precursors of the spinal ganglia, the dorsal spinal nerve roots, and the chromaffin cells, which flank the abdominal aorta (6). The largest of these masses is the adrenal medulla (Fig. 6-1). Most cases of NB occur in an anatomic distribution consistent with the location of neural crest tissue (Fig. 6-2).

The frequency of neuroblastic nodules, resembling NB *in situ,* in the adrenals of autopsied infants who have died of other causes ranges from 1 in 39 to 1 in 600 autopsies, suggesting that most regress by birth (7). This is interpreted to mean that such nodules are embryologic adrenal remnants and are the cells from which adrenal medulla NB may develop.

Several studies using systematic screening of neonates for NB have confirmed the results of earlier autopsy studies by suggesting a much higher incidence of NB than is clinically evident. More than 90% of NBs secrete vanillylmandelic acid (VMA) or homovanillic acid

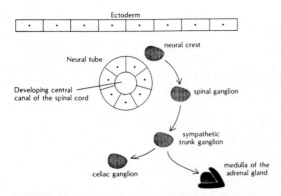

FIG. 6-1. Migration of the neural crest in the human embryo.

(HVA) in the urine, for which rapid quantitative screening methods have been developed that have a high degree of sensitivity and specificity. Urinary catecholamine screening for NB was initially proposed by Woods et al. (8) because

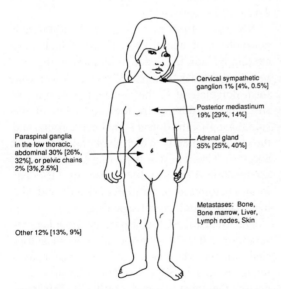

FIG. 6-2. Common locations of neuroblastoma. The first percentage is the overall proportion of cases at the site. The numbers in parentheses are the percentages of cases at a given site in children 1 year of age or younger and older than 1 year of age. (Data are from Bernstein ML, Leclerc JM, Bunin G, et al. A population-based study of neuroblastoma incidence, survival, and mortality in North America. *J Clin Oncol* 1992; 10(2):323–329; and J. Shuster, Ph.D., Pediatric Oncology Group Statistical Office.)

the incidence of 8.7 per 1 million children per year is comparable to or higher than that of other congenital diseases for which screening is already in place, such as hypothyroidism, galactosemia, and phenylketonuria. The poor prognosis for advanced NB in children older than 12 months of age at diagnosis compared with the favorable outcome for those diagnosed in infancy raised the expectation that diagnosis at an earlier age might improve overall outcome. However, the cumulative data from 30 years of screening in Japan, the Quebec Neuroblastoma Screening Project, and screening projects in Europe have shown that screening infants by 6 months of age results in a significant increase in the overall incidence of NB but fails to reduce the incidence of advanced stage disease with poor prognosis (8–12). NBs detected by screening have almost exclusively favorable biologic features (*MYCN* nonamplified, triploid, favorable Shimada histology) (13,14). Thus, screening practices result in the overdiagnosis of tumors that would otherwise have spontaneously regressed. A recent publication from the Quebec project conclusively showed that screening at 3 weeks and 6 months in a cohort of 476,654 infants born over a 5-year period had no impact on overall mortality for the screened cohort compared with multiple control populations from Minnesota, the Delaware Valley, Florida, and the rest of Canada, verifying the results of the earlier studies (9). A second study screened 1,475,773 children at 1 year of age in German states and similarly revealed no impact on outcome (15). The screened group and children in the control area had a similar incidence of stage 4 NB (3.7 cases per 100,000 screened children and 3.8 per 100,000 controls) and a similar rate of death among children with NB (1.3 deaths per 100,000 screened children and 1.2 per 100,000 control subjects). There was a substantial rate of overdiagnosis in the screened group of children without benefit from the screening.

The environmental and inherited factors involved in the pathogenesis of NB are largely unknown, despite extensive epidemiologic and genetic studies. Given the young age at which most NBs present, it has been suggested that environmental exposures before conception or during pregnancy increase the risk of NB. Epidemiologic investigations have implicated fetal exposure to diuretics, tranquilizers, hormones, phenytoin, alcohol, and tobacco as increasing the risk of NB (16–18). However, these studies have lacked the statistical power to convincingly demonstrate that these drugs are etiologic risk factors or have not been confirmed by subsequent studies (19). Environmental exposures are unlikely to be significant, although certain parental occupations have been associated with increased risk of NB, including those involving electrical exposures, gardening, farming, and painting (20–22). However, none of these associations has been seen consistently. A recent report states that infection with a polyoma virus called BK Virus may play a role in the pathogenesis of NB, but this also has not been confirmed (23).

Although NB usually occurs sporadically, 1–2% of patients have a family history of the disease. This is similar to the other embryonal cancers of childhood in which a familial predisposition is observed. Familial NB is inherited in an autosomal dominant Mendelian fashion with incomplete penetrance. Affected children from these families differ from those with sporadic disease in that they are often diagnosed at an earlier age (usually infancy) or they have multiple primary tumors. These clinical characteristics are hallmarks of the two-mutation cancer predisposition model first proposed for retinoblastoma. Therefore, it seems likely that familial NB occurs as a result of a germ line mutation in one allele of a tumor suppressor gene (24). Germ line mutations have rarely been identified, with only rare case reports of familial cases with mutations in 1p36, one of the common areas of allelic loss in sporadic NB. At least 14 other cases of constitutional chromosomal rearrangements in patients with NB have been identified, but the lack of a consistent pattern indicates that many of these rearrangements may be coincidental rather than causal (25–27). A more recent linkage analysis in families of affected patients suggests that some familial cases may be caused by germ line loss of heterozygosity at 16p12–13, an abnormality also noted in 20% of sporadic tumors (28). NB has also been reported in families in conjunction with other neurocristopathies, such as Hirschsprung's disease and central hypoventilation (Ondine's curse) (29). There is surprising heterogeneity among patients with familial NB. Within individual families, the disease can vary from an asymptomatic and spontaneously regressing NB to a rapidly progressive and fatal disease.

BIOLOGY

Cytogenetic and molecular studies in NB are providing new insights into its biology and prognosis. Unfavorable biologic features include amplification of *MYCN*, deletion or loss of heterozygosity of chromosome 1p or 11q, and gains at 17q, and favorable biologic features include hyperdiploidy and overexpression of Trk A (30–34). Recognizing these biologic pathways in NB has improved the ability to treat children with risk-based therapy and may lead to novel therapeutic approaches in the near future.

MYCN amplification was the first and is now the most widely accepted biologic marker of prognosis for NB (31,35–39). *MYCN* is in the family of MYC oncogenes that encode transcriptional regulatory factors involved in the control of other genes. The amplification is generally a consequence of an aberrant gain of multiple copies of the *MYCN* gene. Homogeneously staining regions (HSRs, nonbanding regions of metaphase chromosomes that stain homogeneously) and double-minute chromatin bodies (fragments of HSRs) are a manifestation of gene amplification (Fig. 6-3). They are derived from the distal short arms of chromosome 2, which contains the proto-oncogene *MYCN*. The excess number of *MYCN* genes leads to overexpression of the n-myc protein and subsequent overproduction of growth-promoting signals and stimulation of proliferation and tumorigenesis. Mice with aberrant overexpression of *MYCN* develop NB, providing evidence that *MYCN* plays a prominent role in NB development (40). *MYCN* amplification is most easily detected on fluorescent *in situ* hybridization of fresh tumor imprints, although it may also be tested by immunohistochemistry, Southern blot, or polymerase chain reaction.

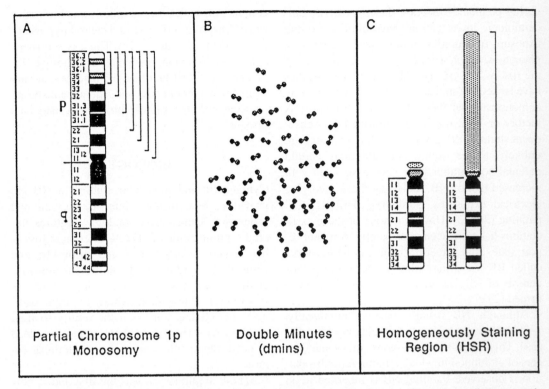

FIG. 6-3. Common cytogenetic abnormalities in human neuroblastomas. Shown are diagrammatic representations of the three most common cytogenetic abnormalities seen in human neuroblastomas. **(A)** Deletions of the short arm of chromosome 1. The brackets indicate that the region deleted in different tumors is variable in terms of its proximal breakpoint, but the distal short arm appears to be deleted in all cases, resulting in partial 1p monosomy. **(B)** Extrachromosomal double-minute chromatin bodies (dmins). These are seen in about 30% of primary neuroblastoma and are a cytogenetic manifestation of gene amplification. **(C)** Homogeneously staining region (HSR). A representative HSR on the short arm of chromosome 13 is shown in this example. HSRs are a cytogenetic manifestation of gene amplification in which the amplified sequences are chromosomally integrated. (From Bernstein ML, Leclerc JM, Bunin G, et al. A population-based study of neuroblastoma incidence, survival, and mortality in North America. *J Clin Oncol* 1992;10(2):323–329; and Powis MR, Imeson JD, Holmes SJ. The effect of complete excision on stage III neuroblastoma: a report of the European Neuroblastoma Study Group. *J Pediatr Surg* 1996;31(4):516–519, with permission.)

Amplification of *MYCN* in primary NB has been shown to correlate with advanced stage and a poor prognosis. Such amplification occurs in 30–40% of advanced-stage NB but in only 5–10% of low-stage or IV-S disease and not at all in benign ganglioneuromas (41). Children who have *MYCN* amplification in their tumor need more intensive or novel therapy to control the disease. *MYCN* usually is an independent prognostic factor such that amplification por-

tends an unfavorable outcome, even in disease settings that would otherwise be favorable. *MYCN* amplification is seldom identified in localized stage disease (stages 1 and 2) but may predict a poor outcome in these patients when present (42). Amplification of *MYCN* is also uncommon in infants with stage 4S disease but predicts a less favorable survival (44% vs. 90%) (39). Amplified *MYCN* was more common in tumors from children older than 1 year with advanced stage and elevated ferritin, neuron-specific enolase, lactate dehydrogenase, and chromosome 1p deletion (35,43).

DNA ploidy is also an important discriminator of response to chemotherapy for NB (19). In 1984, Look et al. (44) described 23 children with unresectable NB. Of the 17 patients with hyperdiploid status, 15 were complete responders to chemotherapy and two were partial responders. None of the six patients with diploid tumors responded ($p = 0.0001$). In a 1991 report, Look et al. (34) evaluated 298 children. In infants with metastatic disease the progression-free survival (PFS) was more than 90% for those with hyperdiploid tumors and 0% in diploid cases. In children 12 to 24 months of age with stage D, the distinction was also striking (50–60% in hyperdiploid cases and 0% in diploid, $p < 0.001$). A subsequent Pediatric Oncology Group (POG) study of infants with unresectable or metastatic NB reported an overall 3-year survival of 94% for patients with hyperdiploid tumors and 55% for diploid (33). Ploidy probably is not useful as a prognostic marker in children older than 24 months, in whom most tumors are diploid.

Specific chromosomal deletions often are present in NB. Deletion of the short arm of chromosome 1 occurs in 30–50% of primary tumors and usually lies at the distal end of chromosome 1 in the area of 1p36 (45,46). Loss of chromosome 1p strongly correlates with *MYCN* amplification and is also associated with a poor prognosis. Whether loss of heterozygosity of 1p and *MYCN* amplification are independent prognostic markers of outcome remains controversial (30,47–49).

Loss of heterozygosity has also been reported for chromosome 11q and is identified in nearly half of the NB samples analyzed (50,51). Unbalanced loss of chromosome 11q is associated with a worse prognosis and inversely related to *MYCN* amplification (51,52). Chromosomal deletion may result in the loss of a suppressor gene. Several candidate genes for the NB suppressor gene have been mapped to 1p36 and 11q; however, none have been shown to have mutations in the nondeleted allele. An alternative pathway for tumorigenesis from one of the candidate genes may relate to dosage effect, with the allelic loss causing a reduction in the level of an important protein.

Partial gains at chromosome 17q are another common genetic alteration and are associated with an adverse outcome. Gains on chromosome 17q have been linked to several prognostic factors: age greater than 1 year, advanced-stage disease, deletion of chromosome 1p, and amplification of *MYCN*. It is the most common genetic alteration found in NB, occurring in 50% of cases (53). In one study, patients with the gain of 17q had a 5-year relapse-free survival of 16%, compared with 75% in patients without this genetic alteration (54). Again, whether 17q gain is an important independent marker of prognosis must be verified in a larger prospective study.

In addition to gains and losses of genetic material, other genes that have been identified as prognostically important include nerve growth factor receptor expression, telomerase activity, and genes involved in invasion and metastasis. The neurotrophins and their receptors are important in nervous system development and hence NB tumorigenesis. Expression of Trk A and Trk C has been found to correlate with lower stage and the absence of *MYCN* amplification. Conversely, expression of Trk B correlates with amplification of *MYCN*. The balance of Trk expression may influence the spontaneous regression of NB or the differentiation into benign ganglioneuromas (26). High levels of telomerase activity may also predict an aggressive tumor phenotype (55). Integrins are also important in NB. The majority of NB tumors express high levels of *CD44,* except for tumors of advanced stage and *MYCN* amplification. Lack of *CD44* expression is strongly associated with *MYCN* amplification and in multivariate analysis is an independent predictor of overall survival (56,57). Another integrin, alphaVbeta3, appears to be expressed predominantly in undifferentiated and high-risk NB (58,59), with an antiangiogenic integrin alphaV antagonist able to inhibit growth of NB in a syngeneic murine tumor model by working synergistically with an anti-GD2 antibody (60). The metalloproteinases

MMP2 (gelatinase A) and *MMP9* (gelatinase B) are expressed in primary NB tumors, with increased expression associated with more advanced stage and *MMP2* correlating with worse outcome (61). The angiogenic vascular endothelial growth factor has been found in both NB cell lines and in primary tumors, with higher expression in high-risk disease (62,63).

PATHOLOGY

NB is one of the small blue round cell tumors, along with non-Hodgkin's lymphoma, Ewing's sarcoma, undifferentiated soft tissue sarcomas including rhabdomyosarcoma, and primitive neuroectodermal tumors. The classic histologic subtypes of neuroblastic tumors include NB, ganglioneuroblastoma, and ganglioneuroma, reflecting a pattern of increasing maturation and differentiation (64). The cells of NB are small and uniformly sized, with dense hyperchromatic nuclei and scant cytoplasm (Fig. 6-4). The cells may be densely packed, separated by thin fibrils or bundles, and necrosis and calcification can occur. Neuritic processes can be demonstrated in most cases, and pseudorosettes can be seen in 15–50% of cases. The other end of the spectrum, ganglioneuroma, has mature ganglion cells, neuritic processes, and Schwann cells and has more fibrillary material. Any immature cells or nuclear atypia negates this diagnosis. Patients with ganglioneuroma or ganglioneuroblastoma generally have localized tumors with favorable biologic characteristics, explaining the excellent associated prognosis.

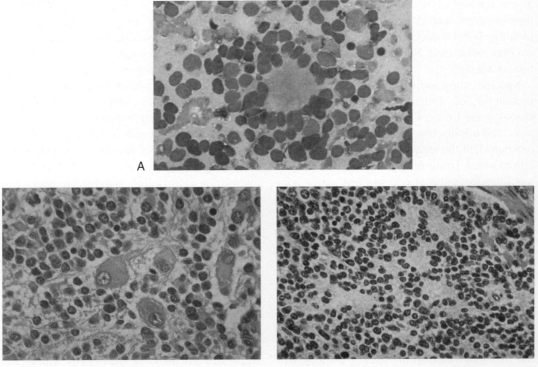

FIG. 6-4. (A) Fine-needle aspirate of neuroblastoma, showing typical Homer–Wright pseudorosettes with neurofibrillary material in the center. **(B)** Differentiating neuroblastoma, Schwannian stroma–poor. **(C)** Neuroblastoma (Schwannian stroma–poor), poorly differentiated subtype, composed of undifferentiated neuroblastic cells with clearly recognizable neuropil. (From Shimada H, Ambros IM, Dehner LP, et al. Terminology and morphologic criteria of neuroblastic tumors: recommendations by the International Neuroblastoma Pathology Committee. *Cancer* 1999;86(2):349–363, with permission.) (See color plate)

NB has a mixture of neuroblastic and mature ganglion cells and cells intermediate in their differentiation. Various immunohistochemical techniques and electron microscopy are used for diagnosis. Immunohistochemical stains recognize neuron-specific enolase (NSE), synaptophysin, chromogranin A, and neuronal filaments (65). Electron microscopy reveals neurofilaments, neurotubules, and neurosecretory granules that contain catecholamines.

Three systems have been proposed to assess the influence of pathology on prognosis: the Shimada classification, the Joshi classification (also called the Joshi modification of the Shimada classification), and the International Neuroblastoma Pathology Committee Classification (66–68). The major aspects of these three systems are summarized in Table 6-1. Shimada et al. formulated a highly prognostic system based on patient age, the presence of stroma ("rich" or "poor") and nodularity, the degree of differenti-

ation, and the mitosis–karyorrhexis index. Joshi et al. (70,71) attempted to combine conventional terminology with criteria used by Shimada and others. The terms *neuroblastoma* and *ganglioneuroblastoma* are retained rather than stroma-poor and stroma-rich NB. Undifferentiated NB, poorly differentiated NB. and differentiating NB are considered distinct, based on degree of cellular density and the number of tumor cells and mitotic karyorrhectic cells per high-power field (Fig. 6-4) (72). The International NB Classification, based largely on the Shimada system, is now being used in protocols worldwide to facilitate comparisons of patient groups (64,66). A retrospective analysis of the Children's Cancer Group (CCG) validated the prognostic value of this system combined with age (73).

CLINICAL PRESENTATION AND EVALUATION

The clinical presentation of NB depends on the site along the sympathetic nervous system chain from which the primary tumor develops (Fig. 6-2) and on the manifestations of metastatic disease. This varies according to patient age. The abdomen is the most common primary tumor location (50–80% of cases). Intra-abdominal primary tumors arise in the adrenals or in a paraspinal location. The paraspinal tumors may have a dumbbell configuration wherein tumor extends through the neural foramina and presents with a mass lesion in the spinal canal; extradural spinal cord compression may occur. Extra-abdominal locations of the primary tumor include sympathetic ganglia in the neck (often initially thought to be lymphadenitis), posterior mediastinum, and pelvis.

The earliest symptoms or signs of NB may be a palpable abdominal mass (often large, firm, irregular, and crossing the midline), a unilateral neck mass often causing Horner's syndrome, spinal cord compression, respiratory compromise caused by thoracic disease or hepatic metastases placing upward pressure on the diaphragm, or bowel and bladder disturbances caused by compression from a pelvic mass. About 60% of children with NB have metastatic disease (either lymphatic or hematogenous) at

TABLE 6-1. *Three major histopathologic classification systems for neuroblastoma*

Shimada system
 Favorable prognosis is associated with
  Stroma rich, all ages, no nodular pattern
  Stroma poor, age 1.5–5 yr, differentiated,
   MKI < 100
  Stroma poor, age <1.5 yr, MKI < 200
 Unfavorable prognosis is associated with
  Stroma rich, all ages, nodular pattern
  Stroma poor, age >5 yr
  Stroma poor, age 1.5–5 yr, undifferentiated
  Stroma poor, age 1.5–5 yr, differentiated,
   MKI > 100
  Stroma poor, age <1.5 yr, MKI > 200
Joshi system
 Favorable prognosis is associated with grade 1, all
  ages; grade 2, <1 yr
 Unfavorable prognosis is associated with grade 2,
  age >1 yr, grade 3, all ages
International Neuroblastoma Pathology Committee
 system
 Classification of neuroblastoma is based on
  Degree of differentiation toward ganglion cells
  Amount of Schwann cell stroma present
  Whether the tumor is nodular, noting particularly
   macronodules (which tend to be associated
   with a poor prognosis compared with
   intermixed nodules)
  Degree of calcification
  MKI

MKI, mitosis–karyorrhexis index.
Based on references 67, 70, and 73.

the time of clinical presentation. The symptoms in this setting are those of systemic illness: fever, weight loss, weakness, or a general failure to thrive. In a few patients, the presenting symptoms are related to secretory products of the tumor. For example, intractable diarrhea (from vasoactive intestinal polypeptide) may rarely occur, usually in children with ganglioneuroblastoma or ganglioneuroma. In another rare paraneoplastic syndrome, seen in about 3% of patients, a child with NB presents with the opsoclonus (rapid multidirectional eye movements)–myoclonus–truncal ataxia syndrome. This paraneoplastic syndrome is associated with early-stage NB, it is probably caused by development of antineuronal antibodies, and neurologic deficits usually persist despite cure of the tumor (74–77). Bone metastases present as pain, refusal to walk, skull masses, or proptosis with orbital ecchymosis. Skin metastases are common in neonates and generally have a blue tinge (the "blueberry muffin" sign). When a skin me-

tastasis is manually compressed, one may observe blanching of the surrounding skin secondary to liberation of vasoconstrictive catecholamine. NB may infiltrate the marrow and cause pancytopenia with resulting complications (infection, pallor, lethargy, bleeding). Intracranial metastatic disease usually is meningeal, and in infants it may cause cranial suture separation.

The standard diagnostic evaluation of NB (Table 6-2) includes imaging and laboratory testing with the goals of determining disease extent and prognosis and identifying markers of disease activity. The primary tumor typically is imaged radiographically and with computed tomography (CT) scan or magnetic resonance imaging (MRI). The classic radiographic sign of adrenal NB is calcification in a suprarenal soft tissue mass. In the thorax, a plain radiograph demonstrates a posterior mediastinal mass. In both abdomen and chest, CT scan and MRI are helpful in assessing possible lymph node metastases and intraspinal extension (2).

TABLE 6-2. *Clinical evaluation of neuroblastoma (international neuroblastoma staging system's minimum recommended studies to determine the extent of disease)*

Tumor site	Tests
Primary	CT, ultrasound, or MRI with three-dimensional measurements
Metastases	Bilateral posterior iliac bone marrow aspirates and core biopsies (four adequate specimens necessary to exclude tumor)
	Bone radiographs and scintigraphy by ^{99m}Tc-diphosphonate, with or without ^{131}I-MIBG or ^{123}I-MIBG
	Abdominal and liver imaging by CT, ultrasound, or MRI
	Chest radiograph (anteroposterior and lateral) and chest CT
Markers	Urinary catecholamine metabolites (vanillylmandelic acid and homovanillic acid)

CT, computed tomography; MIBG, metaiodobenzylguanidine; MRI, magnetic resonance imaging.

From Brodeur GM, Pritchard J, Berthold F, et al. Revisions of the international criteria for neuroblastoma diagnosis, staging, and response to treatment. *J Clin Oncol* 1993;11(8):1466–1477; and Brodeur GM, Seeger RC, Barrett A, et al. International criteria for diagnosis, staging, and response to treatment in patients with neuroblastoma. *J Clin Oncol* 1988;6(12):1874–1881, with permission.

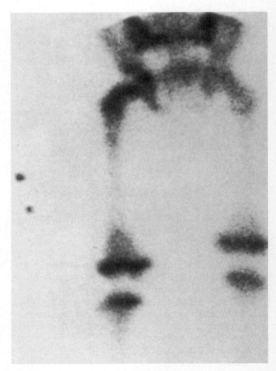

FIG. 6-5. Femoral metastases from neuroblastoma.

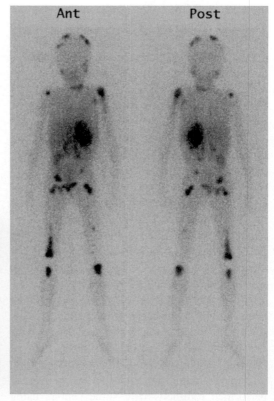

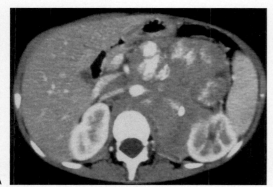

A
B

FIG. 6-6. A 4-year-old boy presented with fever, abdominal pain, and leg pain. **(A)** The computed tomography scan shows a large retroperitoneal neuroblastoma that encases the abdominal aorta and displaces the inferior vena cava. The left kidney is pushed laterally, and calcifications are evident. **(B)** This ^{123}I-metaiodobenzylguanidine scan shows intense localization in the primary retroperitoneal mass. Widespread bone metastases are evident, with large lesions in the distal right femur and proximal left humerus, but multiple other lesions are seen on the dome of the skull, right humerus, right rib, pelvis, and both femurs and tibias, and in a few retroperitoneal areas, probably representing nodal spread. Physiologic uptake is seen in the salivary glands, liver, and thyroid gland, which was insufficiently blocked with potassium iodide drops.

The search for distant, usually bony metastasis must include scanning with ^{123}I-metaiodobenzyl-guanidine (MIBG) and a technetium (Tc) radionuclide bone scan, with conventional radiographs as indicated. Bone metastases are most often periorbital, metaphyseal, and axial in location (Fig. 6-5). Bone scintigraphy is more sensitive than conventional radiographs but is sometimes difficult to interpret in infants younger than 1 year old. MIBG is a guanethidine derivative that is similar in structure to norepinephrine and epinephrine. The compound is taken up by catecholaminergic cells and stored in the chromaffin granules. It is highly sensitive and specific for skeletal and soft tissue metastases of NB, taken up in more than 90% of primary and metastatic tumors. The MIBG is labeled with an isotope of iodine (either ^{131}I or ^{123}I), and scintigraphy is performed for imaging. Because MIBG depends on functional uptake by tumor cells, it is also useful in distinguishing residual active tumor after treatment from masses composed of scar tissue and may complement CT scans (Fig. 6-6) (78,79). More recently, early response by MIBG scan has been shown to be a useful prognostic marker of response and survival (80). ^{99m}Tc-diphosphonate bone scans continue to be used to detect metastatic foci in the skeleton, even in patients who are negative by MIBG (81). Positron emission tomography scans with ^{18}F-fluorodeoxyglucose are a new modality that may complement MIBG for determination of tumor viability. Several studies have demonstrated that positron emission tomography scanning can visualize NB, even in some cases where MIBG is negative, although in other cases the converse is true (82,83).

Liver involvement may be evaluated by CT, ultrasound, or radionuclide liver scan in older children because it is usually focal or nodular. In infants it may be diffuse and not apparent by imaging. For this reason, some authorities recommend liver biopsies for diagnostic workup of infants. Pulmonary parenchymal metastases rarely occur at diagnosis in NB, although at relapse they may be seen in 7% of cases and should be sought with CT scan (84,85).

There may be extensive involvement of the bone marrow by tumor without a change in the peripheral blood counts, with some bone marrow tumor present at diagnosis in 80–90% of children with metastatic disease (84). Therefore, bilateral bone marrow aspiration and biopsy are performed routinely, with some centers using four to ten core biopsies to minimize sampling error (86). Small amounts of NB cells may be difficult to distinguish from hematopoietic elements. The diagnosis of NB in the bone marrow can be confirmed when only small amounts of tumor are present with immunohistochemical stains on the core biopsy, often using NSE as a marker, or with immunostaining on a concentrated cytology specimen from the aspirate. This technology clearly is more sensitive than conventional analyses, detecting one tumor cell per 10^5 to 10^6 normal mononuclear marrow cells (87). The extent of tumor involvement detected by immunocytology at diagnosis in marrow or peripheral blood provides prognostic information (88). At present, tumor detected by immunocytology that is not extensive enough to be diagnosed by conventional bone marrow microscopy does not affect staging (89). Reverse transcriptase polymerase chain reaction (RT-PCR) is being used in a number of prospective studies to further quantitate the prognostic impact of minimal residual disease detected in blood or bone marrow (90,91).

NB is associated with elevated or abnormal production, secretion, and catabolism of catecholamines (or metabolites) in 90% of cases (92). Catecholamines and metabolites may be measured in the urine: norepinephrine, VMA, 3-methoxy-4-hydroxyphenylglycol, or HVA. Dopamine may be measured in urine or serum. Urinary catecholamines typically are presented as ratios to urinary creatinine. The symptoms associated with excess catecholamine production include flushing and sweating, pallor, headache, and hypertension. Diarrhea may occur and has been attributed to the excretion of vasoactive intestinal peptide (VIP). Both VIP and somatostatin can be quantified by radioimmunoassay in NB cells and may relate to prognosis (discussed later in this chapter) (93).

STAGING AND PROGNOSTIC FACTORS

The criteria for diagnosis of NB recommended by the second International Neuroblastoma Staging System (INSS) Conference are unequivocal pathologic diagnosis from tumor tissue by light microscopy, with or without immunohistology, electron microscopy, elevated urine or serum catecholamines or metabolites (dopamine, HVA, or VMA greater than 3.0 SD above the mean per-milligram creatinine for age); or bone marrow aspirate or biopsy containing unequivocal tumor cells (e.g., syncytia or immunocytologically positive clumps of cells) and elevated urine or serum catecholamines or metabolites (89). A diagnosis of NB based only on compatible radiographic findings and elevated urinary catecholamine metabolites is insufficient because of possible confusion with ganglioneuroma or pheochromocytoma or even other solid tumors (e.g., primitive neuroectodermal tumor, rhabdomyosarcoma), which can have false positive urinary findings.

Staging

Four systems have been used for the staging of NB: the international tumor, node, and metastasis system (rarely used in pediatric tumors), the definition by Evans et al. (94) adopted by the

CCG, the surgical staging system of St. Jude's adopted by the POG, and the system internationally developed and in current use, the INSS (Table 6-3A), an attempt to improve and unify the previous definitions. Understanding the nuances of these systems is important for interpreting and accurately comparing data from various reports and determining therapy. Evans et al. (95,96) proposed a clinical system based on the extent of the primary tumor and the presence or absence of distant metastases. A special stage (IV-S) is allotted to infants younger than 1 year old with a small primary tumor and metastases to the liver, skin, or bone marrow. Most children with bona fide stage 4S disease have up to 10% tumor cells in marrow.

The Evans system was criticized because its definition of stage I disease is problematic (Table 6-3B) because primary NB arising from sympathetic ganglia often are small and not well encapsulated. In addition, tumor resectability did not influence staging, and lymph node sampling was not required, although it does influence staging. Hayes et al. (97) proposed an alternative staging system based on initial resectability of the primary tumor and lymph node involvement. The POG staging system reflects this surgical evaluation for local or regional disease and regional node involvement. However, the nature of the lymph node involvement may be confusing because of distinctions between adherent and nonadherent nodes. In fact, the importance of local and regional lymph node status in staging NB is uncertain, with contradictory results in different studies according to lymph node involvement (42,97,98).

TABLE 6-3A. *International neuroblastoma staging system*

Stage	Definition
1	Localized tumor with complete gross excision, with or without microscopic residual disease; representative ipsilateral lymph nodes negative for tumor microscopically.
2A	Localized tumor with incomplete gross excision; representative ipsilateral lymph nodes negative for tumor microscopically.
2B	Localized tumor with or without complete gross excision, with ipsilateral lymph nodes positive for tumor; enlarged contralateral lymph nodes must be negative microscopically.
3	Unresectable unilateral tumor infiltrating across the midline, with or without regional lymph node involvement; localized unilateral tumor with contralateral regional lymph node involvement; or midline tumor with bilateral extension by infiltration (unresectable) or lymph node involvement.
4	Any primary tumor with dissemination to distant lymph nodes, bone, bone marrow, liver, and other organs (except as defined for stage 4S).
4S	Localized primary tumor (as defined as stage 1, 2A, or 2B), in patient <1 yr, with dissemination limited to skin, liver, or bone marrow (marrow involvement should be minimal with malignant cells <10% of total nucleated cells).

Based on Brodeur GM, Pritchard J, Berthold F, et al. Revisions of the international criteria for neuroblastoma diagnosis, staging, and response to treatment. *J Clin Oncol* 1993;11(8):1466–1477; and Brodeur GM, Seeger RC, Barrett A, et al. International criteria for diagnosis, staging, and response to treatment in patients with neuroblastoma. *J Clin Oncol* 1988;6(12):1874–1881.

TABLE 6-3B. *Evans and children's cancer group staging system*

Stage	Definition
I	Tumor confined to the organ or structure of origin.
II	Tumor extending in continuity beyond the organ or structure of origin but not crossing the midline; regional lymph nodes on the ipsilateral side possibly involved.
III	Tumor extending in continuity beyond the midline; regional lymph nodes may be involved bilaterally.
IV	Remote disease involving the bone, bone marrow, soft tissue, or distant lymph node groups.
IV-S	As defined by stage I or II except for the presence of remote disease confined to the liver, skin, or marrow, without bone metastases.

Based on Evans AE. Staging and treatment of neuroblastoma. *Cancer* 1980;45(7 Suppl):1799–1802.

TABLE 6-3C. *St. Jude and Pediatric Oncology Group staging system*

Stage	Definition
A	Complete gross resection of primary tumor, with or without microscopic residual disease. Intracavitary lymph nodes not adherent to the primary tumor are histologically negative; nodes adhering to the surface or within the primary tumor can be positive; liver histologically free of tumor.
B	Grossly unresected primary tumor; lymph nodes are the same as in stage A; liver histologically free of tumor.
C	Complete or incomplete resection of primary tumor; intracavitary lymph nodes not adhering to the primary tumor are histologically positive; liver histologically free of tumor.
D	Dissemination of disease beyond intracavitary nodes (i.e., distant lymph nodes, bone, bone marrow, liver, or skin)
DS	Infants <1 year of age with stage IV-S disease (see Table 6-3B).

Based on Castleberry RP, Shuster JJ, Smith EI. The Pediatric Oncology Group experience with the international staging system criteria for neuroblastoma. *J Clin Oncol* 1994;12(11):2378–2381.

Two international conferences have finalized a consensus for a new NB staging system (INSS), now generally accepted for risk stratification of NB and for reporting of results. The INSS is a postsurgical staging system with substantial reliance on the assessment of tumor resectability and surgical examination of lymph node involvement (99). In classifying tumors that cross the midline, infiltration (extending by contiguous invasion to or beyond the opposite side of the vertebral bodies) was chosen to identify tumors presumably less favorable than those that are pedunculated and simply drape over the midline (Table 6-3). The INSS uses Arabic numbers to distinguish it from the letters and Roman numerals of the other systems. The definition of stage 1 was clarified at the second INSS conference such that nodes attached to the primary (adherent to or in direct continuity with, and re-moved with, the primary) may be positive (89). Because gross resection of a localized tumor is associated with a favorable outcome regardless of microscopic residual disease or involvement of attached lymph nodes, even such tumors that arise in or cross the midline may be stage 1.

An international consensus has also developed the International Neuroblastoma Response Criteria (INRC) (89), shown in Table 6-4, which takes into account some of the unique characteristics of this tumor, such as MIBG uptake, catecholamine excretion, and propensity for bone and bone marrow involvement. This is currently the best accepted method for reporting response to treatment, which supplements the National Institutes of Health criteria generally used for evaluating response in phase I and II studies, the Response Evaluation Criteria in Solid Tumors Group criteria (100).

TABLE 6-4. *International neuroblastoma response criteria*

Response	Primary tumor	Metastatic sites
CR	No tumor.	No tumor; catecholamines normal.
VGPR	Decreased by 90–99%.	No tumor; catecholamines normal; residual ^{99}Tc bone changes allowed.
PR	Decreased by >50%.	All measurable sites decreased by >50%. Bones and bone marrow: number of positive bone sites decreased by >50%, no more than 1 positive bone marrow site allowed.
MR	No new lesions; >50% reduction of any measurable lesion with <50% reduction in any other; <25% increase in any existing lesion.	
NR	No new lesions; <50% reduction but <25% increase in any existing lesion.	
PD	Any new lesion; increase of any measurable lesion by >25%; previous negative marrow positive for tumor.	

CR, complete remission; VGPR, very good partial response; PR, partial response; MR, mixed response; NR, no response; PD, progressive disease.

Based on Brodeur GM, Pritchard J, Berthold F, et al. Revisions of the international criteria for neuroblastoma diagnosis, staging, and response to treatment. *J Clin Oncol* 1993;11(8):1466–1477.

Prognostic Factors

Clinical

Several clinical and biologic characteristics of NB are associated with prognosis. Various cooperative groups and investigators have attempted to select certain variables and group them to identify patients with good, intermediate, or bad prognoses. The differences in various studies probably result from differences in patient characteristics, treatment, study endpoints, and so on. As cytogenetic data are accumulated and interpreted, genetic subsets of NB that reflect clinical behavior are being identified (26).

Stage and age continue to be extremely important determinants of outcome, as originally reported by Breslow and McCann (101–104). The disease stage strongly influences prognosis (Fig. 6-7). With surgery as primary therapy, more than 90% of children with stage 1 and 2 disease survive and 85% of children with stage 4S survive, whereas with multimodality therapy, the survival is 60–90% for INSS 3 but only 40% for stage 4 disease (2). However, age at diagnosis is another strong determinant of outcome, which must be factored in with stage. Infants younger than 18 months of age do better than older children with the same disease stage, an effect that is dramatic for patients with advanced stage 3 and 4 disease (33,38,101,105–109). Adults and adolescents

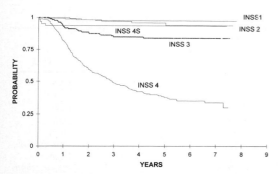

FIG. 6-7. Overall survival according to International NB Staging System (INSS) stage of 1,034 children with neuroblastoma treated on Children's Cancer Group protocols from 1991 to 1995. INSS 1, *n* = 195; INSS 2, *n* = 117, INSS 3, *n* = 184; INSS 4S, *n* = 64; INSS 4, *n* = 474. (Courtesy of the Children's Cancer Group Statistical Office.)

with NB have a particularly poor long-term survival, even with disease presenting without metastases, although their course may be prolonged (110,111). On the other hand, infants with stage 4 disease have more than 70% survival with modest chemotherapy, whereas children older than 1 year at diagnosis with stage 4 have less than 40% survival with very intensive therapy. This may be related to a higher rate of spontaneous tumor regression or tumor maturation in infants (112).

There is no sex difference in survival. Although the survival of patients with thoracic primary tumors is better than that of patients with abdominal primaries, the tumor site is not an independent prognostic factor. Patients with thoracic primary tumors are generally younger children with lower-stage disease (113,114). Metastatic sites at diagnosis are also a prognostic factor, with shorter event-free survival (EFS) for bone, bone marrow, central nervous system (CNS), intracranial or orbital, lung, and pleural metastases, and longer EFS in those with liver and skin metastases (both common features of 4S disease) (84,88,115,116).

Biologic

Ferritin may be produced by NB cells and thus reflects tumor burden or growth, or it may be necessary for NB cell growth. An elevated serum ferritin level (more than 143 ng/mL) is found in up to half of patients with advanced-stage disease but rarely in children with localized disease. PFS is lower for children with elevated levels (117–120).

Neuron-specific enolase is a glycolytic enzyme found in neurons. The enzyme is associated with worse survival when serum levels are elevated (greater than 100 ng/mL). Elevation is more common in patients with advanced-stage disease (121). Neuron-specific enolase may be useful as a marker for following the response to treatment.

Lactate dehydrogenase elaboration may reflect tumor cell burden or turnover, and serum elevations (750–1,500 IU/mL) have been found to be independently associated with a worse prognosis (102,103)

Certain neuropeptides (vasoactive intestinal peptide and somatostatin) have been observed to correlate with neuroblastic cellular differentiation and favorable disease stage (93,122).

The *MDRI* gene encodes P-glycoprotein, which acts as an adenosine triphosphate–dependent drug efflux pump. Its expression before treatment may predict efficacy of therapy (123). This also implies that agents capable of reversing P-glycoprotein–mediated multidrug resistance may be useful in NB. Another gene that encodes for multidrug resistance–associated protein has been reported to correlate with N-*myc* amplification and poor outcome (124). However, the data on this point are contradictory, and not all authorities agree that P-glycoprotein is of prognostic importance.

Genetic factors, including DNA index, *MYCN* amplification, nerve growth factor receptors *CD44, MMP2,* VEGF and its receptors, and genetic gains and losses were discussed earlier under "Biology." In addition, high expression of the *Ha-ras p21* gene has been correlated with lower clinical stage of tumor at diagnosis and increased patient survival; its expression was inversely associated with *MYCN* expression (125).

Ganglioside GD2 is a sialic acid–containing glycosphingolipid found mainly in the cell surface membrane. Elevated circulating levels may be another marker of disease activity and response to treatment (favorable prognosis level is less than 103 pmol/mL, unfavorable prognosis level is greater than 568 pmol/mL). Shed gangliosides may accelerate tumor progression, and anti-GD2 antibodies may be useful in treating NB (126–128).

Chromogranin A is an acidic protein co-stored and co-released with catecholamines from storage vesicles. Its serum concentration is elevated in patients with peptide-producing endocrine neoplasia. The survival rate for patients with lower serum chromogranin A levels (less than 190 ng/mL at the time of diagnosis) was 69%, whereas it was 30% for those with higher chromogranin A levels ($p < 0.05$). Furthermore, when subjects were additionally stratified by age or stage, chromogranin A was an effective prognostic tool in patients who were older than 1 year ($p < 0.005$) or had more advanced disease (stage III or IV; $p < 0.05$) (129,130).

The large number of prognostic factors and the fact that many of them are available only on a research basis has precluded a comprehensive prospective study or multivariate analysis. However, those that have appeared to be consistent over many years and readily available to the clinician have been combined to form a framework for risk stratification in current therapeutic studies. Age, INSS stage, histopathology, tumor cell ploidy, and *MYCN* gene copy number are the

TABLE 6-5. *Children's oncology group neuroblastoma risk groups for treatment*

International neuroblastoma staging system	Age (days)	MYCN	Histology	Ploidy	Risk
1	Any	Any	Any	Any	Low
2A/2B	<365	Any	Any	Any	Low
	≥365	Nonamplified	Any	—	Low
	≥365	Amplified	Favorable	—	Low
	≥365	Amplified	Unfavorable	—	High
3	<365	Nonamplified	Any	Any	Intermediate
	<365	Amplified	Any	Any	High
	≥365	Nonamplified	Favorable	—	Intermediate
	≥365	Nonamplified	Unfavorable	—	High
	≥365	Nonamplified	Any	—	High
4	<365	Nonamplified	Any	Any	Intermediate
	<365	Amplified	Any	Any	High
	≥365	Any	Any	—	High
4S	<365	Nonamplified	Favorable	DI > 1	Low
	<365	Nonamplified	Favorable	DI = 1	Intermediate
	<365	Nonamplified	Unfavorable	Any	Intermediate
	<365	Amplified	Any	Any	High

DI, DNA index.

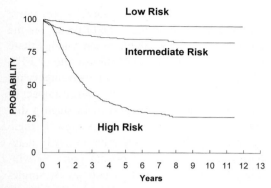

FIG. 6-8. Survival in 2,196 consecutive patients with neuroblastoma treated on Children's Cancer Group and Pediatric Oncology Group protocols according to clinical risk groups (Table 6-5) assigned according to International Neuroblastoma Staging System stage, age, histopathology, *MYCN* copy number, and DNA ploidy. Low risk, n = 916; intermediate risk, n = 431; high risk, n = 849. (Courtesy of the Children's Oncology Group statistical Office.)

factors used in risk stratification and therapy assignment for the Children's Oncology Group (COG) in North America, with very similar guidelines used internationally (Table 6-5). The survival for low-risk patients by this classification is more than 90%, that of intermediate-risk patients is more than 80%, and that of the high-risk group remains at about 30–40% (Fig. 6-8).

SELECTION OF THERAPY

Low-risk tumors are managed with surgery alone unless symptomatic cord compression or respiratory compromise necessitates a short course of chemotherapy. Patients in the low-risk group with stage 1 or 2 disease have an expected 4-year survival of more than 95% with surgery only (42,131,132), whereas infants with INSS 4S have more than 90% survival with supportive care or a short course of chemotherapy (107). The smaller intermediate-risk group consists of infants with stage 4 disease (but no tumor *MYCN* amplification), favorable biology stage 3, or INSS 4S with unfavorable histology or DNA index. Patients in this group are expected to have an estimated survival of more than 80% with standard dosages of chemotherapy for 4 to 8 months and primary tumor resection. Radio-

therapy (RT) is rarely used in the low- or intermediate-risk groups because of their favorable prognosis and the fact that many of these patients are younger than 1 year old. It is reserved for use in life- or function-threatening situations. It is occasionally needed for cases of unresectable primary disease remaining after chemotherapy or regional recurrences not controlled with chemotherapy.

The high-risk group in NB consists primarily of patients with stage 4 disease who are more than 1 year old at diagnosis but also includes stage 3 with either tumor *MYCN* amplification or those older than 1 year with unfavorable histopathology, stage 2 above 1 year of age with *MYCN* amplification, and stage 3, 4, and 4S infants with *MYCN* gene amplification. Despite the use of increasingly aggressive combined-modality treatments, which have higher remission rates and durations, the long-term survival for INSS stage 4 disease in children who are older than 1 year at diagnosis has remained less than 15% until recently (2). The most recent phase III studies indicate that the 3-year EFS of this group has increased in the past decade to 30–40% with the use of myeloablative therapy and treatment for minimal residual disease but is still far below the desired outcome (133). Therapy for high-risk NB is divided into three phases: intensive induction treatment, marrow ablative therapy, and management of minimal residual disease. The goal of induction therapy is to achieve maximum reduction of tumor burden, including reduction of bone marrow tumor (*in vivo* purging), within a timeframe that will minimize the risk of resistant tumor clones and clinical progression. During or at the end of this phase, local control of bulky disease is accomplished with delayed surgery and local RT. Subsequently, very high-dose marrow ablative therapy may be used to try to overcome residual and potentially resistant tumor, followed by hematopoietic cell transplant (HCT). The relapse rate of more than 40% even after such treatment (134) has led to the approach of using tumor-targeted therapies after myeloablative treatment to try to eliminate microscopic resistant clones (minimal residual disease).

Chemotherapy

As indicated earlier, chemotherapy is used in low-risk disease only for recurrence or for symptomatic patients with compromised organ function. Intermediate-risk patients can achieve long-term survival with moderate combination chemotherapy for 4 to 8 months (2,38, 135,136). The most effective induction regimens for obtaining complete or partial response are combination platinum-based regimens including other active drugs such as cyclophosphamide, doxorubicin, etoposide, vincristine, and ifosfamide. Induction regimens used in recent large cooperative studies are shown in Table 6-6, with overall response rates ranging from about 60% to 96% at the end of 5 to 6 months of treatment. Additional variations on these schedules but with the same drugs have

been tested recently by large cooperative groups in the United States and Europe, but the results are not yet available to see whether there is any further impact on response rate or EFS. Most of these regimens also include surgery for residual disease, although the overall impact of complete resection on survival in stage 4 disease is still contradictory. Some newer single agents have also been effective in newly diagnosed NB, using the "up-front phase II window" approach. After two courses of single-agent therapy before induction treatment, response rates for effective agents (more than 30% response) were easily detectable, including ifosfamide, carboplatin, iproplatin (137), and topotecan (138). Two agents that were less effective in this setting were epirubicin (137) and paclitaxel (138). There was no evidence

TABLE 6-6. *Induction regimens for high-risk neuroblastoma since 1985 (more than 50 patients)*

Group and reference	Year	Regimen	N	CR + PR (%)
Pediatric Oncology Group 8742, regimen 1 (137)	1987–1991	Days 1–5, CDDP 40 mg/m^2/day Days 2–4, VP16 100 mg/m^2/day This alternates q 21 days with Days 1–7, CPM p.o. 150 mg/m^2/day Day 8, DOX 35 mg/m^2	111	77%
Pediatric Oncology Group 8742, regimen 2 (137)	1987–1991	Day 1, CDDP 90 mg/m^2 Day 2, VP16 100 mg/m^2 Days 3–10, CPM 150 mg/m^2/day p.o. Day 11, DOX 35 mg/m^2 Repeat q 21 days	115	68%
SFOP CADO/PE (317)	1987–1992	Days 1–5, CPM 300 mg/m^2/day Days 1 and 5, VCR 1.5 mg/m^2/day Day 5, DOX 60 mg/m^2/day Alternates q 21 days for 2 cycles each with Days 1–5, CDDP 40 mg/m^2/day Days 1–5, VP16 100 mg/m^2/day	183	64%
Study Group of Japan (318)	1985–1997	Day 1, CPM 1,200 mg/m^2, VCR 1.5 mg/m^2 Day 3, THP-ADR 40 mg/m^2 Day 5, CDDP 90 mg/m^2 Repeat q 28 days × 6 cycles	168	92%
Children's Cancer Group 3891 (133)	1991–1996	Day 1, CDDP 60/m^2 Day 3, DOX 30 mg/m^2 Days 3 and 6, VP16 100 mg/m^2/day Days 4 and 5, CPM 900 mg/m^2/day Repeat q 28 days × 5 cycles	539	78%
Memorial Sloan–Kettering Cancer Center (319)	1990–2002	Days 1 and 2, CPM 70 mg/kg/day Days 1–3, VCR 0.067 mg/kg/day Days 1–3, DOX 25 mg/m^2/day Days 21–24, CDDP 50 mg/m^2/day and VP16 150 mg/m^2/day	90	96%

DOX, doxorubicin.

Modified from Matthay KK, Yamashiro D. Neuroblastoma. In: Holland, JF, Frei, E, Bast RC et al., eds. *Cancer medicine.* London: BC Decker, 2000:2185–2197.

that such a design adversely affected the subsequent outcome of patients when compared with the outcome of patients treated with similar induction without the phase II window.

Myeloablative Therapy with Hematopoietic Stem Cell Support

Myeloablative high-dose chemotherapy with or without total body irradiation (TBI) has been incorporated as consolidation treatment for high-risk NB for the past two decades, beginning with early studies using melphalan ablation. Numerous single-arm studies using varying myeloablative regimens from 1985 to about 1995 showed an apparent improvement in EFS, usually reported from time of transplantation. The 3-year EFS ranged from 26% to 62%, with an average of about 40% for the large studies (more than 20 patients) shown in Table 6-7 (134,139–147). This approach introduced some bias into the interpretation of results because only patients who

survived for 5 to 6 months and responded to induction chemotherapy were able to receive the high-dose myeloablative treatment with autologous or allogeneic transplantation.

Several retrospective comparisons of concomitant and similar groups of patients treated with standard dosages of chemotherapy and those treated with high-dose therapy and autologous bone marrow transplantation (ABMT) have been performed, with conflicting assessments of the value of myeloablative therapy. The CCG treated children with high-risk NB with either monthly cycles of four-drug chemotherapy over 1 year or, at investigator discretion, with myeloablative therapy with cisplatin, etoposide, melphalan, and TBI followed by purged ABMT. In a retrospective, nonrandomized comparison of ABMT and traditional chemotherapy, EFS of patients who were progression free at 8 months from diagnosis was significantly superior for patients receiving ABMT (40% vs. 19%). An even more significant advantage for ABMT was seen

TABLE 6-7. *EFS for high-risk neuroblastoma in first remission using myeloablative therapy and hematopoietic cell transplant for studies of more than 20 patients*

Reference	Regimen	N	Toxic death	3-Year EFS
321	BCNU, teniposide, melphalan (total of one ($n = 15$) or two ($n = 18$) courses)	33		49% (2-year EFS)
143	Melphalan	24	1	40%
140	Melphalan, TBI	54	7	32%
146, 322	Cisplatin, VM-26, Doxorubicin, melphalan, TBI	45	7	42%
	Cisplatin, VP16, melphalan, TBI	54	5	50%
	Carboplatin, VP16, melphalan, TBI	48	4	41%
147	Vincristine, melphalan, TBI	62	13	30%
323	Vincristine, melphalan, TBI	34	1	29%
324	Cisplatin, BCNU, melphalan (or thiotepa), VP16	25	6	40%
242	Etoposide, melphalan or cisplatin, etoposide, THP-adriamycin, melphalan, with ($n = 6$) or without TBI	31	3	50%
325	VM-26 (or VP16), thiotepa, TBI	27	4	41%
142	Melphalan with or without VP16, vincristine, cisplatin, BCNU	39	7	35%
144	European Bone Marrow Registry Data	439	60	24% (5-year EFS)
326	Cyclophosphamide, thiotepa	51	1	48%
133	Carboplatin, VP16, melphalan, TBI	129	12	43%
245	Carboplatin, VP16, melphalan, local radiation	77	4	62%
116	Busulfan, melphalan	116	7	47%
327	Cyclophosphamide, carboplatin	49	4	33%

Unless otherwise stated, event-free survival (EFS) measured from time of transplantation.
BCNU, carmustine; TBI, total body irradiation; THP, adriamycin; VM-26, teniposide; VP16, etoposide.
Modified from Matthay KK. Hematopoietic stem cell transplantation for neuroblastoma. In: Blume KG, Forman SJ, Appelbaum FR, eds. *Thomas hematopoietic cell transplantation,* 3rd ed. Oxford: Blackwell, 2003.

for patients who were only in partial, as opposed to complete, remission at the end of induction and for those with tumor *MYCN* amplification (146). These results were consistent with results from the Lyon group, in which Philip et al. (139) showed a difference in 2-year survival of 39% versus 12% for concomitant patients treated with myeloablative therapy and ABMT or with standard chemotherapy. In contrast, a retrospective comparison from the POG of 116 patients achieving complete or partial remission did not show any significant difference in outcome for those undergoing bone marrow transplantation before progression (145). A smaller study by the German cooperative group evaluated 39 patients undergoing megatherapy and HCT with a variety of conditioning regimens and either allogeneic or autologous bone marrow, all with a melphalan "backbone," compared with 49 patients receiving continued chemotherapy by investigator choice. All patients achieved complete or partial remissions. EFS was significantly better in the transplanted patients than in the chemotherapy group, although the curves nearly converged by 6 years (142).

A randomized prospective trial was necessary to eliminate the bias inherent in such retrospective comparisons. Pinkerton (143) reported the first attempt at a randomized trial of high-dose therapy with autologous bone marrow support for NB, with a suggestion of improvement noted for ABMT. However, this report included only 65 randomized patients, with widely varying times to ABMT. The CCG conducted the first large prospective, randomized study comparing a single course of myeloablative chemoradiotherapy supported by purged ABMT with three cycles of a dose-intensive, nonmyeloablative, continuous-infusion consolidation chemotherapy. Of 379 eligible patients who were randomized, 85% had INSS stage 4 tumors. Randomized patients were assigned equally to ABMT ($n = 189$) or consolidation chemotherapy ($n = 190$), and 118 were nonrandomly assigned to consolidation chemotherapy because of parental or investigator refusal. Overall toxicity and total mean hospital days were similar between the two randomized arms. The 3-year EFS was 27% for all patients, 34% ± 4% for those assigned to

ABMT, and 22% ± 4% for the cases randomly assigned to consolidation chemotherapy ($p = 0.034$) (Fig. 6-9). The outcome advantage noted with ABMT was also significant in the subgroups of patients with *MYCN*-amplified tumors and in those who were more than 2 years old at diagnosis. The 3-year EFS from time of transplantation for those 129 patients actually receiving ABMT (as-treated analysis) is shown to be 43% ± 6%, similar to that of previous single-arm studies and significantly higher than the 27% ± 5% EFS of the 150 patients receiving the chemotherapy consolidation (133). Although caution is necessary because no significant difference in long-term survival has been shown, myeloablative therapy with stem cell support is considered standard treatment for high-risk NB.

Different myeloablative regimens have been used, although most are melphalan-based. The very first myeloablative regimen used to treat NB was high-dose melphalan alone. This progressed to various combinations of other agents, including cisplatin, etoposide, and doxorubicin, melphalan with busulfan, and melphalan with carboplatin and etoposide. Other centers used a thiotepa base coupled with cyclophosphamide, or etoposide, or busulfan combined with cyclophosphamide. More recently, attempts have been made to incorporate topotecan into the conditioning regimen in combination with thiotepa and etoposide (148). Few studies have tried to compare two myeloablative regimens in a randomized fashion. However, the retrospective analysis by the European Group for Blood and Marrow Transplantation failed to show any difference in EFS using different high-dose regimens (144,149, 150). Only one analysis, from the Institut Gustave-Roussy, has shown that patients treated with busulfan and cyclophosphamide appeared to have better EFS than those on other conditioning regimens at a single institution (116). These data may depend on the chronology of the protocols and the fact that the busulfan regimen was compared with a combination of a variety of other regimens. The European Neuroblastoma Study Group is testing this hypothesis in a randomized study, comparing the COG

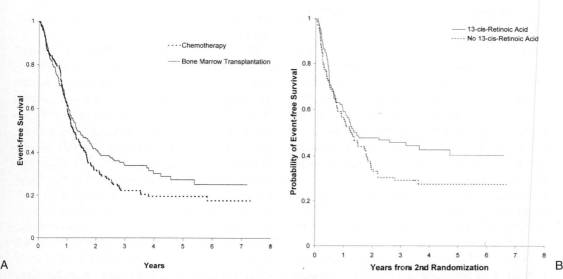

FIG. 6-9. Results of CCG 3891, a randomized study comparing myeloablative chemoradiotherapy and purged autologous bone marrow transplantation with intensive nonmyelcablative therapy. A second randomization was performed on all consenting patients completing the consolidation therapy without progression to test the efficacy of 13-*cis*-retinoic acid for minimal residual disease. **(A)** Superior event-free survival (EFS) with myeloablative therapy compared with standard-dose chemotherapy. The difference in 3-year EFS for the 379 randomized patients was 34% versus 22% (*p* = 0.034). **(B)** 3-year EFS with 13-*cis*-retinoic acid for the 258 randomized patients from the time of second randomization was 46% versus 29% (*p* = 0.027). (From Matthay KK, Villablanca JG, Seeger RC, et al. Treatment of high-risk neuroblastoma with intensive chemotherapy, radiotherapy, autologous bone marrow transplantation, and 13-*cis*-retinoic acid. Children's Cancer Group. *N Engl J Med* 1999; 341(16):1165–1173, with permission.)

regimen of melphalan, etoposide, and carboplatin with the busulfan and melphalan regimen. Other pilot studies are testing whether additional benefit may be obtained from double or triple tandem transplants (151,152).

Bone marrow involvement is present in 70–90% of patients at diagnosis, and residual tumor cells can still be detected in bone marrow samples by sensitive immunodetection methods even after several cycles of induction therapy. For this reason, allogeneic bone marrow transplantation (BMT) has been proposed as an alternative to ABMT. It is also hoped that the allogeneic cells will provide a further "graft-versus-NB" effect, although the rationale for this concept is weak because NB cells express little human leukocyte antigen (HLA) class I. To date, lack of evidence of any immunologic benefit, coupled with the problems with frequent lack of an HLA-compatible sibling donor and the significantly higher toxic death rates, have discouraged extensive use of allogeneic BMT. Two reports directly compared allogeneic and autologous transplantation in NB. A CCG study compared 36 patients receiving an autologous purged BMT and 20 patients receiving the same induction who received allogeneic matched-sibling BMT. There was no significant difference in relapse rate and an apparently higher toxicity in the allogeneic group. Four of 20 patients died of causes other than relapse in the allogeneic group, compared with 3 of 36 in the autologous group (not significant); the estimated PFS was 25% for the allogeneic group versus 49% for the autologous group (*p* = 0.051) (153). In a comparison from the European Bone Marrow Transplant Registry, 17 allogeneic transplant and 34 ABMT cases were matched based on a number of prognostic factors. The PFS was not significantly different: 35% for autologous and 41% for allogeneic at 2 years, respectively (154).

The other way to overcome the problem of possible tumor contamination of autologous bone marrow or stem cells is with *ex vivo* purging of the hematopoietic cells. Although bone marrow and peripheral blood often show gross disappearance of tumor cells after a few courses of chemotherapy, sensitive methods of detection with immunocytology and RT-PCR have shown persistence of low levels of tumor in 10–40% of hematopoietic cell collections (88,91,155–158). Methods tested for *ex vivo* tumor cell removal from bone marrow in patients with NB include physical methods (sedimentation and filtration) (159); chemical purging with 6-hydroxydopamine (160,161), deferoxamine mesylate (162,163), or mafosfamide (164,165); and immunologic methods with direct antibody plus complement (166,167) or immunomagnetic beads (168). CD34 selection has also been shown to reduce tumor cell content but may lead to later lymphoproliferative disorders (169, 170). The most widely tested and validated method with 4 to 6 logs of tumor cell removal and no impairment of engraftment is immunomagnetic purging. This technique has been used in multi-institutional cooperative studies (133,140). CCG studies showed that bone marrow can be successfully harvested; shipped at room temperature overnight; purged using sedimentation, filtration, and immunomagnetic bead separation; and cryopreserved without injury and with successful tumor cell removal and engraftment (133). Future randomized studies, such as that under way in the COG (A3973), will be needed to test whether *ex vivo* tumor cell depletion improves the survival for metastatic NB.

THERAPY FOR MINIMAL RESIDUAL DISEASE

Despite improvements in EFS using myeloablative therapy, the relapse rate, even for patients transplanted in complete response, remains high (133). For this reason, it has become increasingly important to find new approaches to eliminate minimal residual disease with agents that will be tolerable after myeloablative therapy. Immediately after HCT, when disease is likely to be minimal, is the ideal window of time to eradicate resistant clones that are still present using novel therapies not dependent on standard cytotoxic mechanisms.

In vitro, both all-trans retinoic acid and 13-*cis*-retinoic acid cause decreased proliferation and differentiation in NB cell lines, including some established from refractory tumors (171–173). A phase II trial in children with relapsed NB using 13-*cis*-retinoic acid on a single daily administration schedule of 100 mg/m^2 showed only 2 of 22 responses (174). However, based on *in vitro* experiments with higher intermittent dosing, a phase I trial in children with high-risk NB after HCT determined that a high-dose intermittent schedule of 13-*cis*-retinoic acid after BMT had minimal toxicity, achieved levels that were effective against NB cell lines *in vitro,* and resulted in complete bone marrow responses in three of ten patients (175). A subsequent phase III randomized trial by the CCG of children with high-risk NB completing consolidation chemotherapy or ABMT showed that the 3-year EFS from time of randomization was significantly better for the patients randomized to receive 13-*cis*-retinoic acid (46% ± 6%) than for those randomized to receive no further therapy (29% ± 5%; $p = 0.03$) (Fig. 6-9) (133). A European randomized trial of very low-dose continuous 13-*cis*-retinoic acid given after transplant did not show any benefit (176). Other retinoids, such as fenretinide, are under investigation for use in minimal residual disease (177).

Another approach to minimal residual disease after transplant is the use of antibody-targeted therapy. Antibody therapy in relapsed NB using murine, chimeric, and humanized antibodies against the membrane ganglioside GD$_2$ has provided promising response and toxicity profiles that warrant further investigation of these agents in randomized studies (178–182). With granulocyte-macrophage colony-stimulating factor (GM-CSF) or interleukin-2 (IL-2), anti-GD$_2$ seems to be tolerated in patients who have undergone ABMT (179,182). A new randomized prospective trial of the use of chimeric anti-GD2 antibody with GM-CSF and IL-2 is under way in the COG. Patients who are in remission after high-dose therapy and HCT are randomized to receive either 13-*cis*-retinoic acid alone or the retinoid along with chimeric anti-GD2 antibody

(Ch14.18), GM-CSF, and IL-2. Further improvements are being tested in phase I trials using a fusion protein of the humanized form of the antibody Hu14.18 and IL-2. This immunocytokine has the advantage of working simultaneously through both antibody-dependent cytotoxicity and natural killer cell mechanisms. A murine NB model showed superior activity of the immunocytokine to the physical mixture of the antibody and cytokine (183).

Other approaches to minimal residual disease in the future may use genetically engineered vaccines to generate immune response (184–189). Another possible avenue would use antiangiogenic therapy after transplantation. Angiogenesis appears to play a major role in progression of NB in that multiple proteins associated with angiogenesis have been shown to be associated with more advanced disease or worse prognosis (62,190,191). Testing in animal models suggests responsiveness to angiogenic inhibitors, particularly in minimal disease states (192).

Surgery

Surgery has both a diagnostic and a therapeutic role. If the diagnosis has not been established by bone marrow aspirate, biochemical testing, or skin biopsy, surgery provides histologic confirmation of malignancy. Even in the presence of a clear, non–surgically determined diagnosis of NB, a tissue sample is important for biologic analysis.

As previously stated, 20–40% of children present with localized disease. In children without evidence of metastatic disease, an attempt at resection is warranted if substantial morbidity (sacrifice of vital structures) can be avoided. Complete gross excision of the primary tumor in localized disease is associated with a very high likelihood of cure irrespective of the patient's age. For patients with stage 1 or 2 disease, the cure rate exceeds 90% (42,131,132). If the tumor is localized but unresectable (INSS 3) because of its intimate relationship with major blood vessels or other characteristics, the proper extent of surgery may depend on tumor biology. In a study of 228 patients with stage 3 NB, for children who had elevated serum ferritin or tumors with unfa-

vorable histopathology or *MYCN* amplification, the EFS was improved by complete gross resection, whereas the extent of resection did not appear to affect the children with biologically favorable tumors (135). The optimal timing of the surgery is still under debate; it is possible that the advantages of early resection are outweighed by a higher complication rate before chemotherapy reduction followed by delayed surgery (193–195). However, even when the primary tumor is unresectable, defining its extent remains important for staging and determining optimal additional local therapy with radiation.

Recurrence in the local or regional area of primary disease is a component of relapse in a large proportion of children with high-risk NB, at rates ranging from 20% to 80% in reports that often include local RT and myeloablative therapy (133,134,196). Both single-arm studies and one randomized study demonstrate the benefit of local control measures for children with advanced but nonmetastatic NB (135,193,197–201), but the impact of resection in stage 4 disease has been mixed (202–204). It is possible that problems with control of metastatic disease have obscured the potential value of local resection.

Second-look surgical procedures are commonly used in NB. Chemotherapy and irradiation may produce significant interval regression of a bulky primary tumor (193,194,205). For patients with residual tumor, surgery may then be performed to achieve a complete response (193,194,206). Children who have localized NB converted to a resectable status by interval therapy and who undergo complete excision have a reasonable prognosis. Completely resecting the primary tumor also appears feasible for patients with advanced disease; eventual complete excision can be accomplished in up to 65% of patients (207). In this situation, resection after chemotherapy appears to be associated with fewer complications than resection before chemotherapy (193,194,208). The Italian Cooperative Group for Neuroblastoma has reported 145 patients with localized inoperable NB or primary tumor excised with a tumor residue more than 2 mL. Ninety-four of the 145 (65%) achieved a complete or partial response with chemotherapy, and 75 (52%) subsequently underwent complete resection (113).

Although the prognostic value of lymph nodes has been controversial, and nodes adherent to or removed with the primary tumor do not appear to predict prognosis, lymph nodes that are distinct (usually superior or inferior, but especially if bilateral or contralateral) from the tumor are ideally sampled for complete staging (42,89,106,209–213). However, this may be difficult for some patients with cervical or thoracic tumors or infiltrative unresectable abdominal primaries. The utility of other prognostic factors suggests that aggressive attempts to acquire this information are unwarranted. A liver biopsy should be done at the time of surgery for intraabdominal primary tumors because hepatic involvement may remain undetected by current imaging techniques, although a report of children older than 1 year with POG stage C disease (INSS stage 2B and 3) questions this rationale (201). If RT is contemplated, clips should be used to mark the tumor.

If treated surgically, dumbbell tumors are dealt with by a two-stage procedure. The extraspinal component of the tumor is removed at a first operation. The extradural, intraspinal portion of the tumor is removed later. However, if there is evidence of spinal cord compression and surgery is used, the laminectomy is performed first. Osteoplastic laminotomy is preferable to minimize later deformity (214). Many institutions prefer to treat spinal cord compression with chemotherapy, as discussed elsewhere in this chapter.

On occasion, infants with a small primary tumor and extensive liver metastases (stage 4S) warrant special surgical considerations. The enlarging liver may compromise respiratory function from upward pressure on the diaphragm or compress the inferior vena cava or renal vein. If chemotherapy or local irradiation does not adequately reduce hepatic size, a silastic sheet may be inserted in the abdominal wall to allow room for liver expansion and reduce compression of vital structures (107,215). Resection of the primary tumor does not influence survival in stage 4S (39,107,112).

Radiation Therapy

Indications concerning the use of RT in children with NB continue to be refined by progress in devising effective chemotherapy and the desire to avoid unnecessarily aggressive treatment regimens in young children, all on the backdrop of the recalcitrant nature of NB in many children. NB cells in culture are generally radiosensitive (216–219), although radiation responsiveness of NB in patients is less predictable. In the prechemotherapy era, Lingley et al. (220) reported that irradiation to local residual disease in patients with stage 2 and 3 NB resulted in survival in 13 of 13 patients. In discerning the optimal use of RT in NB, reports must be interpreted cautiously because of the differences in staging systems used and thus the differences in patient populations treated.

LOW-RISK DISEASE

Postoperative RT is unnecessary in INSS 1 and 2 NB, as shown by the more than 90% survival with surgery alone or surgery with chemotherapy, as found in recent cooperative studies. Gross surgical excision cures the majority of these children, regardless of age, urinary VMA and HVA ratios, or histologic patterns (42,131, 132). A prospective POG study of 101 children with POG stage A disease treated with surgery alone demonstrated a 2-year disease-free survival of 89% and overall survival (with salvage therapy) of 97% (221). Most recurrences were noted within 1 year of diagnosis, and six of the nine children who relapsed were cured with chemotherapy. Matthay et al. (222) reported outcomes in 156 patients with INSS stage 2A. No significant benefit was associated with the use of chemotherapy or irradiation. The outcome for 75 patients treated with surgery alone was similar to that of 66 patients receiving RT with 6-year PFS of 89% versus 94%, respectively. For the subgroup of patients with residual (postsurgical) gross or microscopic disease, survival was not influenced by the use of irradiation. A subsequent prospective CCG study by Perez et al. (42) demonstrated more than 98% survival for 374 children with stage 1 and 2 NB with surgery alone as primary therapy. Kushner et al. (223) reported ten disease-free survivors of INSS stage 1 NB treated with surgery alone. Six had positive margins. Some patients' tumors were diploid or *MYCN* amplified. Thus, cooperative group studies of localized NB dictate surgery as the primary treatment modality. Chemotherapy is generally reserved for recurrent or progressive tumors that cannot be resected successfully. RT is reserved for the very rare instances of local recurrence in spite of surgery and chemotherapy or for instances in which function is threatened, such as in spinal cord compression or in respiratory insufficiency caused by hepatomegaly.

STAGE 4S AND HEPATOMEGALY

Stage 4S NB was initially proposed as separate from stage 4 in light of the observation that infants with a localized primary NB with metastases to liver, bone marrow, or skin without cortical bone involvement had a surprisingly good outcome compared with other infants with metastatic disease and might need little or no therapy (224). In fact, patients with stage 4S NB who have favorable biology have an excellent prognosis, with 85–90% needing little or no therapy (107,112,136,225). Therefore, RT should be reserved for palliation of life-threatening conditions such as marked, symptomatic hepatomegaly (226,227). The indication for radiation must be balanced against the need for such therapy and the risk of late sequelae of irradiation in infancy (200,228,229). Certainly, routine RT is inappropriate in stage 4S disease and should be instituted only when disease progression threatens vital organ function (227). This occurs most commonly in infants 1 to 2 months old, a risk factor for death in several series (107,226,227). An enlarging liver may induce respiratory compromise from upward pressure on the diaphragm, produce inferior vena cava obstruction, compromise renal perfusion, and occasionally result in gastrointestinal compromise or disseminated intravascular coagulation. When symptoms are early, low-dose chemotherapy can be attempted for symptom reduction. However, often in very young infants the progression is too rapid, and local irradiation in stage 4S NB is indicated for acute reduction of hepatic enlargement (230). Two to 6 Gy of radiation usually is sufficient to reduce hepatic tumor burden and is well within the accepted limit of hepatic radiation tolerance.

INTERMEDIATE-RISK DISEASE

For children with regional NB on the less favorable end of the spectrum (i.e., INSS 3), several reports support a survival advantage from the use of RT (Table 6-8). Unfortunately, because of the previous multiple staging systems, many reports have combined INSS 2B and INSS 3, making it difficult to discern whether radiation is beneficial in both these groups (209,231–234). The recent studies quoted earlier suggest that INSS 2B does not necessitate RT, despite the older reports showing survival with RT. Patients with stage 3 disease who are more than 1 year old with *MYCN* amplification or unfavorable pathology need additional treatment. For these children the EFS is only 50–60%, even with aggressive multimodality therapy (135, 233). Well before the period of biologic staging, Koop and Johnson (235) found that in patients with stage III disease, postoperative irradiation improved survival (six of seven vs. one of nine patients alive with and without postoperative irradiation, respectively). Only one randomized study of RT has clearly delineated results for unresectable nonmetastatic disease. This POG study randomized patients more than 1 year old with stage C NB to receive postoperative chemotherapy or chemotherapy with regional RT (24 to 30 Gy, 16 to 20 fractions) (201). Of 62 eligible patients, in the chemotherapy arm 45% and 31% achieved complete remission and remained disease-free, respectively, at a median of 35 months, and in the chemotherapy and RT arm 67% and 58% achieved complete remission and remain disease-free, respectively, at a median of 23 months. Unfortunately, the chemotherapy used in this 10-year study was much less dose intensive than current protocols, and there were no biologic risk factors reported, making these results difficult to interpret in light of current therapy. However, current reports seem to support the importance of local control in INSS 3 disease, although no further random-

TABLE 6-8. *Effect of radiation in local control of advanced (INSS 3 and 4) neuroblastoma*

References		Local relapse rate		Local radiation dosage median (range), in Gy	Total body irradiation
		With local EBRT	Without local EBRT		
271		32%	81%	12–37.5	None
201	Stage C	24%	54%	24–30	None
233	Stage C	8%	33%	14–36	None
134		26%[a]	31%	Intra-abdominal: 10 Other sites: 20	10 (3.33 q.d.)
314		15%	NA[b]	21 (1.5 b.i.d.)	None
196		18%[a]	14%	10 (7.5–22)	12 (2 b.i.d.)
240		10%	21%	10 (8–24)	12 (2 b.i.d.)
243		10%	NA[b]	21 (1.5 b.i.d.)	None
207	ABMT	22%[a]	35%	Intra-abdominal: 10	10 (3.33 q.d.)
	CC	52%[a]	50%	Other sites: 20	

ABMT, autologous bone marrow transplantation; CC, continuation chemotherapy; EBRT, external beam radiation therapy.
[a]EBRT administered only to patients with residual disease at primary site.
[b]All patients received EBRT.

ized trials have been performed. All current protocols prescribe RT for residual disease after chemotherapy, with the possible exception of infants with favorable biology.

In Evans stage III or with positive lymph nodes (POG stage C), a body of evidence suggests that RT may increase the probability of survival and local tumor control. However, the most recent available trials indicate that patients with *MYCN* nonamplified and favorable ploidy do reasonably well with surgery and chemotherapy. Patients with amplified *MYCN* clearly need improved methods of local and systemic control. It remains to be determined whether more aggressive irradiation will help these patients. Until prospective data are available based on INSS staging, no unequivocal recommendations can be made regarding the efficacy of RT in children with stage 3 disease.

The most recent COG study for intermediate-risk disease, including INSS 3 with favorable biology and infant INSS 4, uses surgery to provide diagnostic material at diagnosis and to attempt maximal safe resection of the primary tumor after chemotherapy. Chemotherapy includes cyclophosphamide, doxorubicin, carboplatin, and etoposide. The duration of chemotherapy is based on the biologic risk factors. RT is limited to situations in which there is clinical deterioration despite chemotherapy and surgery or persistent tumor after chemotherapy and second-look surgery (COG protocol A3961).

HIGH-RISK DISEASE

Nearly half of all patients diagnosed with NB present with high-risk disease. Despite concerted clinical and scientific efforts, the prognosis of children with high-risk NB remains poor. Less than 30% of patients with high-risk disease who are more than 1 year old survive more than 5 years. Historically, early attempts to use radiation to cure children with advanced NB focused on large-volume RT, "segmental" or "sequential" fields administered as fractionated or single doses (236–239). Mixed results in the face of significant toxicities diminished enthusiasm for such radiation approaches, and they ultimately fell out of favor.

Although large-field RT has not proven efficacious, the concept of aggressive systemic therapy has prevailed and has proven successful at improving outcomes for high-risk patients (2). The recently reported randomized CCG 3891 trial showed superior clinical outcomes for patients with high-risk NB who were treated with myeloablative chemotherapy and TBI with transplantation of purged autologous bone marrow. Indeed, TBI has played a prominent role in many myeloablative regimens. Table 6-7 summarizes studies that use autologous or allogeneic BMT either with or without TBI as a component of their preparatory regimens. For most reports EFS rates are on the order of 20–40%, although mortality continues to increase as follow-up lengthens. As with older TBI protocols, trends in conditioning regimens for stem cell transplantation have favored omitting TBI because it limits dosages of myeloablative chemotherapy that can be administered and because of the increase in late effects in young children.

Although the use of TBI for NB is nearly obsolete, an enlarging body of evidence supports the use of local RT to the primary site and bulky metastatic sites. Disease recurrence after BMT for NB is most common at previous sites of disease. Local irradiation delivered either in preparation for the transplant or afterwards appears to reduce the risk of relapse at these sites (207, 240,241). Indeed, the current standard of care dictates that patients with high-risk disease receive radiation to the primary disease site regardless of the extent of surgical resection and to sites of metastatic disease that display persistent ^{131}I-MIBG avidity on the pre–stem cell transplant scans.

Several reports have specifically tackled the role of radiation to the primary tumor site in uniform cohorts of patients with advanced NB. Such results strongly support the administration of radiation to the primary site in high-risk disease. These single-institution and small consortium studies have reported excellent local control rates after treatment regimens that consist of induction chemotherapy, delayed primary surgery with attempted resection of primary and bulky metastatic lesions, external beam radiation to the primary tumor site and persistent metastatic areas, myeloablative chemotherapy, and infusion of stem cells. A report from Japan describes a program of intensive chemotherapy and treatment of primary disease with surgery and radiation for a group of children more than 1 year old with stage 4 disease, although a few patients with stage 3 disease and children younger than 1 year old were included. The 5-year EFS was 39% (242). CCG protocol 321P3 used a dose-intensive combination of four chemotherapeutic agents followed by autologous purged BMT and enrolled 99 children more than 1 year old with stage 4 and high-risk stage 3 disease. The 4-year PFS was 40% (146). Despite TBI and local RT to residual disease, the primary site was involved in more than 50% of the relapses (134). Better primary control was seen at Memorial Sloan–Kettering Cancer Center in patients with stage 4 NB, who received higher-dose local radiation to primary tumor sites regardless of resection and had an actuarial locoregional control rate of 84% at 5 years (241). An update of this single-institution experience reported a 10.1% probability of primary site failure among 99 patients, 92 of whom had no evidence of disease in the primary site at the time of irradiation (2–3). Children received 1.5 Gy twice a day to 21 Gy to the prechemotherapy, presurgery primary tumor volume and regional lymph nodes. Among seven patients with disease at the primary site at the time of irradiation, three had disease that recurred locally. A similar treatment regimen was used by the German multicenter NB trial in which 14 of 26 patients with advanced disease had disease that relapsed, with four (29%) including the primary sites (244). Comparable regimens have resulted in decreased local relapse rates, ranging from 0% to 17% (240,245).

Although favorable local control rates have been reported in single-institution and small consortium studies, large multi-institutional studies have lower rates of complete total resections and differing chemotherapy regimens that limit direct comparisons of clinical results. Therefore, it is not surprising that large, modern multi-institutional trials report higher rates of local relapse. The CCG trial (CCG 3891) showed superior EFS for patients with high-risk NB who were treated with myeloablative chemotherapy and TBI with transplantation of purged autologous bone marrow, followed by treatment with 13-*cis*-retinoic acid. External beam RT (EBRT) was prescribed for all patients with gross residual disease after induction chemotherapy and surgery. Patients randomly assigned to the transplantation arm received additional TBI as a component of the ablative regimen (133).

In CCG 3891, recurrence at the primary disease site was a major component of relapse. Among 539 patients, 349 had recurrences, including 31 with isolated locoregional relapses, 148 with simultaneous local and distant recurrences, and 150 with distant relapses. At 5 years, the estimated regional recurrence rate was 51% ± 5% among patients who received continuation chemotherapy and 33% ± 7% among patients who received transplantation. The difference in local relapses between the continuation chemotherapy and ABMT groups was most pronounced in patients with *MYCN*-amplified tumors. Among patients with *MYCN* amplification, the estimated 5-year local recurrence rate was 70% ± 10% for those who received continuation chemotherapy and 25% ± 15% for patients who received ABMT (207).

Although CCG 3891 did not examine the benefit of local EBRT in a randomized fashion, some conclusions were evident from an analysis of RT administered in this trial. For patients who received 10 Gy of EBRT to the primary site, the addition of 10 Gy of TBI and ABMT resulted in lower local recurrence rates than continuation chemotherapy. The benefit of RT was particularly evident when systemic treatment was optimized with myeloablative therapy and 13-*cis*-retinoic acid (207). For patients with high-risk NB, we recommend EBRT to the primary tumor site in the context of a myeloablative regimen that does not include TBI but incorporates post-transplant therapy for minimal residual disease.

CNS METASTASES

Some controversy exists regarding whether increasingly aggressive multimodality therapy for stage 4 disease has altered patterns of metastatic sites. Some metastatic sites, although perhaps rare in NB patients, pose unique therapeutic challenges, exemplified by CNS metastases. The incidence of CNS metastases in children with high-risk stage 4 NB varies widely in the literature, with crude values of 2–25% reported (84,246–252).

In a recent study, all 648 patients with stage 4 NB in CCG 3881 and 3891 were analyzed for sites of metastases. At diagnosis, the most common sites of metastases were bone marrow, bone, lymph nodes, and liver. The distribution of metastatic sites differed between patients at diagnosis and those at first progression. Whereas the frequencies of bone, bone marrow, liver, lymph nodes, and skin metastases were lower at first progression than at diagnosis, frequencies of adrenal, lung, and CNS metastases exhibited the opposite propensity (84). Whereas CNS involvement was almost never seen at diagnosis, at first progression, CNS metastases were more common in all age groups. For patients with stage 4 disease who relapsed, 11% of children younger than 1 year old, and 3% of children 1 year or older had CNS metastases. Although the number of patients with CNS metastases was small, a few trends were evident. All patients with CNS metastases were more than 1 year old, died within 1 year of diagnosis, and had both *MYCN* amplification (among those tested) and unfavorable Shimada histopathology. Among patients with CNS metastases at diagnosis and those younger than 1 year old who progressed with CNS metastases, hematogenous spread to parenchymal sites was nearly absent. In contrast, for patients older than 1 year, CNS metastases at progression appeared to result from hematogenous routes of spread (84).

A similar analysis at the Institute Curie and Institute Gustave-Roussy confirmed that CNS metastases at diagnosis are extremely rare but revealed an estimated 3-year risk of CNS recurrence of 8% among patients with stage 4 disease, a rate that was stable over 15 years (253). Patients with CNS recurrences were equally distributed among those with parenchymal lesions, those with only meningeal involvement, and those with a combination thereof. Of note, ^{131}I-MIBG scans did not reliably identify CNS recurrences, detecting lesions in only 43% of those with known CNS metastases (253).

In contrast to the aforementioned studies, investigators at Memorial Sloan–Kettering Cancer Center found more CNS metastases associated with increased intensity of curative protocols for patients with stage 4 disease (250). In patients treated with earlier, N4–5 protocols, 2% recurred in the CNS, whereas in those treated with more intensive N6–7 protocols, 12% experienced CNS metastases, perhaps reflecting the longer median survival times in patients treated on N6–7. As patients live longer, metastases to sanctuary sites such as the CNS may become more evident.

Although prospective head CT or MRI scans may better quantify the true incidence of CNS metastases, the infrequent occurrence of such metastases does not justify routine CNS imaging. Furthermore, although most studies do not support an increase in frequency of CNS metastases in the past two decades, it is unclear whether the movement away from TBI for stage 4 NB will result in increased metastases to sanctuary sites such as the CNS. The rarity of CNS metastases does not justify prophylactic CNS radiation; however, for a patient with CNS recurrence the appropriate field of radiation remains unclear.

METASTATIC DISEASE TREATED WITH PALLIATIVE INTENT

Most children with NB have metastatic disease at presentation, which may occasionally threaten function, such as an orbital metastasis affecting vision, an epidural metastasis causing cord compression, or severe pain caused by bone lesions. RT is effective in palliating symptoms secondary to bone and soft tissue metastases, although in a newly diagnosed, chemotherapy-naive patient, systemic treatment usually is initiated first, except in extreme circumstances. A Duke study assessed the value of palliative RT for NB by retrospectively studying 40 irradiated bony sites. Pain completely or partially responded at 65% of treated sites. A subsequent recurrence of pain was seen in 23% of initially responding sites. Complete or partial palliation of soft tissue mass effect was seen in 67% of treated sites. A subsequent relapse of mass effect was seen in 28% of initially responding sites (200). Palliative RT for pain or other symptoms in the refractory relapsed patient can generally be administered rapidly with good relief. There are also extensive phase I and II data concerning palliative treatment of metastatic disease with ^{131}I-MIBG.

ADOLESCENT AND ADULT NEUROBLASTOMA

NB occurs only rarely in adolescents and adults. More than one-third of patients are diagnosed before the age of 1 year (254), whereas fewer than 5% of patients present after the age of 10 years (254). NB in adolescents and adults presents unique challenges that necessitate distinct analyses and therapeutic approaches.

NB in adolescents and adults is characterized by an indolent course, persistent disease, multiple recurrences, and poor outcome. In studies examining patients who were diagnosed with NB between the ages of 15 and 75 years, fewer than 5% of patients are long-term survivors, without evidence of disease (255–253). Most aspects of clinical presentation are similar to those of younger patients. For example, sites of metastatic disease are similar in adolescents and younger children, most commonly found in bone marrow, lymph nodes, bone, and liver. However, distinct differences occur between younger patients and adolescents with NB. Such differences in tumor histology and secretion of catecholamine metabolites may reflect the unique entity of NB in adolescents and adults. The lower frequency of *MYCN* amplification and secretion of catecholamine metabolites probably go hand in hand with the more chronic nature of the disease in this age group (110).

Franks et al. (110) reported the experience of the CCG with NB in adults and adolescents. This study examined 16 patients from the University of California, San Francisco (UCSF), and 38 patients registered in the CCG, all 13 years or older. They found that older patients experienced multiple recurrences; chronic, prolonged courses; and poor outcome regardless of stage or site of disease. For example, although 25% of patients in the UCSF series had pelvic primaries, a site that in younger patients is associated with more favorable outcome, pelvic primaries were associated with outcomes as poor as those for adults and adolescents with other primary sites (110). The indolent, chronic nature of NB in adults and adolescents was reflected with a long median time to progression of 32 months. Although stage IV disease recurred within a year from diagnosis in most patients, late recurrences were observed, as long as 83 months after diagnosis. Furthermore, although younger patients with stage IV NB have only a 3- to 4-month median survival after their first recurrence, similarly staged adolescents experienced multiple recurrences and persistent disease after their first recurrence. After their first recurrence, adolescents and adults had a median survival of 17 months, with a significant proportion surviving more than 4 years after recurrence (110).

Whereas the CCG and UCSF experiences demonstrate poor outcome for all adolescents, regardless of stage, the French Society of Pediatric Oncology found that patients with stage I to II disease fared well and had survival rates comparable to those of younger patients with early stage disease (111). None of six patients with stage I to II disease experienced recurrence. In contrast, adolescents with stage III disease experienced multiple recurrences, with prolonged and chronic clinical courses. This is reflected in discordant PFS and OS rates at 5 years, which were 28% and 86%, respectively. Adolescents with metastatic NB had low PFS and OS rates of 18% and 27%, respectively (111), and exhibited poor responses to intensive chemotherapy.

The poor outcome for adults and adolescents, even with localized disease, calls into question the usual risk-based treatment in this age group. Aggressive multimodality therapy may be appropriate even for patients with low-stage disease but certainly for patients with INSS stage 3 and 4 disease. Specifically, higher radiation dosages are appropriate. Dosages to the primary tumor site should be maximized, tailored to the individual disease sites, and constrained by tolerance of adjacent normal tissues. For example, abdominal primary tumors should be treated with 45 Gy, which constitutes small bowel tolerance, as long as the dosage to the kidneys can be kept within tolerance. Given the poor clinical outcome for adults and adolescents with NB, creative approaches are warranted in the treatment of such patients, including immunotherapy, differentiating agents, targeted RT using ^{131}I-MIBG, and biologic agents.

RADIOTHERAPEUTIC MANAGEMENT

Volume

The volume for irradiation of regional NB is determined by imaging studies and by the operating surgeon's description. If lymph node involvement is suspected or proven, a wide field that covers the primary tumor site and nodal drainage areas is appropriate. If the field must cover a portion of the vertebral body, the full width of the bone should be encompassed. This will reduce the severity of subsequent scoliosis and ensure coverage of the regional lymph nodes (200,264). Some controversy surrounds the issue of whether next-echelon lymph nodes (i.e., mediastinal lymph nodes with an upper abdominal primary tumor) need to be irradiated. Relapse in nonirradiated next-echelon nodes can occur, albeit usually in conjunction with local or distant failure. In the Duke experience of 33 patients with stages A to C, 12 relapsed. Only one of the 21 irradiated patients (5%) experienced an infield failure, whereas seven of the 12 not receiving RT (58%) experienced local failures at the time of recurrence ($p = 0.001$). Routine next-echelon nodal irradiation was not given. Five of the 12 patients who suffered a relapse had next-echelon nodal failure as a component of relapse; only one case was an isolated next-echelon nodal failure (264). Extensive nodal fields may contribute to late morbidity and limit the ability to give chemotherapy, so most radiotherapists cover only the primary tumor volume and adjacent nodal groups. With a dumbbell-shaped tumor, careful attention must be paid to the intraspinal and extravertebral components of the tumor to ensure full coverage.

As previously discussed, RT may be used for INSS 4S–associated hepatomegaly that is symptomatic. The entire liver need not be irradiated to induce tumor regression. The therapist may use portals designed to avoid the kidneys and, in girls, the ovaries. One may use two lateral fields, parallel opposed or slightly angled anteriorly, to treat the majority of the liver but spare the kidneys. Placing the posterior border of the lateral field at the anterior aspect of the vertebral body accomplishes this objective. The ovaries are generally avoided by keeping the inferior border of the field at or above the superior iliac crest. Irradiation dosages for stage 4S hepatomegaly are low, usually 2 to 6 Gy in two to four fractions, so it could be argued that the kidneys are in little danger of chronic injury and that the liver could be treated with parallel, opposed anterior and posterior fields or a single anterior field. Although these are acceptable field arrangement options, the infant kidney is more sensitive to irradiation than kidneys in older children (265). Children with stage 4S disease have high likelihood of survival and, if possible, should not be subjected to the risks of lifetime reductions of glomerular filtration rates. Stage 4 NB with hepatomegaly may also be treated for palliation with ports designed to cover the entire liver, using the anterior–posterior parallel, opposed beams. NB metastases occur in a wide variety of locations. Bone and soft tissue sites are irradiated with moderate margins.

Dosage

Classic radiobiologic analyses reflect the relative radiosensitivity of NB cell lines *in vitro* but produce conflicting results regarding the most appropriate fractionation schedules. The D_0 for most mammalian tumor cell lines is between 1.3 and 1.5 Gy. The n usually is between 1.5 and 10. The n is the extrapolation number and measures the width of the survival curve shoulder. The D_0 describes the final slope of the cell survival curve and is the dose required to reduce survival from 0.1 to 0.037. Collated data on 11 NB cell lines derived from seven patients indicate moderate cellular radiosensitivity beyond that seen for many other mammalian tumors. The median n for NB is 1.36, and the D_0 is 1.04 Gy (217–219,266). This low repair capacity for radiation damage implies that little sparing would result from dose fractionation. Wheldon et al. (219) used human NB grown as multicellular tumor spheroids (MTS) to confirm this hypothesis. There was no significant difference in the killing ability of single-dose and split-dose irradiation. The absence of substantial interfraction repair capacity of MTS may provide a radiobiologic rationale for treating NB with multiple fractions per day. Some NB cell lines have a

rapid doubling time. This would also suggest that the overall treatment time of a fractionated course of radiation should be kept short to prevent tumor repopulation between fractions. However, Deacon et al. (267) performed *in vitro* split-dose irradiation of a NB cell line and found a small but finite capacity for sublethal damage repair. There may be intrinsic variability in repair capabilities between NB cell lines.

Although NB is radiosensitive in the laboratory, its clinical response to irradiation is variable, and in-field recurrences, although rare, do occur. Possible reasons for this discrepancy include the following. First, the *in vitro* data may not indicate clinical NB because cell culture techniques may select more radiosensitive cell lines (268). Second, NB, characterized by certain microscopic and biochemical characteristics, may actually be a spectrum of diseases. Genomic amplification of *MYCN* has been correlated with the stage and prognosis of NB, suggesting that *MYCN* may have a role in determining the aggressiveness of human NB. Perhaps clinical variability in radiosensitivity reflects the variation in oncogene amplification in NB (268).

In defining the role of radiation for high-risk NB, adequate dosages have been defined empirically. Studies on patients now known not to have needed radiation shaped standard radiation dosages that were then translated into dosages adequate for high-risk disease. Historically, RT was administered to most patients with NB, with the exception of those with stage I tumors (95). Radiation dosages ranged from 10 to 45 Gy and were dictated by patient age rather than stage of disease (269). In this era, in which patients with early stage disease received radiation, two studies examined the radiation dosage of NB (231,270). Dosages below 20 Gy were deemed sufficient to achieve local control. However, the majority of patients included in both studies probably would not receive RT in the current era. Nonetheless, the adequacy of dosages of less than 20 Gy was adopted for all stages of disease.

Emerging data suggest that although 20 Gy may be adequate for controlling completely resected tumors, gross residual disease may necessitate higher dosages. Joint Center for Radiation Therapy analyzed radiation dosage and local control and concluded that higher dosages are necessary for local control of NB in older patients (271). The protocol design of CCG 3891 also allowed a limited dose–response analysis, suggesting that the combined effect of external beam radiation and TBI improved local control (207).

Whereas the majority of patients on CCG 3891 had mediastinal and intra-abdominal tumors and therefore received 10 Gy to the primary site, a subgroup of patients received 20 Gy delivered to extra-abdominal primary tumors. Of 36 patients with extra-abdominal primaries, six patients received 20 Gy EBRT (two also received TBI), and 30 patients received no EBRT (ten of these received TBI). Local relapse rates at 5 years were $0\% \pm 0\%$ and $44\% \pm 15\%$ for patients with and without EBRT, respectively ($p = 0.09$). Thus the data suggest a dose–response relationship for local EBRT, although the optimal dosage to primary tumor sites has not been established (207).

As a basic guide for patients with high-risk NB, a minimum dosage of 21 Gy, in either 1.8 Gy daily fractions or 1.5 Gy twice-daily fractions, should be delivered to the tumor volume present before surgical resection. This dosage should be adequate for patients with a complete surgical resection, but patients with incomplete surgical resections may benefit from higher radiation dosages directed at gross residual disease in an attempt to improve on poor local control rates reported in the literature.

Several investigators have published recommendations for time and dose fractionation schedules for the irradiation of metastatic NB in bone or soft tissues with a wide range of daily fractions of 2 to 8.5 Gy and total dosages of 4 to 32 Gy. In a retrospective evaluation of palliative RT for NB at Duke, there was no evidence of a dose–response relationship (200). However, all total dosages used in this study were low. The clinician must avoid selecting too low a dosage for palliation of painful bony or soft tissue lesions. Although most children with stage 4 NB die from the malignancy, some live for 1 year or more after palliative local treatment. The dosage should be adequate to control the symptom for the remainder of the patient's lifetime yet not be so high as to have a significant likelihood of complications. Fractionation depends on volume. Small fields may be treated with 16 to 20 Gy in four or five fractions, whereas large volumes are better treated with 2 to 3 Gy per fraction to 20 to 30 Gy. In the preterminal case, where timely pain control is desired with minimal trips to the RT department, one may administer 6 to 8 Gy once or twice with moderate success.

Palliation of hepatomegaly in stage 4S disease usually can be accomplished by 2 to 6 Gy in two to four fractions. However, regression of the liver may be slow. It is occasionally necessary to repeat the dose. If possible, one should allow a 2- to 3-week interval to gauge response. If the dose is repeated such that the cumulative dosage reaches 12 Gy, the infant's kidney should be out of the field of irradiation.

TECHNIQUES OF IRRADIATION

Some abdominal and pelvic sites are best treated with parallel-opposed anterior and posterior portals. When possible, multiple fields should be used to spare normal tissues. We have often found three-dimensional reconstruction of bulky localized disease useful. After reconstruction of the tumor volume, conformal fields or intensity-modulated RT may be used. In our experience, the principal benefit of computer planning in the treatment of abdominal NB is related to the ability to localize the kidneys and liver. Field position and blocking is used to minimize the dosage to normal tissue. However, after anteroposterior/posteroanterior or minimally obliqued fields prove to be best. A posterior mediastinal volume may be irradiated with an angled wedged posterior pair of fields. Caution should be exercised in the use of a wedge pair of fields adjacent to the spinal column, however. The "hot spot" in such therapy may result in an inhomogeneous dosage across the growth plate of the bone, with a resulting spinal curvature.

INTRAOPERATIVE RADIATION THERAPY

Patients with high-risk disease often present with large abdominal primary tumors, abutting or invading many dose-limiting normal tissues. External beam radiation to these tumors often entails treatment of a large volume of normal tissue, including bowel, liver, kidney, bony structures, and spinal cord. RT to NB occurring at other primary sites, including the thorax and pelvis, similarly exposes normal tissues to the risk of long-term side effects. Long-term toxicities associated with EBRT are particularly severe in children (229,264,272–274). Furthermore, EBRT may decrease renal function, resulting in diminished tolerance to high-dose chemotherapy with stem cell transplant.

Although EBRT plays a key role in NB treatment, several institutions have explored intraoperative RT (IORT) (Table 6-9) as an effective radiation modality that may minimize acute and long-term side effects. In contrast to EBRT, IORT allows treatment of high-risk areas at the time of primary resection. Critical structures can be directly visualized and manipulated at the time of surgery, allowing their exclusion from the radiation field if they are at low risk for microscopic disease. A high radiation dosage can be delivered to residual tumor and areas at high risk for microscopic disease with minimal radiation dosage to nearby normal tissues. A small number of studies have established the potential for IORT as a treatment modality in infants and children, including patients with NB (275–279).

IORT in these studies is extremely well tolerated and may improve local disease control.

A recent update from UCSF reported on a cohort of 28 consecutive patients treated with IORT for newly diagnosed high-risk NB. With follow-up ranging from 19 to 200 months (median 45 months), none of the 20 patients who had gross total resections experienced local recurrences. In contrast, three of eight patients who had subtotal resections experienced local recurrence, despite the addition of 20 Gy of EBRT to the primary site postoperatively. Only one late complication was reported: an atrophic kidney with narrowing of the abdominal aorta (280).

IORT at the time of primary resection achieves excellent local control in patients with high-risk NB and is well tolerated. IORT achieves control and survival rates comparable to those of historical controls while avoiding the use of systematic EBRT. Additional therapy with EBRT may not be warranted in high-risk patients with gross total resection treated with IORT who have only microscopic residual disease, although more conclusive evidence requires larger patient numbers and longer follow-up. Higher local failure rates in patients with high-risk NB after incomplete resections or multiple positive lymph nodes warrant additional therapy with EBRT.

TABLE 6-9. *Intraoperative radiotherapy for neuroblastoma*

Reference	Stage	Local control/total patients	IORT dosage median (range), in Gy	EBRT given (n)	IORT for persistent or recurrent disease	IORT toxicity
275	III: 7 IV: 18	18/25	10 (10–15)	8	25	None identifiable
277	2B: 1 3: 2 4: 5	7/8	10 (3–15)	4	0	None identifiable
276	II: 2 III: 12 IV: 10	13/24	10 (7–15)	6	10	Transient pancreatitis (1) Postoperative intussusception (2)
280	3: 6 4: 17	6/23	10 (7–16)	3	3	Narrowing of abdominal aorta (1)
315	3: 1 4: 26	24/27	10 (7–16)	6	0	None identifiable

EBRT, external beam radiation therapy; IORT, intraoperative radiotherapy.

COMPLICATIONS

Patients with high-risk NB often present with large abdominal primaries, abutting or invading many dose-limiting normal tissues. EBRT to these tumors often entails treating a large volume of normal tissue, including bowel, liver, kidney, bony structures, and spinal cord. RT to NB occurring at other primary sites, including the thorax and pelvis, similarly exposes normal tissues to the risk of long-term side effects. Long-term toxicities associated with radiation are particularly severe in children (272–274). Furthermore, EBRT may decrease renal function, resulting in diminished tolerance to high-dose chemotherapy with stem cell transplant.

Acute side effects during RT depend on the precise normal tissues included in the radiation field. In the treatment of most primary tumors, whether thoracic or abdominal, radiation to the gastrointestinal tract, particularly the small bowel, may cause nausea and vomiting. Antiemetic medications are very effective in ameliorating such symptoms. Diarrhea and abdominal pain occur less often, and dietary counseling is generally sufficient to control such side effects. Some primary tumors and metastatic sites necessitate the inclusion of significant regions of bone marrow, resulting in a fall in blood counts that necessitates regular monitoring.

Long-term sequelae of radiation are of particular concern because most patients with NB are very young and prone to such toxicities (272–274). Dosages of approximately 20 Gy to bones produce only minimal deficits, although specific effects depend on the type of bone growth: Radiation to epiphyses of tubular bones leads to bone shortening, whereas radiation to diaphyses impairs bone modeling and thickness. Effects on bone are highly dependent on patient age and radiation dosage (229). Substantial impairment in bone growth has been reported for dosages greater than 30 Gy, and although dosages of 10 to 20 Gy probably affect all cell types in maturing bones, such lower dosages probably will produce more subtle clinical sequelae. For all patients, regardless of delivered dosage, shielding of bone growth centers will minimize potential growth arrest and skeletal abnormalities. When one is treating regions close to vertebrae, irradiation of the entire vertebral bodies reduces the risk of scoliosis and other musculoskeletal abnormalities.

A high incidence of spinal deformity has been seen in long-term survivors of NB. Among the most common abnormalities are postsurgery or postirradiation kyphosis or scoliosis (200, 281–284). The incidence of these abnormalities in 5-year survivors of NB with paraspinal tumors ranges from 25% to 50% (285). Factors associated with development of spinal deformity include irradiation at a very young age, orthovoltage irradiation, asymmetric irradiation of the spine, epidural spread of tumor, and laminectomy. In young children, a laminectomy may result in growth abnormality, gibbus formation, and instability of the spine. Therefore, the young child with a dumbbell-shaped tumor is at risk for spinal deformity, and every effort should be made to minimize this and other late sequelae with use of chemotherapy when possible as first-line treatment for cord compression or surgical decompression using osteoplastic laminotomy rather than traditional laminectomy (42,214,283,284, 286,287).

In addition to musculoskeletal toxicities, local radiation may cause organ dysfunction if tolerance dosages are exceeded. Whole organ tolerance levels generally are presented as dosages that cause a severe complication rate of 5% within 5 years of radiation completion. These include the lungs (17.5 Gy), kidneys (20 Gy), liver (30 Gy), small bowel (40 Gy), ovaries (10 Gy), and testes (2 Gy). These tolerance dosages are general guidelines and may be lower in children and in patients who are also receiving chemotherapy. Skull and orbital metastases are common in NB, often necessitating irradiation of normal brain tissue. The risks of neurocognitive dysfunction and endocrine abnormalities increase with higher dosages of radiation, larger volumes of irradiated normal brain, and younger age at time of radiation. Lens tolerance is as low as 10 Gy, and dosages to the lens should be minimized to prevent cataract formation. Permanent alopecia is extremely rare after dosages of 21

Gy or less, but permanent hair thinning may occur in a small proportion of children.

Whereas side effects of local radiation depend on the exposed normal structures, TBI carries inherent toxicities that, like local radiation, worsen with increasing radiation dosage and decreasing patient age. Long-term side effects of TBI include risks of impaired growth, chronic interstitial lung disease, cataracts, neurocognitive deficits, chronic renal insufficiency, dental disturbances, and endocrinopathies (288–296). After fractionated TBI, a majority of patients experience diminished height and endocrine deficits, most commonly manifest by delayed puberty, but only a minority of patients experience other major organ toxicities (289,292).

Both local RT and TBI carry the risk of second malignancies. Reliable risk estimates of second malignancies after RT for NB are not available. In the treatment of a malignancy with guarded prognosis such as high-risk NB, the risk of death from recurrent disease clearly outweighs the risk of death from a second malignancy. One may extrapolate from a large body of literature in pediatric Hodgkin's disease survivors and assume that children who are cured after receiving radiation for NB will develop additional cancers 10 to 20 years later (297). Common radiation-related malignancies include breast cancer, sarcomas, lymphomas, and other solid tumors. Long-term survivors of NB need lifelong screening for late sequelae of RT.

TARGETED RADIONUCLIDES

Targeted radioisotope therapy using anti-GD2 antibody or MIBG for delivery of radiation in the form of ^{131}I has also been tested extensively in clinical trials in relapsed and newly diagnosed NB. Cheung et al. (298–301) reported on the use of [131]I-3F8 to treat refractory NB with documented responses and now have an ongoing study for newly diagnosed patients using [131]I-3F8 in myeloablative dosages followed by bone marrow rescue and further treatment with cold antibody after transplant (302). MIBG is a guanethidine derivative that is structurally similar to norepinephrine and therefore concentrates in the neurosecretory granules of catecholamine-secreting cells. Radiolabeled MIBG provides very sensitive and specific visualization of primary and metastatic NB by scintigraphy (79). In an attempt to deliver higher dosages of tumor-specific radiotherapy and avoid normal organ toxicity, ^{131}I-MIBG therapy has been used in pilot trials since the mid-1980s, with more than 500 children reported in the literature. Initially, it was shown to induce a 30–40% response rate in highly refractory relapsed patients, without significant nonhematologic toxicity (303–305). At low and moderate dosages, up to 12 mCi/kg of ^{131}I, the main toxicity has been thrombocytopenia, usually self-limited. Phase I dosage escalation studies showed that higher dosages, up to 18 mCi/kg, could be administered with bone marrow or peripheral blood stem cell support to mitigate the neutropenia and thrombocytopenia, but still without other organ toxicity, excepting a 10–15% incidence of hypothyroidism caused by uptake of some free iodide by the thyroid gland (304,306). There are a few reports of patients with secondary leukemia developing after MIBG therapy, but the estimated risk of this problem at 5 years after therapy is only 4%, lower than with some chemotherapy regimens (307,308). Recent studies are investigating the use of low-dose ^{131}I-MIBG at diagnosis before surgical resection (309) or in combination with standard (310) or high-dose myeloablative chemotherapy (311, 312). New phase I studies are open in a multi-institution phase I consortium, New Approaches to Neuroblastoma Therapy, to study the use of double infusions of ^{131}I-MIBG with stem cell support or further combination with myeloablative chemotherapy and stem cells. Additional investigations are needed to determine the optimal timing and use of this targeted approach.

FUTURE INVESTIGATIONS

Current treatment regimens for NB are risk based; that is, the biologic characteristics of the tumor are considered together with traditional clinical prognostic factors in determining optimal therapy. As data are accumulated, the most powerful independent prognostic determinants will be clarified. Areas of active investigation include the following:

- Efforts to develop chemotherapeutic agents with new mechanisms of action.
- Megatherapy (high-dose chemotherapy with or without radiotherapy) followed by hematopoietic stem cell rescue.
- Targeted therapy using radiolabeled MIBG or monoclonal antibodies.
- The use of biologic response modifiers or immunotherapy, such as IL-2, IL-12, or dendritic cells and vaccines. The retinoids, such as 13-*cis*-retinoic acid and fenretinide, can decrease tumor cell proliferation, morphologic differentiation, decreased expression of N-*myc,* or apoptosis.
- Clinical studies are in progress to assess the potential benefit of these agents.

REFERENCES

References particularly recommended for further reading are indicated by an asterisk.

1. Cushing H, Wolbach SB. The transformation of a malignant paravertebral sympathicoblastoma into a benign ganglioneuroma. *Am J Pathol* 1927;3: 203–216.
2. Matthay KK. Neuroblastoma: biology and therapy. *Oncology* 1997;11(12):1857–1866, 1869–1872, 1875.
3. Goodman MT, Gurney JG, Smith MA, et al. Sympathetic nervous system tumors. In: Ries LAG, Smith MA, Gurney JG, et al., eds. *Cancer incidence and survival among children and adolescents: United States SEER program 1975–1995.* Bethesda, MD: National Cancer Institute, SEER Program, 1999: 65–72.
4. Young JL Jr, Ries LG, Silverberg E, et al. Cancer incidence, survival, and mortality for children younger than age 15 years. *Cancer* 1986;58(2 Suppl):598–602.
5. Bernstein ML, Leclerc JM, Bunin G, et al. A population-based study of neuroblastoma incidence, survival, and mortality in North America. *J Clin Oncol* 1992;10(2):323–329.
6. Williams PL, Wendell-Smith CP, Treadgold S. *Basic human embryology.* Philadelphia: JB Lippincott, 1984:98–99.
7. Guin GH, Gilbert EF, Jones B. Incidental neuroblastoma in infants. *Am J Clin Pathol* 1969;51(1): 126–136.
8. Woods WG, Tuchman M, Robison LL, et al. A population-based study of the usefulness of screening for neuroblastoma. *Lancet* 1996;348(9043):1682–1687.
*9. Woods WG, Gao RN, Shuster JJ, et al. Screening of infants and mortality due to neuroblastoma. *N Engl J Med* 2002;346(14):1041–1046.
10. Woods WG. Screening for neuroblastoma: the final chapters. *J Pediatr Hematol Oncol* 2003;25(1):3–4.
11. Yamamoto K, Hanada R, Tanimura M, et al. Natural history of neuroblastoma found by mass screening [letter; comment]. *Lancet* 1997;349(9058):1102.
12. Suita S, Zaizen Y, Sera Y, et al. Mass screening for neuroblastoma: quo vadis? A 9-year experience from the Pediatric Oncology Study Group of the Kyushu area in Japan. *J Pediatr Surg* 1996;31(4):555–558.
13. Nakagawara A, Zaizen Y, Ikeda K, et al. Different genomic and metabolic patterns between mass screening-positive and mass screening-negative later-presenting neuroblastomas. *Cancer* 1991;68(9): 2037–2044.
14. Takeuchi LA, Hachitanda Y, Woods WG, et al. Screening for neuroblastoma in North America. Preliminary results of a pathology review from the Quebec Project. *Cancer* 1995;76(11):2363–2371.
15. Schilling FH, Spix C, Berthold F, et al. Neuroblastoma screening at one year of age. *N Engl J Med* 2002;346(14):1047–1053.
16. Kramer S, Ward E, Meadows AT, et al. Medical and drug risk factors associated with neuroblastoma: a case-control study. *J Natl Cancer Inst* 1987;78(5): 797–804.
17. Michalek AM, Buck GM, Nasca PC, et al. Gravid health status, medication use, and risk of neuroblastoma. *Am J Epidemiol* 1996;43(10):996–1001.
18. Schwartzbaum JA. Influence of the mother's prenatal drug consumption on risk of neuroblastoma in the child. *Am J Epidemiol* 1992;135(12):1358–1367.
19. Olshan AF, Smith J, Cook MN, et al. Hormone and fertility drug use and the risk of neuroblastoma: a report from the Children's Cancer Group and the Pediatric Oncology Group. *Am J Epidemiol* 1999;150(9): 930–938.
20. Olshan AF, De Roos AJ, Teschke K, et al. Neuroblastoma and parental occupation. *Cancer Causes Control* 1999;10(6):539–549.
21. De Roos AJ, Olshan AF, Teschke K, et al. Parental occupational exposures to chemicals and incidence of neuroblastoma in offspring. *Am J Epidemiol* 2001; 154(2):106–114.
22. De Roos AJ, Teschke K, Savitz DA, et al. Parental occupational exposures to electromagnetic fields and radiation and the incidence of neuroblastoma in offspring. *Epidemiology* 2001;12(5):508–517.
23. Flaegstad T, Andresen PA, Johnsen JI, et al. A possible contributory role of BK virus infection in neuroblastoma development. *Cancer Res* 1999;59(5): 1160–1163.
24. Kushner BH, Gilbert F, Helson L. Familial neuroblastoma. Case reports, literature review, and etiologic considerations. *Cancer* 1986;57(9):1887–1893.
25. Laureys G, Versteeg R, Speleman F, et al. Characterisation of the chromosome breakpoints in a patient with a constitutional translocation t(1;17)(p36.31–p36.13;q11.2–q12) and neuroblastoma. *Eur J Cancer* 1995;31A(4):523–526.
*26. Maris JM, Matthay KK. Molecular biology of neuroblastoma. *J Clin Oncol* 1999;17(7):2264–2279.
27. Tonini GP, Longo L, Coco S, et al. Familial neuroblastoma: a complex heritable disease. *Cancer Lett* 2003;197(1–2):41–45.

28. Maris JM, Weiss MJ, Mosse Y, et al. Evidence for a hereditary neuroblastoma predisposition locus at chromosome 16p12–13. *Cancer Res* 2002;62(22): 6651–6658.

29. Maris JM, Chatten J, Meadows AT, et al. Familial neuroblastoma: a three-generation pedigree and a further association with Hirschsprung disease. *Med Pediatr Oncol* 1997;28(1):1–5.

30. Caron H, van Sluis P, de Kraker J, et al. Allelic loss of chromosome 1p as a predictor of unfavorable outcome in patients with neuroblastoma. *N Engl J Med* 1996;334(4):225–230.

31. Seeger RC, Brodeur GM, Sather H, et al. Association of multiple copies of the N-*myc* oncogene with rapid progression of neuroblastomas. *N Engl J Med* 1985; 313(18):1111–1116.

32. Nakagawara A, Arima Nakagawara M, Scavarda NJ, et al. Association between high levels of expression of the TRK gene and favorable outcome in human neuroblastoma. *N Engl J Med* 1993;328:847–854.

33. Bowman LC, Castleberry RP, Cantor A, et al. Genetic staging of unresectable or metastatic neuroblastoma in infants: a Pediatric Oncology Group study. *J Natl Cancer Inst* 1997;89(5):373–380.

34. Look AT, Hayes FA, Shuster JJ, et al. Clinical relevance of tumor cell ploidy and N-myc gene amplification in childhood neuroblastoma: a Pediatric Oncology Group study. *J Clin Oncol* 1991;9(4): 581–591.

35. Tonini GP, Boni L, Pession A, et al. *MYCN* oncogene amplification in neuroblastoma is associated with worse prognosis, except in stage 4s: the Italian experience with 295 children. *J Clin Oncol* 1997;15(1):85–93.

36. Shimada H, Stram DO, Chatten J, et al. Identification of subsets of neuroblastomas by combined histopathologic and N-myc analysis. *J Natl Cancer Inst* 1995;87(19):1470–1476.

37. Rubie H, Hartmann O, Michon J, et al. N-Myc gene amplification is a major prognostic factor in localized neuroblastoma: results of the French NBL 90 study. *J Clin Oncol* 1997;15(3):1171–1182.

38. Schmidt ML, Lukens JN, Seeger RC, et al. Biologic factors determine prognosis in infants with stage IV neuroblastoma: a prospective Children's Cancer Group study. *J Clin Oncol* 2000;18(6):1260–1268.

*39. Katzenstein HM, Bowman LC, Brodeur GM, et al. Prognostic significance of age, *MYCN* oncogene amplification, tumor cell ploidy, and histology in 110 infants with stage D S neuroblastoma: the pediatric oncology group experience—a Pediatric Oncology Group study. *J Clin Oncol* 1998;16(6):2007–2017.

40. Weiss WA, Aldape K, Mohapatra G, et al. Targeted expression of *MYCN* causes neuroblastoma in transgenic mice. *EMBO J* 1997;16(11):2985–2995.

41. Brodeur GM, Maris JM, Yamashiro DJ, et al. Biology and genetics of human neuroblastomas. *J Pediatr Hematol Oncol* 1997;19(2):93–101.

*42. Perez CA, Matthay KK, Atkinson JB, et al. Biologic variables in the outcome of stages I and II neuroblastoma treated with surgery as primary therapy: a Children's Cancer Group study. *J Clin Oncol* 2000; 18(1):18–26.

43. Brodeur GM, Nakagawara A. Molecular basis of clinical heterogeneity in neuroblastoma. *Am J Pediatr Hematol Oncol* 1992;4(2):111–116.

44. Look AT, Hayes FA, Nitschke R, et al. Cellular DNA content as a predictor of response to chemotherapy in infants with unresectable neuroblastoma. *N Engl J Med* 1984;311:231–235.

45. Gilbert F. Chromosome abnormalities, gene amplification, and tumor progression. *Prog Clin Biol Res* 1985;175:151–159.

46. Maris JM, White PS, Beltinger CP, et al. Significance of chromosome 1p loss of heterozygosity in neuroblastoma. *Cancer Res* 1995;55(20):4664–4669.

47. Gehring M, Berthold F, Edler L, et al. The 1p deletion is not a reliable marker for the prognosis of patients with neuroblastoma. *Cancer Res* 1995;55(22):5366–5369.

48. Maris JM, Weiss MJ, Guo C, et al. Loss of heterozygosity at 1p36 independently predicts for disease progression but not decreased overall survival probability in neuroblastoma patients: a Children's Cancer Group study. *J Clin Oncol* 2000;18(9):1888–1899.

49. Maris JM, Guo C, Blake D, et al. Comprehensive analysis of chromosome 1p deletions in neuroblastoma. *Med Pediatr Oncol* 2001;36(1):32–36.

50. Guo C, White PS, Weiss MJ, et al. Allelic deletion at 11q23 is common in *MYCN* single copy neuroblastomas. *Oncogene* 1999;18(35):4948–4957.

51. Maris JM, Guo C, White PS, et al. Allelic deletion at chromosome bands 11q14-23 is common in neuroblastoma. *Med Pediatr Oncol* 2001;36(1):24–27.

52. Plantaz D, Vandesompele J, Van Roy N, et al. Comparative genomic hybridization (CGH) analysis of stage 4 neuroblastoma reveals high frequency of 11q deletion in tumors lacking *MYCN* amplification. *Int J Cancer* 2001;91(5):580–686.

53. Plantaz D, Mohapatra G, Matthay KK, et al. Gain of chromosome 17 is the most frequent abnormality detected in neuroblastoma by comparative genomic hybridization. *Am J Pathol* 1997;150(1):81–89.

54. Bown N, Cotterill S, Lastowska M, et al. Gain of chromosome arm 17q and adverse outcome in patients with neuroblastoma. *N Engl J Med* 1999; 340(25):1954–1961.

55. Hiyama E, Hiyama K, Yokoyama T, et al. Correlating telomerase activity levels with human neuroblastoma outcomes. *Nat Med* 1995;1(3):249–255.

56. Combaret V, Gross N, Lasset C, et al. Clinical relevance of CD44 cell-surface expression and N-myc gene amplification in a multicentric analysis of 121 pediatric neuroblastomas. *J Clin Oncol* 1996;14(1): 25–34.

57. Combaret V, Gross N, Lasset C, et al. Clinical relevance of TRKA expression on neuroblastoma: comparison with N-MYC amplification and CD44 expression. *Br J Cancer* 1997;75(8):1151–1155.

58. Gladson CL, Hancock S, Arnold MM, et al. Stage-specific expression of integrin alphaVbeta3 in neuroblastic tumors. *Am J Pathol* 1996;148(5):1423–34.

59. Erdreich-Epstein A, Shimada H, Groshen S, et al. Integrins alpha(v)beta3 and alpha(v)beta5 are expressed by endothelium of high-risk neuroblastoma and their inhibition is associated with increased endogenous ceramide. *Cancer Res* 2000;60(3): 712–721.

60. Lode HN, Moehler T, Xiang R, et al. Synergy between an antiangiogenic integrin alphav antagonist and an antibody–cytokine fusion protein eradicates spontaneous tumor metastases. *Proc Natl Acad Sci U S A* 1999;96(4):1591–1596.

61. Sugiura Y, Shimada H, Seeger RC, et al. Matrix metalloproteinases-2 and -9 are expressed in human neuroblastoma: contribution of stromal cells to their production and correlation with metastasis. *Cancer Res* 1998;58(10):2209–2216.

62. Eggert A, Ikegaki N, Kwiatkowski J, et al. High-level expression of angiogenic factors is associated with advanced tumor stage in human neuroblastomas. *Clin Cancer Res* 2000;6(5):1900–1908.

63. Fukuzawa M, Sugiura H, Koshinaga T, et al. Expression of vascular endothelial growth factor and its receptor Flk-1 in human neuroblastoma using in situ hybridization. *J Pediatr Surg* 2002;37(12):1747–1750.

*64. Shimada H, Ambros IM, Dehner LP, et al. Terminology and morphologic criteria of neuroblastic tumors: recommendations by the International Neuroblastoma Pathology Committee. *Cancer* 1999;86(2): 349–363.

65. Triche TJ. Neuroblastoma and other childhood neural tumors: a review. *Pediatr Pathol* 1990;10(1–2): 175–193.

66. Shimada H, Ambros IM, Dehner LP, et al. The International Neuroblastoma Pathology Classification (the Shimada system). *Cancer* 1999;86(2):364–372.

67. Shimada H, Chatten J, Newton WA Jr, et al. Histopathologic prognostic factors in neuroblastic tumors: definition of subtypes of ganglioneuroblastoma and an age-linked classification of neuroblastomas. *J Natl Cancer Inst* 1984;73(2):405–416.

68. Joshi VV, Silverman JF. Pathology of neuroblastic tumors. *Semin Diagn Pathol* 1994;11(2):107–117.

69. Chatten J, Shimada H, Sather HN, et al. Prognostic value of histopathology in advanced neuroblastoma: a report from the Children's Cancer Study Group. *Hum Pathol* 1988;19(10):1187–1198.

70. Joshi VV, Cantor AB, Altshuler G, et al. Age-linked prognostic categorization based on a new histologic grading system of neuroblastomas. A clinicopathologic study of 211 cases from the Pediatric Oncology Group. *Cancer* 1992;69(8):2197–2211.

71. Joshi VV, Cantor AB, Brodeur GM, et al. Correlation between morphologic and other prognostic markers of neuroblastoma. A study of histologic grade, DNA index, N-myc gene copy number, and lactic dehydrogenase in patients in the Pediatric Oncology Group. *Cancer* 1993;71(10):3173–3181.

72. Joshi VV, Cantor AB, Altshuler G, et al. Recommendations for modification of terminology of neuroblastic tumors and prognostic significance of Shimada classification. A clinicopathologic study of 213 cases from the Pediatric Oncology Group. *Cancer* 1992;69(8):2183–96.

*73. Shimada H, Umehara S, Monobe Y, et al. International neuroblastoma pathology classification for prognostic evaluation of patients with peripheral neuroblastic tumors: a report from the Children's Cancer Group. *Cancer* 2001;92(9):2451–2461.

74. Antunes NL, Khakoo Y, Matthay KK, et al. Antineuronal antibodies in patients with neuroblastoma and paraneoplastic opsoclonus–myoclonus. *J Pediatr Hematol Oncol* 2000;22(4):315–320.

75. Hayward K, Jeremy RJ, Jenkins S, et al. Long-term neurobehavioral outcomes in children with neuroblastoma and opsoclonus–myoclonus–ataxia syndrome: relationship to MRI findings and anti-neuronal antibodies. *J Pediatr* 2001;139(4):552–559.

76. Rudnick E, Khakoo Y, Antunes NL, et al. Opsoclonus–myoclonus–ataxia syndrome in neuroblastoma: clinical outcome and antineuronal antibodies—a report from the Children's Cancer Group Study. *Med Pediatr Oncol* 2001;36(6):612–622.

77. Russo C, Cohn SL, Petruzzi MJ, et al. Long-term neurologic outcome in children with opsoclonus–myoclonus associated with neuroblastoma: a report from the Pediatric Oncology Group. *Med Pediatr Oncol* 1997;28(4):284–288.

78. Hadley GP, Rabe E. Scanning with iodine-131 MIBG in children with solid tumors: an initial appraisal. *J Nucl Med* 1986;27(5):620–626.

79. Shulkin BL, Shapiro B. Current concepts on the diagnostic use of MIBG in children. *J Nucl Med* 1998;39(4):679–688.

80. Matthay KK, Edeline V, Lumbroso J, et al. Correlation of early metastatic response by ^{123}I-metaiodobenzylguanidine scintigraphy with overall response and event-free survival in stage IV neuroblastoma. *J Clin Oncol* 2003;21(13):2486–2491.

81. Gordon I, Peters AM, Gutman A, et al. Skeletal assessment in neuroblastoma: the pitfalls of iodine-123-MIBG scans. *J Nucl Med* 1990;31(2):129–134.

82. Shulkin BL, Hutchinson RJ, Castle VP, et al. Neuroblastoma: positron emission tomography with 2-(fluorine-18)-fluoro-2-deoxy-D-glucose compared with metaiodobenzylguanidine scintigraphy. *Radiology* 1996;199(3):743–750.

83. Kushner BH, Yeung HW, Larson SM, et al. Extending positron emission tomography scan utility to high-risk neuroblastoma: fluorine-18 fluorodeoxyglucose positron emission tomography as sole imaging modality in follow-up of patients. *J Clin Oncol* 2001;19(14): 3397–3405.

84. DuBois SG, Kalika Y, Lukens JN, et al. Metastatic sites in stage IV and IVS neuroblastoma correlate with age, tumor biology, and survival. *J Pediatr Hematol Oncol* 1999;21(3):181–189.

85. Kammen BF, Matthay KK, Pacharn P, et al. Pulmonary metastases at diagnosis of neuroblastoma in pediatric patients: CT findings and prognosis. *AJR Am J Roentgenol* 2001;176(3):755–759.

86. Cheung NK. Detecting neuroblastoma using bone marrow aspiration and bone marrow biopsy [Letter]. *J Pediatr Hematol Oncol* 2000;22(1):86–88.

87. Moss TJ, Reynolds CP, Sather HN, et al. Prognostic value of immunocytologic detection of bone marrow metastases in neuroblastoma. *N Engl J Med* 1991; 324:219–226.

88. Seeger RC, Reynolds CP, Gallego R, et al. Quantitative tumor cell content of bone marrow and blood as a predictor of outcome in stage IV neuroblastoma: a Children's Cancer Group Study. *J Clin Oncol* 2000; 18(24):4067–4076.

89. Brodeur GM, Pritchard J, Berthold F, et al. Revisions

of the international criteria for neuroblastoma diagnosis, staging, and response to treatment. *J Clin Oncol* 1993;11(8):1466–1477.

90. Cheung IY, Lo Piccolo MS, Kushner BH, et al. Quantitation of GD2 synthase mRNA by real-time reverse transcriptase polymerase chain reaction: clinical utility in evaluating adjuvant therapy in neuroblastoma. *J Clin Oncol* 2003;21(6):1087–1093.

91. Burchill SA, Lewis IJ, Abrams KR, et al. Circulating neuroblastoma cells detected by reverse transcriptase polymerase chain reaction for tyrosine hydroxylase mRNA are an independent poor prognostic indicator in stage 4 neuroblastoma in children over 1 year. *J Clin Oncol* 2001;19(6):1795–1801.

92. LaBrosse EH, Comoy E, Bohuon C, et al. Catecholamine metabolism in neuroblastoma. *J Natl Cancer Inst* 1976;57(3):633–638.

93. Qualman SJ, O'Dorisio MS, Fleshman DJ, et al. Neuroblastoma. Correlation of neuropeptide expression in tumor tissue with other prognostic factors. *Cancer* 1992;70(7):2005–2012.

94. Evans AE, D'Angio GJ, Sather HN, et al. A comparison of four staging systems for localized and regional neuroblastoma: a report from the Children's Cancer Study Group. *J Clin Oncol* 1990;8(4):678–688.

95. Evans AE. Staging and treatment of neuroblastoma. *Cancer* 1980;45(7 Suppl):1799–1802.

96. Evans AE, D'Angio GJ, Randolph J. A proposed staging for children with neuroblastoma. Children's Cancer Study Group A. *Cancer* 1971;27:374–378.

97. Hayes FA, Green A, Hustu HO, et al. Surgicopathologic staging of neuroblastoma: prognostic significance of regional lymph node metastases. *J Pediatr* 1983;102:59–62.

98. Ninane J, Pritchard J, Morris Jones PH, et al. Stage II neuroblastoma. Adverse prognostic significance of lymph node involvement. *Arch Dis Child* 1982;57(6):438–442.

99. Brodeur GM, Seeger RC, Barrett A, et al. International criteria for diagnosis, staging, and response to treatment in patients with neuroblastoma. *J Clin Oncol* 1988;6(12):1874–1881.

100. Therasse P, Arbuck SG, Eisenhauer EA, et al. New guidelines to evaluate the response to treatment in solid tumors. *J Natl Cancer Inst* 2000;92(3):205–216.

101. Breslow N, McCann B. Statistical estimation of prognosis for children with neuroblastoma. *Cancer Res* 1971;31:2098–2103.

102. Shuster JJ, McWilliams NB, Castleberry R, et al. Serum lactate dehydrogenase in childhood neuroblastoma. A Pediatric Oncology Group recursive partitioning study. *Am J Clin Oncol* 1992;15(4):295–303.

103. Berthold F, Kassenbohmer R, Zieschang J. Multivariate evaluation of prognostic factors in localized neuroblastoma. *Am J Pediatr Hematol Oncol* 1994;16(2):107–115.

104. Cotterill SJ, Pearson AD, Pritchard J, et al. Clinical prognostic factors in 1277 patients with neuroblastoma: results of the European Neuroblastoma Study Group "Survey" 1982–1992. *Eur J Cancer* 2000;36(7):901–908.

105. Oppedal BR, Storm-Mathisen I, Lie SO, et al. Prognostic factors in neuroblastoma. Clinical, histopathologic, and immunohistochemical features and DNA ploidy in relation to prognosis. *Cancer* 1988;62(4):772–780.

106. Castleberry RP, Shuster JJ, Altshuler G, et al. Infants with neuroblastoma and regional lymph node metastases have a favorable outlook after limited postoperative chemotherapy: a Pediatric Oncology Group study. *J Clin Oncol* 1992 10(8):1299–1304.

107. Nickerson HJ, Matthay KK, Seeger RC, et al. Favorable biology and outcome of stage IV-S neuroblastoma with supportive care or minimal therapy: a Children's Cancer Group study. *J Clin Oncol* 2000;18(3):477–486.

108. Nickerson HJ, Nesbit ME, Grosfeld JL, et al. Comparison of Stage IV and IV-S neuroblastoma in the first year of life. *Med Pediatr Oncol* 1985;13:261–268.

109. Rubie H, Plantaz D, Coze C, et al. Localised and unresectable neuroblastoma in infants: excellent outcome with primary chemotherapy. Neuroblastoma Study Group, Société Française d'Oncologie Pediatrique. *Med Pediatr Oncol* 2001;36(1):247–250.

110. Franks LM, Bollen A, Seeger RC, et al. Neuroblastoma in adults and adolescents: an indolent course with poor survival. *Cancer* 1997;79(10):2028–2035.

111. Gaspar N, Hartman O, Munzer C, et al. Neuroblastoma in adolescents. *Cancer* 2003;98(2):349–355.

112. Haas D, Ablin AR, Miller C, et al. Complete pathologic maturation and regression of stage IVS neuroblastoma without treatment. *Cancer* 1988;62(4):818–825.

113. Garaventa A, De Bernardi B, Pianca C, et al. Localized but unresectable neuroblastoma: treatment and outcome of 145 cases. Italian Cooperative Group for Neuroblastoma. *J Clin Oncol* 1993;11(9):1770–1779.

114. Rubie H, Hartmann O, Giron A, et al. Nonmetastatic thoracic neuroblastomas: a review of 40 cases. *Med Pediatr Oncol* 1991;19(4):253–257.

115. Labreveux de Cervens C, Hartmann O, Bonnin F, et al. What is the prognostic value of osteomedullary uptake on MIBG scan in neuroblastoma patients under one year of age? *Med Pediatr Oncol* 1994;22(2):107–114.

116. Hartmann O, Valteau-Couanet D, Vassal G, et al. Prognostic factors in metastatic neuroblastoma in patients over 1 year of age treated with high-dose chemotherapy and stem cell transplantation: a multivariate analysis on 218 patients treated in a single institution. *Bone Marrow Transplant* 1999;23(8):789–795.

117. Evans AE, D'Angio GJ, Propert K, et al. Prognostic factors in neuroblastoma. *Cancer* 1987;59(11):1853–1859.

118. Hann HW, Stahlhut MW, Evans AE. Basic and acidic isoferritins in the sera of patients with neuroblastoma. *Cancer* 1988;62(6):1179–1182.

119. Hann HW, Evans AE, Siegel SE, et al. Prognostic importance of serum ferritin in patients with Stages III and IV neuroblastoma: the Children's Cancer Study Group experience. *Cancer Res* 1985;45(6):2843–2848.

120. Silber JH, Evans AE, Fridman M. Models to predict

outcome from childhood neuroblastoma: the role of serum ferritin and tumor histology. *Cancer Res* 1991; 51(5):1426–1433.

121. Zeltzer PM, Marangos PJ, Evans AE, et al. Serum neuron-specific enolase in children with neuroblastoma. Relationship to stage and disease course. *Cancer* 1986;57(6):1230–1234.

122. Kropp J, Hofmann M, Bihl H. Comparison of MIBG and pentetreotide scintigraphy in children with neuroblastoma. Is the expression of somatostatin receptors a prognostic factor? *Anticancer Res* 1997;17(3B): 1583–1588.

123. Chan HS, Haddad G, Thorner PS, et al. P-glycoprotein expression as a predictor of the outcome of therapy for neuroblastoma. *N Engl J Med* 1991;325(23):1608–1614.

124. Norris MD, Bordow SB, Marshall GM, et al. Expression of the gene for multidrug-resistance–associated protein and outcome in patients with neuroblastoma. *N Engl J Med* 1996;334(4):231–238.

125. Tanaka T, Slamon DJ, Shimada H, et al. A significant association of Ha-ras p21 in neuroblastoma cells with patient prognosis. A retrospective study of 103 cases. *Cancer* 1991;68(6):1296–1302.

126. Ladisch S, Wu ZL, Feig S, et al. Shedding of GD2 ganglioside by human neuroblastoma. *Int J Cancer* 1987;39(1):73–76.

127. Wu ZL, Schwartz E, Seeger R, et al. Expression of GD2 ganglioside by untreated primary human neuroblastomas. *Cancer Res* 1986;46(1):440–443.

128. Valentino L, Moss T, Olson E, et al. Shed tumor gangliosides and progression of human neuroblastoma. *Blood* 1990;75(7):1564–1567.

129. Hsiao RJ, Seeger RC, Yu AL, et al. Chromogranin A in children with neuroblastoma. Serum concentration parallels disease stage and predicts survival. *J Clin Invest* 1990;85(5):1555–1559.

130. Ferrari L, Seregni E, Bajetta E, et al. The biological characteristics of chromogranin A and its role as a circulating marker in neuroendocrine tumours. *Anticancer Res* 1999;19(4C):3415–3427.

131. Alvarado CS, London WB, Look AT, et al. Natural history and biology of stage A neuroblastoma: a Pediatric Oncology Group study. *J Pediatr Hematol Oncol* 2000;22(3):197–205.

132. De Bernardi B, Conte M, Mancini A, et al. Localized resectable neuroblastoma: results of the second study of the Italian Cooperative Group for Neuroblastoma. *J Clin Oncol* 1995;13(4):884–893.

*133. Matthay KK, Villablanca JG, Seeger RC, et al. Treatment of high-risk neuroblastoma with intensive chemotherapy, radiotherapy, autologous bone marrow transplantation, and 13-*cis*-retinoic acid. Children's Cancer Group. *N Engl J Med* 1999;341(16): 1165–1173.

134. Matthay KK, Atkinson JB, Stram DO, et al. Patterns of relapse after autologous purged bone marrow transplantation for neuroblastoma: a Children's Cancer Group pilot study. *J Clin Oncol* 1993;11(11): 2226–2233.

*135. Matthay KK, Perez C, Seeger RC, et al. Successful treatment of stage III neuroblastoma based on prospective biologic staging: a Children's Cancer Group study. *J Clin Oncol* 1998;16(4):1256–1264.

136. Strother D, Shuster JJ, McWilliams N, et al. Results

of pediatric oncology group protocol 8104 for infants with stages D and DS neuroblastoma. *J Pediatr Hematol Oncol* 1995;17(3):254–259.

137. Castleberry RP, Cantor AB, Green AA, et al. Phase II investigational window using carboplatin, iproplatin, ifosfamide, and epirubicin in children with untreated disseminated neuroblastoma: a Pediatric Oncology Group study. *J Clin Oncol* 1994;12(8):1616–1620.

138. Kretschmar CS, Kletzel K, Murray K, et al. Phase II therapy with taxol and topotecan in untreated children (>365 days) with disseminated (INSS stage 4) neuroblastoma (NB). A POG study. *Med Pediatr Oncol* 1995;24:243.

139. Philip T, Bernard JL, Zucker JM, et al. High-dose chemoradiotherapy with bone marrow transplantation as consolidation treatment in neuroblastoma: an unselected group of stage IV patients over 1 year of age. *J Clin Oncol* 1987;5(2):266–271.

140. Pole JG, Casper J, Elfenbein G, et al. High-dose chemoradiotherapy supported by marrow infusions for advanced neuroblastoma: a Pediatric Oncology Group study (erratum appears in *J Clin Oncol* 1991; 9(6):1094). *J Clin Oncol* 1991;9(1):152–158.

141. Dini G, Lanino E, Garaventa A, et al. Unpurged ABMT for neuroblastoma: AIEOP-BMT experience. *Bone Marrow Transplant* 1991;7(Suppl 2):92.

142. Hero B, Kremens B, Klingebiel T, et al. Does megatherapy contribute to survival in metastatic neuroblastoma? A retrospective analysis. German Cooperative Neuroblastoma Study Group. *Klin Padiatr* 1997;209(4):196–200.

143. Pinkerton CR. ENSG 1-randomised study of high-dose melphalan in neuroblastoma. *Bone Marrow Transplant* 1991;7(Suppl 3):112–113.

144. Ladenstein R, Philip T, Lasset C, et al. Multivariate analysis of risk factors in stage 4 neuroblastoma patients over the age of one year treated with megatherapy and stem-cell transplantation: a report from the European Bone Marrow Transplantation Solid Tumor Registry. *J Clin Oncol* 1998;16(3):953–965.

145. Shuster JJ, Cantor AB, McWilliams N, et al. The prognostic significance of autologous bone marrow transplant in advanced neuroblastoma. *J Clin Oncol* 1991;9(6):1045–1049.

146. Stram DO, Matthay KK, O'Leary M, et al. Consolidation chemoradiotherapy and autologous bone marrow transplantation versus continued chemotherapy for metastatic neuroblastoma: a report of two concurrent Children's Cancer Group studies. *J Clin Oncol* 1996;14(9):2417–2426.

147. Philip T, Zucker JM, Bernard JL, et al. Improved survival at 2 and 5 years in the LMCE1 unselected group of 72 children with stage IV neuroblastoma older than 1 year of age at diagnosis: is cure possible in a small subgroup? *J Clin Oncol* 1991;9(6):1037–1044.

148. Park JR, Slattery J, Gooley T, et al. Phase I topotecan preparative regimen for high-risk neuroblastoma, high-grade glioma, and refractory/recurrent pediatric solid tumors. *Med Pediatr Oncol* 2000;35(6):719–723.

149. Dini G, Philip T, Hartmann O, et al. Bone marrow transplantation for neuroblastoma: a review of 509 cases. EBMT Group. *Bone Marrow Transplant* 1989;4(Suppl 4):42–46.

150. Philip T, Ladenstein R, Lasset C, et al. 1070 my-

eloablative megatherapy procedures followed by stem cell rescue for neuroblastoma: 17 years of European experience and conclusions. European Group for Blood and Marrow Transplant Registry Solid Tumour Working Party. *Eur J Cancer* 1997;33(12): 2130–2135.

151. Grupp SA, Stern JW, Bunin N, et al. Tandem high-dose therapy in rapid sequence for children with high-risk neuroblastoma. *J Clin Oncol* 2000; 18(13):2567–2575.

152. Kletzel M, Katzenstein HM, Haut PR, et al. Treatment of high-risk neuroblastoma with triple-tandem high-dose therapy and stem-cell rescue: results of the Chicago Pilot II Study. *J Clin Oncol* 2002;20(9): 2284–2292.

153. Matthay KK, Seeger RC, Reynolds CP, et al. Comparison of autologous and allogeneic bone marrow transplantation for neuroblastoma. *Prog Clin Biol Res* 1994;385:301–307.

154. Ladenstein R, Lasset C, Hartmann O, et al. Comparison of auto versus allografting as consolidation of primary treatments in advanced neuroblastoma over one year of age at diagnosis: report from the European Group for Bone Marrow Transplantation. *Bone Marrow Transplant* 1994;14(1):37–46.

155. Moss TJ, Sanders DG, Lasky LC, et al. Contamination of peripheral blood stem cell harvests by circulating neuroblastoma cells. *Blood* 1990;76:1879–1883.

156. Moss TJ, Cairo M, Santana VM, et al. Clonogenicity of circulating neuroblastoma cells: implications regarding peripheral blood stem cell transplantation. *Blood* 1994;83(10):3085–3089.

157. Moss TJ. Tumor contamination in stem cell products from patients with neuroblastoma and breast cancer. *Bone Marrow Transplant* 1996;18(Suppl 1):S17.

158. Miyajima Y, Horibe K, Fukuda M, et al. Sequential detection of tumor cells in the peripheral blood and bone marrow of patients with stage IV neuroblastoma by the reverse transcription–polymerase chain reaction for tyrosine hydroxylase mRNA. *Cancer* 1996; 77(6):1214–1219.

159. Figdor CG, Voute PA, de Kraker J, et al. Physical cell separation of neuroblastoma cells from bone marrow. *Prog Clin Biol Res* 1985;175:459–470.

160. Kushner BH, Gulati SC, Kwon JH, et al. High-dose melphalan with 6-hydroxydopamine-purged autologous bone marrow transplantation for poor-risk neuroblastoma. *Cancer* 1991;68(2):242–247.

161. Reynolds CP, Seeger RC, Vo DD, et al. Model system for removing neuroblastoma cells from bone marrow using monoclonal antibodies and magnetic immunobeads. *Cancer Res* 1986;46(11):5882–5886.

162. Hruba A, Skala JP, Matejckova S, et al. Purging of hemopoietic progenitor cells in autologous transplantation. *Cas Lek Cesk* 1997;136(5):151–153.

163. Skala JP, Rogers PC, Chan KW, et al. Deferoxamine as a purging agent for autologous bone marrow grafts in neuroblastoma. *Prog Clin Biol Res* 1992;377: 71–78.

164. Hartmann O, Valteau-Couanet D, Benhamou E, et al. Stage IV neuroblastoma in patients over 1 year of age at diagnosis: consolidation of poor responders with combined busulfan, cyclophosphamide and melphalan followed by in vitro mafosfamide-purged autolo-gous bone marrow transplantation. *Eur J Cancer* 1997;33(12):2126–2129.

165. Beaujean F, Hartmann O, Benhamou E, et al. Hemopoietic reconstitution after repeated autologous transplantation with mafosfamide-purged marrow. *Bone Marrow Transplant* 1989;4(5):537–541.

166. Saarinen UM, Coccia PF, Gerson SL, et al. Eradication of neuroblastoma cells in vitro by monoclonal antibody and human complement: method for purging autologous bone marrow. *Cancer Res* 1985;45(11 Pt 2):5969–5975.

167. Duerst RE, Ryan DH, Frantz CN. Variables affecting the killing of cultured human neuroblastoma cells with monoclonal antibody and complement. *Cancer Res* 1986;46(7):3420–3425.

168. Treleaven JG, Gibson FM, Ugelstad J, et al. Removal of neuroblastoma cells from bone marrow with monoclonal antibodies conjugated to magnetic microspheres. *Lancet* 1984 1(8368):70–73.

169. Handgretinger R, Greil J, Schurmann U, et al. Positive selection and transplantation of peripheral CD34+ progenitor cells: feasibility and purging efficacy in pediatric patients with neuroblastoma. *J Hematother* 1997;6(3):235–242.

170. Ringhoffer M, Dohner K, Scheil S, et al. Fatal outcome in a patient developing Epstein–Barr virus–associated lymphoproliferative disorder (EBV-LPD) without measurable disease. *Bone Marrow Transplant* 2001;28(6):615–618.

171. Melino G, Thiele CJ, Knight RA, et al. Retinoids and the control of growth/death decisions in human neuroblastoma cell lines. *J Neurooncol* 1997;31(1–2): 65–83.

172. Melino G, Draoui M, Bellincampi L, et al. Retinoic acid receptors alpha and gamma mediate the induction of "tissue" transglutaminase activity and apoptosis in human neuroblastoma cells. *Exp Cell Res* 1997;235(1):55–61.

173. Reynolds CP, Kane DJ, Einhorn PA, et al. Response of neuroblastoma to retinoic acid in vitro and in vivo. *Prog Clin Biol Res* 1991;366:203–211.

174. Finklestein JZ, Krailo MD, Lenarsky C, et al. 13-*cis*-retinoic acid (NSC 122758) in the treatment of children with metastatic neuroblastoma unresponsive to conventional chemotherapy: report from the Children's Cancer Study Group. *Med Pediatr Oncol* 1992;20(4):307–311.

175. Villablanca JG, Khan AA, Avramis VI, et al. Phase I trial of 13-*cis*-retinoic acid in children with neuroblastoma following bone marrow transplantation. *J Clin Oncol* 1995;13(4):394–901.

176. Kohler JA, Imeson J, Ellershaw C, et al. A randomized trial of 13-*cis*-retinoic acid in children with advanced neuroblastoma after high-dose therapy. *Br J Cancer* 2000;83(9):1124–1127.

177. Reynolds CP, Lie S. Retinoid therapy of neuroblastoma. In: Brodeur GM, Tsuchida Y, Voute PA, eds. *Neuroblastoma.* Amsterdam: Elsevier Science, 2000:519–540.

178. Cheung NK, Kushner BH, Cheung IY, et al. Anti-G(D2) antibody treatment of minimal residual stage 4 neuroblastoma diagnosed at more than 1 year of age. *J Clin Oncol* 1998;16(9):3053–3060.

179. Frost JD, Hank JA, Reaman GH, et al. A phase I/IB trial of murine monoclonal anti-GD2 antibody

14.G2a plus interleukin-2 in children with refractory neuroblastoma: a report of the Children's Cancer Group. *Cancer* 1997;80(2):317–333.

180. Handgretinger R, Baader P, Dopfer R, et al. A phase I study of neuroblastoma with the anti-ganglioside GD2 antibody 14.G2a. *Cancer Immunol Immunother* 1992;35(3):199–204.

181. Yu AL, Uttenreuther-Fischer MM, Huang CS, et al. Phase I trial of a human–mouse chimeric anti-disialoganglioside monoclonal antibody ch14.18 in patients with refractory neuroblastoma and osteosarcoma. *J Clin Oncol* 1998;16(6):2169–2180.

182. Ozkaynak MF, Sondel PM, Krailo MD, et al. Phase I study of chimeric human/murine anti-ganglioside G(D2) monoclonal antibody (ch14.18) with granulocyte–macrophage colony-stimulating factor in children with neuroblastoma immediately after hematopoietic stem-cell transplantation: a Children's Cancer Group Study. *J Clin Oncol* 2000;18(24):4077–4085.

183. Lode HN, Xiang R, Varki NM, et al. Targeted interleukin-2 therapy for spontaneous neuroblastoma metastases to bone marrow. *J Natl Cancer Inst* 1997; 89(21):1586–1594.

184. Pertl U, Wodrich H, Ruehlmann JM, et al. Immunotherapy with a posttranscriptionally modified DNA vaccine induces complete protection against metastatic neuroblastoma. *Blood* 2003;101(2):649–654.

185. Bowman L, Grossmann M, Rill D, et al. IL-2 adenovector-transduced autologous tumor cells induce antitumor immune responses in patients with neuroblastoma. *Blood* 1998;92(6):1941–1949.

186. Bowman LC, Grossmann M, Rill D, et al. Interleukin-2 gene-modified allogeneic tumor cells for treatment of relapsed neuroblastoma. *Hum Gene Ther* 1998;9(9):1303–1311.

187. Davidoff AM, Kimbrough SA, Ng CY, et al. Neuroblastoma regression and immunity induced by transgenic expression of interleukin-12. *J Pediatr Surg* 1999;34(5):902–906; discussion 906–907.

188. Hock RA, Reynolds BD, Tucker-McClung CL, et al. Murine neuroblastoma vaccines produced by retroviral transfer of MHC class II genes. *Cancer Gene Ther* 1996;3(5):314–320.

189. Lode HN, Xiang R, Duncan SR, et al. Tumor-targeted IL-2 amplifies T cell–mediated immune response induced by gene therapy with single-chain IL-12. *Proc Natl Acad Sci U S A* 1999;96(15):8591–8596.

190. Canete A, Navarro S, Bermudez J, et al. Angiogenesis in neuroblastoma: relationship to survival and other prognostic factors in a cohort of neuroblastoma patients. *J Clin Oncol* 2000;18(1):27–34.

191. Meitar D, Crawford SE, Rademaker AW, et al. Tumor angiogenesis correlates with metastatic disease, N-myc amplification, and poor outcome in human neuroblastoma. *J Clin Oncol* 1996;14(2):405–414.

192. Stern JW, Fang J, Shusterman S, et al. Angiogenesis inhibitor TNP-470 during bone marrow transplant: safety in a preclinical model. *Clin Cancer Res* 2001; 7(4):1026–1032.

193. Haase GM, O'Leary MC, Ramsay NK, et al. Aggressive surgery combined with intensive chemotherapy improves survival in poor-risk neuroblastoma. *J*

Pediatr Surg 1991;26(9):1119–1123; discussion 1123–1124.

194. Shamberger RC, Allarde-Segundo A, Kozakewich HP, et al. Surgical management of stage III and IV neuroblastoma: resection before or after chemotherapy? *J Pediatr Surg* 1991;26(9):1113–1117; discussion 1117–1118.

195. Shamberger RC, Smith EI, Joshi VV, et al. The risk of nephrectomy during local control in abdominal neuroblastoma. *J Pediatr Surg* 1998;33(2):161–164.

196. Ikeda H, August CS, Goldwein JW, et al. Sites of relapse in patients with neuroblastoma following bone marrow transplantation in relation to preparatory "debulking" treatments. *J Pediatr Surg* 1992;27(11): 1438–1441.

197. Powis MR, Imeson JD, Holmes SJ. The effect of complete excision on stage III neuroblastoma: a report of the European Neuroblastoma Study Group. *J Pediatr Surg* 1996;31(4):516–519.

198. Haase GM, Atkinson JB, Stram DO, et al. Surgical management and outcome of locoregional neuroblastoma: comparison of the Children's Cancer Group and the International staging systems. *J Pediatr Surg* 1995;30:289–295.

199. Kaneko M, Ohakawa H, Iwakawa M. Is extensive surgery required for treatment of advanced neuroblastoma? *J Pediatr Surg* 1997;32(11):1616–1619.

200. Halperin EC, Cox EB. Radiation therapy in the management of neuroblastoma: the Duke University Medical Center experience 1967–1984. *Int J Radiat Oncol Biol Phys* 1986;12(10):1829–1837.

201. Castleberry RP, Kun LE, Shuster JJ, et al. Radiotherapy improves the outlook for patients older than 1 year with Pediatric Oncology Group stage C neuroblastoma. *J Clin Oncol* 1991;9(5):789–795.

202. La Quaglia MP, Kushner BH, Heller G, et al. Stage 4 neuroblastoma diagnosed at more than 1 year of age: gross total resection and clinical outcome. *J Pediatr Surg* 1994;29(8):1162–1165; discussion 1165–1166.

203. Matsumura M, Atkinson JB, Hays DM, et al. An evaluation of the role of surgery in metastatic neuroblastoma. *J Pediatr Surg* 1988;23(5):448–453.

204. Shorter NA, Davidoff AM, Evans AE, et al. The role of surgery in the management of stage IV neuroblastoma: a single institution study. *Med Pediatr Oncol* 1995;24(5):287–291.

205. Evans AE, D'Angio GJ, Koop CE. Diagnosis and treatment of neuroblastoma. *Pediatr Clin North Am* 1976;23(1):161–170.

206. Nitschke R, Smith EI, Altshuler G, et al. Postoperative treatment of nonmetastatic visible residual neuroblastoma: a Pediatric Oncology Group study. *J Clin Oncol* 1991;9(7):1181–1188.

*207. Haas-Kogan DA, Swift PS, Selch M, et al. Impact of radiotherapy for high-risk neuroblastoma: a Children's Cancer Group study. *Int J Radiat Oncol Biol Phys* 2003;56(1):28–39.

208. Von Schweinitz D, Hero B, Berthold F. The impact of surgical radicality on outcome in childhood neuroblastoma. *Eur J Pediatr Surg* 2002;12(6):402–409.

209. Rosen EM, Cassady JR, Kretschmar C, et al. Influence of local-regional lymph node metastases on prognosis in neuroblastoma. *Med Pediatr Oncol* 1984;12(4):260–263.

210. Hayes FA, Green A, Hustu HO, et al. Surgicopatho-

logic staging of neuroblastoma: prognostic significance of regional lymph node metastases. *J Pediatr* 1983;102(1):59–62.

211. Contador MP, Johnston S, Smith EI, et al. Lymph node sampling in localized neuroblastoma: a Pediatric Oncology Group study. *J Pediatr Surg* 1999; 34(6):967–974.

212. Nakagawara A, Morita K, Okabe I, et al. Proposal and assessment of Japanese tumor node metastasis postsurgical histopathological staging system for neuroblastoma based on an analysis of 495 cases. *Jpn J Clin Oncol* 1991;21(1):1–7.

213. Ninane J, Wese FX. Treatment of localized neuroblastoma. *Am J Pediatr Hematol Oncol* 1986;8(3): 248–252.

214. Plantaz D, Rubie H, Michon J, et al. The treatment of neuroblastoma with intraspinal extension with chemotherapy followed by surgical removal of residual disease. A prospective study of 42 patients: results of the NBL 90 Study of the French Society of Pediatric Oncology. *Cancer* 1996;78(2):311–319.

215. Roberts S, Creamer K, Shoupe B, et al. Unique management of stage 4S neuroblastoma complicated by massive hepatomegaly: case report and review of the literature. *J Pediatr Hematol Oncol* 2002;24(2): 142–144.

216. Ohnuma N, Kasuga T, Nojiri I, et al. Radiosensitivity of human neuroblastoma cell line (NB-1). *Gann* 1977;68(5):711–712.

217. Wheldon TE, O'Donoghue JA, Gregor A. Radiobiological rationale for hyperfractionation in the radiotherapy of neuroblastoma. *Int J Radiat Oncol Biol Phys* 1987;13(9):1430–1431.

218. Wheldon TE, O'Donoghue J, Gregor A, et al. Radiobiological considerations in the treatment of neuroblastoma by total body irradiation. *Radiother Oncol* 1986;6(4):317–326.

219. Wheldon TE, Wilson L, Livingstone A, et al. Radiation studies on multicellular tumour spheroids derived from human neuroblastoma: absence of sparing effect of dose fractionation. *Eur J Cancer Clin Oncol* 1986;22(5):563–566.

220. Lingley JF, Sagerman RH, Santulli TV, et al. Neuroblastoma. Management and survival. *N Engl J Med* 1967;277(23):1227–1230.

221. Nitschke R, Smith EI, Shochat S, et al. Localized neuroblastoma treated by surgery: a Pediatric Oncology Group study. *J Clin Oncol* 1988;6(8):1271–1279.

222. Matthay KK, Sather HN, Seeger RC, et al. Excellent outcome of stage II neuroblastoma is independent of residual disease and radiation therapy. *J Clin Oncol* 1989;7(2):236–244.

223. Kushner BH, Cheung NK, LaQuaglia MP, et al. International neuroblastoma staging system stage 1 neuroblastoma: a prospective study and literature review. *J Clin Oncol* 1996;14(7):2174–2180.

224. Evans AE, Baum E, Chard R. Do infants with stage IV-S neuroblastoma need treatment? *Arch Dis Child* 1981;56:271–274.

225. Suarez A, Hartmann O, Vassal G, et al. Treatment of stage IV-S neuroblastoma: a study of 34 cases treated between 1982 and 1987. *Med Pediatr Oncol* 1991; 19(6):473–477.

226. van Noesel MM, Heahlen K, Hakvoort-Cammel FG,

et al. Neuroblastoma 4S: a heterogeneous disease with variable risk factors and treatment strategies. *Cancer* 1997;80(5):834–843.

227. Hsu LL, Evans AE, D'Argio GJ. Hepatomegaly in neuroblastoma stage 4s: criteria for treatment of the vulnerable neonate. *Med Pediatr Oncol* 1996;27(6): 521–528.

228. Blatt J, Deutsch M, Wollman MR. Results of therapy in stage IV-S neuroblastoma with massive hepatomegaly. *Int J Radiat Oncol Biol Phys* 1987; 13(10):1467–1471.

229. Paulino AC, Mayr NA. Simon JH, et al. Locoregional control in infants with neuroblastoma: role of radiation therapy and late toxicity. *Int J Radiat Oncol Biol Phys* 2002;52(4):1025–1031.

230. Evans AE, Chatten J. D'Angio GJ, et al. A review of 17 IV-S neuroblastoma patients at the Children's Hospital of Philadelphia. *Cancer* 1980;45:833–839.

231. Jacobson GM, Sause WT, O'Brien RT. Dose response analysis of pediatric neuroblastoma to megavoltage radiation. *Am J Clin Oncol* 1984;7(6): 693–697.

232. McGuire WA, Simmons D, Grosfeld JL, et al. Stage II neuroblastoma: does adjuvant irradiation contribute to cure? *Med Pediatr Oncol* 1985;13(3): 117–121.

233. West DC, Shamberger RC, Macklis RM, et al. Stage III neuroblastoma over 1 year of age at diagnosis: improved survival with intensive multimodality therapy including multiple alkylating agents. *J Clin Oncol* 1993;11(1):84–90.

234. de Bernardi B, Rogers D, Carli M, et al. Localized neuroblastoma. Surgical and pathologic staging. *Cancer* 1987;60(5):1056–1072.

235. Koop CE, Johnson DG. Neuroblastoma: an assessment of therapy in reference to staging. *J Pediatr Surg* 1971;6(5):595–600.

236. Green AA, Hustu HO, Palmer R, et al. Total-body sequential segmental irradiation and combination chemotherapy for children with disseminated neuroblastoma. *Cancer* 1976;38(6):2250–2257.

237. Helson L, Jereb B, Vogel R. Sequential hemi-body irradiation (HBI) in treatment of advanced neuroblastoma: a pilot study. *Int J Radiat Oncol Biol Phys* 1981;7(4):531–534.

238. Kun LE, Casper JT, Kline RW, et al. Fractionated total body irradiation for metastatic neuroblastoma. *Int J Radiat Oncol Biol Phys* 1981;7(11):1599–1602.

239. Sagerman RS. Primary management of disseminated neuroblastoma by sequential segmental irradiation. *Radiology* 1968;90(2):352–353.

*240. Sibley GS, Mundt AJ, Goldman S, et al. Patterns of failure following total body irradiation and bone marrow transplantation with or without a radiotherapy boost for advanced neuroblastoma. *Int J Radiat Oncol Biol Phys* 1995;32(4):127–1135.

241. Wolden SL, Gollamudi SV, Kushner BH, et al. Local control with multimodality therapy for Stage 4 neuroblastoma. *Int J Radiat Oncol Biol Phys* 2000;46(4): 969–974.

242. Ohnuma N, Takahashi H, Kaneko M, et al. Treatment combined with bone marrow transplantation for advanced neuroblastoma: an analysis of patients who were pretreated intensively with the protocol of the

Study Group of Japan. *Med Pediatr Oncol* 1995; 24(3):181–187.

243. Kushner BH, Wolden S, LaQuaglia MP, et al. Hyperfractionated low-dose radiotherapy for high-risk neuroblastoma after intensive chemotherapy and surgery. *J Clin Oncol* 2001;19(11):2821–2828.

244. Kremens B, Klingebiel T, Herrmann F, et al. High-dose consolidation with local radiation and bone marrow rescue in patients with advanced neuroblastoma. *Med Pediatr Oncol* 1994;23(6):470–475.

245. Villablanca JG, Matthay KK, Swift PS, et al. Phase I trial of carboplatin, etoposide, melphalan and local irradiation (CEM-LI) with purged autologous bone marrow transplantation for children with high risk neuroblastoma. *Med Pediatr Oncol* 1999;33:170.

246. Bouffet E, Doumi N, Thiesse P, et al. Brain metastases in children with solid tumors. *Cancer* 1997; 79(2):403–410.

247. Kellie SJ, Hayes FA, Bowman L, et al. Primary extracranial neuroblastoma with central nervous system metastases characterization by clinicopathologic findings and neuroimaging. *Cancer* 1991;68(9): 1999–2006.

248. Shaw PJ, Eden T. Neuroblastoma with intracranial involvement: an ENSG Study. *Med Pediatr Oncol* 1992;20(2):149–155.

249. Rohrlich P, Hartmann O, Couanet D, et al. Secondary metastatic neuromeningeal localization of neuroblastoma in children. *Arch Fr Pediatr* 1989;46(1):5–10.

250. Kramer K, Kushner B, Heller G, et al. Neuroblastoma metastatic to the central nervous system. The Memorial Sloan–Kettering Cancer Center experience and a literature review. *Cancer* 2001;91(8):1510–1519.

251. Astigarraga I, Lejarreta R, Navajas A, et al. Secondary central nervous system metastases in children with neuroblastoma. *Med Pediatr Oncol* 1996;27(6): 529–533.

252. Blatt J, Fitz C, Mirro J Jr. Recognition of central nervous system metastases in children with metastatic primary extracranial neuroblastoma. *Pediatr Hematol Oncol* 1997;14(3):233–241.

253. Matthay KK, Brisse H, Couanet D, et al. Central nervous system metastases in neuroblastoma: radiologic, clinical, and biologic features in 23 patients. *Cancer* 2003;98(1):155–165.

254. Matthay KK. Neuroblastoma. In: Pochedly C, ed. *Neoplastic diseases in childhood*. London: Harwood Academic Publishers, 1994:735–778.

255. Tang CK, Hajdu SI. Neuroblastoma in adolescence and adulthood. *N Y State J Med* 1975;75(9): 1434–1438.

256. Aleshire SL, Glick AD, Cruz VE, et al. Neuroblastoma in adults. Pathologic findings and clinical outcome. *Arch Pathol Lab Med* 1985;109(4):352–356.

257. Allan SG, Cornbleet MA, Carmichael J, et al. Adult neuroblastoma. Report of three cases and review of the literature. *Cancer* 1986;57(12):2419–2421.

258. Dosik GM, Rodriguez V, Benjamin RS, et al. Neuroblastoma in the adult: effective combination chemotherapy. *Cancer* 1978;41(1):56–63.

259. Grubb BP, Thant M. Neuroblastoma in an adult. *South Med J* 1984;77(9):1180–1182.

260. Kaye JA, Warhol MJ, Kretschmar C, et al. Neuroblas-

toma in adults. Three case reports and a review of the literature. *Cancer* 1986;58(5):1149–1157.

261. Krikke AP, van der Jagt EJ. Adult neuroblastoma: a report of two cases. *Rofo Fortschr Geb Rontgenstr Nuklearmed* 1989;150(2):138–141.

262. Lopez R, Karakousis C, Rao U. Treatment of adult neuroblastoma. *Cancer* 1980;45(5):840–844.

263. Prestidge BR, Donaldson SS. Treatment results among adults with childhood tumors: a 20-year experience. *Int J Radiat Oncol Biol Phys* 1989;17(3): 507–514.

264. Halperin EC. Long-term results of therapy for stage C neuroblastoma. *J Surg Oncol* 1996;63(3):172–178.

265. Peschel RE, Chen M, Seashore J. The treatment of massive hepatomegaly in stage IV-S neuroblastoma. *Int J Radiat Oncol Biol Phys* 1981;7(4):549–553.

266. O'Neill JA, Littman P, Blitzer P, et al. The role of surgery in localized neuroblastoma. *J Pediatr Surg* 1985;20(6):708–712.

267. Deacon JM, Wilson P, Steel GG. Radiosensitivity of neuroblastoma. *Prog Clin Biol Res* 1985;175: 525–531.

268. Livingstone A, Mairs RJ, Russell J, et al. N-myc gene copy number in neuroblastoma cell lines and resistance to experimental treatment. *Eur J Cancer* 1994;30A(3):382–389.

269. Evans AR, Brand W, de Lorimier A, et al. Results in children with local and regional neuroblastoma managed with and without vincristine, cyclophosphamide, and imidazolecarboxamide: a report from the Children's Cancer Study Group. *Am J Clin Oncol* 1984;7:3–7.

270. Jacobson HM, Marcus RB Jr, Thar TL, et al. Pediatric neuroblastoma: postoperative radiation therapy using less than 2000 rad. *Int J Radiat Oncol Biol Phys* 1983;9(4):501–505.

271. Rosen EM, Cassady JR, Frantz CN, et al. Neuroblastoma: the Joint Center for Radiation Therapy/ Dana–Farber Cancer Institute/Children's Hospital experience. *J Clin Oncol* 1984;2(7):719–732.

272. Donaldson SS. Lessons from our children. *Int J Radiat Oncol Biol Phys* 1993;26(5):739–749.

273. Hawkins MM. Second primary tumors following radiotherapy for childhood cancer. *Int J Radiat Oncol Biol Phys* 1990;19(5):1297–1301.

274. Meadows AT. Second malignant neoplasms in childhood cancer survivors. *J Assoc Pediatr Oncol Nurses* 1989;6(1):7–11.

275. Haase GM, Meagher DP Jr, McNeely LK, et al. Electron beam intraoperative radiation therapy for pediatric neoplasms. *Cancer* 1994;74(2):740–747.

276. Leavey PJ, Odom LF, Poole M, et al. Intra-operative radiation therapy in pediatric neuroblastoma. *Med Pediatr Oncol* 1997;28(6):424–428.

277. Aitken DR, Hopkins GA, Archambeau JO, et al. Intraoperative radiotherapy in the treatment of neuroblastoma: report of a pilot study. *Ann Surg Oncol* 1995;2(4):343–350.

278. Merchant TE, Zelefsky MJ, Sheldon JM, et al. High-dose rate intraoperative radiation therapy for pediatric solid tumors. *Med Pediatr Oncol* 1998;30(1): 34–39.

279. Nag S, Retter E, Martinez-Monge R, et al. Feasibility of intraoperative electron beam radiation therapy in

the treatment of locally advanced pediatric malignancies. *Med Pediatr Oncol* 1999;32(5):382–384.

*280. Haas-Kogan DA, Fisch BM, Wara WM, et al. Intraoperative radiation therapy for high-risk pediatric neuroblastoma. *Int J Radiat Oncol Biol Phys* 2000; 47(4):985–992.

281. Hoover M, Bowman LC, Crawford SE, et al. Long-term outcome of patients with intraspinal neuroblastoma. *Med Pediatr Oncol* 1999;2(5):353–359.

282. Mayfield J, Al E. Spinal deformity in children treated for neuroblastoma. *J Bone Joint Surg* 1981;63: 183–193.

283. De Bernardi B, Pianca C, Pistamiglio P, et al. Neuroblastoma with symptomatic spinal cord compression at diagnosis: treatment and results with 76 cases. *J Clin Oncol* 2001;19(1):183–190.

284. Katzenstein HM, Kent PM, London WB, et al. Treatment and outcome of 83 children with intraspinal neuroblastoma: the Pediatric Oncology Group experience. *J Clin Oncol* 2001;19(4):1047–1055.

285. Plantaz D, Hartmann O, Kalifa C, et al. Localized dumbbell neuroblastoma: a study of 25 cases treated between 1982 and 1987 using the same protocol. *Med Pediatr Oncol* 1993;21:249–253.

*286. Sanderson IR, Pritchard J, Marsh HT. Chemotherapy as the initial treatment of spinal cord compression due to disseminated neuroblastoma. *J Neurosurg* 1989;70(5):688–690.

287. Bertsch H, Rudoler S, Needle MN, et al. Emergent/urgent therapeutic irradiation in pediatric oncology: patterns of presentation, treatment, and outcome. *Med Pediatr Oncol* 1998;30(2):101–105.

288. Cardozo BL, Zoetelief H, van Bekkum DW, et al. Lung damage following bone marrow transplantation: I. The contribution of irradiation. *Int J Radiat Oncol Biol Phys* 1985;11(5):907–914.

289. Chou RH, Wong GB, Kramer JH, et al. Toxicities of total-body irradiation for pediatric bone marrow transplantation. *Int J Radiat Oncol Biol Phys* 1996;34(4):843–851.

290. Appelbaum FR. The influence of total dose, fractionation, dose rate, and distribution of total body irradiation on bone marrow transplantation. *Semin Oncol* 1993;20(Suppl 4):3–10.

291. Deeg HJ. Acute and delayed toxicities of total body irradiation. Seattle Marrow Transplant Team. *Int J Radiat Oncol Biol Phys* 1983;9(12):1933–1939.

292. Barrett A, Nicholls J, Gibson B. Late effects of total body irradiation. *Radiother Oncol* 1987;9(2):131–135.

293. Tarbell NJ, Guinan EC, Chin L, et al. Renal insufficiency after total body irradiation for pediatric bone marrow transplantation. *Radiother Oncol* 1990; 18(Suppl 1):139–142.

294. Holtta P, Alaluusua S, Saarinen-Pihkala UM, et al. Long-term adverse effects on dentition in children with poor-risk neuroblastoma treated with high-dose chemotherapy and autologous stem cell transplantation with or without total body irradiation. *Bone Marrow Transplant* 2002;29(2):121–127.

295. Fleitz JM, Wootton-Gorges SL, Wyatt-Ashmead J, et al. Renal cell carcinoma in long-term survivors of advanced stage neuroblastoma in early childhood. *Pediatr Radiol* 2003;33(8):540–545.

296. Donnelly LF, Rencken IO, Shardell K, et al. Renal cell carcinoma after therapy for neuroblastoma. *AJR Am J Roentgenol* 1996;167(4):915–917.

297. Wolden SL, Lamborn KR, Cleary SF, et al. Second cancers following pediatric Hodgkin's disease. *J Clin Oncol* 1998;16(2):536–544.

298. Cheung NK, Landmeier B, Neely J, et al. Complete tumor ablation with iodine 131-radiolabeled disialoganglioside GD2-specific monoclonal antibody against human neuroblastoma xenografted in nude mice. *J Natl Cancer Inst* 1986;77(3):739–745.

299. Cheung NK, Miraldi FD. Iodine 131 labeled GD2 monoclonal antibody in the diagnosis and therapy of human neuroblastoma. *Prog Clin Biol Res* 1988;271: 595–604.

300. Cheung NK, Munn D, Kushner BH, et al. Targeted radiotherapy and immunotherapy of human neuroblastoma with GD2 specific monoclonal antibodies. *Int J Radiat Appl Instrum* (B), 1989;16(2):111–120.

301. Cheung NK, Yeh SD, Gulati S, et al. [131]I-3F8: clinical validation of imaging studies and therapeutic applications. *Prog Clin Biol Res* 1991;366:409–415.

*302. Kushner BH, Kramer K, LaQuaglia MP, et al. Curability of recurrent disseminated disease after surgery alone for local–regional neuroblastoma using intensive chemotherapy and anti-G(D2) immunotherapy. *J Pediatr Hematol Oncol* 2003;25(7):515–519.

303. Klingebiel T, Berthold F, Treuner J, et al. Metaiodobenzylguanidine (mIBG) in treatment of 47 patients with neuroblastoma: results of the German Neuroblastoma Trial. *Med Pediatr Oncol* 1991;19(2): 84–88.

304. Matthay KK, DeSantes K, Hasegawa B, et al. Phase I dose escalation of ^{131}I-metaiodobenzylguanidine with autologous bone marrow support in refractory neuroblastoma. *J Clin Oncol* 1998;16:229–236.

305. Voute PA, Hoefnagel CA, de Kraker J, et al. Results of treatment with ^{131}I-metaiodobenzylguanidine (^{131}I-MIBG) in patients with neuroblastoma. Future prospects of zetotherapy. *Prog Clin Biol Res* 1991; 366:439–445.

306. Lashford LS, Lewis I, Fielding SL, et al. Phase I/II study of iodine 131 metaiodobenzylguanidine in chemoresistant neuroblastoma: a United Kingdom Children's Cancer Study Group investigation. *J Clin Oncol* 1992;10(12):1889–1896.

307. Garaventa A, Gambini C, Villavecchia G, et al. Second malignancies in children with neuroblastoma after combined treatment with ^{131}I-metaiodobenzylguanidine. *Cancer* 2003;97(5):1332–1338.

308. Weiss B, Vora A, Huberty J, et al. Secondary myelodysplastic syndrome and leukemia following ^{131}I-metaiodobenzylguanidine therapy for relapsed neuroblastoma. *J Pediatr Hematol Oncol* 2003;25(7): 543–547.

309. Troncone L, Rufini V, Luzi S, et al. The treatment of neuroblastoma with (^{131}I)MIBG at diagnosis. *Q J Nucl Med* 1995;39(4 Suppl 1):65–68.

310. Mastrangelo S, Tornesello A, Diociaiuti L, et al. Treatment of advanced neuroblastoma: feasibility and therapeutic potential of a novel approach combining 131-I-MIBG and multiple drug chemotherapy. *Br J Cancer* 2001;84(4):460–464.

311. Yanik GA, Levine JE, Matthay KK, et al. Pilot study

of iodine-131-metaiodobenzylguanidine in combination with myeloablative chemotherapy and autologous stem-cell support for the treatment of neuroblastoma. *J Clin Oncol* 2002;20(8):2142–2149.

312. Klingebiel T, Bader P, Bares R, et al. Treatment of neuroblastoma stage 4 with ^{131}I-metaiodo-benzylguanidine, high-dose chemotherapy and immunotherapy. A pilot study. *Eur J Cancer* 1998; 34(9):1398–1402.

313. Castleberry RP, Shuster JJ, Smith EI. The Pediatric Oncology Group experience with the international staging system criteria for neuroblastoma. *J Clin Oncol* 1994;12(11):2378–2381.

314. Kremens B, Klingebiel T, Herrmann F, et al. High-dose consolidation with local radiation and bone marrow rescue in patients with advanced neuroblastoma. *Med Pediatr Oncol* 1994;23(6):470–475.

315. DeWitt KD, Matthay KK, Weinberg V, et al. *Intraoperative radiation therapy for high-risk pediatric neuroblastoma.* Aachen, Germany: International Society of Intraoperative Radiation Therapy, 2002.

316. Matthay KK, Yamashiro D. Neuroblastoma. In: Holland, JF, Frei, E, Bast RC et al., eds. *Cancer medicine.* London: BC Decker, 2000:2185–2197.

317. Coze C, Hartmann O, Michon J, et al. NB87 induction protocol for stage 4 neuroblastoma in children over 1 year of age: a report from the French Society of Pediatric Oncology. *J Clin Oncol* 1997;15(12): 3433–3440.

318. Kaneko M, Tsuchida Y, Uchino J, et al. Treatment results of advanced neuroblastoma with the first Japanese study group protocol. Study Group of Japan for Treatment of Advanced Neuroblastoma. *J Pediatr Hematol Oncol* 1999;21(3):190–197.

319. Kushner BH, Yeh SD, Kramer K, et al. Impact of metaiodobenzylguanidine scintigraphy on assessing response of high-risk neuroblastoma to dose-intensive induction chemotherapy. *J Clin Oncol* 2003;21(6): 1082–1086.

320. Matthay KK. Hematopoietic stem cell transplantation for neuroblastoma. In: Blume KG, Forman SJ, Appelbaum FR, eds. *Thomas hematopoietic cell transplantation,* 3rd ed. Oxford: Blackwell, 2003.

321. Hartmann O, Benhamou E, Beaujean F, et al. Repeated high-dose chemotherapy followed by purged autologous bone marrow transplantation as consolidation therapy in metastatic neuroblastoma. *J Clin Oncol* 1987;5(8):1205–1211.

322. Seeger RC, Villablanca JG, Matthay KK, et al. Intensive chemoradiotherapy and autologous bone marrow transplantation for poor prognosis neuroblastoma. *Prog Clin Biol Res* 1991;366:527–533.

323. Dini G, Lanino E, Garaventa A, et al. Myeloablative therapy and unpurged autologous bone marrow transplantation for poor-prognosis neuroblastoma: report of 34 cases. *J Clin Oncol* 1991;9(6):962–969.

324. Kushner BH, O'Reilly RJ, Mandell LR, et al. Myeloablative combination chemotherapy without total body irradiation for neuroblastoma. *J Clin Oncol* 1991;9(2):274–279.

325. Kamani N, August CS, Bunin N, et al. A study of thiotepa, etoposide and fractionated total body irradiation as a preparative regimen prior to bone marrow transplantation for poor prognosis patients with neuroblastoma. *Bone Marrow Transplant* 1996;17(6): 911–916.

326. Kletzel M, Abella EM, Sandler ES, et al. Thiotepa and cyclophosphamide with stem cell rescue for consolidation therapy for children with high-risk neuroblastoma: a phase I/II study of the Pediatric Blood and Marrow Transplant Consortium. *J Pediatr Hematol Oncol* 1998;20(1):49–54.

327. Castel V, Canete A, Navarro S, et al. Outcome of high-risk neuroblastoma using a dose intensity approach: improvement in initial but not in long-term results. *Med Pediatr Oncol* 2001;37(6):537–542.

7

Hodgkin's Disease

Melissa M. Hudson, M.D., and Louis S. Constine, M.D.

In 1832, Thomas Hodgkin (1) described seven patients with enlarged absorbent (lymphatic) glands not thought to result from inflammation. At the turn of the century, Sternberg and Reed each described the multinucleated giant cell characteristic of Hodgkin's disease (HD) (2). Shortly after the discovery of X-rays, in 1902 Pusey (3) demonstrated the radioresponsiveness of HD. In the 1930s, Gilbert (4) laid the foundation for its definitive treatment with radiotherapy (RT), and Peters (5) provided additional definition of important principles. During World War I and World War II, the lympholytic effects of nitrogen mustard were recognized (6), and over the next two decades progress in safely combining multiple chemotherapeutic agents to treat HD led to De Vita's (7) report on the use of nitrogen mustard, vincristine (Oncovin), procarbazine, and prednisone (MOPP) chemotherapy. Kaplan (2) systematically studied the role of RT for HD during these decades. Concurrently, advances were made in identifying different pathologic subtypes, determining staging criteria, improving diagnostic imaging capabilities, and developing effective chemotherapeutic regimens. When the clonality of the Reed–Sternberg (RS) cell was finally established in the 1960s, controversy over the malignant or inflammatory nature of HD abated (8).

Although the biology and natural history of HD in children are similar to that in adults, when irradiation techniques and dosages suitable for controlling disease in adults were translated to the pediatric setting, substantial morbidities (primarily musculoskeletal growth inhibition) were produced (9,10). It is in this context that new strategies for the treatment of pediatric HD were developed by Donaldson and others (11–19). Historically, children were thought to have a worse prognosis than adults (2). It is now apparent that the converse is true (20–23).

BIOLOGY AND EPIDEMIOLOGY

For many years, the rarity and distribution of malignant cells in pathologic material precluded elucidation of the origin and evolution of the RS cell. Advances in immunohistology and molecular biology subsequently revealed that the RS cell and its variants most commonly derive from a neoplastic clone that originates from B lymphocytes in lymphoid germinal centers. Clonality can be demonstrated at diagnosis and relapse through detection of unique nucleotide sequences, which molecularly fingerprint the RS cell clone; these sequences represent rearrangements of immunoglobulin variable-region (V) genes, which are B-cell derived (24,25). Complicating this scenario is the finding by Kanzler et al. (25) that flawed V genes, which would be lethal for normal B cells, are present in RS cells and prevent them from expressing immunoglobulin. Such cells would be expected to die of apoptosis. Therefore, the genesis of classic Hodgkin's disease (CHD) probably involves evasion by the RS cell of the apoptotic pathway. Deregulation of the nuclear transcription factor (NFκB) in the RS cells has been hypothesized as a mechanism that prevents apoptosis (26). Epstein-Barr virus (EBV) and genes that monitor cell damage, such as p53, may play a role in the rescue and repair of the RS cells (25,27). EBV genome fragments can be found in RS cells in 30–50% of HD specimens, most commonly in the mixed-cellularity (MCHD) subtype and rarely in the lymphocyte-predominant type (LPHD) (28–30). The EBV genome is temporally stable because it can be found at diagnosis and relapse. Finally, the RS cell can also have characteristics of T lymphocytes and the interdigitating reticulum cell. Such evidence of a multilineage origin of the RS cell may be explicable by postulating that the RS cell is a hybridoma resulting from fusion of different cell lines, provoked by a virus or other agent. Cytogenetic data also show an unexpected frequency of B-cell translocation (14:18) and bcl-2 gene involvement in HD, but these may derive from bystander normal lymphocytes rather than the RS cell (31,32). A pathogenetic model for HD is depicted in Fig. 7-1, which suggests that the RS cells arises in a germinal lymphoid center from a clone of antigen-stimulated B cells and through genetic changes achieves immortality and malignant properties (33).

A curious characteristic of HD is the rarity (about 1%) of the malignant RS cell in specimens and the abundant reactive cellular infiltrate of lymphocytes, macrophages, granulocytes, and eosinophils. The histologic features and clinical symptoms of HD have been attributed to the numerous cytokines secreted by the RS cells,

which include interleukin-1 and interleukin-6, and tumor necrosis factor (34,35). Interleukin-5 could be responsible for the eosinophilia in MCHD, and transforming growth factor β could be responsible for the fibrosis in the nodular sclerosis subtype. These cytokines also enable the cells to evade immunologic surveillance and promote their own replication (34).

Evidence that HD comprises a family of diseases includes the observation that RS cells can rarely be derivatives of cytotoxic T cells and that nodular lymphocyte-predominant HD (NLPHD) is a distinctive and uncommon lymphoproliferative disorder. The lymphocytic and histiocytic (L&H) cells characteristic of NLPHD have folded and lobate nuclei and among small lymphocytes and histiocytes. The L&H cells are also B cell–derived but harbor V gene alterations, which differ from those in RS cells; whether the L&H cells are monoclonal is unclear (36,37). The clinical characteristics of NLPHD differ from those of the subtypes of CHD by virtue of its indolence, excellent prognosis, epidemiology,

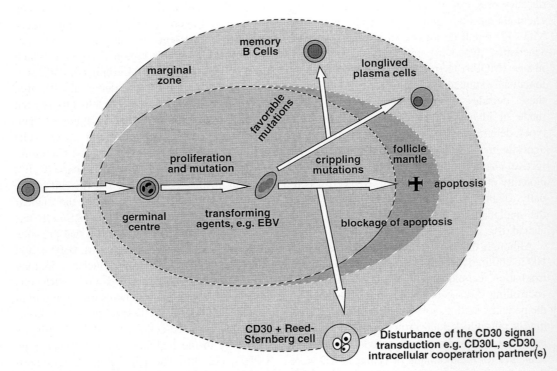

FIG. 7-1. Pathogenetic model for Hodgkin's disease. (From Jox A, Zander T, Diehl V, et al. Clonal relapse in Hodgkin's disease. *N Engl J Med* 1997;337(7):499, with permission).

and response to chemotherapy. The Revised European–American Classification of Lymphoid Neoplasia (REAL) has proposed a schema that reflects the distinction of NLPHD from CHD (38).

EPIDEMIOLOGY

HD makes up 6% of childhood cancers. A striking male:female predominance is found among children, with a ratio of 4:1 for 3- to 7-year-olds, 3:1 for 7- to 9-year-olds, and 1.3:1 (a ratio more similar to that of adults) for older children (20,39–41). The age-specific incidence curves for HD in the United States are bimodal, peaking in the 20s and then again after age 50 (42). The disease is uncommon before age 5 and, among children, is most common in adolescence.

Although evidence that HD is infectious or contagious was suggested by reports of case clusters (43), confirmatory data are lacking (44). However, the role of EBV in its pathogenesis is well established. In a recent report, EBV early RNA1 was expressed in RS cells in 58% of childhood cases (45). Of particular interest, expression was age dependent: 75% of children under age 10 years compared with 20% of older children. In addition, a history of infectious mononucleosis increases the risk for HD, and anti-EBV titers are elevated before diagnosis of HD.

Evidence of a genetic predisposition exists and is relevant when counseling families. The incidence of HD is two to five times higher in the siblings of affected children and nine times higher in same-sex siblings than in the general population. Parent–child associations have been reported (42,44,46). Mack et al. (47) reported a 99-fold increased risk in monozygotic twins of patients but no increased risk in dizygotic twins. The status of the immune system in patients with HD also deserves comment. A complex deficiency in cellular immunity exists, which includes a deficiency in naive T cells and an elevated sensitivity of effector T cells to suppressor monocytes and T-suppressor cells (48,49). Of interest is that radiation results in a long-term dysregulation of T-cell subset homeostasis. Finally,

it is unclear whether HD is more common in patients with either congenital (e.g., ataxia–telangiectasia) or acquired immunodeficiency states, including acquired immunodeficiency syndrome (43,50), but HD is rarely seen as a second malignancy. In patients with the human immunodeficiency virus, the disease more commonly presents in an advanced stage with systemic symptoms, extranodal involvement, and a poor response to therapy (51).

CLINICAL PRESENTATION

HD appears to be unifocal in origin, with 90% of patients presenting in a pattern that suggests contiguous lymphatic spread (2,52). Most children are diagnosed on the basis of supradiaphragmatic lymph nodes, with painless cervical adenopathy in 80%. The nodes are generally firm and may be tender. Mediastinal involvement occurs in 76% of adolescents but in only 33% of 1- to 10-year-olds. Mediastinal disease may produce symptoms such as dyspnea, cough, and superior vena cava syndrome. Axillary adenopathy is less common (2). Associations exist between the mediastinum and neck, the neck and ipsilateral axilla, the mediastinum and hilum, and the spleen and abdominal lymph nodes (52). Isolated mediastinal or infradiaphragmatic HD is rare, occurring in fewer than 5% of patients. About one-third of the patients have systemic "B" symptoms, as defined in Table 7-1 (2,53).

PATHOLOGIC CLASSIFICATION

The RS cell is the essential malignant cell in HD (Fig. 7-2). It is large, with abundant cytoplasm, two or three nuclei, and a prominent nucleolus. However, its frequency in pathologic specimens is greatly variable because of the presence of numerous reactive cells including lymphocytes, eosinophils, and plasma cells. Moreover, the RS cell, particularly its mononuclear variant, is not pathognomonic for HD because cells simulating it can be found in other disorders that are reactive, infectious, or malignant (54). The diagnosis of HD must be established by lymph node biopsy. Aspiration cytology alone is not recommended

TABLE 7-1. *Ann Arbor Staging System with Cotswold modifications for Hodgkin's lymphoma*

Stage	Description
I	Involvement of a single lymph node region or lymphoid structure (e.g., spleen, thymus, Waldeyer's ring, or single extralymphatic site [IE]).
II	Involvement of two or more lymph node regions on the same side of the diaphragm or localized contiguous involvement of only one extranodal organ or site and lymph node region on the same side of the diaphragm (IIE). The number of anatomic sites is indicated by a subscript (e.g., II_3).
III	Involvement of lymph node regions on both sides of the diaphragm (III), which may be accompanied by involvement of the spleen (III_S) or by localized contiguous involvement of only one extranodal organ site (III_E) or both (III_{SE}).
III_1	With or without involvement of splenic hilar, celiac, or mesenteric nodes.
III_2	With involvement of para-aortic, iliac, or mesenteric nodes.
IV	Diffuse or disseminated involvement of one or more extranodal organs or tissues, with or without associated lymph node involvement.
Designations applicable to any stage	
A	No symptoms.
B	Fever (temperature >38°C), drenching night sweats, unexplained loss of >10% of body weight in the preceding 6 months.
X	Bulky disease (a widening of the mediastinum by more than one-third or the presence of a nodal mass with a maximal dimension >10 cm).
E	Involvement of a single extranodal site that is contiguous or proximal to the known nodal site.
CS	Clinical stage.
PS	Pathologic stage (as determined by laparotomy).

Modified from Kaplan H. *Hodgkin's disease.* Cambridge, MA: Harvard University Press, 1980; and Grufferman S, Delzell E. Epidemiology of Hodgkin's disease. *Epidemiol Rev* 1984;6:76–106, with permission.

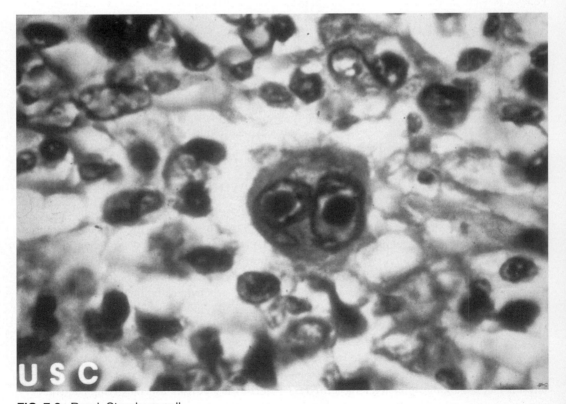

FIG. 7-2. Reed–Sternberg cell.

because of the lack of stromal tissue, the small number of cells present in the specimen, and the difficulty of classifying HD into one of the four categories of the Rye classification. The Rye classification subcategorizes HD into nodular sclerosing (NSHD), mixed-cellularity (MCHD), lymphocyte-predominant (LPHD), and lympho-cyte-depleted (LDHD) types. With modern treatment the prognostic significance of these subtypes has diminished, although the presenting characteristics and natural history remain evident, particularly for the nodular subtype of LPHD. The importance of distinguishing NLPHD from the other types has led to the REAL classification (Table 7-2) (38). The clinicopathologic characteristics are the same as those in adults and are briefly described here.

- NLPHD (55): The distinctive cell is the L&H "popcorn" cell, which is CD20+ (B-lympho-cyte marker), CD15−. Classic RS cells (which are usually CD15+ and CD30+) are rare, as is the detection of EBV. Progressive transformation of the germinal centers of lymph nodes is often seen, and, in fact, can occur in the absence of NLPHD. Therefore, it is important to distinguish these entities. NLPHD has a long natural history, in its time to diagnosis and to relapse, reminiscent of that of indolent non-Hodgkin's lymphomas. It is more common in young children (33% of all patients are younger than 15 years old), has a high male:female ratio (4:1), and commonly involves a single lymph node region with sparing of the mediastinum (56–58).

- Lymphocyte-rich (classic) HD: RS cells (CD15+) are identifiable against a background predominantly of lymphocytes. Clinical behavior is similar to that of mixed-cellularity HD.

- Mixed-cellularity (classic) HD: RS cells (CD15+) are common against a background of abundant normal reactive cells (lymphocytes, plasma cells, eosinophils, histiocytes). This subtype can be confused with peripheral T-cell lymphoma. MCHD is less common in children, often accompanied by "B" symptoms, and more often involves infradiaphragmatic nodes.

- Nodular sclerosis (classic) HD: This subtype is distinctive because of the presence of collagenous bands that divide the lymph node into nodules, which often contain an RS cell variant called the lacunar cell. NSHD often occurs in children, involves supradiaphragmatic nodes, and spreads in an orderly manner along contiguous nodal chains.

- Lymphocyte-depleted (classic) HD: This subtype is rare and commonly confused with non-Hodgkin's lymphoma, particularly of the anaplastic large cell type. RS and pleomorphic variants are common relative to the number of background lymphocytes. LDHD often is advanced at diagnosis and has a poor prognosis.

TABLE 7-2. *Comparison of Revised European–American Classification of Lymphoid Neoplasia (REAL) and Rye classification of Hodgkin's disease*

REAL Classification	Rye Classification
Lymphocyte predominance, nodular	Lymphocyte predominance, nodular (most cases)
Classic Hodgkin's disease	
Lymphocyte-rich	Lymphocyte predominance, diffuse (most cases)
Nodular sclerosing	Lymphocyte predominance, nodular (some cases)
Mixed cellularity	Mixed cellularity
Lymphocyte depletion	Lymphocyte depletion

Modified from Klein G. Epstein–Barr virus–carrying cells in Hodgkin's disease. *Blood* 1992;80(2):299–301, with permission.

Although the pathologic and immunohisto-chemical characteristics of HD generally are sufficiently clear to establish a diagnosis, confusion with select subtypes of non-Hodgkin's lymphoma is problematic. In particular, CHD and NLPHD can be confused with anaplastic large cell lymphoma, and LPHD can be confused with T cell–rich B-cell lymphoma (Fig. 7-3) (33,38).

The relative distribution of the subtypes in younger children differs from that in adolescents and adults, as reported from Stanford University (20). LPHD is more common (13%) in

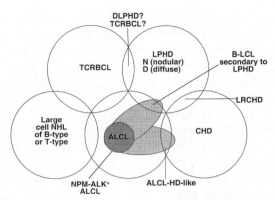

FIG. 7-3. Morphologic overlaps of Hodgkin's disease with anaplastic large cell lymphoma and other lymphomas. (From Jox A, Zander T, Diehl V, et al. Clonal relapse in Hodgkin's disease. *N Engl J Med* 1997;337(7):499, with permission.)

younger children (younger than 10 years), whereas LDHD is exceedingly rare. Although NSHD is the most common subtype in all age groups, it is more common in adolescents (77%) and adults (72%) than in younger children (44%). Conversely, MCHD is more common in younger children (33%) than in adolescents (11%) or adults (17%).

STAGING

Using anatomic groups of regional lymph nodes, the staging system was designed for all age groups, according to a modification of the system devised at the 1970 Ann Arbor Symposium. This was subsequently revised at the Cotswolds Meeting, although not all suggestions from those recommendations are consistently used (53). In this system patients are assigned a clinical stage, and if staging laparotomy is performed, the patient is assigned a pathologic stage (Table 7-1) (2).

A weakness of the Ann Arbor system is its failure to consider disease bulk (either dimension or number of involved sites) or specific patterns of involvement. For this reason, subclassifications of the Ann Arbor staging system have been proposed, particularly for patients with large mediastinal adenopathy (LMA) or stage IIIA disease. LMA, most commonly defined as a mass exceeding one-third the transverse diameter of the chest (intrathoracic width measured at the dome of the diaphragm) on a standard

posteroanterior chest radiograph, places a patient at a greater risk for disease recurrence after radiation alone. Patients with pathologic stage (PS) III disease limited to the spleen or splenic, celiac, or portal nodes are denoted anatomic substage III1 and considered to have a more favorable prognosis than patients with involvement of para-aortic, iliac, or mesenteric nodes, denoted as III2 (59). However, this system has not proven useful in some centers.

The distribution of stages observed in children is somewhat different from that observed in adults. Table 7-3 summarizes the demographic and clinical features of children, adolescents,

TABLE 7-3. *Demographic and clinical characteristics at presentation of pediatric Hodgkin's disease*

	Children[a,b] (%)	Adults[b] (%)
Number of patients	1,985	1,912
<10 yr old	360 (18.1)	
≥10 yr old	1,615 (81.4)	
>17 yr old	10 (0.5)	1,912 (100)
Sex		
Male	1,100 (55.4)	1,147 (60.0)
Female	885 (44.6)	765 (40.0)
Histology		
Lymphocyte predominant	192 (9.7)	96 (5.0)
Mixed cellularity	307 (15.5)	325 (17.0)
Nodular sclerosing	1,431 (72.1)	1,376 (72.0)
Not classified and lymphocyte depleted	55 (2.8)	115 (6.0)
Stage[c]		
I	229 (11.5)	210 (11.0)
II	1,078 (54.3)	899 (47.0)
III	391 (19.7)	593 (31.0)
IV	287 (14.5)	210 (11.0)
B symptoms		
Present	564 (28.4)	612 (32.0)
Absent	1,421 (71.6)	1,300 (68.0)

[a]Data from Nachman JB, Sposto R, Herzog P, et al. Randomized comparison of low-dose involved-field radiotherapy and no radiotherapy for children with Hodgkin's disease who achieve a complete response to chemotherapy. *J Clin Oncol* 2002;20(18):3765–3771; and Ruhl U, Albrecht M, Dieckmann K, et al. Response-adapted radiotherapy in the treatment of pediatric Hodgkin's disease: an interim report at 5 years of the German GPOH-HD 95 trial. *Int J Radiat Oncol Biol Phys* 2001;51(5):1209–1218.
[b]Data from Cleary SF, Link MP, Donaldson SS. Hodgkin's disease in the very young. *Int J Radiat Oncol Biol Phys* 1994;28(1):77–83.
[c]Data derived from both pathological and clinically staged patients.

and young adults presenting with HD at three pediatric centers (20,60,61). Among 3,571 consecutive patients with HD treated at three pediatric centers, 18.1% were younger than 10 years old and 81.4% were 11 to 16 years old. Stage I or II disease was present in 65.8% of children.

DIAGNOSTIC EVALUATION

After pathologic confirmation, the patient undergoes an extensive clinical staging. This begins with a detailed history of systemic symptoms and evidence of cardiorespiratory compromise or organ dysfunction. The physical examination carefully records the location and size of all palpable lymph nodes. An evaluation of Waldeyer's ring, cardiorespiratory status, and organomegaly is vital. Laboratory studies include complete blood count with platelets and biochemical evaluation of renal and liver function. Acute phase reactants, including erythrocyte sedimentation rate, serum copper, and ferritin, may be elevated at diagnosis and can be used as nonspecific marker of disease activity. Elevated serum CD30 and CD25 have been correlated with advanced stage, the presence of constitutional symptoms, and poor prognosis; however, these studies have not been widely used to stage and monitor patients during therapy (62,63). C-reactive protein, another acute phase protein produced in the liver, holds promise as a diagnostic and prognostic index for both Hodgkin's and cardiovascular disease (64). Patients with "B" symptoms or stage III to IV disease should undergo bone marrow biopsy (65). The low yield of a bone marrow evaluation in asymptomatic patients with localized disease (stages I and III) does not support routine use of the procedure.

Imaging studies of the thorax should include a chest radiograph with a posteroanterior and lateral view. The criterion for LMA is the ratio of the measurement of the mediastinal lymph nodes to the maximal measurement of the chest cavity on an upright chest radiograph; those with mediastinal ratios of 33% or more are considered bulky. Computed tomography (CT) scans help delineate the status of intrathoracic lymph node groups (including the hila and cardiophrenic angle), lung parenchyma, pericardium, pleura, and the chest wall, demonstrating abnormalities in about one-half of patients with unremarkable chest radiographs (23,66,67). Definition of disease involvement of intrathoracic tissues by CT often dictates more aggressive therapy than would otherwise have been administered. Distinguishing normal (or hyperplastic) thymus from nodes in children can be problematic.

Imaging of the abdomen and pelvis may involve an abdominal and pelvic CT scan, magnetic resonance imaging (MRI), or a bilateral lower-extremity lymphangiogram (LAG). If CT is used, oral and intravenous contrast administration is needed to accurately distinguish retroperitoneal and pelvic lymph nodes from other infradiaphragmatic structures. In cases with suboptimal contrast resolution of the bowel, MRI may provide a better evaluation of the fat-encased retroperitoneal nodes (68). In previous German and Pediatric Oncology Group (POG) trials using CT or MRI for staging, the size of abdominal and pelvic lymph nodes was used to predict disease involvement. Abdominal nodes less than 1.5 cm in diameter and pelvic nodes less than 2.0 cm were considered negative, whereas abdominal nodes more than 2 cm in diameter and pelvic nodes more than 3 cm were considered positive. Nodal biopsies were undertaken in equivocal nodes falling in between these sizes. The LAG uniquely provides information about nodal architecture that can help distinguish reactive and malignant nodes; residual nodal contrast also helps the radiation therapist design abdominal radiation fields. However, the procedure is invasive, and specific expertise is needed to perform and interpret it. For these reasons, LAG is no longer used as a staging modality in most pediatric centers.

HD involving the liver and spleen is suggested by CT or MRI findings of organomegaly with areas of abnormal density. Organ size alone does not reliably predict lymphomatous involvement because tumor deposits may be less than 1 cm in diameter and not visualized by diagnostic imaging studies. In a POG analysis of 216 children, intrinsic spleen lesions and abnormal portohepatic and celiac nodal areas were highly predictive CT findings but were infrequently observed (69). Therefore, only histologic assessment can definitively evaluate the liver and spleen, but the indications for surgical staging of these organs are limited.

Nuclear imaging with gallium-67 is widely used to stage and monitor treatment response in children with HD. Gallium has limitations because of its low resolution and physiologic biodistribution, which cause difficulties in evaluating abdominal and pelvic lymph nodes and necessitate delayed imaging. Persistence of gallium avidity in patients with mediastinal disease that has not completely regressed after therapy may indicate residual disease (70). Positron emission tomography (PET) is becoming increasingly recognized as a useful staging modality for lymphoma (71–76). Uptake of the radioactive glucose analog fluorodeoxyglucose (FDG) correlates with proliferative activity in tumors undergoing anaerobic glycolysis. FDG-PET has advantages over gallium-67 because the scan is a 1-day procedure with higher resolution, better dosimetry, and less intestinal activity and has a quantitation potential. Gallium-67 and FDG-PET both provide full-body imaging in which areas of abnormal avidity have been correlated with treatment outcomes. Both also have limitations in the pediatric setting (e.g., tracer avidity in nonmalignant thymic rebound commonly observed after completion of therapy for HD). To date, prospective trials evaluating FDG-PET in pediatric HD have not been reported.

Historically, surgical staging includes splenectomy, inspection and wedge biopsy of the liver, multiple lymph node biopsies, and, in the presence of disease, oophoropexy in girls. Staging laparotomy was popularized in the 1970s and 1980s through investigations indicating an unusually high number of patients with clinically unsuspected splenic involvement at presentation. Subsequently, a variety of factors prompted the shift to clinical staging, including advances in diagnostic imaging technology, the standard use of systemic therapy in young children, and appreciation of late complications after splenectomy. Surgical staging is rarely performed and is limited to evaluation of equivocal disease sites identified during clinical staging if the findings will significantly alter the treatment plan.

PROGNOSTIC FACTORS

As the treatment of HD has improved, characteristics that influence outcome have diminished in importance. However, several factors continue to influence the success and certainly the choice of therapy. These factors are interrelated in the sense that disease stage, bulk, and biologic aggressiveness often are codependent (77). Also complicating the determination of prognostic factors is that relevant variables often depend on staging evaluation and treatment. Most data are based on reports that include primarily adults.

The disease stage persists as the most important prognostic variable. Patients with advanced stage disease, especially stage IV, have a worse outlook than those with early stage disease (78,79).

The bulk of disease is reflected by the disease stage and is determined more specifically by the volume of distinct areas of involvement and the number of disease sites. LMA places a patient at a greater risk for disease recurrence when treated with RT alone. However, overall survival remains high because of the effectiveness of salvage chemotherapy (2,23,80–83), although patients with LMA have a somewhat lower survival rate (2,23,81). Patients (at least those staged only clinically) with several sites of involvement, generally defined as more than four, fare less well (23,81,83–85). Patients with extensive splenic involvement (more than five nodules) have a worse prognosis if treated with primary irradiation (86). Patients with stage IV disease who have multiple organs involved fare especially poorly.

Systemic ("B") symptoms, which result from cytokine secretion, reflect biologic aggressiveness and confer a worse prognosis. The constellation of symptoms appears to be relevant to this observation. That is, patients with night sweats only (at least among patients with PS I and II disease) appear to fare as well as patients with PS I to IIA, and those with both fever and weight loss have the worst prognosis (87).

Laboratory studies, including the erythrocyte sedimentation rate, serum ferritin, hemoglobin level, serum albumin, and serum CD8 antigen levels have been reported to predict a worse outcome (62,63,77,88,89). This could reflect disease biology or bulk. Other investigational serum markers associated with an adverse outcome include soluble vascular cell adhesion molecule-1 (90), tumor necrosis factor (91), soluble CD (30,92), β_2-microglobulin (93), transferrin, and serum interleukin-10 (94,95). High levels of caspase 3 in Hodgkin–Reed–Sternberg cells have been correlated with a favorable outcome (96).

Histologic subtype is relevant, at least among adults. Patients with clinical stage I or II MCHD have a higher frequency of subdiaphragmatic relapse, and disease subtype independently influences survival in some reports (23,85). Grade 2 NSHD histology has conferred poor outcome in some but not all studies (97). Patients with LDHD fare poorly. A recent report from the United Kingdom Children's Cancer Study Group, assessing the relevance of histology in 331 children, is revealing. Fewer than 1% had LDHD, obviating any meaningful assessment of its prognostic significance. For patients with other histologies treated with combined therapy, no difference in outcome was observed (98). As previously discussed, patients with NLPHD have distinctive differences in disease-free and overall survival.

Age is a significant prognostic factor in some studies. Survival rates for children with HD approach 95%. In a report from Stanford, the 5- and 10-year survival for children younger than 10 years old with HD is 94% and 92%, respectively, compared with 93% and 86% for adolescents (11 to 16 years old) and 84% and 73% for adults (20). Several features of the youngest patient group may improve their prognosis, including higher frequency of LPHD and MCHD subtypes and of stage I disease, a lower frequency of systemic symptoms, and the more common use of combined modality therapy. Multivariate analysis of these data showed that age, stage, histology, and treatment modality (combined radiation and chemotherapy vs. radiation alone) were all independent prognostic variables for survival (20). Although children younger than 4 years old with HD are uncommon, even these children appear to have an excellent prognosis (22).

The rapidity of response to initial therapy is an important prognostic variable in many forms of cancer, including Hodgkin's lymphoma. In some trials, the rapidity of response to chemotherapy is used to determine subsequent therapy (99). Early response to therapy as measured by gallium-67 or FDG-PET imaging is under investigation as a possible marker of prognosis.

Although prognostic factors will continue to be influenced by choice of therapy, parameters such as disease, bulk, number of involved sites, and systemic symptoms are likely to remain relevant to outcome. Nonetheless, as therapy becomes increasingly tailored to prognostic factors and therapeutic response, overall outcome should become less affected by those parameters.

SELECTION OF THERAPY

HD is one of the pediatric malignancies that has an adult counterpart with a similar natural history and biology. Devising the optimal therapeutic approach for children with this disease is complicated by their greater risk of adverse effects. In particular, RT dosages and fields used in adults can cause profound musculoskeletal retardation, including intraclavicular narrowing, shortened sitting height, decreased mandibular growth, and decreased muscle development in the treated volume (see Chapter 19) (9,10). Therefore, whereas adults with early-stage HD may be treated with full-dose radiation as a single modality (23,81), in prepubertal children, despite a similar success rate, this approach produces unacceptable sequelae (10,19,82,100–102). Additionally complicating the treatment of children are sex-specific differences in chemotherapy-induced gonadal injury. The desire to cure young children with minimal side effects has stimulated attempts to reduce staging procedures, the intensity and types of chemotherapy, and the radiation dosage and volume. Because of the differences in the age-related developmental status of children and the sex-related sensitivity to chemotherapy, no single treatment method is ideal for all children.

Important studies using chemotherapy and low-dose radiation in children to effect cure with tolerable sequelae were first undertaken at Stan-

TABLE 7-4. *Treatment results for early, favorable pediatric Hodgkin's disease*

Group or institution	Patients (n)	Stage	Chemotherapy	Radiation (Gy), field	Survival (%) Overall	Survival (%) DFS, EFS, or RFS	Follow-up interval (yr)	Reference
Radiation therapy alone								
Joint Center/Harvard	50	PS I, IIA	None	36–44, IF	97	82	11	10
Intergroup Hodgkin's	39 (IF)	PS I–II	None	35–40, IF	95	41	5	102
	58 (EF)	PS I, II	None	35, EF	96	67	5	
Bart's/GOS	28	CS I, II	None	35–40, IF	95.5	79	10	101
Stanford	48	PS‡ I, II	None	40–44, IF	86	82	10	101
Toronto	8 (EF)	CS, PS I	None	35, IF	95	87	10	19
	23 (IF)							
Gustave-Roussy	42 (EF)	PS IIA, IIIA	None	40, IF	85	45	10	141
Royal Marsden	33	PS I	None	35, IF	80	33	5	
	99	CS I	None		92	70	10	98
Combined-modality trials								
Stanford	27	PS‡ I, II	6 MOPP	15–25, IF	100	96	5	12
Stanford	44	CS/PS I–III	3 MOPP/3 ABVD	15–25.5, IF	100	100	10	103
St. Jude	58	CS II and III	4–5 COPP/3–4 ABVD	20, IF	96/100	96/97	5	146
Stanford St. Jude Dana Farber Consortium	110	CS I and II†	4 VAMP	15–25.5, IF	99	93	5	135
Intergroup Hodgkin's	97	PS I–II	6 MOPP	35, IF	90	95	5	102
U.S. CCG	294	CS IA/B, IIA	4 COPP/ABV	21, IF	100	97	3	60
Germany–Austria HD-82	100	IA/IB–IIA	2 OPPA	35, IF	100	98	9	104
	53	IIB–IIIA	2 OPPA/2 COPP	30, IF	96	94	9	
Germany–Austria HD-85	53	IA/IB–IIA	2 OPA	35, IF	98	85	6	104
	21	IIB–IIIA	2 OPA/2 COMP	30, IF	95	55	6	
Germany–Austria HD-90	275	IA/IB–IIA	2 OEPA/OPPA	25, IF	99	94/95	5	15, 16
	124	IIB–IIIA	2 OEPA/OPPA + 2 COPP	25, IF	97	90/96	5	
Germany–Austria HD-95	326	I, IIA	2 OEPA/OPPA	20–35, IF for PR; no RT if CR	97	91	3	61
	224	IIB, IIIA	2 OEPA/OPPA + 2 COPP		97	94	3	

Royal Marsden	46	I–III	8 VEEP	30–35, IF	93	82	5	129
Royal Marsden	125	II	6–10 ChlVPP	35, IF	92	85	10	98
Hôpital St. Louis, Paris	72	CS IA–II$_2$A	3 MOPP	35–40, IF	} 91.6	87.6	6.8	143
		PS II$_{3+}$A–IIB	6 MOPP or 3 MOPP or 3 CVPP	35–40, IF				
SFOP MDH-82	79	CS I–IIA	4 ABVD	20–40, IF		90	6	139
	67	CS I–IIA	2 MOPP/2 ABVD	20–40, IF		87	6	
	31	CS IB–IIB	3 MOPP/3 ABVD	20–40, EF	92		6	
SFOP MDH-90	171	I–II	4 VBVP, good responders	20, IF		91	5	136
	27	I–II	4 VBVP + 1–2 OPPA, poor responders	20, IF	97.5	78	5	
AEIOP MH-83	83	Group 1	Group 1	Group 1	95	86	7	140
	83	IA	3 ABVD	20–40, IF				
		IIA (M/T < 0.33)	3 ABVD	20–40, R				
		Group 2	Group 2	Group 2	81		7	
		IIA (M/T ≥ 0.33)	3 MOPP/3 ABVD	20–40, R				
		IIIA	3 MOPP/3 ABVD	20–40, EF				
Chemotherapy alone								
USA-CCG	106	CS IA/B, IIA	4 COPP/ABV	None	100	91	3	60
The Netherlands	21	CS I–II	6 MOPP (<4 cm node)	None	100	90	5	120
	16	CS I–II	6 MOPP (≥4 cm node)	None	100	87.5	5	
GATLA	10	CS IA, IIA	3 CVPP	None	100	86	6.7	123
	16	CS IB, IIB	6 CVPP	None		87	6.7	
Costa Rica	52	CS IA–IIIA	6 CVPP	None	100	90	5	121
Nicaragua	14	CS I, IIA	6 COPP	None	100	100	3	126
Madras, India	10	CS I–IIA	6 COPP/ABV	None		89	5	127
Uganda	18	CS I–IIIA	6 MOPP	None	75	75	5	122

† Mediastinal thoracic ratio <0.33, lymph node <6 cm
‡ Some patients were clinically staged.

ABVD, adriamycin, bleomycin, vinblastine, and dacarbazine; AEIOP, Italian Association of Hematology and Pediatric Oncology; Bart's/GOS, St. Bartholomew's Hospital/Great Ormond Street; CCG, Children's Cancer Group; ChlVPP, chlorambucil, vinblastine, procarbazine, and prednisolone; COMP, cyclophosphamide, vincristine (Oncovin), methotrexate, and prednisolone; COPP, cyclophosphamide, vincristine (Oncovin), procarbazine, and prednisone; COPP/ABV, cyclophosphamide, vincristine (Oncovin), procarbazine, prednisone, adriamycin, bleomycin, and vinblastine; CR, complete response; CS, clinical stage; CVPP, cyclophosphamide, vinblastine, procarbazine, and prednisone; DFS, disease-free survival; EF, extended field; EFS, event-free survival; GATLA, Grupo Argentino de Tratamiento de Leucemia Aguda; HD, Hodgkin's disease; IF, involved field; MDH, multicenter trial; MH, multicenter Hdogkin's trial; MOPP, nitrogen mustard, vincristine (Oncovin), procarbazine, and prednisone; M/T, mediastinal/thoracic ratio; OEPA, vincristine (Oncovin), etoposide, prednisone, and adriamycin; OPA, vincristine (Oncovin), prednisone, and adriamycin; OPPA, vincristine (Oncovin), procarbazine, prednisone, and adriamycin; PR, partial response; PS, pathologic stage; R, regional; RFS, relapse-free survival; RT, radiotherapy; SFOP, French Society of Pediatric Oncology; VAMP, vinblastine, adriamycin, methotrexate, and prednisone; VBVP, vinblastine, bleomycin, etoposide (VP-16), and prednisone; VEEP, vincristine, etoposide, epirubicin, and prednisolone.

TABLE 7-5. *Treatment results for advanced, unfavorable pediatric Hodgkin's disease*

Group or institution	Patients (n)	Stage	Chemotherapy	Radiation (Gy), field	Survival, % Overall	Survival, % DFS, EFS, or RFS	Follow-up interval (yr)	Reference
Combined-modality trials								
Germany–Austria HD-82	50	II_EB, III_EA/B, IIIB, IVA/B	2 OPPA/4 COPP	25, IF	85	86	9	104
Germany–Austria HD-85	24	II_EB, III_EA/B, IIIB, IVA/B	2 OPA/4 COMP	25, IF	100	49	6	15, 16
Germany–Austria HD-90	179	II_EB, III_EA/B, IIIB, IVA/B	2 OEPA/OPPA + 4 COPP	20, IF	98/89	83/91	5	15, 16
Germany–Austria HD-95	280	II_EB, III_EA/B, IIIB, IVA/B	2 OEPA/OPPA + 4 COPP	20–35, IF for PR; no RT if CR	97	84	3	61
Gustave-Roussy	60	I–IV	3–6 MOPP	40, IF	93	86	5	17
SFOP MDH-82	40	CS III	3 MOPP/3 ABVD	20–40, EF		82	6	139
	21	CS IV	3 MOPP/3 ABVD	20–40, EF		62	6	
AEIOP MH-83	49	IIIB–IV	Group 3 / 5 MOPP/5 ABVD	20–40, EF	60		7	140
GATLA			Intermediate					123
	43	I–IV	6 CVPP	30–40, IF		87	5	
	21	I–IV	6 AOPE	30–40, IF		67	5	
			Unfavorable					
	24	I–IV	CCOPP/CAPTe	30–40, IF		83	5	
Royal Marsden	80	III	6–10 ChlVPP	35, IF	84	73	10	98
	27	IV	6–10 ChlVPP	35, IF	71	38	10	
Royal Marsden	8	IV	8 VEEP/ChlVPP if NR or PR to VEEP	30–35, IF	50	44	5	129
Toronto	57	CS IIA–IV	6 MOPP	25–30, EF	85	80	10	19
U.S. POG	62	CS/PS IIB, $IIIA_2$, IIIB, IV	4 MOPP/4 ABVD	21, TLI	91	77	3	70, 115
U.S. POG	80	CS/PS IIB, $IIIA_2$, IIIB, IV	4 MOPP/4 ABVD	21, EF	87	80	5	128
Stanford	28	III–IV	6 MOPP	15–25.5, IF	78	84	7.5	12
Stanford	13	III–IV	3 MOPP/3 ABVD	15–25.5, IF	85	69	10	103
St. Jude	27	CS IV	4–5 COPP/3–4 ABVD	20 Gy, IF	86	85	5	146
Joint Center/Harvard	83	IA–IIIB	6 MOPP	25–40	95	77	11	10
Stanford, St. Jude, Dana Farber Consortium	56	CS I/II bulky (n = 26), CS III/IV (n = 30)	6 VEPA	15–25.5, IF	81.9	67.8	5	134

234

Group	No.	Stage	Chemotherapy	Radiation			Yr	Ref.
U.S. CCG	64	PS III–IV	12 ABVD	21, R	89	87	3	111
U.S. CCG	54	PS III–IV	6 ABVD	21, EF	90	87	4	110
U.S. CCG	394	CS I/II‡, CS IIB, CS III	6 COPP/ABV	21, IF	95	87	3	60
U.S. CCG	141	CS IV	COPP/ABV + CHOP + AraC/VP-16	21, IF	100	90	3	
Chemotherapy alone								
UKCCSG	67	CS IV	6–8 ChlVPP	None‡	80.8	55.2	5	147
Australia/New Zealand	53	CS IV	6–8 MOPP or 6 ChlVPP	None	94	92	4	116
Australia/New Zealand	25	CS I–IV	3 EVAP/ABV	None	100	79	3	124
Australia/New Zealand	53	CS I–IV	5–6 VEEP	None	92	78	5	125
Uganda	10	CS IIIB, IV	6 MOPP	None		60	5	122
Nicaragua	23	CS IIIB, IV	8–10 COPP/ABV	None		75	3	126
Costa Rica	24	CS IIIB, IV	6 CVPP/6 EBO	None	81	60	5	121
Madras, India	43	CS IIB–IVB	6 COPP/ABV	None		90	5	127
The Netherlands	21	CS I–IV (<4 cm node)	6 MOPP	None	100	91	5	118, 119, 148
	17	CS I–IV	6 ABVD		94	70		
	21	CS I–IV	3 MOPP/3 ABVD		91	91		
U.S. CCG	57	PS III/IV	6 MOPP/6 ABVD	None	84	77	4	110
U.S. CCG	394	CS I/II†, CS IIB, CS III	6 COPP/ABV	None	100	83	3	60
U.S. CCG	141	CS IV	COPP/ABV + CHOP + AraC/VP-16	None	94	81	3	
U.S. POG	81	CS IIB, III_2A, IIIB, IV	4 MOPP/4 ABVD	None	96	79	5	128

† Presence of adverse features = (t)hila, >4 nodal sites, bulk

‡ 12 patients received 20–35 Gy, IF; 2 received whole lung irradiation

ABVD, adriamycin, bleomycin, vinblastine, and dacarbazine; AEIOP, Italian Association of Hematology and Pediatric Oncology; AOPE, adriamycin, vincristine (Oncovin), prednisone, and etoposide; AraC, cytosine arabinoside; CAPTe, cyclophosphamide, adriamycin, prednisone, and teniposide; CCG, Children's Cancer Group; CCOPP, CCNU, vincristine (Oncovin), procarbazine, and prednisone; ChlVPP, chlorambucil, vinblastine, procarbazine, and prednisone; CHOP, cyclophosphamide, hydroxydavnamycin, vincristine (Oncovin), and prednisone; COMP, cyclophosphamide, vincristine (Oncovin), methotrexate, and prednisolone; COPP, cyclophosphamide, vincristine (Oncovin), prednisone, and procarbazine; COPP/ABV, cyclophosphamide, vincristine (Oncovin), procarbazine, prednisone, adriamycin, bleomycin, and vinblastine; CR, complete response; CS, clinical stage; CVPP, cyclophosphamide, vinblastine, procarbazine, and prednisone; DFS, disease-free survival; EBO, epirubicin, bleomycin, and vincristine (Oncovin); EF, extended field; EFS, event-free survival; EVAP/ABV, etoposide, vinblastine, cytarabine, cisplatin, adriamycin, bleomycin, and vincristine; GATLA, Grupo Argentino de Tratamiento de Leucemia Aguda; HD, Hodgkin's disease; IF, involved field; MDH, multicenter trial; MH, multicenter Hodgkin's trial; MOPP, nitrogen mustard, vincristine (Oncovin), procarbazine, and prednisone; NR, no response; OEPA, vincristine (Oncovin), etoposide, prednisone, and adriamycin; OPA, vincristine (Oncovin), prednisone, and adriamycin; OPPA, vincristine (Oncovin), procarbazine, prednisone, and adriamycin; POG, Pediatric Oncology Group; PR, partial response; PS, pathologic stage; R, regional; RFS, relapse-free survival; RT, radiotherapy; SFOP, French Society of Pediatric Oncology; TLI, total lymphoid irradiation; UKCCSG, United Kingdom Children's Cancer Study Group; VEEP, vincristine, etoposide, epirubicin, and prednisolone; VEPA, vinblastine, etoposide, prednisone, and adriamycin.

ford University. These trials used chemotherapy in combination with lower dosages of RT for young children with early-stage disease (2, 11,12). Donaldson and Link (12) reported excellent results with low-dose irradiation combined with MOPP. Radiation dosages were 15 Gy for patients with bone age less than 5 years, 20 Gy for those 6 to 10 years, and 25 Gy for those 11 to 14 years old. Additional boosts were given to those who did not achieve a complete remission or in those with bulky disease (nodes larger than 6 cm or LMA if mediastinal disease was present). The overall local control was 97% (12). Although growth deformity was decreased, full-course MOPP is associated with a high risk of sterility and secondary leukemia (discussed in Chapters 19 and 20). Therefore, alternative regimens were used subsequently (14,16,47,103, 104).

An important sequence of studies performed by the German–Austrian Pediatric Hodgkin's Disease Study Group progressively refined the extent of staging and the intensity of chemotherapy and radiation (14,16,104). The nature and results of these studies (HD-82, HD-85, HD-87, HD-90, and HD-95) are summarized in Tables 7-4 and 7-5. Staging was reduced from systematic use of laparotomy (HD-78) to selective laparotomy and splenectomy (HD-82), to infrequent laparotomy without splenectomy (HD-90), to routine clinical staging (HD-95). Stage-dependent chemotherapy and radiation dosage and volume were also used. In the early studies, vincristine (Oncovin), procarbazine, prednisone, and doxorubicin (adriamycin) (OPPA) were used, as were cyclophosphamide, vincristine (Oncovin), procarbazine, and prednisone (COPP). In HD-85 and HD-87, OPA (eliminating procarbazine) was used for boys to reduce testicular toxicity, but event-free survival (EFS) declined. In HD-90, girls received OPPA plus COPP (depending on stage), whereas boys received vincristine (On-

TABLE 7-6. *Treatment recommendations in pediatric Hodgkin's disease*

Clinical Presentation	Stage	Recommended Treatment Approach
Early (favorable): localized disease involving <4 nodal regions in absence of "B" symptoms, bulk, or extranodal extension	IA, IIA	Recommended therapy: 2–4 cycles non–cross-resistant chemotherapy without alkylators (ABVD or derivative) plus low-dose, involved-field radiation (1,500–2,550 cGy) Other considerations: 6 cycles non–cross-resistant chemotherapy alone (alternating COPP and ABVD or derivative) In clinical trial setting only: 4 cycles of chemotherapy alone
Localized unfavorable (intermediate): localized disease involving ≥3 nodal regions in presence of bulky lymphadenopathy (mediastinal ratio ≥33%; lymph node mass ≥610 cm)	IA, IIA, IIB*, IIIA	Recommended therapy: 4–6 cycles (3–5 compacted, dose-intensive cycles) non–cross-resistant chemotherapy (alternating COPP and ABVD or derivative with or without etoposide) plus low-dose, involved-field radiation (1,500–2,550 cGy) Other considerations: 6–8 cycles (5 compacted, dose-intensive) non–cross-resistant chemotherapy alone (alternating COPP and ABVD or derivative with or without etoposide)
Advanced (unfavorable): stage II disease with constitutional symptoms of fever or weight loss and any advanced disease	IIB^a, IIIB, IV	Recommended therapy: 6–8 cycles (5–6 compacted, dose-intensive cycles) of non–cross-resistant chemotherapy (alternating COPP and ABVD or derivative with or without etoposide) plus low-dose, involved-field radiation (1,500–2,550 cGy) Other considerations: 8 cycles (6–7 compacted, dose-intensive cycles) non–cross-resistant chemotherapy alone (alternating COPP and ABVD or derivative with or without etoposide)

ABVD, adriamycin, bleomycin, vinblastine, and dacarbazine; COPP, cyclophosphamide, vincristine (Oncovin), prednisone, and procarbazine.

^{a}Patients with stage IIB disease have been variably treated as having intermediate or unfavorable risk. Some studies use associated factors (e.g., weight loss, bulk disease, or extranodal extension) for further risk stratification.

covin), etoposide, prednisone, and adriamycin (OEPA) with COPP, adding etoposide to OPA. These studies served as the paradigm for the risk-adapted treatment approach that is currently used at most pediatric treatment centers.

In general, the use of radiation and chemotherapy broadens the spectrum of potential toxicities while reducing the severity of individual (drug- or radiation-related) toxicities. Current approaches include chemotherapy alone and in conjunction with lower radiation dosages. The volume of radiation and the intensity and duration of chemotherapy are risk adapted, or determined by prognostic factors at presentation, including presence of constitutional symptoms, disease stage, and bulk. Results for patients with early (favorable) and advanced (unfavorable) HD are summarized in Tables 7-4 and 7-5, and our therapeutic recommendations are summarized in Table 7-6.

COMBINATION CHEMOTHERAPY

MOPP was the standard chemotherapy regimen used in the United States for many years after DeVita et al.'s 1972 report (105). The major toxicities include an associated risk of acute myeloid leukemia, azoospermia in more than 90% of boys treated at any age, and a risk of sterility in girls, which increases with age (106,107). Subsequently, the effectiveness of adriamycin, bleomycin, vinblastine, and dacarbazine (ABVD) as front-line chemotherapy was established (108–111). Second malignancies and sterility were less common with ABVD than with MOPP (112). The predominant adverse effects of ABVD are pulmonary toxicity related to bleomycin and cardiovascular toxicity secondary to adriamycin. These side effects may be exacerbated by the addition of mediastinal or mantle irradiation (113). Consequently, ABVD and MOPP were combined with the aim of improving disease control and reducing the risk of leukemogenesis and sterility related to the alkylating agents in the MOPP regimen. This alternating combination proved to be more effective than MOPP chemotherapy alone (18, 103,110,114,115). Its use in pediatric patients also diminished the risk of cardiopulmonary

dysfunction predisposed by the anthracycline and bleomycin in the ABVD regimen. Over the years, the MOPP and ABVD regimens have undergone a variety of modifications, but the majority of the chemotherapeutic regimens used today are derived from these two combinations.

COMBINED MODALITIES VERSUS CHEMOTHERAPY ALONE

The arguments that favor treatment with chemotherapy alone for all stages propose that this treatment approach obviates surgical staging and avoids the dysmorphic and carcinogenic consequences of irradiation. The disadvantages of the use of chemotherapy alone are the risks of treatment-related fatality, cardiopulmonary toxicity, infertility, and leukemogenesis caused by the higher cumulative dosages of anthracyclines, alkylating agents, and bleomycin (116) and a greater likelihood of disease recurrence in sites of bulk disease (78,117). Generalization of treatment outcomes after these trials has been limited because most studies include small numbers of patients assigned to treatments in a nonrandom fashion. Also, long-term follow-up related to disease control and late treatment sequelae has not been reported.

Early chemotherapy trials used MOPP or similar regimens derived from MOPP and prescribed 6 to 12 months of chemotherapy (116,118–123). The longest follow-up data are from the Uganda experience, with only a 67% 9-year survival (122). Subgroups included clinical stage (CS) I–IIIA, with a 75% survival rate, and CS IIIB–IV, with 60% and 47% survival at 5 and 10 years, respectively. Ekert et al. (116) reported a 90% 5-year survival for children with CS I and II disease treated with MOPP or a similar program that substitutes chlorambucil for nitrogen mustard and vinblastine for vincristine (ChlVPP) (Table 7-5), but the disease-free and overall survival were 40% and 55%, respectively, for children with advanced disease. A report from the Netherlands described 37 children treated with six cycles of MOPP for small (up to 4 cm in diameter) lymph node disease, with the addition of 25 Gy involved-field RT (IFRT) for children with large lymph node disease. The disease-free survival with a median follow-up of more than 62 months is 90% for the former (21 children) and 85.5% for the latter (16 children) (120).

In an effort to avoid treatment complications associated with alkylating agent chemotherapy, contemporary chemotherapy-alone trials have alternated MOPP-type regimens with ABVD or similar derivatives or used combinations without alkylating agents (60,110,119,121,124–129). Across all stages, EFS rates after treatment with 6 to 12 months of alternating MOPP and ABVD chemotherapy alone range from 77% at 4 years to 91% at 10 years; several of these investigations included pathologic staging to confirm eligibility for reduced therapy (110,128,130). Nicaraguan investigators used 8 to 10 cycles of COPP and adriamycin, bleomycin, and vinblastine (ABV) hybrid chemotherapy alone in clinically staged patients; 3-year EFS was 100% for the 25 patients with stages I, II, and IIIA but only 74.9% for the 23 patients with stages IIIB or IV (126). Similarly, Costa Rican investigators observed inferior outcomes for patients with stage IV disease treated with 12 months of cyclophosphamide, vincristine, procarbazine, and prednisone (CVPP) and epirubicin, bleomycin, and vincristine (Oncovin) (EBO) chemotherapy (60% 5-year relapse-free survival) (121). The use of ABVD or ABVD-derivative chemotherapy combinations produced unsatisfactory outcomes in advanced-stage patients treated with six cycles of ABVD chemotherapy alone (71% 8-year disease-free survival) and five or six cycles of vincristine, etoposide, epirubicin, and prednisolone (VEEP) chemotherapy alone (78% 5-year disease-free survival) (119,125).

Only three randomized controlled trials have prospectively compared chemotherapy alone with combined-modality therapy in children and adolescents with HD (60,110,128). The Children's Cancer Group (CCG) compared 12 cycles of alternating MOPP and ABVD with six cycles of ABVD and low-dose (21 Gy) radiation. The trend in event-free and overall survival suggested a survival advantage for the combined-modality group (90% 4-year EFS) over the chemotherapy-alone group (84%

4-year EFS), but this difference was not statistically significant (110). The POG evaluated the benefit of adding low-dose radiation to four cycles each of MOPP and ABVD (Table 7-6) (128); the addition of RT did not improve disease-free or overall survival. However, statistical and quality assurance issues complicate interpretation of this data (131). Long-term follow-up will be necessary to assess the toxicity from these two trials, but cardiopulmonary and neoplastic sequelae were observed in early follow-up and could potentially increase with the cumulative dosages of alkylating agent chemotherapy, anthracyclines, and bleomycin.

In a recent CCG trial reported by Nachman et al. (60), chemotherapy alone using the COPP and ABV hybrid regimen was compared with combined-modality therapy including low-dose IFRT. Treatment assignment was risk adapted based on the presence of clinical features including the presence of "B" symptoms, hilar adenopathy, mediastinal and peripheral lymph node bulk, and the number of involved nodal regions. Patients with favorable disease presentations received four cycles of COPP and ABV; those with unfavorable risk features received six cycles of COPP and ABV. Patients with stage IV HD received sequential cycles of high-dose cytarabine and etoposide, COPP and ABV, and cyclophosphamide, vincristine, doxorubicin, and methylprednisolone. Patients achieving a complete response to chemotherapy were eligible for randomization to receive low-dose IFRT or no further therapy. The trial was terminated prematurely because results indicated a significantly higher number of relapses among patients treated with chemotherapy alone. The 3-year EFS estimates according to patient randomization were 92% for patients treated with combined-modality therapy and 87% for those treated with chemotherapy alone; the benefit of IFRT remained significant in the as-treated analysis. The difference was most marked in patients with stage IV disease, who had 90% EFS if randomized to receive IFRT and 81% if randomized to receive chemotherapy alone. Because of successful salvage therapy after relapse, estimates of overall survival do not differ between the randomized groups in early follow-up. However, other investigations of long-term outcomes after treatment for pediatric HD implicate retrieval therapy after relapse as a significant risk factor for neoplastic complications and early mortality (132,133). Finally, in the recent German-Austrian Pediatric Hodgkin's Disease Study Group (GPOH) HD-95 trial, relapse-free survival rates were higher for patients treated with RT after partial response (93%) than for those without RT after complete response (89%) (61). The difference was significant for patients treated for advanced-stage but not early-stage disease.

In summary, numerous investigations have confirmed that chemotherapy alone is an effective treatment approach for pediatric HD. However, the higher cumulative dosages used in these protocols predispose survivors to greater risks of acute and late toxicity associated with alkylating agents, anthracyclines, and bleomycin. Conversely, these protocols avoid radiation-associated treatment complications including musculoskeletal growth impairment, cardiopulmonary dysfunction, and solid tumor carcinogenesis. Current information suggests that children with advanced and unfavorable symptomatic or bulky disease at presentation have better outcomes using a combined-modality approach. Identifying the prognostic features of patients who need radiation to optimize disease control is a focus of many ongoing pediatric trials.

RISK-ADAPTED THERAPY

Numerous investigations published in the 1990s supported the use of a risk-adapted treatment assignment based on clinical features at disease presentation (14,16,56,60,61,104,123,128,134–140). Parameters have varied according to individual studies, but those used most often in risk assessments include the presence of "B" symptoms, mediastinal and peripheral lymph node bulk, extranodal extension of disease to contiguous structures, hilar lymph node involvement, number of involved nodal regions, and Ann Arbor stage. These studies uniformly evaluated treatment outcomes using a lower number of multiagent chemotherapy cycles in clinically staged patients with favorable clinical presentations (Tables 7-5 and 7-6). Novel treatment approaches have been explored in patients with intermediate- and high-risk features in an effort to improve long-term disease control and reduce late therapy-related complications. The results of these studies are summarized in Tables 7-4 and 7-5.

Treatment of Early-Stage Disease

Early-stage disease may present with favorable or unfavorable features. A favorable clinical presentation is typically defined as localized (stage I or II) nodal involvement in the absence of "B" symptoms and nodal bulk. LMA is designated as bulky when the ratio of the maximum measurement of the mediastinal lymphadenopathy to intrathoracic cavity or upright chest radiograph is greater than 33%. The criterion for peripheral lymph node bulk has varied across studies from 4 to 10 cm. The presence of extranodal extension to contiguous sites, hilar lymphadenopathy, or involvement of more than three nodal regions typically moves the patient into an intermediate- or high-risk group. Children and adolescents with early-stage, favorable presentations of HD are excellent candidates for reduced therapy. Several multiagent regimens and a variety of nonalkylator regimens have proved effective (Table 7-4) (10,12,14,16,56,60,61,98,101–104,120–123,126–128,135–143). Treatment for patients with a favorable clinical presentation typically involves two to four cycles of chemotherapy and low-dose IFRT. In some regimens, the radiation dosage has been reduced based on a favorable response to chemotherapy.

The GPOG pioneered the use of risk- and sex-adapted therapy featuring the OPPA regimen. After the efficacy of two cycles of OPPA chemotherapy in combination with 35 Gy IFRT was demonstrated in patients with favorable clinical presentations (104), the regimen was modified to OEPA for boys and the radiation dosage reduced to 25 Gy for boys and girls achieving a sufficient remission after two cycles of OEPA or OPPA chemotherapy (16). The current GPOH HD-95 trial is investigating whether RT can be omitted in patients achieving a complete response to chemotherapy. Early results (median follow-up time of 38 months) indicate a

94% EFS for favorable-risk patients and no difference in outcome in favorable-risk patients treated with chemotherapy alone or combined-modality therapy (61). Notably, bulky lymphadenopathy is not used in the GPOH risk assessment because bulk has not influenced outcome in the German trials, which prescribe a 5- to 10-Gy boost in cases with an insufficient remission after chemotherapy (144).

French investigators initially determined that treatment outcomes were not compromised in patients with early, favorable clinical presentations whose therapy was reduced to four cycles of chemotherapy (two MOPP and two ABVD or four ABVD) and 20 Gy IFRT (139). Their next trial evaluated a novel regimen without alkylators or anthracyclines, vinblastine, bleomycin, etoposide, and prednisone (VBVP), which produced a 91% 5-year EFS in patients achieving a good response after four cycles of chemotherapy and 20 Gy to involved fields (136). Similarly, Italian investigators demonstrated comparable outcomes (91% 7-year freedom from progression) using reduced therapy with three cycles of ABVD and 20 Gy IFRT (140).

Several North American investigators have observed excellent treatment results in combined-modality trials for favorable-risk HD. Pediatric Hodgkin's Consortium investigators from Stanford, St. Jude Children's Research Hospital, and Dana Farber Cancer Institute recently reported treatment results using a novel nonalkylator regimen, vinblastine, adriamycin, methotrexate, and prednisone (VAMP), for children with clinical stage I or II, nonbulky HD (135). Patients received four cycles of VAMP chemotherapy and IFRT; the radiation dosage was determined by early response after two cycles of chemotherapy. Patients achieving a complete response received 15 Gy, and those achieving a partial response received 25.5 Gy. At a median follow-up of 5.6 years (range, 1.1 to 10.4 years), 5-year EFS was 93%. Very good early treatment results have also been observed by POG investigators using response-based doxorubicin, bleomycin, vincristine, and etoposide (DBVE) chemotherapy and low-dose (25.5 Gy) IFRT (145). Two-year EFS for the entire cohort is 91%, with 93% EFS for rapid early responders treated with two cycles of DBVE and 89% EFS for slower responders treated with four cycles of DBVE.

Treatment of Advanced and Unfavorable Disease

In risk-adapted treatment regimens, early disease presenting with unfavorable features sometimes is treated similarly to advanced stage disease. Alternatively, an intermediate designation is given in some risk categorizations to patients with localized (stage IA, IIA) disease presentations that have one or more of the unfavorable features and to patients with stage IIIA disease. For example, the GPOH studies prescribe four cycles of chemotherapy (two OPPA or two OEPA and two COPP) for patients with intermediate risk (designated as stage IIEA, IIB, or IIIA) and six cycles (two OPPA or two OEPA and four COPP) for patients with unfavorable and advanced disease (16,61). The criteria for unfavorable clinical presentations vary between investigations but typically include the presence of "B" symptoms, bulky lymphadenopathy, hilar lymphadenopathy, involvement of three or more nodal regions, extranodal extension to contiguous structures, or advanced stage (IIIB–IV). Chemotherapy used for this group includes MOPP and ABVD or derivative combinations that incorporate etoposide in many cases. As illustrated in Table 7-5, RT for unfavorable and advanced HD is variable and protocol dependent. Although IFRT remains the standard in patients treated with combined-modality therapy, restricting RT to areas of initial bulky disease (generally defined as larger than 5 cm at the time of disease presentation) or postchemotherapy residual disease (generally defined as larger than 2 cm, or residual PET avidity) is under investigation (10,12,15–17,19, 60,61,98,103,104,110,111,115,116,119,12–129, 134,139,140,146–148).

Two primary treatment approaches have been used for patients with unfavorable and advanced disease presentations. A conventional treatment approach prescribes chemotherapy on a twice-monthly schedule for 6 to 8 months (61,134). An alternative strategy administers treatment over 3 to 5 months to increase dosage intensity and reduce the risk of developing resistant disease (60,145). This is accomplished by alternating myelosuppressive and nonmyelosuppressive agents in a weekly schedule and using colony-stimulating factor to support neutrophil recovery. A summary of treatment results of published trials is provided in Table 7-5, which demonstrates EFS rates ranging from 70% to 90%. Long-term follow-up is not yet available to determine whether the abbreviated, dose-intensive treatment approach is superior to a conventional treatment administration in maintaining disease control.

SUMMARY RECOMMENDATIONS FOR PRIMARY DISEASE

Optimal treatment planning involves a multidisciplinary approach beginning at diagnosis. This is best accomplished if the pediatric and radiation oncologist can meet to review staging studies after examining the patient. The treatment approach should consider host factors, such as age and sex, which may increase the risk of specific treatment complications, and disease factors (e.g., presence of "B" symptoms, bulky lymphadenopathy, and stage). Recommended treatment approaches for favorable localized, intermediate, and advanced unfavorable disease presentations are summarized in Table 7-6.

REFRACTORY AND RELAPSED DISEASE

HD may still be cured even after initial treatment programs fail. Relapse usually occurs within 4 years, but late relapse is not rare. The choice of therapy for such patients depends on the initial treatment and the disease characteristics at the time of relapse. A spectrum of treatment options exist, including those outlined here (149). This section focuses on the role of radiation in the setting of refractory or relapsed therapy.

- Standard-dose chemotherapy with either the same initial regimen or an alternative regimen, which could be third line (depending on

previous regimens). If possible, RT can be added.
- RT alone.
- High-dose chemotherapy (with or without RT), followed by stem cell support. The source of the stem cells can be allogeneic or autologous bone marrow or peripheral stem cells.
- Experimental therapy (e.g., radiolabeled antiferritin, immunotherapy).
- Palliative therapy.

For patients who were initially treated with RT alone, salvage chemotherapy is effective, increasing disease-free and overall survival in 55–80% (150–152). If RT can be safely added to chemotherapy as salvage treatment, the outcome may be superior (149,152). Factors that independently predict a more favorable outcome include the following:

- Site of relapse (nodal better than extranodal)
- The stage that could be assigned at relapse (early better than advanced)
- The histology (LPHD and NSHD better than MCHD)

For children who relapse after treatment that includes chemotherapy, conventional (standard-dose) salvage chemotherapy regimens are of limited success, increasing disease-free and overall survival in only 10–50% (149,151). Fortunately, other strategies can be effective. The selection of the most appropriate salvage regimen is based on several considerations, including the following:

- Did the patient achieve a complete remission, or was the disease refractory?
- If a complete response was achieved, was it durable (longer than 1 year)?
- Did the relapse occur in nodal or extranodal sites, and, as a corollary, was the stage at relapse early or advanced?

The patients with the most favorable prognosis are those who have disease recurrence only at a prolonged interval after an initial complete response and in a limited nodal pattern. Some of these patients can be cured by RT alone, often administered as standard-dose total lymphoid irradiation (TLI) (153–156). However, TLI is difficult to administer in patients who have had a significant marrow insult from aggressive chemotherapy. Moreover, the toxicities associated with standard-dose therapy are unacceptable in growing children, and too few children have been treated with this approach to provide adequate outcome data. In fact, even these patients may have a superior outcome (EFS as high as 80%) if treated with high-dose chemotherapy and autologous stem cell rescue (157,158). On the opposite end of the spectrum are patients who have chemotherapy-refractory disease, who are never cured by conventional salvage chemotherapy.

Patients who relapse after regimens that include chemotherapy have been treated with high-dose chemotherapy and hematopoietic stem cell rescue (149,157,159,160). Three- to 5-year survival probabilities of 25–80%, depending on characteristics at relapse, have been reported (primarily in adults) after such treatment (158,159,161). Only one prospective study randomizing refractory or relapsed patients with HD to high-dose chemotherapy and stem cell rescue or conventional-dose chemotherapy has been performed. The British National Lymphoma Investigation Group randomized 40 patients to carmustine (BCNU), etoposide, cytarabine (arabinosylcytosine), and melphalan (BEAM) with stem cell support or lower-dose (mini) BEAM (162). Progression-free survival at 3 years was 53% and 10%, respectively. Recently, investigators at Stanford compared patients with recurrent or relapsed HD who were treated with high-dose chemotherapy and autologous bone marrow transplantation (ABMT) (EFS 53%) with a matched group treated with conventional-dose chemotherapy (EFS 27%) (163). Consistent with previous data, patients refractory or relapsing within 12 months of therapy benefited the most; conversely, an advantage was not observed for patients with a durable (longer than 1 year) first remission. Data specific to children with recurrent HD are limited. However, an analysis of 81 pediatric patients with HD who underwent ABMT and were reported to the European Bone Marrow Transplant Group demonstrated a similar outcome to a case-matched group of adults similarly treated (Fig. 7-4) (164). Prognostic factors for a favorable outcome include the duration of initial response to chemotherapy, "B" symptoms at relapse, disseminated pulmonary or bone marrow disease at relapse, and more than minimal dis-

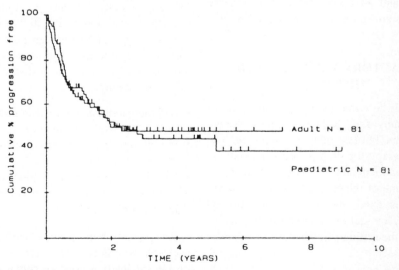

FIG. 7-4. Progression-free survival after allogeneic bone marrow transplant for Hodgkin's disease: comparison between pediatric and matched adult patients. $x = 0.2194$, $p = 0.6395$. (From Yahalom J. Management of relapsed and refractory Hodgkin's disease. *Semin Radiat Oncol* 1996;6(3):210–224, with permission.)

ease at the time of transplantation (158,165). A variety of preparative regimens provide similar outcome (160,165–167).

What are the possible roles for RT in the setting of high-dose chemotherapy and stem cell rescue for HD? The basis for including RT is twofold: These aggressive salvage programs still fail to cure a large proportion of patients, and ample data show that many patients with progressive, recurrent HD after chemotherapy do not exhibit a cross-resistance to radiation (149,153–156). Moreover, most patients relapse in sites of previous involvement, mostly nodal (158,166). RT can be administered, in combination with chemotherapy conditioning regimens, as total body irradiation (TBI), involved-field RT, and TLI. Typical preparative regimens that include TBI or TLI are cyclophosphamide with or without etoposide (149,165,168). The rationale for TBI (e.g., 12 to 14 Gy in 4 to 5 days at 1.5 to 2.5 Gy twice daily) or TLI (e.g., 18 Gy in 2 weeks at 0.9 Gy twice daily) is the associated tumor cell kill and immunosuppressive effects. However, TBI and TLI programs for patients who have previously been treated with mediastinal RT are associated with a significant increase in pulmonary complications (168,169). Pneumonitis and pulmonary alveolar hemorrhage often are fatal. Because there appears to be no difference in relapse-free survival between TBI or TLI preparative regimens and those that do not use magna field irradiation, it is reasonable to avoid TBI or TLI if prior mediastinal irradiation has been given or is contemplated as boost treatment.

In considering the role of IFRT in the setting of high-dose chemotherapy and stem cell rescue, three essential questions must be answered: Does RT to sites of recurrent or refractory HD diminish relapse at these sites? If so, then what is the impact on freedom from relapse, EFS, and overall survival? Is the associated morbidity of IFRT acceptable? Data from several series support an affirmative answer to these questions (149,160,167,170–172). In a Stanford report, patients with stages I to III disease at relapse who received ABMT and IFRT had a 3-year freedom from relapse of 100% and overall survival of 85%, compared with 67% and 60%, re-

spectively, for patients not receiving IFRT (172). For patients not previously irradiated, IFRT was associated with an improved freedom from relapse of 85% and overall survival of 93%, in contrast to 57% and 55%, respectively, for those previously irradiated. Morbidity was similar to that of those not irradiated, although RT may have contributed to the peritransplant death of two patients.

Central issues relating to the use of IFRT are the dosage, target volume, and timing with respect to transplantation. RT dosages generally are 20 to 36 Gy, in 1.5- to 2.0-Gy fractions. This variation relates to potential normal tissue toxicity and the value of higher radiation dosages in patients with identifiable tumor that demonstrates radiation responsiveness (160,173). Radiation volume can vary and include treatment to all sites of initial disease, recurrent disease, persistent disease after salvage chemotherapy, persistent disease after the preparative regimen for transplantation, or all nodal sites (149, 157,160). TLI administered before transplantation has been an effective program at Memorial Sloan–Kettering (168). IFRT can be administered before high-dose chemotherapy to place patients in a minimal disease state. RT can also be administered after high-dose chemotherapy to decrease the potential for disease progression elsewhere while RT is being administered and for RT-related peritransplant morbidity such as esophagitis, pneumonitis, cardiomyopathy, and veno-occlusive disease. Possible disadvantages of this approach include the loss of the pretransplant cytoreductive effect and the theoretical carcinogenic effect of RT on the newly proliferating hematopoietic system (149,157,160).

Because of the historically high transplant-related mortality associated with allogeneic transplantation, autologous hematopoietic stem cell transplantation has been preferred for patients with relapsed HD. However, recent investigations of reduced-intensity allogeneic transplantation have demonstrated acceptable rates of transplant-related mortality (174,175). Nonmyeloablative conditioning regimens have varied, but most often they use fludarabine or low-dose TBI to provide a nontoxic immunosuppression. If successful, the procedure establishes a graft-versus-lymphoma effect and provides a platform for adoptive cellular immunotherapy. Evaluation of the effectiveness of this approach has been limited by reports describing treatment outcomes in small heterogeneous patient cohorts assigned to a variety of conditioning regimens in a nonrandom fashion. A longer follow-up period is needed to determine the efficacy of this approach.

RADIOTHERAPEUTIC MANAGEMENT

The curability of pediatric HD, the complexity of current treatment approaches, and the vulnerability of the developing child to radiation and chemotherapy require the involved radiation oncologist to thoroughly understand the role of radiation and to deliver it with skill. As discussed earlier, most newly diagnosed children are treated with risk-adapted chemotherapy alone or combined-modality therapy including low-dose IFRT. In the past, fully grown adolescents with favorable early-stage disease were considered for full-dose extended field RT using techniques that are standard for adults. This approach has been abandoned because of concerns about cardiac toxicity and second malignant neoplasms, which are discussed in Chapters 19 and 20, respectively. Historically, the Patterns of Care studies (176–178) guided the definition of RT standards of practice. Results of treatment with RT alone were statistically better at institutions that treated a large number of patients with HD. Factors associated with a higher risk of relapse included the use of inappropriate radiation field volume with inadequate margins, cobalt-60 machines with a source–skin distance of less than 80 cm, and treating without simulation. Certainly the last two inadequacies should not occur in the current era. Although different institutions and radiation oncologists may use slightly different treatment techniques, the underlying principles and most of the technical details remain constant (2,179–181). Because most children are treated in institutional (or multi-institutional) studies, the radiation oncologist should confirm all aspects of the diagnostic workup and staging and must also understand study requirements in order to deliver appropriate radiation. In a recent review of the DAL-HD-90

trial (German–Austrian pediatric multicenter trial), up-front centralized review of patients in the study altered the treatment approach in a large number of children (182). Unpublished data from the POG also support the superior outcome of children treated with appropriate radiation fields and dosages, in contrast to cases in which protocol violations occurred.

VOLUME CONSIDERATIONS

Most children with HD are treated with combined chemotherapy and low-dose IFRT. Meticulous and judiciously designed fields are necessary for optimizing disease control and tissue damage. The definitions of such fields depend on the anatomy of the region in terms of lymph node distribution, patterns of disease extension into regional areas, and consideration for match line problems should disease recur. Involved fields typically should include not just the identifiably abnormal lymph nodes but the entire lymph node region containing the involved nodes (Table 7-7). The traditional definitions of lymph node regions can be helpful but are not necessarily sufficient. For example, the cervical and supraclavicular lymph nodes generally are treated when abnormal nodes are located anywhere in this area; this is consistent with the

TABLE 7-7. *Involved-field radiation guidelines*

Involved nodes	Radiation field
Cervical	Neck and or supraclavicular[a]/infraclavicular
Supraclavicular	Supraclavicular/infraclavicular and lower neck
Axilla	Axilla with or without supraclavicular/infraclavicular
Mediastinum	Mediastinum, hila, and infraclavicular/supraclavicular[a,b]
Hila	Hila, mediastinum
Spleen	Spleen with or without para-aortic
Para-aortic	Para-aortic with or without spleen
Iliac	Iliac, inguinal, femoral
Inguinal	External iliac, inguinal, femoral
Femoral	External iliac, inguinal, femoral

[a]Upper cervical region not treated if supraclavicular involvement is extension of the mediastinal disease.

[b]Prechemotherapy volume is treated except for lateral borders of the mediastinal field.

anatomic definition of lymph node regions used for staging purposes (183). However, the hila are irradiated when the mediastinum is involved, despite the fact that the hila and mediastinum are separate lymph node regions. Similarly, the supraclavicular volume often is treated when the axilla or the mediastinum is involved, and the ipsilateral external iliac nodes often are treated when the inguinal nodes are involved. However, in both these situations care must be taken to shield relevant normal tissues such as the breast in the former situation and ovaries in the latter. Moreover, it might be appropriate to treat the axilla or mediastinum without the supraclavicular volume and the inguinal nodes without the iliacs depending on the size and distribution of involved nodes at presentation. Field definitions often are protocol specific, but excessively small fields usually are inappropriate. In a very young child (younger than 5 years), consideration may be given to treating bilateral areas (e.g., both sides of the neck) to avoid growth asymmetry. However, this is less of a concern with low radiation dosages, so unilateral fields usually are appropriate if the disease is unilateral. Every effort should be made to exclude unnecessary normal tissues (e.g., breast tissue in a child with isolated mediastinal disease and no axillary involvement). Treatment of involved supradiaphragmatic fields or a mantle field requires precision because of the distribution of lymph nodes and the critical adjacent normal tissues. These fields can be simulated with the arms up over the head or down with hands on the hips. The former pulls the axillary lymph nodes away from the lungs, allowing greater lung shielding. However, the axillary lymph nodes then move into the vicinity of the humeral heads, which should be blocked in growing children. Therefore, the position chosen involves weighing concerns regarding lymph nodes, lung, and humeral heads. Attempts should be made to exclude or position breast tissue under the lung and axillary blocking. When the decision is made to include some or all of a critical organ in the radiation field, such as liver, kidney, or heart, then normal tissue constraints, depending on the chemotherapy used and patient age, are critical.

Equally weighted anterior and posterior fields are used for daily treatment. Anteriorly weighted fields excessively irradiate the anterior heart, with associated cardiac morbidity (184). Dosage calculations should be based on the patient separation at the central axis. When a full mantle field is treated, nodes in the neck and axilla receive a higher dosage because the patient's body is thinner than at the midthorax. Therefore, separate axillary, neck, and low mediastinal dosimetry should be performed, and compensating filters or other modifications should be used to minimize inhomogeneity. Extended source-to-skin distances decrease dosage inhomogeneity in these different areas. Because of the increased dosage to the neck and cervical spinal cord, a posterior cervical spine block extending from the top of the field to below the level of the larynx may be added at a neck dosage of 20 Gy if midline disease is not present. Blocking the thoracic cord is not recommended because mediastinal nodes may be underdosed (181). Lung blocks should be carefully drawn, allowing adequate (1- to 2-cm) margins around mediastinal disease. If chemotherapy has been given, then the width of the field generally is based on the postchemotherapy residual disease, whereas the cephalad–caudad dimension respects the original disease extent. As previously stated, humeral head blocks are appropriate unless bulky axillary adenopathy would thereby be shielded. Laryngeal and occipital blocks are also used unless disease is located in the vicinity of these structures; these blocks can be placed at the beginning of treatment or after some portion of it. Depending on the response of the disease to chemotherapy and the dosage administered, field reductions may be possible. Because 10- to 15-Gy dosages can cytoreduce HD, increasing the size of lung or cardiac blocks often is possible once or twice during the course of therapy; however, it is uncommon to use RT when large disease bulk has not already been treated with chemotherapy. The entire heart and lungs are rarely treated above dosages of 10 to 16 Gy, depending on the distribution of disease and chemotherapy used. More specifically, the indications for whole heart irradiation include pericardial involvement as suggested by a pericardial effusion or frank pericardial invasion with tumor; such patients generally receive combined-modality therapy and 10 to 15 Gy to the entire heart. Whole lung irradiation with partial transmission blocks is an option in the setting of overt pulmonary nodules or hilar involvement. Again, this is protocol dependent because some children treated for advanced-stage HD receive RT only to areas of initial bulk disease or postchemotherapy residual disease. However, this approach remains investigational, and IFRT may remain the appropriate treatment approach. For children with pulmonary nodules at diagnosis, whole lung irradiation of 10 to 15 Gy is an option. A gap should be calculated in matching the para-aortic field (179,183).

When the subdiaphragmatic region is being treated, the spleen or pedicle must be included in patients who have splenic or para-aortic involvement, and the radiation dosage to the kidneys must be minimized. Usually the upper pole of the left kidney is within the irradiated volume. An intravenous pyelogram performed at the time of the simulation, a treatment planning CT, and diagnostic information obtained from the CT or MRI (coronal slices from a thoracic MRI will reveal the relationship of the spleen to the kidney) are helpful in drawing the blocks. When the pelvis is being treated, special attention must be given to the ovaries and testes. The ovaries should be relocated, marked with surgical clips, laterally along the iliac wings or centrally behind the uterus. In this manner, appropriate shielding may be used. The testes receive 5–10% of the administered pelvic dosage, which is sufficient to cause transient or permanent azoospermia, depending on the total pelvic dosage. The greatest shielding can be afforded to the testes if the patient is placed in a frog-legged position with an individually fitted testes shield. If multileaf collimation is available, the multileaf can be placed over the testes, additionally decreasing the transmitted dosage. Clearly, careful planning and judgment are necessary. As previously stated, RT for unfavorable and advanced HD is variable and protocol dependent. Although IFRT remains the standard when patients are treated with combined-modality therapy, restricting RT to areas of initial bulky disease (generally defined as larger than 5 cm at the time of disease presentation) or postchemother-

apy residual disease (generally defined as larger than 2 cm or residual PET avidity) is under investigation.

ENERGY

Megavoltage energies are necessary. A 4- to 6-MV linear accelerator should be used for supradiaphragmatic fields, thereby ensuring adequate dosages to the superficial nodes in the build-up region and to deep nodal areas such as the mediastinum. Higher-energy machines (8 to 15 MV) may be appropriate for treating para-aortic nodes. If high-energy machines must be used to treat the mantle field, some therapists use a beam spoiler or bolus on the neck and supraclavicular regions. Cobalt-60 units can underdose the field edge, and orthovoltage units are absolutely inappropriate. Distances of less than 80 cm are also contraindicated because of suboptimal depth–dosage characteristics.

DOSAGE CONSIDERATIONS

Kaplan (2) constructed a radiation dose–response curve for HD, but limitations of its current applicability include its use of kilovoltage data. Reports demonstrate that lower radiation dosages provide excellent local control, with variables including tumor size and fractionation schedule (176–178,180,185,186). In the absence of chemotherapy, subclinical disease is reliably (95%) controlled with 25 to 30 Gy, small bulk disease (variously defined but less than 5 cm in most reports) necessitates 30 to 35 Gy, and large bulk disease an additional 5 to 10 Gy. The dosages per fraction should be 1.5 to 1.8 Gy daily, five times a week. Patients treated with large volumes may tolerate only 1.5-Gy fractions. In the setting of combined therapy, certainly the intensity of the chemotherapy is important to consider in the choice of the radiation dosage and volume. However, dosages of 15 to 25 Gy are typical, with shrinking fields and boosts individualized. In Tables 7-4 and 7-5, the radiation dosages selected to complement the chemotherapy regimen are provided. In general, dosages of more than 25 Gy are uncommon in pediatrics. Of interest in this regard is the recently analyzed DAL-HD-90 trial, in which dosages of 20 to 25 Gy were administered in combination with OEPA or OPPA, with or without COPP. The radiation dosages administered were 20 to 25 Gy, with a local boost of 5 to 10 Gy for insufficient remission after chemotherapy. Tumor burden, indicated by bulky disease or number of involved nodes, proved not to be prognostically significant (144). Also of interest is the reported randomized trial by the German Hodgkin Lymphoma Group (187), in which adults with stage I to IIIA disease with intermediate prognosis received 20, 30, or 40 Gy to nonbulky or uninvolved sites after 4 months of chemotherapy. Bulky (larger than 7.5 cm) disease always received 40 Gy. With this constraint, no difference was observed for the various dosages.

SEQUENCE OF THERAPY

The most effective sequence of therapy in the setting of combined chemotherapy and irradiation has not been established. However, chemotherapy usually is the first modality. This allows assessment of drug response, maximization of the amount of drug treatment, and shrinkage of disease and more limited fields of irradiation. Occasionally, focal irradiation before chemotherapy is necessary because of airway obstruction.

RESULTS

In assessing the results of therapy for HD, specific reports must be evaluated for the following:

- Definitions of survival (e.g., event-free, relapse-free, freedom from progression, overall)
- Characteristics of the patient population regarding evaluation and prognostic factors
- Treatment regimens and techniques, including chemotherapy dosage intensity
- Morbidity and mortality of therapy

The actuarial 10-year survival for children with early-stage disease is 85–95%, and for children with advanced-stage disease it is 70–90% (Tables 7-4 and 7-5). The data for early-stage patients (Table 7-4) indicate a similar overall survival for patients treated with full-dose RT, combined full-dose RT and chemotherapy, and low-dose RT and chemotherapy. This was illustrated in a report by Donaldson et al. (101) comparing results in early-stage disease from Stanford (pathologic staging, extended-field RT alone or combined chemotherapy and IFRT) with those from St. Bartholomew's/Great Ormond Street (clinical staging, involved or regional-field full-dose RT). Overall survival from each institution was 91% at 10 years, although the disease-free survival for stage I patients at St. Bartholomew's/Great Ormond Street was somewhat lower than that at Stanford. However, the toxicities vary greatly between the treatment strategies, which underlie the recommendations present in Table 7-6.

Size of mediastinal disease is an important prognostic factor. Historically, the overall relapse-free survival is 53% for patients with LMA treated with RT alone, in contrast to 86% for small or no mediastinal disease. Overall survival is not significantly different (88% and 93%, respectively) because of the use of salvage chemotherapy. However, this high rate of relapse makes the use of initial chemotherapy with consolidative RT a more rational approach in patients with LMA. Regardless, combined modality therapy would currently be the standard of care. Although relapse-free and overall survival are excellent for patients with favorable, early-stage disease, patients with unfavorable disease continue to fare less well (Table 7-6). This is highlighted by the results from the GPOG HD-95 study of 830 children treated with two to six chemotherapy cycles and 20-Gy IFRT. The contrasting results for patients with favorable, intermediate, and unfavorable risk are depicted in Fig. 7-5 (61).

It is critical to appreciate the extent to which death from causes other than recurrence of HD compromises overall survival. Several investigators have observed a greater risk of mortality in long-term survivors of pediatric HD than in the general population (132,133,188). In the first 10 years after diagnosis, deaths were most commonly attributable to HD; with subsequent follow-up, subsequent cancers and cardiovascular disease contributed to higher mortality rates than in age- and sex-matched population control

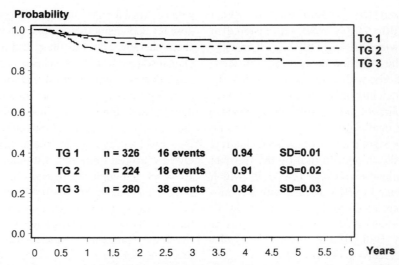

FIG. 7-5. Comparison of treatment outcomes on the German Pediatric Oncology Group HD-95 trial according to treatment risk group (TG) at a median follow-up time of 38 months. (From Wolden SL, Lamborn KR, Cleary SF, et al. Second cancers following pediatric Hodgkin's disease. *J Clin Oncol* 1998;16(2):536–544, Fig. 3, p. 1214, with permission.)

subjects. This is illustrated in Fig. 7-6, which demonstrates the cumulative incidence functions for cause-specific deaths among survivors of pediatric HD treated at St. Jude Children's Research Hospital (132). Standardized inci-

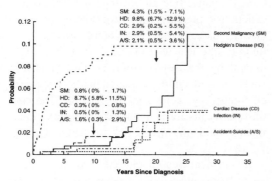

FIG. 7-6. Cumulative incidence functions for cause-specific deaths among St. Jude Children's Research Hospital cohort with Hodgkin's disease from second malignancy, Hodgkin's disease, cardiac disease, infection, and accident or suicide. Ten- and 20-year estimates are shown, with 95% confidence intervals in parentheses. (From Hudson MM, Poquette CA, Lee J, et al. Increased mortality after successful treatment for Hodgkin's disease. *J Clin Oncol* 1998; 16(11):3592–3600, with permission.)

dence ratios in this cohort showed a 12-fold elevated risk for all second malignancies, 11-fold elevated risk for a second solid tumor, and 33-fold elevated risk of breast cancer in female patients. Standardized mortality ratios also indicated greater mortality from cardiovascular disease (22; 95% CI, 8–48) and infection (18; 95% CI, 7–38). Importantly, HD consistently accounts for the majority of events in studies of long-term survivors; furthermore, relapse of HD is associated with a higher risk of subsequent events, including second cancers and cardiovascular disease. These findings underscore the need to proceed cautiously with therapeutic modifications because a reduced treatment intensity or duration may compromise disease control and promote late treatment complications.

COMPLICATIONS

Acute Side Effects

Acute side effects seen during mantle irradiation include temporary loss or change in taste, low posterior scalp epilation, xerostomia, skin erythema (particularly on the neck and shoulders), and occasional nausea and vomiting necessitating antiemetics. Acute effects of para-aortic irradiation are uncommon, but nausea and vomiting can occur. Late effects of para-aortic irradiation are also uncommon. Small bowel obstruction is rare because of the infrequency of surgical staging. For the few patients who have had abdominal surgery and irradiation, small bowel obstruction necessitating surgical intervention is related to the total dosage given: 1% for dosages less than 35 Gy and 3% for dosages greater than 35 Gy (176).

Long-Term Side Effects

Long-term adverse sequelae of greatest concern that are specific to irradiation in children include impairment of muscle and bone development (9,189–191) and injury to the lungs (192–195), heart (170,188,196–199), thyroid gland (200,201), and reproductive organs (107,202–211). Survivors who underwent surgical staging with splenectomy also have a lifelong risk of overwhelming sepsis from encapsulated bacterial organisms (212,213). Cardiovascular dysfunction and secondary carcinogenesis may result in early mortality in long-term survivors (132,170,198). Pulmonary fibrosis can compromise the quality of life in survivors. Long-term complications are discussed extensively in Chapter 20 and are briefly outlined here. Fortunately, these effects are less common with the use of modern treatment programs (60,103, 146).

Chronic pneumonitis and pulmonary fibrosis should be rare in the current era of treatment for primary HD. Predisposing therapies include thoracic radiation and ABVD chemotherapy (111, 169,192–195). The bleomycin in ABVD can cause both acute pulmonary compromise and late pulmonary fibrosis and can be augmented by the fibrosis that can be associated with pulmonary radiation. A "radiation recall" phenomenon can be seen when RT is administered after doxorubicin. Asymptomatic pulmonary dysfunction that improves over time has is observed after contemporary combined-modality treatment (194,195).

Cardiovascular disease is a major concern in survivors of pediatric HD. Cardiac dysfunction is most commonly observed after anthracycline therapy, particularly doxorubicin (196,197–199, 214). Young children may be at greater risk for anthracycline injury than adults because of an adverse effect on cardiac myocyte growth. This is suggested by studies of childhood leukemia survivors who demonstrate a high frequency of abnormalities of afterload and contractility (215). Mediastinal irradiation and other chemotherapeutic agents (e.g., cyclophosphamide) may predispose patients with pediatric HD to anthracycline-related myocardiopathy (197–199). The risk at very delayed time points (more than 20 years) has not been established.

Radiation also injures the pericardium and myocardium in a dose-related fashion (196, 199,214). High-dose (35- to 44-Gy) mantle irradiation produces cardiac injury in 13% of children and adults, most commonly manifest as constrictive pericarditis or accelerated coronary atherogenesis. Stanford investigators reported that the actuarial risk of developing cardiac disease necessitating pericardectomy was 4% at 17 years in a series of long-term survivors of childhood HD (199). Most patients with severe pericardial complications were irradiated before the introduction of subcarinal shielding and received little or no cardiac blocking. Premature coronary artery disease and acute myocardial infarction may also increase mortality risk in patients treated with mediastinal radiation in dosages of more than 30 Gy before 20 years of age (198). With the introduction of techniques that reduce the radiation dosage to the heart, the rates of radiation-associated cardiac injury have declined dramatically. Likewise, myocardial infarctions have not been systematically reported in children treated with combined-modality regimens using lower radiation dosages and volumes and protective cardiac shielding. Again, the impact of subclinical cardiac injury after low-dose RT may not become apparent until larger cohorts of survivors treated with these regimens begin to age.

Thyroid sequelae are common after RT for pediatric HD. Hypothyroidism, hyperthyroidism, thyroid nodules, and thyroid cancer have been observed in long-term survivors (200,201). Of these, hypothyroidism, particularly compensated hypothyroidism, defined as thyroid-stimulating hormone (TSH) elevation in the presence of a normal thyroxine (T4) level, is the most common thyroid abnormality. Risk factors for hypothyroidism include younger age at treatment and higher cumulative radiation dosage. As many as 78% of patients treated with radiation dosages greater than 26 Gy demonstrate thyroid dysfunction, as indicated by elevated TSH levels (195,201). Because persistent TSH elevation most often signals impending gland failure and may be a carcinogenic stimulus to the gland, thyroid hormone replacement therapy should be instituted. Gland suppression with thyroid hormone replacement is also recommended for patients who develop thyroid nodules after radiation. Replacement therapy should suppress gland function, as indicated by a TSH of 0.5 to 1.5 μIU/mL. Periodic withdrawal of hormonal therapy in asymptomatic patients permits assessment of gland recovery, which has been observed in some patients serially monitored after RT. Persistent and enlarging nodules should be monitored with ultrasound and periodic biopsies for malignant degeneration because thyroid carcinoma is a common second malignancy after HD (200). The risk of gonadal injury after HD is related to the type and intensity of treatment. In boys, high-dose pelvic radiation may produce a transient oligospermia or azoospermia, but spermatogenesis typically recovers (210,216). Six to eight cycles of MOPP (or similar hybrid chemotherapy-containing alkylators) produces irreversible sterility in 80–90% of male patients; fertility may be preserved if treatment is limited to three or fewer cycles (206). Recovery of gonadal function 10 to 15 years after MOPP chemotherapy has been rarely reported. Anthracycline-based regimens such as ABVD (or similar hybrid) usually are associated with full recovery of spermatogenesis after a temporary period of azoospermia (203,217). In contrast, testicular Leydig cell function is more resistant to the effects of antineoplastic treatment, so growth and puberty are adversely affected only in boys treated with very high cumulative dosages of alkylating agent chemotherapy. Risk-adapted therapies reducing or eliminating gonadotoxic

alkylating agent chemotherapy offer young men with newly diagnosed HD excellent prospects to maintain fertility (204).

Young women have a higher chance of maintaining regular menses after treatment for HD than older women. The risk of ovarian failure after pelvic radiation is high but can be reduced by midline ovarian transposition (oophoropexy) (202). Although most young women maintain or resume menses after MOPP (or similar hybrid) chemotherapy, they are predisposed to early menopause, particularly if they also received abdominal–pelvic radiation (107,205,211). In a report of female HD survivors by the Late Effects Study Group, 42% of women treated with alkylating agent chemotherapy and subdiaphragmatic radiation had experienced menopause by age 31 years, compared with 5% of control subjects (205). Reports by other groups have not indicated an excessive risk of premature menopause in young women treated with supradiaphragmatic RT alone (211).

The overall cumulative risk of developing a subsequent malignancy after treatment for pediatric HD ranges from 7% to 8% at 15 years from diagnosis and rises to 16–28% by 20 years (133,142,218–227). Tumor histologies comprise two main types: acute myeloid leukemia (including a pancytopenic myelodysplastic syndrome) and solid tumors. Secondary leukemias exhibit a brief latency with a peak frequency in the first 5 to 10 years after treatment. The risk decreases to less than 2% after 10 years from diagnosis. Clinical and treatment factors correlated with secondary leukemogenesis include older age at treatment, history of splenectomy, presentation with advanced disease, treatment with high cumulative dosages of alkylating agents, and history of relapse (133,142,219, 221–229). In contrast to secondary hematopoietic malignancies, the risk of developing a second solid tumor increases with the passage of time from diagnosis, with a latency usually exceeding 10 years from diagnosis. A variety of solid tumors have been observed, most commonly involving the breast, thyroid, bone, and soft tissues (39,133,142,218–220,223–228,230, 231).

FUTURE INVESTIGATIONS

Devising new strategies to treat children with HD is problematic because of the overall success of current treatment regimens. However, grouping patients into different risk categories allows investigators to construct protocols intended to diminish therapy-induced toxicity for patients with favorable prognoses, improve treatment effectiveness for patients with unfavorable prognoses, and aim for both goals in patients who are intermediate in their prognosis. Unfortunately, the ability to conduct clinical trials in which the differences in survival between treatment arms are likely to be small is compromised by the large patient numbers necessary to detect such differences. If a reduction in treatment toxicity is the intended goal of a new regimen, then many years of follow-up are necessary to prove effectiveness. Some generalizations regarding ongoing efforts in clinical trials for pediatric HD are as follows:

- Patients with early-stage disease (I, IIA without bulk disease, and perhaps IIB disease with sweats as the only systemic symptom) have an excellent prognosis. Therefore, can the intensity and duration of chemotherapy be decreased, and can agents be used that are associated with less severe side effects? Concomitantly, can the volume and perhaps dosage of RT be reduced? Can the amount of chemotherapy be based on the response to the initial cycles? Will chemoprotectants and radioprotectants prove useful?
- Patients with disease of an intermediate stage or with characteristics indicating that their prognosis is intermediate (II with bulky disease, IIB with fevers or weight loss, IIIA) are appropriate for studies that intend to increase efficacy without increasing toxicity. Generally, this entails modification of existing chemoradiotherapy programs.
- Patients with advanced-stage disease (IIIB, IV) need more effective treatment regimens. These might include increasing dosage intensity or the rate of drug delivery and combining agents into new regimens. The use of hematopoietic growth factors may assist in

drug delivery. Defining the role of RT in such trials will continue to be an important objective.

Of interest, ongoing trials are evaluating the paradigm of early response using functional imaging as a prognostic factor for therapy reduction or intensification.

Finally, immunotherapeutic approaches are under development and investigation, such as the use of antiferritin antibody jointed with yttrium-90 (232), EBV-specific cytotoxic T lymphocytes (233), and monoclonal antibody immunotherapy targeting cell surface antigens (e.g., CD20, CD30) (234,235). If effective, these novel approaches will provide an alternative to cytotoxic treatment approaches with potentially fewer adverse long-term treatment effects.

REFERENCES

References particularly recommended for further reading are marked with an asterisk.

1. Hodgkin T. On some morbid appearances of the absorbent gland and spleen. *Med Chir Trans* 1832; 17:68–114.
2. Kaplan H. *Hodgkin's disease.* Cambridge, MA: Harvard University Press, 1980.
3. Pusey W. Cases of sarcomas and of Hodgkin's disease treated by exposures to X rays: a preliminary report. *JAMA* 1902;38:166–170.
4. Gilbert R. Radiotherapy in Hodgkin's disease (malignant granulomatosis): anatomic and clinical foundations, governing principles, results. *AJR* 1939;41: 198–241.
5. Peters M. A study of survival in Hodgkin's disease treated radiologically. *AJR* 1950;63:299–311.
6. Goodman L, Wintrobe M, Dameshe W, et al. Nitrogen mustard therapy: use of methyl-bis-(chloroethyl)amine hydrochloride for Hodgkin's disease, lymphosarcoma, leukemia and certain allied and miscellaneous disorders. *JAMA* 1946;132:126–131.
7. De Vita VTJ, Canellos G, Moxley J. A decade of combination chemotherapy of advanced Hodgkin's disease. *Cancer* 1972;30:1495–1504.
8. Seif G, Spriggs A Chromosome changes in Hodgkin's disease. *J Natl Cancer Inst* 1967;39: 557–570.
9. Donaldson SS, Kaplan HS. Complications of treatment of Hodgkin's disease in children. *Cancer Treat Rep* 1982;66(4):977–989.
10. Mauch PM, Weinstein H, Botnick L, et al. An evaluation of long-term survival and treatment complications in children with Hodgkin's disease. *Cancer* 1983;51(5):925–932.

11. Donaldson SS, Glatstein E, Rosenberg SA, et al. Pediatric Hodgkin's disease. II. Results of therapy. *Cancer* 1976;37(5):2436–2447.

12. Donaldson SS, Link MP. Combined modality treatment with low-dose radiation and MOPP chemotherapy for children with Hodgkin's disease. *J Clin Oncol* 1987;5(5):742–749.

13. Donaldson SS, Link MP. Hodgkin's disease. Treatment of the young child. *Pediatr Clin North Am* 1991;38(2):457–473.

14. Schellong G, Bramswig JH, Hornig-Franz I, et al. Hodgkin's disease in children: combined modality treatment for stages IA, IB, and IIA. Results in 356 patients of the German/Austrian Pediatric Study Group. *Ann Oncol* 1994;5[Suppl 2]:113–115.

15. Schellong G. The balance between cure and late effects in childhood Hodgkin's lymphoma: the experience of the German–Austrian Study Group since 1978. *Ann Oncol* 1996;7[Suppl 4]:67–72.

16. Schellong G. Treatment of children and adolescents with Hodgkin's disease: the experience of the German–Austrian Paediatric Study Group. *Baillieres Clin Haematol* 1996;9(3):619–634.

17. Oberlin O, Boilletot A, Leverger G, et al. Clinical staging, primary chemotherapy and involved field radiotherapy in childhood Hodgkin's disease. *Eur Paediatr Haematol Oncol* 1985;2:65–70.

18. Dionet C, Oberlin O, Habrand JL, et al. Initial chemotherapy and low-dose radiation in limited fields in childhood Hodgkin's disease: results of a joint cooperative study by the French Society of Pediatric Oncology (SFOP) and Hôpital Saint-Louis, Paris. *Int J Radiat Oncol Biol Phys* 1988;15(2):341–346.

19. Jenkin D, Doyle J, Berry M, et al. Hodgkin's disease in children: treatment with MOPP and low-dose, extended field irradiation without laparotomy. Late results and toxicity. *Med Pediatr Oncol* 1990;18(4):265–272.

20. Cleary SF, Link MP, Donaldson SS. Hodgkin's disease in the very young. *Int J Radiat Oncol Biol Phys* 1994;28(1):77–83.

21. Kennedy BJ, Loeb V Jr, Peterson V, et al. Survival in Hodgkin's disease by stage and age. *Med Pediatr Oncol* 1992;20(2):100–104.

22. Kung FH. Hodgkin's disease in children 4 years of age or younger. *Cancer* 1991;67(5):1428–1430.

23. Mauch P, Tarbell N, Weinstein H, et al. Stage IA and IIA supradiaphragmatic Hodgkin's disease: prognostic factors in surgically staged patients treated with mantle and paraaortic irradiation. *J Clin Oncol* 1988;6(10):1576–1583.

24. Jox A, Zander T, Diehl V, et al. Clonal relapse in Hodgkin's disease. *N Engl J Med* 1997;337(7):499.

25. Kanzler H, Kuppers R, Hansmann ML, et al. Hodgkin and Reed–Sternberg cells in Hodgkin's disease represent the outgrowth of a dominant tumor clone derived from (crippled) germinal center B cells. *J Exp Med* 1996;184(4):1495–1505.

26. Fiumara P, Snell V, Li Y, et al. Functional expression of receptor activator of nuclear factor kappaB in Hodgkin disease cell lines. *Blood* 2001;98(9):2784–2790.

27. Gupta RK, Patel K, Bodmer WF, et al. Mutation of p53 in primary biopsy material and cell lines from Hodgkin disease. *Proc Natl Acad Sci U S A* 1993;90(7):2817–2821.

28. Ambinder RF, Browning PJ, Lorenzana I, et al. Epstein–Barr virus and childhood Hodgkin's disease in Honduras and the United States. *Blood* 1993;81(2):462–467.

29. Klein G. Epstein–Barr virus–carrying cells in Hodgkin's disease. *Blood* 1992;80(2):299–301.

30. Weiss LM, Movahed LA, Warnke RA, et al. Detection of Epstein–Barr viral genomes in Reed–Sternberg cells of Hodgkin's disease. *N Engl J Med* 1989;320(8):502–506.

31. Gupta RK, Whelan JS, Lister TA, et al. Direct sequence analysis of the t(14;18) chromosomal translocation in Hodgkin's disease. *Blood* 1992;79(8):2084–2088.

32. Poppema S, Kaleta J, Hepperle B. Chromosomal abnormalities in patients with Hodgkin's disease: evidence for frequent involvement of the 14q chromosomal region but infrequent bcl-2 gene rearrangement in Reed–Sternberg cells. *J Natl Cancer Inst* 1992;84(23):1789–1793.

33. Stein H, Hummel M, Durkop H, et al. Biology of Hodgkin's disease. In: Canellos GLT, Lister TA, Sklar JL, Lampert R, eds. *The lymphomas.* Philadelphia: W.B. Saunders, 1998:287–304.

34. Gruss HJ, Pinto A, Duyster J, et al. Hodgkin's disease: a tumor with disturbed immunological pathways. *Immunol Today* 1997;18(4):156–163.

35. Schwartz RS. Hodgkin's disease: time for a change. *N Engl J Med* 1997;337(7):495–496.

36. Marafioti T, Hummel M, Anagnostopoulos I, et al. Origin of nodular lymphocyte–predominant Hodgkin's disease from a clonal expansion of highly mutated germinal-center B cells. *N Engl J Med* 1997;337(7):453–458.

37. Ohno T, Stribley JA, Wu G, et al. Clonality in nodular lymphocyte-predominant Hodgkin's disease. *N Engl J Med* 1997;337(7):459–465.

*38. Harris NL, Jaffe ES, Stein H, et al. A revised European–American classification of lymphoid neoplasms: a proposal from the International Lymphoma Study Group. *Blood* 1994;84(5):1361–1392.

39. Tarbell NJ, Gelber RD, Weinstein HJ, et al. Sex differences in risk of second malignant tumours after Hodgkin's disease in childhood. *Lancet* 1993;341(8858):1428–1432.

40. Spitz MR, Sider JG, Johnson CC, et al. Ethnic patterns of Hodgkin's disease incidence among children and adolescents in the United States, 1973–82. *J Natl Cancer Inst* 1986;76(2):235–239.

41. Miller RW. Mortality in childhood Hodgkin's disease. An etiologic clue. *JAMA* 1966;198(11):1216–1217.

42. MacMahon B. Epidemiological evidence on the nature of Hodgkin's disease. *Cancer* 1957;10:1045–1054.

43. Vianna NJ, Polan AK. Epidemiologic evidence for transmission of Hodgkin's disease. *N Engl J Med* 1973;289(10):499–502.

44. Grufferman S, Delzell E. Epidemiology of Hodgkin's disease. *Epidemiol Rev* 1984;6:76–106.

45. Razzouk BI, Gan YJ, Mendonca C, et al. Ep-

stein–Barr virus in pediatric Hodgkin disease: age and histiotype are more predictive than geographic region. *Med Pediatr Oncol* 1997;28(4):248–254.

46. Robertson SJ, Lowman JT, Grufferman S, et al. Familial Hodgkin's disease. A clinical and laboratory investigation. *Cancer* 1987;59(7):1314–1319.

47. Mack TM, Cozen W, Shibata DK, et al. Concordance for Hodgkin's disease in identical twins suggesting genetic susceptibility to the young-adult form of the disease. *N Engl J Med* 1995;332(7):413–418.

48. Slivnick DJ, Nawrocki JF, Fisher RI. Immunology and cellular biology of Hodgkin's disease. *Hematol Oncol Clin North Am* 1989;3(2):205–220.

49. Watanabe N, De Rosa SC, Cmelak A, et al. Long-term depletion of naive T cells in patients treated for Hodgkin's disease. *Blood* 1997;90(9):3662–3672.

50. Filipovich AH, Mathur A, Kamat D, et al. Primary immunodeficiencies: genetic risk factors for lymphoma. *Cancer Res* 1992;52[Suppl 19 Suppl]:5465s–5467s.

51. Rubio R. Hodgkin's disease associated with human immunodeficiency virus infection. A clinical study of 46 cases. *Cancer* 1994;73(9):2400–2407.

52. Mauch PM, Kalish LA, Kadin M, et al. Patterns of presentation of Hodgkin disease. Implications for etiology and pathogenesis. *Cancer* 1993;71(6):2062–2071.

53. Lister TA, Crowther D, Sutcliffe SB, et al. Report of a committee convened to discuss the evaluation and staging of patients with Hodgkin's disease: Cotswolds meeting. *J Clin Oncol* 1989;7(11):1630–1636.

54. Jackson H, Parker F. Hodgkin's disease II: pathology. *N Engl J Med* 1994:35.

55. Ferry JA, Harris NL. The pathology of Hodgkin's disease: what's new? *Semin Radiat Oncol* 1996;6(3):121–130.

56. Pellegrino B, Terrier-Lacombe MJ, Oberlin O, et al. Lymphocyte-predominant Hodgkin's lymphoma in children: therapeutic abstention after initial lymph node resection—a study of the French Society of Pediatric Oncology. *J Clin Oncol* 2003;21(15):2948–2952.

57. Sandoval C, Venkateswaran L, Billups C, et al. Lymphocyte-predominant Hodgkin disease in children. *J Pediatr Hematol Oncol* 2002;24(4):269–273.

58. Karayalcin G, Behm FG, Gieser PW, et al. Lymphocyte predominant Hodgkin disease: clinico-pathologic features and results of treatment—the Pediatric Oncology Group experience. *Med Pediatr Oncol* 1997;29(6):519–525.

59. Farah R, Weichselbaum RR. Substaging of stage III Hodgkin's disease. *Hematol Oncol Clin North Am* 1989;3(2):277–286.

*60. Nachman JB, Sposto R, Herzog P, et al. Randomized comparison of low-dose involved-field radiotherapy and no radiotherapy for children with Hodgkin's disease who achieve a complete response to chemotherapy. *J Clin Oncol* 2002;20(18):3765–3771.

*61. Ruhl U, Albrecht M, Dieckmann K, et al. Response-adapted radiotherapy in the treatment of pediatric Hodgkin's disease: an interim report at 5 years of the German GPOH-HD 95 trial. *Int J Radiat Oncol Biol Phys* 2001;51(5):1209–1218.

62. Pui CH, Ip SH, Thompson E, et al. High serum inter-leukin-2 receptor levels correlate with a poor prognosis in children with Hodgkin's disease. *Leukemia* 1989;3(7):481–484.

63. Gause A, Pohl C, Tschiersch A, et al. Clinical significance of soluble CD30 antigen in the sera of patients with untreated Hodgkin's disease. *Blood* 1991;77(9):1983–1988.

64. Wieland A, Kerbl R, Berghold A, et al. C-reactive protein (CRP) as tumor marker in pediatric and adolescent patients with Hodgkin disease. *Med Pediatr Oncol* 2003;41(1):21–25.

65. Mahoney DH Jr, Schreuders LC, Gresik MV, et al. Role of staging bone marrow examination in children with Hodgkin disease. *Med Pediatr Oncol* 1998;30(3):175–177.

66. Castellino RA, Blank N, Hoppe RT, et al. Hodgkin disease: contributions of chest CT in the initial staging evaluation. *Radiology* 1986;160(3):603–605.

67. Rostock RA, Giangreco A, Wharam MD, et al. CT scan modification in the treatment of mediastinal Hodgkin's disease. *Cancer* 1982;49(11):2267–2275.

68. Hanna SL, Fletcher BD, Boulden TF, et al. MR imaging of infradiaphragmatic lymphadenopathy in children and adolescents with Hodgkin disease: comparison with lymphography and CT. *J Magn Reson Imaging* 1993;3(3):461–470.

69. Mendenhall NP, Cantor AB, Williams JL, et al. With modern imaging techniques, is staging laparotomy necessary in pediatric Hodgkin's disease? A Pediatric Oncology Group study. *J Clin Oncol* 1993;11(11):2218–2225.

70. Weiner M, Leventhal B, Cantor A, et al. Gallium-67 scans as an adjunct to computed tomography scans for the assessment of a residual mediastinal mass in pediatric patients with Hodgkin's disease. A Pediatric Oncology Group study. *Cancer* 1991;68(11):2478–2480.

71. Bar-Shalom R, Valcivia AY, Blaufox MD. PET imaging in oncology. *Semin Nucl Med* 2000;30(3):150–185.

72. Bar-Shalom R, Yefremov N, Haim N, et al. Camera-based FDG PET and 67Ga SPECT in evaluation of lymphoma: comparative study. *Radiology* 2003;227(2):353–360.

73. Hueltenschmid B, Sautter-Bihl ML, Lang O, et al. Whole body positron emission tomography in the treatment of Hodgkin disease. *Cancer* 2001;91(2):302–310.

74. Jadvar H, Connolly L, Shulkin B, et al. Positron-emission tomography in pediatrics. In: Leonard M, Freeman MD, eds. *Nuclear medicine annual 2000*. Philadelphia: Lippincott Williams & Wilkins, 2000.

75. Jerusalem G, Beguin Y, Fassotte MF, et al. Whole-body positron emission tomography using ^{18}F-fluorodeoxyglucose for posttreatment evaluation in Hodgkin's disease and non-Hodgkin's lymphoma has higher diagnostic and prognostic value than classical computed tomography scan imaging. *Blood* 1999;94(2):429–433.

76. Wirth A, Seymour JF, Hicks RJ, et al. Fluorine-18 fluorodeoxyglucose positron emission tomography, gallium-67 scintigraphy, and conventional staging for Hodgkin's disease and non-Hodgkin's lymphoma. *Am J Med* 2002;112(4):262–268.

77. Specht L. Prognostic factors in Hodgkin's disease. *Semin Radiat Oncol* 1996;6(3):146–161.

78. Bader SB, Weinstein H, Mauch P, et al. Pediatric stage IV Hodgkin disease. Long-term survival. *Cancer* 1993;72(1):249–255.

79. Smith R, Chen Q, Hudson M. Prognostic factors in pediatric Hodgkin's disease. *Int J Radiat Oncol Biol Phys* 2001;51(3):199.

80. Behar RA, Hoppe RT. Radiation therapy in the management of bulky mediastinal Hodgkin's disease. *Cancer* 1990;66(1):75–79.

81. Hoppe RT. Stage I–II Hodgkin's disease: current therapeutic options and recommendations. *Blood* 1983;62(1):32–36.

82. Maity A, Goldwein JW, Lange B, et al. Mediastinal masses in children with Hodgkin's disease. An analysis of the Children's Hospital of Philadelphia and the Hospital of the University of Pennsylvania experience. *Cancer* 1992;69(11):2755–2760.

83. Specht L, Nordentoft AM, Cold S, et al. Tumor burden as the most important prognostic factor in early stage Hodgkin's disease. Relations to other prognostic factors and implications for choice of treatment. *Cancer* 1988;61(8):1719–1727.

84. Hoppe RT, Coleman CN, Cox RS, et al. The management of stage I–II Hodgkin's disease with irradiation alone or combined modality therapy: the Stanford experience. *Blood* 1982;59(3):455e465.

85. Tubiana M, Henry-Amar M, Carde P, et al. Toward comprehensive management tailored to prognostic factors of patients with clinical stages I and II in Hodgkin's disease. The EORTC Lymphoma Group controlled clinical trials: 1964–1987. *Blood* 1989; 73(1):47–56.

86. Hoppe RT, Cox RS, Rosenberg SA, et al. Prognostic factors in pathologic stage III Hodgkin's disease. *Cancer Treat Rep* 1982;66(4):743–749.

87. Crnkovich MJ, Leopold K, Hoppe RT, et al. Stage I to IIB Hodgkin's disease: the combined experience at Stanford University and the Joint Center for Radiation Therapy. *J Clin Oncol* 1987;5(7):1041–1049.

88. Friedman S, Henry-Amar M, Cosset JM, et al. Evaluation of erythrocyte sedimentation rate as predictor of early relapse in posttherapy early-stage Hodgkin's disease. *J Clin Oncol* 1988;6(4):596–602.

89. Pui CH, Ip SH, Thompson E, et al. Increased serum CD8 antigen level in childhood Hodgkin's disease relates to advanced stage and poor treatment outcome. *Blood* 1989;73(1):209–213.

90. Christiansen I, Sundstrom C, Enblad G, et al. Soluble vascular cell adhesion molecule-1 (sVCAM-1) is an independent prognostic marker in Hodgkin's disease. *Br J Haematol* 1998;102(3):701–709.

91. Warzocha K, Bienvenu J, Ribeiro P, et al. Plasma levels of tumour necrosis factor and its soluble receptors correlate with clinical features and outcome of Hodgkin's disease patients. *Br J Cancer* 1998; 77(12):2357–2362.

92. Nadali G, Tavecchia L, Zanolin E, et al. Serum level of the soluble form of the CD30 molecule identifies patients with Hodgkin's disease at high risk of unfavorable outcome. *Blood* 1998;91(8):3011–3016.

93. Chronowski GM, Wilder RB, Tucker SL, et al. An elevated serum beta-2-microglobulin level is an adverse prognostic factor for overall survival in patients with early-stage Hodgkin disease. *Cancer* 2002; 95(12):2534–2538.

94. Hann HW, Lange B, Stahlhut MW, et al. Prognostic importance of serum transferrin and ferritin in childhood Hodgkin's disease. *Cancer* 1990;66(2): 313–316.

95. Bohlen H, Kessler M, Sextro M, et al. Poor clinical outcome of patients with Hodgkin's disease and elevated interleukin-10 serum levels. Clinical significance of interleukin-10 serum levels for Hodgkin's disease. *Ann Hematol* 2000;79(3):110–113.

96. Dukers DF, Meijer CJ, ten Berge RL, et al. High numbers of active caspase 3–positive Reed–Sternberg cells in pretreatment biopsy specimens of patients with Hodgkin disease predict favorable clinical outcome. *Blood* 2002;100(1):36–42.

97. von Wasielewski S, Franklin J, Fischer R, et al. Nodular sclerosing Hodgkin disease: new grading predicts prognosis in intermediate and advanced stages. *Blood* 2003;101(10):4063–4069.

98. Shankar AG, Ashley S, Radford M, et al. Does histology influence outcome in childhood Hodgkin's disease? Results from the United Kingdom Children's Cancer Study Group. *J Clin Oncol* 1997;15(7): 2622–2630.

99. Carde P, Koscielny S, Franklin J, et al. Early response to chemotherapy: a surrogate for final outcome of Hodgkin's disease patients that should influence initial treatment length and intensity? *Ann Oncol* 2002;13[Suppl 1]:86–91.

100. Barrett A, Crennan E, Barnes J, et al. Treatment of clinical stage I Hodgkin's disease by local radiation therapy alone. A United Kingdom Children's Cancer Study Group study. *Cancer* 1990;66(4): 670–674.

*101. Donaldson SS, Whitaker SJ, Plowman PN, et al. Stage I–II pediatric Hodgkin's disease: long-term follow-up demonstrates equivalent survival rates following different management schemes. *J Clin Oncol* 1990;8(7):1128–1137.

102. Gehan EA, Sullivan MP, Fuller LM, et al. The intergroup Hodgkin's disease in children. A study of stages I and II. *Cancer* 1990;65(6):1429–1437.

103. Hunger SP, Link MP, Donaldson SS. ABVD/MOPP and low-dose involved-field radiotherapy in pediatric Hodgkin's disease: the Stanford experience. *J Clin Oncol* 1994;12(10):2160–2166.

104. Schellong G, Bramswig JH, Hornig-Franz I. Treatment of children with Hodgkin's disease: results of the German Pediatric Oncology Group. *Ann Oncol* 1992;3[Suppl 4]:73–76.

105. DeVita V, Mauch P, Harris NL. Hodgkin's disease. In: DeVita VT Jr, Hellman S, Rosenberg SA, eds. *Cancer: principles and practice of oncology*. Philadelphia: Lippincott–Raven Publishers, 1997: 2242–2283.

106. Longo DL, Young RC, Wesley M, et al. Twenty years of MOPP therapy for Hodgkin's disease. *J Clin Oncol* 1986;4(9):1295–1306.

107. Horning SJ, Hoppe RT, Kaplan HS, et al. Female reproductive potential after treatment for Hodgkin's disease. *N Engl J Med* 1981;304(23):1377–1382.

108. Bonadonna G, Zucali R, Monfardini S, et al. Combination chemotherapy of Hodgkin's disease with adriamycin, bleomycin, vinblastine, and imidazole car-

boxamide versus MOPP. *Cancer* 1975;36(1):252–259.

109. Santoro A, Bonadonna G, Valagussa P, et al. Long-term results of combined chemotherapy–radiotherapy approach in Hodgkin's disease: superiority of ABVD plus radiotherapy versus MOPP plus radiotherapy. *J Clin Oncol* 1987;5(1):27–37.

110. Hutchinson R, Krailo M, Fryer C. Prognostic factor analysis in advanced Hodgkin's disease (stages III and IV). Results of the CCG 521 trial. *Med Pediatr Oncol* 1993;61.

111. Fryer CJ, Hutchinson RJ, Krailo M, et al. Efficacy and toxicity of 12 courses of ABVD chemotherapy followed by low-dose regional radiation in advanced Hodgkin's disease in children: a report from the Children's Cancer Study Group. *J Clin Oncol* 1990; 8(12):1971–1980.

112. Bonadonna G, Valagussa P, Santoro A. Alternating non–cross-resistant combination chemotherapy or MOPP in stage IV Hodgkin's disease. A report of 8-year results. *Ann Intern Med* 1986;104(6): 739–746.

113. LaMonte CS, Yeh SD, Straus DJ. Long-term follow-up of cardiac function in patients with Hodgkin's disease treated with mediastinal irradiation and combination chemotherapy including doxorubicin. *Cancer Treat Rep* 1986;70(4):439–444.

114. Maity A, Goldwein JW, Lange B, et al. Comparison of high-dose and low-dose radiation with and without chemotherapy for children with Hodgkin's disease: an analysis of the experience at the Children's Hospital of Philadelphia and the Hospital of the University of Pennsylvania. *J Clin Oncol* 1992;10(6):929–935.

115. Weiner MA, Leventhal BG, Marcus R, et al. Intensive chemotherapy and low-dose radiotherapy for the treatment of advanced-stage Hodgkin's disease in pediatric patients: a Pediatric Oncology Group study. *J Clin Oncol* 1991;9(9):1591–1598.

116. Ekert H, Waters KD, Smith PJ, et al. Treatment with MOPP or ChlVPP chemotherapy only for all stages of childhood Hodgkin's disease. *J Clin Oncol* 1988;6(12):1845–1850.

117. Yahalom J, Ryu J, Straus DJ, et al. Impact of adjuvant radiation on the patterns and rate of relapse in advanced-stage Hodgkin's disease treated with alternating chemotherapy combinations. *J Clin Oncol* 1991;9(12):2193–2201.

118. van den Berg H. Hodgkin's disease. *Ned Tijdschr Geneeskd* 1997;141(39):1877–1878.

119. van den Berg H, Zsiros J, Behrendt H. Treatment of childhood Hodgkin's disease without radiotherapy. *Ann Oncol* 1997;8[Suppl 1]:15–17.

120. Behrendt H, Van Bunningen BN, Van Leeuwen EF. Treatment of Hodgkin's disease in children with or without radiotherapy. *Cancer* 1987;59(11):1870–1873.

121. Lobo-Sanahuja F, Garcia I, Barrantes JC, et al. Pediatric Hodgkin's disease in Costa Rica: twelve years' experience of primary treatment by chemotherapy alone, without staging laparotomy. *Med Pediatr Oncol* 1994;22(6):398–403.

122. Olweny CL, Katongole-Mbidde E, Kiire C, et al. Childhood Hodgkin's disease in Uganda: a ten year experience. *Cancer* 1978;42(2):787–792.

123. Sackmann-Muriel F, Zubizarreta P, Gallo G, et al.

Hodgkin disease in children: results of a prospective randomized trial in a single institution in Argentina. *Med Pediatr Oncol* 1997;29(6):544–552.

124. Ekert H, Fok T, Dalla-Pozza L, et al. A pilot study of EVAP/ABV chemotherapy in 25 newly diagnosed children with Hodgkin's disease. *Br J Cancer* 1993;67(1):159–162.

125. Ekert H, Toogood I, Downie P, et al. High incidence of treatment failure with vincristine, etoposide, epirubicin, and prednisolone chemotherapy with successful salvage in childhood Hodgkin disease. *Med Pediatr Oncol* 1999;33(4):255–258.

126. Baez F, Ocampo E, Conter V, et al. Treatment of childhood Hodgkin's disease with COPP or COPP-ABV (hybrid) without radiotherapy in Nicaragua. *Ann Oncol* 1997;8(3):247–250.

127. Sripada PV, Tenali SC, Vasudevan M, et al. Hybrid (COPP/ABV) therapy in childhood Hodgkin's disease: a study of 53 cases during 1989–1993 at the Cancer Institute, Madras. *Pediatr Hematol Oncol* 1995;12(4):333–341.

*128. Weiner MA, Leventhal B, Brecher ML, et al. Randomized study of intensive MOPP-ABVD with or without low-dose total-nodal radiation therapy in the treatment of stages IIB, IIIA2, IIIB, and IV Hodgkin's disease in pediatric patients: a Pediatric Oncology Group study. *J Clin Oncol* 1997;15(8): 2769–2779.

129. Shankar AG, Ashley S, Atra A, et al. A limited role for VEEP (vincristine, etoposide, epirubicin, prednisolone) chemotherapy in childhood Hodgkin's disease. *Eur J Cancer* 1998;34(13):2058–2063.

130. Behrendt H, Brinkhuis M, Van Leeuwen EF. Treatment of childhood Hodgkin's disease with ABVD without radiotherapy. *Med Pediatr Oncol* 1996;26(4): 244–248.

131. Donaldson SS, Lamborn KR. Radiation in pediatric Hodgkin's disease. *J Clin Oncol* 1998;16(1): 391–393.

132. Hudson MM, Poquette CA, Lee J, et al. Increased mortality after successful treatment for Hodgkin's disease. *J Clin Oncol* 1998;16(11):3592–3600.

133. Wolden SL, Lamborn KR, Cleary SF, et al. Second cancers following pediatric Hodgkin's disease. *J Clin Oncol* 1998;16(2):536–544.

134. Friedmann AM, Hudson MM, Weinstein HJ, et al. Treatment of unfavorable childhood Hodgkin's disease with VEPA and low-dose, involved-field radiation. *J Clin Oncol* 15 2002;20(14):3088–3094.

*135. Donaldson SS, Hudson MM, Lamborn KR, et al. VAMP and low-dose, involved-field radiation for children and adolescents with favorable, early-stage Hodgkin's disease: results of a prospective clinical trial. *J Clin Oncol* 2002;20(14):3081–3087.

136. Landman-Parker J, Pacquement H, Leblanc T, et al. Localized childhood Hodgkin's disease: response-adapted chemotherapy with etoposide, bleomycin, vinblastine, and prednisone before low-dose radiation therapy. Results of the French Society of Pediatric Oncology Study MDH90. *J Clin Oncol* 2000;18(7):1500–1507.

137. Lemerle J, Oberlin O, Schaison G, et al. Hodgkin's disease in children: adaptation of treatment to risk factors. *Recent Results Cancer Res* 1989;117:214–221.

138. Oberlin O, Habrand JL, Schaison G, et al. Hodgkin's

disease in children. Current therapeutic strategies. *Bull Cancer* 1988;75(1):53–60.

139. Oberlin O, Leverger G, Pacquement H, et al. Low-dose radiation therapy and reduced chemotherapy in childhood Hodgkin's disease: the experience of the French Society of Pediatric Oncology. *J Clin Oncol* 1992;10(10):1602–1608.

140. Vecchi V, Pileri S, Burnelli R, et al. Treatment of pediatric Hodgkin disease tailored to stage, mediastinal mass, and age. An Italian (AIEOP) multicenter study on 215 patients. *Cancer* 1993;72(6):2049–2057.

141. Bayle-Weisgerber C, Lemercier N, Teillet F, et al. Hodgkin's disease in children. Results of therapy in a mixed group of 178 clinical and pathologically staged patients over 13 years. *Cancer* 1984;54(2): 215–222.

142. Beaty O III, Hudson MM, Greenwald C, et al. Subsequent malignancies in children and adolescents after treatment for Hodgkin's disease. *J Clin Oncol* 1995;13(3):603–609.

143. Cramer P, Andrieu JM. Hodgkin's disease in childhood and adolescence: results of chemotherapy–radiotherapy in clinical stages IA–IIB. *J Clin Oncol* 1985;3(11):1495–1502.

144. Dieckmann K, Potter R, Hofmann J, et al. Does bulky disease at diagnosis influence outcome in childhood Hodgkin's disease and require higher radiation doses? results from the German–Austrian Pediatric Multicenter Trial DAL-HD-90. *Int J Radiat Oncol Biol Phys* 2003;56(3):644–652.

145. Schwartz CL, Constine LS, London W, et al. POG 9425: response-based, intensively timed therapy for intermediate/high stage pediatric Hodgkin's disease. *Proc Am Soc Clin Oncol* 2002;21:389a.

146. Hudson MM, Greenwald C, Thompson E, et al. Efficacy and toxicity of multiagent chemotherapy and low-dose involved-field radiotherapy in children and adolescents with Hodgkin's disease. *J Clin Oncol* 1993;11(1):100–108.

147. Atra A, Higgs E, Capra M, et al. ChlVPP chemotherapy in children with stage IV Hodgkin's disease: results of the UKCCSG HD 8201 and HD 9201 studies. *Br J Haematol* 2002;119(3):647–651.

148. van den Berg H, Stuve W, Behrendt H. Treatment of Hodgkin's disease in children with alternating mechlorethamine, vincristine, procarbazine, and prednisone (MOPP) and adriamycin, bleomycin, vinblastine, and dacarbazine (ABVD) courses without radiotherapy. *Med Pediatr Oncol* 1997;29(1):23–27.

149. Yahalom J. Management of relapsed and refractory Hodgkin's disease. *Semin Radiat Oncol* 1996;6(3): 210–224.

150. Biti GP, Cimino G, Cartoni C, et al. Extended-field radiotherapy is superior to MOPP chemotherapy for the treatment of pathologic stage I–IIA Hodgkin's disease: eight-year update of an Italian prospective randomized study. *J Clin Oncol* 1992;10(3):378–382.

151. Healey EA, Tarbell NJ, Kalish LA, et al. Prognostic factors for patients with Hodgkin disease in first relapse. *Cancer* 1993;71(8):2613–2620.

152. Roach M III, Brophy N, Cox R, et al. Prognostic factors for patients relapsing after radiotherapy for early-stage Hodgkin's disease. *J Clin Oncol* 1990; 8(4):623–629.

153. Pezner RD, Lipsett JA, Vora N, et al. Radical radio-

therapy as salvage treatment for relapse of Hodgkin's disease initially treated by chemotherapy alone: prognostic significance of the disease-free interval. *Int J Radiat Oncol Biol Phys* 1994;30(4):965–970.

154. Roach M III, Kapp DS, Rosenberg SA, et al. Radiotherapy with curative intent: an option in selected patients relapsing after chemotherapy for advanced Hodgkin's disease. *J Clin Oncol* 1987;5(4):550–555.

155. Uematsu M, Tarbell NJ, Silver B, et al. Wide-field radiation therapy with or without chemotherapy for patients with Hodgkin disease in relapse after initial combination chemotherapy. *Cancer* 1993; 72(1):207–212.

156. Wirth A, Corry J, Laidlaw C, et al. Salvage radiotherapy for Hodgkin's disease following chemotherapy failure. *Int J Radiat Oncol Biol Phys* 1997;39(3): 599–607.

157. Yahalom J. Do not miss a second (and possibly last) chance to cure Hodgkin's disease. *Int J Radiat Oncol Biol Phys* 1997;39(3):595–597.

158. Reece DE, Connors JM, Spinelli JJ, et al. Intensive therapy with cyclophosphamide, carmustine, etoposide +/− cisplatin, and autologous bone marrow transplantation for Hodgkin's disease in first relapse after combination chemotherapy. *Blood* 1994;83(5): 1193–1199.

159. Bierman PJ, Vose JM, Armitage JO. Autologous transplantation for Hodgkin's disease: coming of age? *Blood* 1994;83(5):1161–1164.

160. Constine LS, Rapoport AP. Hodgkin's disease, bone marrow transplantation, and involved field radiation therapy: coming full circle from 1902 to 1996. *Int J Radiat Oncol Biol Phys* 1996;36(1):253–255.

161. Desch CE, Lasala MR, Smith TJ, et al. The optimal timing of autologous bone marrow transplantation in Hodgkin's disease patients after a chemotherapy relapse. *J Clin Oncol* 1992;10(2):200–209.

162. Leverger G, Oberlin O, Schaison G, et al. Treatment of Hodgkin's disease in children with chemotherapy and low-dose radiation. *Nouv Rev Fr Hematol* 1987;29(1):83–85.

163. Yuen AR, Rosenberg SA, Hoppe RT, et al. Comparison between conventional salvage therapy and high-dose therapy with autografting for recurrent or refractory Hodgkin's disease. *Blood* 1997;89(3):814–822.

164. Williams CD, Goldstone AH, Pearce R, et al. Autologous bone marrow transplantation for pediatric Hodgkin's disease: a case-matched comparison with adult patients by the European Bone Marrow Transplant Group Lymphoma Registry. *J Clin Oncol* 1993;11(11):2243–2249.

165. Horning SJ, Negrin RS, Hoppe RT, et al. High-dose therapy and autologous bone marrow transplantation for follicular lymphoma in first complete or partial remission: results of a phase II clinical trial. *Blood* 2001;97(2):404–409.

166. Anderson JE, Litzow MR, Appelbaum FR, et al. Allogeneic, syngeneic, and autologous marrow transplantation for Hodgkin's disease: the 21-year Seattle experience. *J Clin Oncol* 1993;11(12):2342–2350.

167. Rapoport AP, Rowe JM, Kouides PA, et al. One hundred autotransplants for relapsed or refractory Hodgkin's disease and lymphoma: value of pretransplant disease status for predicting outcome. *J Clin Oncol* 1993;11(12):2351–2361.

168. Yahalom J, Gulati S, Shank B, et al. Total lymphoid irradiation, high-dose chemotherapy and autologous bone marrow transplantation for chemotherapy-resistant Hodgkin's disease. *Int J Radiat Oncol Biol Phys* 1989;17(5):915–922.

169. Jules-Elysee K, Stover DE, Yahalom J, et al. Pulmonary complications in lymphoma patients treated with high-dose therapy autologous bone marrow transplantation. *Am Rev Respir Dis* 1992;146(2): 485–491.

*170. Hancock SL, Hoppe RT. Long-term complications of treatment and causes of mortality after Hodgkin's disease. *Semin Radiat Oncol* 1996;6(3):225–242.

171. Mundt AJ, Sibley G, Williams S, et al. Patterns of failure following high-dose chemotherapy and autologous bone marrow transplantation with involved field radiotherapy for relapsed/refractory Hodgkin's disease. *Int J Radiat Oncol Biol Phys* 1995;33(2): 261–270.

172. Poen JC, Hoppe RT, Horning SJ. High-dose therapy and autologous bone marrow transplantation for relapsed/refractory Hodgkin's disease: the impact of involved field radiotherapy on patterns of failure and survival. *Int J Radiat Oncol Biol Phys* 1996;36(1): 3–12.

173. Brasacchio R, Constine L, Rapoport AP. Dose escalation of consolidation radiation therapy (involved field) following autologous bone marrow transplant for recurrent Hodgkin's disease and lymphoma. *Int J Radiat Oncol Biol Phys* 1996:171.

174. Carella AM, Cavaliere M, Lerma E, et al. Autografting followed by nonmyeloablative immunosuppressive chemotherapy and allogeneic peripheral-blood hematopoietic stem-cell transplantation as treatment of resistant Hodgkin's disease and non-Hodgkin's lymphoma. *J Clin Oncol* 2000;18(23):3918–3924.

175. Robinson SP, Goldstone AH, Mackinnon S, et al. Chemoresistant or aggressive lymphoma predicts for a poor outcome following reduced-intensity allogeneic progenitor cell transplantation: an analysis from the Lymphoma Working Party of the European Group for Blood and Bone Marrow Transplantation. *Blood* 2002;100(13):4310–4316.

176. Coia LR, Hanks GE. Complications from large field intermediate dose infradiaphragmatic radiation: an analysis of the patterns of care outcome studies for Hodgkin's disease and seminoma. *Int J Radiat Oncol Biol Phys* 1988;15(1):29–35.

177. Hanks GE, Herring DF, Kramer S. Patterns of care outcome studies. Results of the national practice in cancer of the cervix. *Cancer* 1983;51(5):959–967.

178. Kinzie JJ, Hanks GE, MacLean CJ, et al. Patterns of care study: Hodgkin's disease relapse rates and adequacy of portals. *Cancer* 1983;52(12):2223–2226.

179. Hoppe RT. Treatment planning in the radiation therapy of Hodgkin's disease. *Front Radiat Ther Oncol* 1987;21:270–287.

180. Nautiyal J, Weichselbaum RR, Vijayakumar S. Radiation therapy techniques in the treatment of Hodgkin's disease. *Semin Radiat Oncol* 1996;6(3): 172–184.

181. Prosnitz LR, Brizel DM, Light KL. Radiation techniques for the treatment of Hodgkin's disease with combined modality therapy or radiation alone. *Int J Radiat Oncol Biol Phys* 1997;39(4):885–895.

182. Dieckmann K, Potter R, Wagner W, et al. Up-front centralized data review and individualized treatment proposals in a multicenter pediatric Hodgkin's disease trial with 71 participating hospitals: the experience of the German–Austrian pediatric multicenter trial DAL-HD-90. *Radiother Oncol* 2002;62(2):191–200.

183. Kaplan HS, Rosenberg SA. The treatment of Hodgkin's disease. *Med Clin North Am* 1966;50(6): 1591–1610.

184. Gottdiener JS, Katin MJ, Borer JS, et al. Late cardiac effects of therapeutic mediastinal irradiation. Assessment by echocardiography and radionuclide angiography. *N Engl J Med* 1983;308(10):569–572.

185. Schewe KL, Reavis J, Kun LE, et al. Total dose, fraction size, and tumor volume in the local control of Hodgkin's disease. *Int J Radiat Oncol Biol Phys* 1988;15(1):25–28.

186. Sears JD, Greven KM, Ferree CR, et al. Definitive irradiation in the treatment of Hodgkin's disease. Analysis of outcome, prognostic factors, and long-term complications. *Cancer* 1997;79(1):145–151.

187. Loeffler M, Diehl V, Pfreundschuh M, et al. Dose–response relationship of complementary radiotherapy following four cycles of combination chemotherapy in intermediate-stage Hodgkin's disease. *J Clin Oncol* 1997;15(6):2275–2287.

188. Green DM, Gingell RL. Regarding cardiac function and morbidity in long-term survivors of Hodgkin's disease. *Int J Radiat Oncol Biol Phys* 1998;41(4):971.

189. Probert JC, Parker BR, Kaplan HS. Growth retardation in children after megavoltage irradiation of the spine. *Cancer* 1973;32(3):634–639.

*190. Probert JC, Parker BR. The effects of radiation therapy on bone growth. *Radiology* 1975;114(1):155–162.

191. Willman KY, Cox RS, Donaldson SS. Radiation induced height impairment in pediatric Hodgkin's disease. *Int J Radiat Oncol Biol Phys* 1994;28(1):85–92.

192. Tarbell N, Mauch P, Hellman S. Pulmonary complications of Hodgkin's disease treatment: radiation pneumonitis, fibrosis, and the effect of cytotoxic drugs. In: Lacher MJ, Redman JR, eds. *Hodgkin's disease: the consequences of survival.* Philadelphia: Lea & Febiger, 1990.

193. Mertens AC, Yasui Y, Liu Y, et al. Pulmonary complications in survivors of childhood and adolescent cancer. A report from the Childhood Cancer Survivor Study. *Cancer* 2002;95(11):2431–2441.

194. Marina NM, Greenwald CA, Fairclough DL, et al. Serial pulmonary function studies in children treated for newly diagnosed Hodgkin's disease with mantle radiotherapy plus cycles of cyclophosphamide, vincristine, and procarbazine alternating with cycles of doxorubicin, bleomycin, vinblastine, and dacarbazine. *Cancer* 1995;75(7):1706–1711.

195. Mefferd JM, Donaldson SS, Link MP. Pediatric Hodgkin's disease: pulmonary, cardiac, and thyroid function following combined modality therapy. *Int J Radiat Oncol Biol Phys* 1989;16(3):679–685.

196. Adams MJ, Hardenbergh PH, Constine LS, et al. Radiation-associated cardiovascular disease. *Crit Rev Oncol Hematol* 2003;45(1):55–75.

197. Green DM, Gingell RL, Pearce J, et al. The effect of mediastinal irradiation on cardiac function of patients treated during childhood and adolescence for Hodgkin's disease. *J Clin Oncol* 1987;5(2):239–245.

198. Green DM, Hyland A, Chung CS, et al. Cancer and cardiac mortality among 15-year survivors of cancer diagnosed during childhood or adolescence. *J Clin Oncol* 1999;17(10):3207–3215.

199. Hancock SL, Donaldson SS, Hoppe RT. Cardiac disease following treatment of Hodgkin's disease in children and adolescents. *J Clin Oncol* 1993;11(7): 1208–1215.

200. Sklar C, Whitton J, Mertens A, et al. Abnormalities of the thyroid in survivors of Hodgkin's disease: data from the Childhood Cancer Survivor Study. *J Clin Endocrinol Metab* 2000;85(9):3227–3232.

201. Constine LS, Donaldson SS, McDougall IR, et al. Thyroid dysfunction after radiotherapy in children with Hodgkin's disease. *Cancer* 1984;53(4):878–883.

202. Le Floch O, Donaldson SS, Kaplan HS. Pregnancy following oophoropexy and total nodal irradiation in women with Hodgkin's disease. *Cancer* 1976;38(6): 2263–2268.

203. Anselmo AP, Cartoni C, Bellantuono P, et al. Risk of infertility in patients with Hodgkin's disease treated with ABVD vs MOPP vs ABVD/MOPP. *Haematologica* 1990;75(2):155–158.

204. Bramswig JH, Heimes U, Heiermann E, et al. The effects of different cumulative doses of chemotherapy on testicular function. Results in 75 patients treated for Hodgkin's disease during childhood or adolescence. *Cancer* 1990;65(6):1298–1302.

205. Byrne J, Fears TR, Gail MH, et al. Early menopause in long-term survivors of cancer during adolescence. *Am J Obstet Gynecol* 1992;166(3):788–793.

206. da Cunha MF, Meistrich ML, Fuller LM, et al. Recovery of spermatogenesis after treatment for Hodgkin's disease: limiting dose of MOPP chemotherapy. *J Clin Oncol* 1984;2(6):571–577.

207. Gerres L, Bramswig JH, Schlegel W, et al. The effects of etoposide on testicular function in boys treated for Hodgkin's disease. *Cancer* 1998;83(10): 2217–2222.

208. Green DM, Hall B. Pregnancy outcome following treatment during childhood or adolescence for Hodgkin's disease. *Pediatr Hematol Oncol* 1988; 5(4):269–277.

209. Hassel JU, Bramswig JH, Schlegel W, et al. Testicular function after OPA/COMP chemotherapy without procarbazine in boys with Hodgkin's disease. Results in 25 patients of the DAL-HD-85 study. *Klin Padiatr* 1991;203(4):268–272.

210. Pedrick TJ, Hoppe RT. Recovery of spermatogenesis following pelvic irradiation for Hodgkin's disease. *Int J Radiat Oncol Biol Phys* 1986;12(1):117–121.

211. Ortin TT, Shostak CA, Donaldson SS. Gonadal status and reproductive function following treatment for Hodgkin's disease in childhood: the Stanford experience. *Int J Radiat Oncol Biol Phys* 1990;19(4): 873–880.

212. Kaiser CW. Complications from staging laparotomy for Hodgkin disease. *J Surg Oncol* 1981;16(4): 319–325.

213. Jockovich M, Mendenhall NP, Sombeck MD, et al. Long-term complications of laparotomy in Hodgkin's disease. *Ann Surg* 1994;219(6):615–621.

214. Scholz KH, Herrmann C, Tebbe U, et al. Myocardial infarction in young patients with Hodgkin's disease: potential pathogenic role of radiotherapy, chemotherapy, and splenectomy. *Clin Invest* 1993;71(1):57–64.

215. Lipshultz SE, Colan SD, Gelber RD, et al. Late cardiac effects of doxorubicin therapy for acute lymphoblastic leukemia in childhood. *N Engl J Med* 1991;324(12):808–815.

216. Kinsella TJ, Trivette G, Rowland J, et al. Long-term follow-up of testicular function following radiation therapy for early-stage Hodgkin's disease. *J Clin Oncol* 1989;7(6):718–724.

217. Viviani S, Santoro A, Ragni G, et al. Gonadal toxicity after combination chemotherapy for Hodgkin's disease. Comparative results of MOPP vs ABVD. *Eur J Cancer Clin Oncol* 1985;21(5):601–605.

218. Wolden SL, Hancock SL, Carlson RW, et al. Management of breast cancer after Hodgkin's disease. *J Clin Oncol* 2000;18(4):765–772.

219. van Leeuwen FE, Klokman WJ, Veer MB, et al. Long-term risk of second malignancy in survivors of Hodgkin's disease treated during adolescence or young adulthood. *J Clin Oncol* 2000;18(3):487–497.

220. Tucker MA, D'Angio GJ, Boice JD Jr, et al. Bone sarcomas linked to radiotherapy and chemotherapy in children. *N Engl J Med* 1987;317(10):588–593.

221. Schellong G, Riepenhausen M, Creutzig U, et al. Low risk of secondary leukemias after chemotherapy without mechlorethamine in childhood Hodgkin's disease. German–Austrian Pediatric Hodgkin's Disease Group. *J Clin Oncol* 1997;15(6):2247–2253.

222. Sankila R, Garwicz S, Olsen JH, et al. Risk of subsequent malignant neoplasms among 1,641 Hodgkin's disease patients diagnosed in childhood and adolescence: a population-based cohort study in the five Nordic countries. *J Clin Oncol* 1996;14(5):1442– 1446.

223. Metayer C, Lynch CF, Clarke EA, et al. Second cancers among long-term survivors of Hodgkin's disease diagnosed in childhood and adolescence. *J Clin Oncol* 2000;18(12):2435–2443.

224. Meadows AT, Baum E, Fossati-Bellani F, et al. Second malignant neoplasms in children: an update from the Late Effects Study Group. *J Clin Oncol* 1985;3(4):532–538.

225. Meadows AT, Obringer AC, Marrero O, et al. Second malignant neoplasms following childhood Hodgkin's disease: treatment and splenectomy as risk factors. *Med Pediatr Oncol* 1989;17(6):477–484.

*226. Green DM, Hyland A, Barcos MP, et al. Second malignant neoplasms after treatment for Hodgkin's disease in childhood or adolescence. *J Clin Oncol* 2000;18(7):1492–1499.

227. Bhatia S, Robison LL, Oberlin O, et al. Breast cancer and other second neoplasms after childhood Hodgkin's disease. *N Engl J Med* 1996;334(12):745–751.

228. Swerdlow AJ, Barber JA, Hudson GV, et al. Risk of second malignancy after Hodgkin's disease in a collaborative British cohort: the relation to age at treatment. *J Clin Oncol* 2000;18(3):498–509.

229. Tucker MA, Meadows AT, Boice JD Jr, et al. Leukemia after therapy with alkylating agents for childhood cancer. *J Natl Cancer Inst* 1987;78(3): 459–464.

230. Travis LB, Hill DA, Dores GM, et al. Breast cancer following radiotherapy and chemotherapy among

young women with Hodgkin disease. *JAMA* 2003; 290(4):465–475.

231. Gilbert ES, Stovall M, Gospodarowicz M, et al. Lung cancer after treatment for Hodgkin's disease: focus on radiation effects. *Radiat Res* 2003;159(2): 161–173.

232. Bierman PJ, Vose JM, Leichner PK. et al. Yttrium 90–labeled antiferritin followed by high-dose chemotherapy and autologous bone marrow transplantation for poor-prognosis Hodgkin's disease. *J Clin Oncol* 1993;11(4):698–703.

233. Rooney CM, Smith CA, Ng CY. et al. Use of gene-modified virus-specific T lymphocytes to control Epstein–Barr virus–related lymphoproliferation. *Lancet* 1995;345(8941):9–13

234. Younes A, Carbone A. CD30/CD30 ligand and CD40/CD40 ligand in malignant lymphoid disorders. *Int J Biol Markers* 1999;14(3):135–143.

235. Younes A, Consoli U. Snell V, et al. CD30 ligand in lymphoma patients with CD30+ tumors. *J Clin Oncol* 1997;15(11):3355–3362.

8

Non-Hodgkin's Lymphoma

Nancy J. Tarbell, M.D., and Howard J. Weinstein, M.D.

Malignant lymphoma was described by Hodgkin in 1832 (1) and was distinguished from leukemia by Virchow in 1845 (2). Progress in treating children with non-Hodgkin's lymphoma (NHL) mirrors the recognition of the systemic nature of the disease and underlying biology. Response to therapy and overall prognosis depend on the underlying histologic subtype, primary site, and the extent of disease (3,4). Historically, local therapy resulted in an overall survival of 10–30% (4). New multiagent protocols result in overall survivals of 70–90% (5–8).

Childhood NHL is distinguished from adult NHL by differing frequencies of histopathologic types and by the greater frequency of extranodal presentations (9,10). The pediatric NHLs are mostly (more than 95%) high grade and include the following four major subtypes: precursor B and precursor T lymphoblastic, Burkitt's or atypical Burkitt's, diffuse large B cell, and anaplastic large-cell lymphoma (Fig. 8-1). Many of these high-grade lymphomas disseminate noncontiguously, evolve into a leukemic phase, and involve the central nervous system (CNS) (10). The more common low-grade lymphomas seen in adults, such as follicular and marginal zone, are rare in children (9).

EPIDEMIOLOGY AND ETIOLOGY

The lymphomas are the third most common malignancy in children younger than 15 years of age. They are rare under the age of 3 years, peaking in incidence from age 7 to 11 years. There is approximately a 3:1 male:female ratio (3,4,6). Lymphomas account for approximately 10% of all childhood cancers; 60% are NHL, and 40% are Hodgkin's disease (11). There is geographic variation in the incidence of the NHLs. For example,

in equatorial Africa, Burkitt's lymphoma accounts for almost 50% of all childhood cancers. In this setting, endemic Burkitt's lymphoma is invariably positive for Epstein–Barr virus (EBV), in contrast to about 10% of cases of sporadic Burkitt's lymphoma. However, both endemic and sporadic cases of Burkitt's lymphoma have the same chromosomal translocations involving the immunoglobin heavy chain gene and myc oncogene t(8;14) or the immunoglobulin light chain genes and myc t(2;8) or t(8;22). EBV is also associated with other tumors, including nasopharyngeal carcinoma, and leiomyosarcomas in children with human immunodeficiency virus (HIV). The exact role of EBV in the pathogenesis of Burkitt's lymphoma and other malignancies is unknown. NHL occurs in association with congenital immunodeficiency syndromes such as X-linked lymphoproliferative syndrome, ataxia telangiectasia, Wiscott–Aldrich syndrome, and common variable immune deficiency disease, presumably caused by host defects in immunoregulation or gene rearrangement (12,13). Immunosuppressive therapy and acquired immunologic disorders including HIV also increase the risk of developing NHL (13). These are predominantly diffuse large B cell or Burkitt's subtypes. Screening for HIV should be considered for all children with NHL, especially for those with B-cell lymphomas.

CLINICAL PRESENTATION

Several subtypes of NHL in children are associated with distinct clinical manifestations and sites of disease (Table 8-1). Symptoms leading to diagnosis usually are of short duration. Approximately 25% of children with NHL have an anterior mediastinal mass (usually precursor T lymphoblastic or large B cell) and present with

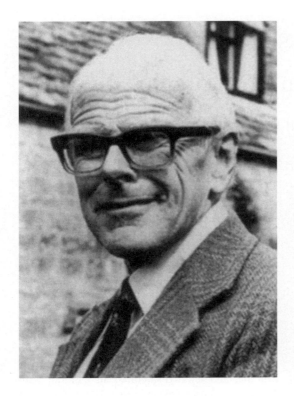

FIG. 8-1. Denis Parsons Burkitt (1911–1993) was the son of an engineer. A Protestant raised in Northern Ireland, he lost an eye in a fight as a schoolboy. He graduated as a physician in 1935 and trained in surgery but had difficulty in obtaining surgical positions because of his visual loss. Eventually he was posted as an Army physician in Africa and subsequently worked as a missionary physician. He characterized a previously undescribed aggressive head and neck cancer of childhood. Michael Epstein attended one of Burkitt's lectures in England, suspected a viral origin, and requested a tissue sample. Epstein and Yvonne M. Barr isolated the virus (Epstein–Barr virus). Burkitt also described the crucial influence of dietary fiber on health and disease.

TABLE 8-1. *Clinical and biologic features of Non-Hodgkin's lymphoma in children*

WHO and REAL classification	Percentage of cases	Primary site	Immunophenotype	Chromosomal changes	Genes affected
Burkitt's lymphoma	40	Abdomen or H/N	sIgM with K or high light chains, CD10, CD19, CD20	t(8;14), t(2;8), or t(8;22)	Ig heavy- or light-chain genes and MYC
Diffuse large B-cell lymphoma (includes mediastinal)	20	Mediastinum, H/N, bone	sIgM > G (75%) CD10, CD19, CD20, CD22	3g27 and t(14;18) in adults	bcl-2 (adult, bcl-6)
Precursor B-lymphoblastic lymphoma	5	Bone, skin, H/N	Td++, CD10, CD19, CD79a	Hyperdiploid > 50 (ALL)	TEL/AML1 (mostly in ALL)
Precursor T-lymphoblastic lymphoma	25	Mediastinum	Td++, CD2, CD3, CD4, CD5, CD7, and CD8, CD13 or CD33	14q11.2, 7q35, 7p14–15	TALI, TCR receptors, HOX 11, RBTN1
Anaplastic large-cell lymphoma	10	Skin, soft tissue, bone, mediastinum	CD30, EMA	t(2;5) or variant translocation	NPM-ALK

ALL, acute lymphoblastic leukemia; EMA, epithelial membrane antigen; H/N, head and neck; Ig, immunoglobulin; REAL, Revised European–American Classification of Lymphoid Neoplasia; TCR, T cell receptor; WHO, World Health Organization.

Adapted from Percy C, Smith M, Linet M, et al. Lymphomas and reticuloendothelial neoplasms. In: Ries LAG, Smith MA, Gurney JG, et al. *Cancer incidence and survival among children and adolescents: United States SEER Program 1975–1995*. Bethesda, MD: National Cancer Institute, 1999:35–50.

wheezing, stridor, and cough progressing to dyspnea. The majority of these patients are adolescents, and their presentation may pose a medical emergency (14). Patients with large anterior mediastinal masses are at risk of cardiac or respiratory arrest during general anesthesia or deep sedation. A careful workup including a chest computed tomography (CT) scan and airway measurements is essential (15). The least invasive procedures (bone marrow aspirate, thoracentesis, biopsy of a peripheral node) should be carried out. If these procedures are not successful in providing a diagnosis, then a CT-guided needle biopsy of the mediastinal mass should be considered (16). In some clinical situations, preoperative or preprocedure steroids should be considered. Localized irradiation is rarely used. Primary gastrointestinal involvement occurs in about 30% (usually Burkitt histology), commonly presenting as an abdominal mass with ascites, an acute abdomen, intussusception, or a malnutrition syndrome with colitis symptoms (6,17). Many children presenting with an acute abdomen or intussusception have limited gastrointestinal involvement that is completely resectable (Murphy stage 2 or group A). In 20–30% of children, the head and neck, including Waldeyer's ring or cervical lymph nodes, is the site of origin. The remainder of patients have miscellaneous primary sites, including bone, breast, skin, epidural space, or noncervical lymph nodes (6). Involvement of the bone marrow at diagnosis is common, occurring in 10–30% of Burkitt's and lymphoblastic subtypes. Overt CNS involvement at diagnosis is not common but is most common in children with advanced-stage Burkitt's and lymphoblastic lymphomas and occasional head and neck sites. Endemic or African Burkitt's lymphoma usually presents in the jaw, in contrast to the abdominal presentation typical of nonendemic Burkitt's lymphoma.

EVALUATION

Surgical biopsy establishes the diagnosis. Although histology continues to be the primary determinant of therapy, morphologic analysis is supplemented by immunophenotypic, cytogenetic, and molecular genetic studies. The workup includes complete blood cell count with differential, routine chemistries with electrolytes, calcium, phosphorus, magnesium, uric acid, liver and renal function tests, lactate dehydrogenase (LDH), chest radiograph, bone scan, bone marrow aspirate and biopsy (which may obviate lymph node biopsy) (18), and a lumbar puncture with cytocentrifugation. Abdominal, thoracic, and head and neck CT scans should be obtained depending on the presenting site (19). Gallium and positron emission tomography scans are now part of the initial staging for most patients with NHL and are particularly helpful in assessing response to induction therapy for large B-cell and anaplastic large-cell lymphomas. Laparotomy is not indicated for staging and is performed only for abdominal presentations necessitating surgical intervention. There is no role for surgical debulking of NHL in children.

STAGING AND CLASSIFICATION

Originally, the Ann Arbor staging system for Hodgkin's disease was used for NHL (see Chapter 7, Table 7-1) (20). The usefulness of this system in pediatric NHL is limited, and an alternative staging system proposed by Murphy has become widely accepted (Table 8-2). This system recognizes typical patterns of disease presentation and has greater prognostic utility than the Ann Arbor system. In Burkitt's lymphoma and large B-cell lymphomas, another staging system developed by Patte et al. (21) is used (Table 8-3). It classifies patients according to tumor burden and surgical resection.

As previously discussed, the pediatric NHLs are high grade and fall into four major histologic subtypes. Several classification systems have been used for NHL. These include the Rappaport system, the Lukes–Collins classifications, the Kiel system, and the Working Formulation (22–25). The Revised European–American Classification of Lymphoid Neoplasia (REAL) in conjunction with the recent World Health Organization classification is gaining increased acceptance as the preferred classification system (26).

TABLE 8-2. *Murphy and St. Jude Children's Research Hospital staging system for childhood NHL*[a]

Stage I	A single tumor (extranodal) or single anatomic area (nodal), with the exclusion of mediastinum or abdomen
Stage II	A single tumor (extranodal) with regional node involvement
	Two or more nodal areas on the same side of the diaphragm
	Two single (extranodal) tumors with or without regional node involvement on the same side of the diaphragm
	A primary gastrointestinal tract tumor, usually in the ileocecal area, with or without involvement of associated mesenteric nodes only[b]
Stage III	Two single tumors (extranodal) on opposite sides of the diaphragm
	Two or more nodal areas above and below the diaphragm
	All the primary intrathoracic tumors (mediastinal, pleural, thymic)
	All extensive primary intra-abdominal disease[b]
	All paraspinal or epidural tumors, regardless of other tumor sites
Stage IV	Any of the preceding stages with initial central nervous system or bone marrow involvement[c]

[a]See references 6, 10, 41, and 61.
[b]A distinction is made between apparently localized gastrointestinal tract lymphoma and more extensive intra-abdominal disease. Stage II disease typically is limited to a segment of the gut with or without the associated mesenteric nodes only, and the primary tumor can be completely removed grossly by segmental excision. Stage III disease typically exhibits spread to para-aortic and retroperitoneal areas by implants and plaques in mesentery or peritoneum or by direct infiltration of structures adjacent to the primary tumor. Ascites may be present, and complete resection of all gross tumor is not possible.
[c]If marrow involvement is present initially, the number of abnormal cells must be 25% or less in an otherwise normal marrow aspirate with normal peripheral blood picture.

The most common subtypes of NHL in children include precursor T-lymphoblastic lymphoma and precursor B-lymphoblastic lymphoma, also called *diffuse lymphoblastic lymphoma* (30% of cases; precursor T-cell is the more common type); Burkitt's lymphoma and high-grade B-cell, Burkitt-like lymphoma, also called *diffuse small noncleaved-cell lymphoma* (derived from germinal center B cells; 35–40% of cases); diffuse large B-cell lymphoma, also including mediastinal thymic large B-cell lymphoma (20% of cases); and anaplastic large-cell lymphoma (CD30+ lymphoma [T-cell and null-cell types; 10% of cases]).

Precursor B-lymphoblastic lymphoma consists of cells with round or convoluted nuclei, fine chromatin, inconspicuous nuclei, and scant, faintly basophilic cytoplasm. In precursor B-lymphoblastic lymphoma, the tumor cells are characteristically TdT+, CD10+, CD19+, and CD79a+, which is identical to the most common immunophenotype of precursor B acute lymphoblastic leukemia (ALL) in childhood (27). The precursor T-lymphoblastic lymphomas are TdT+ and express a combination of T-cell antigens (CD2, CD3, CD4, CD5, and CD8) similar to that of precursor T ALL. Lymphoblastic lymphomas share many clinical and biologic features with ALL (28,29). When the bone marrow is involved with lymphoblasts, the distinction between lymphoma and leukemia is difficult and generally determined by the percentage of blast cells in the bone marrow, with 25% considered leukemia (28). There are no distinct biologic differences between the blasts in precursor T-lymphoblastic leukemia and precursor T-lymphoblastic lymphoma.

Burkitt's lymphoma tumor cells are monomorphic, medium-sized cells with round nuclei, multiple nucleoli, and basophilic cytoplasm. A "starry-sky" pattern is the result of benign

TABLE 8-3. *Clinical staging of B-cell lymphomas*

Stage	Extent of Tumor
A	Resected stage 1 and abdominal stage 2
B	Multiple extra-abdominal sites; nonresected stage I, II, III, and IV (CNS BM < 25%)
C	Intra-abdominal tumor stage IV (CNS+), BM > 25% (mature B acute lymphoblastic leukemia)

BM, bone marrow; CNS, central nervous system.

macrophages that have ingested apoptotic tumor cells. Cells are typically sIgM+, CD19+, CL20+, CD22+, CD79a+, and CD10+. High-grade B-cell lymphoma, or Burkitt-like or atypical Burkitt's lymphoma, has features intermediate between those of large-cell and Burkitt's lymphoma (27).

Diffuse large B-cell lymphoma consists of large cells with vesicular nuclei, basophilic cytoplasm, and a moderate to high proliferation fraction (27). The nuclear size is equal to or greater than that of a normal macrophage. Large B-cell lymphomas presenting in the mediastinum typically are associated with sclerosis. These large B-cell lymphomas express CD19, CD20, CD22, and CD50 to 75% express surface immunoglobulin G or M.

Anaplastic large-cell lymphoma (ALCL) consists of lymphoid cells that are usually large with abundant cytoplasm and pleomorphic, often horseshoe-shaped nuclei. The cells are CD30+, and the majority of pediatric cases are also positive for the anaplastic lymphoma kinase (ALK) protein. Most case of ALCL express T-cell antigens, but some do not express B- or T-cell markers and are called null-cell lymphoma.

PROGNOSTIC FACTORS

The most prominent prognostic determinant in childhood NHL is the clinical stage. Tumor burden, as measured in part by serum LDH, has been predictive of outcome in some series, especially for Burkitt's lymphoma (6,30–34). In general, patients with localized stage I and II lymphomas have a better prognosis than those with more extensive stage III and IV. Site of involvement has also been prognostic. For example, mediastinal primaries in lymphoblastic and large B-cell lymphomas have been higher-risk sites. In the past, bone marrow involvement was associated with a poor prognosis, but with intensive chemotherapy it no longer carries prognostic significance (31–33). Before the use of preventive CNS therapy, CNS relapse developed in 30–40% of children with stage III and IV Burkitt's and lymphoblastic lymphomas. CNS relapses were also noted, albeit in a much lower percentage, in children who had head and neck primary sites of

NHL (6,35,36). However, overt CNS involvement at diagnosis is rare and is associated with a poorer prognosis. In this situation, cranial irradiation plus intrathecal (IT) chemotherapy is necessary for children with lymphoblastic but not Burkitt's lymphomas.

SELECTION OF THERAPY

Chemotherapy

Because of the high likelihood of disseminated disease, all children, regardless of stage or histology, receive systemic chemotherapy. Childhood NHL responds to a wide range of agents, but different combinations and schedules are optimal for particular histologies. Active drugs include adriamycin, methotrexate, vincristine, prednisone, mercaptopurine, cyclophosphamide, ifosfamide, etoposide, and cytosine arabinoside. Tables 8-4 and 8-5 list some of the commonly used regimens and treatment outcomes.

For stages I and II Burkitt's lymphoma, short-duration therapy with cyclophosphamide, vincristine (Oncovin), methotrexate, and prednisone (COMP); cyclophosphamide, doxorubicin, vincristine (Oncovin), and prednisone (CHOP); or COPAD results in excellent (5,31,37–40) relapse-free survivals of 90–95%. Both CHOP (three cycles) and COPAD (two cycles) are also effective for early-stage large B-cell lymphomas, with disease-free survival of 85–90% (41). CHOP is similarly effective for early-stage anaplastic large-cell lymphoma. For stages I and II lymphoblastic lymphoma, the use of ALL therapy is effective, with approximately 90% disease-free survival (31,42). An alternative to an ALL regimen for these children is CHOP followed by maintenance with mercaptopurine and methotrexate. This results in about 50% disease-free survival but an overall survival of 90% through successful salvage.

In patients with stages III or IV lymphoblastic lymphoma, fewer than 40% were cured with standard-risk ALL treatment regimens (31). The adriamycin, prednisone, and vincristine (Oncovin; APO) and LSA2-L2 regimens were two of the early successful protocols for children with high-risk ALL and advanced-stage lymphoblastic

TABLE 8-4. *Survival for early stage (Murphy I, II, or group A) non-Hodgkin's lymphoma*

WHO/REAL	Regimen	Event-free survival (%)
Burkitt's	CHOP, COPAD COMP[a], COPADM	90–95
Lymphoblastic (mostly precursor B)	CHOP with methotrexate and mercaptopurine BFM-90,[b] COMP[a]	60 90
Large B cell	CHOP, COPADM[a]	90–95
Anaplastic large cell	CHOP[a]	90

BFM, Berlin–Frankfurt–Munster; CHOP, cyclophosphamide, doxorubicin, vincristine (Oncovin), and prednisone; COMP, cyclophosphamide, vincristine (Oncovin), methotrexate, and prednisone; COPADM, cyclophosphamide, doxorubicin, prednisolone, methotrexate, vincristine, hydrocortisone; COPAD without methotrexate; REAL, Revised European–American Classification of Lymphoid Neoplasia; WHO, World Health Organization.
[a]Central nervous system prophylaxis: intrathecal methotrexate for head and neck.
[b]BFM-90: Initial treatment is cyclophosphamide and prednisone. Based on histology and stage, this is followed by dexamethasone, ifosfamide, methotrexate, cytarabine, prednisolone, etoposide, cyclophosphamide, doxorubicin, or these drugs with vincristine or vindesine instead of etoposide.

TABLE 8-5. *Survival for advanced-stage (Murphy III, IV, Group B, C) NHL*

WHO/REAL	Regimen	Event-free survival (%)
Burkitt	COPADM Modified total B	80–90
Lymphoblastic (mostly precursor T)	NHL-BFM 90	80–90
Large B cell	APO COPADM	70–80
Anaplastic large cell	APO, NHL-BFM 90	70

APO, adriamycin, prednisone, and vincristine (Oncovin); BFM, Berlin–Frankfurt–Munster; COPAD without methotrexate; HMDXx, high dose methotrexate; IT, intrathecal; NHL, non-Hodgkin's lymphoma; REAL, Revised European–American Classification of Lymphoid Neoplasia; WHO, World Health Organization.
Central nervous system prophylaxis: Burkitt, high-dose methotrexate, IT chemotherapy; lymphoblastic, cranial + IT or HMDXx + IT chemotherapy; large B cell, IT chemotherapy; anaplastic large cell, IT chemo.

lymphoma (31,40). Both protocols included preventive CNS therapy. These protocols resulted in approximately 65% survival. The use of more intensive ALL chemotherapy regimens has further improved outcomes for these children (disease-free survival of 85–90%) (7,21,42). As mentioned previously, the least toxic and most effective method of CNS prophylaxis for these patients is under investigation. Cranial irradiation and IT methotrexate have been very effective but are associated with neurocognitive late effects. The use of intensive IT chemotherapy with or without systemic high-dose methotrexate is being evaluated in prospective clinical trials.

Large-cell lymphoma constitutes approximately 30% of childhood NHL and includes large B-cell, anaplastic large-cell, and other rare peripheral T-cell lymphomas. In some centers and cooperative groups, children with both large B-cell lymphoma and Burkitt's lymphoma are treated with similar protocols. The lymphoma malignant B type (LMB)-89 protocol, a multiagent intensive

chemotherapy regimen for B-cell lymphoma, has resulted in about 80% disease-free survival. LMB-89 includes 4 to 5 months of intensive cycles of cyclophosphamide, vincristine, prednisone, high-dose methotrexate, doxorubicin, cytosine arabinoside (AraC), and etoposide (43). The APO protocol does not include an alkylating agent but features intensive doxorubicin. This protocol has also been effective for advanced-stage large B-cell lymphoma (ALCL) in children but is not used for Burkitt's lymphoma (42,44–47).

Most protocols for children with ALCL do not include involved-field radiotherapy, but no controlled trials have addressed this issue (48, 49). The APO regimen has also been effective for ALCL in children (disease-free survival 70%). Other regimens for ALCL have been modeled after B-cell protocols and report similar results. The risk of an isolated CNS relapse for large B-cell lymphoma and ALCL is rare, but pediatric protocols include IT chemotherapy for these patients.

Children with Burkitt's and atypical Burkitt's lymphomas have been treated with the same protocols with identical results (17,39,50). Current protocols include rapid sequencing of high dosages of active drugs (usually including cyclophosphamide, methotrexate, and AraC) given over a short duration of 3 to 5 months. There is no benefit for maintenance therapy in these patients. Result of therapy for stage III and IV or group B and C Burkitt's lymphoma have markedly improved in the past decade. Overall disease-free survival ranges from 80% to 90%, including children with mature B-cell ALL and stage IV Burkitt's lymphoma. CNS prophylaxis is necessary and includes intensive triple IT chemotherapy with methotrexate, AraC, hydrocortisone, and systemic high-dose methotrexate (39,43,51).

In the course of treatment for Burkitt's lymphoma, a tumor lysis syndrome may develop. This can result in elevated serum uric acid, uric acid nephropathy, hypocalcemia, and hyperkalemia and renal failure necessitating the temporary use of dialysis. Careful management of hydration with urinary alkalinization, allopurinol, and monitoring of uric acid and electrolyte balance is needed (52,53). The risk of renal failure and electrolyte disturbances has been markedly decreased with the use of urate oxidase. Urate oxidase is a recombinant product that has been shown to be superior to allopurinol for patients at high risk for tumor lysis syndrome (53).

Radiotherapy

The role of radiotherapy in the management of all childhood NHL has decreased as chemotherapeutic regimens have become more effective (5,6,44). As treatment programs were developed, it was clear that the combination of chemotherapy and irradiation significantly increased survival rates (31). Clinical trials assessing the need for radiotherapy followed. Reports from the Pediatric Oncology Group (POG) demonstrated successful local and systemic control with chemotherapy alone for children with Murphy stages I and II NHL regardless of histology (5). It also became evident that there was no benefit to adding radiation therapy to the primary site or for CNS prophylaxis in Burkitt's lymphoma (28,35,36,54). The addition of localized radiation therapy to chemotherapy has also shown no benefit for patients with advanced-stage lymphoblastic lymphoma (6).

In the past 10 years, it has also become clear that primary NHL of bone in children can be treated successfully with chemotherapy alone. The major subtypes of primary bone NHL in children are large B-cell and anaplastic large cell lymphoma, but Burkitt's and lymphoblastic lymphoma occasionally present as isolated lesions in bone (55,55).

The current indications for radiation therapy outside the CNS in pediatric NHL are emergency treatment for mediastinal disease or spinal cord compression, treatment for patients who do not obtain a complete remission after induction chemotherapy, palliation of pain or mass effect, and consolidation to regions of local disease before or after bone marrow transplantation in patients with recurrent disease.

Emergency radiation therapy for superior vena cava syndrome, acute airway compromise, or spinal cord compression can provide rapid symptom relief. The response is particularly dramatic with lymphoblastic lymphoma. Symptoms usually are relieved within 48 hours of treatment. Usually 1.5 to 2 Gy per fraction for a total dosage of 6 to 7.5 Gy is adequate to relieve symptoms. Hyperfractionated regimens (1.2 to 1.5 Gy per fraction twice a day for a total dosage of 6 to 10 Gy) can also be used. On rare occasions emergency radiotherapy is appropriate in the absence of a histologic diagnosis. Because of the rapid response to radiation, the histologic diagnosis may be lost, and selection of the appropriate definitive therapy depends on biopsy of other disease or on a presumed diagnosis (16).

As previously discussed, prophylactic CNS treatment is needed in the majority of children with NHL, thereby reducing the otherwise high risk of CNS relapse (36). The approach for all nonlymphoblastic histologies includes systemic and IT chemotherapy. The current CNS preventive regimens for advanced-stage lymphoblastic lymphoma include either cranial irradiation and IT chemotherapy or IT chemotherapy and systemic chemotherapy only. The Berlin–Frankfurt–Munster (BFM) group safely reduced the dosage of cranial radiation therapy to 12 Gy for lymphoblastic lymphoma and eliminated it entirely from BFM-95 without increasing the CNS relapse rate. Cranial irradiation (18 to 24 Gy) is still warranted for the rare patient with lymphoblastic lymphoma with initial CNS disease or a CNS relapse. Patients with cranial nerve palsies at diagnosis, independent of cerebrospinal fluid findings, are treated in a similar fashion as children with initial CNS lymphoma.

Some patients are irradiated to regions of local residual disease after failing to achieve a complete remission on chemotherapy, or for relapse with local disease only. Both of these situations are rare. Care should be taken to use modest fractionation schedules and to avoid exceeding normal tissue tolerance dosages because patients may be eligible for subsequent bone marrow transplantation necessitating total body irradiation (TBI) as a component of the preparative regimen.

Children with refractory or relapsed NHL can experience prolonged disease-free survival after treatment with high-dose chemotherapy or high-dose chemoradiotherapy followed by autologous or allogeneic bone marrow transplant (51,57–60). When TBI is a component of the preparatory regimen, fractionated courses to total dosages of 12 to 14 Gy are common (see Chapter 2). Disease recurrence rather than the morbidity of transplant is the predominant cause of failure in this setting. The strategy of irradiating the local sites of initial disease recurrence before or after transplant, whether or not TBI is used, has proved to be effective in adults and should be considered (19,57). Dosages to these sites (usually at least 20 Gy) are constrained by normal tissue tolerances.

RESULTS OF THERAPY

Before 1975, when therapy was directed to the identifiable gross tumor, few children survived. The small number of patients who did survive had favorable presentations, including limited resectable abdominal disease or involvement of a single nodal region or extranodal site. With current intensive multiagent regimens, survival is generally excellent for all patients, including those with disseminated disease and adverse prognostic factors such as bone marrow involvement, CNS involvement, and high serum LDH. Most relapses occur within 12 months of diagnosis for Burkitt's lymphomas and within the

first 2 to 4 years for the other histologic subtypes. Late relapse has been reported with ALCL and precursor B-lymphoblastic lymphoma.

Children with stage I to II disease have 2-year disease-free survival rates of 85–95% (5,6,31, 37–39). Children with stage III disease have an 85–90% 2-year disease-free survival. Those with stage IV disease and marrow involvement have an 85–90% disease-free survival, and those with CNS disease (Burkitt's) have an 80% event-free survival. Deaths from second malignancies can occur after prolonged time intervals and modify survival curves (61).

Patients undergoing transplantation early in their disease course (i.e., after first relapse or second complete remission) have 2-year disease-free survival approaching 50%, whereas those with refractory disease fare less well (5–20%) (57,58).

REFERENCES

References particularly recommended for further reading are indicated with an asterisk.

1. Hodgkin T. On some morbid appearances of the absorbent gland and spleen. *Med Chir Trans* 1832; 17:68–114.
2. Virchow R. *Weisses Blu, neue Notizen aus dem Gebiete der Natur and Heilkunde (Frorip's neue Notizen).* 1845;36:151–156.
3. Sandlund JT, Downing JR, Crist WM. Non-Hodgkin's lymphoma in childhood. *N Engl J Med* 1996;334: 1238–1248.
4. Lemerle M, Gerard-Marchant R, Sancho H, et al. Natural history of non-Hodgkin's malignant lymphomata in children: a retrospective study of 190 cases. *Br J Cancer* 1975;31:324–331.
5. Link M, Donaldson S, Berard C, et al. Results of treatment of childhood localized non-Hodgkin's lymphoma with combination chemotherapy with or without radiotherapy. *N Engl J Med* 1990;322:1169–1174.
6. Murphy S, Fairclough D, Hutchison R, et al. Non-Hodgkin's lymphomas of childhood: an analysis of the histology, staging and response to treatment of 338 cases at a single institution. *J Clin Oncol* 1989;7: 186–193.
*7. Reiter A, Schrappe M, Parwaresch R, et al. Non-Hodgkin's lymphomas of childhood and adolescence: results of a treatment stratified for biologic subtypes and stage—a report of the Berlin–Frankfurt–Munster Group. *J Clin Oncol* 1995;13:359–372.
8. Percy C, Smith M, Linet M, et al. Lymphomas and reticuloendothelial neoplasms. In: Ries LAG, Smith

MA, Gurney JG, et al. *Cancer incidence and survival among children and adolescents: United States SEER Program 1975–1995*. Bethesda, MD: National Cancer Institute, 1999:35–50.

9. Frizzera G, Murphy SB. Follicular (nodular) lymphoma in childhood: a rare clinical-pathological entity. Report of eight cases from four cancer centers. *Cancer* 1979;44:2218–2235.

10. Murphy SB. Classification, staging and end results of treatment of childhood non-Hodgkin's lymphomas: dissimilarities from lymphomas in adults. *Semin Oncol* 1980;7:332–339.

11. Young JL Jr, Ries LG, Silverberg E, et al. Cancer incidence, survival, and mortality for children younger than age 15 years. *Cancer* 1986;58:598–602.

12. Taylor AM, Metcalfe JA, Thick J, et al. Leukemia and lymphoma in ataxia telangiectasia. *Blood* 1996;87:423–438.

13. Reynolds P, Saunders L, Lavefsky M, et al. The spectrum of acquired immunodeficiency syndrome (AIDS) associated malignancies in San Francisco, 1980–1987. *Am J Epidemiol* 1993;137:19–30.

14. Weinstein H, Vance Z, Jaffe N, et al. Improved prognosis for patients with mediastinal lymphoblastic lymphoma. *Blood* 1979;53:687–694.

15. Shamberger RC, Holzman RS, Griscom NT, et al. Prospective evaluation by computed tomography and pulmonary function tests of children with mediastinal masses. *Surgery* 1995;118:468–471.

*16. Loeffler JS, Leopold KA, Recht A, et al. Emergency prebiopsy radiation for mediastinal masses: impact on subsequent pathologic diagnosis and outcome. *J Clin Oncol* 1986;4:716–721.

17. Magrath IT, Shiramizu B. Biology and treatment of small non-cleaved cell lymphoma. *Oncology (Huntingt)* 1989;3:41–53.

18. Haddy TB, Parker RI, Magrath IT. Bone marrow involvement in young patients with non-Hodgkin's lymphoma: the importance of multiple bone marrow samples for accurate staging. *Med Pediatr Oncol* 1989;17:418–423.

19. Freedman AS, Takvorian T, Anderson KC, et al. Autologous bone marrow transplantation in B-cell non-Hodgkin's lymphoma: very low treatment-related mortality in 100 patients in sensitive relapse. *J Clin Oncol* 1990;8:784–791.

20. Carbone P, Kaplan H, Musshoff K, et al. Report of the Committee on Hodgkin's Disease staging classification. *Cancer Res* 1971;31:1860–1861.

21. Patte C, Kalifa C, Flamant F, et al. Results of the LMT81 protocol, a modified LSA2-L2 protocol with high dose methotrexate, on 84 children with non-B-cell (lymphoblastic) lymphoma. *Med Pediatr Oncol* 1992;20:105–113.

22. Griffith RC, Kelly DR, Nathwani BN, et al. A morphologic study of childhood lymphoma of the lymphoblastic type. The Pediatric Oncology Group experience. *Cancer* 1987;59:1126–1131.

23. Lukes RJ, Collins RD. Immunologic characterization of human malignant lymphomas. *Cancer* 1974;34[Suppl]:1488–1503.

24. Nathwani BN, Kim H, Rappaport H, et al. Non-Hodgkin's lymphomas: a clinicopathologic study comparing two classifications. *Cancer* 1978;41:303–325.

25. Wilson JF, Jenkin ED, Anderson JR, et al. Studies on the pathology of non-Hodgkin's lymphoma of childhood. I. The role of routine histopathology as a prognostic factor. A report from the Children's Cancer Study Group. *Cancer* 1984;53:1695–1704.

26. Harris NL, Jaffe ES, Diebold J, et al. World Health Organization classification of neoplastic diseases of the hematopoietic and lymphoid tissues: report of the Clinical Advisory Committee meeting—Airlie House, Virginia, November 1997. *J Clin Oncol* 1999;17:3835–3849.

*27. Harris NL, Jaffe ES, Stein H, et al. A revised European–American classification of lymphoid neoplasms: a proposal from the International Lymphoma Study Group. *Blood* 1994;84:1361–1392.

28. Duque-Hammershaimb L, Wollner N, Miller DR. LSA2-L2 protocol treatment of stage IV non-Hodgkin's lymphoma in children with partial and extensive bone marrow involvement. *Cancer* 1983;52:39–43.

29. Bernard A, Boumsell L, Reinherz EL, et al. Cell surface characterization of malignant T cells from lymphoblastic lymphoma using monoclonal antibodies: evidence for phenotypic differences between malignant T cells from patients with acute lymphoblastic leukemia and lymphoblastic lymphoma. *Blood* 1981;57:1105–1110.

30. Magrath IT, Janus C, Edwards BK, et al. An effective therapy for both undifferentiated (including Burkitt's) lymphomas and lymphoblastic lymphomas in children and young adults. *Blood* 1984;63:1102–1111.

31. Anderson JR, Jenkin RD, Wilson JF, et al. Long-term follow-up of patients treated with COMP or LSA2-L2 therapy for childhood non-Hodgkin's lymphoma: a report of CCG-551 from the Children's Cancer Group. *J Clin Oncol* 1993;11:1024–1032.

32. Patte C, Philip T, Rodary C, et al. Improved survival rate in children with stage III and IV B cell non-Hodgkin's lymphoma and leukemia using multi-agent chemotherapy: results of a study of 114 children from the French Pediatric Oncology Society. *J Clin Oncol* 1986;4:1219–1226.

33. Pullen DJ, Sullivan MP, Falletta JM, et al. Modified LSA2-L2 treatment in 53 children with E-rosette-positive T-cell leukemia: results and prognostic factors (a Pediatric Oncology Group study). *Blood* 1982;60:1159–1168.

34. Pui CH, Ip SH, Kung P, et al. High serum interleukin-2 receptor levels are related to advanced disease and a poor outcome in childhood non-Hodgkin's lymphoma. *Blood* 1987;70:624–628.

*35. Mandell LR, Wollner N, Fuks Z. Is cranial radiation necessary for CNS prophylaxis in pediatric NHL? *Int J Radiat Oncol Biol Phys* 1987;13:359–363.

36. Murphy SB, Bleyer WA. Cranial irradiation is not necessary for central-nervous-system prophylaxis in pediatric non-Hodgkin's lymphoma. *Int J Radiat Oncol Biol Phys* 1987;13:467–468.

37. Meadows AT, Sposto R, Jenkin RD, et al. Similar efficacy of 6 and 18 months of therapy with four drugs (COMP) for localized non-Hodgkin's lymphoma of children: a report from the Children's Cancer Study Group. *J Clin Oncol* 1989;7:92–99.

38. Nachman J. Therapy for childhood non-Hodgkin's lymphomas, nonlymphoblastic type. Review of recent

studies and current recommendations. *Am J Pediatr Hematol Oncol* 1990;12:359–366.

39. Schwenn MR, Blattner SR, Lynch E, et al. HiC-COM: a 2-month intensive chemotherapy regimen for children with stage III and IV Burkitt's lymphoma and B-cell acute lymphoblastic leukemia. *J Clin Oncol* 1991;9:133–138.

40. Weinstein HJ, Cassady JR, Levey R. Long-term results of the APO protocol (vincristine, doxorubicin (adriamycin), and prednisone) for treatment of mediastinal lymphoblastic lymphoma. *J Clin Oncol* 1983;1: 537–541.

41. Murphy SB, Bowman WP, Abromowitch M, et al. Results of treatment of advanced-stage Burkitt's lymphoma and B cell (SIg+) acute lymphoblastic leukemia with high-dose fractionated cyclophosphamide and coordinated high-dose methotrexate and cytarabine. *J Clin Oncol* 1986;4:1732–1739.

*42. Reiter A, Schrappe M, Ludwig WD, et al. Intensive ALL-type therapy without local radiotherapy provides a 90% event-free survival for children with T-cell lymphoblastic lymphoma: a BFM group report. *Blood* 2000;95:416–421.

43. Patte C, Auperin A, Michon J, et al. The Société Francaise d'Oncologie Pediatrique LMB89 protocol: highly effective multiagent chemotherapy tailored to the tumor burden and initial response in 561 unselected children with B-cell lymphomas and L3 leukemia. *Blood* 2001;97:3370–3379.

44. Camitta BM, Lauer SJ, Casper JT, et al. Effectiveness of a six-drug regimen (APO) without local irradiation for treatment of mediastinal lymphoblastic lymphoma in children. *Cancer* 1985;56:738–741.

45. Hvizdala EV, Berard C, Callihan T, et al. Nonlymphoblastic lymphoma in children: histology and stage-related response to therapy: a Pediatric Oncology Group study. *J Clin Oncol* 1991;9:1189–1195.

*46. Laver JH, Mahmoud H, Pick TE, et al. Results of a randomized phase III trial in children and adolescents with advanced stage diffuse large cell non-Hodgkin's lymphoma: a Pediatric Oncology Group study. *Leuk Lymphoma* 2001;42:399–405.

47. Thomas DA, Kantarjian HM. Lymphoblastic lymphoma. *Hematol Oncol Clin North Am* 2001;15: 51–95, vi.

48. Sandlund JT, Santana V, Abromowitch M, et al. Large cell non-Hodgkin lymphoma of childhood: clinical characteristics and outcome. *Leukemia* 1994;8: 30–34.

49. Lones MA, Perkins SL, Sposto R, et al. Large-cell lymphoma arising in the mediastinum in children and adolescents is associated with an excellent outcome: a Children's Cancer Group report. *J Clin Oncol* 2000;18:3845–3853.

50. Hutchison RE, Murphy SB, Fairclough DL, et al. Diffuse small noncleaved cell lymphoma in children, Burkitt's versus non-Burkitt's types. Results from the Pediatric Oncology Group and St. Jude Children's Research Hospital. *Cancer* 1989;64:23–28.

51. Reiter A, Schrappe M, Tiemann M, et al. Improved treatment results in childhood B-cell neoplasms with tailored intensification of therapy: a report of the Berlin–Frankfurt–Munster Group Trial NHL-BFM 90. *Blood* 1999;94:3294–3306.

52. Stapleton FB, Strother DR, Roy S III, et al. Acute renal failure at onset of therapy for advanced stage Burkitt lymphoma and B cell acute lymphoblastic lymphoma. *Pediatrics* 1988;82:863–869.

53. Pui CH, Mahmoud HH, Wiley JM, et al. Recombinant urate oxidase for the prophylaxis or treatment of hyperuricemia in patients with leukemia or lymphoma. *J Clin Oncol* 2001;19:697–704.

54. Ziegler JL, DeVita VJ, Graw R, et al. Combined modality treatment of American Burkitt's lymphoma. *Cancer* 1976;38:2225–2231.

55. Haddy TB, Keenan AM, Jaffe ES, et al. Bone involvement in young patients with non-Hodgkin's lymphoma: efficacy of chemotherapy without local radiotherapy. *Blood* 1988;72:1141–1147.

*56. Lones MA, Perkins SL, Sposto R, et al. Non-Hodgkin's lymphoma arising in bone in children and adolescents is associated with an excellent outcome: a Children's Cancer Group report. *J Clin Oncol* 2002;20:2293–2301.

57. Armitage JO. Bone marrow transplantation in the treatment of patients with lymphoma. *Blood* 1989;73: 1749–1758.

58. Kurtzberg J, Graham ML. Non-Hodgkin's lymphoma. Biologic classification and implication for therapy. *Pediatr Clin North Am* 1991;38:443–456.

59. Kobrinsky NL, Sposto R, Shah NR, et al. Outcomes of treatment of children and adolescents with recurrent non-Hodgkin's lymphoma and Hodgkin's disease with dexamethasone, etoposide, cisplatin, cytarabine, and l-asparaginase, maintenance chemotherapy, and transplantation: Children's Cancer Group Study CCG-5912. *J Clin Oncol* 2001;19:2390–2396.

60. Gordon BG, Warkentin PI, Weisenburger DD, et al. Bone marrow transplantation for peripheral T-cell lymphoma in children and adolescents. *Blood* 1992; 80:2938–2942.

61. Murphy SB. Childhood non-Hodgkin's lymphoma. *N Engl J Med* 1978;299:1446–1448.

9

Ewing's Sarcoma

Karen J. Marcus, M.D., and Nancy J. Tarbell, M.D.

James Ewing (1866–1943) first described the bone tumor that bears his name in 1921 (1). Ewing characterized the tumor as either an endothelioma or endothelial myeloma of bone. He observed that the malignancy was most common in teenagers, occurred in the metaphyseal and diaphyseal region of long bones or in the flat bones, was associated with pain and often fever, had a histologic appearance of highly vascular sheets of small round cells, and was quite sensitive to radiation (Fig. 9-1) (2).

Ewing was a leading authority on cancer. He became professor and chair of pathology at Cornell Medical School in New York City at 33 years of age and went on to serve as director of the Memorial Hospital, playing a crucial role in the growth of what is now known as the Memorial Sloan–Kettering Cancer Center (2).

Ewing's sarcoma is the second most common childhood primary bone tumor. The tumor is slightly less common than osteosarcoma and represents 3% of pediatric cancers. Approximately 200 cases occur annually in the United States. Although it presents in the pubertal age range in 40% of patients, the age at diagnosis is more variable than that of osteosarcoma: 30% of cases occur in children younger than 10 years old and 5% occur in young adults older than 20 years old. Boys are affected more often than girls, at a ratio of 1.5 to 2:1. Age at diagnosis parallels the earlier onset of puberty in girls, with a median time of onset 3 to 4 years younger than in boys. Ewing's sarcoma is rare in children of Asian or African descent (3).

PATHOLOGY

Ewing's sarcoma consists of monomorphic sheets of small, round malignant cells with hyperchro-

matic nuclei and little cytoplasm. There is a dearth of associated stroma. Cells usually are periodic acid–Schiff (PAS) positive, indicating the presence of glycogen granules. Glycogen in the tumor cells and the demonstration of the MIC2 gene product on the tumor cell membrane help identify Ewing's sarcoma (4,5). The tumor cells are also uniformly vimentin positive and often cytokeratin positive, indicating origin from epithelial and neuronal elements (6).

There has been much debate over the cell of origin of Ewing's sarcoma. Ewing contended that the tumor was of endothelial origin. The current opinion is that Ewing's sarcoma derives from neural crest progenitors (7). Primitive neural features have been described in peripheral primitive neuroectodermal tumors (PNETs) of soft tissue and Ewing's sarcoma (8). The recognition of the characteristic 11:22 chromosomal translocation associated with Ewing's sarcoma was a major step in recognizing Ewing's sarcoma and PNET as a distinct clinicopathologic entity. PNETs typically are neuron-specific enolase positive, S100 positive, and vimentin positive, in contrast to classic Ewing's, which is neuron-specific enolase negative, S100 variable, and vimentin positive (4–6,9–13).

Ewing's sarcoma and PNETs are considered a single family of tumors with variable phenotypic expression. The Ewing's and PNET family of tumors has become a model for the nonmorphologic approaches to diagnosis. Although no routinely used immunohistochemical stains can positively distinguish Ewing's sarcoma and PNET from other undifferentiated childhood tumors, the majority of Ewing's and PNET tumors have been shown to express high levels of the MIC2 glycoprotein (4). The detection of membrane-associated MIC2 expression is a sensitive

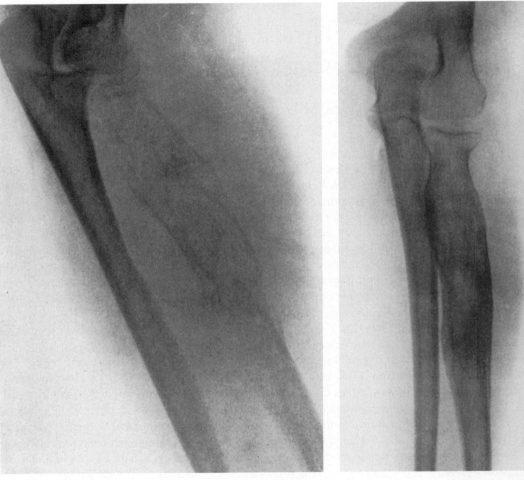

A

B

FIG. 9-1. (A) In the fourth edition of his textbook *Neoplastic Diseases* (1940), James Ewing of the Memorial Hospital, New York, described a "diffuse endothelioma of radius. Diffuse absorption without destruction of shaft. Spontaneous fracture. Wide invasion of muscle. Duration 1 year." Ewing wrote that "the first indication is for treatment by radiation in full doses, and over considerable periods. This recommendation is based on the reported cure of certain cases . . . by radiation alone, and on the clinical disappearance of the disease by variable periods in many more cases. The response to radiation also confirms the diagnosis. The danger of metastases occurring while this treatment is in progress is probably negligible, since the tumor tissue generally undergoes rapid liquefaction and necrosis." **(B)** Ewing illustrated the excellent response of the tumor to radiotherapy.

marker for Ewing's sarcoma and PNET, but it is not specific in that many other tumors and some normal tissues are immunoreactive with anti-MIC2 antibodies.

Ewing's sarcoma and PNET have been linked to the specific chromosomal abnormalities involving a reciprocal translocation between chromosome 11 and 22: t(11;22)(q24;q12). This genetic rearrangement is detectable in 86–90% of tumors. Approximately 5–10% of Ewing's sarcomas do not contain t(11;22) but instead have a translocation between chromosome 21 and 22: t(21;22)(q21;q12). However, this alternate rearrangement has molecular consequences similar to those of t(11;22) (14).

The 11;22 translocation juxtaposes the EWS gene with the FLI gene, a member of the ETS transcription factor family. The 21;22 translocation juxtaposes the EWS gene to another ETS family member, ERG. There are structural similarities between these two translocations, suggesting that they bind to similar DNA target sites. EWS/FLI can produce malignant transformation of some but not all cell lines. The EWS/FLI gene appears to act as an transcription factor. Its mechanism of action appears to be a modulation of transcription of target genes. The Ewing's sarcoma and PNET translocation seems to fall in a developing class of tumor-associated chromosomal translocations that form chimeric transcription factors (14). The formation of aberrant transcription factors is associated with many human malignancies. We may conclude that the probable mechanism of carcinogenesis in Ewing's sarcoma is a translocation that produces an aberrant transcription factor. These factors can cause deregulation of pathways, resulting in tumorigenesis. Using retroviral systems to biologically screen cDNA from cells transformed by EWS/FLI-1, PDGF-C has been identified as the target of EWS/ETS transcriptional deregulation (15). Therefore, Ewing's sarcoma cytogenetics may help us to understand oncogenic mechanisms.

Recent publications have shown that the t(11;22) breakpoint location and therefore the exact amino acid composition of the resultant EWS-FLI fusion oncoproteins might have prognostic relevance (10,13,16). Therefore, the importance of the availability of specimens for genetic analysis cannot be overemphasized (16).

CLINICAL PRESENTATION

Pain is the most common presenting symptom, noted in approximately 90% of cases. Local swelling or mass effect related to the bone tumor is apparent in a majority of children. A distinct soft tissue mass can be appreciated clinically in one-third of cases. Significant limitation of movement has been described in 25% of presentations. Neurologic symptoms or signs occur in 15% of children, either as spinal cord compression or peripheral nerve compression. The latter is most often apparent with lesions of the pelvis or about the knee. Fever is present in 10%

of cases and has been related to tumor size and metastatic disease at diagnosis.

The diagnostic evaluation of the patient with Ewing's sarcoma is shown in Table 9-1. Laboratory findings may include high leukocyte count, a nonspecific finding indicative of tumor bulk or extensive disease. A high leukocyte count has been related to increased risk of tumor recurrence (16,17). Pretreatment serum lactate dehydrogenase (LDH) is of prognostic significance, and the degree of LDH elevation has been related to tumor volume (17). Positron emission tomography using fluorine-18 fluorodeoxyglucose is being studied for detection of osseous metastases in bone tumors and appears to be a sensitive and specific modality in Ewing's sarcoma and PNET.

The diagnostic features of Ewing's sarcoma are radiographically defined as a permeative, destructive lesion of bone. In long bones, the tumor most often presents along the metaphyseal region or within the diaphysis (i.e., at the midshaft level). The periosteum often is displaced by the underlying tumor, resulting in the clinical sign of Codman's triangle, representing a bone expansile lesion. Although bone expansion is common, new bone formation beyond the periosteal margin is rare. An associated soft tissue mass is typical, occurring in more than 50% of long bone neoplasms (18,19). Both computed tomography (CT) and magnetic resonance imaging (MRI) appear necessary for most sites and are complementary. Using both studies has added substantially to the determination of dis-

TABLE 9-1. *Clinical evaluation of the patient with Ewing's sarcoma*

Pathology
  Biopsy with routine histology
  Electron microscopy
  Immunohistochemistry
  Cytogenetics
Radiography
  Computed tomography and magnetic resonance
    imaging of the local tumor extent
  Chest computed tomography
  Bone scan
  Bone marrow aspirate and biopsy
Laboratory
  Routine chemistries, including lactate
    dehydrogenase

ease extent, identifying extraosseous involvement and the degree of marrow infiltration linearly (Fig. 9-2). CT has been valuable in outlining the bone and soft tissue extent of central Ewing's sarcoma (Fig. 9-3), and more accurate definition of tumor extent by CT scans is credited with improvement in control of pelvic Ewing's sarcoma (20). MRI has added to this definition of tumor (Fig. 9-4) (21). Radionuclide bone scan may also be of value, although it may exaggerate the linear tumor extent. MRI may show edema. Whether direct microscopic exten-

sion of tumor is associated with the edema is unknown at present.

Approximately 53% of Ewing's sarcomas have a primary site in an extremity, and 47% have central primaries. Ewing's sarcoma presents in the proximal extremities in 20–30% and distal extremities in 30–40% of cases (22–24). Metastases are present at diagnosis in approximately 20–25% of patients.

Primary lesions of the rib are associated with direct pleural extension and significant extraosseous soft tissue mass in a majority of cases (25,26). The original description of thoracopulmonary malignant tumors by Askin et al. in 1979 (27) characterized small round cell tumors in this location as a separate clinicopathologic entity, often called Askin's tumor. He described a female predominance and a short median survival (8 months). These tumors tend to have a large soft tissue component that can displace most of one lung with or without much rib involvement. This patient group has special management issues (28,29).

The frequency of overt metastasis is estimated at 25–30% for pelvic primaries and less than 10% for tumors of the extremities or ribs. The sites of metastatic disease at diagnosis parallel the distribution noted with treatment failure, most often involving the lungs (40%) or bones (40%), with less common disease involving the bone marrow, lymph nodes, soft tissue, visceral sites, or, rarely, the central nervous system (30). No formal staging system has been recognized for Ewing's sarcoma. The disease factors most recognized as prognostically significant include the bone of origin or primary site, older age, tumor size, presence or degree of soft tissue extension, and identification of hematogenous metastasis at diagnosis (Table 9-2). Smaller tumors (less than 200 mL in volume) and distal extremity tumors tend to be favorable (24,31). At present, the most important prognostic factor at diagnosis appears to be the presence of metastasis (32,33). Reports suggest that the response to initial chemotherapy is significant as well (34). The prognostic importance of the EWS-FLI fusion in Ewing's sarcoma warrants additional study (10,13).

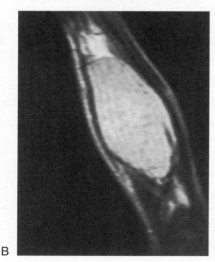

FIG. 9-2. (A) Ewing's sarcoma of the left radius with **(B)** extensive infiltration of the surrounding soft tissue.

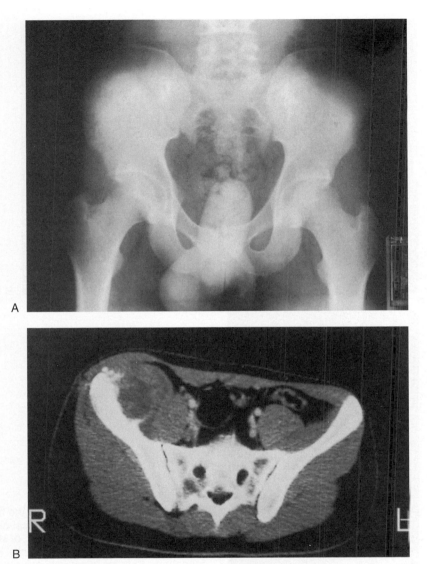

FIG. 9-3. Pelvic Ewing's sarcoma, involving the right ileum. **(A)** Plain films show only mottled destruction of the lateral aspect of the right ilium. **(B)** Computed tomography shows the extensive associated soft tissue mass.

TABLE 9-2. *Prognostic factors in Ewing's sarcoma: disease-related parameters*

Disease factors	Favorable prognosis	Unfavorable prognosis	References
Site	Distal extremity (tibia, fibula, radius, ulna, hands, feet)	Central lesions (especially pelvic bones) less favorable: proximal extremity (humerus, femur), ribs	6, 18, 34, 62, 86, 93, 94
Size	<8 cm in greatest diameter or <200 mL estimated volume	Larger tumors	18, 59, 67, 95
Soft tissue extension	Absence of radiographically identifiable soft tissue extension	Presence of soft tissue extension by radiograph or significant extension by computed tomography	18, 23

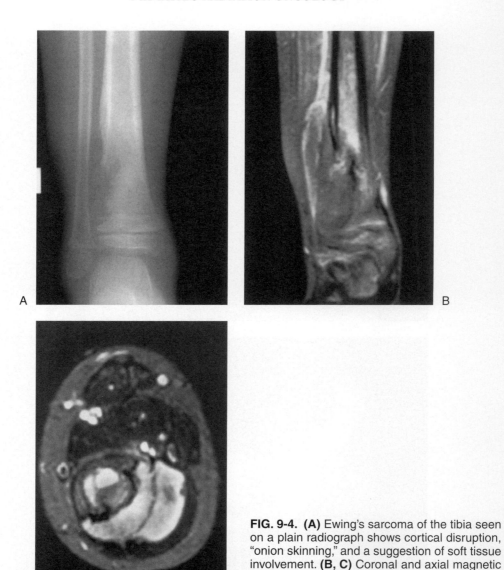

FIG. 9-4. (A) Ewing's sarcoma of the tibia seen on a plain radiograph shows cortical disruption, "onion skinning," and a suggestion of soft tissue involvement. **(B, C)** Coronal and axial magnetic resonance imaging show extensive soft tissue infiltration.

SELECTION OF TREATMENT

Local Control

The relative roles of surgery and radiation therapy for local treatment of Ewing's sarcoma have long been debated. In 1953, Wang and Schulz (35) reported 5-year survival in six of 36 children treated with wide-field irradiation, as compared to one of 14 treated by primary surgical resection. Using 50 Gy to the entire bone, Phillips and Sheline (36) documented survival

in five of 21 cases in 1969. After these reports, Ewing's sarcoma was generally treated with radiation therapy except for small tumors in expendable bones. Reviews have indicated an overall rate of local tumor control of 75% to almost 95% after primary radiation therapy (3,22, 37–41).

Historically, radiotherapy has been the local treatment of choice. However, the role of surgery has increased because of several developments. These important developments include the recognition that the local failure rate of radiotherapy for Ewing's sarcoma ranges from 9% to 25%. This is shown by a survey of the literature in Table 9-3. In addition, the development of innovative surgical techniques allowing preservation of limb and structural bone function has promoted surgery as an alternative to radiation. The routine use of cytoreductive chemotherapy, as discussed later in this chapter, often produces a significant decrease in the soft tissue component, rendering tumors more readily resectable. In addition, the concern over second malignancies from radiation therapy has prompted the reevaluation of the role of surgery as well (42).

However, the data concerning local control with radiotherapy alone are difficult to interpret. Difficulties in assessing response to radiation therapy are evident in the slow rate of resolution of CT, MRI, and radionuclide bone scan findings after irradiation. The significance of residual soft tissue abnormalities and persistent areas of increased uptake on technetium scans is uncertain (22,23,34,43). In patients who have hematologic metastasis, the implication of residual recurrent tumor at the primary site confirmed by biopsy or autopsy is uncertain because of the possibility of reseeding from the primary tumor (20,44).

Several other fundamental factors make it difficult to interpret the data comparing surgery and radiotherapy for local treatment. The local recurrence rate after radiotherapy is strongly correlated with the primary tumor site. Local failure of extremity lesions is on the order of 5–10%, compared with a local failure rate for pelvic lesions of 15–70%. Local recurrence after radiotherapy of pelvic lesions is expected to improve with improved tumor imaging and the widespread use of computerized radiotherapy treatment planning. Therefore, old data may be of more limited use in contemporary management. One must also note that tumor size affects local control. Local control for tumors more than 8 cm in diameter is on the order of 80%, compared with 90% for those less than 8 cm in diameter. The fact that larger tumors are more likely to be treated with radiotherapy instead of surgery influences the clinical results of these modalities.

Some patients are treated with a combination of surgery and radiotherapy. Several factors make it difficult to interpret this data. These include the important effect of quality of radiotherapy on local control. In many "surgical" series, one is not really comparing surgery with radiotherapy but rather radiotherapy with radiotherapy and surgery. This is analogous to the

TABLE 9-3. *The roles of surgery and radiation therapy in the local management of Ewing's sarcoma*

Series (reference)	Number of patients	Relapse-free survival	Local failure	Percentage of patients treated with surgical resection
IESS-1 (16)	333	47%	15%	6%
IESS-2 (55,60)	214 (nonpelvic)	65%	9%	43% (complete resection 27%)
	59 (pelvic)	55%	12%	33% (complete resection 19%)
National Cancer Institute (86)	94	44%	17%	
Memorial Sloan–Kettering Cancer Center (5)	67	79%	21% radiotherapy, 0% surgery	50%
Massachusetts General Hospital (46)	45	50%	21%	25%

IESS, Intergroup Ewing's Sarcoma Group Study.
Modified from Horowitz ME, Neff JR, Kun LE. Ewing's sarcoma. Radiotherapy versus surgery for local control. *Pediatr Clin North Am* 1991;38:365–380.

treatment of many other cell tumors with radiotherapy with resection.

Many surgical series include patients who are at lower risk. They include people who have undergone ray resection of the hands and feet, removal of the wing of the ileum, lower sacrum (lower than the S3 bone), ribs, clavicle, or body of the scapula. One must also consider the relative functional deficits that will be experienced during high-dose irradiation, surgery alone, and surgery with irradiation. In this context, when selecting local treatment for childhood Ewing's sarcoma one must consider the rehabilitation capacity and the psychological adjustment of the patient with these local treatments (25,45,46).

Fundamentally, when attempting to compare surgery with radiotherapy in the management of Ewing's sarcoma, one faces the problem of case selection. Studies are not strictly comparable, so surgery and radiotherapy can be seen not as competitive but as complementary. One additional matter must be considered in comparing radiotherapy with surgery, however: the risk of second malignant neoplasms. As we will describe later in this chapter, radiotherapy and alkylating agents combine to increase the risk of second malignant neoplasms after the treatment of Ewing's sarcoma. Studies indicate that the relative risk of sarcomas in the treatment field is related to the radiotherapy dosage and the extent of exposure to alkylating agents.

The relative functional deficits that will be experienced during high-dose irradiation, surgery alone, and surgery with irradiation must also be considered. In this context, when one is selecting local treatment for childhood Ewing's sarcoma, the patient's rehabilitation capacity and psychological adjustment should be considered (4,40,47).

Surgery

The role of surgical resection in combined-modality treatment was addressed by the Memorial Sloan–Kettering Cancer Center (23,48). With overall disease-free survival approaching 80% at 3.5 years, Rosen et al. (49) described local treatment failure in 34 (21%) patients after

radiation therapy and aggressive multiagent chemotherapy, compared with zero of 33 patients who underwent surgical resection in addition to chemotherapy. In an influential review of the Mayo Clinic experience with Ewing's sarcoma, Wilkins et al. (50) related a significant impact of surgical resection on overall survival: 74% at 5 years, compared with 27% in patients treated without surgery. Other reports have also described improvement in local control with the addition of surgery (22,25,40,45,51–53). However, the studies reflected *selected* surgical intervention. For example, in a review by Wilkins et al. (50) of 27 children with microscopically complete resection in a total series of 65 cases, the analysis included 11 patients treated with radiotherapy and no adjuvant chemotherapy. These 11 were included in the analysis of the "non-operated group" and were compared with the patients receiving surgery plus chemotherapy, clearly biasing the results to favor the surgical group. In a more balanced comparison, Brown et al. (22) described improvement in local control with surgery in extremity lesions. There were local recurrences in zero of five resected cases, compared with three of 15 treated with primary radiation therapy. Brown et al.'s analysis pointed out the selected use of surgery in 35 of 67 patients, clearly selecting cases with distal and smaller lesions for surgery.

Treatment results after surgical resection when combined with chemotherapy have been excellent, even considering the selection factors inherent in surgical subsets. In cases with complete or good partial response to preoperative chemotherapy, Hayes et al. (54) described disease-free survival in 11 of 11 cases with negative operative margins and no added irradiation. Most other series addressing the impact of surgery have incorporated postoperative radiation therapy, often at reduced dosage levels (25,45, 47,49,50,53,55). The addition of surgery for "dispensable bones" (e.g., fibula, rib, smaller lesions of the hands or feet) often is considered a significant addition to therapy with little attendant functional deficit, although excellent results have also been reported with irradiation (44). Options for surgical management have also been considered primarily in the very young population, in whom radiation late effects would be more significant (55–58).

Appropriate comparison of surgical results for Ewing's sarcoma entails attention to the adequacy of radiation therapy in the control arm (23,43). The German Cooperative Ewing's Sarcoma Study (CESS) reported a significant difference in local control and survival favoring the cases operated on in the CESS-81 trial (20,40, 55). On review, the high rate of local failure in the radiation therapy group was attributed to a substantial number of cases with inadequate irradiation volume. In fact, a report by Sauer et al. (55), on the same cohort, showed equivalent results of surgery or radiation therapy in small lesions. In addition, the CESS initiated a quality assurance program in 1984. The results of the subsequent study (CESS-86) demonstrate a marked improvement in local control with irradiation compared to the previous trial. From 1986 to 1991, 177 patients with localized Ewing's sarcoma were treated with chemotherapy plus radical surgery or surgery plus radiation (45 Gy) or irradiation alone (60 Gy total), with a central treatment planning review for quality assurance. Results are now comparable to those of the surgery group (3-year relapse-free survival 67% after irradiation, 65% after surgery, and 62% after resection plus irradiation) (37,41,43, 51,59,60). If the functional results are similar, the potential for second malignancies in patients treated with irradiation for Ewing's sarcoma would favor surgery as the treatment of choice for small extremity lesions, dispensable bones, or very young children. High-risk lesions may benefit from combined surgery and radiotherapy (37,61).

Chemotherapy

Early studies established the role of chemotherapy in primary management of Ewing's sarcoma (17,50,62). Multiagent regimens incorporating cyclophosphamide and vincristine with actinomycin and adriamycin (VACA) resulted in overall survival rates of 50–75% for patients without metastasis at diagnosis (17,22,39,54,63). The Intergroup Ewing's Sarcoma Group Study (IESS) 1 (1973–1978) demonstrated the importance of combining alkylating agents and anthracyclines. The IESS-2 (1978–1982) showed that early and intensive chemotherapy combined with local treatment of the primary tumor was beneficial (17,38,64,65).

The 5-year relapse-free survival and overall survival improved from IESS-1 to IESS-2 (Table 9-3). The local control rate improved as well, with a local failure rate of 15% on IESS-1 and 9% on IESS-2.

The German Cooperative Ewing's Sarcoma study, CESS-81, was conducted from 1981 to 1985 (40,59,66,67). Patients received VACA for two cycles followed by local therapy and two additional cycles of the four-drug chemotherapy program. The result of this study of local therapy, which was not randomized, showed a 5-year relapse-free survival of 54% for the patients treated with surgery only, 68% for those treated with surgery and postoperative irradiation, and 43% for those treated with radiotherapy alone. The local failure rate was strikingly different: 6% for surgery alone, 17% for surgery and postoperative irradiation, and 50% for radiotherapy alone. The high local failure rate in the radiotherapy alone arm was clearly secondary to major radiotherapy volume deviations. The local failure rate declined after institution of central radiotherapy treatment planning reviewed midway through the trial.

The response of the primary tumor to chemotherapy as an important prognostic factor has been demonstrated in patients undergoing surgery after initial chemotherapy (68). Picci et al. (58) studied 118 patients between 1983 and 1993 and graded the surgical specimens from grade I to III, with grade I having gross visible tumor, grade II microscopic tumor, and grade III specimens with total necrosis. The 5-year disease-free survival ranged from 34% for grade I to 95% in the grade III group (58). Others have confirmed that tumor necrosis after induction chemotherapy carries a favorable prognosis (32,68).

The proportion of patients with distant metastasis is another measure of chemotherapeutic responsiveness. Marcus et al. (21) analyzed the impact of tumor size on survival; the dominant pattern of failure for large tumors remained distant metastasis despite aggressive chemotherapy. Jurgens et al. (40) described distant metastasis in 29% of the CESS-I cases; isolated distant metastasis occurred in 10%. The updated results of IESS-II demonstrated a 63% survival at 5 years, with 25% of patients developing distant metastases only (65).

The substitution of ifosfamide for cyclophosphamide was tested in the CESS-86, which included 177 patients from 1986 to 1991 (20,40, 59,66,67,69,70). Patients whose primary tumors were judged to be smaller than 100 cm^3 received induction VACA. Those with larger tumors received vincristine, actinomycin, ifosfamide, and adriamycin (VAIA). Local therapy, at the discretion of the treating physician, was given at week 10. This was followed by four courses of VACA for the smaller tumors and four courses of VAIA for the larger tumors. When a curative resection was conducted, no additional radiation was given if there were no significant risk factors for local recurrence, such as positive margins. However, if the operative bed was at risk for local persistence of tumor, patients were randomized to once or twice per day postoperative irradiation. For patients in whom a curative resection was possible but there was only small residual disease after induction chemotherapy, surgery was not performed and patients were randomized to once- or twice-a-day radiation. When a tumor resection was not undertaken and there was substantial tumor, patients were randomized to receive either 45 Gy of conventional irradiation once per day to a larger field with a 15-Gy cone-down boost to a total of 60 Gy or 44.8 Gy of twice-daily radiation to a larger field followed by a 16-Gy boost with twice-daily irradiation.

In CESS-86, 22% of the patients were treated locally with surgery, 53% with surgery and radiotherapy, and 25% with radiotherapy. The results of this trial are shown in Table 9-4. Although the patients treated with surgery alone had a low rate of local failure, they had a higher rate of distant metastases. Local treatment did not influence survival. In addition, there appeared to be no difference between once- and twice-daily irradiation. Tumor volume greater than 200 mL and poor histologic response to chemotherapy had a negative effect on outcome by both univariate and multivariate analysis (69).

The impact of local therapy modality for the 1,058 patients enrolled in the CESS and the European Intergroup Cooperative Ewing's Sarcoma Study (EICESS) trials was reported. After induc-

TABLE 9-4. *Cooperative Ewing's Sarcoma Study 86 (CESS-86)*

Patient group	Survival	Local failure	Distant metastases
Entire patient population	57%		
The 22% of the patients treated locally with surgery[a]		0%	26%
The 53% of the patients treated locally with surgery and radiotherapy[a]		5%	29%
The 25% of the patients treated locally with radiotherapy		14%	16%
Of the patients treated locally with radiotherapy only, a comparison of once-daily and twice-daily irradiation[a]	63% q.d. 65% b.i.d.	18% q.d.	
Of the patients treated locally with surgery and radiotherapy, a comparison of once-daily and twice-daily irradiation	69% q.d. 71% b.i.d.	14% b.i.d.	

[a]Local therapy was not randomized. Therefore, the results are a function of case selection.
From Dunst J, Jurgens H, Sauer R, et al. Radiation therapy in Ewing's sarcoma: an update of the CESS 86 trial. *Int J Radiat Oncol Biol Phys* 1995;32:919–930; and Dunst J, Sauer R, Burgers JM, et al. Radiation therapy as local treatment in Ewing's sarcoma. Results of the Cooperative Ewing's Sarcoma Studies CESS 81 and CESS 86. *Cancer* 1991;67:2818–2825, with permission.

tion chemotherapy patients with resectable tumors had excellent local control, with a local relapse rate of 7.5%. Comparable local control was achieved in patients given preoperative radiotherapy in the EICESS-92 trial to patients for whom there was a high likelihood of close resection margins or in whom further tumor reduction was expected to allow function-preserving surgery. For patients treated with definitive radiotherapy, local relapse was 26%, significantly higher than for those able to undergo resection; however, this cohort represented a negatively selected group of patients with unfavorable tumor sites.

The synergistic effectiveness of etoposide in combination with alkylators was studied in the Children's Cancer Group (CCG) Study 7881 and Pediatric Oncology Group (POG) Study 8850 (70). This trial evaluated the use of VACA with and without ifosfamide and etoposide to treat newly diagnosed Ewing's sarcoma or primitive neuroectodermal tumors. This phase III randomized trial was open from 1983 to 1994. Patients were randomly assigned to receive 49 weeks of standard chemotherapy with VACA or the experimental treatment, which alternated VACA with the ifosfamide-etoposide combination. The trial demonstrated, in terms of both increased survival and overall survival, the superiority of six-drug chemotherapy to four-drug chemotherapy for localized disease (Table 9-5). However, no benefit was attributable to six-drug chemotherapy for metastatic disease.

Intensification of chemotherapy to improve the outcome is being tested in more recent trials for the management of Ewing's sarcoma and PNET. Two sequential prospective randomized trials have been testing the hypothesis that intensification of chemotherapy can improve the outcome over standard-dose chemotherapy. The first such trial was open from 1995 to 1998, and the second opened in 2001. Both trials use interval compression as the method of dosage intensification and are limited to patients with newly diagnosed localized disease. The analyses of these studies include event-free and overall survival, toxicity, and the relationship between the intensification achieved and outcome. When the

TABLE 9-5. *National Cancer Institute Protocol INT-0091 (Children's Cancer Group Study 7881 and Pediatric Oncology Group Study 8850)*

Characteristic	Distribution
Primary site	Pelvic 20%
	Femur 18%
	Rib 13%
	Tibia 10%
	Humerus 7%
	Other 29%
Local therapy	Surgery 38%
	Radiotherapy 39%
	Both 23%
5-year event-free survival for patients with local disease	4 drugs 54% vs. 6 drugs 69%, $p = 0.0005$
5-year overall survival for patients with local disease	4 drugs 61% vs. 6 drugs 72%, $p = 0.0007$
Event-free survival for patients with metastatic disease	22%, no difference between the two arms

Biopsy patients were randomized to receive either vincristine, adriamycin, cyclophosphamide, and actinomycin D or these four drugs plus ifosfamide and etoposide. The therapy lasted ~51 weeks. Local therapy was administered at weeks 9 to 15.

From Grier HE, Krailo MD, Tarbell NJ, et al. Addition of ifosfamide and etoposide to standard chemotherapy for Ewing's sarcoma and primitive neuroectodermal tumor of bone. *N Engl J Med* 2003;348:694–701, with permission.

local control from these studies is analyzed, further insight into the impact of chemotherapy on local control will be gained.

In the management of metastatic disease at presentation, little progress appears to have been made during serial studies. For example, in IESS-1 patients with metastatic disease were treated with VACA for a 5-year survival of 30%. In IESS-2 drugs were VACA plus 5-fluorouracil, and the 5-year survival was 28%. In the aforementioned CCG-POG trial recently completed, the 2-year survival was 22%.

Radiotherapeutic Management

The role of radiation therapy in primary management of Ewing's sarcoma is generally evaluated in each patient with a team including surgeons, medical oncologists, and radiation oncologists. As previously discussed, there is controversy concerning the relative advantages of irradiation and surgery with preoperative or postoperative irradiation (21,43,51,60,71).

Volume

Local control of tumor with irradiation improved after the general acceptance of a target volume encompassing the entire medullary cavity to moderately high dosage levels (30,72). Suit (73) summarized the experience of the 1950s and 1960s in recommending irradiation to the entire involved bone with a higher-dose boost to the primary tumor site. He noted few instances of marginal or distant intramedullary recurrence with such treatment. However, subsequent studies have reported irradiation results based largely on treatment techniques that have not included the opposite epiphysis, noting no marginal recurrences despite high variable rates of local tumor control (21,51,74).

The importance of adequate treatment volume and radiotherapy quality cannot be overemphasized. The results of the CESS-I study indicated an excessive rate of local recurrence attributed to poor quality control for radiation therapy. Protocol modification to include central planning for radiation therapy diminished the frequency of local failure (55,74).

Brown et al. (22) analyzed the sites of local recurrence, describing consistent failure in the primary tumor volume for patients with lesions of the extremities and pelvis. Marginal failures occurred infrequently, limited to patients with rib primaries. In a study reducing treatment volume and dosage, Hayes et al. (54) found a high rate of local recurrence (25% isolated, 35% overall). However, treatment failures were localized within the primary target volume in 13 of 14 instances using a limited, postchemotherapy tumor extent to define the soft tissue component of the irradiation fields.

Data addressed the efficacy of diminished treatment volumes (31,75). Local or tailored fields encompassing the primary tumor with a 3- to 5-cm margin rather than the whole bone have been studied (Fig. 9-5). Marcus (31) reported excellent local control using tailored fields, noting the ability to spare a component of the long

bones in tumors less than 8 cm in diameter, whereas full-bone irradiation often is needed to achieve a 4-cm margin around larger tumors. Despite the higher overall rates of local failure in the St. Jude Children's Research Hospital study, Hayes et al. (54) also noted local control in 12 of 14 patients with lesions less than 9 cm in diameter using smaller target volumes.

A seminal study in the determination of the proper field size for the irradiation of localized Ewing's sarcoma was POG-8346. Between 1983 and 1988, 184 children were studied. Of this group, 179 were truly eligible for the study; 79% had localized disease, and 21% had metastases. Induction treatment was cyclophosphamide and adriamycin followed by local treatment with either surgery or radiation therapy. This was followed by actinomycin D and vincristine. Patients treated to the local site with radiotherapy were randomized to receive whole bone irradiation to 39.6 Gy with a 16.2-Gy boost or involved-field irradiation to 55.8 Gy. For the 104 patients with localized disease who were irradiated, the 5-year event-free survival was 42%, with no difference in event-free survival between those randomized to receive large or small fields. The local control rate was only 45% for those not treated to the protocol-specified volume (76).

The current recommendations for treatment volume mandate the use of MRI whenever possible to identify the tumor extent. The entire bony abnormality and soft tissue mass are included, identified at diagnosis before either surgery or chemotherapy as the gross tumor volume (GTV), with a 1.5- to 2-cm margin added to cover potential occult tumor. An additional margin, generally determined by the institution, is then added. This results in the planning target volume (PTV) to account for daily setup, patient movement, and an additional margin for dosimetric considerations. The exception to this method is the case of a large soft tissue mass that protrudes into a body cavity at diagnosis and is responding to chemotherapy and allowing normal tissues to move back to their normal position. In this circumstance, the initial GTV excludes the prechemotherapy volume if that volume previously extended into the body cavity. The vol-

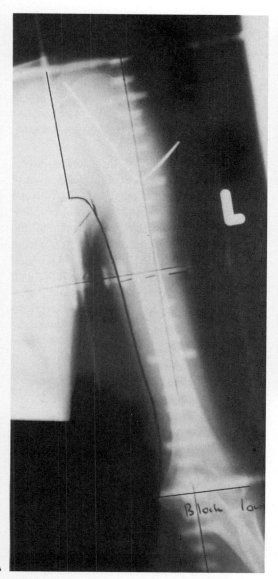

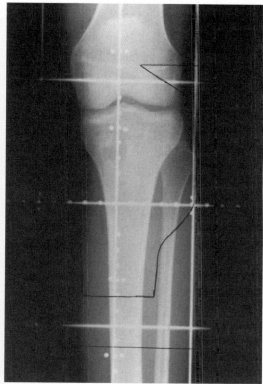

FIG. 9-5. Changes in treatment volume for Ewing's sarcoma. **(A)** Field encompassing the entire length of the medullary cavity for a tumor involving the proximal left humerus. **(B)** Tailored field encompassing only the proximal aspect of the leg for a limited tumor of the left tibia; there is a 5-cm distal margin beyond known bone involvement as demonstrated by all imaging procedures. In recent years, national protocols have called for a 2- to 3-cm margin.

ume of infiltrative soft tissue disease is not modified. The entire original bony abnormality is always treated.

In postoperative irradiation, the appropriate target volume has not been adequately defined. Based on the data supporting local volume for primary radiation therapy, one would recom-

mend treatment to the preoperative tumor bed with adequate margins, later reducing the treatment fields to documented sites of tumor residual in incompletely resected lesions. In all cases with residual tumor in the operative specimen, encompassing the surgical incision appears to be important.

Dosage

Early reports established the efficacy of radiation dosages of 50 to 60 Gy at 180 to 200 cGy per fraction, describing better local control than is achieved with a total dosage of less than 45 Gy (6,77). Dosage recommendations have included 40 to 45 Gy to the entire medullary cavity, with a boost to the primary site to cumulative levels of 55 to 60 Gy (73).

The IESS-I results indicated no dose-response relationship between 40 and 68 Gy (48). Using 50 Gy in 25 fractions, the National Cancer Institute reported clinically apparent local recurrence in 20% of cases (39). Whether the lower frequency of local recurrence in the IESS and selected single-institution series using 60 Gy reflects a dose-response relationship is uncertain based on available data (43,48).

Alterations in total dosage and the time-dose relationship were found in University of Florida research using hyperfractionated irradiation (31,78,79). Patients were treated with 120 cGy twice daily to 36 Gy for initial target volumes encompassing the primary tumor in 4-cm margins. Subsequent reduced fields were used to cumulative levels of 50.4 Gy (with total resolution of the soft tissue component by preirradiation chemotherapy) and 55.2 Gy (with no response to chemotherapy). For patients with a lesion less than 8 cm in diameter, local recurrence was documented in only 1 of 11 children (80). In a review of the University of Florida series of patients treated between 1969 and 1987, those with tumors 8 cm or smaller treated with twice-daily irradiation had a local control rate of 88%, compared with 92% for once-daily radiation. However, for those with tumors larger than 8 cm, the local control rate for twice-daily radiation was 88%, compared with 58% for once-daily irradiation. Evaluation of this data must be tempered by the previously cited randomized trial of CESS, which did not show a benefit to multiple-daily-fraction irradiation (40,59). With larger lesions, some have used more aggressive systemic therapy and total body irradiation (TBI; 400 cGy twice daily) with reported improved local and overall disease control (21).

The current dosage recommendations are 55.8 Gy for gross residual disease and 50.4 Gy for microscopic disease. Lesions of the vertebral body are treated with 45 Gy. Standard, once-per-day fractionation is generally used. No dosage modifications are recommended for smaller tumors, although normal tissues should be protected whenever possible. The shielding of critical structures must also be weighed against the possibility of underdosing known tumor-bearing tissue.

Chemotherapy influences local control. Aforementioned studies suggested a local control benefit from the addition of adriamycin, and more recent reports address the prognostic implications of the histologic response of the primary tumor to chemotherapy. The recent randomized trial CCG-7881 and POG-8850 showed a local control benefit of VACA with ifosfamide and etoposide compared with VACA alone (Table 9-6) (70). It is likely that along with improved imaging (MRI and functional MRI) for tumor identification, improvements in chemotherapy will increase local control of the primary tumor.

Technique

Multiple imaging studies must be interpreted carefully to accurately outline both the osseous and the soft tissue extent when defining the primary target volume. The minimal target volume generally should encompass the primary lesion,

TABLE 9-6. *Influence of chemotherapy on local control of Ewing's sarcoma in CCG-7881 and POG-8850*

	VACA	VACA-IE	p
5-year cumulative incidence of local failure	15%	9%	<0.01
Systemic failure	21%	20%	0.92
Local and systemic failure	5%	2%	0.1
Any local failure	20%	11%	

IE, ifosfamide and etoposide; VACA, vincristine, actinomycin D, cyclophosphamide, and adriamycin.
From Grier HE, Krailo MD, Tarbell NJ, et al. Addition of ifosfamide and etoposide to standard chemotherapy for Ewing's sarcoma and primitive neuroectodermal tumor of bone. *N Engl J Med* 2003;348:694–701, with permission.

with 1.5- to 2-cm margins around the bone and soft tissue.

Sophisticated radiation therapy techniques will achieve maximal local tumor control while minimizing treatment-related complications. For extremity lesions, sparing a strip of linear soft tissue is fundamental. Avoiding circumferential irradiation decreases the likelihood of significant late fibrosis and limitation of function (43,81). To achieve adequate coverage, treatment plans incorporating oblique opposed fields or angled pairs with compensating wedges may be necessary. Conventional opposed anterior-posterior or lateral field configurations may be ideal if adequate soft tissue can be spared. Immobilizing casts or molds are important for daily reproducibility and accuracy during treatment (see Chapter 22).

Large extremity lesions often necessitate irradiation of the adjacent joint. With the same attention to normal tissue sparing, the major late problem associated with joint irradiation appears to be greater growth alterations if both epiphyses of the joint are included, particularly at the knee (41,81).

Lesions of the distal extremities, including the ankle, feet, and hands, present individualized problems regarding treatment planning. The use of tissue compensation, immobilizing devices, and detailed attention to dosimetry are critical to achieving excellent tumor control and functional integrity (23,77). The use of a water bath to achieve dosage homogeneity has been suggested. Alternatively, a single-photon beam incident on the contralateral surface of the hand or foot may be combined with an ipsilateral electron field.

For pelvic lesions, techniques to avoid full-dose irradiation of the bladder often are possible with oblique or multifield configurations. Carefully including the soft tissue extent, often more impressive on CT or MRI studies, will ensure maximal tumor control. For vertebral Ewing's sarcoma, uniform irradiation of the adjacent vertebrae will minimize late effects. The use of weighted opposed anterior-posterior fields or a wedged-pair technique generally ensures adequate coverage of the vertebrae, of necessity including the spinal canal.

There is a limited experience with brachytherapy for Ewing's sarcoma. Potter et al. (82) described six patients treated with chemotherapy, external beam irradiation, and intraoperative high-dose rate brachytherapy for close surgical resection margins. All six children are alive and well.

Improvements in imaging modalities, particularly the routine use of MRI scans to assess tumor extent, provide more accurate target definition. Technologic advances in radiation therapy treatment delivery will also allow greater sparing of normal tissue without compromising tumor treatment. Such technologic advances may include the use of intensity-modulated radiation therapy and the use of protons.

Rib lesions (Askin's tumor) are generally large tumors, often with extension to the pleural surfaces. This site warrants special consideration because it is often associated with a large soft tissue component (67). The surgeon must not attempt to remove the tumor initially before chemotherapy. After biopsy, chemotherapy should be given for large lesions because it induces tumor shrinkage (28,83). In thoracic rib and soft tissue primaries, the postchemotherapy volume appears adequate to define the irradiation volume. If resection is done first, margins may be positive and may necessitate a much larger volume of irradiation. The radiation volume often is limited by organ toxicity such as the heart in left-sided lesions. Resection after chemotherapy may be adequate if operative margins are clearly negative after nearly complete response to chemotherapy. If the resection margins are positive or the tumor is incompletely resected, local irradiation is indicated to increase the likelihood of local tumor control (22,26,28,54,83). Inclusion of the pleural cavity in patients with cytologically positive effusions has been recommended because the pattern of failure as described by Askin et al. (27) included the pleura in a significant number of cases. There is also a risk of pleural relapse in patients with Askin's tumor and no initial pleural effusion. Some clinicians attempt to treat the pleural surface but spare the lung by using external beam electrons. An alternative technique is intrapleural radioisotope application. A small amount of dye is placed in the pleural cavity with saline and the patient is rotated. Free flow is confirmed by fluo-roscopy. As an alternative, a tracer amount of ra-dioactivity may be used to confirm free flow in the pleural space with a gamma camera. After free flow is confirmed, a therapeutic dose of ^{32}P is instilled to irradiate the pleural surface. The pa-tient is turned periodically to distribute the iso-tope (83). The treatment of the entire pleural sur-face in the absence of a positive pleural effusion is controversial.

Radiation Therapy for Metastatic Disease

The efficacy of low-dose irradiation in control-ling pulmonary micrometastases is documented in the IESS-I study. The frequency of pul-monary relapse was lower and survival rates were higher with prophylactic pulmonary irradi-ation in comparison to triple-drug chemother-apy alone (17,48,57,84).

For patients with metastatic Ewing's sarcoma of the lung, local irradiation to the lungs and pri-mary site are valuable in overall disease control (30,66). An interesting review addressed the role of lung irradiation for Ewing's sarcoma with pulmonary metastases at diagnoses (66). Of patients accessioned to CESS studies from 1981 to 1992, 42 presented with pulmonary metastases. One died of progressive disease be-fore irradiation. The other patients either had a complete radiographic remission after chemo-therapy ($n = 25$) or chemotherapy with resec-tion of the lung metastases ($n = 4$). Twenty-two patients received bilateral lung irradiation at doses of 12 to 21 Gy. Six had no additional treatment after chemotherapy or surgery, and one underwent bone marrow transplantation. Of the ten patients in complete remission, nine had received lung irradiation and one had undergone complete resection of lung metastases. Overall, one of six patients was in complete remission without lung irradiation, compared with four of ten who received 12 to 16 Gy and five out of six who received 18 to 21 Gy. These data suggest the value of lung irradiation for a patient with pulmonary metastases at diagnosis of Ewing's sarcoma, and they appear consistent with the suggestion from IESS-1 that pulmonary irradia-tion may sterilize micrometastatic disease in the well-oxygenated lungs.

The treatment strategy for patients presenting with bone metastases is under investigation. Treatment of the primary site using a tailored field is recommended.

Total Body Irradiation and Bone Marrow Transplantation

TBI has been used in advanced Ewing's sar-coma since the late 1960s (44). Improvement in survival using TBI led the Princess Margaret Hospital group to studies incorporating sequen-tial hemibody irradiation with an attenuated three-drug chemotherapy regimen (85). The use of low-dose, fractionated TBI (15 cGy twice weekly to cumulative levels of 150 cGy) at the National Cancer Institute (NCI) has been fol-lowed by studies using "intensification TBI" (400 cGy twice daily), both at NCI and the Uni-versity of Florida (21,39). These initial reports have yielded different results, with a positive impact in the University of Florida series (86) and little or no impact in the NCI series. The NCI series has been updated, and the long-term results continue to demonstrate no benefit to this approach (87).

Burdach et al. (88) reported using TBI (12 Gy, 1.5 twice daily) and simultaneous high-dose melphalan, followed by etoposide and stem cell rescue. Their results (17 patients) are encour-aging, with seven of 17 patients disease free, $45\% \pm 12\%$ at 6 years, compared with $2\% \pm 2\%$ for the historic control group. Two recent re-ports using a non-TBI regimen appeared to yield similar results (19,84). Overall, reports of im-provements in overall survival for patients with advanced local or metastatic disease have been mixed (89,90).

CURE RATES AND SIDE EFFECTS OF TREATMENT

Current experience with Ewing's sarcoma indi-cates 5-year disease-free survival in 50–75% of patients with localized disease at diagnosis (17,25,53,65). There have been late relapses, and the 10-year survival is decidedly worse than the 5-year survival. A limited number of single-institution reports indicate higher disease-free survival (21,40,49). Survival clearly parallels initial disease extent (38). Disease-free survival greater than 75% has been documented for limited-volume Ewing's sarcoma involving the distal extremities. Survival rates of only 25–35% are achieved with large central lesions (22,38, 40,53).

Overall functional results after treatment of Ewing's sarcoma have correlated closely with the degree of attention to detailed local management. Selection of primary surgery for lesions permitting function-preserving resection with negative or microscopically positive margins may decrease late effects of high-dose irradiation, particularly in prepubertal youngsters (25, 52,53).

With appropriate radiation therapy, patients treated for Ewing's sarcoma of the extremities had excellent functional results in more than 60% of cases. The NCI late effects review noted minor alterations in leg length or minimal symptoms of soft tissue change in another 20% of cases (81). Significant treatment-related morbidity occurred in 20% of the NCI cases and was related primarily to larger primary lesions or posttreatment fracture of the femur. Significantly higher morbidities have been reported in series combining systemic chemotherapy with dosages greater than 60 Gy (22,53,81). In a limited number of patients treated with 70 Gy to the primary site, severe functional deterioration was reported in 26% of patients (49).

The risk of posttreatment fracture has also been related to total dosage. Fracture appears to correlate more directly with the extent of cortical disruption at the time of biopsy, in addition to tumor size and younger age at presentation (17,20,52,56).

Limited changes have been reported after primary irradiation of tumors of the upper extremities. Some degree of hip dysfunction and potential growth disturbances are documented in long-term follow-up of patients with pelvic Ewing's sarcoma. Combined cyclophosphamide-irradiation cystopathy has also been noted in such cases (22,41). One of the primary concerns regarding irradiation is the impact on bone growth. Morphologic changes of the irradiated epiphysis have been reviewed in the NCI series (81). Quantitatively, reduction and subsequent growth relates to the sites of epiphyseal irradia-

tion and the age at treatment. Overall functional results are less favorable in very young children (41,81). (See Chapter 19.)

The high incidence of secondary tumors in Ewing's sarcoma was originally suggested in the combined reporting of the Late Effect Study Group (LESG), assessing the frequency of secondary bone sarcomas in 9,170 children surviving more than 2 years after treatment for cancer. The rate of carcinogenesis in patients with Ewing's sarcoma was second only to that in patients with retinoblastoma in this study. There was a sharp dose-response relationship after dosages to the bone of more than 60 Gy. With the current standard in Ewing's of 45 to 55 Gy, this risk of second tumors appears to be less than in the original reports. In contrast to the 22% actuarial risk of second tumors reported by LESG (90), more recent data demonstrate a cumulative incidence of 9.2% for any second malignancy and 6.5% for secondary sarcoma (46). Here again, a dose-response relationship was demonstrated, with no secondary sarcomas seen with a dosage of less than 48 Gy. The risk of secondary leukemia may be greater with high-dose regimens as well (91).

In an overall review of second malignancies after treatment for Ewing's sarcoma in CESS-81 and CESS-86, the addition of radiotherapy to surgery or treatment with radiotherapy alone was associated with a higher cumulative risk of second malignancies (Table 9-7) (92). The Childhood

TABLE 9-7. *Second malignancies after treatment for Ewing's sarcoma in patients treated in the German Cooperative Ewing's Sarcoma Studies CESS-81 and CESS-86*

Type of local treatment in a total population of 674 patients followed for a median of 7 years	Cumulative risk of any second malignancy after 15 years
All patients	4.6%
Local treatment with surgery alone	0.9%
Local treatment with surgery and postoperative irradiation to 36–46 Gy	6.1%
Local treatment with definitive irradiation to 46–60 Gy	6.7%

From Ahrens S, Dunst J, Rube C, et al. Second malignancy after treatment for Ewing's sarcoma. *Int J Radiat Oncol Biol Phys* 1997;39:142, with permission.

Cancer Survivor Study, a retrospective study of 13,581 children diagnosed with cancer before age 21 and surviving at least 5 years, reported a 5% cumulative incidence of secondary malignancies at 25 years for the entire cohort (42). The incidence continued to increase over the follow-up period. Survivors of Ewing's sarcoma were at higher risk of developing second malignant tumors than others in the cohort. Other factors in addition to radiotherapy were found to play a role in the development of a second malignant tumor. The use of anthracycline increased the risk of soft tissue sarcoma, and the use of alkylators increased the risk of secondary bone tumors. Although children treated for Ewing's sarcoma and PNET must be followed up over the long term, the success in treatment should not be overshadowed by these adverse sequelae.

REFERENCES

References particularly recommended for further reading are indicated by an asterisk.

1. Ewing J. Diffuse endothelioma of bone. *Proc NY Pathol Soc* 1921;21:17–24.
2. Roberts KB. Ewing's sarcoma. *N C Med J* 1991; 52:319.
3. Miller RW. Contrasting epidemiology of childhood osteosarcoma, Ewing's tumor, and rhabdomyosarcoma. *Natl Cancer Inst Monogr* 1981;9–15.
4. Ambros IM, Ambros PF, Strehl S, et al. MIC2 is a specific marker for Ewing's sarcoma and peripheral primitive neuroectodermal tumors. Evidence for a common histogenesis of Ewing's sarcoma and peripheral primitive neuroectodermal tumors from MIC2 expression and specific chromosome aberration. *Cancer* 1991;67: 1886–1893.
5. Delattre O, Zucman J, Melot T, et al. The Ewing family of tumors: a subgroup of small-round-cell tumors defined by specific chimeric transcripts. *N Engl J Med* 1994;331:294–299.
6. Moll R, Lee I, Gould VE, et al. Immunocytochemical analysis of Ewing's tumors. Patterns of expression of intermediate filaments and desmosomal proteins indicate cell type heterogeneity and pluripotential differentiation. *Am J Pathol* 1987;127:288–304.
7. Arvand A, Denny CT. Biology of EWS/ETS fusions in Ewing's family tumors. *Oncogene* 2001;20:5747–5754.
8. Whang-Peng J, Triche TJ, Knutsen T, et al. Chromosome translocation in peripheral neuroepithelioma. *N Engl J Med* 1984;311:584–585.
9. Kretschmar CS. Ewing's sarcoma and the "peanut" tumors. *N Engl J Med* 1994;331:325–327.
10. de Alava E, Kawai A, Healey JH, et al. EWS-FLI1 fusion transcript structure is an independent determinant

of prognosis in Ewing's sarcoma. *J Clin Oncol* 1998;16:1248–1255.
11. Schmidt D, Herrmann C, Jurgens H, et al. Malignant peripheral neuroectodermal tumor and its necessary distinction from Ewing's sarcoma. A report from the Kiel Pediatric Tumor Registry. *Cancer* 1991;68:2251–2259.
12. Shimada H, Newton WA Jr, Soule EH, et al. Pathologic features of extraosseous Ewing's sarcoma: a report from the Intergroup Rhabdomyosarcoma Study. *Hum Pathol* 1988;19:442–453.
13. Zoubek A, Dockhorn-Dworniczak B, Delattre O, et al. Does expression of different EWS chimeric transcripts define clinically distinct risk groups of Ewing tumor patients? *J Clin Oncol* 1996;14:1245–1251.
14. Denny CT. Gene rearrangements in Ewing's sarcoma. *Cancer Invest* 1996;14:83–88.
15. Zwerner JP, May WA. PDGF-C is an EWS/FLI induced transforming growth factor in Ewing family tumors. *Oncogene* 2001;20:626–633.
16. Fletcher JA. Ewing's sarcoma oncogene structure: a novel prognostic marker? *J Clin Oncol* 1998;16: 1241–1243.
*17. Nesbit ME Jr, Gehan EA, Burgert EO Jr, et al. Multimodal therapy for the management of primary, nonmetastatic Ewing's sarcoma of bone: a long-term follow-up of the First Intergroup study. *J Clin Oncol* 1990;8:1664–1674.
18. Braun BS, Frieden R, Lessnick SL, et al. Identification of target genes for the Ewing's sarcoma EWS/FLI fusion protein by representational difference analysis. *Mol Cell Biol* 1995;15:4623–4630.
19. Ladenstein R, Lasset C, Pinkerton R, et al. Impact of megatherapy in children with high-risk Ewing's tumours in complete remission: a report from the EBMT Solid Tumour Registry. *Bone Marrow Transplant* 1995;15:697–705.
20. Jenkin RD. Ewing's sarcoma: radiation treatment at the primary site: regarding Dunst et al., IJROBP 32:919–930; 1995. *Int J Radiat Oncol Biol Phys* 1995; 32:1253–1254.
21. Marcus RB Jr, Graham-Pole JR, Springfield DS, et al. High-risk Ewing's sarcoma: end-intensification using autologous bone marrow transplantation. *Int J Radiat Oncol Biol Phys* 1988;15:53–59.
22. Brown AP, Fixsen JA, Plowman PN. Local control of Ewing's sarcoma: an analysis of 67 patients. *Br J Radiol* 1987;60:261–268.
23. Kinsella TJ, Loeffler JS, Fraass BA, et al. Extremity preservation by combined modality therapy in sarcomas of the hand and foot: an analysis of local control, disease free survival and functional result. *Int J Radiat Oncol Biol Phys* 1983;9:1115–1119.
24. Mendenhall CM, Marcus RB Jr, Enneking WF, et al. The prognostic significance of soft tissue extension in Ewing's sarcoma. *Cancer* 1983;51:913–917.
25. Anne P, Efird J, Spiro I, et al. Ewing's sarcoma: comparison of local treatment with radiation or radiation plus surgery. *Int J Radiat Oncol Biol Phys* 1993;27: 295–296.
26. Thomas PR, Foulkes MA, Gilula LA, et al. Primary Ewing's sarcoma of the ribs. A report from the intergroup Ewing's sarcoma study. *Cancer* 1983;51:1021–1027.
27. Askin FB, Rosai J, Sibley RK, et al. Malignant small

cell tumor of the thoracopulmonary region in child-hood: a distinctive clinicopathologic entity of uncertain histogenesis. *Cancer* 1979;43:2438–2451.

28. Shamberger R, LaQuaglia M, Gebhardt M, et al. Ewing sarcoma/primitive neuroectodermal tumor of the chest wall: the impact of initial versus delayed resection on tumor margins, survival, and use of radiation therapy. *Ann Surg* 2003;238:563–567.

29. Shamberger RC, Laquaglia MP, Krailo MD, et al. Ewing sarcoma of the rib: results of an intergroup study with analysis of outcome by timing of resection. *J Thorac Cardiovasc Surg* 2000;119:1154–1161.

*30. Vietti TJ, Gehan EA, Nesbit ME Jr, et al. Multimodal therapy in metastatic Ewing's sarcoma: an Intergroup Study. *Natl Cancer Inst Monogr* 1981;56:279–284.

31. Marcus RB Jr. Current controversies in pediatric radiation oncology. *Orthop Clin North Am* 1996;27:551–557.

*32. Cotterill SJ, Ahrens S, Paulussen M, et al. Prognostic factors in Ewing's tumor of bone: analysis of 975 patients from the European Intergroup Cooperative Ewing's Sarcoma Study Group. *J Clin Oncol* 2000;18:3108–3114.

33. Bacci G, Ferrari S, Bertoni F, et al. Prognostic factors in nonmetastatic Ewing's sarcoma of bone treated with adjuvant chemotherapy: analysis of 359 patients at the Istituto Ortopedico Rizzoli. *J Clin Oncol* 2000;18:4–11.

34. Murphy WA Jr. Imaging bone tumors in the 1990s. *Cancer* 1991;67:1169–1176.

35. Wang C, Schultz M. Ewing's sarcoma. *N Engl J Med* 1953;248:571–576.

36. Phillips TL, Sheline GE. Radiation therapy of malignant bone tumors. *Radiology* 1969;92:1537–1545.

*37. Dunst J, Jurgens H, Sauer R, et al. Radiation therapy in Ewing's sarcoma: an update of the CESS 86 trial. *Int J Radiat Oncol Biol Phys* 1995;32:919–930.

38. Evans RG, Nesbit ME, Gehan EA, et al. Multimodal therapy for the management of localized Ewing's sarcoma of pelvic and sacral bones: a report from the second intergroup study. *J Clin Oncol* 1991;9:1173–1180.

39. Horowitz ME, Kinsella TJ, Wexler LH, et al. Total-body irradiation and autologous bone marrow transplant in the treatment of high-risk Ewing's sarcoma and rhabdomyosarcoma. *J Clin Oncol* 1993;11:1911–1918.

40. Jurgens H, Exner U, Gadner H, et al. Multidisciplinary treatment of primary Ewing's sarcoma of bone. A 6-year experience of a European Cooperative Trial. *Cancer* 1988;61:23–32.

41. Thomas PR, Perez CA, Neff JR, et al. The management of Ewing's sarcoma: role of radiotherapy in local tumor control. *Cancer Treat Rep* 1984;68:703–710.

42. Neglia JP, Friedman DL, Yasui Y, et al. Second malignant neoplasms in five-year survivors of childhood cancer: childhood cancer survivor study. *J Natl Cancer Inst* 2001;93:618–629.

43. Kinsella TJ, Lichter AS, Miser J, et al. Local treatment of Ewing's sarcoma: radiation therapy versus surgery. *Cancer Treat Rep* 1984;68:695–701.

44. Jenkin RD, Rider WD, Sonley MJ. Ewing's sarcoma: adjuvant total body irradiation, cyclophosphamide and vincristine. *Int J Radiat Oncol Biol Phys* 1976;1:407–413.

45. Bacci G, Picci P, Gitelis S, et al. The treatment of lo-calized Ewing's sarcoma: the experience at the Istituto Ortopedico Rizzoli in 163 cases treated with and without adjuvant chemotherapy. *Cancer* 1982;49:1561–1570.

46. Kuttesch JF Jr, Wexler LH, Marcus RB, et al. Second malignancies after Ewing's sarcoma: radiation dose-dependency of secondary sarcomas. *J Clin Oncol* 1996;14:2818–2825.

47. Aurias A, Rimbaut C, Buffe D, et al. Chromosomal translocations in Ewing's sarcoma. *N Engl J Med* 1983;309:496–497.

48. Perez CA, Tefft M, Nesbit ME Jr, et al. Radiation therapy in the multimodal management of Ewing's sarcoma of bone: report of the Intergroup Ewing's Sarcoma Study. *Natl Cancer Inst Monogr* 1981;263–271.

49. Rosen G, Caparros B, Nirenberg A, et al. Ewing's sarcoma: ten-year experience with adjuvant chemotherapy. *Cancer* 1981;47:2204–2213.

50. Wilkins RM, Pritchard DJ, Burgert EO Jr, et al. Ewing's sarcoma of bone. Experience with 140 patients. *Cancer* 1986;58:2551–2555.

51. Barbieri E, Emiliani E, Zini G, et al. Combined therapy of localized Ewing's sarcoma of bone: analysis of results in 100 patients. *Int J Radiat Oncol Biol Phys* 1990;19:1165–1170.

52. Neff JR. Nonmetastatic Ewing's sarcoma of bone: the role of surgical therapy. *Clin Orthop* 1986;204:111–118.

53. Sailer SL, Harmon DC, Mankin HJ, et al. Ewing's sarcoma: surgical resection as a prognostic factor. *Int J Radiat Oncol Biol Phys* 1988;15:43–52.

54. Hayes FA, Thompson EI, Meyer WH, et al. Therapy for localized Ewing's sarcoma of bone. *J Clin Oncol* 1989;7:208–213.

*55. Sauer R, Jurgens H, Burgers JM, et al. Prognostic factors in the treatment of Ewing's sarcoma. The Ewing's Sarcoma Study Group of the German Society of Paediatric Oncology CESS 81. *Radiother Oncol* 1987;10:101–110.

56. Hayes FA, Thompson EI, Parvey L, et al. Metastatic Ewing's sarcoma: remission induction and survival. *J Clin Oncol* 1987;5:1199–1204.

57. Newton WA Jr, Meadows AT, Shimada H, et al. Bone sarcomas as second malignant neoplasms following childhood cancer. *Cancer* 1991;67:193–201.

58. Picci P, Bohling T, Bacci G, et al. Chemotherapy-induced tumor necrosis as a prognostic factor in localized Ewing's sarcoma of the extremities. *J Clin Oncol* 1997;15:1553–1559.

59. Dunst J, Sauer R, Burgers JM, et al. Radiation therapy as local treatment in Ewing's sarcoma. Results of the Cooperative Ewing's Sarcoma Studies CESS 81 and CESS 86. *Cancer* 1991;67:2818–2825.

60. Horowitz ME, Neff JR, Kun LE. Ewing's sarcoma. Radiotherapy versus surgery for local control. *Pediatr Clin North Am* 1991;38:365–380.

61. Scully SP, Temple HT, O'Keefe RJ, et al. Role of surgical resection in pelvic Ewing's sarcoma. *J Clin Oncol* 1995;13:2336–2341.

62. Hayes FA, Thompson EI, Hustu HO, et al. The response of Ewing's sarcoma to sequential cyclophosphamide and adriamycin induction therapy. *J Clin Oncol* 1983;1:45–51.

63. Fellinger EJ, Garin-Chesa P, Triche TJ, et al. Immunohistochemical analysis of Ewing's sarcoma cell sur-

face antigen p30/32MIC2. *Am J Pathol* 1991;139: 317–325.

64. Tefft M, Razek A, Perez C, et al. Local control and survival related to radiation dose and volume and to chemotherapy in non-metastatic Ewing's sarcoma of pelvic bones. *Int J Radiat Oncol Biol Phys* 1978;4: 367–372.

65. Burgert EO Jr, Nesbit ME, Garnsey LA, et al. Multimodal therapy for the management of nonpelvic, localized Ewing's sarcoma of bone: intergroup study IESS-II. *J Clin Oncol* 1990;8:1514–1524.

66. Dunst J, Paulussen M, Jurgens H. Lung irradiation for Ewing's sarcoma with pulmonary metastases at diagnosis: results of the CESS studies. *Strahlenther Onkol* 1993;169:621–623.

67. Jurgens H, Bier V, Harms D, et al. Malignant peripheral neuroectodermal tumors. A retrospective analysis of 42 patients. *Cancer* 1988;61:349–357.

68. Wunder JS, Paulian G, Huvos AG, et al. The histological response to chemotherapy as a predictor of the oncological outcome of operative treatment of Ewing sarcoma. *J Bone Joint Surg Am* 1998;80:1020–1033.

*69. Ahrens S, Hoffmann C, Jabar S, et al. Evaluation of prognostic factors in a tumor volume-adapted treatment strategy for localized Ewing sarcoma of bone: the CESS 86 experience. *Med Pediatr Oncol* 1999;32: 186–195.

*70. Grier HE, Krailo MD, Tarbell NJ, et al. Addition of ifosfamide and etoposide to standard chemotherapy for Ewing's sarcoma and primitive neuroectodermal tumor of bone. *N Engl J Med* 2003;348:694–701.

71. Marcove RC, Rosen G. Radical en bloc excision of Ewing's sarcoma. *Clin Orthop* 1980;153:86–91.

72. Pomeroy T, Johnson R. Integrated therapy of Ewing's sarcoma. *Front Radiat Ther Oncol* 1975;10:152–166.

73. Suit HD. Role of therapeutic radiology in cancer of bone. *Cancer* 1975;35:930–935.

74. Prindull G, Jurgens H, Jentsck F, et al. Radiotherapy of non-metastatic Ewing's sarcoma. *J Cancer Res Clin Oncol* 1985;110:127–130.

75. Arai Y, Kun LE, Brooks MT, et al. Ewing's sarcoma: local tumor control and patterns of failure following limited-volume radiation therapy. *Int J Radiat Oncol Biol Phys* 1991;21:1501–1508.

*76. Donaldson SS, Torrey M, Link MP, et al. A multidisciplinary study investigating radiotherapy in Ewing's sarcoma: end results of POG #8346. *Int J Radiat Oncol Biol Phys* 1998;42:125–135.

77. Shirley SK, Askin FB, Gilula LA, et al. Ewing's sarcoma in bones of the hands and feet: a clinicopathologic study and review of the literature. *J Clin Oncol* 1985;3:686–697.

*78. Bolek TW, Marcus RB Jr, Mendenhall NP, et al. Local control and functional results after twice-daily radiotherapy for Ewing's sarcoma of the extremities. *Int J Radiat Oncol Biol Phys* 1996;35:687–692.

*79. Marcus RB Jr, Cantor A, Heare TC, et al. Local control

and function after twice-a-day radiotherapy for Ewing's sarcoma of bone. *Int J Radiat Oncol Biol Phys* 1991;21:1509–1515.

80. Kushner BH, Meyers PA, Gerald, WL et al. Very–high-dose short-term chemotherapy for poor-risk peripheral primitive neuroectodermal tumors, including Ewing's sarcoma, in children and young adults. *J Clin Oncol* 1995;13:2796–2804.

81. Jentzsch K, Binder H, Cramer H, et al. Leg function after radiotherapy for Ewing's sarcoma. *Cancer* 1981; 47:1267–1278.

82. Potter R, Knocke TH, Kovacs G, et al. Brachytherapy in the combined modality treatment of pediatric malignancies. Principles and preliminary experience with treatment of soft tissue sarcoma (recurrence) and Ewing's sarcoma. *Klin Padiatr* 1995;207:164–173.

83. Shamberger RC, Grier HE, Weinstein HJ, et al. Chest wall tumors in infancy and childhood. *Cancer* 1989; 63:774–785.

84. Ozkaynak MF, Matthay K, Cairo M, et al. Double-alkylator non–total-body irradiation regimen with autologous hematopoietic stem-cell transplantation in pediatric solid tumors. *J Clin Oncol* 1998;16:937–944.

85. Berry MP, Jenkin RD, Harwood, AR et al. Ewing's sarcoma: a trial of adjuvant chemotherapy and sequential half-body irradiation. *Int J Radiat Oncol Biol Phys* 1986;12:19–24.

86. Hartman KR, Triche TJ, Kinsella TJ, et al. Prognostic value of histopathology in Ewing's sarcoma. Long-term follow-up of distal extremity primary tumors. *Cancer* 1991;67:163–171.

87. McKeon C, Thiele CJ, Ross RA, et al. Indistinguishable patterns of protooncogene expression in two distinct but closely related tumors: Ewing's sarcoma and neuroepithelioma. *Cancer Res* 1988;48:4307–4311.

88. Burdach S, Jurgens H, Peters C, et al. Myeloablative radiochemotherapy and hematopoietic stem-cell rescue in poor-prognosis Ewing's sarcoma. *J Clin Oncol* 1993;11:1482–1488.

89. Meyers PA, Krailo MD, Ladanyi M, et al. High-dose melphalan, etoposide, total-body irradiation, and autologous stem-cell reconstitution as consolidation therapy for high-risk Ewing's sarcoma does not improve prognosis. *J Clin Oncol* 2001;19:2812–2820.

90. Tucker MA, D'Angio GJ, Boice JD Jr, et al. Bone sarcomas linked to radiotherapy and chemotherapy in children. *N Engl J Med* 1987;317:588–593.

91. Kushner BH, Meyers PA. How effective is dose-intensive/myeloablative therapy against Ewing's sarcoma/primitive neuroectodermal tumor metastatic to bone or bone marrow? The Memorial Sloan–Kettering experience and a literature review. *J Clin Oncol* 2001; 19:870–880.

92. Ahrens S, Dunst J, Rube C, et al. Second malignancy after treatment for Ewing's sarcoma. *Int J Radiat Oncol Biol Phys* 1997;39:142.

10

Osteosarcoma

Edward C. Halperin, M.D.

Osteosarcoma is the most common primary malignant bone tumor in children. The tumor derives from bone-forming mesenchyme (1–9). The majority of cases occur in the second decade of life, and there is a male predominance. The incidence is one to three new cases per million per year (Fig. 10-1) (10).

Inactivation of the retinoblastoma (Rb) gene may be important for osteosarcoma formation. Rb is a tumor suppressor gene that is discussed in detail in Chapter 5. A common karyotype change in osteosarcoma is deletion of the short arm of chromosome 17, where the p53 gene is localized; p53 is a nuclear phosphoprotein with properties of a tumor suppressor gene (11). Second malignant neoplasms can occur in patients with osteosarcoma treated with surgery alone or with surgery and chemotherapy, perhaps as a result of these genetic abnormalities (12–14). Osteosarcoma may develop in long-term survivors of heritable retinoblastoma. These secondary osteosarcomas may arise in or outside the irradiated field and in children treated without radiotherapy (also see Chapters 5 and 20).

SIGNS, SYMPTOMS, EVALUATION, AND STAGING

Osteosarcoma usually occurs in the metaphyses of the long bones, especially around the knee joint. The bones most commonly involved are the femur (approximately 40% of cases), tibia (15%), and humerus (15%) (Fig. 10-2) (1,3,4,10,15). The usual clinical presentation is swelling or pain. A few patients present with a pathologic fracture.

The tumor has a typical appearance on conventional radiographs. There are poorly defined margins, interrupted periosteal new bone, and soft tissue invasion. Where the bony cortex is

penetrated at the edge of a tumor, there may be a periosteal elevation and vertical spicule formation (Codman's triangle) (3,4,15). Computed tomography (CT) and magnetic resonance imaging (MRI) help delineate the intramedullary extent of tumor as it tracks along the marrow cavity and the soft tissue extent of tumor (4,16). The bone scan has nearly 100% sensitivity for the presence of malignant bone tumor, although the specificity is less. On the bone scan one may observe osteoblastic activity in the shaft of the long bone proximal to the primary tumor. This may represent reactive change and not indicate the presence of malignancy (4). Thallium scintigraphy also aids in tumor localization. A surgeon may order an angiogram to determine tumor vascularity, detect vascular displacement, determine the relationship to vessels to the tumor, and identify vascular anomalies. The most common sites of dis-

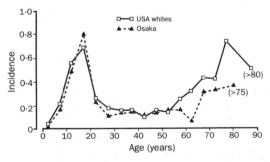

FIG. 10-1. Osteosarcoma incidence per 100,000 population per year by age. The peak for older people is associated with Paget's disease. (Reproduced from Ishikawa Y, Tsukuma, H, Miller RW, et al. Low rates of Paget's disease of bone and osteosarcoma in elderly Japanese. *Lancet* 1996;347:1559, with permission.)

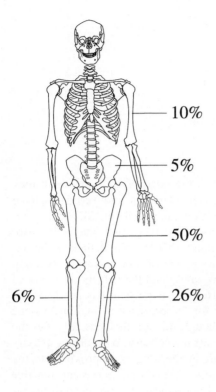

FIG. 10-2. Skeletal distribution of primary osteosarcomas in patients treated on the Neoadjuvant Cooperative Osteosarcoma Study Group protocols of the Cooperative German–Austrian–Swiss Osteosarcoma Study Group. (Modified from Bielack S, Kempf-Bielack B, Delling G, et al. Prognostic factors in high-grade osteosarcoma of the extremities or trunk: an analysis of 1,702 patients treated on Neoadjuvant Cooperative Osteosarcoma Study Group protocols. *J Clin Oncol* 2002;20:776–790, with permission.)

tant metastases are the lungs and bones (3,6, 15–19). To evaluate pulmonary metastases, a plain chest radiograph is used to identify chest nodules or cannonball lesions. A CT of the chest can be used to assess the presence or absence of small nodules (19).

If we are to improve the treatment of osteosarcoma, it will be important to adapt therapy to the individual patient's prognostic factors (20). The conventional means of doing this is a staging system. The presence or absence of metastases and the use of histologic subtyping do help predict prognosis. A system for subclassification by histopathologic evaluation and site of tumor origin is shown in Table 10-1. A variety of factors have been investigated as potential prognostic factors. As will be discussed later in this chapter, histologic response to neoadjuvant chemotherapy is useful in predicting outcome. However, information of this type is available only after chemotherapy and surgery. Clinical features with predictive value in determining outcome include the duration of presenting symptoms (shorter is worse), tumor size (larger is worse), location of the primary tumor (head, spine, rib, and pelvic sites are worse), and weight loss of more than 10 lb. Tumor size seems strongly predictive of outcome and may be calculated as either absolute tumor length (more than 10 cm), relative tumor length given as the proportion of tumor length to the overall length of the involved bone (more than one-third of the involved bone), or absolute tumor volume (more than 70 or 150 cm^3) (2–22).

There is no widely used staging system for osteosarcoma. Some clinicians simply separate patients into those with localized disease and those with metastatic disease. The system developed by Enneking and adopted by the Musculoskeletal Tumor Society is used by some orthopedic oncologists. However, there are few low-grade osteosarcomas, so in this system most tumors are stage II or III (Table 10-2). One study from the European Osteosarcoma Intergroup suggested that patients with

TABLE 10-1. *A system for osteosarcoma subclassification by histology and origin*

Centrally located tumor
Primary tumors
  Conventional: About 75% of patients fall in this category. This group may be additionally subdivided based on the predominant matrix pattern into the following three subgroups:
    Osteoblast, **14.4**
    Chondroblastic, **9.6**
    Fibroblastic (spindle cell stroma with a herringbone pattern similar to that seen in fibrosarcoma), **10.7**
  Telangiectatic (characterized by a purely lytic radiographic appearance and a macroscopic and microscopic resemblance to aneurysmal bone cyst), **14.5**
  Small cell
  Malignant fibrous histiocytoma subtype
  Low-grade intraosseous (a rare low-grade fibro-osseous lesion often confused with fibrous dysplasia)
  Multicentric
  Gnathic
Secondary tumors
  Associated with Paget's disease, **64.2**
  Radiation-induced
  Associated with other benign preexisting condition (i.e., fibrous dysplasia)
Juxtacortical tumor, **1.0**
Parosteal (often arises from the posterior distal femur in older patients. Generally it is a low-grade spindle cell tumor with well-formed, parallel trabecular bone. Some patients may dedifferentiate into a higher grade lesion.)
Periosteal (typically involves femur or tibia)
High-grade surface

The death rates per 100 patient-years, correlated with histologic group and calculated by Taylor et al. (149), are shown in bold type. The death rates for the three subtypes of conventional osteosarcoma are similar. There is some controversy in the literature concerning the prognostic importance of the telangiectatic variant. Most authorities now believe that with aggressive therapy, there is no prognostic difference attached to this diagnosis variant. It is generally agreed that the prognosis for patients with juxtacortical tumors is better and that the prognosis for tumor associated with Paget's disease, an entity seen in adults, is decidedly worse.
From references 1, 4, 7, 9, 28, and 149, with permission.

chondroblastic tumors had a slightly superior survival to those with other histologies, but this difference did not reach statistical significance and awaits confirmation in other research (23).

TABLE 10-2. *The Enneking staging system for osteosarcoma*

Stage I: Low grade
  IA. Confined to bone of origin
  IB. Extension beyond bone of origin
Stage II: High grade
  IIA. Confined to bone of origin
  IIB. Extension beyond bone of origin
Stage III: Metastatic disease
  IIIA. Confined to bone of origin
  IIIB. Extension beyond bone of origin

Modified from Damaron JA, Pritchard DJ. Current combined treatment of high-grade osteosarcomas. *Oncology* 1995;9:327–350, and Ennedking WF, Spanier SS, Goodman MA. A system for the surgical staging of musculoskeletal sarcoma. *Clin Orthop* 1980;153: 106–120.

The Cooperative German–Austrian–Swiss Osteosarcoma Study Group (COSS) has provided an extensive evaluation of prognostic factors in high-grade osteosarcoma of the extremities or trunk. In an evaluation of 1,702 patients treated on neoadjuvant osteosarcoma protocols, the investigators found that the long-term survival of patients with limb primaries was superior to that of those with axial primaries, patients who presented without metastases had higher survival rates than those who presented with metastases, patients with extremity sarcomas occupying less than one-third of the bone had higher survival rates than those with sarcomas occupying more than one-third, and distal extremity tumors had a superior outcome to proximal tumors. The response to chemotherapy (i.e., the amount of tumor necrosis at the time of resection in a setting of neoadjuvant chemotherapy) also was a highly important predictor of outcome along with the extent of surgical resection (Table 10-3) (24–26).

TABLE 10-3. *Influence of the histologic response to neoadjuvant chemotherapy on survival in osteosarcoma*

Group (reference)	Response	n	Survival	p
Istituto Ortopedico Rizzoli (114)	≥90% necrosis	621	76% 5-yr OS	0.0001
	<90% necrosis	437	48% 5-yr OS	
Pediatric Oncology Group 8651 (120)	≥90% necrosis	26	73% 5-yr EFS	0.027
	<90% necrosis	16	44% 5-yr EFS	

EFS, event-free survival; OS, overall survival.

SELECTION OF THERAPY

Surgery

Local Disease

The biopsy site should be selected to allow access to the infiltrating edge of the tumor. In general, either minimal or no cortical bone should be removed in order to reduce the risk of pathologic fracture (27–31).

The classic definitive operative procedure is an amputation above the region of the affected bone or a disarticulation at the joint above the lesion. Traditional teaching is that if one resects the bone beyond the site defined by all radiographs as the most proximal extent of disease and if the margins are pathologically negative, the chance of stump recurrence is negligible (29,30). In recent years surgical treatment for local osteosarcoma has changed. New limb salvage procedures have been performed with gratifying results (32).

Limb-sparing operations may be selected if there is no evidence of neurologic or vascular compromise by the local tumor, if the surgeon believes that he or she can obtain an adequate margin around the primary osteosarcoma, and if there is a plan for reconstruction that will provide better function than amputation. Relative contraindications to limb sparing include the presence of a pathologic fracture, a poor response to neoadjuvant chemotherapy, or skeletal immaturity that will lead to significant limb growth discrepancies (33).

What is an adequate surgical margin for local management of osteosarcoma? A radical margin entails removal of the entire bone of origin with accompanying soft tissue involvement, as is achieved by a hip disarticulation for a distal femoral tumor. A wide margin is defined as excision of the tumor with a cuff of surrounding normal tissue, and a marginal margin entails excision of the tumor and its surrounding reactive pseudocapsule. Local control is improved by the adequacy of the surgical margin and the response to neoadjuvant chemotherapy (Table 10-3). It is generally accepted that limb-sparing surgery has a slightly greater risk of local tumor recurrence than does amputation. Amputation has a slightly greater risk of local recurrence than does disarticulation (Table 10-4). A good chemotherapeutic response may allow the surgeon to have a tighter margin on the primary tumor and exclude more normal tissue from the resection. However, to know before surgery whether a marginal excision is reasonable, one must have an idea of what tumor response was achieved by chemotherapy. Unfortunately, no single imaging study can reliably provide this information, although plain radiographs, CT,

TABLE 10-4. *Local recurrence rates for osteosarcoma as a function of the extent of surgery*

Site (reference)	Type of operation	Local recurrence rate
Distal femur (36)	Limb sparing	11%
	Above-the-knee amputation	8%
	Hip disarticulation	0%
Pelvis (57)	Radical or wide	48%
	Marginal	70%
	Intralesional[a]	92%

[a]Some patients were irradiated.

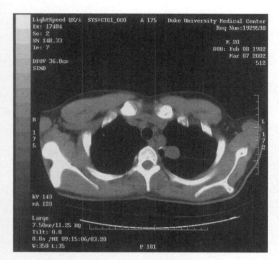

FIG. 10-3. An 18-year-old right-handed high school senior presented to medical attention when his tennis game and weight-lifting activities were inhibited by pain in his left shoulder. Diagnostic images showed a mixed sclerotic and lytic mass in the proximal left humerus. Incisional biopsy made the diagnosis of osteosarcoma. The patient was treated with induction chemotherapy in the hope of producing a substantial tumor response eventually leading to limb-sparing surgery. Unfortunately, within 2 years of the initial diagnosis widespread pulmonary metastases developed, refractory to chemotherapy, which led to the patient's death.

bone scan, and MRI can be used to make a reasonable prediction (33).

The reconstruction technique elected after limb-sparing procedures depends on the location of the osteosarcoma, whether there is joint involvement, the extent of bone and soft tissue resection, the patient's age, the functional demands of the patient and the family, and the prospects for rehabilitation. When the excision is intra-articular (within or involving a joint), reconstruction options include custom segmental total joint replacement, whole segment osteoarticular allograft (i.e., from a cadaveric donor), allograft–prosthetic composite reconstruction, arthrodesis (surgical fixation of a joint; artificial ankylosis) with autologous or allogeneic bone, or arthrodesis with a porous prosthesis allowing host bone ingrowth and bone graft. If a joint is not involved, one can re-

construct with autologous or allogeneic bone, a prosthesis, or a segmental prosthetic spacer. Rotation plasty is also an option in certain situations (2,34–36).

It is gratifying that in modern pediatric oncology practice, the child with osteosarcoma may be offered limb-sparing options for local treatment beyond the traditional amputation or hip disarticulation. The previous discussion has cited indications and relative contraindications to limb-sparing surgery, the risk of local recurrence after various forms of surgery, options for reconstruction after tumor resection, and the need for adequate surgical margins. Although it is reasonably clear that limb function after limb-sparing surgery is better for patients than that achieved after amputation, limb-sparing surgery is not for everyone faced with osteosarcoma. Case selection by a skilled orthopedic oncologist, invocation of sound oncologic principles, and adequate rehabilitative services postoperatively are all necessary to achieve the best possible function and cancer control.

Metastatic Disease

Surgery also plays a role in treating osteosarcoma metastatic to the lung. Some patients present with a primary tumor along with limited pulmonary involvement. Aggressive multiagent chemotherapy, surgical management of the primary tumor, and thoracotomy for resection of pulmonary metastases appear to have significantly increased survival in cases that seemed hopeless (Table 10-5) (37).

The most common sites of metastases in the relapse of initially localized osteosarcoma are lung and bone (Fig. 10-4). When tumor relapses in the lung, surgical resection of pulmonary nodules may result in a prolonged disease-free interval and occasional cures (6,12,18,29,30,39). In some patients, repeated thoracotomies appear to have prolonged survival in the face of multiple episodes of pulmonary metastases (40). By diagnosing pulmonary recurrences earlier and with limited tumor bulk, thoracic CT may either open the possibility for a beneficial effect of surgery or simply create a lead-time bias (37).

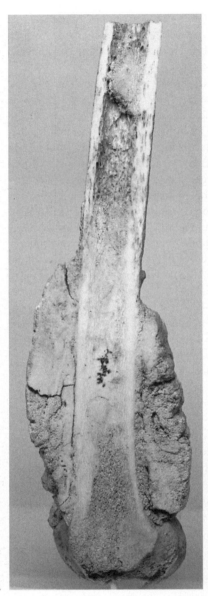

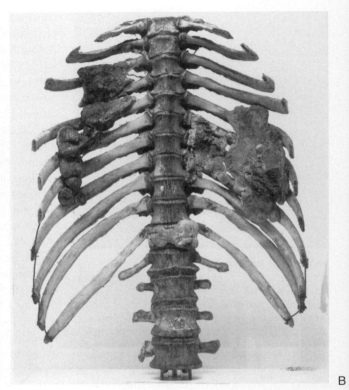

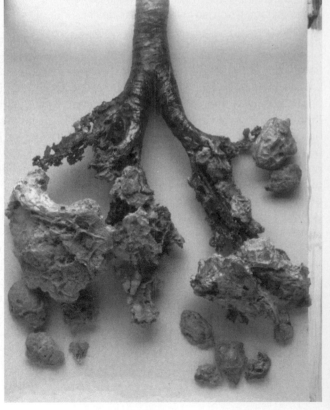

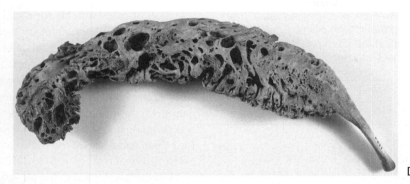

D

FIG. 10-4. John Hunter (1728–1793) was an extraordinary surgeon, anatomist, teacher, and collector. His magnificent collection of scientific specimens was purchased by Parliament and placed in the custody of the Company of Surgeons, renamed the Royal College of Surgeons in 1800. These illustrations of osteosarcoma, taken from the Hunterian Museum, Lincoln's Inn Fields, London, appear by permission of the president and council of the Royal College of Surgeons of England. In November 1786, Hunter encountered a patient with "a hard swelling of the lower part of the thigh, as it were beginning from the knee . . . the part began evidently to enlarge . . . and was attended with more pain as it enlarged . . . and the pain was now exhausting him much." An amputation was done. Hunter described an "osteoid sarcoma" of the distal femur **(A)** and also noted the intramedullary spread of the tumor: "A short distance below the site of amputation there is a second hemispherical tumour in the medullary canal . . . above the main growth, the disease having extended within the canal, in this case, for an unusual distance beyond the limits of the external swelling." Four weeks after the amputation the patient "began to complain of a difficulty in breathing, but not attended with the least pain . . . he began to lose his flesh and sink gradually, his breathing being more and more difficult . . . he died; living only seven weeks after the operation." On autopsy, "bony tumors were found in the cellular membrane of the lungs, upon the pericardium, and some very large ones of the pleura, adhering to the ribs, and upon the anterior surface of the vertebrae of the back" **(B, C).** Hunter noted that "when the leg was amputated he had not the least symptom of any disease in the chest" but deduced that the lung metastases "had taken place a considerable time before the symptoms took place." As for the osteoid appearance of the tumor, Hunter wrote that "one can figure to themselves a reason why the tumour which formed on the outer surface of the thigh-bone might become bony, because it might acquire that disposition from the bone it surrounded; but, from these tumours formed in the chest becoming bone, shows it was the nature of the tumours themselves." The remaining figure **(D)** is "the osseous part of an osteosarcomatous tumour" from "the rib of a Horse" from Hunter's collection. (Descriptions of this material are found in Descriptive catalogue of the pathological series in the Hunterian Museum of the Royal College of Surgeons of England. Edinburgh and London: E. & S. Livingstone, 1972; Part I:133–138; Part II:75–77. Biographical material is from Allen E. Hunterian Museum [pamphlet], Royal College of Surgeons, 1974.)

Several variables must be considered when one uses metastasectomy for pulmonary metastases. These include the aggressiveness of the proposed operation, whether they are unilateral or bilateral, the interval between the development of the metastases and the treatment of the primary, the extent of vascular invasion, the presence or absence of hilar lymph node involvement, and whether additional salvage chemotherapy is available after surgery (33,41,42). The role of the bony metastasectomy is not well defined, undoubtedly because the occurrence of bony metastases in the setting of potentially salvageable osteosarcoma is far less common than that of pulmonary metastases (33).

Radiation Therapy

Prebiopsy

Sweetnam (29) administered low-dose irradiation before the initial biopsy (approximately 10 Gy) to 29 patients in the hope of reducing the viability of cells that might be disseminated into the bloodstream by the biopsy. The 20% overall survival rate, no different from that of historic

TABLE 10-5. *Factors predicting event-free survival in patients with primary metastatic osteosarcoma in the German–Swiss–Austrian Cooperative Osteosarcoma Study Group clinical trials*

Factor	n	5-year event-free survival	p
Primary site			
Extremity	181	20%	<0.001
Trunk	21	5%	
Number of metastatic organ systems			
1	160	21%	<0.006
>1	42	10%	
Number of metastases			
1	38	55%	<0.001
2–5	69	19%	
>5	91	2%	
Isolated lung metastases			
Unilateral	46	45%	<0.001
Bilateral	70	4%	
1	24	58%	<0.001
2–5	41	23%	
>5	57	3%	

From Kager L, Zoubek A, Potschger U, et al. Cooperative German–Austrian–Swiss Osteosarcoma Study Group. Primary metastatic osteosarcoma: presentation and outcome of patients treated on neoadjuvant Cooperative Osteosarcoma Study Group protocols. *J Clin Oncol* 2003;21(10):2011–2018, with permission.

controls, discouraged additional investigation. Only two of 19 patients survived when treated with amputation without prior biopsy.

Primary and Preoperative Treatment

The Cade Technique

In the era before adjuvant therapy, physicians were distressed by the practice of treating the primary lesion with amputation or disarticulation, only to have the young patient die within 6 months of pulmonary metastases. Because the survival rate with surgical ablation alone was only 20%, many limbs were sacrificed in vain. Surgeons and radiotherapists reasoned that if high-dose local irradiation could obtain at least temporary control of the primary tumor, a time interval would be obtained that would allow the selection of cases suitable for a radical surgery. Patients who develop pulmonary metastasis in a 4- to 6-month waiting period after irradiation would be spared an unnecessary amputation. Those who did not develop pulmonary metastasis after the waiting period would undergo extirpation of the primary tumor. This philosophy was promulgated by English physician Sir Stanford Cade and is called the Cade technique. The 5-year survival rates of 15% to 20% were equivalent to those achieved in the pre–adjuvant therapy era with immediate surgical ablation. The delay in surgery appears to have cost no lives (10,39,43–51). There generally was a reduction in pain and swelling at the tumor site after the first 20 Gy. This response tended to continue for several weeks after completion of radiotherapy. In patients who underwent limb ablation after radiotherapy, a histologic analysis could be performed to assess the presence or absence of viable tumor. The majority of patients had a good or excellent local response (Table 10-6). There were some long-term survivors after aggressive treatment with radiation therapy alone (6,50).

Modern Series of Primary Photon Radiation Therapy

In modern radiotherapy practice, it is rare to be asked to use radiotherapy as the primary local treatment for osteosarcoma except for lesions in inaccessible sites. However, the data acquired with the Cade technique make it reasonable to consider the use of radiation in certain situations. Preoperative radiotherapy has been given in the context of a research protocol to reduce tumor viability before surgery, increase the probability of performing limb-sparing surgery instead of amputation, or reduce the risk of local recurrence (39,51). In patients with nonresectable primary tumors such as difficult pelvic bone sites, vertebral column, frontal bones, or base of skull and in patients who refuse definitive surgery, consideration should be given to precision high-dose irradiation. Modern photon techniques use three-dimensional computerized treatment planning and intensity-modulated radiation therapy. Neutron or proton beams can improve local control in certain circumstances

TABLE 10-6. *The Cade technique: management of osteosarcoma with primary irradiation or primary irradiation and selected delayed amputation (excluding parosteal tumors)*

Authors (listed in order of increasing dosage)	Dosage (Gy)	Clinical or pathologic local response	Survival
Jenkin et al. (48, 49)	50–60	Complete 11% Partial 63% None 26%	2-yr: 16%
van den Brenk et al. (131)	60–70, then 40–50 every 6 mo	Severe limb deformity in long-term survivors	5-yr: 12% (includes cases of chondrosarcoma and fibrosarcoma)
Lee et al. (39,50)	70–80	33% totally destroyed 33% doubtful viability 33% capable of growth and perhaps dissemination	5-yr: 22%
Poppe et al. (10)	70–80	70% considerable radiation effect 19% moderate effect	5-yr: 18%
Gaitan-Yanguas (47)	10–100	11% slight or no effect 44% no residual tumor 44% no residual tumor	
Allen and Stevens (44)	79–100	56% residual tumor 86% pain relief 60% reclassification 86% tumor sterilization	60% NED at 30–114 mo
Caceres and Zaharia (45)	80–120	16% remaining viable tumor 56% severe radiation damage 28% total tumor destruction 35% no tumor destruction	5-yr: 18% (no difference from historical surgical controls, 22%)
Phillips and Sheline (51)	50–120	65% tumor in specimen	

NED, no evidence of disease.

and are discussed later in this chapter (52). There is also precedent for high-dose preoperative irradiation and rapid surgery, preoperative radiotherapy with local hyperthermic perfusion (53), intraoperative electron beam therapy (54), and radiotherapy with intra-arterial infusion of a radiosensitizer (55).

Data on photon irradiation as primary treatment for osteosarcoma, in lieu of surgery and in conjunction with aggressive chemotherapy, are available from Albrecht et al. from Berlin (43). They described seven patients with osteosarcoma who were treated from 1977 to 1992 according to contemporary COSS protocols (Table 10-7). Six patients refused the appropriate amputation or rotation plasty. One had a primary tumor described as inoperable. Each patient received 50 to 70 Gy of conventionally fractionated photon irradiation. The patient with the inoperable tumor died within 1 year of initiation of treatment. The remaining six patients are alive without evidence of recurrent disease 2 to

18 years after treatment (mean follow-up, 11 years). Three of the six survivors ultimately suffered a pathologic fracture 8 to 12 months after 50 to 70 Gy, and one of these subsequently had an amputation. This small clinical series suggests that photon radiotherapy in conjunction with chemotherapy may be used to manage osteosarcoma if appropriate surgery is impossible or refused (43). Whether such patients are best treated with photons, neutrons, or protons is a matter for debate.

Some patients with unresectable osteosarcomas are treated with conventional external beam irradiation. The COSS described a series of patients with osteosarcoma of the spine who were treated with intralesional or marginal resections and also received photon irradiation, neutron beam treatment, or samarium. In the analysis of patients who underwent either incomplete surgery or no surgery, seven received postoperative irradiation and ten did not. The seven patients who received irradiation had a slightly higher

TABLE 10-7. *Significant recent cooperative group trials addressing the management of localized osteosarcoma*

Study name and number of eligible patients	Primary objective	Treatment arms	Results	Comments (reference)
Pediatric Oncology Group (POG)				
POG-8651 ($n = 100$)	To determine whether chemotherapy administered before and after definitive surgery is superior to surgery followed by adjuvant chemotherapy.	Arm A: HDMTX + AP, then surgery, then HDMTX + BCD + ADR + AP. Arm B: surgery, then HDMTX + AP + BCD.	The 5-yr survival is 76% for patients assigned to neoadjuvant chemotherapy and 79% for patients treated with the more traditional approach ($p = 0.6$).	There is no evidence of an advantage in event-free survival or survival for either treatment arm (119, 120).
European Osteosarcoma Intergroup (EOI, a combination of the European Organization for Research and Treatment of Cancer and the Medical Research Council)				
EOI-80831 ($n = 307$ registered, 207 evaluable, 163 completed allotted chemotherapy)	This study began as a randomized phase II toxicity and response trial of two short, intensive chemotherapy programs.	Surgery, randomization of chemotherapy of AP vs. AP + MTX.	6-yr survival: AP 65% + MTX 50% ($p = 0.10$). 6-yr disease-free survival: AP 58% vs. AP + MTX 40% ($p = 0.02$).	The dosage intensity of AP was greater in the two-drug arm than the three-drug arm. This may have produced the superior outcome. Disease-free survival was better for patients planned for conservation surgery than amputation (122).
EOI-80861 ($n = 407,391$ eligible)	To compare short, intensive chemotherapy with complex, longer-duration program based on the Rosen T10 program.	Arm A: AP 3 cycles, then surgery, then 3 more cycles Arm B: ADR + V + HDMTX, then surgery, then BCD + ADR + V + HDMTX + AP.	The median follow-up is 5.6 years. Survival in both groups is almost identical. 5-yr progression-free survival is 44%.	AP appears to be as effective as the more complicated program at a lower cost (118, 119).
Scandinavian Sarcoma Group (SSG)				
SSG-VIII	To increase the number of good responders to neoadjuvant therapy with intensified therapy.	HDMTX + AP, then surgery; good responders get HDMTX + AP postoperatively, poor responders get EI.	The median follow-up is 6.9 yr. The year event-free survival is 61%.	Female sex, small tumor volume, and high serum MTX levels predict better outcome (22).

Children's Cancer Group (CCG)

CCG-741 (n = 166)	To compare HDMTX with moderate-dose MTX in the context of a multiagent chemotherapy program.	Surgery, ADR, then randomize to arm: Arm A, HDMTX + AV; Arm B, moderate-dose MTX + AV.	38% disease-free survival at 48 mo. No difference between the two arms ($p > 0.5$).	Lower disease-free survival was associated with the presence of spontaneous tumor necrosis at presentation (123).
CCG-782 (n = 232)	To use histologic response of the primary tumor to neoadjuvant chemotherapy to determine postoperative chemotherapy.	Biopsy, then HDMTX + AV + BCD, then surgery. All patients without local progression received BCD + AV + HDMTX. Then, if <95% necrosis, receive BCD + HDMTX + AV.	5-yr event-free survival was 53%. Patients with local disease progression in the induction phase had 48% 3-yr event-free survival.	A poor prognosis is associated with an evaluated alkaline phosphatase at diagnosis or a primary tumor in the proximal humerus or proximal femur (113,114,122).

Cooperative Osteosarcoma Study (COSS) Group of the German Society of Pediatric Oncology

COSS-77 (n = 68)	Improved survival from adjuvant chemotherapy.	Surgery, then HDMTX + AV.	46% 14-yr metastasis-free survival.	Event-free survival was 48% for good responders and 48% for poor responders (108,150).
COSS-80 (n = 101)	Improved survival with neoadjuvant chemotherapy.	Arm A: ADR + HDMTX + P, then surgery, then ADR + HDMTX + P. Arm B: ADR + HDMTX + BCD ± β-IFN.	5-yr event-free survival: Arm A = 66%, Arm B = 64%.	There was no difference in outcome between the two chemotherapy arms. There was no difference associated with the use of β-IFN (108, 113,114,150).
COSS-86 (n = 153)	Stratified by risk group. High risk was large tumor, chondroid matrix, or poor bone scan response at week 5.	Low risk: ADR + HDMTX + P, then surgery, then ADR + HDMTX + P. High-risk Arm A: ADR + HDMTX + intra-arterial IP, then surgery, then ADR + HDMTX + IP. High-risk Arm B: Same as Arm A except IP is intravenous.	77% 5-yr metastasis-free survival, 66% 10-yr metastasis-free survival, 72% 10-yr overall survival	Response rate is >76%, better than in previous COSS studies (117).

ADR, adriamycin; AP, adriamycin and cisplatinum; AV, adriamycin and vincristine; BCD, bleomycin, cyclophosphamide, and actinomycin D; β-IFN, beta-interferon; EI, etoposide and ifosfamide; HDMTX, high-dose methotrexate; IP, ifosfamide and cisplatinum; MTX, methotrexate; P, cisplatinum; V, vincristine.

long-term survival (~50%) than those who did not (~10%, $p = 0.059$) (56).

In 2003, COSS investigators described a group of patients with pelvic osteosarcomas treated between 1979 and 1998. Of 30 patients with intralesional surgery or no primary surgery, 11 received radiotherapy (65 to 68 Gy with photons, two were treated with neutrons, and one also received ^{153}Sm). The 5-year overall survival of the irradiated patients (16%) was superior to that of those not irradiated (0%, $p = 0.0033$) (57).

Machak et al. (58) from Russia also recently reported a retrospective review of 31 patients with limb osteosarcoma who refused definitive surgery and were treated with cisplatin, doxorubicin (IV or IA), or both. All patients received 40 to 68 Gy at 2.5 to 3 Gy per fraction, one fraction per day, or 1.25 to 1.5 Gy twice daily. With a median follow-up of 39 months, the predicted 5-year overall survival was 61%. Local progression-free survival was 56% (40% for 50 Gy or less, 77% for more than 50 Gy). There were five fractures, one skin necrosis, and one osteomyelitis. It is conceivable that use of neoadjuvant radiotherapy with chemotherapy increased the proportion of good responders of the time of surgery (59).

Hirano et al. (35) from Nagasaki University sandwiched 30 Gy (2 to 3 Gy per fraction) in the midst of preoperative chemotherapy in 15 patients with osteosarcoma. Histology of the resected specimens showed a tumoricidal effect in nine patients and a lesser effect in three.

Maxilla and Mandible

Some surgeons believe that a wide surgical excision of osteosarcoma of the maxilla or mandible is risky because of the functional consequences. Local recurrence and death after intralesional resection or resection with a positive margin are typical (60,61). Chambers and Mahoney (62) reported 33 patients treated with preoperative brachytherapy. Implantation was accomplished by drilling holes in the mandible and placing radium needles. The dosage was 100 to 160 cGy. Wide surgical excision of the involved hemimandible and adjacent soft tissue was performed 2 to 4 weeks after irra-

diation. Ten of 11 children were long-term survivors with follow-up from 4 to 15 years. Suit (27,28) reported an additional three cases (two of the mandible and one of the maxilla) locally controlled with a similar technique. Heroic brachytherapy is rarely necessary in modern practice. With radical surgical resection of the tumor, followed by reconstruction, local control of facial bone osteosarcoma is to be expected (63).

Lung

Historically, the propensity of osteosarcoma to metastasize to the lungs stimulated interest in the use of prophylactic lung irradiation (Table 10-8). The fundamental problem with thoracic irradiation is that pulmonary tolerance may be exceeded before necessary tumoricidal dosages are achieved (71). Abbatucci et al. (72), working from radiobiologic principles, showed that the exponential kill of clonogenic cells produced by fractionated radiotherapy, in principle, could eradicate subclinical metastases in a highly oxygenated lung. Visible tumor deposits, detectable on chest radiograph, measure 6 to 10 mm in diameter and contain 10^8 to 10^9 cells. If one assumes that the dosage needed to reduce the number of viable clonogenic cells in a tumor to 10% (D_{10}) is 4 Gy for osteosarcoma, then 20 Gy of fractionated irradiation should be able to prevent the growth of metastases containing 10^4 or 10^5 cells. Breur (73,74), analyzing 13 patients with microscopic pulmonary metastasis and extrapolating backward in time, showed that about one in four patients with subclinical metastasis have tumors containing about 10^5 cells. In principle, these small metastatic deposits would be curable by adjuvant pulmonary irradiation. This argument has been criticized by Baeza et al. (75).

The technique of prophylactic pulmonary irradiation involves parallel opposed anterior and posterior fields encompassing both the apices and posterior costophrenic angles of the lungs. Some physicians use a customized anterior cardiac shield, particularly if concurrent cardiotoxic chemotherapy is used. The dosimetry conventions at many institutions do not make corrections for the increased transmission of radiation

TABLE 10-8. *Prophylactic lung irradiation in the treatment of osteogenic sarcoma*

Authors	Technique	Number of patients	Survival	Comment
Breur et al. (17)	Local therapy of surgery, Cade technique, or radiotherapy, then randomized:		5-yr:	$p = 0.18$; metastasis-free survival 43% versus 28% ($p = 0.059$).
	17.5 Gy WLI	44	55%	
	Control	42	40%	
Burgers et al. (64)	Local therapy of surgery, Cade technique, or radiotherapy; then randomized:		5-yr:	No difference between the treatment arms.
	Chemotherapy	65	30%	
	20 Gy WLI	25	25%	
Ellis et al. (65) Springfield et al. (21)	Local surgical therapy; 16 Gy WLI with partial heat block, adriamycin	53 or 57	60% metastasis-free survival	Follow-up duration not clear.
Jenkin et al. (48, 49)	Cade technique; 15 Gy WLI ± actinomycin			All six developed lung metastases in 2–6 mo.
Lougheed et al. (67)	15 Gy irradiation to one lung only; actinomycin	8		Four patients developed metastases in the untreated lung, one in the treated lung.
Newton (68)	Radiation and delayed amputation for primary tumor; 19.5 Gy adjuvant WLI	14	43%	Minimum 52 mo follow-up; survival better than that of historical controls.
Rab et al. (69)	Local therapy of surgery, Cade technique, or radiotherapy; then randomized:			WLI did not influence survival.
	15 Gy WLI + actinomycin	26	42%	
	Control	27	38%	
Zaharia et al. (70)	Local therapy of surgery, nonrandomized:			$p < 0.33$.
	20 Gy WLI	7	241 d median	
	20 Gy WLI + adriamycin	29	843 d survival	

WLI, whole lung irradiation.

through healthy lung tissue. Uncorrected prescriptions, based on the inaccurate assumption that the lungs have the same density as normal tissue, underestimate the actual dosage given to the center of the lungs by about 14% (71).

The Role of Adjuvant Whole Lung Irradiation in Osteosarcoma in Nonrandomized Studies

Lougheed et al. (67) thought that elective prophylactic lung irradiation of clinically normal lungs might delay the development of pulmonary metastases in osteosarcoma. They treated only one of the lungs, giving 15 Gy in combination with actinomycin D. Four of eight patients devel-

oped metastases in the untreated lung, but only one patient progressed in the irradiated lung.

Newton (68) reported that fewer patients developed pulmonary metastases in the early follow-up after elective pulmonary irradiation than nonirradiated patients. Only four of 13 irradiated patients progressed after prophylactic irradiation, although the effect was short lived. Caldwell (76) performed sequential elective bilateral whole lung irradiation (WLI) in 38 patients with a variety of tumors, including seven with osteosarcoma. Seventeen had no detectable metastases. Twenty-one, who had pulmonary nodules, received WLI followed by surgical resection or a local boost radiation field to a higher dosage. Three of the four patients with osteosarcoma had no detectable metastases at presentation and were alive and well with no active disease at 2- to 4-year follow-up.

Caceres et al. (77) treated seven evaluable patients with 20 Gy of prophylactic lung irradiation. Ten patients received adjuvant doxorubicin. After 13 months of follow-up, three of seven irradiated patients were free of disease, compared with six of ten on the chemotherapy arm.

Evaluating 62 patients with osteosarcoma in Toronto, Jenkin et al. (78) included six patients who received 15 Gy of prophylactic lung irradiation and actinomycin. All six developed diffuse pulmonary metastases in 2 to 6 months. The French Bone Tumor Study Group (79) published studies on a nonrandomized series of 41 evaluable cases of extremity osteosarcoma treated with chemotherapy and 20 Gy of prophylactic lung irradiation. The 5-year disease-free survival was 58%, and the overall survival was 66%. This compared well with historic control, but there was marked lung toxicity including restrictive ventilatory effects, five life-threatening infections, and one death from *Pneumocystis carinii* pneumonia. A study by Gilchrist et al. (80) from the Mayo Clinic showed no benefit of prophylactic pulmonary irradiation in osteosarcoma.

Evidence from Randomized Studies

In 1976 Rab et al. (69) described a randomized trial of 53 patients from the Mayo Clinic. They were randomized to receive 15 Gy prophylactic lung irradiation (uncorrected) while receiving 100% oxygen with intravenous actinomycin D. The control group did not undergo prophylactic lung irradiation. The median survival time was 42 months in the irradiated arm and 25 months in the unirradiated arm. However, there was no significant difference in overall survival or disease-free survival. The European Organization for Research and Treatment of Cancer (EORTC) conducted the two most important initial trials of WLI. The first study, Study O2, enrolled six patients. The use of local therapy plus 17.5 Gy of WLI achieved a superior but not statistically significant improvement in 5-year survival over local therapy alone. The subsequent trial permitted patients to undergo either definitive surgery, delayed technique, or radiotherapy. Among the 205 patients, 19% underwent radiotherapy as treatment for the primary tumor, 52% underwent amputation, and 29% underwent disarticulation. In the first arm of the study, adjuvant chemotherapy consisting of adriamycin, vincristine, and methotrexate was given every 2 weeks for the first 12 weeks. This was followed by a consolidation phase in which these drugs were alternated with cyclophosphamide every 4 weeks for 6 months. The total adjuvant chemotherapy period was 41 weeks. The second treatment arm was identical to that of Study O2 with no chemotherapy but with WLI to a total dosage of 20 Gy after air correction. In the third treatment arm, the chemotherapy of Arm 1 was used, followed after 12 weeks by WLI. The 5-year overall survival for this study was 43%, with no significant difference between the three treatment arms. The disease-free survival at 5 years was 24%. An unpublished analysis cited by Burgers (81) asserts that "the localization of pulmonary metastases was mainly behind the dome of the diagram behind the heart and mediastinum in those patients who were irradiated. These areas had received a smaller dose, as the irradiation passes partly through non-aerated tissue." No other assertions similar to this appear in the literature. Subgroup analysis showed that the 5-year disease-free survival in patients younger than 17 years old was 50% in the irradiated patients and 31% in the unirradiated patients ($p = 0.074$) (17).

As chemotherapy became more popular for osteosarcoma, the EORTC and the International Society for Pediatric Oncology (SIOP) jointly launched the O3 trial in 1978. Two-hundred forty patients younger than 30 years old were randomized to receive treatment with adjuvant chemotherapy, prophylactic lung irradiation to 20 Gy, or chemotherapy with prophylactic irradiation. The type of adjuvant treatment did not significantly alter the overall survival, disease-free survival, or metastasis-free survival. The patterns of relapse were no different in the three groups. Acute toxicity was greater with chemotherapy and resulted in three deaths. The prophylactic lung irradiation was well tolerated, although more irradiated patients developed a late but symptomatic deterioration in pulmonary function (81,82).

Between 1979 and 1984, approximately 57 patients with osteogenic sarcoma were enrolled in a University of Florida protocol in which patients had definitive surgical treatment of the primary tumors. Within 7 days of the surgery, all patients received WLI to a total dosage of 16 Gy in ten fractions with parallel opposed anterior and posterior fields with 8-MV photons. An anterior heart block was used. After WLI, patients received five courses of adriamycin. Detailed results of the efficacy of this program have not been published. In reports published 4 and 8 years after the study was closed to patient accrual, the crude survival was approximately 67%, and the crude metastasis-free survival was about 56% (65).

Cases of breast cancer developing in long-term survivors after elective WLI for osteosarcoma have been reported (83,84). There may also be a higher risk of breast cancer in women who have had osteosarcoma but never underwent WLI (85). In light of the association of osteosarcoma with abnormalities of tumor suppressor genes, concern is warranted about radiation-induced malignancy.

WLI for Advanced Osteosarcoma

Thoracotomy offers a chance of cure for some patients with pulmonary metastatic disease. Patients more likely to be cured by thoracotomy include those with fewer than four lesions completely removed at the first thoracotomy, unilateral disease, and a prior disease-free interval of at least 18 months (86–89).

When WLI is used for overt pulmonary metastases one would expect little effect. Individual lung lesions may respond to high-dose "rifle shot" fields (30,49). Weichselbaum et al. (82) reported an aggressive program for treating metastatic osteosarcoma with chemotherapy, WLI, and boost irradiation to individual metastases. Three of ten patients were alive without evidence of disease. Equivalent or better results have been achieved with chemotherapy, thoracotomy, and no WLI (37).

Giritsky et al. (90) failed to show a benefit of prethoracotomy or postthoracotomy irradiation. However, the O3 study suggested that successful metastasectomy was possible more often after previous prophylactic lung irradiation than after adjuvant chemotherapy (81).

Extracorporeal Irradiation

Among the more innovative uses of radiotherapy in osteosarcoma treatment has been extracorporeal irradiation. Limb conservation has been changed from being an exception to standard practice in the primary management of osteosarcoma of the extremities. Bony defects created by limb-sparing procedures may be treated with custom-made prostheses with mobile joints, osteoarticular allografts, allograft-prosthesis composites, or intracalary segments filled with autografts. The complication rates from some of these procedures can be high.

Reimplantation of a bone autograph after tumor-ablative extracorporeal irradiation has several theoretical advantages. A major advantage is the precise anatomic fit of the reimplanted bone segment. This may increase the probability of joint mobility. In skeletally immature patients, limb-sparing surgery must be performed carefully to avoid later limb length discrepancy. Extracorporeal irradiation can avoid the growth discrepancy commonly seen in prosthetic replacements by avoiding resection of the normal growth plate and appositional bone growth from surrounding healthy bones. The reimplantation of irradiated bone avoids some of the other problems associated with allografts such as dependence on a bone bank, graft rejection, and the risk of viral transmission. It is also theoretically possible that dead tumor cells in the irradiated bone may stimulate a desirable immunologic response (91,92).

Hong et al. (92) from New South Wales, Australia, have described four patients with osteosarcoma who received a single dose of 50 Gy delivered to bone extracorporeally using a linear accelerator or blood product irradiator. The bone was wrapped in a sterile wrapping, taken for irradiation, and then returned to the operating room. After reimplantation, it appears that the reimplanted bone serves as the framework for appositional bone growth from surrounding healthy bones. There is no evidence of local tumor recurrence at a median follow-up of 19.5 months. For the most part, the functional outcome appears to have been good. Yamamoto et al. (91) described the use of extracorporeal irradiation to treat a distal radius osteosarcoma. This patient received 60 Gy in a single fraction. Araki et al. (93) used 50 Gy to treat 20 patients with primary bone tumors, including osteosarcoma and malignant fibrous histiocytoma. At a median follow-up of 45 months, there was no evidence of local recurrence or symptoms of graft failure such as severe pain or severe fracture.

Chemotherapy

For many years it was accepted that the long-term survival of patients with osteosarcoma treated with radical surgical ablation alone was approximately 20%. A 1978 M. D. Anderson Cancer Center trial used cyclophosphamide, vincristine, melphalan, and adriamycin and achieved a 2-year survival rate of 50% (59). Subsequent pediatric trials from M. D. Anderson used the T7 protocol of preoperative intra-arterial cisplatin, surgery, and postoperative programs of adriamycin, methotrexate, cisplatin, and cyclophosphamide in various combinations. Patients undergoing limb salvage had a 58% 110-month disease-free survival. Patients undergoing amputation had a 54% disease-free survival (difference not significant). Optimum survival (80%) was found in patients with more than 90% tumor necrosis, induced by the preoperative chemotherapy, at the time of amputation. Survival was also correlated with smaller primary tumor volumes (94). Patients with a poor histologic response had a 33% disease-free survival rate (95–97).

In a separate report from the M. D. Anderson group covering the years 1979 to 1982, reporting 37 patients 16 years old or older with extremity lesions, preoperative adriamycin and intra-arterial cisplatin were followed postoperatively by the same drugs. Patients who suffered cisplatin toxicity received dacarbazine as a substitute.

Based on these results, the T7 protocol was modified by the use of cisplatinum, doxorubicin, bleomycin, cyclophosphamide, and dactinomycin in the postoperative period. This was called the T10 protocol (95,97). Sixty additional patients, treated from 1983 to 1988, received intensified preoperative intraarterial cisplatin. Postoperatively, complete responders received adriamycin and cisplatin (or dacarbazine), and partial or poor responders were changed to an alternating program of methotrexate, adriamycin or dacarbazine, and bleomycin, cyclophosphamide, or actinomycin. Patients treated from 1979 to 1982 had a 54% 5-year disease-free survival. Those treated from 1983 to 1988 had a 69% 3-year disease-free survival (94).

In an attempt to confirm the preliminary good results of the T10 protocol, the Children's Cancer Group (CCG) undertook a single-arm trial of neoadjuvant chemotherapy that based the postoperative therapy on the histologic response of the preoperative chemotherapy. The protocol, CCG-782, accrued 268 patients with nonmetastatic osteosarcoma of the extremity between 1983 and 1986. Preoperative chemotherapy consisted of four courses of high-dose methotrexate and one course of bleomycin, cyclophosphamide, and dactinomycin. Good histologic responders (i.e., those with less than 5% residual viable tumor) were treated postoperatively with methotrexate, bleomycin, cyclophosphamide, dactinomycin, and doxorubicin. Poor histologic responders were treated with bleomycin, cyclophosphamide, dactinomycin, doxorubicin, and cisplatinum. The 8-year event-free survival was 53%. The overall survival rate was 60%. Good histologic responders had an 8-year postoperative event-free survival rate of 81% and a survival rate of 87%, whereas those with a poor histologic response had an 8-year postoperative event-free survival of 46% and a survival rate of 52% (99).

Pratt et al. (100) from St. Jude Children's Research Hospital, in studies open from 1973 to 1981, reported 76 patients who received adriamycin, cyclophosphamide, and methotrexate at two different dosage levels after amputation. The actuarial 10-year survival was 46% and 56% for two chemotherapy protocols, compared with 18% to 25% for historic controls who received ineffective or no chemotherapy after amputation ($p < 0.001$).

Sequential chemotherapy trials were conducted at New York's Memorial Sloan–Kettering Cancer Center from 1976 to 1986. Patients received preoperative high-dose methotrexate with leucovorin rescue (some patients were randomized to additionally receive vincristine) and postoperative cyclophosphamide, bleomycin, adriamycin, and actinomycin D. In recent years, patients who had a poor response to methotrexate received adriamycin and cisplatin. The 10-year survival of 279 patients was 73%. As in the M. D. Anderson studies and other series, histologic response of the primary tumor to neoadjuvant chemotherapy was an important predictor of survival (64,98,101–108).

The apparent successes of adjuvant chemotherapy trials were challenged by a research team at the Mayo Clinic. This group suggested that there might be a change in the natural history of osteosarcoma. Whereas the Mayo Clinic noted a 20% survival rate from ablative surgery in patients treated from 1963 to 1965, a comparable group treated from 1972 to 1974 without chemotherapy had a 50% overall survival rate (109). A randomized prospective trial reported by the Mayo Clinic

Group showed that high-dose methotrexate as adjuvant therapy, in comparison to no chemotherapy, offered no benefit: Survival in both groups was 52% (98,110–112).

Two randomized prospective trials attempted to resolve the argument over the value of adjuvant chemotherapy. The University of California at Los Angeles (UCLA) trial randomized 59 patients with nonmetastatic osteosarcoma. All patients received preoperative adriamycin. Thirty-two patients were randomized to receive adjuvant postoperative high-dose methotrexate, adriamycin, bleomycin, cyclophosphamide, and actinomycin D. Twenty-seven patients received no adjuvant chemotherapy. Of the patients who received adjuvant chemotherapy, 55% remained disease free at a median of 2 years after excision of the primary tumor. Of the patients who received no adjuvant chemotherapy, only 20% remained free of disease ($p < 0.01$). Of 18 control patients treated before the trial, the overall disease-free survival was not significantly different from that of the 27 randomized control patients treated without chemotherapy from 1981 to 1984. Overall survival for randomized patients did not differ significantly between the two arms (115). When the larger group of patients who chose their therapy

TABLE 10-9. *Literature review of the local control rates for osteosarcomas after neutron therapy*

Year of report	Reference	Reporting institution	Number of patients	Local control
1979	137a	MANTA	1	1/1
1980	138	Texas A&M Variable Energy Cyclotrol	1	0/1
1981	139a	Amsterdam	3	0/3
1982	140	National Institute of Radiological Sciences, Chiba, Japan	41	33/41
1984	135	Fermilab, Batavia, Illinois	9	2/9
1986	136	Western General Hospital, Edinburgh	5	1/5[a]
1989	133	University of Washington, Seattle	3	3/13[b]
1994	141a	Centre Hospitalier d'Orléans, France	4	4/4[c]
1994	152	Beijing Medical University	5	1/5[c]
2002	56	Cooperative Osteosarcoma Study Group	1	1/1
2003	57	Cooperative Osteosarcoma Study Group	2	0/2

MANTA, Mid-Atlantic Neutron Therapy Facility.
[a]A persistent mass and calcification were considered a local failure. For this reason, local control rates may be underestimated.
[b]These are 2-year actuarial data.
[c]These patients received combined local therapy with photons and neutrons.
Based on material found in the cited references and on references 132, 133, and 134.

was combined with the randomized group, there was a significant overall survival benefit favoring chemotherapy at 6 years.

Link et al. (105,116,123,125) reported a randomized chemotherapy trial involving 36 patients. At 2 years, the actuarial relapse-free survival was 17% in the control group and 66% in the group receiving adjuvant cyclophosphamide, bleomycin, actinomycin, methotrexate with leucovorin rescue, doxorubicin, and cisplatin ($p <$ 0.001). A similar benefit to chemotherapy was observed among 77 patients who declined to undergo randomization but elected observation or chemotherapy.

The long-term results of the COSS-86 protocol included 171 eligible patients; 128 were stratified into the high-risk group. "Low risk" was defined as a tumor length of less than one-third of the involved bone, less than 20% chondroid brown substance in the biopsy specimen, and more than 20% reduction of early- or late-phase activity in sequential bone scans. Other patients were con-

sidered to be at high risk. Doxorubicin, high-dose methotrexate, and cisplatinum were given to all patients. Patients who met one of the high-risk criteria received early systemic treatment intensification with ifosfamide added as a fourth agent. Postoperatively, the high-risk patients received cisplatinum intra-arterially or intravenously. In the total group of 171 patients, which included the high- and low-risk patients, overall event-free survival rates at 10 years were 72% and 66%, respectively. No benefit from intra-arterial cisplatinum was seen (117).

A randomized trial of two chemotherapy regimens in operable osteosarcoma was conducted by the European Osteosarcoma Intergroup and reported in the *Lancet* in 1997 (118). Patients with operable, nonmetastatic osteosarcoma were randomly assigned to receive doxorubicin and cisplatinum preoperatively or vincristine, methotrexate, and doxorubicin preoperatively and postoperative bleomycin, cyclophosphamide, dactinomycin, vincristine, methotrexate,

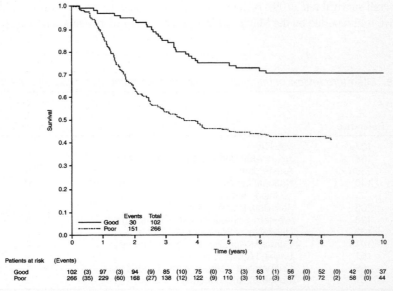

FIG. 10-5. A Kaplan–Meier survival curve for patients in two consecutive trials of the European Osteosarcoma Intergroup shows improved survival for patients with at least 90% necrosis after preoperative chemotherapy ($p < 0.01$ with one degree of freedom). (From Hauben EI, Weeden S, Pringle J, et al. Does the histological subtype of high-grade central osteosarcoma influence the response to treatment with chemotherapy and does it affect overall survival? A study on 570 patients of two consecutive trials of the European Osteosarcoma Intergroup. *Eur J Cancer* 2002;38(9):1218–1225, with permission.)

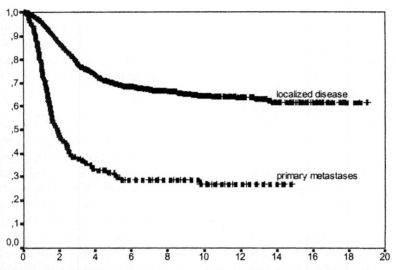

FIG. 10-6. Overall survival for patients with localized disease, compared with those with metastases at diagnosis, in patients treated on Cooperative German–Austrian–Swiss Osteosarcoma Group protocols. (From Bielack S, Kempf-Bielack B, Delling G, et al. Prognostic factors in high-grade osteosarcoma of the extremities or trunk: an analysis of 1,702 patients treated on Neoadjuvant Cooperative Osteosarcoma Study Group protocols. *J Clin Oncol* 2002;20:776–790, with permission.)

doxorubicin, and cisplatinum. Of the 407 randomized patients, 391 were eligible and were followed up for at least 4 years. The proportion showing more than 90% tumor necrosis in response to preoperative chemotherapy was about 29% in both regimens and was a strong predictor for survival. Overall survival was 65% at 3 years and 55% at 5 years in both groups. Thus, there was no difference between the two-drug and multidrug regimens. The two-drug regimen was shorter in duration and better tolerated (118).

In Table 10-7 we summarize studies by several cooperative groups. The data indicate that surgery plus modern chemotherapy should achieve a 60% to 70% 5-year event-free survival (Figs. 10-5 and 10-6). It is not clear that neoadjuvant chemotherapy is superior to postoperative chemotherapy.

RADIOTHERAPEUTIC TECHNIQUE

Dosage

Osteosarcoma has a reputation of being radioresistant. However, this reputation is unjustified. Because radiotherapy was formerly used to treat bulky tumors, it is no surprise that local failures were common. The Do values of human and rodent osteosarcoma cell lines are reported to be similar to those of most other mammalian tumors, perhaps with a higher Dq (51,126).

Canine osteosarcoma has been treated with a variety of dosage and fractionation schemes including 8 Gy three times at 0, 7, and 21 days and 8 Gy four times at 0, 7, 14, and 21 days. Radiotherapy is generally used to palliate the dog's pain and dysfunction. High response rates are achieved, albeit with short follow-up because most animals are euthanized for metastatic disease (126).

In a dose-response study of patients treated with the Cade technique, Gaitan-Yanguas (47) produced uniform tumor sterilization with dosages of 80 to 100 Gy and always found persistent tumor at 50 Gy or less. Phillips and Sheline (51) found viable tumor in one of ten patients receiving less than 100 Gy and in two of seven patients receiving at least 100 Gy.

Lombardi et al. (128) administered 36 Gy at 6 Gy per fraction, with three fractions per week for 2 weeks to 21 osteosarcoma sites irradiated for palliation in 14 patients. There was a clinical response (disappearance of pain, decrease in tumor size, improvement in function) or radiologic response at 18 of the 21 sites. Of eight primary sites irradiated because of synchronous metastases, all showed a clinical or radiographic response. In five patients, radiotherapy was given where preoperative chemotherapy had not rendered the patient suitable for limb-sparing surgery. Surgery after radiotherapy revealed 95–100% tumor necrosis in all cases. Limb-sparing surgery was performed in three of five cases, but because of infectious complications related to soft tissue damage, all limbs were amputated eventually.

Caceres et al. (102) from Peru gave 60 Gy in 6 weeks to 15 patients in conjunction with chemotherapy. Postradiotherapy biopsy showed no evidence of active tumor in 12 of 15 (80%) patients. The whole specimen was studied, because of amputation or autopsy, in five patients. No viable tumor was found. Complications were common, including pathologic fracture, soft tissue fibrosis or necrosis, local infection, and moist desquamation. The degree of tumor necrosis seen by Caceres et al. is inconsistent with an earlier report from the same group of less impressive tumor destruction after 80 to 120 Gy at 10 to 12 Gy per fraction (Table 10-6) (45). If radiotherapy is to be used alone as definitive treatment for a small (less than 5 cm) osteosarcoma in an unresectable location such as the base of skull or vertebral body, or if a patient refuses surgery, the dosage should be as high as normal tissue tolerance allows, that is, 60 to 75 Gy at conventional fractionation with progressive shrinking-field technique (129,130).

When radiotherapy is used for prophylactic treatment of the lungs, the dosage is 13.5 to 19.5 Gy at 1.5 Gy per fraction. These dosages generally have been reported without lung correction factors being applied (17,40,69,70).

Volume

The treatment volume is determined by plain radiographs, bone scan, CT, and MRI. It is customary to define the tumor volume based on the largest volume of these studies (the "worst-case volume"). A margin is then allowed.

Prophylactic WLI is directed to the entire substance of the lung. Particular attention must be paid to coverage of the apices of the lung and to the areas of the lung that curve over the surfaces of the diaphragms.

Technique

An immobilization device is generally needed. The field should be contoured specifically to the anatomic problem for the individual patient. In most cases, multiple fields are used. To maintain a functional limb after irradiation, a strip of skin should be spared, and one should avoid high-dose irradiation to the full width of the joint.

Some investigators have attempted to improve the local control rates of osteosarcoma by altering tumor and normal tissue oxygenation. In the past, the tourniquet technique attempted to produce anoxia in both tumor and normal limb tissues to remove any advantage the tumor might gain from hypoxic areas. Using this technique, patients received fractionated irradiation up to total dosages of 75 to 160 Gy. In patients who were long-term survivors, the functional result was poor (106). One group reported local response rates of approximately 70% and reasonable limb function with tourniquet anoxia and high-dose-per-fraction treatment (i.e., three doses of 25 Gy). Radiation treatment under hyperbaric oxygen conditions was also investigated (131). A group of investigators from Stanford University reported a series of patients who had unresectable osteosarcomas or who refused amputation, treated with 42 to 48 Gy at 6 Gy per fraction, one fraction every 5 days, and pulsed 5′-bromodeoxyuridine infused as a radiosensitizer (52). Local control was achieved in seven of nine patients, four of whom were long-term survivors. Significant soft tissue injury occurred in five patients (55).

Neutron Therapy

Neutrons are a form of high linear energy transfer radiation. They offer several advantages over conventional photon or electron radiotherapy. First, neutrons are better able to kill hypoxic cells than photons. The oxygen enhancement ratio for neutrons is on the order of 1.6, compared with 2.5 to 3.0 for photons. Second, repair of radiation-induced sublethal and potentially lethal damage is less readily accomplished after neutron irradiation than after conventional irradiation. Third, neutrons are toxic throughout the phases of the cell cycle (M, G1, S, G2), whereas photons are more toxic in late G2/M (132,133).

Kubota et al. (127) compared the biologic effects of 13-MeV neutrons with those of ^{137}Cs gamma rays in MG-63 human osteosarcoma cells in plateau phase growth and in multicellular spheroids. The relative biologic effectiveness varied slightly with the measurement technique but was in the range of 1.9 to 2.29. If one accepts the assertion that osteosarcomas are rapidly growing tumors with areas of necrosis and potentially hypoxic areas and that they are resistant to photon irradiation, then one might conclude that they would be more effectively irradiated by neutrons.

There is a small clinical experience with the use of neutrons for local control of osteosarcomas. Many of the patients treated had inoperable tumors or refused amputations (134). The results of neutron treatment are shown in Table 10-9. The 77 patients cited have an overall local control rate of 44 of 77 (58%). There are clearly risks from combining the results of 11 series to draw a conclusion. The local control rates of the individual series range from 0% to 100%, and these series include patients with tumors at a variety of locations. Dense fibrotic reactions can occur after neutron treatment, leading to severe complications and, in some patients, to amputation (135,136). For a patient with osteosarcoma who refuses definitive surgery or is medically or technically inoperable, it is reasonable to consider the use of neutrons. However, part of the informed consent for such treatment must include a discussion of the potential for serious late ill effects of such treatment.

Charged Particle Therapy

Osteosarcoma of the skull base and axial skeleton pose a particularly difficult problem for the pediatric radiation oncologist. These tumors are more difficult to extirpate at surgery. An initial gross and microscopic tumor resection is inhibited by the proximity of brainstem, spinal cord, cranial nerves, nerve roots, or vessels. However, these normal tissue structures also prevent the oncologist from using radiation as an alternative to surgery because tumoricidal dosages for osteosarcoma exceed the tolerance of critical neural tissue (137). Although three-dimensional or intensity-modulated treatment planning with multiple noncoplanar photon beams may be used in an attempt to achieve an acceptable dosage distribution, the penetrance and divergence of photons present significant limitations.

Protons and other charged particle beams (such as neon, helium, and carbon ions) have a finite dosage range with steep dosage fall-off beyond the Bragg peak. This property engenders a treatment beam that has little exit dosage beyond the deposition of energy in the target volume, making these beams distinctly different from photons. The advantage of protons resides solely in this physical difference because proton beams have no significant biologic advantage over megavoltage photons. Other charged particle beams have both the advantage of rapid Bragg peak dosage fall-off and an increase in relative biologic effectiveness (126). Charged particles can be used to shape a dosage distribution around an osteosarcoma of the skull base or vertebral body with the possibility of maintaining the dosage to the adjacent brain or spinal cord within acceptable limits.

The Radiation Oncology Department at the Massachusetts General Hospital, in collaboration with the Harvard Cyclotron Laboratory, treated 15 patients with osteosarcoma with combined proton and photon irradiation (anatomic sites were base of skull, seven; cervical spine, three; lumbar spine, two; sacrum, three). Dosages of 61.1 to 80 cobalt Gray equivalent were administered, and 14 of the 15 patients also received chemotherapy. At 5 years, the actuarial local control rate was 59%, and the overall survival rate was 44% (137). In a series that includes skull base tumors of various histologies, Castro et al. (138a) reported that 20% of disease-free survivors after charged particle therapy had grade III, IV, or V complications such as cranial nerve or vascular injuries.

Intraoperative Therapy

A combined specialty team at the Universidad de Navarra, Spain, treated 22 patients with osteosarcoma with preoperative chemotherapy, surgical excision, a 15- to 20-Gy intraoperative radiation therapy (IORT) electron beam boost to the tumor bed area, and postoperative chemotherapy (54). Five patients also received preoperative and postoperative external beam radiotherapy. There was only one local recurrence among the 22 patients, with a median follow-up of 18 months. Local recurrence after definitive surgery for osteosarcoma is uncommon, and it is not clear that the IORT was helpful.

An additional 32 patients with osteosarcoma were treated with IORT by Yamamuro and Kotoura (139). Before 1984, treatment consisted solely of exposing the primary tumor site and administering 50 to 60 Gy of IORT with 12- to 26-MeV electron beams. After 1984, patients received cisplatinum and adriamycin in combination with IORT. The clinical results from this small series, spread out over many years (1978 to 1990), must be interpreted with caution. Ten patients underwent limb amputation or prosthetic replacement 2 to 10 months after IORT. Eight patients had complete necrosis of the tumor cells throughout the specimen except for a "few scattered, markedly altered, presumably non-viable tumor cells in small clusters" (139). Two patients showed local regional tumor recurrence in nonirradiated areas, and one showed recurrence in the radiation field (a juxtacortical osteosarcoma). Joint function was reported as being satisfactory; five patients had some evidence of moderate to severe skin necrosis, but "among the patients who underwent neither limb amputation nor prosthetic replacement and survived longer than one year after IORT, about 58% sustained pathologic fracture through the lesions. All attempts of osteo synthesis failed to fuse the fracture site" (139).

Oya, Tsuboyama, and colleagues (140a,141) from Kyoto University in Japan described 39 patients with osteosarcoma of the extremities who were treated with definitive IORT. The tumor and a margin were treated with 45 to 80 Gy of electrons or X-rays in a single fraction while major vessels and nerves were retracted out of the treatment field. Nine local recurrences developed in these 39 patients. Eight were considered to be marginal recurrences or occurrences from unirradiated surrounding normal tissue. Complications included associated transient skin reaction attributable to radiation and two cases of mild peroneal palsy, possibly caused by irradiation. Post-IORT fractures occurred in 13 patients. The problem seems to have been solved by the use of preventive nailing in more recent patients.

These series must be interpreted cautiously. It is possible that IORT, in combination with surgery and chemotherapy, may reduce the already low local recurrence rate for most cases of osteosarcoma. This is a testable hypothesis. The use of IORT as the definitive local control measure, as described by Yamamuro and Kotoura (139), must be considered investigational therapy with, apparently, a high risk of subsequent fracture.

Radioisotope Therapy

Bone-seeking radiopharmaceuticals are at an early stage of investigation in the treatment of osteoblastic osteosarcoma. The uptake of radiopharmaceuticals in adult skeletal metastatic lesions such as breast and prostate cancer results from an osteoblastic response in the normal bones surrounding the metastases. However, osteosarcoma often produces bone matrix within the target. A radioisotope that hones into bone and gives off radioactivity for a sufficiently long period of time may produce a therapeutic benefit.

Samarium-153 ethylene diamine tetramethylene phosphonate is a bone-seeking radiopharmaceutical. It is produced by neutron capture from ^{153}Sm to yield a radioisotope of high purity that has both a medium-energy beta emission for therapeutic purposes and gamma emission, which is useful for conventional gamma camera scintigraphic imaging. Compared with technetium-99m methylene diphosphonate preparations, which are used for routine bone imaging, ^{153}Sm has comparable or better bone:blood and bone:muscle ratios. Because of these favorable bone-seeking characteristics, ^{153}Sm has been used for palliative treatment of bone metastases (142).

In pilot studies of the use of ^{153}Sm to irradiate patients with osteosarcoma and bone metastases, all patients receiving high-dose samarium experienced severe pancytopenia, and some needed transfusions. Stem cell infusion was needed. It appears that samarium treatment can reduce bone pain in some patients, albeit with significant toxicity. There also appears to be one long-term survivor, a patient with a large pelvic osteosarcoma and multiple primary pulmonary metastases who was treated with external beam radiotherapy to the pelvic lesion, multiagent chemotherapy, and samarium (142–146).

Palliation

It is reasonable to consider radiotherapy to palliate painful bony sites and treat spinal cord compression (Fig. 10-7) (48,49,128,147). Unfortunately, the literature documenting the palliative efficacy of radiotherapy in osteosarcoma is sparse. The 1963 report by Lee and MacKenzie (50) of the Westminster Hospital, London, describes the results with the administration of 7,000 to 8,000 R with a 2-MeV Van de Graaff electrostatic generator. The authors note that "clinical response of the tumour was very variable. Sometimes there was apparent worsening: there might be sudden increase in the size of the tumor, with more pain. Such changes might be the result of hemorrhage, or fracture, or disintegration of bone. More often there was a gradual reduction of pain and swelling, starting after some 2,000 R (sometimes much later) and continuing for several weeks after completion of treatment" (50). In 1975, deMoor (148) from Johannesburg described the use of radiation for palliation and noted that "pain relief or reduction in swelling was experienced generally, and often within the first two to three weeks of treatment."

The series of Beck et al. (147) from the University of California at San Francisco included 44 patients with adequate information "to assess whether the treatment represented even a short term subjective gain for the patient. In 19 (43%) there was definite palliation. Twenty-five (57%) had either no change or worsening of symptoms. Those who survived experienced relief only after surgery." These authors used conventionally fractionated radiation with total dosages ranging from 5,000 to 8,000 cGy. In contrast,

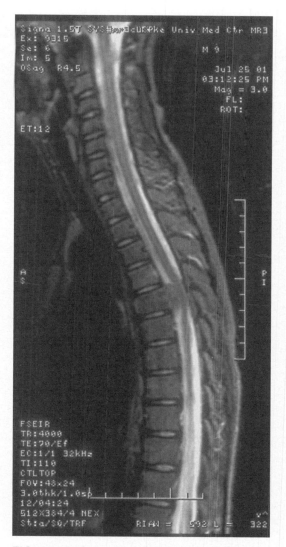

FIG. 10-7. When osteosarcoma metastasizes to bone, radiotherapy may be used for palliation. This 9-year-old boy presented with osteosarcoma of the left femur. Bone metastases were diagnosed a year and a half after the primary tumor was identified. When the child complained of pain in the spine, both magnetic resonance imaging and bone scan identified metastatic disease in conjunction with pulmonary metastasis. For spinal cord compression, palliative radiation therapy was administered.

Lombardi et al. (128) administered 6 Gy three times per week for a total of 36 Gy in six fractions over 2 weeks. In 14 patients with 21 evaluable sites, there was a clinical response in 18 (86%).

Machak et al. (58), describing 31 patients treated with curative intent with chemotherapy, reported "a clinical response and limb function restoration" in 24 of the 31 (77%) of patients but a good imaging and biochemical response in only 11. Of the 20 nonresponders, 15 (75%) improved after radiotherapy, supporting a palliative role for radiotherapy.

REFERENCES

References particularly recommended for further reading are indicated with an asterisk.

1. Carter JR, Abdul-Karim FW. Pathology of childhood osteosarcoma. *Perspect Pediatr Pathol* 1987;9:133–170.
2. Chung EB, Enzinger FM. Extraskeletal osteosarcoma. *Cancer* 1987;60:1132–1142.
3. Kumar R, David R, Madwell JE, et al. Radiographic spectrum of osteogenic sarcoma. *AJR* 1978;148:767–772.
4. Miller JH, Ettinger LJ. Osteosarcoma. In: Miller JH, ed. *Imaging in pediatric oncology.* Baltimore: Williams & Wilkins, 1985:378–388.
5. Spjut HJ, Ayala AG. Skeletal tumors in childhood and adolescence. In: Finegold M, ed. *Pathology of neoplasia in children and adolescents.* Philadelphia: WB Saunders, 1986:265–281.
6. Sweetnam R. Osteosarcoma. *BMJ* 1979;2:536–537.
7. Ueda Y, Roessner A, Grundmann E. Pathological diagnosis of osteosarcoma: the validity of the subclassification and some new diagnostic approaches using immunohistochemistry In: Humphrey GB, Koops HS, Mclenaar WM, et al., eds. *Osteosarcoma in adolescents and young adults: new developments and controversies.* Boston: Kluwer, 1993:109–124.
8. Unni KK, Dahlin DC. Osteosarcoma: pathology and classification. *Semin Roentgenol* 1989;25:143–152.
9. Ushigome S, Nakamori K, Nikaido T, et al. Histologic subclassification of osteosarcoma: differential diagnostic problems and immunohistochemical aspects. In: Humphrey GB, Koops HS, Molenaar WM, et al, eds. *Osteosarcoma in adolescent and young adults: new developments and controversies.* Boston: Kluwer, 1993:125–137.
10. Poppe E, Liverrud K, Efskind J. Osteosarcoma. *Acta Chir Scand* 1968;134:549–556.
11. Diller L, Kassel J, Nelson CE, et al. p53 Functions as a cell cycle control protein in osteosarcoma. *Mol Cell Biol* 1990;10:5772–5781.
12. Beattie EJ, Harvey JC, Marcove R, et al. Results of multiple pulmonary resections for metastatic osteogenic sarcoma after two decades. *J Surg Oncol* 1991;46:154–155.
13. Glasser DB, Lne JM, Nuvos AG, et al. Survival, prognosis, and therapeutic response in osteogenic sarcoma. *Cancer* 1991;69:698–708.
14. Tillotson C, Rosenberg A, Gebhardt M, et al. Postradiation multicentric osteosarcoma. *Cancer* 1988;62:65–71.
15. Jaffe N, Link MP, Cohen D, et al. High-dose methotrexate in osteogenic sarcoma. *Natl Cancer Inst Monogr* 1981;56:201–206.
16. Aisen AD, Martell W, Braunstein EM, et al. MRI and CT evaluation of primary bone and soft issue tumors. *AJR* 1986;146:749–756.
*17. Breur K, Cohen P, Schwiesguth O, et al. Irradiation of the lungs as an adjuvant therapy in the treatment of osteosarcoma of the limbs. An EORTC randomized study. *Eur J Cancer* 1978;14:461–471.
18. Marion J, Burgers V, Breur K, et al. Role of metastasectomy without chemotherapy in the management of osteosarcoma in children. *Cancer* 1980;45:1664–1668.
19. Wittig J, Bickels J, Priebat D, et al. Osteosarcoma: a multidisciplinary approach to diagnosis and treatment. *Am Fam Physician* 2002;65:1123–1132, 1135–1136.
20. Beiling P, Rehan N, Winkler P, et al. Tumor size and prognosis in aggressively treated osteosarcoma. *J Clin Oncol* 1996;14:848–858.
21. Springfield DS, Schmidt R, Graham-Pole J, et al. Surgical treatment for osteosarcoma. *J Bone Joint Surg* 1988;70-A:1124–1130.
22. Smeland S, Muller C, Alvegard TA, et al. Scandinavian Sarcoma Group Osteosarcoma Study SSGVIII: prognostic factors for outcome and the role of replacement salvage chemotherapy for poor histological responders. *Eur J Cancer* 2003;39(4):488–494.
23. Hauben EI, Weeden S, Pringle J, et al. Does the histological subtype of high-grade central osteosarcoma influence the response to treatment with chemotherapy and does it affect overall survival? a study on 570 patients of two consecutive trials of the European Osteosarcoma Intergroup. *Eur J Cancer* 2002;38(9):1218–1225.
*24. Bielack S, Kempf-Bielack B, Delling G, et al. Prognostic factors in high-grade osteosarcoma of the extremities or trunk: an analysis of 1,702 patients treated on neoadjuvant Cooperative Osteosarcoma Study Group protocols. *J Clin Oncol* 2002;20:776–790.
25. Ferrari S, Mercuri M, Bacci G. Comment on "Prognostic factors in high-grade osteosarcoma of the extremities on trunk: an analysis of 1,702 patients treated on neoadjuvant Cooperative Osteosarcoma Study Group protocols." *J Clin Oncol* 2002;20:2910.
26. Bielback SS, Jurgens H. Letter to the editor. *J Clin Oncol* 2002;20:2911–2912.
27. Suit HD. Radiotherapy in osteosarcoma. *Clin Orthop* 1975;111:271–275.
28. Suit HD. Radiation therapy for osteosarcoma, chordoma and chondrosarcoma. In: Kumar S, ed. *Advances in medical oncology, research, and education.* Vol. 10: *Clinical cancer principle sites 1.* New York: Pergamon, 1979:181–185.
29. Sweetnam R. Tumors of bone and their management. *Ann R Coll Surg Engl* 1974;54:63–66.
30. Sweetnam R. The surgical management of primary osteosarcoma. *Clin Orthop* 1975;111:57–64.
31. White VA, Fanning CV, Ayala AG, et al. Osteosarcoma and the role of fine-needle aspiration: a study of 51 cases. *Cancer* 1988;62:1238–1246.
32. Wong ACW, Akahoshi Y, Takeuchi S. Limb-salvage

procedures for osteosarcoma: an alternative to amputation. *Int Orthop* 1986;109:245–251.

33. Damaron JA, Pritchard DJ. Current combined treatment of high-grade osteosarcomas. *Oncology* 1995;9: 327–350.

34. Button S. Rotation plasty for childhood osteosarcoma. *Nurs Times* 1987;83:49–51.

35. Hirano T, Iwasaki K, Kimashiro T, et al. Low dose irradiation for limb salvage in malignant bone tumors. *Int Orthop* 1991;115:381–385.

36. Simon MA, Asxhliman MA, Thomas N, et al. Limb-salvage treatment versus amputation for osteosarcoma of the distal end of the femur. *J Bone Joint Surg* 1986;68-A:1331–1337.

37. Marina NM, Pratt CB, Rao BN, et al. Improved prognosis of children with osteosarcoma metastatic to the lung at the time of diagnosis. *Cancer* 1992;70: 2722–2727.

38. Ennedking WF, Spanier SS, Goodman MA. A system for the surgical staging of musculoskeletal sarcoma. *Clin Orthop* 1980;153:106–120.

39. Lee ES. Treatment of bone sarcoma. *Proc R Soc Med* 1971;64:1179–1181.

40. Marcove RC, Martini N, Rosen G. The treatment of pulmonary metastasis in osteogenic sarcoma. *Clin Orthop* 1975;111:65–70.

41. Meyer WH, Schell MJ, Kumar APM, et al. Thoracotomy for pulmonary metastatic osteosarcoma: an analysis of prognostic indicators of survival. *Cancer* 1987;59:374–379.

42. Suttow WW, Herson J, Perez C. Survival after metastasis in osteosarcoma. *Cancer Inst Monogr* 1981;56: 227–231.

43. Albrecht MR, Henze G, Habermalz HJ, et al. Osteosarcoma: a radioresistant tumor? Long term evaluation after multidrug chemotherapy and definitive irradiation of the primary instead of radical surgery. Unpublished scientific meeting presentation, Philadelphia: Radiation Therapy for Children with Cancer, July 24, 1994.

44. Allen CF, Stevens KR. Preoperative irradiation for osteogenic sarcoma. *Cancer* 1973;31:1364–1366.

45. Caceres E, Zaharia M. Massive preoperative radiation therapy in the treatment of osteogenic sarcoma. *Cancer* 1972;30:634–638.

46. Farrell C, Raventos A. Experience in treating osteosarcoma at the Hospital of the University of Pennsylvania. *Radiology* 1964;83:1080–1083.

47. Gaitan-Yanguas M. A study of the response to osteogenic sarcoma and adjacent normal tissues to radiation. *Int J Radiat Oncol Biol Phys* 1981;7:593–595.

48. Jenkin RDT. Radiation treatment of Ewing's sarcoma and osteogenic sarcoma. *Can J Surg* 1977;20:530–536.

49. Jenkin RDT, Allt WEC, Fitzpatrick PJ. Osteosarcoma: an assessment of management with particular reference to primary irradiation and selective delayed amputation. *Cancer* 1972;30:393–400.

50. Lee ES, MacKenzie DH. Osteosarcoma: a study of the value of preoperative megavoltage radiotherapy. *Br J Surg* 1963;51:252–274.

51. Phillips TL, Sheline GE. Radiation therapy of malignant bone tumors. *Radiology* 1969;92:1537–1545.

52. Goffinet DR, Kaplan HS, Donaldson SS, et al. Combined radiosensitizer infusion and irradiation of osteogenic sarcomas. *Radiology* 1975;117:211–214.

53. Cavaliere R. Hyperthermic treatment of osteogenic sarcoma. *Chemother Oncol* 1978;2:190–196.

54. Calvo FA, de Urbina DO, Sierrasesumaga L, et al. Intraoperative radiotherapy in the multidisciplinary treatment of bone sarcomas in children and adolescents. *Med Pediatr Oncol* 1991;19:478–485.

55. Martinez A, Goffinet DR, Donaldson SS, et al. Intra-arterial infusion of radiosensitizer (RUdr) combined with hypofractionated irradiation and chemotherapy for primary treatment of osteogenic sarcoma. *Int J Radiat Oncol Biol Phys* 1985;11:123–128.

56. Ozaki I, Flege S, Lijenqvist U, et al. Osteosarcoma of the spine: experience of the Cooperative Osteosarcoma Study Group. *Cancer* 2002;94(4):1069–1077.

57. Ozaki T, Flege S, Kevric M, et al. Osteosarcoma of the pelvis: experience of the Cooperative Osteosarcoma Study Group. *J Clin Oncol* 2003;21(2): 334–341.

*58. Machak GN, Tkachev SI, Solovyev YN, et al. Neoadjuvant chemotherapy and local radiotherapy for high-grade osteosarcoma of the extremities. *Mayo Clin Proc* 2003;78(2):147–155.

*59. Anderson PM. Effectiveness of radiotherapy for osteosarcoma that responds to chemotherapy. *Mayo Clin Proc* 2003;78(2):145–146.

60. Bieling F, Dallera P, Bacchini P, et al. The Instituto Rizzoli-Beretta experience with osteosarcoma of the jaw. *Cancer* 1991;68:1555–1563.

61. Panizzoni GA, Gasparini G, Clauser L, et al. Osteosarcoma of the facial bones. *Ann Oncol* 1992;3: S47–S50.

62. Chambers RG, Mahoney WD. Osteogenic sarcoma of the mandible: current management. *Am Surg* 1970; 36:463–471.

63. Saunders WM, Chen GTY, Austin-Seymour M, et al. Precision high dose radiotherapy. II. Helium ion treatment of tumors adjacent to critical central nervous system structures. *Int J Radiat Oncol Biol Phys* 1985;11:1339–1347.

64. Burgers JM, van Glabbeke M, Bussan A, et al. Osteosarcoma of the limbs. Report of the EORTC-SIOP 03 trial 20781 investigating the value of adjuvant treatment with chemotherapy and/or prophylactic lung irradiation. *Cancer* 1988;61:1024–1031.

65. Ellis ER, Marcus RB Jr, Cicale MJ, et al. Pulmonary function tests after whole-lung irradiation and doxorubicin in patients with osteogenic sarcoma. *J Clin Oncol* 1992;10:459–463.

66. Springfield DS, Schakel ME Jr, Spanier SS. Spontaneous necrosis in osteosarcoma. *Clin Orthop* 1991; 263:233–237.

67. Lougheed MN, Palmer JD, Henderson I, et al. Radiation and regional chemotherapy in osteogenic sarcoma. *Excerpta Med Int Cong Ser* 1965;105:1124–1128.

68. Newton KA. Prophylactic irradiation of the lung in bone sarcoma. In: Price CHG, Ross FGM, eds. *Bone: certain aspects of neoplasia.* London: Butterworth-Heinemann, 1972:307–311.

69. Rab GT, Ivins JC, Childs DS Jr, et al. Elective whole lung irradiation in the treatment of osteogenic sarcoma. *Cancer* 1976;38:939–942.

70. Zaharia M, Caceres E, Valdivia S, et al. Postoperative

whole lung irradiation with or without adriamycin in osteogenic sarcoma. *Int J Radiat Oncol Biol Phys* 1986;12:907–910.

*71. Whelan JS, Burcombe RJ, Jamims J, et al. A systematic review of the role of pulmonary irradiation in the management of primary bone tumours. *Ann Oncol* 2002;13(1):23–30.

72. Abbatucci JS, Fourre D, Quint R, et al. Possibilities of radiotherapy in pulmonary metastases. Apropos of 150 cases. *Ann Radiol* 1973;16:385–392.

73. Breur K. Prophylactische longbestraling bij bottumoren. *Jaarboek van Kankeronderzoek en Kanker Bestreiding in Nederland* 1973;22:27–43.

74. Breur K. Growth rate and radiosensitivity of human tumours. *Eur J Cancer* 1966;2:157–160.

75. Baeza MR, Barkley HT Jr, Fernandez CH. Total lung irradiation in the treatment of pulmonary metastases. *Radiology* 1975;116:151–154.

76. Caldwell W. Elective whole lung irradiation. *Radiology* 1976;120:659–666.

77. Caceres E, Zaharia M, Moran M, et al. Adjuvant whole lung radiation with or without adriamycin treatment in osteogenic sarcoma. *Cancer Treat Rep* 1978;62:297–299.

78. Jenkin RD, Allt WE, Fitzpatrick PJ. Osteosarcoma. An assessment of management with particular reference to primary irradiation and selective delayed amputation. *Cancer* 1972;30:393–400.

79. French Bone Tumor Study Group. Age and dose of chemotherapy as major prognostic factors in a trial of adjuvant therapy of osteosarcoma combining two alternating drug combinations and early prophylactic lung irradiation. *Cancer* 1988;61:1304–1311.

80. Gilchrist GS, Pritchard DJ, Dahlin DC, et al. Management of osteogenic sarcoma: a perspective based on the Mayo Clinic experience. *Natl Cancer Inst Monogr* 1981;56:193–199.

81. Burgers JMV. Experience of the EORTC radiotherapy/chemotherapy group in osteosarcoma trials. In: Humphrey GB, Koops HS, Molenaar WM, et al, eds. *Osteosarcoma in adolescent and young adults: new developments and controversies.* Boston: Kluwer, 1993:173–175.

82. Burgers JM, van Glabbeke M, Busson A, et al. Osteosarcoma of the limbs. Report of the EORTC-SIOP O₃ trial 20781 investigating the value of adjuvant treatment with chemotherapy and/or prophylactic lung irradiation. *Cancer* 1988;61:1024–1031.

83. Ivins JC, Taylor WF, Wold LE. Elective whole-lung irradiation in osteosarcoma treatment: appearance of bilateral breast cancer in two long-term survivors. *Skeletal Radiol* 1987;16:133–135.

84. Thompson DK, Li FP, Cassady JR. Breast cancer in a man 30 years after radiation for metastatic osteogenic sarcoma. *Cancer* 1979;44:2362–2365.

85. Russo CL, McIntyre J, Goorin AM, et al. Secondary breast cancer in patients presenting with osteosarcoma: possible involvement of germline p53 mutations. *Med Pediatr Oncol* 1994;23:354–358.

86. Weichselbaum RR, Cassady JR, Jaffe N, et al. Preliminary results of aggressive multimodality therapy for metastatic osteosarcoma. *Cancer* 1977;40:78–83.

87. Marion J, Burgers V, Breur K, et al. Role of metastasectomy without chemotherapy in the management

of osteosarcoma in children. *Cancer* 1980;45:1664–1668.

88. Winkler K. Surgical treatment of pulmonary metastases in childhood. *Thorac Cardiovasc Surg* 1986;34:133–136.

89. Heij HA, Vos A, deKraker J, et al. Prognostic factors in surgery for pulmonary metastases in children. *Surgery* 1994;115:687–693.

90. Giritsky AS, Etucubanas E, Mark JB. Pulmonary resection in children with metastatic osteogenic sarcoma: improved survival with surgery, chemotherapy, and irradiation. *J Thorac Cardiovasc Surg* 1978;75:354–362.

91. Yamamoto T, Akisue T, Marui T, et al. Osteosarcoma of the distal radius treated by intraoperative extracorporeal irradiation. *J Hand Surg [Am]* 2002;29(1):160–164.

92. Hong A, Stevens G, Stalley P, et al. Extracorporeal irradiation for malignant bone tumors. *Int J Radiat Oncol Biol Phys* 2001;50(2):441–447.

93. Araki N, Myoui A, Kuratsus, et al. Intraoperative extracorporeal autogenous irradiated bone graft in tumor surgery. *Clin Orthop* 1999;368:196–206.

94. Hudson M, Jaffe MR, Jaffe N, et al. Pediatric osteosarcoma: therapeutic strategies, results, and prognostic factors derived from a 10-year experience. *J Clin Oncol* 1990;12:1988–1997.

95. Rosen G, Caparros B, Huvos AG, et al. Preoperative chemotherapy for osteosarcoma: selection of postoperative adjuvant chemotherapy based on the response of the primary tumor to preoperative therapy. *Cancer* 1982;49:1221–1230.

96. Rosen G, Marcove RC, Caparros B, et al. Primary osteogenic sarcoma: the rationale for preoperative chemotherapy and delayed surgery. *Cancer* 1979;43:2163–2177.

97. Rosen G, Caparros B, Huvos AG, et al. Perioperative chemotherapy for osteosarcoma: selection of postoperative adjuvant chemotherapy based on the response of the primary tumor to preoperative therapy. *Cancer* 1982;49:1221–1230.

98. Benjamin RS, Chawla SP, Carrasco CH, et al. Preoperative chemotherapy for osteosarcoma with intravenous adriamycin and intra-arterial therapy in the treatment of osteosarcoma. *Radiology* 1976;120:163–165.

99. Provisor AJ, Ehinger LJ, Nachman JB, et al. Treatment of nonmetastatic osteosarcoma of the extremity with preoperative and postoperative chemotherapy: a report from the Children's Cancer Group. *J Clin Oncol* 1997;15:76–84.

100. Pratt CB, Champion JE, Fleming ID, et al. Adjuvant chemotherapy for osteosarcoma of the extremity. *Cancer* 1976;38:939–942.

101. Bacci G, Springfield D, Capanna R, et al. Neoadjuvant chemotherapy for osteosarcoma of the extremity. *Clin Orthop* 1987;224:268–276.

102. Caceres E, Zaharia M, Valdivia S, et al. Local control of osteogenic sarcoma by radiation and chemotherapy. *Int J Radiat Oncol Biol Phys* 1984;10:35–39.

103. Silberman A, Elber FR, Giuliano AE, et al. Adjuvant chemotherapy of osteosarcoma. *J Clin Oncol* 1987;5:982–984.

104. Goorin AM, Perrz-Atayade A, Gebhardt M, et al.

Weekly high-dose methotrexate and doxorubicin for osteosarcoma: the Dana Farber Cancer Institute/The Children's Hospital, Study III. *J Clin Oncol* 1987;15: 381–385.

105. Link MP, Goorin M, Miser AW, et al. The effect of adjuvant chemotherapy on relapse-free survival in patients with osteosarcoma of the extremity. *N Engl J Med* 1986;314:1600–1606.

106. Saeter G, Alvegard TA, Elomaa I, et al. Treatment of osteosarcoma of the extremities with the T-10 protocol, with emphasis on the effects of preoperative chemotherapy with a single-agent high-dose methotrexate: a Scandinavian Sarcoma Group Study. *J Clin Oncol* 1991;9:1766–1775.

107. Thorpe WP, Reilly JJ, Rosenberg SA. Prognostic significance of alkaline phosphative measurements in patients with osteogenic sarcoma receiving chemotherapy. *Cancer* 1979;43:2178–2181.

108. Winkler K, Beran G, Delling G, et al. Neoadjuvant chemotherapy of osteosarcoma: results of a randomized cooperative trial (COSS-82) with salvage chemotherapy based on histological tumor response. *J Clin Oncol* 1988;6:329–337.

109. Taylor WF, Ivins JC, Pritchard DJ, et al. Trends and variability in survival among patients with osteosarcoma: 7 year update. *Mayo Clin Proc* 1985;60: 91–104.

110. Bentzen SM, Paulsen HS, Kaae S, et al. Prognostic factors in osteosarcomas: a regression analysis. *Cancer* 1988;62:194–202.

111. Edmonson JH, Green SJ, Ivins JC, et al. A controlled pilot study of high-dose methotrexate as post surgical adjuvant treatment for primary osteosarcoma. *J Clin Oncol* 1987;5:21–26.

112. Holland JF. Adjuvant chemotherapy of osteosarcoma: no runs, no hits, two men left on base. *J Clin Oncol* 1987;5:4–5.

113. Ferguson WS, Goorin AM. Current treatment of osteosarcoma. *Cancer Invest* 2001;19(3):292–315.

114. Bacci G, Lari S. Current treatment of high grade osteosarcoma of the extremity review. *J Chemother* 2001;13(3):225–243.

115. Eilber F, Giuliano A, Eckardt J, et al. Adjuvant chemotherapy for osteosarcoma: a randomized prospective trial. *J Cancer Clin Oncol* 1987;5:21–26.

116. Link MP, Goorin AM, Horowitz M, et al. Adjuvant chemotherapy of high-grade osteosarcoma of the extremity. Updated results of the Multi-Institutional Osteosarcoma Study. *Clin Orthop* 1991;270:8–14.

117. Fuchs N, Bielack SS, Epler D, et al. Long-term results of the Co-Operative German–Austrian–Swiss Osteosarcoma Study Group's Protocol cross-86 of intensive multidrug chemotherapy and surgery for osteosarcoma of the limbs. *Ann Oncol* 1998;9:893–899.

118. Souhami RL, Craft AW, Vander EI, et al. Randomized trial of two regimens of chemotherapy in operable osteosarcoma: a study of the European osteosarcoma intergroup. *Lancet* 1997;350:911–917.

119. Anonymous. Osteosarcoma chemo regimens debated. *Oncol News Int* 1995;4:1–26.

120. Goorin AM, Schwartzentruber DJ, Devidas M, et al. Presurgical chemotherapy compared with immediate surgery and adjuvant chemotherapy for nonmetastatic osteosarcoma: Pediatric Oncology Group

Study POG-8651. *J Clin Oncol* 2003;21(8):1574–1580.

121. Craft AW, Burgers JMW. The European osteosarcoma intergroup (E.O.I.) studies in 1980–1991. In: Humphrey GB, Koops HS, Molenaar WM, et al, eds. *Osteosarcoma in adolescents and young adults: new developments and controversies.* Boston: Kluwer, 1993:279–286.

*122. Miser JS, Krailo M. The children's cancer group (CCG) studies. In: Humphrey GB, Koops HS, Molenaar WM, et al, eds. *Osteosarcoma in adolescents and young adults: new developments and controversies.* Boston: Kluwer, 1993:287–291.

123. Link MP. Commentary of the use of presurgical chemotherapy. In: Humphrey GB, Koops HS, Molenaar WM, et al., eds. *Osteosarcoma in adolescents and young adults: new developments and controversies.* Boston: Kluwer, 1993:383–385.

124. Kager L, Zoubek A, Potschger U, et al. Cooperative German–Austrian–Swiss Osteosarcoma Study Group. Primary metastatic osteosarcoma: presentation and outcome of patients treated on neoadjuvant Cooperative Osteosarcoma Study Group protocols. *J Clin Oncol* 2003;21(10):2011–2018.

*125. Link MP. The multi-institutional osteosarcoma study: an update. In: Humphrey GB, Koops HS, Molenaar WM, et al., eds. *Osteosarcoma in adolescents and young adults: new developments and controversies.* Boston: Kluwer, 1993:261–267.

126. Kubota N, Suzuke M, Furusawa Y, et al. A comparison of biological effects of modulate carbon ions and fast neutrons in human osteosarcoma cells. *Int J Radiat Oncol Biol Phys* 1995;33:135–141.

127. Green EM, Adams WM, Forrest LJ. Four fraction palliation radiotherapy for osteosarcoma in 24 dogs. *J Am Anim Hosp Assoc* 2002;38:445–451.

128. Lombardi F, Gandola L, Fossati-Bellani F, et al. Hypofractionated accelerated radiotherapy in osteogenic sarcoma. *Int J Radiat Oncol Biol Phys* 1991;24: 761–765.

129. Suit HD. Role of therapeutic radiology in cancer of bone. *Cancer* 1975;35:930–935.

130. Urtasun RC, McConnachie PR. Disappearance of osteogenic sarcoma after irradiation: immunologic observations. *J Assoc Can Radiol* 1976;27:80–83.

131. van den Brenk HAS, Kerr RC, Madigan JP, et al. Results from tourniquet anoxia and hyperbaric oxygen techniques combined with megavoltage treatment of sarcomas of bone and soft tissues. *AJR* 1966;96: 760–776.

132. Chauvel P. Osteosarcomas and adult soft tissue sarcomas: is there a place for high LET radiation therapy? *Ann Oncol* 1992;3:S107–S110.

133. Laramore GE, Griffith JT, Boespflug M, et al. Fast neutron radiotherapy for sarcomas of soft tissue, bone, and cartilage. *Am J Clin Oncol* 1989;12: 320–326.

134. Wambersie A. Fast neutron therapy at the end of 1988: a survey of the clinical data. *Strahlenther Onkol* 1990;166:52–60.

135. Cohen L, Hendrickson F, Mansell J, et al. Response of sarcomas of bone and soft tissue to neutron beam therapy. *Int J Radiat Oncol Biol Phys* 1984;10: 821–824.

136. Duncan W, Arnott SJ, Jack WJL. The Edinburgh experience of treating sarcomas of soft tissues and bone with neutron irradiation. *Clin Radiol* 1986;37:317–320.

137. Hug EB, Fitzek MM, Liebsch NJ, et al. Locally challenging osteo- and chondrogenic tumors of the axial skeleton: results of combined proton and photon radiation therapy using three-dimensional treatment planning. *Int J Radiat Oncol Biol Phys* 1995;31: 467–476.

137a. Ornitz R, Herskovic A, Schell M, et al. Treatment experience: locally advanced sarcomas with 15 MeV fast neutrons. *Cancer* 1980;45:2712–2716.

138. Salinas R, Hussey DH, Fletcher GH, et al. Experience with fast neutron therapy for locally advanced sarcomas. *Int J Radiat Oncol Biol Phys* 1980;6: 267–272.

138a. Castro JR, Linstadt DE, Bahary JP, et al. Experience in charged particle irradiation of tumors of the skull base: 1977–1992. *Int J Radiat Oncol Biol Phys* 1994;29:647–655.

139. Yamamuro T, Kotoura Y. Intraoperative radiation therapy for osteosarcoma. In: Humphrey GB, Koops HS, Molenaar WM, et al., eds. *Osteosarcoma in adolescents and young adults: new developments and controversies.* Boston: Kluwer, 1993:177–183.

139a. Batterman JJ, Bruer K. Fast neutron therapy for locally advanced sarcomas. *Int J Radiat Oncol Biol Phys* 1981;7:1051–1053.

140. Tsunemoto H, Arai T, Morita S, et al. Japanese experience with clinical trials of fast neutrons. *Int J Radiat Oncol Biol Phys* 1982;8:2169–2172.

140a. Oya N, Kokubo M, Mizowaki T, et al. Definitive intraoperative very high-dose radiotherapy for localized osteosarcoma in the extremities. *Int J Radiat Oncol Biol Phys* 2001;51(1):87–93.

141. Tsuboyama T, Toguchida J, Kotoura Y, et al. Intraoperative radiation therapy for osteosarcoma in the extremities *Int Orthop* 2000;24:202–207.

141a. Carrie C, Bretau N, Negrier S, et al. The role of fast neutron therapy in unresectable pelvic osteosarcoma: preliminary report. *Med Pediatr Oncol* 1994;22: 355–357.

142. Anderson PM, Wiseman GA, Dispenzieri A, et al. High dose samarium-153 ethylene diamine tetramethylene phosphonate: low toxicity of skeletal irradiation in patients with osteosarcoma and bone metastases. *J Clin Oncol* 2002;20(1):189–196.

142a. Ozaki T, Flege S, Liljenqvist U, et al. Osteosarcoma of the spine: experience of the Cooperative Osteosarcoma Study Group. *Cancer* 2002;94(4):1069–1077.

143. Franziusc, Bielack S, Flee S, et al. High activity samarium-153–EDTMP therapy followed by autologous peripheral blood stem cell support in unresectable osteosarcoma. *Nuckleomedizin* 2001;40: 215–220.

144. Franzius C, Schuka A, Bielack SS. High dose samarium tetramethylene phosphonate: low toxicity of skeletal irradiation in patients with osteosarcoma and bone metastases. *Clin Oncol* 2002;20:1953–1954.

145. Bruland OS, Skretting A, Solhein OP, et al. Targeted radiotherapy of osteosarcoma using ^{153}Sm-EDTMP: a new promising approach. *Acta Oncol* 1996;35: 381–384.

146. Blake GM, Zivanovic MA, McEwan AJ, et al. Strontium-89 therapy: strontium kinetics and dosimetry in two patients treated for metastasizing osteosarcoma. *Br J Radiol* 1987;60:253–259.

147. Beck JC, Wara WM, Bovil EG Jr, et al. The role of radiation therapy in the treatment of osteosarcoma. *Radiology* 1976;120:163–165.

148. deMoor NG. Osteosarcoma: a review of 72 cases treated by megavoltage radiation therapy with or without surgery. *S Afr J Surg* 1975;13:137–146.

149. Taylor WF, Ivins JC, Unni KK, et al. Prognostic variables in osteosarcoma: a multi-institutional study. *J Natl Cancer Inst* 1989;81:21–30.

*150. Winkler K, Bielack SS, Belling G, et al. Treatment of osteosarcoma: experience of the cooperative osteosarcoma study group (COSS). In: Humphrey GB, Koops HS, Molenaar WM, et al., eds. *Osteosarcoma in adolescents and young adults: new developments and controversies.* Boston: Kluwer, 1993:269–277.

151. Li HG, Ma ZT, He Q. Fast neutron treatment osteosarcoma. *Zhanhua Zhong Liu Za Zhi* 1994;16: 199–202.

11

Rhabdomyosarcoma

Alison M. Friedmann, M.D., Nancy J. Tarbell, M.D.,
and Louis S. Constine, M.D.

Rhabdomyosarcoma (RMS) is a highly malignant neoplasm that arises from embryonic mesenchyme with the potential for differentiating into striated muscle (1). Although the cells show differentiation along rhabdomyoblastic lines, RMS is not limited to cells with recognizable muscle cross-striations (2,3). Although RMS was initially described in 1854 by Weber (4), progress in our understanding and treatment of this complex neoplasm accelerated with Stout's (5) landmark descriptive series in 1946 and the delineation by Horn and Enterline (6) in 1958 of the four classic forms of RMS. It can arise almost anywhere in the body, is locally invasive, and rapidly disseminates early in its course. Early in this century, the only cures were accomplished with radical surgery, and these cures were possible only in the few fortunate children without metastases. Significant disfigurement and loss of function were common sequelae. High-dose radiation therapy increased the potential for local control but caused a different set of morbidities (7–11). As chemotherapy has become increasingly effective in eliminating micrometastatic disease and assisting in local control, the need for aggressive surgery and large-volume irradiation has diminished, although surgery and radiation therapy still play pivotal roles in the curative treatment of RMS (12). Overall survival rates have concomitantly increased from 15–25% to more than 70% (1,12–22).

RMS is a rare tumor with clinical and biologic heterogeneity. Consequently, multi-institutional trials were necessary to develop and refine treatment approaches. A paramount role in this progress has been played by North American investigators of the Intergroup Rhabdomyosarcoma Study Group (IRSG), which is now in its fifth generation of protocols. The difficulty of this undertaking is clear in view of the myriad sites, stages, and histologies of RMS, which are associated with different natural histories and prognoses (23). Beyond this, advances in imaging, changes in end-points, and the need for mature data all increased the difficulty in conducting and comparing randomized, controlled clinical studies of patients with RMS. With this view, the IRSG was established through the collaboration of three multidisciplinary cancer treatment study groups (Cancer and Leukemia Group B, Children's Cancer Study Group, and the Pediatric Branch of the Southwest Oncology Group, which later became the Pediatric Oncology Group). Intergroup Rhabdomyosarcoma Study I (IRS-I) was open for patient entry from 1972 to 1978 (19). With an overall 5-year survival rate of 55% in IRS-I, IRS-II was designed to improve survival for the patient subgroups with poor outcomes and to refine treatment for the remaining patients (18). IRS-II ran from 1978 to 1984, IRS-III from 1984 to 1991, and IRS-IV from 1991 to 1997; IRS-V opened in 1997 and is still in progress. Although the previous generations of IRS studies were based on a surgically oriented clinical grouping system dependent on the tumor that remained after initial surgery, IRS-IV and IRS-V were based on a more biologically oriented staging system, discussed later in this chapter. These studies, each based on the results of its predecessor, have provided a database of approximately 4,000 patients. Other multi-institutional group studies have also provided important data (24). Of particular note are the European-based International Society of Pediatric Oncology (SIOP) and the United Kingdom–based Children's Solid Tumor Group (CSTG) (16,25). Finally, many single-institution studies have also been quite informative regarding RMS (7,12,26,27). The progress in

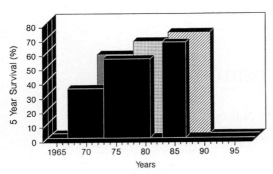

FIG. 11-1. Improvement in 5-year survival of children with RMS treated between 1967 and 1991 in IRS trials (*light dots,* IRS-I; *heavy dots,* IRS-II; *diagonal slashes,* IRS-III) and compared with data from the Epidemiology and End Results Section of the National Cancer Institute *(solid bars).* (From Wexler L, Helman LJ. Rhabdomyosarcoma and the undifferentiated sarcomas. In: Pizzo P, Poplack D, eds. *Principles and practice of pediatric oncology.* Philadelphia: Lippincott-Raven, 1997:799–829, with permission.)

treating RMS is exemplified by the improvement in overall 5-year survival in the IRS studies: 56% in IRS-I, 63% in IRS-II, and 71% in IRS-III (Fig. 11-1) (13,14,18,19). Early results from IRS-IV show an overall 3-year survival rate of 86% for patients with nonmetastatic disease and 39% for patients with metastatic disease (22,28).

EPIDEMIOLOGY

RMS accounts for about 3.5% of all malignant disease in children younger than 15 years of age and 2% of cancer cases among adolescents and young adults 15 to 19 years old (29,30). RMS is the most common soft tissue sarcoma of childhood, representing about half of this otherwise very heterogeneous group of tumors. The annual incidence of RMS is 4.4 per million in white children and 1.3 per million in black children. There is a slight male predominance (1.4:1). Seventy percent of cases occur before the age of 10 years, with a peak incidence at 2 to 5 years of age (Fig. 11-2). Congenital anomalies have been identified in as many as one-third of children with RMS, most commonly involving the gastrointestinal,

genitourinary, cardiovascular, and central nervous systems (31).

Environmental factors in the development of RMS are undefined, but some suggestive influences are under study. For example, a national case control report of 332 children with RMS enrolled in IRS-III demonstrated an association of RMS with maternal and paternal marijuana and cocaine use (32). Although the majority of cases of RMS occur sporadically, a small proportion are associated with genetic conditions, including the Li–Fraumeni syndrome (in which germ line mutations of p53 exist), neurofibromatosis type 1, and Beckwith–Wiedemann syndrome (33,34).

BIOLOGY

Although the origin and genetics of RMS remain unclear, clinical observations can provide direction for additional understanding of this tumor. If we can determine the tumor characteristics that predict radiochemotherapy responsiveness or, conversely, tumor resistance to therapy and a propensity to disseminate, then we can select the patients in whom more or less toxic therapy should be used. Moreover, we may devise novel biologic maneuvers to treat such tumors that minimize normal tissue damage. Reducing the toxicity of therapy becomes increasingly important as the cure rate continues to improve. Areas in which progress has been made include the genetic control of myogenesis, tumor suppressor genes, and molecular diagnostics (35,36).

Cytogenetics

Alveolar RMS usually is characterized by one of two translocations, both of which involve the FKHR gene on chromosome 13 (37–39). The most common translocation, t(2;13)(p35;q14), fuses the PAX3 gene, a transcription regulator, to the FKHR transcription factor. This translocation is present in about 70% of children with alveolar RMS. The less common translocation, t(1;13)(p36;q14), fuses the PAX7 transcription regulator to FKHR and is involved in about 20% of cases. This latter translocation seems to occur in younger patients and to be associated with a

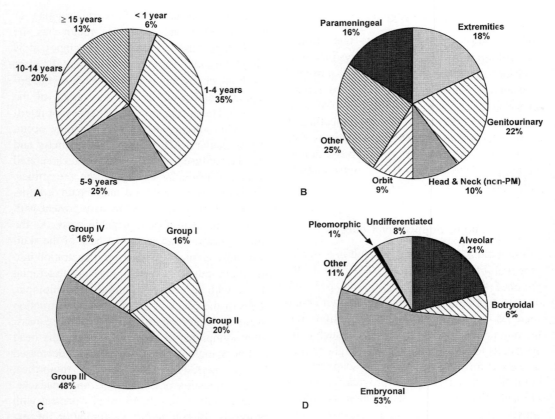

FIG. 11-2. Clinical features of RMS from IRS-I, IRS-II, and IRS-III pooled data. **(A)** Age at presentation. **(B)** Site of primary tumor. **(C)** Clinical group. **(D)** Histology. (Modified from Wexler L, Helman LJ. Rhabdomyosarcoma and the undifferentiated sarcomas. In: Pizzo P, Poplack D, eds. *Principles and practice of pediatric oncology.* Philadelphia: Lippincott-Raven, 1997:799–829, with permission.)

higher event-free survival rate than the PAX3 gene rearrangement. In the future, monitoring for these fusion products with sensitive techniques such as reverse transcriptase polymerase chain reaction may be useful for detecting minimal residual disease during or after treatment and for guiding therapy (37,40,41).

Embryonal RMS often is characterized by loss of heterozygosity at 11p15.5, suggesting the presence of a tumor suppressor gene (38).

Genomic amplification also differs in alveolar and embryonal RMS. It is rare in embryonal RMS, whereas gains of whole chromosomes (particularly of chromosomes 2, 8, 12, and 13) and hyperdiploidy are common (42–45). In alveolar RMS, gene amplification is common, as is near-tetraploidy.

Cell Cycle Control

Myogenesis involves differentiation of the mesenchymal fibroblast into skeletal muscle and is under the control of a series of gene products including the MyoD protein family (myogenin, MYF5, and MYF6). These gene products also halt cell cycling. Expression of the MyoD proteins, which can be determined by an anti-MyoD antibody, has demonstrated that malignant cells have characteristics of skeletal muscle differentiation and therefore represent RMS. It is possible that some tumor suppressor factor is present in the normal fibroblast that, when combined with the RMS cell and the MyoD gene product, can drive the cell toward differentiation and halt cell proliferation.

Proto-Oncogenes

The *myc* gene can contribute to uncontrolled cell proliferation via several pathways including insertion mutations, translocations, retroviral transductions, and amplification. Two reports involving 20 patients showed that 50% of those with alveolar RMS had n-*myc* amplification, in contrast to its uniform absence in patients with embryonal RMS (46,47). Impressively, among the patients with alveolar RMS, n-*myc* amplification predicted a fatal outcome.

Tumor Suppressor Genes

p53 mutations can be demonstrated in a significant proportion of childhood RMS (48). In the presence of damaged DNA, normal p53 produces G1 arrest and prevents the cell with damaged DNA from undergoing any proliferation. In conjunction with *myc,* p53 drives such damaged cells toward apoptosis. This might explain why some forms of RMS, which escape cure by radiochemotherapy, become progressively more virulent: they generate resistant clones of tumor cells.

CLINICAL PRESENTATION

RMS occurs in any anatomic location where there is skeletal muscle and in some locations where skeletal muscle is not normally found (Fig. 11-2) (18). The most common locations are the genitourinary sites and the head and neck. Genitourinary sites include the bladder, prostate, vagina, uterus, urethra, and paratesticular region. Head and neck lesions are divided into parameningeal sites (nasopharynx, nasal cavity, paranasal sinuses, middle ear and mastoid region, infratemporal fossa, and pterygopalatine and parapharyngeal areas) and other head and neck sites (parotid region, cheek, masseter muscle, oral cavity, oropharynx, larynx, hypopharynx, scalp, face, and pinna) (49).

RMS commonly presents as a mass with poorly defined margins, but specific presentations relate to the primary disease site. A mass in the genitourinary system may cause urinary tract or rectal obstruction. On occasion, the mass may protrude from the cervix, vagina, or urethra. When the protruding tumor has the gross appearance of a cluster of grapes, it is called botryoid (grapelike) sarcoma. Prostate and bladder RMS may also have a botryoid appearance and protrude into the lumen of the bladder. Hematuria, urinary frequency, or retention with subsequent renal failure may occur. Paratesticular RMS presents with a mass and may be confused with a hydrocele, incarcerated hernia, or testicular torsion. In the extremities, RMS often is palpable and causes pain or limits motion. Parameningeal RMS may present with airway obstruction or a palpable mass. As the tumor grows, it can erode the base of the skull and cause cranial nerve palsies. Penetration into the brain can occur and mimic an intracranial mass, with headache, vomiting, and diplopia. RMS of the cheek or larynx causes obstruction of the aerodigestive track or a discernible mass; other symptoms or signs referable to the head and neck include hoarseness, polyps, decreased hearing, persistent otitis, otorrhea, rhinorrhea, nasal congestion or obstruction, and headache. Patients with orbital RMS usually present with proptosis, discoloration, or limitation of extraocular motion. RMS of the trunk can present as a mass simulating a hernia or hematoma, or causing a classic superior vena cava syndrome. In the retroperitoneum, RMS can cause gastrointestinal discomfort or other mass-related symptoms.

Diagnostic Evaluation

The history and physical examination should focus on the extent of local disease and the possible presence of metastases. RMS may extend locally and infiltrate along fascial planes and into surrounding tissues. Tumor margins often are indistinct. Depending on the site, the local tumor generally is imaged by some combination of computed tomography (CT), magnetic resonance imaging (MRI), and plain radiography. Genitourinary RMS often is investigated initially by ultrasound and barium enema, and voiding cystourethrogram, cystoscopy, or pelvic examination under anesthesia occasionally is indicated. The draining lymphatics, in genitourinary primary sites, are evaluated with CT (50,51). The most common sites of metastases are lung, bone, bone marrow, and locoregional lymph nodes (51). Chest CT is the optimal imaging method for lung metastases. A nuclear medicine bone scan is performed to detect bony metastases but is not reliable to determine skull base involvement in parameningeal tumors, which is evaluated with CT or MRI. Bone marrow aspirate and biopsy are performed, and examination of cerebrospinal fluid (CSF) cytology is indicated if the tumor is in a parameningeal site (52). MRI or myelography is used to evaluate spinal cord–related symptoms.

Prognostic Features

Histology

Most RMSs are soft, fleshy tumors with variation in the extent of invasion and necrosis. Cross-striations and periodic acid–Schiff positivity (from cytoplasmic glycogen) may be seen on light microscopy, whereas intracytoplasmic filaments and Z band material may be seen on electron microscopy. Immunohistochemical stains, including antidesmin, antivimentin, and anti–muscle-specific actin, are used routinely to help ascertain the muscle origin of the tumor cells (3), and the detection of the muscle regulatory gene MyoD1 may be even more sensitive than desmin.

Four histologic subtypes of RMS are classically described: embryonal, alveolar, pleomorphic, and mixed (Fig. 11-2). However, the lack of agreement in classification among pathologists and the need to develop a single prognostically significant system prompted formation of an international panel to devise a new system, the International Classification of Rhabdomyosarcoma (Table 11-1) (53–55).

Favorable: Embryonal, Botryoid, and Spindle Cell Variants

Embryonal RMS is the most common histologic subtype. Embryonal RMS accounts for 60–70% of RMS in childhood and typically arises in the head and neck region and genitourinary tract

TABLE 11-1. *International Classification of Rhabdomyosarcoma*

	Frequency (%)	Actuarial 5-year survival (%)
I. Superior prognosis		
a. Botryoid rhabdomyosarcoma	6	95
b. Spindle cell rhabdomyosarcoma	3	88
II. Intermediate prognosis		
a. Embryonal rhabdomyosarcoma	79	66
III. Poor prognosis		
a. Alveolar rhabdomyosarcoma	32	54
b. Undifferentiated sarcoma	1	40
Other	9	

Data from Newton WA Jr, Gehan EA, Webber BL, et al. Classification of rhabdomyosarcomas and related sarcomas. Pathologic aspects and proposal for a new classification: an Intergroup Rhabdomyosarcoma Study. *Cancer* 1995;76:1073–1085.

(55). This form is composed of blastemal mesenchymal cells that tend to differentiate into cross-striated muscle cells. Although it resembles normally developing skeletal muscle in the 7- to 10-week fetus, great variation in the degree of differentiation can exist. Cellularity is moderate, and the stroma is loose and myxoid in most cases. The cells are generally fusiform or stellate, often admixed with primitive round cell forms. Cross-striations are present in about one-third of cases (2). Periodic acid–Schiff staining, actin/desmin positive reactivity, and Z band material usually are present. Loss of heterozygosity at 11p15.5 may be identifiable. The pathologic differential diagnosis often includes lymphoma, Ewing's sarcoma, and neuroblastoma (other small, round, blue cell tumors of childhood that have in common their light microscopic appearance and necessitate immunohistochemical evaluation for further characterization).

The botryoid polypoid variant of embryonal RMS represents about 10% of all RMS cases and occurs in mucosa-lined organs including the bladder, vagina, nasopharynx, nares, middle ear, and biliary tree. The stroma is loose with a myxoid character, and a condensed tumor cell or cambial layer must be identifiable. The tumor cells may be small or large, with varying degrees of myogenesis. These tumors are generally localized and noninvasive (2,53,54).

The spindle cell variant is composed exclusively of spindle-shaped cells and has a low cellularity. It can be collagen rich or poor, with the former having a storiform pattern. Its most common site is paratesticular.

Unfavorable: Alveolar and Undifferentiated

About 20% of children with RMS have the alveolar subtype, and it is increasingly common in adolescents and in tumors involving the extremities, trunk, and perianal and perineal region. The alveolar form resembles developing skeletal muscle in the 10- to 20-week-old fetus. The cells are round, with scanty eosinophilic cytoplasm that is occasionally vacuolated. Cross-striations are quite rare. The name *alveolar* is derived from the pattern produced by the tendency of cells to line connective tissue septa reminiscent of alveoli. Variable arrangement of trabeculae may cause the tumor cells to be arranged in strands, clefts, sheets, or clusters (2). The characteristic translocations are discussed in the "Biology" section earlier in this chapter. A "solid" variant has been identified, which grows as solid masses of closely aggregated cells with little or no discernible alveolar arrangement.

Undifferentiated sarcoma is generally diffuse, with no specific features other than primitive noncommitted mesenchymal cells. It is defined by its lack of the common antigenic markers and therefore is a diagnosis of exclusion. Patients with this variant are treated similarly to those with alveolar histology in current IRS protocols. The previously designated "pleomorphic" variant is rare in children and occurs primarily in adults aged 30 to 50 years. Many of these cases would currently be classified as malignant fibrous histiocytoma.

Stage

RMS has been staged according to multiple systems developed in different institutions or multi-institutional groups (16). With the advent of IRS-III, a pretreatment staging system was developed based on the tumor, node, metastasis (TNM) system used by SIOP, which reflected the disease characteristics at diagnosis (Table 11-2). IRS-IV and IRS-V have used this TNM staging system, which incorporates tumor size and invasiveness (a or b, T1 or T2, respectively), nodal status, presence of metastasis, and tumor site. Essentially, stage 1 tumors are in favorable sites. Stage 2 tumors are in unfavorable sites but are small (less than 5 cm) with negative lymph nodes. Stage 3 tumors are in unfavorable sites and are large or with positive lymph nodes.

TABLE 11-2. *Tumor, node, metastasis pretreatment staging classification for IRS-V*

Stage	Sites	Tumor invasiveness	Tumor size	Lymph node status	Metastasis
1	Orbit Head and neck (excluding parameningeal) Genitourinary (nonbladder, nonprostate) Biliary tract	T1 or T2	a or b	Any N	M0
2	Bladder or prostate Extremity Head and neck parameningeal Other (e.g., trunk, retroperitoneum)	T1 or T2	a	N0 or NX	M0
3	Same as stage 2	T1 or T2	a b	N1 Any N	M0
4	All	T1 or T2	a or b	Any N	M1

T1, confined to anatomic site of origin; T2, extension; a, less than 5 cm in diameter; b, more than 5 cm in diameter; NX, clinical status unknown; N0, not clinically involved; N1, clinically involved; M0, no metastasis; M1, metastasis present.

Stage 4 tumors are at any site, with hematogenous metastasis. This staging system has been validated with respect to its relationship to patient outcome (20).

Group

Implicit in the discussion of the grouping and staging systems is the importance of accurately identifying prognostic variables. Most of these variables are interrelated. A wealth of data support the relevance of the clinical group of the patient, which in essence is the postsurgical disease extent at the time chemotherapy is initiated. The clinicopathologic grouping system has been used since the first IRS studies (Table 11-3, Fig. 11-2). The clinical group reflects either the absence (group I, 13% of patients) or presence of microscopic disease (group II, 20% of patients), gross disease (group III, 48% of patients), or metastatic disease (group IV, 18% of patients) (13,14). Clearly, the clinical group also reflects the disease site (in terms of resectability) and the biologic invasiveness of the tumor. Because therapeutic decisions made before study entry affected the assigned group, this system did not accurately reflect the biology of RMS (20,56,57). Moreover, the emphasis on surgical reduction of tumor bulk implicit in this system led surgeons to perform unnecessarily morbid surgeries at inappropriate times. In addition, the surgical approach was not uniformly applied, which obfuscated interpretation of results (56). Data from the three fully an-

alyzed IRS studies support the utility of the grouping system, and it continues to be used in conjunction with stage (Fig. 11-3) (13,14, 18,19).

Primary Site

The primary site is a strong determinant of outcome, as verified by data from IRS-II and IRS-III (Fig. 11-4) (13,14,18,19). This relates, at least in part, to the association of site with other tumor and treatment variables. The primary site generally dictates resectability, which in turn determines the IRS grouping (18). Resectability relates to tumor invasiveness and the morbidity that would attend resection. Most orbital lesions are in group III (73.5% in IRS-I, IRS-II, and

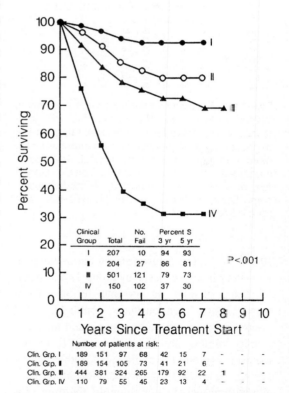

FIG. 11-3. Survival by clinical group for all patients treated in IRS-III. (From Crist W, Gehan EA, Ragab AH, et al. The Third Intergroup Rhabdomyosarcoma Study. *J Clin Oncol* 1995;13: 610–630, with permission.)

TABLE 11-3. *The IRS grouping system*

Group I: Localized disease, completely resected
    a. Confined to muscle or organ of origin
    b. Infiltration outside the muscle or organ
       of origin
Group II: Total gross resection with
    a. Microscopic residual disease
    b. Regional lymphatic spread, resected
    c. Both
Group III: Incomplete resection with gross residual
    disease
    a. After biopsy only
    b. After major resection (more than 50%)
Group IV: Distant metastatic disease present at onset

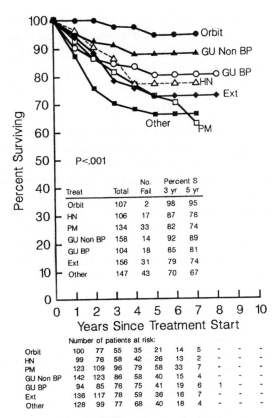

FIG. 11-4. Survival by primary site for all patients treated in IRS-III. Ext, extremities; GU BP, genitourinary tract (bladder or prostate); GU Non BP, genitourinary tract (nonbladder, nonprostate); HN, head and neck, nonparameningeal; PM, parameningeal sites. (From Crist W, Gehan EA, Ragab AH, et al. The Third Intergroup Rhabdomyosarcoma Study. *J Clin Oncol* 1995;13:610–630, with permission.)

is also related to tumor site through presenting symptoms and signs. Primary site influences the propensity for lymphatic spread (Table 11-4) (51). Whereas genitourinary, abdominal or pelvic, and extremity tumors commonly involve regional lymph nodes, tumors in the head and neck, trunk, and female genital organs rarely do so. However, the frequency of lymph node involvement is almost certainly underestimated by IRS data because the assessment of nodal status has not been systematic. Data from Stanford and Memorial Sloan–Kettering support the prognostic significance of lymph node involvement (27,59). Pedrick et al. (27) showed that 88% of patients presenting with involved nodes had pri-

TABLE 11-4. *Lymph node metastasis by primary site for 592 patients with visibly resected disease[a] from IRS-I and IRS-II*

Site	Number of patients	Number and percentage with nodal metastases
Extremity		
Upper	74	12 (16%)
Lower	107	10 (9%)
Total	181	22 (12%)
Genitourinary organs		
Paratesticular	107	28 (26%)
		$p = 0.001$[b]
Bladder	29	6 (21%)
Prostate	12	5 (42%)
		$p = 0.03$
Female genital organs	17	1 (6%)
Other	1	—
Total	166	40 (24%)
Head and neck		
Orbit	39	0 (0%)
Other	96	8 (8%)
		$p = 0.06$
Total	135	8 (6%)
Other		
Anus and perineum	15	2 (13%)
Pelvis and retroperitoneum	22	5 (23%)
Trunk	65	2 (3%)
		$p = 0.01$
Abdomen and thorax	8	2 (25%)
Total	110	11 (10%)
Totals	592	81 (14%)

[a]Microscopic or no residual disease.
[b]p values relate to comparison of frequency of nodal metastases for this site compared with the 14% for all 592 patients.
From Lawrence W Jr, Hays DM, Heyn R, et al. Lymphatic metastases with childhood rhabdomyosarcoma. *Cancer* 1987;60:910–915, with permission.

IRS-III) (58); this is also true for parameningeal lesions (which are never in group I) and genitourinary bladder or prostate lesions. Conversely, most genitourinary nonbladder and nonprostate tumors are in group I, and most extremity tumors are in group I or II or are metastatic (group IV) at diagnosis. Other factors are also relevant to the association of primary site with prognosis. For example, the tumor location determines the presenting signs and symptoms, which are often related to the rapidity of diagnosis. Tumor size (up to 5 cm vs. more than 5 cm) is associated with survival time ($p < 0.001$) by multivariate analysis (54). Size

mary tumors that were invasive and extended beyond the site or organ of origin. The more current IRS studies should provide more consistent documentation of lymph node status with improvements in imaging techniques and careful surgical guidelines.

Other Factors

A variety of other factors have prognostic significance, some of which are general and others specific to certain tumor subgroups. IRS data show that lymphocyte count, patient sex, and age are prognostically relevant (13). Although younger age is associated with a better outcome (59), the specific subgroup of children younger than 1 year old with alveolar histology have a significantly poorer survival than do older children, a finding not seen for infants with the embryonal subtype (60,61). Some site-specific variables influence outcome. In the head and neck, risk factors that predict tumor access to the cranial subarachnoid space (skull base erosion, cranial nerve palsy, intracranial extension) decrease the likelihood of disease-free survival (51% vs. 81% if no risk factors) (52,62,63). In extremity sites, the presence of lymph node involvement is strongly associated with a high incidence of relapse in metastatic sites and inferior survival (58).

GENERAL PRINCIPLES OF THERAPY

Currently, the IRS studies (IRS-V) stratify patients into three risk groups (low, intermediate, and high) on the basis of known prognostic factors and historical outcome (23). The prognostic features incorporated into the risk classification scheme include histology, stage (which in turn incorporates site, tumor size, invasiveness, node status, and metastases), clinical group, and patient age. General definitions of the risk groups are as follows:

- *Low risk:* Patients with localized embryonal RMS occurring at favorable sites (stage 1) and patients with embryonal RMS occurring at unfavorable sites with either completely re-

sected disease (group I) or microscopic residual disease (group II)
- *Intermediate risk:* Patients with embryonal RMS occurring at unfavorable sites with gross residual disease (group III), patients with metastatic embryonal RMS who are younger than 10 years old, and patients with nonmetastatic alveolar RMS or undifferentiated sarcoma at any site
- *High risk:* Patients with metastatic RMS or undifferentiated sarcoma at presentation excepting embryonal cases in children younger than 10 years

Clearly, this scheme will continue to evolve as treatments improve and new data emerge regarding particular subsets of patients and biologically based prognostic features. The overall goals are to reduce long-term toxicities in patients with a high likelihood of cure and to develop superior, innovative therapies for patients who continue to fare poorly with modern treatment regimens.

The therapeutic struggle for clinicians managing children with RMS, to cure while minimizing functional and cosmetic deficits, is heightened by the difficulty in eradicating both local and systemic disease. The spectrum of sites and histologies complicates determination of treatment strategies through differences in the propensity for local and systemic control and treatment sequelae. It is clear that multidisciplinary therapy is necessary. Aggressive surgery and radiation therapy alone have been curative in fewer than 25% of children, with the exception of patients with orbital or genitourinary primary sites (64). Conversely, chemotherapy alone is associated with high local failure rates, a lesson learned by attempts to manage orbital or genitourinary tumors without radiation (65,66). The judicious use of chemotherapy to eradicate micrometastatic disease and reduce the extent of local disease and radiation therapy to increase the potential for local control has led to a decrease in aggressive surgery except in selected situations (12). The current challenge is to develop approaches to additionally enhance the complementary actions of all three treatment modalities in terms of intensity and sequence.

Surgery

Before the advent of radiation and chemotherapy, complete resection of RMS was the clear goal of surgical treatment. This may have involved pelvic exenteration, radical prostatectomy, cystectomy, amputations, and orbital exenterations. Even so, fewer than 10% of children were amenable to complete resection and curable because of the absence of metastatic disease. Beyond this, most of these children had severely compromised quality of life functionally, cosmetically, and psychologically. Select sites that were more often curable by aggressive surgery included the orbit and bladder. Using pooled data from IRS-I, IRS-II, and IRS-III, if patients with overt metastatic disease (group IV) are excluded, then 16% of children have RMS that is minimally invasive and in an accessible site such that complete resection is possible (group I); 20% can undergo a subtotal resection leaving microscopic disease (Fig. 11-5). In general, achievement of local control and organ preservation with nonradical surgery, radiotherapy, and chemotherapy is the appropriate goal. Although this is often compatible with a complete surgical resection, qualifications and frank

exceptions now exist. Exenterative surgery remains appropriate in certain situations, particularly for salvage therapy.

Reoperation for microscopic residual disease after an initial excision, or when the first operation was performed without knowledge of the type of neoplasm involved, may be indicated before additional management. This is called pretreatment reexcision in the IRS guidelines and is site dependent. Reoperation after chemotherapy as a second-look procedure has proven to be an attractive option (67). Many of these patients have had a "pathologic" complete response and have a survival similar to that of patients who had an initial complete resection.

The role of lymph node dissection as a component of surgical therapy continues to evolve. Should clinically involved lymph nodes be resected? Should elective dissections of clinically uninvolved regions be performed? Current guidelines are site specific because of the variability in the frequency of lymph node involvement and outcome data relating to its significance. Genitourinary and extremity RMS have a 10–40% incidence of lymph node metastases (Table 11-4) (51). The high frequency of nodal spread for extremity tumors, often without clinical or radiographic evidence of involvement, has both prognostic and therapeutic implications (68,69). Currently, the surgical guidelines of IRS-V include systematic axillary node sampling for upper extremity tumors and inguinal and femoral triangle node sampling for lower extremity tumors. In select patients with paratesticular tumors, routine lymph node sampling and sometimes dissection are advised (70). This topic is considered further in later sections because considerations are site specific.

Overall, the extent and timing of surgical excision depend on the site of tumor and overall treatment strategy, balancing cure with functional outcome.

Chemotherapy

Before the 1960s, chemotherapy in RMS was largely reserved for the treatment of metastatic disease. Several investigators reported responses to vincristine and actinomycin used alone (VA) or in combination with cyclophos-

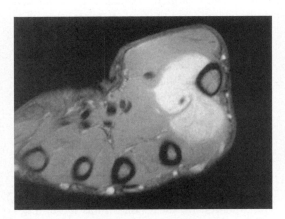

FIG. 11-5. Alveolar rhabdomyosarcoma of the hand, involving the periosteum of the first metacarpal, imaged by magnetic resonance imaging. Sentinel node biopsy was performed after gross excision of the primary tumor with microscopic positive margins.

TABLE 11-5. *Design and results of IRS-I, 1972–1978 (686 patients)*

Clinical group	Chemotherapy regimen	Conventional radiation therapy	5-Year survival	Entire group survival
I	VAC × 2 yr	No	93%	83%
	VAC × 2 yr	Yes	81%	
II	Cyclic sequential VA × 1 yr	Yes	73%	71%
	VAC × 2 yr	Yes	70%	
III	Pulse VAC × 2 yr	Yes	53%	52%
	Pulse VAC + Adr × 2 yr	Yes	51%	
IV	Pulse VAC × 2 yr	Yes	14%	21%
	Pulse VAC + Adr × 2 yr	Yes	26%	
Overall			55%	

A, actinomycin D; Adr, doxorubicin; C, cyclophosphamide; V, vincristine.
Modified from Mandell LR. Ongoing progress in the treatment of childhood rhabdomyosarcoma. *Oncology (Huntingt)* 1993;7:71–83, with permission.

phamide (VAC) (1). Various groups then began to report that the adjuvant administration of chemotherapy for totally or subtotally resected localized disease contributed to an increase in survival probability from 10–40% to 60–80% (71). In 1974, Heyn et al. (12) randomized 32 children with completely resected RMS to adjuvant therapy with VA or no adjuvant therapy. There were eight deaths among the 15 children in the control group and two deaths in the 17 treated children. All children with microscopic residual disease received chemotherapy, and survival rates were excellent.

With the widespread adoption of chemotherapy as part of the therapy of RMS, several trials were undertaken to establish the optimum drug combinations. IRS-I tested whether VAC was superior to VA in group II disease and whether pulse VAC plus adriamycin was superior to pulse VAC alone in groups II and III (Table 11-5). The study found no benefit to cyclophosphamide in group II diseases, nor did it find a benefit to the addition of adriamycin in groups III and IV (19).

IRS-II built on the results of IRS-I (Table 11-6) (18). Patients in group I received VAC or VA. Disease-free survival was similar. IRS-II showed no benefit to pulse VAC compared with cyclic sequential VA for group II. In groups III and IV, pulse VAC was better than a VAC and

TABLE 11-6. *Design and results of IRS-II, 1978–1984 (1,003 patients)*

Clinical group	Chemotherapy	Conventional radiation therapy	5-Year survival	Entire group survival
I[a]	VA × 1 yr	No	85%	81%[b]
	VAC × 2 yr	No	84%	
II[a]	Cyclic sequential VA × 1 yr	Yes	88%	80%[b]
	Repetitive pulse VAC × 1 yr	Yes	79%	
III	Repetitive pulse VAC × 2 yr	Yes	66%	65%
	Repetitive pulse VAdrC-VAC × 2 yr	Yes	65%	
IV	Repetitive pulse VAC × 2 yr	Yes	26%	27%
	Repetitive pulse VAdrC-VAC × 2 yr	Yes	27%	
Overall			62%	63%

A, actinomycin D; Adr, doxorubicin; C, cyclophosphamide; V, vincristine.
[a]Patients with alveolar and extremity tumors excluded in groups I and II; treated with repetitive pulse vincristine, actinomycin D, and cyclophosphamide × 1 to 2 years with or without conventional radiotherapy.
[b]Includes extremity and alveolar tumors treated differently.
Modified from Mandell LR. Ongoing progress in the treatment of childhood rhabdomyosarcoma. *Oncology (Huntingt)* 1993;7:71–83; and Maurer HM, Gehan EA, Beltangady M, et al. The Intergroup Rhabdomyosarcoma Study II. *Cancer* 1993;71:1904–1922, with permission.

adriamycin combination but not statistically significantly better.

IRS-III began in 1984 and ended in 1991; it separated patients by histology into either a favorable (embryonal) or unfavorable (alveolar, anaplastic, and monomorphous cell types) category. The assignment of therapy according to specific subgroups, results, and lessons learned is outlined in Table 11-7 (14). Several drug pairs (adriamycin with imidazole carboxamide [DTIC], actinomycin D with VP-16, and actinomycin D with DTIC) appear to have been associated with gain in survival (14).

IRS-IV began in August 1991 and ended in 1997 and used the new staging system to assign drug therapy. Patients with group I paratesticular tumors and group I or II orbital tumors were treated with VA, and all other nonmetastatic patients except those with preexisting renal abnormalities were randomized to receive one of three chemotherapy regimens: VAC; vincristine, actinomycin D, and ifosfamide (VAI); or vincristine, ifosfamide, and etoposide (VIE) (22). Patients with group III tumors were also randomized to receive conventional radiation therapy (RT) or hyperfractionated RT. VAC, VAI, and VIE were equally effective, and overall, the patients with embryonal tumors who received three-drug therapy benefited in comparison to those in IRS-III, where just VA was given. For patients with metastatic tumors, a pilot IRS study looked at the activity of ifosfamide and doxorubicin in an up-front window and found a response rate of 63% (complete and partial responses) (72). Subsequently, a full randomized IRS trial in 128 patients compared two up-front treatment windows, vincristine and melphalan (VM) and ifosfamide and etoposide (IE), and later therapy consisted of VAC or VAC with the window therapy included if the patient had an initial response (73). Initial response rates were comparable (VM 74% vs. IE 79%, $p = 0.428$), but 3-year failure-free survival (FFS) and overall survival (OS) rates were higher in the patients who received the IE-containing regimen (FFS 33% vs. 19%, OS 55% versus 27%).

IRS-V is under way and uses the risk stratification schema outlined previously to assign pa-

tients to three risk groups (23). VA or VAC is used in a nonrandomized fashion in the low-risk patients. VA is given to patients with tumors in favorable sites with group I or group II disease, to patients with small, group I tumors in unfavorable sites, and to all patients with orbital tumors (including group III). All other patients meeting the low-risk criteria receive VAC. All of the low-risk patients have embryonal histology or one of its variants. For intermediate-risk patients, the gold standard VAC therapy is being compared in a randomized trial to VAC alternating with vincristine, topotecan, and cyclophosphamide (VTC). Previous studies in both untreated and relapsed patients have shown topotecan to be a very active agent, particularly for patients with alveolar histology (74,75). For high-risk patients with metastatic disease who have a poor outcome with current therapy, the combination of irinotecan and vincristine is being tested in an up-front window and is then incorporated into subsequent therapy with VAC for patients who respond. Irinotecan has demonstrated antitumor activity for patients with relapsed RMS in a single institution study (76).

The challenge remains to identify the drug combinations with the most favorable therapeutic ratio when used in combination with the other modalities and to develop innovative therapies for the subset of patients who continue to fare poorly despite the advances in therapy that have been made over the past few decades.

Radiation Therapy

The goal of RT is to provide local and regional control, with or without surgery but, currently, always in conjunction with chemotherapy. The optimal multimodal strategy would coordinate RT with these other therapies so as not to impair surgical healing or drug administration. Therefore, major considerations would include the primary site of the tumor, the extent of surgery, the interaction of RT with chemotherapeutic agents, and any emergent contingencies. An analysis of IRS-II data for group III patients underscores the difficulty that still exists in obtaining local and regional control (21).

TABLE 11-7. *Therapy and outcomes according to specific patient subgroups in IRS-III, 1984–1991 (1,032 patients)*

Risk subgroup	Treatment	5-year progression-free survival	5-year survival	Progress (IRS-II vs. IRS-II)
Group I (favorable histology)	VA × 1 yr	83%	93%	C not necessary.
Group II (favorable histology)	VA × 1 yr + RT	56%	54%	Need for Adr not proven because of small patient numbers and different histologies compared with IRS-I.
Group I and II (unfavorable histology)	VAdrA × 1 yr + RT	77%	89%	Better than IRS-II because of intense chemotherapy.
	VAdrC-VAC + CDDP × 1 yr + RT	71%	80%	
Group II (paratesticular)	VA × 1 yr + RT	81%	81%	C not necessary.
Group II and III (orbit and head)	VA × 1 yr + RT	78%	91%	C not necessary.
Group III (except special pelvic, orbit, and head sites)	VAC × 2 yr + RT	70%	70%	Differences not statistically significant but better than IRS-II because of intense induction chemotherapy, second-look surgery.
	VAdrC-VAC + CDDP × 2 yr[a] + RT	62%	63%	
	VAdrC-VAC + CDDP + VP-16 × 2 yr[a] + RT	56%	64%	
Group III (special pelvic sites)	VAdrAC-VAC + CDDP + VP-16 × 2 yr ± RT ± surgery	74%	83%	Better than IRS-II because of intense chemotherapy, early RT, second-look surgery. The bladder salvage rate more than doubled (60% vs. 25%).
Group IV	VAC × 2 yr + RT	27%	27%	No significant differences and no better than IRS-II.
	VAdrAC-VAC + CDDP × 2 yr + RT	27%	31%	
	VAdrAC-VAC + CDDP + VP-16 × 2 yr + RT	30%	29%	

A, actinomycin D; Adr, doxorubicin; C, cyclophosphamide; CDDP, cisplatin; DTIC, imidazole carboxamide; RT, radiation therapy; V, vincristine; VP-16, etoposide.
[a]Second-look surgery recommended at week 20; if partial response, patients received Adr + DTIC, A + VP-16, or A + DTIC.
Modified from Pappo AS. Rhabdomyosarcoma and other soft tissue sarcomas of childhood. *Curr Opin Oncol* 1995;7:361–366, with permission.

The responsiveness of RMS to radiotherapy was established in the 1940s and 1950s (8). Fifty to 65 Gy was thought to be necessary to achieve local control of the primary tumor regardless of the nature of the surgical procedure. In the setting of postoperative microscopic residual disease, these dosages were demonstrated to achieve local control in 90% of cases (9,64,71,77–79). Because RMS was known to extensively infiltrate tissues, large radiation volumes initially were used, as was appropriate for other soft tissue sarcomas. As the efficacy of chemotherapy for micrometastatic disease became established and the risk of normal tissue damage caused by combined-modality therapy was recognized, investigators considered whether equivalent local control rates could be obtained with lower radiation dosages and volumes (9). Beyond this, the need for any RT after wide local tumor resection with negative margins was questioned. The IRS studies attempted to systematically examine the issues of RT dosage and volume within the limits imposed by the many chemotherapy questions that were also asked.

IRS-I patients in group I were randomized to receive postoperative RT or no RT, whereas all other patients were irradiated (Table 11-5). The dosage was adjusted to the patient's age and ranged from 40 to 60 Gy. Daily fractions were 1.5 to 2 Gy, and RT was administered immediately after surgery and protocol randomization for group I patients and after 6 weeks of chemotherapy for groups III and IV. At 5 years, approximately 80% of the patients in both group I study arms were continuously disease free. Overall survival was 93% (control) versus 81% (irradiated group, $p = 0.67$) (9,19), which prompted the deletion of RT in group I favorable histology cases for IRS-II. Overall, in IRS-I (9), the dosage given for local control was related to patient age and tumor size. A 32% local recurrence rate was seen after dosages less than 40 Gy and a 12% rate was seen after dosages greater than 40 Gy ($p = 0.41$) in the subgroup of children older than 6 years. A dose–response relationship for local control also existed in children who had tumors with a diameter greater than 6 cm (9). These data were corroborated by the Children's Solid Tumor Group (CSTG) (25). IRS-I found no dose–response relationship when patients were stratified solely by clinical group (9). The treatment volume was also analyzed for its impact on local failure. Patients who received RT to less than the entire muscle bundle were compared with those whose RT encompassed the entire bundle. In patients younger than 6 years, local control rates were 84% vs. 92%, respectively, and in older children rates were 91% vs. 85%; these differences were nonsignificant. RT to clinically uninvolved lymph nodes was not encouraged, whereas it was recommended for involved nodal regions. Local control was better in genitourinary sites than in the extremity.

In IRS-II the RT guidelines were modified based on IRS-I results (Table 11-6). The minimum tumor dosages were 40 and 45 Gy for younger (less than 6 years of age) and older children, respectively, but tumors larger than 5 cm received 50 to 55 Gy. The treatment volume was reduced to 5 cm beyond evident tumor. Analyses of local and regional failure have been performed for IRS-II, with local failure defined as initial failure to achieve complete response or local relapse after an initial response (18,21). Regional failure is defined as tumor recurrence in lymph nodes adjacent to the primary site or in the same anatomic compartment. For group I patients, those with an unfavorable alveolar histology had a significantly higher frequency of locoregional recurrence than those with favorable histology (78). Although the frequency of local failure was only 10% in group II, it was at 20% for group III (excluding "special pelvic" sites) and 41% for group IV. When local relapse was analyzed as a percentage of all relapses, it accounted for 46% of relapses in group I (despite "complete" surgical removal of tumor) and 36%, 53%, and 20% of relapses in groups II, III, and IV, respectively (18,21). Moreover, the local relapse rate was greater (and survival rates inferior) for patients with unfavorable versus favorable histologic features (41% vs. 13%) and for lesions larger than 5 cm versus smaller than 5 cm (34% vs. 23%) (77). Locoregional relapse rates were also higher in all groups and greater than distant relapse rates in all but group IV patients (18). In an analysis by Wharam et al. (21), for group III patients, prognostic factors for local failure were identified. Patients with primary tumors in the chest, pelvis, extremity, or trunk, or with tumors larger than 10 cm in diameter had a local failure rate of 35%, compared with 15% for all other patients. Patients at high risk, 23%, for regional (nodal) failure had node involvement at diagnosis and a primary site other than orbit, parameningeal, or trunk; other patients had a 9% rate. The relevance of radiation dosage to local control was suggested by an analysis by Wharam et al. (49) for patients with nonparameningeal head and neck tumors. An increased relapse rate occurred at dosages less than 40 Gy, although these data must be interpreted with caution because this was not a randomized dosage study. Local control for all patients receiving more than 40 Gy was 93%.

In IRS-III, which accrued 1,062 patients between 1984 and 1991, therapy was assigned or randomized not only by clinical group but also by histology (with unfavorable types comprising those with alveolar, anaplastic, and monomorphous cells or patterns) and primary site (Table 11-7). Postoperative RT was administered to all patients except those in group I with favorable histology tumors and those in group III with special pelvic sites in complete pathologic remission after primary chemotherapy.

The RT dosage for group I and II patients was 41.4 Gy. For patients with gross residual disease, the dosage depended on patient age and tumor size: 41.4 Gy was given for children younger than 6 years old with tumors smaller than 5 cm, 50.4 Gy was given for children older than 6 years old with tumors greater than or equal to 5 cm, and an intermediate dosage of 45 Gy was given for children who were either older or had larger tumors, but not both. The overall survival at 5 years was 71%, superior to that in IRS-II (63%) and IRS-I (55%) (14). An update of patients in group I with alveolar or undifferentiated histology confirmed a benefit to the addition of RT for this cohort (80). For group III patients, the rates were 73%, 65%, and 52%, respectively. Although local control rates of 90% were achieved for patients in groups I and II, local recurrence in patients with group III disease remained unacceptably high, as in IRS-II

IRS-IV accrued 1,011 patients between 1991 and 1997 and used the pretreatment TNM staging system to assign chemotherapy and the clinical grouping system to assign radiotherapy. Group II patients did especially well (Table 11-8) (81). Because of the unsatisfactory local control rates for patients with gross residual dis-

TABLE 11-8. *Outcome for patient with group II tumors according to histology, primary site, and IRS study*

	N	5-year failure-free survival %	p	5-year overall survival %	p
Patients with embryonal histology tumors			<.001		0018
IRS-I	105	75		78	
IRS-II	74	73		75	
IRS-III	129	79		86	
IRS-IV	90	93		97	
Patients with alveolar histology or UDS tumors			.11		.24
IRS-I	60	53		58	
IRS-II	85	58		70	
IRS-III	68	65		70	
IRS-IV	44	73		64	
Favorable primary site			.95		
IRS-I and IRS-II	36	75			
IRS-III and IRS-IV	27	71			
Unfavorable primary site			.01		
IRS-I and IRS-II	109	50			
IRS-III and IRS-IV	85	66			

UDS, undifferentiated sarcoma.
From Smith LM, Anderson JR, Qualman SJ, et al. Which patients with microscopic disease and rhabdomyosarcoma experience relapse after therapy? A report from the soft tissue sarcoma committee of the Children's Oncology Group. *J Clin Oncol* 2001;19:4058–4064, with permission.

ease (group III) in IRS-II and IRS-III and because of the normal tissue toxicities associated with radiation dosages higher than those used in the previous studies, hyperfractionated RT was tested in 490 patients in a randomized trial (1.1 Gy twice daily to 59.4 Gy vs. 1.8 Gy daily to 50.4 Gy) (15). Although feasible, no advantage to hyperfractionation was demonstrated in terms of local control, and conventional RT remains the standard of care for treating patients with gross residual disease. The 5-year local recurrence rate for these patients was 13%.

IRS-V is currently open and looks prospectively at using smaller dosages of RT for patients with favorable histology: 36 Gy for patients with microscopic residual disease and no regional node involvement, 45 Gy for patients with orbital tumors and gross residual disease, and 36 to 41.4 Gy for patients with superficial head and neck tumors, biliary tumors, and vulva or uterus tumors who undergo second-look surgery and have either negative margins or microscopic residual tumor. For intermediate-risk patients, IRS-V will determine the rate of local failure in patients with gross residual tumor at diagnosis who, after second-look surgery, have response-adjusted radiation dosage reduction (to 36 Gy for complete response and to 41.4 Gy for microscopic residual). It also aims to determine whether preoperative radiation therapy followed by second-look surgery for patients with group III disease and poor response to induction chemotherapy is feasible. All patients with alveolar group I tumors will receive 36 Gy to the primary site.

Although patients will optimally be treated in appropriate institutional or multi-institutional studies, occasional patients will not be entered into such trials. Until such studies are complete, most cases of bulky local RMS should be treated to at least 50 Gy, and postoperative microscopic disease should be treated to at least 40 Gy (26). A report from St. Jude Children's Research Hospital found that local control was maintained in ten of ten evaluable patients who received a mean and median dosage of 40 Gy for microscopic residual (IRS group II) disease, which had been cytoreduced from gross disease (group III) using chemotherapy with or without delayed surgery (82). The local control rate for orbital

RMS is 93%, and 45 to 50 Gy seems satisfactory (79). In cervical, vaginal, and head and neck sites, brachytherapy will allow the administration of a high local dosage of irradiation, often with an acceptable risk of morbidity (25,83). It is imperative that when radiotherapy is used in this infiltrative tumor, the prechemotherapy tumor volume is covered with an adequate margin to avoid marginal misses. Margins are based on the confidence with which this volume can be identified and on the location of critical normal tissues that should be excluded. In the setting of surgical reduction of gross disease and multiagent chemotherapy, a 1.5- to 2-cm margin as determined by the prechemotherapy CT or MRI scan is generally recommended. However, a recent report suggests that a shrinking field technique can be used, with the boost of radiation given to the postchemotherapy volume. This remains an open area for study because the setup error and improvements in radiation planning may allow smaller fields to be used (84). Every effort is made to shield epiphyses as long as this is consistent with adequate tumor coverage. Brachytherapy may be appropriate in selected situations (85). Other conformal techniques such as proton therapy may also be used to spare normal tissue, especially in young children or when critical areas are adjacent to the tumor (86–88).

SPECIFIC SITES

Bladder

Bladder RMS usually arises as a pedunculated mass in the submucosa. Although the tumor may remain intravesical for some period of time, it ultimately develops a broad base and invades the bladder wall. In most boys, the tumor arises in the bladder neck and then invades the prostate, making it difficult to distinguish between primary bladder and prostate RMS on clinical findings alone. RMS in these two sites accounts for about one-half of pelvic RMS and usually occurs in younger children. Urinary abnormalities, including dysuria, polyuria, and, in particular, retention, are early signs. Ultrasound can greatly assist in defining the tumor, and cystoscopy often allows histologic diagnosis (1).

More than 90% of tumors are embryonal, including the botryoid subtype, which accounts for one-third. Regional lymph node involvement is documented in about 20% (18). The hypogastric or external iliac nodes are most commonly involved, although spread to lumboaortic nodes may occur, even in isolation. Only 15% have demonstrable metastases at diagnosis. It was clearly demonstrated in the prechemotherapy era that 10–40% of patients could be cured by exenteration alone (89). Treatment programs were subsequently designed to improve the cure rate and to increase bladder preservation (50).

The SIOP attempted to achieve local control of bladder (and prostate) RMS with a program emphasizing chemotherapy alone; however, complete responses were not achieved. Small single-institution studies have generally used surgery, chemotherapy, and RT.

IRS-I provided data that suggested that limited surgery (partial cystectomy or "tumorectomy") followed by RT and chemotherapy might allow preservation of the bladder with excellent cure rates (90). Although one-third of patients underwent pelvic exenteration, most patients who underwent bladder-preserving surgery ultimately retained their bladders. IRS-II adopted a strategy using more vigorous primary chemotherapy with the intention of using minimal surgery to remove residual tumor (followed by additional chemotherapy) and avoiding the morbidity of pelvic irradiation. RT was added in the setting of residual (postsurgical) disease or if an exenterative procedure would be needed. Almost all patients eventually needed RT, surgery, or both to achieve a complete remission. Although the 3-year survival for these patients (70%) was similar to that in IRS-I (78%), the 3-year disease-free survival rate was significantly lower (52% vs. 70%). Although the bladder preservation rate was initially higher in IRS-II (97%) than in IRS-I (58%), the percentage of patients who retained their bladders and were alive at 3 years was only 22%, compared with 23% in IRS-I (90,91). The delay of irradiation to week 16 was a negative prognostic factor, reducing the likelihood of local control (9,25).

IRS-III investigators approached the problem of bladder tumors with a view of what appeared to limit successful bladder preservation in IRS-I and IRS-II; therefore, RT was routinely administered to all patients at week 6, after induction chemotherapy, except those in whom complete tumor removal was possible without total cystectomy. Surgery was then performed to document a complete response or to excise residual tumor while attempting to maintain bladder function. The results of IRS-III have been gratifying: the bladder retention rate at 4 years was 60% and survival was 90% for patients presenting with local or regional disease. An analysis of the 28 group III patients by Heyn et al. (92) showed that 15 (54%) ultimately retained their bladders. Induction chemoradiotherapy induced a complete loss of tumor cells in 46%; in cystectomy specimens tumor cellularity was reduced, and tumor cell maturation occurred. Of interest is that cellular maturation was greater in tumor specimens of patients who retained their bladders (92).

Table 11-9 demonstrates how the treatment philosophies of IRS-I, IRS-II, and IRS-III influenced clinical grouping. The number of patients in groups I and II fell significantly during successive studies. This was the result of an increasing emphasis on primary chemotherapeutic approaches in an attempt to preserve the bladder and a move away from aggressive up-front surgery.

In determining the optimum therapeutic approach for bladder tumors, the site of the lesion is relevant; tumors in the dome are more commonly resectable at diagnosis than trigone or bladder neck tumors. IRS-IV recommended bladder-preserving surgery at second look after

TABLE 11-9. *Distribution of patients with localized bladder and prostate tumors by clinical group in IRS-I, IRS-II, and IRS-III*

Study	Group I	Group II	Group III	Total
IRS-I	13 (20%)	21 (32%)	32 (48%)	66
IRS-II	1 (1%)	3 (3%)	91 (96%)	95
IRS-III	9 (9%)	7 (7%)	88 (85%)	104
Total	23 (9%)	31 (12%)	211 (80%)	265

The numbers in parentheses are the percentage of the individual row totals.

From references 14, 43, 44, 65, 89, 93, and 126, with permission.

induction chemoradiotherapy, if possible (65), and IRS-V recommends initial chemotherapy and radiation therapy, with aggressive surgery reserved for patients with biopsy-proven residual tumor after completion of all therapy or with early failure or progression. The RT technique for pelvic tumors is somewhat controversial. Many radiotherapists use a four-field box or arcs similar to those used in adults. In children, however, high-energy megavoltage photon fields with anteroposterior–posteroanterior technique often give good dosimetry. The use of simple anterior and posterior fields allows shielding of the femoral epiphyseal plates and proximal femurs. Multiportal conventional techniques may not improve on the dosage distribution obtained with the simpler technique (25). It is conceivable that intensity-modulated RT may offer an improvement. Careful long-term follow-up of patients is necessary in order to diagnose and manage treatment-related normal tissue damage (93).

Prostate

Whereas bladder RMS occasionally can be cured with radical surgery alone, prostatic RMS is far less amenable to this approach. Not only do primary prostate tumors tend to be more locally invasive, but they also tend to disseminate earlier (25). Symptoms are similar to those of bladder tumors through compression of the base of the bladder and infiltration of the bladder neck and urethra.

In IRS-I, 14 patients had nondisseminated prostatic primary tumors and were treated with exenteration. Only one patient died, and this death was therapy related. Eleven patients were treated with a primary chemotherapy program without radical surgery. Two patients died of RMS, and two of the survivors later needed urinary diversion or exenteration, leaving seven of the 11 with normal bladder function (89).

The treatment strategy in IRS-II was the same as that for patients with bladder RMS, but the 3-year survival was inferior (59%) to that of patients with prostate RMS in IRS-I (82%) and to that of patients with primary bladder RMS in either study (70–81%) (91). In addition, approxi-

mately one-half of all patients had lost their bladder by 3 years. However, it is also noteworthy that patients with pelvic primary tumors who had the botryoid subtype had a higher survival rate than those with the solid embryonal subtype. This is relevant because botryoid tumors were almost exclusively found in patients with vaginal and bladder primaries, and nonbotryoid tumors were found in patients with prostate primaries. Beyond this, the prostatic lesions tended to be larger than their counterparts in the vagina and bladder (91). This experience suggests that children with prostatic RMS have a worse outlook than those with other pelvic primary RMS and that definitive local control measures should not be delayed for primary chemotherapy (Table 11-10).

Paratesticular

Intrascrotal paratesticular RMS usually arises in the distal area of the spermatic cord and may invade the testis or surrounding tissues, although primary RMS of the epididymis or tunics can also occur (1). It often spreads through the lymphatics to the para-aortic nodes, following the course of the spermatic cord into the renal hilar retroperitoneal space. It often presents as a unilateral painless scrotal swelling and may grow large before the patient is diagnosed. An orchiectomy is performed through an inguinal incision, with a high ligation of the spermatic cord at the level of the inguinal ring.

TABLE 11-10. *Three-year treatment results for patients with bladder and prostate tumors in IRS-I, IRS-II, and IRS-III*

Study	Overall survival	Disease-free survival	Alive with functioning bladder
IRS-I	75%	68%	23%
IRS-II	71%	56%	22%
IRS-III	81%	73%	60%[a]

[a]In IRS-III the data are presented as bladder salvage rate, presumably at 5 years, for bladder, prostate, vagina, and other central pelvic sites. A bladder salvage rate of 64% for those cured has been reported for patients with prostate tumors.

From references 14, 65, 89-91, 93, and 126-130, with permission.

Lymphangiography and CT have been used to detect gross nodal involvement but may fail to demonstrate microscopic infiltration in some patients. Consequently, it has been the practice in the United States to perform a unilateral (transabdominal) nerve-sparing retroperitoneal lymph node dissection. Twenty-six percent of patients in IRS-I and IRS-II had retroperitoneal lymph node involvement at diagnosis, and 16% had positive ipsilateral inguinal nodes; contralateral nodal involvement is rare (25,94). A similar percentage of patients in IRS-III had nodal disease (95). Patients with group II disease on the basis of positive nodes receive RT to the nodal areas in the IRS studies, in contrast to patients with negative lymph node dissections.

Currently, the IRS studies recommend thin-cut abdominal and pelvic CT scans with contrast to evaluate nodal involvement for all patients. For patients younger than 10 years old with group I disease and no evidence of nodal involvement by CT scan, a repeat CT scan every 3 months is recommended without retroperitoneal node biopsy or sampling (96,97). For patients younger than 10 years old with concerning or positive CT scans, lymph node sampling without formal node dissection is recommended, with treatment based on the findings of this procedure (94,95). For children 10 years and older, a staging ipsilateral retroperitoneal lymph node dissection is necessary for all children regardless of the CT findings. However, it is not absolutely certain that a lymph node dissection or nodal irradiation in the absence of involvement by imaging studies is necessary. European investigators have relied on radiographic assessment of retroperitoneal lymph node involvement, although the CT scan does not always accurately predict the presence of nodal involvement (70,96).

If a transscrotal biopsy is performed instead of the inguinal approach, then the patient is considered to have group II disease, and the hemiscrotum is irradiated. Resection of the violated scrotal tissue is necessary, and even hemiscrotectomy should be considered. The contralateral testicle can be transposed laterally into the thigh before irradiation and later reimplanted into the scrotum. The 5-year survival of patients treated for paratesticular RMS exceeds 80% (14,25,94).

Vagina and Vulva

RMS of the vagina most commonly occurs in very young children (90% younger than 5 years of age). It commonly presents as a mass or discharge and is almost exclusively the embryonal (usually botryoid) subtype. The mean age of girls with vulvar tumors is 8 years (98). Vulval inflammation and genital bleeding are the most common presenting signs. Vulvar RMS is most commonly found as a firm nodule embedded in the labial folds or in a periclitoric location and is often of the alveolar subtype (1). Vaginal tumors most commonly arise from the anterior wall, are often multicentric, and can invade the vesicovaginal septum or bladder wall. Regional nodal involvement is uncommon (1). The classic surgical technique for treatment of vaginal tumors was an anterior exenteration with urinary diversion. Occasionally, this was accompanied by resection of the adjacent colon. Unfortunately, fewer than 20% of patients could be cured with surgery alone (99) and only 25% with chemotherapy alone. Survival rates improved to 60–80% when chemotherapy was added to extirpative surgery, with or without RT. Attempts to minimize the surgical procedure, in the absence of adjuvant RT, led to an unacceptably high rate of local recurrence. Vulvar tumors often are localized and curable with wide excision, usually hemivulvectomy, followed by chemotherapy with or without RT (100).

To better integrate all three treatment modalities, IRS-II adopted a strategy that included second-look surgery at week 8 or 16, depending on the response to chemotherapy. The use of RT depended on the completeness of the surgical procedure. Limited surgery (partial vaginectomy) was preferred when the procedure was expected to result in the removal of all visible tumor (91). Using this treatment approach, 18 of 21 (86%) patients survived at 3 years (91). IRS-III gave 20 weeks of chemotherapy and then RT to patients who had not achieved a complete remission by that time, whereas IRS-IV gave RT at week 9, and the cure rate remained high

(101). Current guidelines are similar; limited surgery is preferred, and complete vaginectomy is inappropriate except in the setting of persistent or recurrent disease. For vulvar tumors, surgery is currently performed if feasible as a second look at week 12 with reduced dosages of RT for patients with completely resected tumor or only microscopic residual tumor. For vaginal tumors, second look is performed at week 28, with no radiation given for negative biopsies or completely resected disease and lower RT dosages for patients with microscopic residual tumor postoperatively. When radiation is needed, teletherapy is most common, although intracavitary or interstitial brachytherapy may be possible (25,102). This approach has been successful at the Institut Gustave–Roussy (83). Either technique should strive to minimize the RT dosage to the ovaries (which at times should be transposed outside the primary radiation volume), hips, and pelvic organs. More than 90% of children are expected to survive.

Uterus and Cervix

Uterine and cervical RMS is much less common than vaginal RMS, and it tends to occur in adolescent girls near puberty. Patients may present with pedunculated polyps with vaginal extrusion of tumor tissue or with a pelvic mass caused by diffuse intramural involvement; bleeding is common (102,103). When uterine tumors occur in younger children, distinction from a vaginal tumor may be difficult. Sometimes this is possible only after regression of the tumor after chemotherapy.

In IRS-I and IRS-II, 13 patients had uterine (five patients) or cervical (eight patients) primaries. In patients who presented with localized polypoid tumors, polypectomy and adjuvant chemotherapy were highly curative. When hysterectomy or vaginectomy successfully removed all gross tumor, cure was also likely. Conversely, patients with group III or IV RMS died (98,102). Brand et al. (103) reviewed 21 cases of sarcoma botryoides of the uterine cervix. Most patients received chemotherapy, and eight underwent pelvic irradiation. Eighty percent of these patients survived.

Currently, treatment of uterine and cervical RMS is intended to preserve pelvic organs when possible. Patients with initially resectable disease are placed in group I or II by surgery, followed by chemotherapy, and then RT, if microscopic residual disease is proven to persist, or hysterectomy with no RT. For those with group III disease, primary chemotherapy is given, followed by a second-look laparotomy. If there is gross residual that cannot be completely resected with hysterectomy, or if microscopic disease is found after resection, the patient then receives RT and continues on chemotherapy. If the second-look exploration shows no demonstrable tumor or tumor that is completely resected, then no radiotherapy is given, and the patient continues on chemotherapy alone. Survival rates should approximate those of patients with RMS of the vagina and vulva (101,104).

Extremity

Extremity lesions have a poor prognosis (Fig. 11-1). Approximately one-half of these lesions are alveolar RMS with unfavorable histology (Table 11-2). In IRS-I and IRS-II, regional lymph node involvement occurred in 15% and 9% of patients with upper- and lower-extremity lesions, respectively (51,105).

The prognosis for patients with extremity RMS is compromised by the high frequency (50%) of the alveolar subtype, of lymphatic metastasis at diagnosis, and of metastasis to any site at diagnosis (27% vs. 18% in all patients with RMS) (Fig. 11-5) (106). Although there is no evidence that amputation is more often curative than wide local excision, this procedure retains a role in patients where limited excision and high-dose irradiation would produce unacceptable functional results, in patients with distal (alveolar) extremity lesions where gross removal is otherwise impossible, and in patients with massive local recurrences after conservative therapy (1,69,107). The preferred operative procedure for primary management is wide excision with negative margins and adjacent lymph node group sampling. In IRS-V, the axilla or inguinal regions are explored even in the absence of clinically evident nodal involvement.

Sentinel lymph node mapping may also play a role in identifying regional nodes most likely to be involved (108). Chemotherapy is always given. RT is omitted only for patients with completely resected favorable histology tumors with negative nodes. The tumor is treated with a 2-cm margin, and regional lymph nodes are treated only when involved. One should spare a strip of soft tissue along the extremity to avoid late radiation-induced extremity edema.

Parameningeal

Parameningeal (PM) RMSs include those arising in the skull base and therefore can extend intracranially and produce neoplastic meningitis, which occurs in about 35% of cases (44,86). In IRS-III, PM RMS made up 41% of head and neck tumors and 15% of all tumors. Most patients were younger than 10 years old (72%) (14). Middle ear tumors extend through the tegmen tympani to middle cranial fossa meninges or through the posterior mastoid to the posterior cranial fossa. Tumors of the nasal cavity, paranasal sinus, and nasopharynx extend to meninges through the basal foramina or sinus roofs. Nasopharyngeal RMS invades the base of the skull in 35% of patients, involving the cavernous sinus and causing cranial nerve palsies (1,62,109). Although lymph node involvement was previously thought to be common, in IRS-III fewer than 20% were classified as node positive (1,52). The ratio of embryonal to alveolar histology is 4:1. Meningeal penetration and leptomeningeal tumor cell seeding must be assessed in patients with PM RMS. Complete surgical extirpation of the primary with a satisfactory cosmetic and functional result is almost never possible; in IRS-III 76% of patients were group III. Therefore, the role of surgery is confined to establishing a diagnosis with a biopsy or a subtotal excision. Cervical lymph node dissection (radical neck) is rarely appropriate because of the morbidity and low frequency of subclinical nodal involvement; conversely, suspicious nodes should be examined. Before the use of chemotherapy, fewer than 20% of patients survived despite intense irradiation (71,109).

For patients with PM RMS, the volume and timing of RT are critical. The volume of irradiation appropriate for PM lesions been reevaluated in light of the experience in IRS and advances in imaging. Meningeal extension is associated with a high risk of CNS relapse and a 90% chance of death. In IRS-I, meningeal extension after radiotherapy appeared to be associated with inadequate fields and dosages less than 50 Gy (63,109). These findings prompted a call for the use of local treatment with cranial or craniospinal irradiation. Follow-up analysis of the IRS-I patients suggested that part of the risk of CNS relapse was engendered by fields that were too tight but that widespread use of full cranial irradiation did not increase disease control and increased morbidity, a conclusion supported by non-IRS data (110). In IRS-III, if there was no evidence of intracranial extension, CSF cytology was negative, and bone erosion or cranial nerve palsies were absent, then the primary lesion was irradiated with a 5-cm margin, including treatment of the adjacent meninges. Patients not meeting these criteria received intrathecal chemotherapy. If the CT or MRI demonstrated in-continuity intracranial extension of the primary tumor, but the CSF cytology was negative, prophylactic whole brain irradiation results were given along with treatment to the primary tumor. Finally, for positive CSF cytology, craniospinal irradiation was given. Results are as follows: 69% 5-year progression-free survival, 15% local failure for group III patients, and a 4.7% contiguous CNS relapse (52). Based on IRS-II data, three risk factors for tumor access to the cranial subarachnoid space were determined: skull base erosion, cranial nerve palsy, and intracranial extension. Patients with any risk factor had a 51% 3-year progression-free survival, compared with 81% for other patients. In IRS-IV the radiation margin was reduced to 2 cm, and only patients with diffuse intracranial meningeal extension or multiple sites of brain parenchymal disease were treated to the entire cranial cavity (111). Currently, RT is given at the beginning of the treatment course when there is clear evidence of intracranial extension, defined as positive CSF cytology results or any imaging evidence (by MRI) that tumor touches, displaces, invades, distorts, or otherwise causes a signal abnormality of the dura. Otherwise, chemotherapy is given first, with RT given at week 12. RT is omitted only for patients with completely resected, favorable histology tumors with negative nodes. Intrathecal chemotherapy and craniospinal irradiation are no longer used. The extent of surgery is determined by the potential cosmetic and functional outcome, and second-look procedures may be effectively performed (112). Of interest is an analysis comparing outcome for PM RMS treated on IRS and three European cooperative groups. For low-risk patients, 5-year survival was superior in IRS, possibly because of early routine RT, the IRS quality assurance program, and inclusion of patients with smaller tumors without involved lymph nodes (113). Despite its parameningeal location, middle ear RMS has a favorable prognosis (114).

Other Head and Neck Sites

Parotid region, oral cavity, oropharynx, and larynx RMS generally has an embryonal histology. Cheek and scalp lesions have a high frequency of alveolar histology (49). Superficial lesions may be marginally or, at times, widely resected with satisfactory cosmesis and function, a situation that less often pertains for deeper tumors. Narrower resection margins (less than 1 mm) are acceptable because of anatomic restrictions. Optimal cosmesis with excellent disease control may best be obtained with a marginal resection and subsequent RT. For the deeper tumors (oral cavity, buccal mucosa, larynx, parapharyngeal, or parotid region), RT is generally necessary. Because of the favorable outlook for patients with nonparameningeal head and neck tumors, such patients are classified as stage I in IRS-IV and IRS-V and therefore receive less intense chemotherapy than do those with PM head and neck tumors (115). However, if a nonparameningeal head and neck tumor extends to and invades a parameningeal region, then it should be treated as a PM RMS.

Although the early experience with head and neck RMS suggested that lymph node involvement was uncommon (8% in IRS-I and IRS-II), this may have resulted from less than thorough assessments. In fact, lymph nodes were positive in 20% of patients in whom lymph node status was reported (49). Donaldson et al. (71) reported a similar incidence. Involved lymph node groups may be resected as well as irradiated.

Orbit

Because of the accessibility of the orbit to examination and the sensitivity of ocular function to mass effect, orbital RMS often is diagnosed early. Eyelid swelling and globe displacement are common presenting signs. Orbital exenteration was the standard treatment until the mid-1960s but rarely achieved local control or survival. In the late 1960s, Cassady and co-workers (7,64) observed that RT afforded local control in five of five patients after a biopsy. RT has now assumed a major role in the treatment of orbital RMS. Approximately two-thirds of cases are group III. Treatment is with biopsy, chemotherapy, and RT. The volume need not include the entire orbit if the tumor is small. In the IRS study, local control has been 94% with RT and is increased to 98% with surgical salvage (79). Of note, orbital RMS can also invade meninges via erosion of the superior orbital fissure. An analysis of IRS data suggested a relationship of histology to outcome. For the 84% with embryonal histologies, the 5-year survival was 94%. However, for the 10% of children with alveolar RMS, this rate was 74%, and all five infants with alveolar disease died (58). Because of the favorable outcome of patients with orbital RMS, investigators have attempted to use chemotherapy alone (66). Local control was compromised by this strategy.

The late adverse effects of orbital irradiation are considerable because the minimum irradiated volume often includes all bony limits of the orbit, or more if there is extension into adjacent soft tissue or bone (116). The child should be treated with the eye open to avoid the bolus effect of the lids unless the lids are involved. Proton therapy may help decrease late effects in the orbit (86–88).

Trunk

Truncal sites include the chest wall, paraspinal area, and abdominal wall, in decreasing order of frequency. Scapular and buttock lesions are considered to be extensions of the extremity, and retroperitoneal and perineal tumors are considered separately. An early IRS report focused on 30 children with soft tissue sarcoma of the trunk (117). Ten of the 14 children with chest wall primaries had group I or III disease, and five were long-term survivors. None of the four children with metastases at diagnosis survived.

Paraspinal tumors were rare (3.3%) in IRS-I and IRS-II. They tended to be greater than 5 cm in diameter, often invaded the spinal extradural space, and were commonly of an undifferentiated or extraosseous Ewing's subtype. Survival at 5 years was approximately 50% in both studies (118). Local and distant relapses were common, and patients with embryonal subtypes fared no better than others.

Current guidelines include as wide a surgical resection as is feasible, either at diagnosis or after chemoradiotherapy as a second look. For patients with an initial excision that was less aggressive than feasible or of an uncertain nature, a reexcision should be considered. RT is given to all patients except those with completely excised small, favorable histology tumors and uninvolved lymph nodes. RT fields encompass the original disease extent, and chemotherapy is always used (117,118).

Retroperitoneal

Retroperitoneal tumors often are large at diagnosis, probably because there is much room for expansion before they cause symptoms (119). These tumors are technically difficult to resect, and lymph node involvement is common (23% in IRS-I and IRS-II for retroperitoneal pelvic tumors). Therefore, most patients have group III or IV disease. Not only is resection problematic, but the aggressiveness of RT is compromised by the tolerance of normal tissue, in terms both of volume and dosage. In the IRS, 39% of patients with retroperitoneal RMS had difficulties in delivery of the specified RT. All these factors combine to render the prognosis for retroperitoneal RMS worse than for most other sites; 5-year survival was approximately 40% in IRS-II (Fig. 11-1) (18,119). Guidelines are essentially the same as those noted previously for truncal tumors. Because of normal tissue tolerance, RT usually involves multiple reductions in field size.

Perineal

Perineal tumors, in IRS-I and IRS-II, were most commonly alveolar (56%) or embryonal (30%), and patients were equally likely to have negative or microscopic versus gross residual disease after surgery (120). The 3-year survival was 59%, which was somewhat inferior to that of patients with disease in other sites (18,120). The approach to these patients also entails as complete a resection as functionally acceptable, followed by chemotherapy and RT as appropriate.

Hepatobiliary Tree

The common bile duct, the common, right, or left hepatic duct, and the ampulla of Vater may be sites for RMS. A recent IRS report reviewed the experience of the 25 patients in IRS-I–IRS-IV with RMS of the biliary tract (121). The most common presentation included intermittent obstructive jaundice with or without abdominal distention, fever, pain, and loss of appetite. Imaging was inadequate for the identification of regional metastases. Despite aggressive surgery, gross total resection at diagnosis was possible in only six cases, two of which had negative surgical margins. However, the 5-year survival rate was 78%, and much of the mortality was related to infectious complications associated with external biliary drains. The IRS-V schema includes the biliary tract as a favorable site, and current recommendations include conservative surgery (without bile drainage) to establish an accurate diagnosis and determine the extent of regional disease, followed by chemotherapy and RT.

Metastatic Disease

Fewer than 10% of patients with bone marrow metastases at diagnosis achieve long-term survival. Patients with metastatic disease not involving the bone marrow are more likely to survive (25–30%) (14,18,19,28). A recent analysis of IRS-IV patients with metastatic RMS showed a favorable subgroup of patients with embryonal histology and two or fewer metastatic sites with a 3-year failure-free survival of 40% and overall survival of 47% (28).

Chemotherapy is the dominant treatment modality for patients with metastatic disease. Because extirpative surgery usually is not appropriate, RT assumes the major role in obtaining local control of both primary and metastatic lesions, which are imageable and localizable. Respecting normal tissue tolerances, the volume used includes that which existed before chemotherapy, and the dosage is 40 to 50 Gy (although this must often be modified). Low-dose whole-lung irradiation is used as part of the treatment of pulmonary metastasis. If there are a few isolated lung metastases, not encompassing an excessive volume of lung, they may be boosted by a "rifle shot" field. In addition, lung nodules can be resected after chemoradiotherapy if acceptable lung function is preserved.

RECURRENT DISEASE

Unfortunately, the prognosis for most patients with recurrent rhabdomyosarcoma is poor, although there is a subset of patients with favorable salvage rates (122). These patients are those with favorable histology who initially presented with stage 1 or group I disease and whose recurrence is local or regional. The 5-year survival rates are 50–70% for this group, whereas most other children have an extremely poor prognosis. Despite the poor long-term outlook for patients with recurrent disease, many can still achieve a second remission with salvage therapy, and there are several active chemotherapy regimens, including ifosfamide with etoposide and cyclophosphamide with topotecan (123,124). The IRS (now known as the Soft Tissue Sarcoma Committee of the Children's Oncology Group) is investigating a risk-based approach to salvage treatment in which favorable-risk patients are treated with doxorubicin and cyclophosphamide alternating with ifosfamide and etoposide. Unfa-

vorable-risk patients with measurable disease receive vincristine and irinotecan (with a randomization to two different drug administration schedules), followed by the alternating schedule, or the aforementioned regimen with the addition of a new agent, tirapazamine, for patients without measurable disease. RT often is used as palliative treatment of painful or obstructing lesions, and aggressive surgery often is used in this setting of recurrent disease. Unfortunately, high-dose cytotoxic therapy with bone marrow rescue has not proven to be effective for patients with metastatic or recurrent disease (125).

Therapeutic Maneuvers

Identifying settings in which lower RT dosages are effective will decrease late effects, and IRS-V is investigating this strategy in several groups of patients. Optimally sequencing RT and chemotherapy to improve efficacy, safety, and protocol compliance continues to be explored. Administering short, intensive chemotherapy regimens, with growth factor support, is another area of study. RT must strive to improve the local control rates for bulky RMS without engendering high morbidity from damage to normal tissue. Among the areas meriting additional investigation proton therapy are hyperthermia, brachytherapy, intraoperative RT, chemical radiosensitizers, and radioprotectors.

REFERENCES

References particularly recommended for further reading are indicated by an asterisk.

1. Maurer H, Ruymann F, Pochedly C. *Rhabdomyosarcoma and related tumors in children and adolescents.* Boca Raton, FL: CRC Press, 1991.
2. Newton WA Jr, Soule EH, Hamoudi AB, et al. Histopathology of childhood sarcomas, Intergroup Rhabdomyosarcoma Studies I and II: clinicopathologic correlation. *J Clin Oncol* 1988;6:67–75.
3. Parham DM, Webber B, Holt H, et al. Immunohistochemical study of childhood rhabdomyosarcomas and related neoplasms. Results of an Intergroup Rhabdomyosarcoma study project. *Cancer* 1991;67: 3072–3080.
4. Weber C. Anatomische untersuchung einer hypertrophische zunge nebst bemerkungen ueber die neubildung quergestreifter muskelfasem, virchow. *Arch Pathol Anat* 1954;7:115–121.

5. Stout A. Rhabdomyosarcoma of the skeletal muscle. *Ann Surg* 1946;123:447–472.

6. Horn RJ, Enterline H. Rhabdomyosarcoma: a clinicopathologic study and classification of 39 cases. *Cancer* 1958;11:181–199.

7. Cassady JR, Sagerman RH, Tretter P, et al. Radiation therapy for rhabdomyosarcoma. *Radiology* 1968;91: 116–120.

8. Stobbe G, Dargeaon H. Embryonal rhabdomyosarcoma of the head and neck in children and adolescents. *Cancer* 1950;3:826–836.

9. Tefft M, Lindberg RD, Gehan EA. Radiation therapy combined with systemic chemotherapy of rhabdomyosarcoma in children: local control in patients enrolled in the Intergroup Rhabdomyosarcoma Study. *Natl Cancer Inst Monogr* 1981:75–81.

10. Paulino AC, Simon JH, Zhen W, et al. Long-term effects in children treated with radiotherapy for head and neck rhabdomyosarcoma. *Int J Radiat Oncol Biol Phys* 2000;48:1489–1495.

11. Ludin A, Macklis RM. Radiotherapy for pediatric genitourinary tumors. Its role and long-term consequences. *Urol Clin North Am* 2000;27:553–562.

12. Heyn RM, Holland R, Newton WA Jr, et al. The role of combined chemotherapy in the treatment of rhabdomyosarcoma in children. *Cancer* 1974;34:2128–2142.

*13. Crist WM, Garnsey L, Beltangady MS, et al. Prognosis in children with rhabdomyosarcoma: a report of the intergroup rhabdomyosarcoma studies I and II. *J Clin Oncol* 1990;8:443–452.

*14. Crist W, Gehan EA, Ragab AH, et al. The Third Intergroup Rhabdomyosarcoma Study. *J Clin Oncol* 1995;13:610–630.

*15. Donaldson SS, Asmar L, Breneman J, et al. Hyperfractionated radiation in children with rhabdomyosarcoma: results of an Intergroup Rhabdomyosarcoma Pilot Study. *Int J Radiat Oncol Biol Phys* 1995;32:903–911.

16. Kingston JE, McElwain TJ, Malpas JS. Childhood rhabdomyosarcoma: experience of the Children's Solid Tumour Group. *Br J Cancer* 1983;48:195–207.

17. Mandell LR. Ongoing progress in the treatment of childhood rhabdomyosarcoma. *Oncology (Huntingt)* 1993;7:71–83; discussion 84–96, 89–90.

18. Maurer HM, Gehan EA, Beltangady M, et al. The Intergroup Rhabdomyosarcoma Study II. *Cancer* 1993;71:1904–1922.

19. Maurer HM, Beltangady M, Gehan EA, et al. The Intergroup Rhabdomyosarcoma Study I. A final report. *Cancer* 1988;61:209–220.

20. Rodary C, Gehan EA, Flamant F, et al. Prognostic factors in 951 nonmetastatic rhabdomyosarcoma in children: a report from the International Rhabdomyosarcoma Workshop. *Med Pediatr Oncol* 1991;19:89–95.

*21. Wharam MD, Hanfelt JJ, Tefft MC, et al. Radiation therapy for rhabdomyosarcoma: local failure risk for clinical group III patients on Intergroup Rhabdomyosarcoma Study II. *Int J Radiat Oncol Biol Phys* 1997;38:797–804.

*22. Crist WM, Anderson JR, Meza JL, et al. Intergroup Rhabdomyosarcoma Study IV: results for patients with nonmetastatic disease. *J Clin Oncol* 2001;19: 3091–3102.

*23. Raney RB, Anderson JR, Barr FG, et al. Rhabdomyosarcoma and undifferentiated sarcoma in the first two decades of life: a selective review of Intergroup Rhabdomyosarcoma Study Group experience and rationale for Intergroup Rhabdomyosarcoma Study V. *J Pediatr Hematol Oncol* 2001;23:215–220.

24. Koscielniak E, Jurgens H, Winkler K, et al. Treatment of soft tissue sarcoma in childhood and adolescence. A report of the German Cooperative Soft Tissue Sarcoma Study. *Cancer* 1992;70:2557–2567.

25. Plowman P. Radiotherapy of pediatric genitourinary tumors. In: Broeker B, Klein F. *Pediatric tumors of the genitourinary tract.* New York: Alan R. Liss, 1988:263–281.

26. Mandell L, Ghavimi F, Peretz T, et al. Radiocurability of microscopic disease in childhood rhabdomyosarcoma with radiation doses less than 4,000 cGy. *J Clin Oncol* 1990;8:1536–1542.

27. Pedrick TJ, Donaldson SS, Cox RS. Rhabdomyosarcoma: the Stanford experience using a TNM staging system. *J Clin Oncol* 1986;4:370–378.

*28. Breneman JC, Lyden E, Pappo AS, et al. Prognostic factors and clinical outcomes in children and adolescents with metastatic rhabdomyosarcoma: a report from the Intergroup Rhabdomyosarcoma Study IV. *J Clin Oncol* 2003;21:78–84.

29. Gurney JG, Severson RK, Davis S, et al. Incidence of cancer in children in the United States. Sex-, race-, and 1-year age-specific rates by histologic type. *Cancer* 1995;75:2186–2195.

30. Anonymous. *SEER cancer statistics review 1973–1996.* Bethesda, MD: National Cancer Institute, 1999.

31. Ruymann FB, Maddux HR, Ragab A, et al. Congenital anomalies associated with rhabdomyosarcoma: an autopsy study of 115 cases. *Med Pediatr Oncol* 1988;16:33–39.

32. Grufferman S, Schwartz AG, Ruymann FB, et al. Parents' use of cocaine and marijuana and increased risk of rhabdomyosarcoma in their children. *Cancer Causes Control* 1993;4:217–224.

33. Birch JM, Hartley AL, Blair V, et al. Cancer in the families of children with soft tissue sarcoma. *Cancer* 1990;66:2239–2248.

34. McKeen EA, Bodurtha J, Meadows AT, et al. Rhabdomyosarcoma complicating multiple neurofibromatosis. *J Pediatr* 1978;93:992–993.

35. Constine LS, Marcus RB Jr, Halperin EC. The future of therapy for childhood rhabdomyosarcoma: clues from molecular biology. *Int J Radiat Oncol Biol Phys* 1995;32:1245–1249; discussion 1263.

36. Pappo AS, Shapiro DN, Crist WM, et al. Biology and therapy of pediatric rhabdomyosarcoma. *J Clin Oncol* 1995;13:2123–2139.

37. Barr FG. Molecular genetics and pathogenesis of rhabdomyosarcoma. *J Pediatr Hematol Oncol* 1997; 19:483–491.

38. Merlino G, Helman LJ. Rhabdomyosarcoma: working out the pathways. *Oncogene* 1999;18:5340–5348.

39. Sorensen PH, Lynch JC, Qualman SI, et al. PAX3-FKHR and PAX7-FKHR gene fusions are prognostic indicators in alveolar rhabdomyosarcoma: a report from the Children's Oncology Group. *J Clin Oncol* 2002;20:2672–2679.

40. Edwards RH, Chatten J, Xiong QB, et al. Detection

of gene fusions in rhabdomyosarcoma by reverse transcriptase–polymerase chain reaction assay of archival samples. *Diagn Mol Pathol* 1997;6:91–97.

41. Kelly KM, Womer RB, Barr FG. Minimal disease detection in patients with alveolar rhabdomyosarcoma using a reverse transcriptase–polymerase chain reaction method. *Cancer* 1996;78:1320–1327.

42. Weber-Hall S, Anderson J, McManus A, et al. Gains, losses, and amplification of genomic material in rhabdomyosarcoma analyzed by comparative genomic hybridization. *Cancer Res* 1996;56:3220–3224.

43. Shapiro DN, Parham DM, Douglass EC, et al. Relationship of tumor-cell ploidy to histologic subtype and treatment outcome in children and adolescents with unresectable rhabdomyosarcoma. *J Clin Oncol* 1991;9:159–166.

44. Pappo AS, Crist WM, Kuttesch J, et al. Tumor-cell DNA content predicts outcome in children and adolescents with clinical group III embryonal rhabdomyosarcoma. *J Clin Oncol* 1993;11:1901–1905.

45. De Zen L, Sommaggio A, d'Amore ES, et al. Clinical relevance of DNA ploidy and proliferative activity in childhood rhabdomyosarcoma: a retrospective analysis of patients enrolled onto the Italian Cooperative Rhabdomyosarcoma Study RMS88. *J Clin Oncol* 1997;15:1198–1205.

46. Dias P, Kumar P, Marsden HB, et al. N-myc gene is amplified in alveolar rhabdomyosarcomas (RMS) but not in embryonal RMS. *Int J Cancer* 1990;45:593–596.

47. Driman D, Thorner PS, Greenberg ML, et al. MYCN gene amplification in rhabdomyosarcoma. *Cancer* 1994;73:2231–2237.

48. Felix CA, Kappel CC, Mitsudomi T, et al. Frequency and diversity of p53 mutations in childhood rhabdomyosarcoma. *Cancer Res* 1992;52:2243–2247.

49. Wharam MD, Beltangady MS, Heyn RM, et al. Pediatric orofacial and laryngopharyngeal rhabdomyosarcoma. An Intergroup Rhabdomyosarcoma Study report. *Arch Otolaryngol Head Neck Surg* 1987;113:1225–1227.

*50. Breneman JC. Genitourinary rhabdomyosarcoma. *Semin Radiat Oncol* 1997;7:217–224.

51. Lawrence W Jr, Hays DM, Heyn R, et al. Lymphatic metastases with childhood rhabdomyosarcoma. *Cancer* 1987;60:910–915.

*52. Wharam MD Jr. Rhabdomyosarcoma of parameningeal sites. *Semin Radiat Oncol* 1997;7:212–216.

53. Asmar L, Gehan EA, Newton WA, et al. Agreement among and within groups of pathologists in the classification of rhabdomyosarcoma and related childhood sarcomas. Report of an international study of four pathology classifications. *Cancer* 1994;74:2579–2588.

54. Newton WA Jr, Gehan EA, Webber BL, et al. Classification of rhabdomyosarcomas and related sarcomas. Pathologic aspects and proposal for a new classification: an Intergroup Rhabdomyosarcoma Study. *Cancer* 1995;76:1073–1085.

55. Parham DM. Pathologic classification of rhabdomyosarcomas and correlations with molecular studies. *Mod Pathol* 2001;14:506–514.

56. Donaldson SS, Belli JA. A rational clinical staging system for childhood rhabdomyosarcoma. *J Clin Oncol* 1984;2:135–139.

57. Lawrence W Jr, Anderson JR, Gehan EA, et al. Pretreatment TNM staging of childhood rhabdomyosarcoma: a report of the Intergroup Rhabdomyosarcoma Study Group. *Cancer* 1997;80:1165–1170.

58. Kodet R, Newton WA Jr, Hamoudi AB, et al. Orbital rhabdomyosarcomas and related tumors in childhood: relationship of morphology to prognosis—an Intergroup Rhabdomyosarcoma study. *Med Pediatr Oncol* 1997;29:51–60.

59. La Quaglia MP, Heller G, Ghavimi F, et al. The effect of age at diagnosis on outcome in rhabdomyosarcoma. *Cancer* 1994;73:109–117.

60. Ragab AH, Heyn R, Tefft M, et al. Infants younger than 1 year of age with rhabdomyosarcoma. *Cancer* 1986;58:2606–2610.

61. Salloum E, Flamant F, Rey A, et al. Rhabdomyosarcoma in infants under one year of age: experience of the Institut Gustave-Roussy. *Med Pediatr Oncol* 1989;17:424–428.

62. Mandell LR, Massey V, Ghavimi F. The influence of extensive bone erosion on local control in non-orbital rhabdomyosarcoma of the head and neck. *Int J Radiat Oncol Biol Phys* 1989;17:649–653.

*63. Raney RB Jr, Tefft M, Newton WA, et al. Improved prognosis with intensive treatment of children with cranial soft tissue sarcomas arising in nonorbital parameningeal sites. A report from the Intergroup Rhabdomyosarcoma Study. *Cancer* 1987;59:147–155.

64. Sagerman RH, Cassady JR, Tretter P. Radiation therapy for rhabdomyosarcoma of the orbit. *Trans Am Acad Ophthalmol Otolaryngol* 1968;72:849–854.

65. Hays DM, Raney RB, Wharam MD, et al. Children with vesical rhabdomyosarcoma (RMS) treated by partial cystectomy with neoadjuvant or adjuvant chemotherapy, with or without radiotherapy. A report from the Intergroup Rhabdomyosarcoma Study (IRS) Committee. *J Pediatr Hematol Oncol* 1995;17:46–52.

*66. Rousseau P, Flamant F, Quintana E, et al. Primary chemotherapy in rhabdomyosarcomas and other malignant mesenchymal tumors of the orbit: results of the International Society of Pediatric Oncology MMT 84 Study. *J Clin Oncol* 1994;12:516–521.

67. Weiner E. Survival is improved in clinical group III children with complete response established by second look operations in the Intergroup Rhabdomyosarcoma Study III. *Med Pediatr Oncol* 1991;19:399(abst).

68. Mandell L, Ghavimi F, LaQuaglia M, et al. Prognostic significance of regional lymph node involvement in childhood extremity rhabdomyosarcoma. *Med Pediatr Oncol* 1990;18:466–471.

69. Neville HL, Andrassy RJ, Lobe TE, et al. Preoperative staging, prognostic factors, and outcome for extremity rhabdomyosarcoma: a preliminary report from the Intergroup Rhabdomyosarcoma Study IV (1991–1997). *J Pediatr Surg* 2000;35:317–321.

70. Wiener ES, Anderson JR, Ojimba JI, et al. Controversies in the management of paratesticular rhabdomyosarcoma: is staging retroperitoneal lymph node dissection necessary for adolescents with resected paratesticular rhabdomyosarcoma? *Semin Pediatr Surg* 2001;10:146–152.

71. Donaldson SS, Castro JR, Wilbur JR, et al. Rhabdomyosarcoma of head and neck in children. Combination treatment by surgery, irradiation, and chemotherapy. *Cancer* 1973;31:26–35.

72. Sandler E, Lyden E, Ruymann F, et al. Efficacy of ifosfamide and doxorubicin given as a phase II "window" in children with newly diagnosed metastatic rhabdomyosarcoma: a report from the Intergroup Rhabdomyosarcoma Study Group. *Med Pediatr Oncol* 2001;37:442–448.

73. Breitfeld PP, Lyden E, Raney RB, et al. Ifosfamide and etoposide are superior to vincristine and melphalan for pediatric metastatic rhabdomyosarcoma when administered with irradiation and combination chemotherapy: a report from the Intergroup Rhabdomyosarcoma Study Group. *J Pediatr Hematol Oncol* 2001;23:225–233.

74. Womer RB, Daller RT, Fenton JG, et al. Granulocyte colony stimulating factor permits dose intensification by interval compression in the treatment of Ewing's sarcomas and soft tissue sarcomas in children. *Eur J Cancer* 2000;36:87–94.

75. Arndt CA, Nascimento AG, Schroeder G, et al. Treatment of intermediate risk rhabdomyosarcoma and undifferentiated sarcoma with alternating cycles of vincristine/doxorubicin/cyclophosphamide and etoposide/ifosfamide. *Eur J Cancer* 1998;34:1224–1229.

76. Pappo AS, Lyden E, Breneman J, et al. Up-front window trial of topotecan in previously untreated children and adolescents with metastatic rhabdomyosarcoma: an intergroup rhabdomyosarcoma study. *J Clin Oncol* 2001;19:213–219.

77. Tefft M, Wharam M, Gehan E. Local and regional control of rhabdomyosarcoma by radiation in IRS-II. *Int J Radiat Oncol Biol Phys* 1988;15:159(abst).

78. Tefft M, Wharam M, Ruymann F, et al. Radiotherapy for rhabdomyosarcoma in children: a report from the Intergroup Rhabdomyosarcoma Study #2. *Proc ASCO* 1985;4:234(abst).

*79. Wharam M, Beltangady M, Hays D, et al. Localized orbital rhabdomyosarcoma. An interim report of the Intergroup Rhabdomyosarcoma Study Committee. *Ophthalmology* 1987;94:251–254.

80. Wolden SL, Anderson JR, Crist WM, et al. Indications for radiotherapy and chemotherapy after complete resection in rhabdomyosarcoma: a report from the Intergroup Rhabdomyosarcoma Studies I to III. *J Clin Oncol* 1999;17:3468–3475.

81. Smith LM, Anderson JR, Qualman SJ, et al. Which patients with microscopic disease and rhabdomyosarcoma experience relapse after therapy? A report from the soft tissue sarcoma committee of the Children's Oncology Group. *J Clin Oncol* 2001;19:4058–4064.

82. Regine WF, Fontanesi J, Kumar P, et al. A phase II trial evaluating selective use of altered radiation dose and fractionation in patients with unresectable rhabdomyosarcoma. *Int J Radiat Oncol Biol Phys* 1995;31:799–805.

83. Flamant F, Gerbaulet A, Nihoul-Fekete C, et al. Long-term sequelae of conservative treatment by surgery, brachytherapy, and chemotherapy for vulval and vaginal rhabdomyosarcoma in children. *J Clin Oncol* 1990;8:1847–1853.

84. Chen C, Shu HK, Goldwein JW, et al. Volumetric considerations in radiotherapy for pediatric parameningeal rhabdomyosarcomas. *Int J Radiat Oncol Biol Phys* 2003;55:1294–1299.

85. Nag S, Martinez-Monge R, Ruymann F, et al. Innova-tion in the management of soft tissue sarcomas in infants and young children: high-dose-rate brachytherapy. *J Clin Oncol* 1997;15:3075–3084.

86. Hug EB, Adams J, Fitzek M, et al. Fractionated, three-dimensional, planning-assisted proton-radiation therapy for orbital rhabdomyosarcoma: a novel technique. *Int J Radiat Oncol Biol Phys* 2000;47:979–984.

87. Miralbell R, Lomax A, Cella L, et al. Potential reduction of the incidence of radiation-induced second cancers by using proton beams in the treatment of pediatric tumors. *Int J Radiat Oncol Biol Phys* 2002; 54:824–829.

88. Yock T, Schneider R, Sharis C, et al. Proton radiation compared to photon radiation for orbital rhabdomyosarcoma, UICC Oral Presentation. *Int J Cancer* 2002;[Suppl 18;Abstract No. 0159]:120.

89. Hays DM, Raney RB Jr, Lawrence W Jr, et al. Bladder and prostatic tumors in the Intergroup Rhabdomyosarcoma Study (IRS-I): results of therapy. *Cancer* 1982;50:1472–1482.

90. Hays DM, Lawrence W Jr, Crist WM, et al. Partial cystectomy in the management of rhabdomyosarcoma of the bladder: a report from the Intergroup Rhabdomyosarcoma Study. *J Pediatr Surg* 1990;25: 719–723.

91. Raney RB Jr, Gehan EA, Hays DM, et al. Primary chemotherapy with or without radiation therapy and/or surgery for children with localized sarcoma of the bladder, prostate, vagina, uterus, and cervix. A comparison of the results in Intergroup Rhabdomyosarcoma Studies I and II. *Cancer* 1990;66: 2072–2081.

92. Heyn R, Newton WA, Raney RB, et al. Preservation of the bladder in patients with rhabdomyosarcoma. *J Clin Oncol* 1997;15:69–75.

93. Raney B Jr, Heyn R, Hays DM, et al. Sequelae of treatment in 109 patients followed for 5 to 15 years after diagnosis of sarcoma of the bladder and prostate. A report from the Intergroup Rhabdomyosarcoma Study Committee. *Cancer* 1993;71:2387–2394.

94. Raney RB Jr, Tefft M, Lawrence W Jr, et al. Paratesticular sarcoma in childhood and adolescence. A report from the Intergroup Rhabdomyosarcoma Studies I and II, 1973–1983. *Cancer* 1987;60:2337–2343.

95. Wiener ES, Lawrence W, Hays D, et al. Retroperitoneal node biopsy in paratesticular rhabdomyosarcoma. *J Pediatr Surg* 1994;29:171–177; discussion 178.

*96. Ferrari A, Bisogno G, Casanova M, et al. Paratesticular rhabdomyosarcoma: report from the Italian and German Cooperative Group. *J Clin Oncol* 2002;20: 449–455.

97. Ferrari A, Casanova M, Massimino M, et al. The management of paratesticular rhabdomyosarcoma: a single institutional experience with 44 consecutive children. *J Urol* 1998;159:1031–1034.

98. Hays DM, Shimada H, Raney RB Jr, et al. Clinical staging and treatment results in rhabdomyosarcoma of the female genital tract among children and adolescents. *Cancer* 1988;61:1893–1903.

*99. Friedman M, Peretz BA, Nissenbaum M, et al. Modern treatment of vaginal embryonal rhabdomyosarcoma. *Obstet Gynecol Surv* 1986;41:614–618.

100. Andrassy RJ, Hays DM, Raney RB, et al. Conserva-

tive surgical management of vaginal and vulvar pediatric rhabdomyosarcoma: a report from the Intergroup Rhabdomyosarcoma Study III. *J Pediatr Surg* 1995;30:1034–1036; discussion 1036–1037.

101. Arndt CA, Donaldson SS, Anderson JR, et al. What constitutes optimal therapy for patients with rhabdomyosarcoma of the female genital tract? *Cancer* 2001;91:2454–2468.

*102. Hays DM, Shimada H, Raney RB Jr, et al. Sarcomas of the vagina and uterus: the Intergroup Rhabdomyosarcoma Study. *J Pediatr Surg* 1985;20: 718–724.

*103. Brand E, Berek JS, Nieberg RK, et al. Rhabdomyosarcoma of the uterine cervix. Sarcoma botryoides. *Cancer* 1987;60:1552–1560.

104. Corpron CA, Andrassy RJ, Hays DM, et al. Conservative management of uterine pediatric rhabdomyosarcoma: a report from the Intergroup Rhabdomyosarcoma Study III and IV pilot. *J Pediatr Surg* 1995;30:942–944.

105. Heyn R, Beltangady M, Hays D, et al. Results of intensive therapy in children with localized alveolar extremity rhabdomyosarcoma: a report from the Intergroup Rhabdomyosarcoma Study. *J Clin Oncol* 1989;7:200–207.

106. Lawrence W Jr, Hays DM, Heyn R, et al. Surgical lessons from the Intergroup Rhabdomyosarcoma Study (IRS) pertaining to extremity tumors. *World J Surg* 1988;12:676–684.

107. Neville HL, Raney RB, Andrassy RJ, et al. Multidisciplinary management of pediatric soft-tissue sarcoma. *Oncology (Huntingt)* 2000;14:1471–1481; discussion 1482–1486, 1489–1490.

108. Neville HL, Andrassy RJ, Lally KP, et al. Lymphatic mapping with sentinel node biopsy in pediatric patients. *J Pediatr Surg* 2000;35:961–964.

109. Tefft M, Fernandez C, Donaldson M, et al. Incidence of meningeal involvement by rhabdomyosarcoma of the head and neck in children: a report of the Intergroup Rhabdomyosarcoma Study (IRS). *Cancer* 1978;42:253–258.

110. Gasparini M, Lombardi F, Gianni MC, et al. Questionable role of CNS radioprophylaxis in the therapeutic management of childhood rhabdomyosarcoma with meningeal extension. *J Clin Oncol* 1990;8: 1854–1857.

111. Raney RB, Meza J, Anderson JR, et al. Treatment of children and adolescents with localized parameningeal sarcoma: experience of the Intergroup Rhabdomyosarcoma Study Group protocols IRS-II through -IV, 1978–1997. *Med Pediatr Oncol* 2002; 38:22–32.

112. Blatt J, Snyderman C, Wollman MR, et al. Delayed resection in the management of non-orbital rhabdomyosarcoma of the head and neck in childhood. *Med Pediatr Oncol* 1997;28:294–298.

113. Benk V, Rodary C, Donaldson SS, et al. Parameningeal rhabdomyosarcoma: results of an international workshop. *Int J Radiat Oncol Biol Phys* 1996;36:533–540.

*114. Hawkins DS, Anderson JR, Paidas CN, et al. Improved outcome for patients with middle ear rhabdomyosarcoma: a Children's Oncology Group study. *J Clin Oncol* 2001;19:3073–3079.

115. Pappo AS, Meza JL, Donaldson SS, et al. Treatment of localized nonorbital, nonparameningeal head and neck rhabdomyosarcoma: lessons learned from Intergroup Rhabdomyosarcoma Studies III and IV. *J Clin Oncol* 2003;21:638–645.

116. Heyn R, Ragab A, Raney RB Jr, et al. Late effects of therapy in orbital rhabdomyosarcoma in children. A report from the Intergroup Rhabdomyosarcoma Study. *Cancer* 1986;57:1738–1743.

117. Raney RB Jr, Ragab AH, Ruymann FB, et al. Soft-tissue sarcoma of the trunk in childhood. Results of the intergroup rhabdomyosarcoma study. *Cancer* 1982;49:2612–2616.

118. Ortega JA, Wharam M, Gehan EA, et al. Clinical features and results of therapy for children with paraspinal soft tissue sarcoma: a report of the Intergroup Rhabdomyosarcoma Study. *J Clin Oncol* 1991;9:796–801.

119. Crist WM, Raney RB, Tefft M, et al. Soft tissue sarcomas arising in the retroperitoneal space in children. A report from the Intergroup Rhabdomyosarcoma Study (IRS) Committee. *Cancer* 1985;56:2125–2132.

120. Raney RB Jr, Crist W, Hays D, et al. Soft tissue sarcoma of the perineal region in childhood. A report from the Intergroup Rhabdomyosarcoma Studies I and II, 1972–1984. *Cancer* 1990;65:2787–2792.

121. Spunt SL, Lobe TE, Pappo AS, et al. Aggressive surgery is unwarranted for biliary tract rhabdomyosarcoma. *J Pediatr Surg* 2000;35:309–316.

122. Pappo AS, Anderson JR, Crist WM, et al. Survival after relapse in children and adolescents with rhabdomyosarcoma: a report from the Intergroup Rhabdomyosarcoma Study Group. *J Clin Oncol* 1999;17: 3487–3493.

123. Miser JS, Kinsella TJ, Triche TJ, et al. Ifosfamide with mesna uroprotection and etoposide: an effective regimen in the treatment of recurrent sarcomas and other tumors of children and young adults. *J Clin Oncol* 1987;5:1191–1198.

124. Saylors RL III, Stine KC, Sullivan J, et al. Cyclophosphamide plus topotecan in children with recurrent or refractory solid tumors: a Pediatric Oncology Group phase II study. *J Clin Oncol* 2001;19: 3463–3469.

125. Weigel BJ, Breitfeld PP, Hawkins D, et al. Role of high-dose chemotherapy with hematopoietic stem cell rescue in the treatment of metastatic or recurrent rhabdomyosarcoma. *J Pediatr Hematol Oncol* 2001; 23:272–276.

126. Geary ES, Gong MC, Shortliffe LM. Biology and treatment of pediatric genitourinary tumors. *Curr Opin Oncol* 1994;6:292–300.

127. Fryer CJ. Pelvic rhabdomyosarcoma: paying the price of bladder preservation. *Lancet* 1995;345:141–142.

128. Heij HA, Vos A, de Kraker J, et al. Urogenital rhabdomyosarcoma in children: is a conservative surgical approach justified? *J Urol* 1993;150:165–168.

129. Lobe TE, Wiener E, Andrassy RJ, et al. The argument for conservative, delayed surgery in the management of prostatic rhabdomyosarcoma. *J Pediatr Surg* 1996;31:1084–1087.

130. Yeung CK, Ward HC, Ransley PG, et al. Bladder and kidney function after cure of pelvic rhabdomyosarcoma in childhood. *Br J Cancer* 1994;70:1000–1003.

12

Soft Tissue Sarcomas Other Than Rhabdomyosarcoma; Desmoid Tumor

Edward C. Halperin, M.D.

The word *sarcoma* is derived from the Greek word *sarkoma* meaning a fleshy excrescence (1). Soft tissue sarcomas are defined as all malignant tumors of nonepithelial, extraskeletal tissues including the peripheral and autonomic nervous system but excluding the hematopoietic system, glia, and supporting tissues of specific organs and viscera. Soft tissue sarcomas constitute approximately 6.5–7% of childhood cancer. Within this 6.5–7%, approximately one-half are rhabdomyosarcoma (2–4). Therefore, nonrhabdomyosarcoma soft tissue sarcoma (NRSTS) constitutes 3–3.5% of childhood cancers (5).

For most children with NRSTS, the origin of the tumor is unknown. Some cases may be traced to prior radiation exposure (see Chapter 20), chemical exposure, iatrogenic or disease-caused immunosuppression, and neurofibromatosis (NF), with the latter group having a 7–10% lifetime risk of developing malignant neurofibrosarcoma. The association of sarcomas with neurofibromatosis indicates that some sarcomas are associated with chromosomal deletions and translocations and the presence of abnormalities of tumor suppressor genes. Homozygous gene deletions occur in both the long and short arms of chromosome 17 in neurofibromatosis type 1. Candidate tumor suppressor genes include 17q11 (the NF tumor suppressor gene) and p53 (17p13) (2). Rhabdomyosarcoma and NRSTS also occur as part of the familial Li–Fraumeni syndrome.

PATHOLOGY

The frequency of the different histologic subgroups of NRSTS of childhood varies between reporting institutions (Table 12-1). These differences may be attributable to variations in referral patterns and to the small numbers in each series. In addition, NRSTSs often are difficult for pathologists to classify, and there is wide intraobserver variation (6). In an M. D. Anderson Hospital series of sarcomas of the head and neck in children and adolescents, histologic diagnoses were changed in 22% of patients (7). Several other studies have assessed discrepancy rates between the original diagnosis of soft tissue tumors and the diagnosis made by expert reviewers when patients are referred to specialty centers for entry in therapeutic trials. About 5–10% of cases having the original diagnosis of sarcoma are revised to nonsarcoma, and for 16–32% of patients with a sarcoma, the histologic subtype is revised. Where grade was analyzed, there was disagreement in up to 40% of the cases (8). For example, malignant fibrous histiocytoma (MFH) was first described as a separate entity in the 1960s. General recognition of this tumor's existence, distinct from other classifications, followed. Therefore, the reported incidence of MFH in adults sharply increased while that of fibrosarcoma fell (9). MFH is unusual in childhood.

Many of the childhood NRSTSs have characteristic cell types (Table 12-2). *Neurogenic sarcoma* is also known as neurofibrosarcoma, malignant peripheral nerve sheath tumor (PNST), malignant schwannoma, or malignant neurilemmoma. It is a malignant neoplasm that arises in a peripheral nerve sheath. In children, from one-fifth to two-thirds of cases of neurogenic sarcoma are associated with NF (10–12). The morphology is characterized by fascicles of spindle cells with a herringbone or storiform pattern.

TABLE 12-1. *The most common types of childhood nonrhabdomyosarcoma soft tissue sarcoma in recent clinical series*[a]

Histology	St. Jude Children's Research Hospital[b] (4,73,156)	Harvard Joint Center for Radiation Therapy[c] (25)	Children's Hospital of Philadelphia (146)	Baylor/Texas Children's Hospital (5)	Children's Hospital and Medical Center Seattle (2)	M. D. Anderson Hospital Head and Neck Sarcomas (7)	SEER[e] Data (35)	Italian Cooperative Study of Childhood Soft Tissue Sarcoma (147)	Pediatric Oncology Group (148)	Rambam Medical Center (37)	Mayo Clinic (21)
Primitive neuroectodermal tumor and extraosseous Ewing's and Askin's tumor	11%/**18%**	**30%**	**38%**	**32%**	**40%**			**36%**		5%	
Neurogenic sarcoma and neurofibrosarcoma	**28%**/15%		10%	9%			10%	15%	10%	2%	2%
Synovial sarcoma	6%/12%	16%	10%	6%	10%	17%	10%	14%	**42%**	16%	**36%**
Alveolar soft part sarcoma			2%	2%		4%		2%		7%	5%
Sarcoma not otherwise specified		14%	2%	30%		**26%**	15%	8%			
Malignant fibrous histiocytoma	14%/12%	11%	15%			4%		4%	12%	5%	13%
Hemangiopericytoma	—/4%				2%				5%	2%	1%
Liposarcoma	—/4%			2%				1%		2%	3%
Dermatofibrosarcoma protuberans					[d]	4%		5%			1%
Fibrosarcoma	11%	9%	18%	4%	20%	17%	**48%**	14%	13%	**33%**	15%
Mixed mesenchymoma	—/8%		2%	6%							
Angiosarcoma and hemangiosarcoma			2%			4%		3%		<2%	
Epithelioid sarcoma	5%/8%		8%					2%		<2%	12%
Extrarenal rhabdoid sarcoma	—/8%							3%			
Clear cell sarcoma	5%/8%							1%	4%		8%
Leiomyosarcoma								1%		5%	2%
Other	20%/16%		20%		4%				12%		2%

[a] In each series, the most common histologic types are indicated by bold type.

[b] The number to the left of the slash is the number of surgically resectable patients; to the right are patients with metastatic disease.

[c] This series does not include children with metastatic disease.

[d] This series combines dermatofibrosarcoma protuberans with fibrosarcoma.

[e] Survival, epidemiology, and end results.

TABLE 12-2. *Cells of origin of nonrhabdomyosarcoma soft tissue sarcoma of childhood*

Cell of origin	Sarcoma
Fat	Liposarcoma
Blood and lymphatic vessels	Angiosarcoma, hemangiopericytoma
Fibroblasts	Fibrosarcoma, malignant fibrous histiocytoma
Smooth muscle	Leiomyosarcoma
Nervous tissue	Malignant peripheral nerve sheath tumor
Synovial	Synovial sarcoma
Chondrocytic	Extraskeletal chondrosarcoma
Epithelial	Epithelioid sarcoma
Melanocytes	Clear cell sarcoma of tendons and aponeuroses
Myofibroblasts	Myofibrosarcoma

Based on Pappo AS, Parham DM, Rao BN, et al. Soft tissue sarcomas in children. *Semin Surg Oncol* 1999;16:121–143.

One may observe evidence of schwannian differentiation (13). There can be areas of significant nuclear hyperchromatism and abundant mitotic figures (14). These tumors usually are positive for S-100, vimentin, and neuron-specific enolase. In about 2–16% of patients with NF type 1 (NF1), nodular and plexiform neurofibromas transform to malignant peripheral nerve sheath tumors. NF1 is transmitted as an autosomal dominant with variable penetrance. However, almost 50% of cases are sporadic mutations (1). People with NF1 are 1.2 times more likely to have a malignant neoplasm listed on their death certificates than those who do not have the disease. These include malignant PNST, optic gliomas, and pheochromocytomas (15). NF is also called von Recklinghausen's disease. Friedrich von Recklinghausen (1833–1910) was born in Guterslah, Westphalia, Germany, and studied medicine at the Universities of Bonn, Wurzburg, and Berlin. He was a professor in Konigsberg, Wurzburg, and Strasbourg.

Biphasic *synovial sarcoma,* the more common type, also has spindle-shaped cells. These are mixed with oval and keratin-positive epithelial cells. Pseudoglandular spaces or slits and clefts mimic synovium (16–18). About one-third of synovial sarcomas in children are the monophasic type (19). About two-thirds of cases involve the lower extremity and one-third the upper. Synovial sarcomas differ from other NRSTSs in that they have a significant risk of lymph node metastases (19,20). The monophasic type may have a better prognosis, but this is debatable (21,22). Synovial sarcomas commonly have a t(x;18)(p 11.2;q11.2) translocation that may result in two different fusion genes (SYT-SSX1 and SYT-SSX2). The type of fusion gene correlates with histologic subtype and clinical behavior. In a recent small series, the SYT-SSX1 fusion was associated with a 42% 5-year metastasis-free survival, compared with 89% for the SYT-SSX2. The SYT-SSX1 fusion is also associated with a higher cell proliferation rate as assessed by Ki-67 staining (23).

Liposarcomas originate from primitive mesenchymal cells rather than from mature adipose tissue. Some have a myxoid appearance, whereas others resemble benign lipomas. The pleomorphic type may resemble fibroblastic, myoblastic, or synovial sarcoma. *Angiosarcoma* should always be considered high grade with an aggressive behavior, a high rate of local recurrence, a propensity to metastasize, and a poor prognosis (24).

Leiomyosarcoma originates from smooth muscle. The well-differentiated lesions usually have a centrally located blunt-ended nucleus ("cigar-shaped").

Fibrosarcoma is an infiltrative, fibrous neoplasm composed of interlocking bundles of spindle cells (25,26). The tumor usually stains positive for vimentin (19). There are two clinically different forms of fibrosarcoma in children. One is a lesion appearing in the first 5 years of life with a low rate of distant spread. This type of fibrosarcoma, called the congenital type, is generally treated by excision (2,6,25). In children younger than 5 years of age this tumor may also be called infantile fibrosarcoma. The other occurs in children older than 5 years of age and has a more ominous prognosis with behavior similar to that of adult forms (26). This classic or adult-type fibrosarcoma is treated according to the principles outlined for other NRSTSs. Infantile fibrosarcoma has a rapid initial growth but generally indolent behavior. Local recurrence is common, metastases are rare, spontaneous regressions have been reported, and radiotherapy is rarely used. Infantile and adult fibrosarcoma are histologically identical. There is no routine microscopic, immunohisto-chemical, or ultrastructural way of distinguishing the two clinical types (27). *Low-grade fibromyxoid sarcoma* is an indolent tumor that rarely occurs in children. It consists of spindle and stellate cells with uniform nuclei arranged in a whorled pattern with alternating areas of fibrous and myxoid stroma (28). *Malignant fibrous histiocytomas* are pleomorphic sarcomas often characterized by a whorled growth pattern. They are thought to arise from histiocytic cells acting as facultative fibroblasts. *Hemangiopericytomas* arise from pericytes, the modified smooth muscle cell with contractile function located on the internal surface of venous capillaries and postcapillary venules (29). The *malignant mesenchymoma* has two or more cell types, any of which, taken by itself, might be considered a malignant neoplasm (30,31).

There are several childhood NRSTSs that have a characteristic microscopic picture, but the cell of origin is uncertain. The *epithelioid sarcoma* is a tumor of the subcutaneous tissue, tendons, and fascia, usually of the upper extremity, including the hand (29). There is a nodular arrangement of plump, polygonal to round, epithelioid cells interspersed with spindle-shaped cells (32,33). Central degeneration or necrosis is often present. The tumor tends to spread within fascial planes or aponeuroses and may grow along the neurovascular bundle and encroach on large vessels or nerves. Regional lymph node metastasis may occur in association with high-grade tumors and tumors larger than 5 cm (32). The tumor generally stains positive for keratin.

Alveolar soft part sarcomas have a characteristic crystalline material seen with periodic acid–Schiff (PAS) stain (34,35). The tumor tests positive for vimentin on immunohistochemistry. The tumor cells typically have an organoid or nestlike arrangement. Vascular invasion is always seen. Of 11 children with alveolar soft part sarcoma seen at St. Jude Children's Research Hospital in a 32-year period, six had localized disease and five had unresectable or metastatic disease. Recent cytogenetic studies indicate that 17q25 abnormalities are common (35). In 19 patients seen in Italy, four had metastatic disease at presentation. The 5-year survival for all 19 patients was 80% (36). A slow doubling time of the tumor may explain its very late occurrences (sometimes more than 10 years) (37).

Extraskeletal Ewing's sarcoma and *peripheral primitive neuroectodermal tumor* (PNET) are characterized by cohesive, uniform, small hyperchromatic cells in a fibrous background. Dense clumping of chromatin, mitotic figures, and rosette formation are typical of PNET. On immunohistochemistry analysis, extraosseous Ewing's sarcomas are generally positive for vimentin and HBA-17. PNET is generally positive for neuron-specific enolase and other neuron-related markers such as S-100 protein, neurofilament, or HNK-1. Both PNET and extraosseous Ewing's sarcoma are associated with a particular chromosome translocation t(11;22)(q24;q12). The progenitor cell for these two small, round, blue cell NRSTSs is not established. They may arise from neural crest, primordial germ cells, or perhaps mesenchymal stem cells (2,38). When PNET or extraosseous Ewing's sarcoma arises in the thoracic cavity it is called *Askin's tumor*.

Desmoplastic small, round, blue cell tumor is a rare intraperitoneal malignancy occurring predominantly in adolescent boys (Fig. 12-1). It is characterized by a reciprocal translocation t(11;12)(p13;q12) associated with the EWS-WT1 gene fusion transcript. Cells often stain positive for desmin, keratin, and neuron-specific enolase. The predominant pattern of relapse is intraperitoneal. Patients generally are treated with surgical debulking, alkylator chemotherapy, and whole abdomen irradiation or intra-abdominal P32. The relapse-free survival rate is approximately 20% (39,40). *Clear cell sarcoma* is characterized by ovoid or polygonal cells with abundant clear cytoplasm, indistinct borders, large nucleoli, and abundant intracytoplasmic glycogen. Immunocytochemistry often is positive for S-100 protein, neuron-specific enolase, and melanocyte-associated antigen HMB-45. A specific chromosomal translocation t(12;22)(q13;q12) involving the DNA tran-

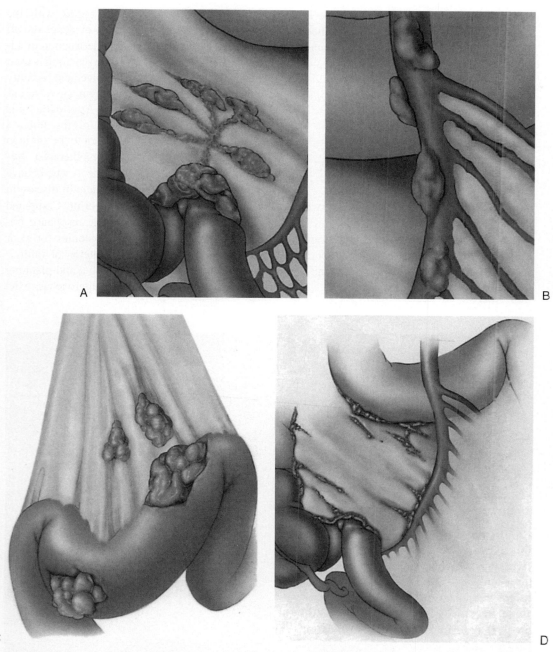

FIG. 12-1. The four major patterns of mesenteric tumor spread are **(A)** along the mesenteric vessels and surrounding fat, **(B)** extension via the mesenteric lymphotics, **(C)** embolic hematogenous spread, and **(D)** intraperitoneal seeding. (From Sheth S, Horton KM, Garland MR, and Fishman EK. Mesenteric neoplasms: CT appearances of primary and secondary tumors and differential diagnosis. *RadioGraphics* 2003;23:457–473, with permission.)

scription factors ATF-1 on chromosome 12 and the EWS gene on chromosome 22 has been described in 60–75% of clear cell sarcoma cases (41,42).

A fair proportion of NRSTSs show no cellular differentiation. These are called *undifferentiated sarcomas* or *sarcomas not otherwise specified*.

PRESENTATION, WORKUP, AND STAGING

Most NRSTSs present as a painless swelling. NRSTS may also present with signs and symptoms of vascular compression, neurologic impairment from nerve compression, or bowel dysfunction when tumors arise from the retroperitoneum.

The radiographic workup begins with the plain radiograph. One looks for evidence of soft tissue mass, calcification, and destruction of adjacent bone. Radionuclide bone scanning is used to assess metastatic bone involvement, activity in bone adjacent to the tumor, and active vascular activity in the tumor itself. Arteriography is advocated for its delineation of the tumor's blood supply, a matter of concern to the surgeon or to the direct infusional chemotherapist. Xeroradiography has a few proponents who believe that its outline of soft tissue extent of disease in the neck or extremities is superior. Computed tomography (CT) and magnetic resonance imaging (MRI) are the essential studies for clear definition of tumor extent, patterns of infiltration, evaluation of adjacent bone, and planning surgical and radiotherapeutic approaches. MRI

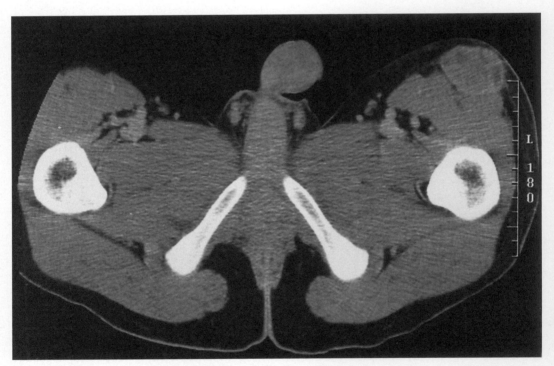

FIG. 12-2. This 17-year-old white boy presented with a 7-month history of a mass, noted on self-examination, of the left thigh. The mass eventually grew to 4 cm in size. Magnetic resonance imaging demonstrated a mass without involvement of bone. Positron emission tomography showed increased metabolic activity. On pathology, the tumor was "hypercellular highly vascularized neoplastic proliferation of generally small round to oval nuclei with evenly distributed chromatin and small nucleoli. Immunohistochemical stains are positive for vimentin, negative for leukocyte antigen; most consistent with extra skeletal Ewing's sarcoma/primitive neuroectodermal tumor." The patient was treated with tumor excision, involved-field irradiation, and systemic chemotherapy.

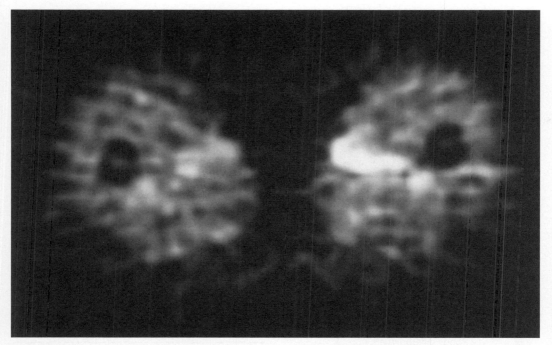

FIG. 12-3. A positron emission tomography scan showing increased metabolic activity in a limb primitive neuroectodermal tumor.

often shows a larger area of involvement than does CT (Fig. 12-2). The evaluation for distant metastasis focuses on the most common site, the lungs, with chest radiograph and thoracic CT scanning (11,12,43–46). Metabolic scanning techniques, such as thallium scans and positron emission tomography (PET), are being used with increasing frequency. Fluorine-1-fluorode-oxyglucose PET measures glucose utilization rate in sarcomas and may be used to assess lesion grade and to monitor neoadjuvant therapeutic response (Fig. 12-3) (47).

NRSTS in childhood may be staged by one of two systems. Some investigators use the rhabdomyosarcoma grouping system, although their number is shrinking (see Table 11-2 in Chapter 11). This system is convenient and relies on surgical resectability as an important prognostic factor. There is no doubt that tumor size and resectability are important in predicting outcome in NRSTS of children. However, the histologic tumor grade is also important and is not directly considered in the rhabdomyosarcoma grouping system (6,48–50). Sarcoma grade assessment

incorporates pleomorphism, spontaneous necrosis, and number of typical and atypical mitoses per ten high-power fields. In the 1940s, Broders and colleagues at the Mayo Clinic developed a grading system for sarcomas based on the degree of nuclear atypia. In 1969, the American Joint Commission (AJC) on Cancer Staging described a staging system for soft tissue sarcoma that uses grade, tumor size, nodal involvement, and presence of metastases as the determinants of stage (Table 12-3). In the AJC system, grade is determined by evaluation of the degree of cellularity, cellular anaplasia or pleomorphism, mitotic activity, expansive or infiltrative growth, and necrosis (33).

Histologic grading is an important way to predict the outcome of NRSTS. There are various strategies for grading. One system, developed by the Pediatric Oncology Group (POG), labeled grade 1 as tumor that has little propensity for malignancy. Grade 2 tumors are those with fewer than five mitoses per ten high-powered fields or less than 15% geographic necrosis, and grade 3 tumors are those known

TABLE 12-3. *The American Joint Committee staging system for sarcoma of soft tissue[a]*

T: Primary tumor		
Tx	Primary tumor cannot be assessed	
T0	No evidence of primary tumor	
T1	Tumor less than 5 cm in greatest dimension	
T1a	Superficial tumor[a]	
T1b	Deep tumor[a]	
T2	Tumor more than 5 cm in greatest dimension	
T2a	Superficial tumor[a]	
T2b	Deep tumor[a]	
N: Regional lymph nodes		
Nx	Regional lymph nodes cannot be assessed	
N0	No regional lymph node metastasis	
N1	Regional lymph nodes metastasis	
M: Distant metastasis		
MX	Distant metastasis cannot be assessed	
M0	No distant metastasis	
M1	Distant metastasis	
G: Histopathologic grading		
Gx	Grade cannot be assessed	
G1	Well differentiated	
G2	Poorly differentiated	
G4	Poorly differentiated or undifferentiated (four-tiered systems only)	
Stage[b]		
Stage I1	G1 T1a–2b N0M0	
Stage II1	G2–3 T1a–2a N0M0	
Stage III	G2–3 T2B N0M0	
Stage IV	Any G, any T, N1, or M1	

[a]Superficial, above superficial fascia without invasion of the fascia; Deep, located either beneath the superficial fascia or superficial to the fascia with invasion of or through the fascia. Retroperitoneal, mediastinal, and pelvic sarcomas are classified as deep.

[b]In a four-tier system, I is G1–2, II G3–4, III is G3–4. From Greene FL Page, DL, Fleming, ID, et al., eds. *AJCC cancer staging manual,* 6th ed. New York: Springer-Verlag, 2002, with permission.

TABLE 12-4. *Grading pediatric nonrhabdomyosarcoma soft tissue sarcomas (NRSTSs)*

Grade	
1	Liposarcoma: myxoid and well differentiated
	Deep-seated dermatofibrosarcoma protuberans
	Fibrosarcoma: well differentiated or infantile (<5 yr)
	Hemangiopericytoma: well differentiated or infantile (<5 yr)
	Well-differentiated malignant peripheral nerve sheath tumor
	Angiomatoid malignant fibrous histiocytoma
2	All NRSTSs not in grades 1 or 3; <15% of tumor shows geographic necrosis, or mitotic index is <5 mitoses/10 high-power fields
3	Fibrosarcoma with >15% of tumor with geographic necrosis or mitotic index >5 mitoses/10 high-power fields
	Liposarcoma: pleomorphic, round cell
	Mesenchymal chondrosarcoma
	Extraskeletal osteosarcoma
	Malignant triton tumor
	Alveolar soft part sarcoma

Based on Pappo AS, Parham DM, Rao BN, et al. Soft tissue sarcomas in children. *Semin Surg Oncol* 1999;16:121–143.

to be clinically aggressive by virtue of histologic diagnosis and with more than four mitoses per ten high-powered fields or more than 15% geographic necrosis (Table 12-4) (51). One review of this POG grading system found a 73% mortality in grade 3 lesions and 15% mortality in grade 1 and 2 tumors (52).

Frequency of distant metastases increases and the survival probability decreases with increasing size of the primary tumor (49). About 15% of patients have metastatic disease at presentation (2).

SELECTION OF THERAPY

Surgery

Every biopsy should be planned to be consistent with the treatment plan. The two techniques for the biopsy are either via needle or open incisional. Needle biopsy techniques include fine-needle aspiration (of variable accuracy and dependent on the experience of the cytopathologist) or core needle biopsy (2). The incision for an open incisional biopsy should be small (the minimum that is technically feasible), and homeostasis should be secure. Incisions on the extremity should be in the long axis (46). Muscle compartments should not be crossed; one does not want to contaminate adjacent areas with tumor. The biopsy should be placed so that the entire surgical tract will be removed at the time of the definitive operation.

Complete surgical excision is the mainstay of therapy. NRSTS may infiltrate widely. Sarcomas tend to expand and infiltrate adjoining tissue spaces, producing a pseudocapsule made up of compressed normal tissue intermingled with microscopic extensions of the tumor. A system for assessing the adequacy of surgical margins in sarcoma surgery was described by Enneking et al. (53). An intralesional surgical margin is through tumor, with gross or microscopic contamination. A margin resection is through the reactive or inflammatory zone. A wide excision is through normal tissue outside the inflammatory zone. A radical excision is outside the anatomic compartment containing the tumor. A wide excision or amputation often is needed to obtain the microscopic-free margin needed for control. Clinical experience, primarily in adults, has shown that the local failure rate for simple excision of malignant soft tissue sarcomas is 60–90% (11,12,43). This failure rate falls to 18–30% when simple excision is replaced by radical resection, radical compartmental resection, or amputation above the proximal joint (4,6,46,54–57). In a pediatric series, the 5-year survival rate was higher for complete tumor excision than for partial excision (37). For low-grade lesions, wide excision with negative margins may be curative as the sole treatment (5,55).

There are some patients for whom limb-sparing treatments may be considered (56–60). Limb-sparing surgery removes a soft tissue sarcoma while preserving the extremity with a satisfactory functional and cosmetic result. To achieve results comparable to those of radical procedures, most limb-sparing procedures involve the planned use of preoperative or postoperative external beam irradiation, brachytherapy, or intra-arterial or systemic chemotherapy. Limb-sparing is clearly not appropriate for some patients. These patients include young children who may deal with an amputation better than with the limb-length discrepancy that may occur with limb-sparing procedures, those with extremity lesions where it is not possible to acquire adequate surgical margins and where radiotherapy may produce major long-term complications, those with lesions that involve major vessels or nerves where resection will severely compromise function, and those in whom a fracture has resulted from tumor and the limb is use-

less and painful (54,60). Simply put, in the skeletally immature patient, due consideration must be given to the possibility that inappropriate or incorrectly administered radiotherapy may produce a stiff, painful, shortened, or disfigured extremity and engender a risk of second malignant neoplasm. Therefore, in some situations amputation may be preferred.

The role of regional node dissection in NRSTS is evolving. Overall, the incidence of nodal involvement is about 4%, ranging from close to 0% for grade 1 to 12% for grade 3 (4,61). It is reasonable to biopsy enlarged regional nodes in high-grade primary tumors.

Surgery also plays a role in managing NRSTS in the treatment of pulmonary metastases. With proper patient selection, long-term survival is possible for those undergoing removal of pulmonary metastases. Preoperative evaluation with chest radiograph and thoracic CT scanning is performed to determine the number and location of the metastases. Tumor may be resected via a median sternotomy or lateral thoracotomy, generally with double-lumen endotracheal anesthesia. Two studies in the literature, both of which included adult and pediatric patients, evaluated the important prognostic factors predicting survival after pulmonary metastasectomy. Higher survival rates appear to be associated with complete resection of all metastases, the presence of few lesions (i.e., one to three), and a long disease-free interval before the development of metastases. Patients rendered free of disease in the series of Jablons et al. (62) had a median survival of 26.8 months. A similar group in the series of Casson et al. (63) had a median survival of 28 months. It is only fair to note that there are no randomized series in the literature comparing surgery with observation or with chemotherapy without resection. Therefore, it cannot be proven that the apparent prolongation of survival after surgery is attributable to the surgical therapy as opposed to good tumor biology (62).

Radiotherapy

We have previously noted that the local control rate for NRSTS increases as the extent of surgical resection increases. This is undoubtedly be-

cause more radical surgery extirpates microscopic extension of tumor. It is well known that
radiation can also sterilize microscopic extensions of tumor (64). We may infer that radiation
can be used to accomplish that which is
achieved by increasing the extent of surgery
(46). The judicious combination of limited surgery and radiotherapy should be able to achieve
local control rates equivalent to those of radical
surgery, with a superior functional result in
many cases. Most of the available data support
this line of reasoning (46,59,64–66).

POG protocol 8653 was designed to study the
role of adjuvant chemotherapy in children with
resectable NRSTS (67). Local therapy was standardized to include surgery only for patients
with wide or radical margins and surgery with
postoperative irradiation for marginal excisions.
Protocol guidelines were imperfectly followed.
The results, shown in Table 12-5, indicate higher
local control rates with radiotherapy for marginal excisions in high-grade tumors (68). There
will be situations in which radical surgery is not
recommended for children or is recommended
and declined because of unacceptable functional,
cosmetic, emotional, or psychological consequences. Radiotherapy may play a crucial role
for these patients by allowing more conservative
surgery with equivalent rates of local control.

In retrospective reviews of adult patients with
NRSTS, treatment with conservative surgery and
postoperative irradiation for microscopic extension of tumor yields local failure rates of
10–20%, comparable to those of radical surgery
(46,56,57). In an analysis of 132 patients, largely
adults, treated with preoperative radiation and
conservative resection at the Massachusetts Gen-

eral Hospital, the local control results were 97%
for patients with negative surgical margins and
82% for those with positive margins (68). In a
series confined to children, the local control rate
for patients who had no or microscopic residual
disease after surgery and who were treated with
postoperative irradiation was 79% (25). Tumor
grade and size are the most important predictors
of local failure in these series. The randomized
prospective National Cancer Institute (NCI) trial,
including adults and children, compared limb-
sparing surgery and postoperative irradiation
with amputation. The 5-year disease-free survival rate for the limb-spared group was 69%
and was 72% for the amputated group ($p = 0.7$).
The local failure rate was higher in the limb conservation group, and several patients had to undergo salvage surgery (57,69). Psychological
tests indicate that the amputees fared as well as
those having limb-sparing surgery (70). In addition to survival as an endpoint, one should also
consider the functional outcome of limb-sparing
surgery with radiotherapy for NRSTS. A retrospective review of a large number of NCI patients who underwent limb-sparing surgery with
radiotherapy for extremity NRSTS indicates that
the most common long-term complications are
contracture, limb edema, decreased range of motion, and decreased muscle strength. Certain radiotherapy technical factors were associated
with a higher risk of complications: inclusion of
more than 50% of a joint in the portal, dosages
over the equivalent of 63 Gy at 1.8 Gy per fraction, and large portals that encompassed more
than 75% of the extremity diameter (71). Bertucio et al. (72) analyzed 30 patients with extremity sarcomas who were younger than 21 years

TABLE 12-5. *POG Protocol 8653: local control by surgical margins and radiotherapy*

		Low grade		High grade	
Surgical margins	IRS group	Surgery alone n (%)	Surgery + radiotherapy n (%)	Surgery alone n (%)	Surgery + radiotherapy n (%)
Marginal	II	2/2 (100%)	10/11 (91%)	1/4 (25%)	10/11 (91%)
Wide	I	18/18 (100%)	3/3 (100%)	14/16 (88%)	2/2 (100%)
Radical	I	1/1 (100%)	No data	6/6 (100%)	No data

Modified from Marcus RJ. Current controversies in pediatric radiation oncology. *Orthop Clin North Am* 1996;27:551–557, with permission.

old at diagnosis and received radiotherapy as part of a limb-sparing treatment. Of the 30 patients, 11 had NRSTS, eight rhabdomyosarcoma, and 11 Ewing's sarcoma. On follow-up 50% of the patients had no limitation of limb function and 40% had full function but had a mild limp or needed a shoe lift, compression device, or pins or rods.

Three retrospective reviews of the St. Jude Children's Research Hospital clinical experience with NRSTS, published in 1999–2000, considered the role of adjuvant radiotherapy (4,73–75). In completely resected disease (clinical group I), postoperative irradiation appeared to reduce local recurrences only in high-grade disease. In patients with positive surgical margins (clinical group II), radiotherapy reduced local recurrences (*p* = 0.001) (Table 12-6). Several retrospective reviews, confined to children, have suggested a role for postoperative irradiation of NRSTS. Radiotherapy has been used, in accordance with the standards of the Intergroup Rhabdomyosarcoma Study, in patients with group II (grossly complete tumor resection with microscopic residual disease or involved but completely resected regional nodes) and group III (incomplete resection with gross residual disease) NRSTS (3,11,12,25,43,50,69,76).

In conclusion, acceptable indications for radiotherapy in childhood NRSTS are localized, incompletely resected tumor with gross residual disease; palliation of metastasis (palliation of pain or compressive syndromes requires 35 to 50 Gy; however, radiotherapy is rarely effective for gross lung metastases) (4,54); as part of a planned limb-sparing procedure; and after an attempt at gross total tumor removal when there is microscopic residual tumor or positive regional lymph nodes.

Chemotherapy

The use of adjuvant chemotherapy in childhood NRSTS initially was defended on the basis of the significant risk of metastatic disease and local recurrence in high-grade lesions, retrospective comparisons, and the success of chemotherapy in rhabdomyosarcoma. The most active single agents are adriamycin and ifosfamide. Other active agents are dacarbazine, actinomycin D, vincristine, etoposide, and cyclophosphamide (4,6, 11,43,50,55,69,76–78). In this portion of the chapter we will review the most pertinent larger-scale studies.

Cooperative Group Studies of Chemotherapy and NRSTS Exclusive of PNET, Extraosseous Ewing's Sarcoma, and Askin's Tumor

POG protocols 8653 and 8654 were open to patients younger than 21 years old at diagnosis with any biopsy-proven soft tissue sarcoma other than rhabdomyosarcoma, extraosseous Ewing's sarcoma, or undifferentiated round cell sarcoma.

TABLE 12-6. *Factors affecting local relapse in NRSTS in the St. Jude Children's Research Hospital retrospective reviews*

Group	Grade	Margin	Radiotherapy	Local recurrence (%)	
I	Low	<1 cm	Yes	1/5 (20%)	
		<1 cm	No	1/5 (20%)	
		≥1 cm	No	2/44 (5%)	
	High	<1 cm	Yes	0/7 (0%)	
		<1 cm	No	3/7 (43%)	
		≥1 cm	No	4/20 (20%)	
II[a]	All	Positive	Yes	DNG/21	*p* = .001
		Positive	No	DNG/19	favoring RT
I–II[a]	All	Negative	Yes	DNG/31(31%)	*p* = .043
		Positive	No	DNG/90(16%)	

DNG, data not given; RT, radiation therapy.
[a]The trend favoring radiotherapy in groups I and II is the result of a likely benefit in high-grade, close margin group I and all group II.
From references 73 and 75.

Children who were treated with surgical resection with complete extirpation of tumor; surgical excision of the tumor with postoperative irradiation; or biopsy, preoperative irradiation, and secondary surgery obtaining complete resection were randomized to receive postoperative adjuvant vincristine, adriamycin, and cyclophosphamide (VAdrC) or observation. This randomization, constituting protocol 8653, would be analogous, were one to use the rhabdomyosarcoma grouping system for NRSTS, to randomizing patients in groups I–III, including those rendered resectable by radiation (67).

Protocol 8654 was for patients who were judged to have inoperable tumors or for those with metastatic disease. These patients were randomized to receive either VAdrC, or those three agents plus dacarbazine. Involved-field radiation was administered to the primary tumor site.

Study 8653 was open from June 1986 to May 1992. Study 8654 was open from June 1986 through April 1994. However, there was approximately a 1-year period in which all patients in

Study 8654 were treated with vincristine, actinomycin, and cyclophosphamide because of a shortage of dacarbazine.

There were 81 eligible patients for protocol 8653. Only 30 patients accepted randomization: 15 received chemotherapy, and 15 were observed. Of the remaining 51 patients, 19 elected adjuvant chemotherapy, and 32 elected observation. For the total group of 81 patients, the 5-year overall survival was 85%, and the event-free survival (EFS) was 72%. The 5-year EFS for randomization patients was 69% for the chemotherapy arm and 87% for the observation arm. A grade 3 tumor conferred a significant disadvantage with respect to EFS. The 3-year EFS for grade 3 was 75% and was 91% for grades 1 and 2 ($p = 0.018$). Therefore, there was no discernible benefit to the use of chemotherapy. For study 8654, the 4-year EFS for patients receiving vincristine, actinomycin D, cyclophosphamide, and adriamycin (VACA) was no different from that for the four drugs plus dacarbazine. The 4-year overall and EFS were 31% and 18%, respectively (Fig. 12-4) (4,79,80).

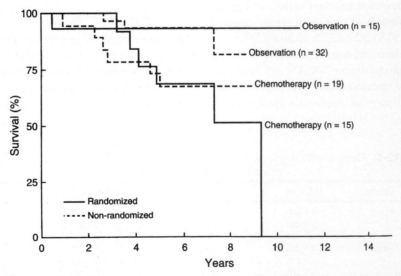

FIG. 12-4. Pediatric Oncology Group protocol 8653 randomized children with Intergroup Rhabdomyosarcoma Study group I–III nonrhabdomyosarcoma soft tissue sarcoma to observation or vincristine, cyclophosphamide, adriamycin, and actinomycin D. Of the 81 eligible patients, 15 were randomized to observation, 15 were randomized to chemotherapy, 19 elected chemotherapy, and 32 elected observation. The four survival curves show no benefit to chemotherapy. (From Pratt CB, Pappo AS, Gieser P, et al. Role of adjuvant chemotherapy in the treatment of surgically resected pediatric nonrhabdomyosarcomatous soft tissue sarcomas: a Pediatric Oncology Group study. *J Clin Oncol* 1999;17:1219–1226, with permission.)

The German soft tissue sarcoma study CWS-81 was initiated in 1981 under the auspices of the German Society of Pediatric Oncology. This study was open to children with rhabdomyosarcoma, undifferentiated sarcoma, extraosseous Ewing's sarcoma, synovial sarcoma, leiomyosarcoma, peripheral PNET, fibrosarcoma, hemangiosarcoma, neurofibrosarcoma, and liposarcoma. For the purposes of this chapter, we will confine our discussion to the results concerning NRSTS exclusive of extraosseous Ewing's sarcoma and PNET. Patients with localized disease, completely resected, received vincristine, actinomycin D, cyclophosphamide, and adriamycin. Patients with grossly resected tumor, microscopic residual disease, and no evidence of regional node involvement received the same chemotherapy but also had involved-field irradiation. These patients were then treated with vincristine, actinomycin D, and cyclophosphamide. Patients with grossly resected tumor with microscopic residual disease and regional nodal involvement or those with incomplete resection or biopsy with gross residual disease received four-drug chemotherapy initially. Those who were good responders continued on this chemotherapy and received involved-field irradiation; ultimately the adriamycin was dropped. Those who were poor initial responders received involved-field irradiation, but ifosfamide was substituted for cyclophosphamide. Patients who had stage IV disease received vincristine, actinomycin D, ifosfamide, and adriamycin. In 1984, ifosfamide was also added for patients with stage III disease who did not respond to preoperative chemotherapy. Detailed information is available concerning the 30 children and adolescents with synovial sarcomas treated on this study (81). A survival rate of 70% was observed, with a median observation time of 34 months. Patients with synovial sarcoma of the extremities had a disease-free survival rate of 88%. Six of eight patients who had their tumors resected with no residual disease are disease-free survivors, seven out of nine patients who had disease resected with microscopic residual are disease-free survivors, six of eight patients who have had their tumor resected with gross residual disease are disease-free survivors, and

three of five patients with metastatic disease at presentation (stage IV) were disease-free survivors. Obviously, the German study was not a head-to-head comparison of chemotherapy and observation, and it is not clear what the survival would have been if patients were treated with local therapy alone.

The International Society of Pediatric Oncology (SIOP) has conducted two protocols for NRSTS. The treatment program consisted of a primary complete tumor excision if feasible without mutilation. For patients who were not resectable initially, neoadjuvant chemotherapy was administered. Initial chemotherapy was ifosfamide, vincristine, and actinomycin D. Second-line chemotherapy on study MMT84 was cyclophosphamide and doxorubicin, and in study MMT89 it was epirubicin, doxorubicin, carboplatin, and VM26. Patients were then taken to surgery if possible. Radiotherapy was used for macroscopic residual tumor after surgery. For patients who had initial primary excision adjuvant chemotherapy was given with ifosfamide, vincristine, and actinomycin D. In nonmetastatic patients an initial complete excision was obtained in 24% of patients, complete response was obtained in 30% of patients by initial partial excision followed by chemotherapy, and a complete response was obtained in 30% of patients by an initial biopsy, neoadjuvant chemotherapy, and second surgery. In 8% of patients a complete tumor response was obtained by surgery, chemotherapy, and radiotherapy, and in another 8% of patients complete response was obtained by surgery, chemotherapy, second surgery, and radiotherapy. Therefore, 16% of patients received radiotherapy. The overall survival rate in study MMT84 was 73% at 5 years for nonmetastatic patients, and in MMT89 it was 84%. Survival was only 15% for metastatic patients. The 5-year survival rate was 60% for fibrosarcoma, leiomyosarcoma, synovial sarcoma, and other classified sarcomas and 50% for PNET and extraosseous Ewing's sarcoma (82,83).

In summary, the small study that randomized patients with NRSTS to chemotherapy or observation showed no benefit to chemotherapy To date, the studies that have randomized patients to various chemotherapy arms have not shown a substantive difference from those results with local therapy alone.

Large-Scale Studies of Adjuvant Chemotherapy in Adults with NRSTS

There are at least 14 randomized prospective trials of mostly adult patients evaluating adjuvant chemotherapy for NRSTS. These studies include comparisons of observation with adriamycin as a single agent; with adriamycin, cyclophosphamide, dacarbazine, and vincristine; with adriamycin, vincristine, cyclophosphamide, dactinomycin, and dacarbazine; with adriamycin, cyclophosphamide, and methotrexate; with adriamycin, cyclophosphamide, vincristine, and dacarbazine; and with adriamycin and ifosfamide. The majority of these studies are equivocal as to the benefit of adjuvant chemotherapy. We will briefly summarize some of the larger ones.

The NCI trial was conducted for patients with stages IIA–IIIB extremity soft tissue sarcoma. Patients underwent either amputation or limb-sparing surgery followed by radiotherapy. They were then randomized to observation or adriamycin and cyclophosphamide. After a maximum cumulative dosage of adriamycin, chemotherapy was switched to methotrexate with leucovorin rescue. At a median follow-up of 7.1 years, the 5-year relapse-free survival is better for patients who receive chemotherapy ($p = 0.04$); however, the difference in overall survival was not significant (55,60,69,83).

The Scandinavian Sarcoma Group randomized 240 patients with high-grade sarcomas to receive either adriamycin or no systemic treatment. No significant difference was seen between the adriamycin and the control group with respect to local recurrence, relapse-free survival, or overall survival for the 181 evaluable patients or the 240 randomized patients (83,84).

The European Organization for the Research and Treatment of Cancer's Soft-Tissue and Bone Sarcoma Group conducted a phase III trial of chemotherapy after local therapy of histologically proven soft tissue sarcoma in adults with either surgery or radiotherapy. Randomization was to treatment with cyclophosphamide, vincristine, adriamycin, and dacarbazine or to observation. Between 1997 and 1998, 468 patients entered the study; 151 patients were considered ineligible. The mean follow-up duration was 80 months. Relapse-free survival with chemotherapy was 56%, compared with 43% for control subjects ($p = 0.006$); local recurrence was lower in the chemotherapy arm (17% vs. 31%, $p = 0.0041$), but overall survival did not differ significantly between the two arms (66% for chemotherapy vs. 55% for observation, $p = 0.64$). In patients with extremity tumors, no significant improvement was seen with chemotherapy in terms of local recurrence, metastases, or survival. In contrast, local recurrence was less with chemotherapy for head, neck, and trunk sarcomas (85).

The remaining 11 randomized trials for adult NRSTS, in general, do not show clear benefits to the use of adjuvant chemotherapy. Between 1991 and 1997, we are aware of four meta-analyses that attempted to derive some information by combining the results of the extant randomized trials. In the 1997 meta-analysis of 1,568 patients included in 14 analyzed trials, fewer than 1% of the patients were younger than 15 years old. The randomized trials accrued patients from 1973 to 1990 and included patients treated, on the chemotherapy arm of the various studies, with adriamycin only or adriamycin with vincristine, actinomycin, cyclophosphamide (VAC); adriamycin with VAC and dacarbazine; adriamycin with cyclophosphamide and methotrexate; adriamycin with cyclophosphamide, vincristine, and dacarbazine; or adriamycin with ifosfamide. About two-thirds of the analyzed patients had high-grade tumors, and one-half received radiotherapy. The meta-analysis indicated that adjuvant chemotherapy statistically significantly improved the local recurrence-free survival from 75% to 81% at 10 years, the distant recurrence-free survival from 60% to 70%, and the overall recurrence-free survival from 45% to 55%. The overall survival increased from 50% to 54%, which was not statistically significant (83,86–90).

After the 1997 meta-analysis an Italian cooperative group compared adjuvant epirubicin, ifosfamide, sodium mercaptoethane sulfonate

(MESNA), and granulocyte colony-stimulating factor (G-CSF) with a control group (91). There was a median disease-free survival of 16 months in the control group, compared with 48 months in the adjuvant group ($p = 0.04$), and an improvement in median survival from 46 to 75 months ($p = 0.03$). There was thought to be an improvement in survival at 4 years in the adjuvant arm on a planned interim analysis of the data. However, a closer analysis of the data showed that the adjuvant chemotherapy group experienced fewer metastatic events at 2 years (28% vs. 45%, $p = 0.08$). By 4 years this difference had disappeared, with 44% of the control group having metastatic disease and 45% in the adjuvantly treated group ($p = 0.94$). The difference in disease-free survival in the groups at 4 years was related to a significantly greater frequency of local failure in the patients in the control group (17% vs. 6% in those receiving chemotherapy).

Patients with metastatic disease are infrequently cured. A recent study of adults with NRSTS from institutions participating in the Scandinavian Sarcoma Group described a highly select group of 38 patients with metastatic NRSTS or locally advanced disease and who had achieved a complete response with chemotherapy alone or chemotherapy followed by surgery. The drug programs used were either vincristine, ifosfamide, MESNA, and G-CSF (VIG), VIG with doxorubicin, or ifosfamide, vincristine, doxorubicin, dacarbazine, and MESNA. The 2-year disease-free survival, even in this select group, was only 34%. In general, the complete response rate to chemotherapy in advanced NRSTS is less than 10%, and the combined complete and partial response rate is less than 50% (92).

The drugs used for the adjuvant treatment of NRSTS, particularly adriamycin, have significant toxicities. With the data currently available, chemotherapy probably is not the appropriate adjuvant therapy for low-grade NRSTS treated with appropriate local therapy. For high-grade lesions, trials are ongoing to evaluate new drug combinations such as adriamycin and ifosfamide. It has been argued that improved staging and better local control techniques have been the major contributing factors to improved survival in NRSTS, as opposed to any benefits of

chemotherapy. Adjuvant therapy for NRSTS is best given in the context of a clinical trial. However, chemotherapy often is given as a component of the treatment of metastatic disease.

RADIOTHERAPEUTIC MANAGEMENT

Radiotherapy for childhood NRSTS may be administered after biopsy but before definitive surgery (preoperatively), postoperatively, or intraoperatively. The arguments for preoperative irradiation include the following. First, preoperative treatment will produce partial regression of the tumor, and the resection may be less extensive than if the surgery had been done initially. Second, preoperative treatment may decrease the risk of autotransplantation of the tumor in the surgical bed and may also decrease the risk of intravascular seeding. Third, in preoperative treatment the clinically and radiographically demonstrable areas of risk are treated. Other tissues are shielded (93,94). In addition, because postoperative treatment must cover all surgically manipulated areas, the irradiated volume often is larger.

Some of the results of preoperative radiotherapy in combined adult and pediatric series of NRSTS are promising. Suit and co-workers (46,56) achieved an 88% 5-year actuarial local control rate and a 66% survival with limited surgery and radiotherapy in 258 patients with extremity and head and neck primaries. These results have been echoed in other studies (48,95). Eilber et al. (59) administered preoperative external beam irradiation and intra-arterial adriamycin (30 mg per day for 3 days) followed by limb-sparing surgery for extremity sarcomas. The local control rate was 96% for patients who received 35 Gy, 90–95% for those who received 28 Gy, and 82% for those who received 17.5 Gy. Preoperative radiotherapy with hyperthermia for NRSTS is being investigated. Local control rates are quite good when thermoradiotherapy is followed by conservative surgery (96). It is not uncommon to find no remaining viable tumor at the time of resection. External microwave hyperthermia generally is appropriate only in older and more cooperative children.

The disadvantages of preoperative therapy include a delay in the start of definitive surgery, loss of ability to examine the whole tumor specimen for stage and grade, and loss of the ability to surgically assess the extent of the disease. Therefore, many radiotherapists and surgeons favor postoperative treatment. Postoperative radiotherapy must be delayed until adequate wound healing has occurred (46,56). A retrospective review comparing preoperative and postoperative external beam irradiation from the University of Minnesota for adults with NRSTS found no significant difference in overall or relapse-free survival or local control. However, wound complications were more common in preoperative radiotherapy patients (31% vs. 8%, $p = 0.0014$) (93). Several other centers have done retrospective comparisons of preoperative and postoperative irradiation in series of largely adult patients. Some studies favor preoperative treatment (46,97); others do not (98).

A randomized trial centered at the Princess Margaret Hospital addressed the timing of radiotherapy in adults. The trial was open from 1994–1997 and included patients with limb MFH, liposarcoma, leiomyosarcoma, and other spindle cell sarcoma histologies. There were 182 patients analyzed, most more than 50 years old. Half received 50 Gy of preoperative radiotherapy and a 16- to 20-Gy postoperative boost for a positive margin. Patients in the postoperative group received 50 Gy and a 16- to 20-Gy boost. The wound complication rate was higher with preoperative treatment (35% vs. 17%; $p = 0.01$), and the local recurrence rate, regional or distant failure rate, and progression-free survival rate did not differ between groups (99).

Most agree that wound complications are higher with preoperative treatment (97,100). When the therapeutic plan includes external beam radiotherapy and surgery for the local treatment of NRSTS, it is generally preferable to completely excise small lesions and treat with postoperative irradiation. In most cases, large lesions are better treated with biopsy, preoperative irradiation, and then excision.

Volume

Extremity NRSTSs tend to grow in a longitudinal fashion by following muscle groups. General

ous proximal and distal margins beyond the tumor volume (5 to 10 cm) are appropriate. Because the lesions usually do not cross muscle compartments, the circumferential margins may be more modest (57). A limb CT or MRI scan, followed by a computerized treatment plan, is extremely helpful. The treatment of sarcomas often is a venue for the demonstration of the benefits of intensity-modulated radiation therapy, three-dimensional treatment planning techniques, tissue compensators, wedges, customized blocking, and rigid immobilization for reproducible treatments. One should avoid high-dose irradiation of the entire width of a limb in order to avoid severe lymphedema (radiation-induced elephantiasis) (54). Blocking should be used to avoid the ankylosis attendant to the high-dose irradiation of the full width of a joint (64). Growth plates should be shielded when possible (although it is usually better to fully treat a growth plate and shorten a limb rather than asymmetrically irradiate a growth plate and angulate a limb). In nonextremity lesions the tumor volume must be covered with as generous a margin as is feasible.

Epithelioid sarcoma and synovial sarcoma may metastasize to lymph nodes in 10–20% of cases (3,43,87,101–103). Some physicians use elective lymph node irradiation for these lesions, particularly high-grade tumors. Its efficacy is unknown.

Dosage

Modern radiobiologic evidence gives little credence to the assertion that NRSTSs are inherently radioresistant. The available retrospective reviews suggest that a minimum of 40 Gy is necessary for the postoperative control of microscopic NRSTS in children (11,12). At these dosages, however, there is a substantial chance of local failure. More aggressive treatment is generally warranted. Most investigators favor a dosage of 50 to 60 Gy using a shrinking field technique (25,46,54). Some clinicians favor the use of twice-a-day irradiation (i.e., 1.1 to 1.2 Gy twice daily to 66 to 72 Gy) (54). Similar dosages are used for preoperative treatment. There were no local failures in POG protocol 8653 or in the

University of Florida series for excised tumors treated with more than 55 Gy (68). When intraoperative boosts with brachytherapy or electrons are given as part of a combined approach, the dosage usually is 10 to 20 Gy. Gross residual sarcoma requires 65 to 72 Gy by external beam and implant (25,56,57). Some adult patients with unresectable lesions have been treated with external beam and intravenous radiosensitizers or external beam plus hyperthermia (5,104).

Brachytherapy and Intraoperative Radiation Therapy

Brachytherapy may play an important role in limb-sparing surgery for NRSTS. Brachytherapy is often but not always given in combination with preoperative or postoperative external beam treatment. Brachytherapy has the following potential advantages: Its radiobiologic effectiveness is increased by the administration of a high dosage of irradiation over a few days rather than several weeks; an intense dose is given deep in the tumor bed; surrounding normal tissue and overlying skin are spared through the rapid falloff of the dosage; and the short treatment time is more convenient, avoiding the problems of travel and housing for protracted external beam therapy (65,105,106).

Conventional afterloading brachytherapy is suitable for children capable of doing self-care. It is more complex, from a nursing standpoint, in younger children. Several techniques are available for brachytherapy for NRSTS in children. The most commonly used type is a manually loaded low–dose rate system. Plastic catheters are inserted into the target volume with the aid of hollow needles. These catheters are subsequently loaded with the radioactive sources. Needles may be placed freehand or with the assistance of a custom-built or standardized template. Intracavitary applicators have been developed for use in treating vaginal sarcomas and lesions of the upper aerodigestive track. Most commonly, iridium-192 or cesium-137 is used. When there is particular concern about radiation exposure to nursing personnel or parents, and if the anatomy of the tumor allows, one should consider using a low-energy radioisotope such as iodine-125 or palladium. When these isotopes are used, thin sheets of lead applied over the treatment area or a standard lead apron provide a measure of protection for visitors.

In a conventional low–dose rate afterloading procedure, the afterloading catheters are placed at the time of surgical excision. After tumor excision, the radiation oncologist and surgeon inspect the operative bed and plan the implant. Parallel plastic catheters are placed approximately 1 cm apart throughout the entire tumor bed, usually with a 1- to 2-cm margin. For extremity lesions, some radiation oncologists place the catheters parallel to the axis of the limb (i.e., parallel to the incision), whereas others place catheters perpendicular to the axis of the incision and limb. Postoperative radiographs are taken with dummy sources to calculate the dose distribution and rate. Initial wound healing is allowed to begin, and the catheters are not loaded with iridium-192 (the most commonly used isotope in this situation) until the sixth postoperative day. Earlier loading is associated with a significant risk of wound complications, up to a 44% incidence (16,107). When the situation warrants it, catheters may be placed adjacent to bone or neurovascular bundles. In general, little irradiation is given via the implant to the superficial incision.

The second general technique of pediatric brachytherapy for NRSTS involves permanent interstitial implant. Low-activity iodine-125, gold-198, or palladium seeds are used. They may be placed with the use of a seed gun (a device used for their implantation), placed through individual needles, or embedded in Vicryl suture material and then sewn into the tumor bed. Although the low energy of these radioactive sources lowers the risk to visitors, these implants often are extremely difficult to perform.

The third form of brachytherapy for pediatric NRSTS is remote afterloading. This may be done at a low dose rate, high dose rate, or pulsed dose rate (intermittent use of a high–dose rate machine). The catheters or applicators are inserted into or placed on the tumor site. They are then connected to the afterloader for remotely controlled radioactive loading. The radioactive sources are retracted into the high–dose rate applicator's vault during planned interruptions. The procedure may be done in an outpatient clinic or operating room. Some departments have specially designated rooms for this purpose. Intraoperative high–dose rate brachytherapy is a modification of this general technique (108–111).

In the treatment of NRSTS, brachytherapy may be used as a boost after or before external beam radiotherapy or as the sole form of irradiation monotherapy. In general, the planning volume for brachytherapy for NRSTS is smaller than for external beam radiotherapy. In brachytherapy the volume treated closely approximates the clinical target volume. There is no need to allow for internal organ movement, patient movement, or setup errors. Because the dosage from the radioisotope falls off rapidly, the volume of normal tissue irradiated outside the planning target volume is minimized.

When brachytherapy is the sole form of irradiation to be given, surgical drain sites usually are not implanted. In adult practice, if 45 to 50 Gy of external irradiation is given as part of a course of treatment, the brachytherapy boost generally is 10 to 20 Gy at about 50 cGy per hour. If brachytherapy is the sole form of irradiation used in combination with surgery, then 40 to 50 Gy in 4 or 5 days is given. The role of brachytherapy in adult NRSTS has been evaluated in several retrospective reviews, but some randomized prospective trials are particularly noteworthy. Between 1982 and 1987, 126 patients, mostly adults, with soft tissue sarcoma were entered into a prospective randomized trial at Memorial Sloan–Kettering Cancer Center (MSKCC). Patients underwent a grossly complete resection with a limb-sparing operation for NRSTS of the extremity or superficial trunk. Intraoperatively, after the resection was complete, patients were randomized to receive either adjuvant brachytherapy or no adjuvant therapy. Patients who received the implant had a dosage of 42 to 45 Gy administered with iridium-192 over a 4- to 6-day period. The median follow-up of this trial was 76 months. The 5-year actuarial local control rate for high-grade tumors was 89% for brachytherapy-treated patients and 66% for control subjects ($p = 0.0025$). There was no local control benefit in the low-grade tumor group.

The improved local control with brachytherapy in high-grade tumors did not translate into an overall decrease in distant metastasis. Even in the high-grade tumor, freedom from distant metastases was approximately 70% at 5 years in both the brachytherapy and control arms (112,113). This trial is of interest not only because it demonstrated a benefit to adjuvant brachytherapy but also because it showed a benefit to a form of therapy that, in contrast to adjuvant external beam irradiation, generally does not irradiate the full surgical scar, does not irradiate the drain site, is shorter in duration (10 to 14 days of hospitalization vs. 6 to 7 weeks of outpatient treatment), and is slightly less costly.

The team from MSKCC elected to explore the use of brachytherapy in low-grade tumors in more detail because their initial randomized trial did not include a large number of patients with low-grade NRSTS. From 1982 to 1992, they randomized 45 patients with low-grade tumors to brachytherapy or observation. There was no benefit to brachytherapy in terms of local recurrence (about 76% local control in each arm, $p = 0.60$) or overall survival ($p = 0.38$) (114). In two studies, patients with high-grade NRSTS with a negative margin had an 89% and 94% local control rate, respectively, when treated with brachytherapy, compared with 59% and 77% in those with a positive margin. In patients with high-grade tumors and positive margins treated with brachytherapy and external beam irradiation, the local control rate was 90% (16,112,114). In the view of the investigators, these two randomized trials argue in favor of adjuvant brachytherapy for resected high-grade tumors, for surgery alone as the treatment for resected low-grade tumors smaller than 5 cm, and for consideration of external beam for resected low-grade tumors larger than 5 cm because of the remaining high risk of local recurrence in these tumors (i.e., 20–25%). In the early years of the MSKCC trials, there was a substantially higher rate of wound complications in the brachytherapy-treated patients than in control subjects (44% vs. 14%, $p = 0.0006$). The higher rate of complications has been alleviated by a policy of not loading patients with radioactivity until the fifth postoperative day

(113). Burmeister et al. (107), in Australia, obtained slightly less satisfactory results with brachytherapy and external beam therapy in patients with large high-grade sarcomas with close or positive margins. When brachytherapy is used as the only form of radiotherapy, some of the local failures result from marginal misses (65,106,112,115). In the Institut Gustave–Roussy series, 14 of 16 local failures were marginal or distant from the high-dose brachytherapy region (68).

Data from approximately 100 to 150 children given brachytherapy for the treatment of rhabdomyosarcoma and NRSTS have been reported. The techniques have included low–dose rate applications, high–dose rate applications, and pulse applications. Although the local control rate is excellent, it is clear from the retrospective reviews that careful patient selection is essential for successful outcomes. In general, brachytherapy seems to be most appropriate for patients who have NRSTS and microscopic small-volume residual disease at an accessible site and who have responded well to chemotherapy, external beam radiotherapy, and surgery. The American Brachytherapy Society's recommendations for brachytherapy of soft tissue sarcomas offer general guidelines as to the appropriate dosage. When brachytherapy alone is used, 45 to 50 Gy is administered over 4 to 6 days. For patients in whom low–dose rate brachytherapy is used in combination with external beam radiotherapy (generally 40 to 50 Gy), a 15- to 25-Gy boost is given. There are few clinical data to invoke in selecting dosages for fractionated high–dose rate brachytherapy. When high–dose rate therapy is used as the sole local control in modality, a dosage of 2.5 to 3 Gy twice daily, to a total dosage of 30 to 36 Gy, may be considered (108,109). If high–dose rate brachytherapy is used as a boost to external beam radiotherapy, then the linear quadratic model can be used to devise a fractionated scheme that generates the equivalent to a low–dose rate brachytherapy dosage of 15 to 25 Gy (108,111).

What are we to conclude, on the basis of these NRSTS studies, concerning the role of brachytherapy in pediatric patients? Brachytherapy should be considered as an option in treating children. It has the ability to deliver a highly localized dose while sparing normal tissue (Fig. 12-5). However, in children brachytherapy poses problems of inpatient management. Can the child provide for his or her own feeding, bodily care, and immediate needs while radioactive? If not, will there be an unacceptable exposure to nursing personnel or to the parents during the implant? Several solutions have been proposed. One is to use a remote afterloading brachytherapy machine. If a high–dose rate remote afterloader is used, the duration of the radiation exposure is short and personnel exposure is minimized. The drawback is that the dose rate is so high that some of the normal tissue–sparing benefits of brachytherapy may be lost. To address this latter concern, some physicians pulse or fractionate the brachytherapy (i.e., use multiple exposures). As an alternative, one can use a remote afterloader with conventional activity sources. In this way, the duration of the implant is no different than with conventional afterloading. However, the sources can be withdrawn whenever nursing personnel or a parent enters the room for a planned feeding, wound care, bathing the child, and so on. A third way to deal with the particular problems of brachytherapy in a child is to use iodine-125 instead of iridium-192. The treatment energy for iodine-125 is 28 keV, compared with 380 keV for iridium-192. The lower energy of iodine-125 reduces exposure to clinical staff and family, allows more efficacious shielding with lead drapes, and reduces exposure to normal tissue at a distance from the implant. The iodine-125 may be embedded in suture material or absorbable mesh (113).

Intraoperative radiation therapy (IORT) has been described for the treatment of NRSTS in adults (116). It can also be used in children. There are two general forms: intraoperative electron beam therapy (IO-ERT) and intraoperative high–dose rate brachytherapy (IO-HDRBT). There are three techniques for administering IO-ERT. Historically, patients underwent surgery in the operating room and then were transported, using specialized sterile techniques, from the operating room to the radiation oncology department. The linear accelerator suite was draped and prepared as a temporary operating room.

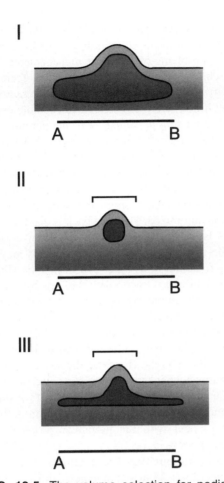

FIG. 12-5. The volume selection for pediatric brachytherapy for NRSTS is highly nuanced. In many cases the patient has been treated with induction chemotherapy or external beam radiotherapy. Often one cannot be sure whether a partial response of gross tumor implies a complete response of all or part of the initial occult disease volume. Consider the following hypothetical example. **(I)** An NRSTS is shown near an epithelial surface. The bulky tumor's left-to-right dimension is noted by line *AB*. Let us assume that the tumor is treated with induction cytotoxic therapy and that it regresses. **(II)** The left-to-right dimension, demarcated in relation to line *AB*, has shrunk. If the brachytherapy volume is denoted by the bracketed area, then the irradiated volume will be adequate. **(III)** On the other hand, assume that the tumor regressed significantly but that the total left-to-right dimension did not change. If the brachytherapy volume is addressed only to the readily palpable or visible tumor, as shown by the bracketed area, then a large portion of the tumor will be missed.

The accelerator was "docked" to a cone used to demarcate the area that the physicians wanted to irradiate. A single large fraction of electrons was administered. Normal tissue was spared by retraction and shielding. A second technique involved placing a conventional linear accelerator in the operating room as a dedicated IO-ERT device. Of course, this necessitated reinforcing the weight-bearing capacity of the floor of the operating room, particularly if it was located in an upper floor of the hospital. The accelerator was only used for its electron-generating capabilities, so the purchase of a conventional linear accelerator with photon and electron capabilities wasted the photon capabilities of the machine. This problem was addressed by the third technique for IO-ERT: the development of an electron-only dedicated linear accelerator for placement in the operating room. Such devices are now available and can be moved from operating room to operating room. Because they generate only electrons, shielding needs for the walls, floor, and ceiling of the operating room are minimal.

Some authorities view IO-HDRBT as an alternative to IO-ERT or an adjunct to it. Intraoperative electrons often cannot treat inaccessible or highly contoured sites such as the base of the skull, the pelvic side wall, the deep pelvic area, or angled areas in the abdomen or thorax. The IO-HDRBT device uses flexible applicators and catheters to treat almost any surface. Retraction and shielding are used to spare critical normal structures. A single high-activity iridium-192 source is used, and one can customize the dose distribution. However, one is constrained by the penetration attendant to iridium-192. There is very limited clinical experience with the use of IORT to treat childhood NRSTS. In small series of highly selected patients, excellent local control rates have been achieved. The generally recommended dosage, if 40 to 50 Gy of external beam radiotherapy is used, is an IORT boost of 10 to 15 Gy (108–111).

Hyperthermia

Hyperthermia has been demonstrated to be an effective radiosensitizer in a variety of clinical situations. Cells that are hypoxic, in S phase, or low pH are particularly sensitive to heating, the converse of conventional radiation. It is not surprising that hyperthermia plus radiation has been evaluated for the preoperative treatment of NRSTS and the primary treatment of inoperable tumors. Uno et al. (117) from Tokyo treated eight patients with NRSTS with external beam irradiation, doxorubicin infusion, and radiofrequency hyperthermia. Five of the eight patients had a gross recurrent tumor after surgical excisions; there were two complete responses and three partial responses. Five of the eight had no local tumor progression until death or last follow-up.

A trial of preoperative radiotherapy plus hyperthermia for NRSTS in adults at Duke University Medical Center was opened in 1984. Forty-four patients with deep nonmetastatic high-grade NRSTS received 50 Gy of radiotherapy and microwave hyperthermia. Negative surgical margins were obtained in 40 patients. The local control rate was 98%, the 3-year overall survival 72%, and 3-year disease-free survival 58%. Patients with tumor median pO_2 less than 10 mm Hg had an 18-month actuarial disease-free survival of 35%, compared with 70% for patients with a median tumor pO_2 of more than 10 mm Hg ($p = 0.01$) (118–120).

Radiotherapy with hyperthermia and surgery seems capable of achieving high local control rates. To date it has not shown an ability to reduce distant metastases. The modality is largely untested in children.

Neutrons

Radiobiologists and clinical radiotherapists have been intrigued by the therapeutic uses of neutrons. High–linear energy transfer neutrons, by virtue of a low oxygen enhancement ratio and lack of cell cycle cytotoxicity preference, are toxic and have been used to treat bulky tumors of various histologies and sites. Data are available from the United States, Europe, and Japan concerning the use of neutrons to treat bulky sarcomas of adults and children. Although definitions of local tumor control vary between reports, the local control rate for neutron treatment of inoperable or residual soft tissue sarcomas is about

50% (121). In a retrospective comparison, Larramore et al. (122) found a higher local control rate of bulky sarcomas with neutrons than with photons and electrons (53% vs. 38%). Between November 1980 and June 1981, 14 patients, presumably adults, were entered in a prospective trial comparing postoperative photons and fast neutrons (15.6 Gy) for NRSTS. Two of the nine patients treated with photons (63 Gy) relapsed locally, as did two of the five patients treated with neutrons. The trial was halted because of unacceptable late tissue damage in the neutron-treated patients.

RESULTS

When NRSTS in children is localized and amenable to definitive surgical excision or limited excision plus radiotherapy, the survival probability is 60–90%. The 5-year event-free survivals in the retrospective reviews from St. Jude Children's Research Hospital are group I, 83%; group II, 65%; group IV, ~9%; groups I and II and less than 5 cm, 92%; groups I and II and more than 5 cm, 55% (4,73). In the Mayo Clinic series the 10-year event-free survival was 76%. A worse prognosis is associated with high stage, high grade, and tumor size greater than 5 cm (21). The 5-year disease-free survival for children with NRSTS of the head and neck in the M. D. Anderson Hospital series was 75% (7). For patients with stage I–III NRSTS treated on SIOP trial MMT84, the 5-year survival rate was 73%; it was 80% for trial MMT89 (35). A multivariate analysis of predictive factors for local tumor recurrence in the Royal Marsden series of NRSTS (adults and children) showed significant worsening of the risk for local recurrence with retroperitoneal versus lower limb tumors, high versus low grade, and inadequate surgical margins. Metastases were predicted by tumor size more than 5 cm, high grade, local recurrence, or the presence of involved lymph nodes (54). In POG Study 8653/8654 the 5-year overall survival for IRS group I–II NRSTS was 82% and event-free survival was 71%; for IRS group III–IV disease the overall survival was 26% and event-free survival was 19% (79). A retrospective review from the Rambam Medical Center, which includes desmoid tumors in the series, showed 5-year overall survival of 72% for IRS group, 75% for group II, 90% for group III, and 40% for group IV (37). A retrospective review of synovial sarcoma treatment in children and adolescents treated with surgery, chemotherapy, and radiotherapy found that progression-free survival was associated with IRS group (I, 79%; II, 82%; III, 38%; IV, 0%), maximum tumor diameter (less than 5 cm, 82%; more than 5 cm, 56%), and histology (monophasic, 86%; biphasic, 54%) (19). A small series of childhood angiosarcomas had a characteristically poor event-free (29%) and overall (22%) survival (41). For fibrosarcomas, because of the difference in behavior between the congential or infantile and adult types, survival is a function of age (younger than 2 years, 79%; older than 2 years, 51%) (123).

Unresectable or metastatic disease carries a dismal prognosis. Unresectable NRSTSs are rarely cured by radiotherapy with chemotherapy, and the local control rate is also poor (68). The 5-year survival rate for children with stage IV NRSTS treated on SIOP trials MMT84 and MMT89 was 15% (35). In a St. Jude Children's Research Hospital review of metastatic NRSTS, the 2-year progression-free survival was 15% (4,74).

DESMOID TUMORS

There are a variety of childhood mesenchymal tumors of fibroblastic and myofibroblastic derivation that are generally regarded as benign in the sense that these tumors have no potential for metastasis. The group includes infantile myofibromatosis, digital fibromatosis, fibromatosis colli, and desmoid tumors (124). In addition to the term *desmoid tumor,* these lesions are called extra-abdominal desmoid, well-differentiated nonmetastasizing fibrosarcoma, aggressive fibromatosis, and grade I fibrosarcoma (desmoid) (33,125). The usual presenting complaint is a deep-seated, firm mass arising in muscles or soft tissues (33,124,126–128). These lesions tend to extend along fascial planes. Histologically, spindle cells with an abundant collagenous background form interlacing bundles and infiltrate surrounding tissue. Mitoses are rare (Fig. 12-6) (10,32,106,107). A small fraction of

desmoid tumors are associated with Gardner's syndrome.

Desmoid tumors almost never metastasize. The goal of treatment is to obtain local control. Desmoid tumors can occur in a wide variety of locations. For this reason, the degree of resectability is quite variable. Tumors in an accessible site, not adjacent to vital structures, are more amenable to gross total excision than those adjacent to major nerves or vessels. In general, about two-thirds of desmoids can undergo gross total excision. The problem of the extent of excision leads us to the first of several controversies in the management of pediatric desmoid tumors.

What is to be done in the child who has undergone an excision but in whom there are positive margins of resection? Several papers from the Massachusetts General Hospital (MGH) argue that such patients ought to be closely observed. In a recent review, Suit and Spiro (126) wrote,

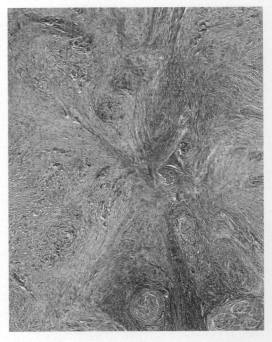

FIG. 12-6. An 8-year-old girl had an extensive desmoid tumor of the left lower leg. She was treated with surgery and chemotherapy. Radiotherapy was not used. The tumor consisted of infiltrative fibroblasts.

Patients with primary desmoid tumors who have had grossly complete resection, but whose surgical margins are positive on pathological examination are exposed to a risk of no local regrowth of at least some 30–40%. This high local control results in margin-positive patients and the fact that salvage treatment of patients who failed locally is usually successful warrant a policy of placing such patients on observation. This policy has been followed at the MGH for approximately 25 years. To date there have been no regrets and a worthwhile number of patients have not been exposed to the risk of radiation-induced damage to normal tissues, including tumor induction. In contrast, margin-positive resection of recurrent desmoid tumors is an unequivocal indication for additional treatment.

In contrast to this argument, one can turn to a recent review by Nuyttens (127) of 22 articles concerning the treatment of desmoid tumors. Table 12-7, derived from this review article, shows that the local control rate for patients with positive margins treated with surgery alone is approximately half that of patients treated with surgery and radiation therapy. Data of this sort may be used to argue for the routine use of postoperative irradiation in patients with positive margins.

If one weighs the conflicting data on this point, several issues ought be considered:

- The long-term ill effects of radiation therapy in children with desmoid tumors can be considerable. Therefore, it would be best to minimize the use of radiation wherever possible.
- Although postoperative irradiation in patients with positive margins reduces the risk of local relapse, most patients with local relapse after surgery alone can be cured by additional surgery and radiation therapy.

- Therefore, it would be reasonable to adopt a policy of watchful waiting in accessible sites, amenable to close follow-up. A significant number of these patients might be locally controlled with surgery alone, even with positive margins. For those who relapse, one could use surgery and radiation therapy to obtain local control.

The probability of local control with surgery alone is highly debatable, and a wide range of local control rates are reported (10,33,124, 125,128,129). A consensus view is that local control in patients with free margins is obtained in about 70% of cases. Several types of patients are at particularly high risk for local recurrence and progression. These include those with unresectable lesions, those who have undergone resection and gross tumor has been left behind, those who have undergone resection with large areas of clearly positive histologic tumor margins, and those who have already suffered one or more local recurrences after primary surgical therapy. With the exception of patients with microscopic positive margins, the remainder should be considered for radiotherapy (Fig. 12-7).

Several retrospective series, combining pediatric and adult patients, have demonstrated that fractionated external beam irradiation or external beam plus brachytherapy can locally control approximately 75% of desmoid tumors (Tables 12-7 and 12-8). Complete or partial resolution may take 2 to 3 years after completion of a course of treatment (125,130). For some patients "local control" means cessation of growth rather than tumor regression. The long-term ill effects of radiation therapy for the treatment of desmoid tumors can include fibrosis in the treated area, paresthesias that are most often as-

TABLE 12-7. *Local control of desmoid tumors with three forms of therapy*

	Surgery alone	Surgery and radiotherapy	Radiotherapy alone
Free margins	72%	94%*	78%
Positive margins	41%	75%*	
Unknown margins	56%		54%

*$p < 0.005$ vs. surgery alone.
Modified from Nuyttens J, Rust PF, Thomas Jr CR, et al. Surgery versus radiotherapy for patients with aggressive fibromatosis or desmoid tumors: a comparative review of 22 articles. *Cancer* 2000;88:1517–1523.

TABLE 12-8. *Local control rates in combined pediatric and adult series of radiotherapy with or without surgery for the management of desmoid tumors*

Institution	Year of the most recent update of the series	Number of patients	Dosage (Gy)	Disease status	Local control
Harvard Joint Center (18)	1981	9	30–68.6	8 gross disease 1 postoperative	87% 100%
University of California San Francisco (147)	1983	19	40.8–61.2	13 gross disease 6 microscopic	69% 67%
Netherlands Cancer Institute (149)	1986	21	60	11 status after subtotal resection 8 status after gross total resection 2 gross disease	91% 87% 100%
Westminster Hospital (66)	1988	38	27–63	29 postoperative 9 gross disease	76% 67%
Institut Curie (150)	1988	16	45–65	3 postoperative for microscopic disease 4 postoperative for macroscopic disease 9 radical radiotherapy for extensive disease	100% 75% 67%
M. D. Anderson Hospital (130)	1990	45	50–76.2	14 gross disease 31 postoperative	71% 77%
Memorial Sloan–Kettering (137)	1991	38	^{192}Ir brachytherapy (20–60.55 Gy) and, often, supplemental external beam radiotherapy		

Institution	Year	No. of patients	Dose (Gy)	Treatment	Local control
Duke (125)	1993	16	49.6–56.2	15 gross disease	93%
				1 postoperative	93%
Groningen University Hospital (151)	1995	17	50–60	14 resection with post-operative treatment	93%
Memorial Sloan–Kettering (142), pediatric patients only	1995	11	30–50	2 gross disease	100%
				1 reexcision with brachytherapy	100%
				2 of 11 were treated preoperatively	64%
Mayo Clinic (152,153)	1996	13	~50.4–64.8	Operation and radiation therapy	100%
				2 wide resection	75%
				4 marginal resection	75%
				4 intralesional resection	33%
				3 radiation therapy only	
University of Florida (136)	1996	53	35–70	29 microscopic residual disease	79%
				24 gross disease	88%
Massachusetts General Hospital (124,129,139)	1997	58	22–70.9	15 radiation therapy alone	92%
				41 radiation therapy and surgery	79% primary tumors, 67% recurrent tumors

Table derived from a concept originally in Acker JC, Bossen EH, Halperin EC. The management of desmoid tumors. *Int J Radiat Oncol Biol Phys* 1993;26:851–858; updated and modified by the author of this chapter.

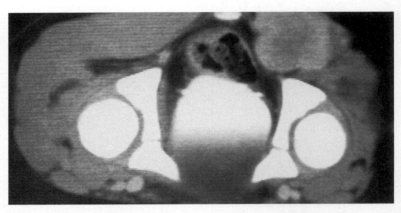

FIG. 12-7. A right buttock desmoid tumor was diagnosed in a 6-year-old boy. The lesion was excised in 1979, 1980, 1982, and 1983 and recurred each time. Postoperative irradiation (49.6 Gy) was given after a reexcision of gross disease. Angled photon fields were used to minimize rectal dosage. The tumor slowly regressed, and local control has been maintained up to the time of this writing (2004). There is partial atrophy of the right buttock musculature, the bones of the right hemipelvis are smaller than those of the left hemipelvis, and the patient walks with a marked limp. Diabetes mellitus was diagnosed in 1994. In 2002, 19 years after radiotherapy, the thin, atrophied tissues gave way and a deep, infected ulcer developed in the right buttock. Plastic surgery with rotation of vascularized flaps was needed for wound closure.

sociated with growth of tumor into a nerve, limb edema, fracture associated with surgical stripping of the ostium or curettage, skin ulcers, cellulitis, and the induction of second malignant neoplasms (Fig. 12-7) (127,131,132).

This risk of late effects raises the question of whether one should be particularly cautious in using radiation therapy in children with desmoid tumors. A recent report by Merchant et al. (131) from St. Jude Children's Research Hospital argued that desmoid tumors in pediatric patients are particularly locally aggressive and often occur after radiation therapy. This adverse biologic behavior, in conjunction with the associated ill effects of radiation, argues against the use of radiation therapy in desmoid tumors. The study by Merchant et al. contains data from only 13 patients collected over a 36-year period. The desmoid tumors arose from a particularly unusual set of locations, such as the paraspinal region in five cases and the nasopharynx and pterygoid fossa in two cases. A wide variety of treatments were used, including surgery and chemotherapy, in addition to radiation therapy. Enzinger and Shiraki (133) and Walther et al. (134) also reported a high risk of failure in adolescents.

On the other hand, as shown in Table 12-8, a large number of patients have been treated successfully with radiation therapy. Most series are a mixture of adults and children. However, they do not report that desmoid tumors in children are more aggressive. Therefore, it seems reasonable to use radiation therapy to treat desmoid tumors in children, albeit with the cautions about positive margins raised earlier in this section.

Desmoids can widely infiltrate. When external beam is used, treatment portals should be generous. Marginal relapses account for a very large number of the relapses after external beam radiation therapy (127,132,135–137). MRI studies of desmoids often show an infiltrative margin. At surgery, microscopic tumor has been found to extend beyond the volume defined by MRI (102). All available evidence from the physical examination, surgical report, CT, and MRI should be integrated to determine the tumor volume. Generous margins (about 5 cm) should then be used around this volume. Daily fractions of 1.8 to 2 Gy are used. There may be a higher local recurrence rate when dosages less than 50 Gy are used. In 1984, Kiel and Suit (124) suggested that dosages greater than 60 Gy may be associated with a greater incidence of local control and have treated some patients with 70 Gy, often using photons and protons. Schultz-Ertner et al. (135) found no benefit of administering more than 50 Gy rather than less than 50 Gy on univariate analysis. Zlotecki et al. (132) found no benefit of hyperfractionated irradiation over standard fractionation. Almost all patients received 50 to 56 Gy. However, Ballo et al. (138) reported a significant difference in local control between dosages less than 50 Gy and dosages more than 50 Gy. They also found greater irradiation-associated morbidity in patients who received dosages less than 56 Gy. Neutron boosts have also been used (130). Evidence indicates that a total dosage of 50 to 55 Gy is appropriate and that higher dosages may increase the risk of complications without commensurate gain in local tumor control (125,129,130). Brachytherapy has been reported as a treatment for desmoids, either alone or with external beam therapy, by one institution (137). Because of concerns about the assessment of tumor margins and their coverage, we believe that the role of brachytherapy is limited in children with desmoids.

In young children with desmoids, radiation's effects on growing bone, the risk for subsequent soft tissue fibrosis, and the potential for secondary malignancy may prompt consideration of alternative therapies. A large range of drugs are available for managing desmoid tumor. Most of these have been used to treat recurrent tumor after surgery and radiation. They include the following:

- Hormonal agents, especially tamoxifen, have been used. Tumor regressions have been observed. However, it is unclear whether this effect is mediated by the interaction of tamoxifen with estrogen receptors.
- There are also anecdotal reports of the regression of desmoid tumors after treatment with nonsteroidal anti-inflammatory agents. It is unclear whether this activity is related to cyclooxygenase inhibition.
- There have been a few reports regarding the use of colchicine.

- Interferons have been described as effective in case reports.
- Cytotoxic chemotherapy has been used both for the primary treatment of desmoids and for recurrences. Combinations used include vinblastine with methotrexate and doxorubicin with dacarbazine. There have been less frequent reports of the use of gemcitabine, liposome-encapsulated doxorubicin, and temozolomide.
- The somatostatin analog octreotide has been labeled with yttrium-90 and used to treat desmoid tumors. (95,124,125,140–147).

REFERENCES

References particularly recommended for further reading are indicated by an asterisk.

1. Andrassy RJ. Advances in the surgical management of sarcomas in children. *Am J Surg* 2002;184(6):484–491.
2. Conrad EU, Bradford L, Chansky HA. Pediatric soft-tissue sarcomas. *Orthop Clin North Am* 1996;17:655–664.
3. Greenberg J. Epithelioid sarcoma. *Med Pediatr Oncol* 1982;10:497–500.
*4. Pappo AS, Parham DM, Rao BN, et al. Soft tissue sarcomas in children. *Semin Surg Oncol* 1999;16:121–143.
5. Hayani A, Mahoney DH Jr, Hawkins HK, et al. Soft-tissue sarcomas other than rhabdomyosarcoma in children. *Med Pediatr Oncol* 1992;20:114–118.
6. Horowitz ME, Pratt CB, Webber BL, et al. Therapy for childhood soft tissue sarcomas other than rhabdomyosarcoma: a review of 62 cases treated at a single institution. *J Clin Oncol* 1986;4:559–564.
7. Lyos AT, Goepfert H, Luna MA, et al. Soft tissue sarcoma of the head and neck in children and adolescents. *Cancer* 1996;77:193–200.
8. Harris M, Hartley AL. Value of peer review of pathology to soft tissue sarcomas. In: Verweij J, Pinedo HM, Suit HD, eds. *Soft tissue sarcomas: present achievements and future prospects.* Boston: Kluwer, 1997:1–8.
9. Scott SM, Reiman HM, Pritchard DJ, et al. Soft tissue fibrosarcoma: a clinicopathologic study of 132 cases. *Cancer* 1989;64:925–931.
10. Coffin CM, Dehner LP. Soft tissue neoplasms in children: a clinicopathologic overview. In: Finegold M, ed. *Pathology of neoplasia in children and adolescents.* Philadelphia: WB Saunders, 1986:223–255.
11. Raney B, Schnaufer L, Ziegler M, et al. Treatment of children with neurogenic sarcoma: experience at the Children's Hospital of Philadelphia, 1958–1984. *Cancer* 1987;59:1–5.
12. Raney RB Jr, Littman P, Jarrett P, et al. Results of multimodal therapy for children with neurogenic sarcoma. *Med Pediatr Oncol* 1979;7:229–236.
13. Ducatman BS, Scheithauer BW, Piepgras DG, et al.

Malignant peripheral nerve sheath tumors: a clinico-pathologic study of 120 cases. *Cancer* 1986;57: 2006–2021.

14. Coffin CM, Dehner LP. Peripheral neurogenic tumors of the soft tissues in children and adolescents: a clin-icopathologic study of 108 examples in 103 patients. *Pediatr Pathol* 1989;11:559–588.

15. Reynolds RM, Browning GGP, Nawroz I, et al. Von Recklinghausen's neurofibromatosis: neurofibroma-tosis type 1. *Lancet* 2003;361:1552–1554.

16. Alekhteyar KM, Leung DH, Brennan MF, et al. The effect of combined external beam radiotherapy and brachytherapy on local control and wound compli-cations in patients with high-grade soft tissue sar-comas of the extremity with positive microscopic margin. *Int J Radiat Oncol Biol Phys* 1996;36: 321–324.

17. Frey E, Niggli F, Stauffer U, et al. Primary resection of soft-tissue sarcomas: yes and no. *Eur J Pediatr Surg* 1997;7:227–229.

18. Greenberg HM, Goebel R, Weichselbaum RR, et al. Radiation therapy in the treatment of aggressive fi-bromatoses. *Int J Radiat Oncol Biol Phys* 1981;7: 305–310.

19. Okcu MF, Despa S, Charozy M, et al. Synovial sar-coma in children and adolescents: thirty three years of experience with multimodal therapy. *Med Pediatr Oncol* 2001;37:90–96.

20. Mazeran JJ, Suit HD. Lymph nodes as sites of metas-tasis from sarcomas of soft tissue. *Cancer* 1987;60: 1800–1808.

*21. McGrary JE, Pritchard DJ, Arndt CA, et al. Nonrhab-domyosarcoma soft tissue sarcomas in children: the Mayo Clinic experience. *Clin Orthop* 2000;374: 247–258.

22. Okcu MF, Despa S, Choroszy M, et al. Synovial sar-coma in children and adolescents: thirty three years of experience with multimodal therapy. *Med Pediatr Oncol* 2001;37(2):90–96.

23. Womer RB, Pressey JG. Rhabdomyosarcoma and soft tissue sarcoma in childhood. *Curr Opin Oncol* 2000;12(4):337–344.

24. Ferrari A, Casanova M, Bisagno G, et al. Malignant vascular tumors in children and adolescents: a report from the Italian and German soft tissue sarcoma co-operative group. *Med Pediatr Oncol* 2002;39: 109–114.

25. Brizel DM, Weinstein H, Hunt M, et al. Failure pat-terns and survival in pediatric soft tissue sarcoma. *Int J Radiat Oncol Biol Phys* 1988;15:37–41.

26. Neifeld JP, Berg JW, Godwin D, et al. A retrospective epidemiologic study of pediatric fibrosarcomas. *J Pe-diatr Surg* 1978;13:735–739.

27. Cecchetto G, Carli M, Alaggio R, et al. Fibrosarcoma in pediatric patients: results of the Italian cooperative group studies (1979–1995). *J Surg Oncol* 2001;78: 225–231.

28. Canpolat C, Evans HL, Corpron C, et al. Fibromyx-oid sarcoma in a four-year old child: case report and review of the literature. *Med Pediatr Oncol* 1996;27: 561–564.

29. Staples JJ, Robinson RA, Wen BC, et al. Heman-giopericytoma: the role of radiotherapy. *Int J Radiat Oncol Biol Phys* 1990;19:445–451.

30. Nash A, Stout AP. Malignant mesenchymomas in children. *Cancer* 1961;14:524–533.

31. Newman PL, Fletcher CDM. Malignant mesenchy-moma: clinicopathologic analysis of a series with ev-idence of low-grade behaviour. *Am J Surg Pathol* 1991;15:607–614.

32. Gross E, Rao BN, Papo A, et al. Epithelioid sarcoma in children. *J Pediatr Surg* 1996;31(12):1663–1665.

33. Enzinger FM, Weiss SW. *Soft tissue sarcomas.* St Louis: CV Mosby, 1983.

34. Kim TH, Bell BA, Mauer HM, et al. Sarcomas of soft tissues and their benign counterparts. In: Fernbach DJ, Vietti TJ, eds. *Clinical pediatric oncology,* 4th ed. St Louis: Mosby–Year Book, 1991:517–544.

35. Pappo AS. Rhabdomyosarcoma and other soft tissue sarcomas in children. *Curr Opin Oncol* 1996;8: 311–316.

36. Casanova M, Ferrari A, Bisogno G, et al. Alveolar soft part sarcoma in children and adolescents: a re-port from the Soft-Tissue Sarcoma Italian Coopera-tive Group. *Ann Oncol* 2000;11(11):1445–1449.

37. Ben Arush MW, Nahum MP, Meller I, et al. The role of chemotherapy in childhood soft tissue sarcomas other than rhabdomyosarcomas: experience of the Northern Israel Oncology Center. *Pediatr Hematol Oncol* 1999;16:397–406.

38. Dehner LP. Primitive neuroectodermal tumor and Ewing's sarcoma. *Am J Surg Pathol* 1993;17:1–13.

39. Goodman KA, Wolden SL, La Quaglia MP, et al. Whole abdominopelvic radiotherapy for desmoplas-tic small round-cell tumor. *Int J Radiat Oncol Biol Phys* 2002;54(1):170–176.

40. Lae ME, Roche PC, Jin L, et al. Desmoplastic small round cell tumor: a clinicopathologic, immunohisto-chemical, and molecular study of 32 tumors. *Am J Surg Pathol* 2002;26(7):823–835.

41. Ferrari A, Casanova M, Bisogno G, et al. Clear cell sarcoma of tendons and aponeuroses in pediatric pa-tients: a report from the Italian and German Soft Tis-sue Sarcoma Cooperative Group. *Cancer* 2002; 94(12):3269–3276.

42. Parasuraman S, Rao BN, Bodner S, et al. Clear cell sarcoma of soft tissues in children and young adults: the St. Jude Children's Research Hospital experience. *Pediatr Hematol Oncol* 1999;16(6):539–544.

43. Raney RB Jr. Synovial sarcoma. *Med Pediatr Oncol* 1981;91:41–45.

44. Raney RB Jr. Chemotherapy for children with aggres-sive fibromatosis and Langerhans' cell history–tosis. *Clin Orthop* 1987;59:1–5.

45. Salloum E, Flamant F, Caillaud JM, et al. Diagnostic and therapeutic problems of soft tissue tumors other than rhabdomyosarcoma in infants under 1 year of age: a clinicopathological study of 34 cases treated at the Institut Gustave–Roussy. *Med Pediatr Oncol* 1991;18:37–43.

46. Suit HD, Mankin HJ, Wood WC, et al. Preoperative, intraoperative, and postoperative radiation in the treatment of primary soft tissue sarcoma. *Cancer* 1985;55:2659–2667.

47. Jones DN, McCowage GB, Sostman HD, et al. Mon-itoring of neoadjuvant therapy response of soft-tissue and musculoskeletal sarcoma using fluorine-18-FDG PET. *J Nucl Med* 1996;37:1438–1444.

48. LeVay J, O'Sullivan B, Cotton C, et al. Outcome and prognostic factors in soft tissue sarcoma. *Int J Radiat Oncol Biol Phys* 1992;24[Suppl 1]:182–183.

49. Miser JS, Triche TJ, Pritchard DJ, et al. Ewing's sarcoma and the nonrhabdomyosarcoma soft tissue sarcomas of childhood. In: Pizzo PA, Poplack DG, eds. *Principles and practice of pediatric oncology.* Philadelphia: JB Lippincott, 1989:659–688.

50. Wenger J, Davidson R. Fibrosarcoma of the leg. *Med Pediatr Oncol* 1984;12:209–211.

51. Parham DM, Webber BL, Jenkins JJ, et al. Nonrhabdomyosarcomatous soft tissue sarcomas of childhood: formulation of a simplified system for grading. *Mod Pathol* 1995;8:705–710.

52. Rao BN. Nonrhabdomyosarcoma in children: prognostic factors influencing survival. *Semin Surg Oncol* 1993;9:524–531.

53. Enneking WF, Spanier SS, Goodman MA. A system for the surgical staging of musculoskeletal sarcomas. *Clin Orthop* 1980;153:106–120.

54. Harmer C. Management of soft tissue sarcomas. In: Selby P, Bailey C, eds. *Cancer and the adolescent.* London: BMJ Publishing Group, 1996:69–89.

55. Mazanet R, Antman KH. Adjuvant therapy for sarcomas. *Semin Oncol* 1991;18:603–612.

56. Suit HD. The George Edelstyn Memorial lecture: radiation in the management of malignant soft tissue tumours. *Clin Oncol* 1989;1:5–10.

57. Tepper JE, Suit HD. The role of radiation therapy in the treatment of sarcoma of soft tissue. *Cancer Invest* 1985;3:587–592.

58. Delaney TF, Stinson SF, Greenberg J, et al. Effects on limb function of combined modality limb-sparing therapy for extremity soft tissue sarcoma. *Proc ASCO* 1991;10:350.

59. Eilber FR, Guiliana AE, Huth J, et al. High grade soft-tissue sarcomas of the extremity: UCLA experience with limb-sparing. *Prog Clin Biol Res* 1985; 201:59–74.

60. National Institutes of Health Consensus Development Conference Statement. Limb-sparing treatment of adult soft-tissue sarcomas and osteosarcomas. Bethesda, MD: NIH, 1985;3:1–8.

61. Mazeron JJ, Suit HD. Lymph nodes as sites of metastases from sarcomas of soft tissue. *Cancer* 1987; 60(8):1800–1808.

62. Jablons D, Steinberg SM, Roth J, et al. Metastasectomy for soft tissue sarcoma: further evidence for efficacy and prognostic indicators. *J Thorac Cardiovasc Surg* 1989;97:695–705.

63. Casson AG, Putman JB, Natarajan G, et al. Efficacy of pulmonary metastasectomy for recurrent soft tissue sarcoma. *J Surg Oncol* 1991;47:1–4.

64. Kalnicki S. Radiation therapy in the treatment of bone and soft tissue sarcomas. *Orthop Clin North Am* 1989;20:505–512.

65. Schray MF, Gunderson LL, Sim FH, et al. Soft tissue sarcoma: integration of brachytherapy, resection, and external irradiation. *Cancer* 1990;66:451–456.

66. Stockdale AD, Casson AM, Coe MA, et al. Radiotherapy and conservative surgery in the management of musculo-aponeurotic fibromatosis. *Int J Radiat Oncol Biol Phys* 1988;15:851–857.

67. Pediatric Oncology Group Protocol 8653/8654. *A study of childhood soft tissue sarcoma other than rhabdomyosarcoma and its variations.* Chicago: Pediatric Oncology Group, 1986.

68. Marcus RJ. Current controversies in pediatric radiation oncology. *Orthop Clin North Am* 1996;27:551–557.

68a. Spiro IJ, Gebhardt MC, Jennings LC, et al. Prognostic factors for local control of sarcomas of the soft tissues managed by radiation and surgery. *Semin Oncol* 1997;24(5):540–546.

69. Rosenberg SA, Glatstein E, Chang AE. The role of adjuvant chemotherapy in the treatment of soft tissue sarcomas: review of the National Cancer Institute studies. In: van Oosteram AT, van Unnik JAM eds. *Management of soft tissue and bone sarcomas.* New York: Raven Press, 1986:201–214.

70. Chang AE, Sugarbaker PH, Rosenberg SA. Quality of life after different treatment modalities for soft tissue sarcoma: review of National Cancer Institute studies. In: van Oosteram AT, van Unnik JAM, eds. *Management of soft tissue and bone sarcomas.* New York: Raven Press, 1986:225–232.

71. Stinson SF, Dellancy TF, Greenberg J, et al. Acute and long-term effects on limb function of combined modality limb sparing therapy for extremity soft tissue sarcoma. *Int J Radiat Oncol Biol Phys* 1991;21:1493–1499.

72. Bertucio CS, Wara WM, Matthay KK, et al. Functional and clinical outcomes of limb-sparing therapy for pediatric extremity sarcomas. *Int J Radiat Oncol Biol Phys* 2001;49(3):763–769.

*73. Spunt SL, Poquette CA, Hurt YS, et al. Prognostic factors for children and adolescents with surgically resected nonrhabdomyosarcoma soft tissue sarcoma: an analysis of 121 patients treated at St. Jude Children's Research Hospital. *J Clin Oncol* 1999;17(12): 3697–3705.

74. Pappo AS, Rao BN, Jenkins JJ, et al. Metastatic nonrhabdomyosarcomatous soft-tissue sarcomas in children and adolescents: the St. Jude Children's Research Hospital experience. *Med Pediatr Oncol* 1999;33(2):76–82.

75. Blaskely ML, Spurbeck WW, Pappo AS, et al. The impact of margin of resection on outcome in pediatric nonrhabdomyosarcoma soft tissue sarcoma. *J Pediatr Surg* 1999;34(5):672–675.

76. Raney RB Jr, Allen A, O'Neill J, et al. Malignant fibrous histiocytoma of soft tissue in childhood. *Cancer* 1991;262:58–63.

77. Horowitz M, Pratt C, Webber B, et al. Childhood malignant soft tissue sarcomas other than rhabdomyosarcoma: results of therapy. *Proc ASCO* 1984;3:84.

78. Meyer WH, Pratt CB, Thompson EI, et al. Ifosfamide/etoposide (Ifos/VP-16) in patients with previously untreated Ewing's sarcoma or primitive neuroectodermal tumors. *Proc ASCO* 1991;10:317.

79. Koscielniak E, Jugens H, Winkler K, et al. Treatment of soft tissue sarcoma in childhood and adolescence. *Cancer* 1992;70:2557–2567.

*80. Pratt CB, Pappo AS, Giesler P, et al. Role of adjuvant chemotherapy in the treatment of surgically resected pediatric nonrhabdomyosarcomatous soft tissue sarcomas: a Pediatric Oncology Group Study. *J Clin Oncol* 1999;17(4):1219.

81. Treuner J, Jurgens H, Winkler K, et al. The treatment of 30 children and adolescents of synovial sarcoma in accordance with the protocol of the German multicenter study for soft tissue sarcoma. *Proc ASCO* 1987;6:215.

82. Sommelet-Olive D. Non-rhabdo malignant mesenchymal tumors in children. *Med Pediatr Oncol* 1995;25:273.

83. Sommelet-Olive D, Oberlin O, Flamant F, et al. Non-rhabdo malignant mesenchymal tumors in children, results of SIOP MMT 84 and 89 protocols. *Proc ASCO* 1995;14:446.

83a. Verweij J, Pinendo HM. Adjuvant chemotherapy of soft tissue sarcomas. In: Verweij J, Pinedo HM, Suit HD, eds. *Soft tissue sarcomas: present achievements and future prospects.* Boston: Kluwer, 1997:173–188.

84. Alvegard TA, Sigurdsson H, Mourdisen H, et al. Adjuvant chemotherapy with doxorubicin and high grade soft tissue sarcoma: a randomized trial of the Scandinavian Sarcoma Group. *J Clin Oncol* 1989;7:1504–1513.

*85. Bramwell V, Rouesse J, Steward W, et al. Adjuvant CYVADIC chemotherapy for adult soft tissue sarcoma: reduced local recurrence but no improvement in survival: a study of the European Organization for Research and Treatment of Cancer Soft Tissue and Bone Sarcoma Group. *J Clin Oncol* 1994;12:1137–1149.

86. Newton WA Jr, Soule EH, Hamoudi AB, et al. A prospective study of nonrhabdomyosarcoma soft tissue sarcomas in the pediatric age group. *J Pediatr Surg* 1992;27:241–245.

87. Womer RB. Problems and controversies in the management of childhood sarcomas. *Br Med Bull* 1996;4:826–843.

*88. Pratt CB, Pappo AS, Gieser P, et al. Role of adjuvant chemotherapy in the treatment of surgically resected pediatric nonrhabdomyosarcomatous soft tissue sarcomas: a Pediatric Oncology Group study. *J Clin Oncol* 1999;17:1219–1226.

*89. Sarcoma Meta-Analysis Collaboration. Adjuvant chemotherapy for localised resectable soft-tissue sarcoma of adults: meta-analysis of individual data. *Lancet* 1997;350:1647–1654.

90. Tierney JF, Mosseri V, Stuart LA, et al. Adjuvant chemotherapy for soft tissue sarcoma: review and meta-analysis of the published results of randomized clinical trials. *Br J Cancer* 1995;72:469–475.

91. Frustaci S, Gherlinzoni F, DePaoli A, et al. Adjuvant chemotherapy for adult soft tissue sarcomas of the extremities and girdles: results of the Italian Cooperative Trial. *J Clin Oncol* 2001;19:1238–1247.

92. Wiklund T, Saeter G, Strander H, et al. The outcome of advanced soft tissue sarcoma patients with complete tumour regression after either chemotherapy alone or chemotherapy plus surgery. The Scandinavian Sarcoma Group Experience. *Eur J Cancer* 1997;33:357–361.

93. Cheng EY, Dusenbery KE, Winters MR, et al. Soft tissue sarcomas: preoperative versus postoperative radiotherapy. *J Surg Oncol* 1996;61:90–99.

94. Tanabe K, Sherman N, Pollock R, et al. Local control of extremity sarcomas treated with preoperative radiotherapy and limb sparing surgery. *Proc ASCO* 1991;10:351.

95. Keus RB, Rutgers EJT, Ho GH, et al. Limb sparing therapy of extremity soft tissue sarcomas: treatment outcome and long-term functional results. *Eur J Cancer* 1994;30A:1459–1463.

96. Hiraoka M, Nishimura Y, Nagata Y, et al. Hyperthermia combined with radiotherapy in the treatment of soft tissue tumors. *Int J Radiat Oncol Biol Phys* 1992;24[Suppl 1]:297–298.

97. Suit HD, Spiro I. Role of radiation in the management of adult patients with sarcoma of soft tissue. *Semin Surg Oncol* 1994;10:347–356.

98. Sawyer TE, Peterson IA, Pritchard DJ, et al. Prognostic factors in extremity soft tissue sarcomas treated with limb salvage therapy. Joint Meeting of European Musculo-skeletal Oncology Society and American Musculo-Skeletal Tumor Society. Florence, Italy, May 8, 1995.

*99. O'Sullivan B, Davis AM, Turcotte R, et al. Preoperative versus postoperative radiotherapy in soft-tissue sarcoma of the limbs: a randomized trial. *Lancet* 2002;359:2235–2241.

100. Barkley H Jr, Martin RG, Romsdahl MM, et al. Treatment of soft tissue sarcomas by preoperative irradiation and conservative surgical resection. *Int J Radiat Oncol Biol Phys* 1988;14:693–699.

101. MacKenzie DH. Synovial sarcoma: a review of 58 cases. *Cancer* 1966;19:169–180.

102. Pratt J, Woodruff JM, Marcove RC. Epithelioid sarcoma: an analysis of 22 cases indicating the prognostic significance of vascular invasion and regional lymph node metastasis. *Cancer* 1978;41:1472–1487.

103. Santavirta S. Synovial sarcoma: a clinicopathological study of 31 cases. *Arch Orthop Trauma Surg* 1992;111:155–159.

103a. Benninghoff D, Robbins R. The nature and treatment of desmoid tumors. *AJR* 1964;91:132–137.

104. Kinsella TJ, Glatstein E. Clinical experience with intravenous radiosensitizers in unresectable sarcomas. *Cancer* 1987;59:908–915.

105. Gerbaulet A, Panis X, Flamant F, et al. Iridium afterloading curietherapy in the treatment of pediatric malignancies: the Institut Gustave–Roussy experience. *Cancer* 1958;56:1274–1279.

106. Shiu MH, Hilaris BS, Harrison LB, et al. Brachytherapy and function-saving resection of soft tissue sarcoma arising in the limb. *Int J Radiat Oncol Biol Phys* 1991;21:1485–1492.

107. Burmeister BH, Dickinson I, Bryant G, et al. Intraoperative implant brachytherapy in the management of soft-tissue sarcomas. *Aust N Z J Surg* 1997;67:5–8.

*108. Nag S, Shasha D, Janjan N, et al. The American Brachytherapy Society recommendations for brachytherapy of soft tissue sarcomas. *Int J Radiat Oncol Biol Phys* 2001;49(4):1033–1043.

*109. Nag S, Tippin D, Ruymann FB. Intraoperative high-dose brachytherapy for the treatment of pediatric tumors: the Ohio State University experience. *Int J Radiat Oncol Biol Phys* 2001;51(3):729–735.

110. Nag S, Fernandes PS, Martinez-Monge R, et al. Use of brachytherapy to preserve function in children with soft-tissue sarcomas. *Oncology* 1999;13(3):361–370, 733–734.

111. Nag S, Gupta N. A simple method of obtaining equivalent doses for use in HDR brachytherapy. *Int J Radiat Oncol Biol Phys* 2000;46:507–513.

*112. Harrison LB, Franzese F, Gaynor J, et al. Long term

results of a prospective randomized trial of adjuvant brachytherapy in the management of completely resected soft tissue sarcoma of the extremity and superficial trunk. *Int J Radiat Oncol Biol Phys* 1993; 27:259–265.

113. Devlin PM, Harrison LB. Brachytherapy for soft tissue sarcomas. In: Verweig J, Pinedo HM, Suit HD, eds. *Soft tissue sarcomas: present achievements and future prospects.* Boston: Kluwer, 1997:107–128.

*114. Pisters PWT, Harrison LB, Woodruff JM, et al. A prospective randomized trial of adjuvant brachytherapy in the management of low-grade soft tissue sarcomas of the extremity and superficial trunk. *J Clin Oncol* 1994;6:1150–1155.

115. Habrand JL, Gerbaulet A, Pejovic MH, et al. Twenty years experience of interstitial iridium brachytherapy in the management of soft tissue sarcomas. *Int J Radiat Oncol Biol Phys* 1991;20:405–411.

116. Willett CG, Suit HD, Tepper JE, et al. Intraoperative electron beam radiation therapy for retroperitoneal soft tissue sarcoma. *Cancer* 1991;68:278–283.

117. Uno T, Itami J, Kato H. Combined chemo-radiation and hyperthermia for locally advanced soft tissue sarcoma: response and toxicity. *Anticancer Res* 1995;15:2655–2658.

118. Brizel DM, Scully SP, Harrelson JM, et al. Radiation therapy and hyperthermia improve the oxygenation of human soft tissue sarcomas. *Cancer Res* 1996;56:5347–5350.

119. Leopold KA, Harrelson J, Prosnitz L, et al. Preoperative hyperthermia and radiation for soft tissue sarcomas: advantage of two vs. one hyperthermia treatments per week. *Int J Radiat Oncol Biol Phys* 1989;16:107–115.

120. Scully SP, Oleson JR, Leopold KA, et al. Clinical outcome after neoadjuvant thermoradiotherapy in high grade soft tissue sarcomas. *J Surg Oncol* 1994;57:143–151.

121. Glaholm J, Harmer C. Soft-tissue sarcoma: neutrons versus photons for postoperative irradiation. *Br J Radiol* 1988;61:829–834.

122. Larramore GE, Griffith JT, Boespflug M, et al. Fast neutron radiotherapy for sarcomas of soft tissue, bone, and cartilage. *Am J Clin Oncol* 1989;12: 320–326.

123. Cecchetto G, Carli M, Scotti G, et al. Importance of local treatment in pediatric soft tissue sarcomas with microscopic residual after primary surgery: results of the Italian Cooperative Study RMS-88. *Med Pediatr Oncol* 2000;34(2):97–101.

124. Kiel KD, Suit HD. Radiation therapy in the treatment of aggressive fibromatoses (desmoid tumors). *Cancer* 1984;54:2041–2055.

125. Acker JC, Bossen EH, Halperin EC. The management of desmoid tumors. *Int J Radiat Oncol Biol Phys* 1993;26:851–858.

*126. Suit H, Spiro I. Radiation in the multidisciplinary management of desmoid tumors. In: Meyer JL, ed. *The radiation therapy of benign disease. Current indicators and techniques. Front Radiat Ther Oncol.* Basel: Karger, 2001;35:107–119.

127. Nuyttens J, Rust PF, Thomas Jr CR, et al. Surgery versus radiotherapy for patients with aggressive fibromatosis or desmoid tumors: a comparative review of 22 articles. *Cancer* 2000;88:1517–1523.

128. Reitamo JJ. The desmoid tumor. *Arch Surg* 1983;118:1318–1322.

129. Suit HD, Spiro IJ, Speer M. Benign and low grade tumors of the soft tissues: role for radiation therapy. In: Verweig J, Pinedo HM, Suit HD, eds. *Soft tissue sarcomas: present achievements and future prospects.* Boston: Kluwer, 1997:95–106.

130. Sherman NE, Romsdahl M, Evans H, et al. Desmoid tumors: a 20 year radiotherapy experience. *Int J Radiat Oncol Biol Phys* 1990;19:37–40.

*131. Merchant TE, Nguyen D, Walter AW, et al. Long-term results with radiation therapy for pediatric desmoid tumor. *Int J Radiat Oncol Biol Phys* 2000; 47:1267–1271.

132. Zlotecki RA, Scarborough MT, Morris CG, et al. External beam radiotherapy for primary and adjuvant management of aggressive fibromatosis. *Int J Radiat Oncol Biol Phys* 2002;54:177–181.

133. Enzinger FM, Shiraki M. Musculoaponeurotic fibromatoma of shoulder girdle (extra abdominal desmoid): analysis of 30 cases. *Cancer* 1967;20:1131–1140.

134. Walther E, Hunig R, Zaled S. Behandlung der aggressiven Fibramatose (desmoid). *Orthopedie* 1988; 17:193–200.

135. Schultz-Ertner D, Zierhut D, Mende U, et al. The role of radiation therapy in the management of desmoid tumors. *Strahlenther Onkol* 2002;178:78–83.

136. McCullough WM, Parson JT, van der Griend R, et al. Radiation therapy for aggressive fibromatosis. *J Bone Joint Surg* 1991;73A(5):717–725.

137. Zelefsky MJ, Harrison LB, Shiu MH, et al. Combined surgical resection and iridium 192 implantation for locally advanced and recurrent desmoid tumors. *Cancer* 1991;67:380–384.

138. Ballo MT, Zagars GK, Pollac A. Radiation therapy in the management of desmoid tumors. *Int J Radiat Oncol Biol Phys* 1998;42:1007–1014.

139. Miralbell R, Suit HB, Mankin H, et al. Fibromatoses: from postsurgical surveillance to combined surgery and radiation therapy. *Int J Radiat Oncol Biol Phys* 1990;18:535–540.

140. De Pas T, Boderi L, Pelasi G, et al. Peptide receptor radiotherapy: a new option for the management of aggressive fibromatosis on behalf of the Italian sarcoma group. *Br J Cancer* 2003;88:645–647.

141. Samuels BL. Management of recurrent desmoid tumor after surgery and radiation: rate of cytotoxic and non-cytotoxic therapies. *Surg Oncol* 1999;8:191–196.

*142. Faulkner LB, Hajdu SI, Kher U, et al. Pediatric desmoid tumor: retrospective analysis of 63 cases. *J Clin Oncol* 1995;13:2813–2818.

143. Lackner H, Urban C, Kerbi R, et al. Noncytotoxic drug therapy in children with unresectable desmoid tumors. *Cancer* 1997;80:334–340.

144. Raney RB. Soft-tissue sarcoma in childhood and adolescence. *Curr Oncol Rep* 2002;4(4):291–298.

145. Raney B Jr. Soft-tissue sarcoma in adolescents. In: Tebbi CK, ed. *Major topics in adolescent oncology.* Mount Kisco, NY: Futura Publishing, 1987:221–240.

146. Carli M, Guglielmi M, Sotti G, et al. Soft tissue sarcoma. In: Pinkerton CR, Plowman PN, eds. *Paediatric oncology: clinical practice and controversies,* 2nd ed. London: Chapman & Hall Medical, 1997: 380–416.

147. Dillon P, Maurer J, Jenkins J, et al. A prospective

study of nonrhabdomyosarcoma soft tissue sarcomas in the pediatric age group. *J Pediatr Surg* 1992;27:241–245.

148. Leibel SA, Wara WM, Hill DR, et al. Desmoid tumors: local control and patterns of relapse following radiation therapy. *Int J Radiat Oncol Biol Phys* 1983;9(8):1167–1171.

149. Keus R, Bartelink H. The role of radiotherapy in the treatment of desmoid tumors. *Radiother Oncol* 1986;7:1–5.

150. Bataini JP, Belloir C, Mazabraud A, et al. Desmoid tumors in adults: the role of radiotherapy in their management. *Am J Surg* 1988;155:754–760.

151. Plukker JT, Oort IV, Vermey A, et al. Aggressive fibromatosis (non-familial desmoid tumour): therapeutic problems and the role of adjuvant radiotherapy. *Br J Surg* 1995;82:510–514.

152. Pritchard DJ, Nascimento AG, Petersen IA. Local control of extra-abdominal desmoid tumors. *J Bone Joint Surg* 1996;78A;848–854.

153. Kamath SS, Parsons JT, Marcus RB, et al. Radiotherapy for local control of aggressive fibromatosis. *Int J Radiat Oncol Biol Phys* 1996;36:325–328.

154. Shin KH, Shin SJ, Lee DH, et al. The role of radiotherapy in the treatment of aggressive fibromatosis. *Yonsei Med J* 1999;40:439–443.

155. Pignatti G, Barbanti-Brodano G, Ferrari D, et al. Extraabdominal desmoid tumor: a study of 83 cases. *Clin Orthop* 2000;375:207–213.

156. Hayes-Jordan AA, Spunt SL, Poquette CA, et al. Nonrhabdomyosarcoma soft tissue sarcomas in children: is age at diagnosis an important variable? *J Pediatr Surg* 2000;35(6):948–954.

13

Wilms' Tumor

Edward C. Halperin, M.D.

HISTORY

The first description of a Wilms' tumor was from Thomas F. Rance (1) in his 1814 report "Case of Fungus Haematodes in Kidnies." In 1828, Dr. Ebenezer Gairdner (2), Fellow of the Royal College of Physicians, Edinburgh, published the second case. The patient was a 3-year-old girl named Agnes B. who died of a left renal tumor that weighed 5 pounds, 3 ounces. In 1879, renowned physician William Osler (3) described two cases of "myo-sarcoma of the kidney," one of which had tumor extension into the right heart and pulmonary artery. Max Wilms (1867–1918), who was trained in pathology, internal medicine, and surgery thoroughly reviewed the pertinent literature and added seven new patients in his 1899 monograph *Die Mischgeschwuelste*. In addition to renal tumors, Wilms described the histologically "mixed tumors" of the ovary, testicle, head and neck, bladder, and other organs (4). It was because of Wilms' exceptional monograph that his name became connected with this childhood tumor (Fig. 13-1) (5).

By the mid-twentieth century, radiation oncologists had developed a large body of clinical experience with Wilms' tumor and began formulating opinions about the role of radiotherapy in the management of the tumor. Ralston Paterson (6), distinguished radiation oncologist of the Christie Hospital and Holt Radium Institute of Manchester, England, wrote in his 1948 textbook,

> We feel that the most promising policy's to start treatment by radiotherapy and not by surgery. X-ray therapy is used and consists of abdominal x-ray baths to cover the entire tumor and any possible intra-abdominal extension. An interval of six weeks to three months is then allowed in which the tumor mass entirely disappears. . . . Two opposing fields, anterior and posterior . . . cover the whole abdomen including the liver. . . . The essential point in the treatment of Wilms' tumor is to remember that even enormous tumors can be made operable and that radiation followed by nephrectomy can undoubtedly obtain cure in some cases.

Dean and Guttmann (7) expressed the predominant viewpoint of U.S. radiation oncologists when they wrote in their 1950 textbook.

> The successful treatment of a Wilms' tumor depends upon the complete removal or complete devitalization of the primary growth before metastasis occurs. No type of treatment given singly or combined with other forms of treatment has proved successful after metastasis has become established. Ladd, working at the Children's Hospital of Boston, has obtained by far the best end results by operating on these infants as soon as possible. We also recommend prompt removal. . . . [When preoperative therapy is necessary] . . . to shrink a Wilms' tumor and thereby facilitate its operable removal, external roentgen therapy is the treatment of choice. Usually, however, after five or six exposures, the tumors become significantly smaller and sometimes at the end of two weeks it is no longer palpable. . . . Following radiation infarction seems to be more widespread.

Dean and Guttmann's views were reinforced by Jacox and Cahill's (8) review of the management of Wilms' tumor. They wrote,

> At present we believe that nephrectomy should be performed as soon as the diagnosis of Wilms' tumor is made, irrespective of the size of the mass. In general, preoperative irradiation is not favored, because we believe that waiting needlessly jeopardizes the patient's chances of survival. Ladd and White and their confreres at the Boston Children's Hospital have made a serious study of the removal of these tumors by the transperitoneal route, with a minimum of handling either for diagnosis or on the opera-

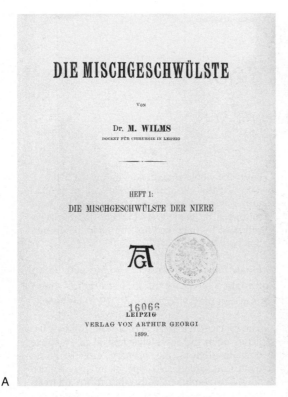

A

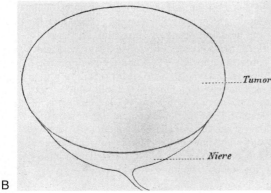

B

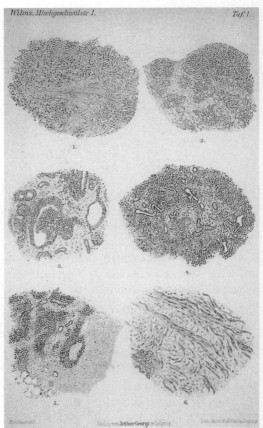

C

FIG. 13-1. (A, B) In his monograph, *Die Mischgeschwulste der Niere* (*The Mixed Tumor of the Kidney*), published in Leipzig in 1899, Max Wilms described, as his first illustrative case, "niven tumor von einem 3 jahrien Madchen" ("renal tumor of a 3-year-old girl"). **(C)** Wilms described the blastemal, epithelial (tubules), and stromal elements seen on microscopic examination of "mixed" renal tumor.

ing table, with ligation of the renal vessels and pedicle before displacement of the tumor. The result has been a much higher proportion free from recurrence that has formerly been reported.

What we can see, in this brief historical review of the origins of radiotherapy for Wilms' tumor, is the divide between U.S. radiation oncologists and their European colleagues. The European literature favored preoperative treatment, and the U.S. literature favored postoperative radiation therapy. We also see the acknowl-

edgment that wide treatment volumes to cover the entire tumor bed are necessary. We will address these themes in more detail later in this chapter.

EPIDEMIOLOGY

Wilms' tumor (nephroblastoma) is an embryonic kidney tumor. It is the most common abdominal tumor in children and represents 6% of childhood cancer. The incidence rate in white children younger than 15 years is 8.1 new cases per million population (9). There are approximately 470 to 500 new cases in the United States per year (10,11). Wilms' tumor is bilateral at presentation in 4–8% of cases (12–14).

The median age at diagnosis is 41.5 months for boys with unilateral tumors and 46.9 months for girls with unilateral tumors. For bilateral tumors, the median age at presentation is 29.5 months for boys and 32.6 months for girls (10). More than 75% of patients present before 5 years of age. The male:female ratio is 0.92 for unilateral tumors and 0.6 for bilateral tumors (10). The incidence rate is approximately three times higher for blacks in the United States and Africa than for East Asians. Rates for the white populations in Europe and North America are intermediate between those of blacks and East Asians. Children tend to present with more advanced disease in less developed nations (15–18).

MOLECULAR BIOLOGY

In Chapter 5 of this text we discussed the Knudson "two-hit" hypothesis of the origins of retinoblastoma. This hypothesis explained the earlier age of onset and bilateral presentation of familial retinoblastoma compared with sporadic cases. Subsequent research confirmed the veracity of the two-hit hypothesis for retinoblastoma and showed that it could be explained by the inactivation of both alleles of a tumor suppressor gene on the long arm of chromosome 13 (13q). After vetting his hypothesis for retinoblastoma, Knudson proposed a similar model for Wilms' tumor in 1972 (19,20).

Like retinoblastoma, Wilms' tumor may be unilateral or bilateral. The 4–8% occurrence of bilateral disease, appearing at an earlier age than unilateral disease and associated with a greater frequency of other hereditary anomalies, supports the concept of a specific predisposing constitutional chromosomal deletion. It should be noted that fewer familial and bilateral cases of Wilms' tumor than retinoblastoma were available for analysis because of the lower incidence of familial Wilms' tumor and the poor disease survival at that time (21–24).

Wilms' tumor is associated with congenital anomalies in 10–13% of cases (16,17,25,26). Aniridia is present in 1% of children with Wilms' tumor; hemihypertrophy is noted in 2–3% (26–28). Other genitourinary malformations are identified in 5% of cases, primarily cryptorchidism, hypospadias, double collecting system, or fused kidney (17,28,29). It seemed reasonable to look for candidate Wilms' tumor genes in association with these congenital anomalies.

The next major clue to the molecular genetics of Wilms' tumor was found from the syndrome of Wilms' tumor with aniridia, genitourinary malformations, and mental retardation (WAGR syndrome). Karyotypic analysis of children with WAGR syndrome showed a deletion on the short arm of chromosome 11, band 13 (11p13). This deletion encompasses the aniridia gene *PAX6* and the Wilms' tumor suppressor gene *WT1*. *WT1* is a developmentally regulated transcription factor of the zinc finger family. However, analysis of sporadic Wilms' tumors shows evidence of *WT1* mutation in only 5–10% of cases. Therefore, although *WT1* appears to be a tumor suppressor gene, it accounts for a minority of Wilms' tumors (21–24).

Wilms' tumor also occurs with greater frequency in the Beckwith–Wiedemann syndrome (30). This familial condition variably includes macrosomia or hemihypertrophy, macroglossia, omphalocele, abdominal organomegaly, and ear pits or creases. The genetic locus of this syndrome is also on the short arm of chromosome 11 (11p15). The putative second Wilms' tumor suppressor gene, located at this site, is called *WT2* (18,19). *WT2*(LP15) has effects on IGF2, the H19 tumor suppressor gene, and the P57 cell cycle regulator (31–35).

In addition to the tumor suppressor genes associated with Wilms' tumor, there is evidence of genetic loci that may be related to more malignant or aggressive Wilms' tumors. In a study of 232 children with Wilms' tumor registered in the National Wilms' Tumor Studies 3 and 4, loss of chromosomal material (called loss of heterozygosity [LOH]) on the long arm of chromosome 16 (16q) was associated with a statistically significantly poorer 2-year relapse-free and overall survival. (If there is no LOH for 16q, 2-year relapse-free survival is 90%, compared with 78% if there is LOH.) The difference remained when the analysis was adjusted for stage or histologic subgroup (31,35). Loss of chromosomal material from the short arm of chromosome 1 (1p) was also associated with poorer relapse-free and overall survival of borderline statistical significance (if chromosomal material from 1p is absent, 2-year relapse-free survival is 88%, compared with 64% if present) (10,31). Recent assessments of the Wilms' tumor 1 gene (11p13) include analyses of the knockout model for this gene. Mice who have the gene knocked out have failure of development of the kidneys and gonads. High levels of *WT1* suppress VGR1, IGF2, and PDFA as well as complex p53 (32,33). These data suggest that the gene acts as a tumor suppressor gene or is a dominant oncogene. The prognostic importance of loss of material on 1p and 16q is prospectively evaluated in National Wilms' Tumor Study 5 (NWTS-5). They are appropriately called *Wilms' tumor progression genes*.

Our current understanding indicates that loss of heterozygosity at 16q and at 1p is associated with a worse outcome. However, it is important to be aware that molecular staging may prove only to be different from, not better than, conventional staging. Molecular staging must be tested and evaluated as any other form of staging should.

It is hoped that identifying the genes associated with Wilms' tumor will add to our knowledge of tumor suppressor genes, allow more precise genetic counseling, help predict outcome of treatment for this tumor, and identify children in need of more aggressive therapy (22,31).

In the future, translational research opportunities may include an assessment of the role of vascular endothelial growth factor (VEGF) in Wilms' tumor management. VEGF seems to promote tumor growth in animals, and anti-VEGF therapy may be promising. Assessing telomerase activity in the tumor and specific antitelomerase drugs may be of value (31–35).

PATHOLOGY

The two popular childhood kidney tumor pathology classification systems are those of the NWTS (Table 13-1) and the International Society of Pediatric Oncology (SIOP) study (Table 13-2).

TABLE 13-1. *Classification of pediatric renal tumors*

International Society of Pediatric Oncology	National Wilms' Tumor Study
I. Low risk	
Cystic partially differentiated Wilms' tumor	Mesoblastic nephroma
Mesoblastic nephroma	
Wilms' tumor with fibroadenomatous structures	
Highly differentiated epithelial Wilms' tumor	
II. Intermediate risk	
Nonanaplastic Wilms' tumor with its variants (excluding low-risk types)	Favorable histology Wilms' tumor
III. High risk	
Anaplastic Wilms' tumor	Anaplastic Focal Diffuse
Clear cell sarcoma	Clear cell sarcoma
Rhabdoid tumor	Rhabdoid tumor

Modified from Schmidt D, Beckwith JB. Histopathology of childhood renal tumor. *Hematol Oncol Clin North Am* 1995;9:1179–1200, with permission.

TABLE 13-2. *Revised International Society of Pediatric Oncology working classification of renal tumors of childhood (2001) for pretreated cases*

Low-risk tumors
Mesoblastic nephroma
Cystic partially differentiated nephroblastoma
Completely necrotic nephroblastoma
Intermediate-risk tumors
Nephroblastoma, epithelial type
Nephroblastoma, stromal type
Nephroblastoma, mixed type
Nephroblastoma, regressive type
Nephroblastoma, focal anaplasia
High-risk tumors
Nephroblastoma, blastemal type
Nephroblastoma, diffuse anaplasia
Clear cell sarcoma of the kidney
Rhabdoid tumor of the kidney

From Vujanic GM, Sandstedt B, Harms D, et al. Revised International Society of Paediatric Oncology (SIOP) working classification of renal tumors of childhood. *Med Pediatr Oncol* 2002;38:79–82, with permission.

Mesoblastic Nephroma

Mesoblastic nephroma is the most common renal tumor encountered in the first month of life. Its median age at presentation is 3 months. It is distinguished from Wilms' tumor by its usually benign behavior, a preponderance of mesenchymal derivatives, and a lack of the malignant epithelial components seen in Wilms'. The tumor consists of spindle-shaped cells in interlacing bundles adjacent to renal parenchyma where there are foci of cystic or dysplastic tubules. The treatment of choice is nephrectomy. Local recurrence is unusual. Nonetheless, adequate margins of resection should be obtained, although recurrence even after operative rupture or positive margins at resection is rare. Distant metastases are also rare. The actuarial 2-year survival is excellent at 98% (35–40).

Nodular Renal Blastemas and Nephrogenic Rests

A spectrum of "pre–Wilms' tumor" entities have been described. Nodular renal blastemas are small but visible subcapsular nodules composed of benign embryonic rests. Nephrogenic rests may be limited to the periphery of the renal cortex (perilobar) or randomly distributed throughout the renal lobe (intralobar). Multifocal or diffuse nephrogenic rests are called nephroblastomatosis.

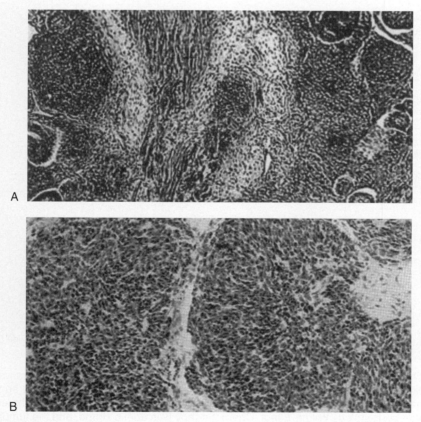

FIG. 13-2. (A, B) James B. Ewing, renowned for the four editions of his book *Pathology of Neoplasia* (Philadelphia: WB Saunders, 1942) and his identification for the tumor now called Ewing's sarcoma, also provided excellent histological descriptions of Wilms' tumor. These slides, from Ewing's book, show the topography of Wilms' embryonal tumor of the kidney with **(A)** epithelial tubules lining in masses of spindle and polyhedral cells and **(B)** the small round cells of the embryonal tumor infiltrating adjacent tissue.

Wilms' Tumor

Wilms' tumor is a triphasic embryonal neoplasm, which includes blastemal, epithelial (tubules), and stromal elements. Each element may exhibit a variety of patterns of aggregation or lines of differentiation (Fig. 13-2) (30,38,39). The proportion of the three components varies from tumor to tumor. If one of the components comprises more than two-thirds of the tumor sample, the pattern is designated according to the predominant component. The mixed type is most common (41% of Wilms' tumor), followed closely by the clinically more aggressive blastemal predominant (39%), the more indolent epithelial predominant (18%), and the stromal predominant (1%), which behaves like the mixed type (Fig. 13-3) (40).

The gross pathologic features of Wilms' tumor include its general occurrence as a single unilateral tumor, although multicentric growth and bilateral disease can occur. The tumor is typically solid, lobulated, and not calcified. However, soft and cystic areas may be encountered.

Histopathologic studies in the NWTS identified factors that correlate with prognosis. In the

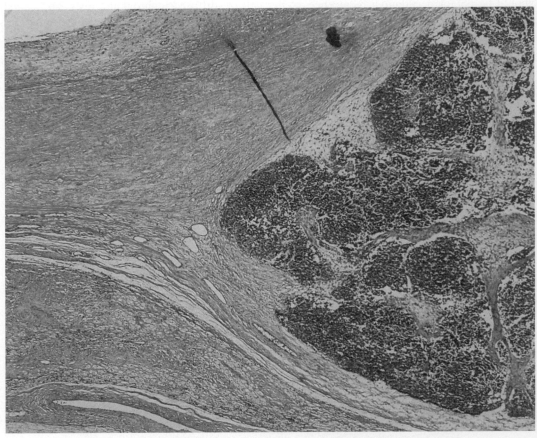

FIG. 13-3. This 4-year-old boy presented with abdominal pain, fever, and vomiting. There was a large right abdominal mass that, on computed tomography, was 10.5 × 13.5 × 18 cm and appeared to arise from the right kidney. There were bilateral pulmonary nodules. Biopsy from the right renal mass indicated favorable histology Wilms' tumor. Chemotherapy was administered, and the tumor partially regressed. A right radical nephrectomy was performed. The 12 × 7 × 9–cm, 530-g kidney had multiple nodules replacing most of the parenchyma. Renal capsular invasion is clearly seen in this photomicrograph. Outside pathology review changed the diagnosis from favorable to unfavorable histology Wilms' tumor. The child received whole lung irradiation and right renal flank irradiation. Chemotherapy was continued. There was no evidence of persistence or recurrent tumor 2 years and 2 months after diagnosis.

first NWTS, 88% of cases were categorized as favorable histology (FH), defined as having typical histologic features of Wilms' tumor without anaplastic or sarcomatous components (41,42). The frequency of this pattern was upheld in the third NWTS, with 89% of cases categorized as FH on central pathology review (43).

Three entities traditionally have been grouped under the general term *unfavorable histology* (UH) in the NWTS: anaplastic Wilms' tumor, clear cell sarcoma, and rhabdoid tumor (39). The latter two are no longer considered to be variants of Wilms' tumor but are distinct entities (30,38).

Anaplasia is defined as significant enlargement of nuclei in the stromal, epithelial, or blastemal cell lines to at least three times the diameter of adjacent nuclei of the same cell type; hyperchromatism of these enlarged nuclei; and multiple mitotic figures (30,38,40,44,45). DNA indices greater than 1.5 are associated with anaplastic histology (37). Anaplasia was noted in 4% of all NWTS-3 entries and in 5% of patients in the SIOP study (38,43,45). Anaplastic tumors are extremely rare in infants, are uncommon before 2 years of age, and make up about 10% of Wilms' tumors diagnosed after 5 years of age

(40). Anaplasia appears to be associated with greater resistance to chemotherapy rather than greater aggressiveness of Wilms' tumor. The 4-year survival in NWTS-3 for patients with anaplastic histology was 82% but was lower in earlier studies (17,42–47).

Anaplastic Wilms' tumor may be focal or diffuse. When this distinction was originally drawn, the term *diffuse anaplasia* was applied to tumors with anaplastic nuclear changes in more than 10% of 400 microscopic fields. *Focal anaplasia* was applied to the remainder of anaplastic tumors. Using this distinction, focal anaplasia was associated with a more favorable outcome than diffuse anaplasia in the first NWTS, but this difference did not obtain statistical significance and was not confirmed in the second and third NWTSs (Fig. 13-4) (48).

The original distinction between focal and diffuse anaplasia did not consider distribution of tumor throughout the kidney, which might affect the likelihood of complete resection. In a recently revised definition, *focal anaplasia* refers to anaplasia that is sharply localized in the primary tumor, without significant nuclear or mitotic atypia in the remainder of the lesion. Diffuse anaplasia is either nonlocalized anaplasia, local-

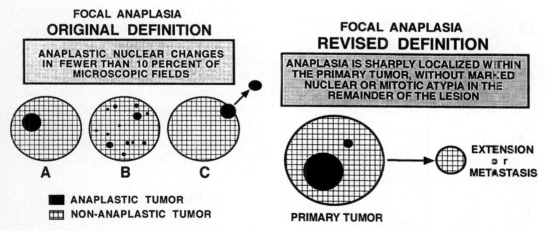

FIG. 13-4. The original definition of focal anaplasia *(left)* included tumors with **(A)** localized anaplasia, **(B)** widely distributed but sparse anaplasia, and **(C)** anaplasia in invasive or metastatic sites but not in most sections of the primary tumor. The revised definition of focal anaplasia *(right)* is more restrictive and includes only localized anaplasia. Black, anaplasia; crosshatch, tumor without anaplasia. (From Faria P, Beckwith JB, Mishra K, et al. Focal versus diffuse anaplasia in Wilms' tumor—new definitions with prognostic significance: a report from the National Wilms' Tumor Study Group. *Am J Surg Pathol* 1996;20:909–920, with permission.)

ized anaplasia with severe nuclear unrest elsewhere in the tumor, anaplasia outside the tumor capsule or in metastases, or anaplasia found in a random biopsy taken from the tumor (Fig. 13-5).

Using the new criteria, and on review of patients in NWTS-3 and NWTS-4, patients with focal anaplasia had a 4-year survival rate statistically significantly higher than that of patients with diffuse anaplasia (97% vs. 50%). This difference did not exist for stage I tumors (100% survival for focal or diffuse) but did exist for stages II (90% vs. 55%), III (100% vs. 45%), and IV (100% vs. 4%) (40,48).

Rhabdoid Tumor of the Kidney

Rhabdoid tumor is a highly malignant tumor characterized by uniform cellular infiltrates initially interpreted as rhabdomyoblastic or sarcomatous elements. The tumor is unrelated to rhabdomyosarcoma or Wilms' tumor and may be of neural crest origin (30,39,49). Rhabdoid cells are characterized by eosinophilic cytoplasm that contains hyaline globular inclusions. On electron microscopy, these inclusions are found to be intermediate filaments; most contain vimentin and cytokeratin. The nuclei are large, round, and vesicular, often containing a centrally placed eosinophilic nucleolus (40).

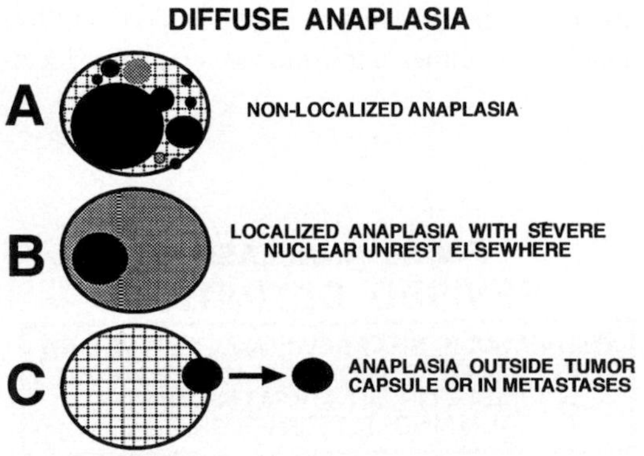

Most rhabdoid tumors of the kidney are diagnosed in the first 2 years of life. Rhabdoid tumors have also been reported as primary extrarenal lesions; there is a known association between rhabdoid tumor of the kidney and primary central nervous system neoplasms (30). Children with rhabdoid tumors have responded poorly to the therapies of the NWTS. The 4-year relapse-free survival for patients treated with vincristine, actinomycin D, and adriamycin on NWTS-3 was 23.1%, and the 4-year overall survival rate was 25% (17,43,50).

Clear Cell Sarcoma of the Kidney

Clear cell sarcoma of the kidney (CCSK) is a primitive mesenchymal neoplasm that makes up 4% of childhood renal tumors. The cell of origin is unknown. The lesion is distinguished by cells with poorly stained cytoplasm. The cell boundaries are indistinct, and cytoplasmic vacuolation may be prominent. The classic histologic pattern has a characteristic arborizing network of thin-walled capillary blood vessels that separates groups of cells (40). In NWTS-3, 23% of children with CCSK developed bone metastases, compared with 0.3% of all other children entered in the study (25).

Response of CCSK to therapy was poor until adriamycin and local irradiation were added to the treatment program. The 4-year relapse-free survival rate for patients with stage I–IV CCSK treated with vincristine, adriamycin, and actinomycin D on NWTS-3 was 71%.

DIFFUSE ANAPLASIA

A — NON-LOCALIZED ANAPLASIA

B — LOCALIZED ANAPLASIA WITH SEVERE NUCLEAR UNREST ELSEWHERE

C — ANAPLASIA OUTSIDE TUMOR CAPSULE OR IN METASTASES

D ? — RANDOM BIOPSY REVEALS ANAPLASIA

FIG. 13-5. Diffuse anaplasia is now defined by any of the four specified criteria. Black, anaplasia; gray, severe nuclear unrest; crosshatch, tumor with neither anaplasia nor severe nuclear unrest. (From Faria P, Beckwith JB, Mishra K, et al. Focal versus diffuse anaplasia in Wilms' tumor—new definitions with prognostic significance: a report from the National Wilms' Tumor Study Group. *Am J Surg Pathol* 1996;20:909–920, with permission.)

CLINICAL PRESENTATION AND WORKUP

As we have already noted, several clinical syndromes are risk factors for the development of Wilms' tumor. These include aniridia, the Beckwith–Wiedemann syndrome (exomphalos, macroglossia, and gigantism), and hemihypertropia.

If somatic changes of these kinds are known to exist, then routine screening in an attempt to make the early diagnosis of Wilms' tumor is appropriate (11,51). A physical examination and periodic ultrasound are indicated. It is interesting to note that in Germany, 10% of patients with Wilms' tumor are diagnosed at infant and childhood screening examinations, conducted for known predisposing syndromes, and at routine well-baby examinations (51).

The majority of children with Wilms' tumor are diagnosed in response to a medical complaint causing a visit to the doctor; the clinical presentation usually is an abdominal mass (83%), fever (23%), or hematuria (21%). Abdominal pain (37%) may be the result of local distention, spontaneous intralesional hemorrhage, or peritoneal rupture. In one major series, abdominal pain correlated with poorer 5-year survival (52). Less common presenting signs and symptoms include hypertension, varicocele, hernia, enlarged testicle, congestive heart failure, hypoglycemia, Cushing's syndrome, hydrocephalus, pleural effusion, and an acute abdomen (53).

The presence and character of the abdominal pain, the previous medical history, and the family history are important aspects of the medical interview. Physical examination is of value in assessing abdominal status and identifying associated congenital anomalies.

The optimum diagnostic imaging workup for Wilms' tumor is a matter of controversy. Evaluation of disease extent classically included intravenous pyelogram (IVP) and chest radiograph. Current imaging protocols largely replace the IVP with abdominal ultrasound. Ultrasound usually allows determination of the origin of a childhood abdominal mass, identifies a contralateral kidney, and demonstrates the presence or absence of tumor extension into the renal vein or inferior vena cava (10).

When an abdominal mass is identified or suspected, abdominal computed tomography (CT) is used to assess the volume of tumor involvement in one or both kidneys, renal function, retroperitoneal lymph nodes, and invasion of the collecting system or renal vein; evaluate the margin between tumor, kidney, and surrounding structures; assess hepatic metastasis (although

many children thought to have invasion of the liver from a right-sided Wilms' tumor are found at surgery to have hepatic compression rather than invasion); and demonstrate lesions in the opposite kidney, which may represent either bilateral Wilms' tumor or nephrogenic rests (Fig. 13-6) (10). The evaluation of the contralateral kidney has become a matter of discussion in the surgical literature. Some authorities believe that preoperative CT and magnetic resonance imaging (MRI) can be used to rule in or rule out bilateral Wilms' tumor. Others believe that imaging is useful but not definitive and that a surgical exploration of the contralateral kidney remains essential during the surgical approach to the primary tumor (24,51).

Plain chest radiographs should be obtained to determine whether pulmonary metastases are present. Some centers recommend thoracic CT to detect pulmonary metastasis that might be missed on chest radiograph. CT-positive, chest radiograph–negative lung metastases do occur, albeit infrequently (10). There has been much uncertainty regarding appropriate therapy for pulmonary disease documented only by CT in the presence of normal plain chest films (54). Data from NWTS-3 show no significant difference in 4-year event-free survival between 18 patients with FH and CT-positive, chest radiograph–negative lungs treated with whole lung irradiation (WLI; 88% event-free survival) and nine patients with FH treated without WLI (88% event-free survival) (55). These results, though interesting, are from a small number of patients. NWTS-4 recommendations were to treat with WLI in CT-positive, chest radiograph–negative FH patients only if disease is unresponsive to chemotherapy. Biopsy proof of intrathoracic disease was recommended for strong consideration (15). NWTS-5 recommendations are that pulmonary nodules not detected on chest radiographs but visible on chest CT do not mandate treatment with WLI. Although the decision to administer WLI is at the discretion of the investigator, excisional biopsy of suspected pulmonary metastatic lesions is strongly recommended to confirm the diagnosis.

Radionuclide bone scan is indicated in CCSK and renal rhabdoid tumor. Bone scan and skele-

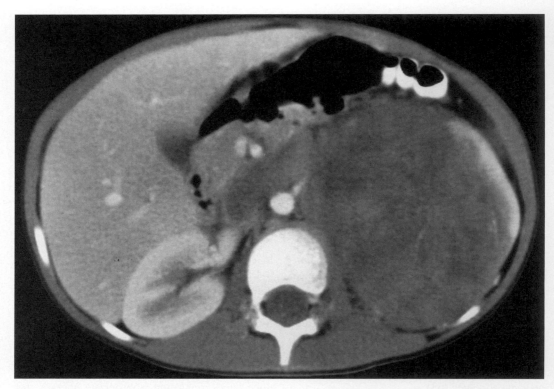

FIG. 13-6. A 5-year-old girl presented with intermittent sharp abdominal pain, nausea, vomiting, weight loss, and hematuria. Abdominal computed tomography showed a 7 × 9 × 12.5–cm mass at the left renal region, beginning immediately subdiaphragmatically and extending to just below the aortic bifurcation. There was a calcified rim superiorly and a heterogeneous parenchymal enhancement. Left renal vein invasion and inferior vena cava thrombosis were observed. On exploratory laparotomy, tumor was palpated in the inferior vena cava. The tumor was resected, with some tumor spillage from a weak point on Gerota's fascia. Tumor thrombus was removed from the inferior vena cava. Pathology showed a favorable histology Wilms' tumor, 13.5 cm in greatest diameter, invading through the renal capsule to the inked surgical margin. Rupture of the renal capsule was identified. Tumor was present at the renal vein margin of the tumor thrombosis with focal invasion of the vein wall. No lymph nodes were involved. For pathologic stage III Wilms' tumor, favorable histology, the child was treated with chemotherapy and flank irradiation. There was no evidence of persistent or recurrent tumor 3 years after diagnosis.

tal survey are complementary in CCSK. If only one technique is used, metastases may be missed (56). Cranial CT is of value in rhabdoid tumors and, perhaps, in Wilms' tumor with overt pulmonary involvement at diagnosis.

STAGING

A staging system for Wilms' tumor was first published by Cassady et al. (58,59) in 1973, building on prognostic factors identified in a review from Garcia et al. (60). The Cassady system remains useful for determining whether young children with early stage disease may be appropriate for therapy with surgery alone. For tumor confined to the kidney and completely excised in children younger than 2 years of age at diagnosis and with tumors that weigh less than 550 g, the prognosis is excellent. Such patients may be treated appropriately with surgery alone and are considered to have stage I disease (57–59). The absence of an inflammatory pseudocapsule, renal sinus invasion, capsular invasion, and intrarenal vessel invasion in such patients are additional factors that mitigate against the risk of relapse when treated with nephrectomy alone (10).

TABLE 13-3. *Grouping system used in National Wilms' Tumor Studies 1 and 2*

Group I.   Tumor limited to the kidney and completely excised (intact surface of the renal capsule, tumor not ruptured before or during removal, no residual tumor apparent beyond excision margins).

Group II. Tumor extending beyond the kidney that is completely excised (penetration into the perirenal soft tissues or para-aortic lymph node involvement, renal vessels outside the kidney infiltrated or contained tumor thrombus, no residual tumor apparent beyond the margins of excision).

Group III. Residual nonhematogenous tumor confined to abdomen (tumor has undergone biopsy or rupture before or during surgery, implants on peritoneal surfaces, lymph nodes involved beyond the periaortic region, tumor incompletely removed because of local infiltration into vital structures).

Group IV. Hematogenous metastasis (deposits beyond group III, e.g., lung, liver, bone, brain).

Group V.   Bilateral renal involvement either initially or subsequently.

The NWTS proposed initial staging criteria to prospectively address tumor-related factors. The first two NWTS studies were based on a system of surgically identified groups (Table 13-3) (11).

Beginning with the third NWTS trial in 1979, a new staging system was adopted (Table 13-4). Specific disease-related parameters noted to be prognostically significant in analyses of NWTS-1 and NWTS-2 led to modifications of the system and the change from groups to stages. A closed or open biopsy permitted categorization as stage II (rather than group III), assuming subsequent total tumor removal. Local spill of tumor during surgery was downstaged from group III to stage II, reflecting data indicating that such cases had excellent tumor control even with limited irradiation and chemotherapy in NWTS-1 and NWTS-2 (29,61).

The more recent NWTS staging system upstages all previous group II cases with lymph node metastasis to stage III, even when all visible disease has been completely resected. The adverse impact of lymph node involvement, both on abdominal recurrence and on ultimate relapse-free survival, has been documented (16,29,47,52,62).

In the SIOP Wilms' Tumor Trial 1, investigators compared preoperative radiotherapy with primary surgery. The staging system used in this trial is shown in Table 13-5. SIOP subsequently began using NWTS grouping and staging, with the proviso that the NWTS systems were not specifically designed for the preoperative ther-

TABLE 13-4. *Staging system used in National Wilms' Tumor Studies 3 and 4*

Stage I.   Tumor is limited to kidney and completely excised. The surface of the renal capsule is intact. Tumor was not ruptured before or during removal. No residual tumor is apparent beyond the margins of resection.

Stage II. Tumor extends beyond the kidney but is completely removed. There is regional extension of the tumor, that is, penetration through the outer surface of the renal capsule into perirenal soft tissues.
Vessels outside the kidney substance are infiltrated or contain tumor thrombus. The tumor may have been biopsied, or there has been local spillage of tumor confined to the flank. No residual tumor is apparent at or beyond the margins of excision.

Stage III. Residual nonhematogenous tumor is confined to the abdomen. Any one or more of the following occur:
   a. Lymph nodes on biopsy are found to be involved in the hilus, the periaortic chains, or beyond.
   b. There has been diffuse peritoneal contamination by tumor such as by tumor spillage beyond the flank before or during surgery or by tumor growth that has penetrated through the peritoneal surface.
   c. Implants are found on the peritoneal surfaces.
   d. The tumor extends beyond the surgical margins either microscopically or grossly.
   e. The tumor is not completely resectable because of local infiltration into vital structures.

Stage IV. Hematogenous metastases; deposits beyond stage III (e.g., lung, liver, bone, and brain).

Stage V.   Bilateral renal involvement at diagnosis. An attempt should be made to stage each side on the basis of disease extent before biopsy.

Staging, which is on the basis of gross and microscopic tumor distribution, is the same for tumors with favorable and unfavorable histologic features. The patient should be characterized by a statement of both criteria, such as "stage II (favorable histologic features)" or "stage III (unfavorable histologic features)."
Tumors of unfavorable type are those with focal or diffuse anaplasia or those of sarcomatous histology.

TABLE 13-5. *Staging system used in SIOP Wilms' tumor trial 1*

Stage I. The tumor is limited to the kidney and is completely excised.

Stage II. The tumor extends outside the kidney but is completely excised.

Stage III. Incomplete excision of the tumor but without hematogenous metastatic spread.

Stage IV. Hematogenous metastases are present.

Stage V. Bilateral renal tumors.

apy often used by SIOP (63,64). For this reason, outcomes between NWTS and SIOP studies should not be compared stage-for-stage (46, 65–69). In addition, SIOP uses a "stage II, node negative" and "stage II, node positive" distinction and therefore includes some NWTS stage III tumors in the stage II infradiaphragmatic SIOP stage.

NWTS, SIOP, AND THE MANAGEMENT OF WILMS' TUMOR

The NWTS, SIOP, and the United Kingdom Children's Cancer Study Group have compiled a large body of information concerning the clinical management of Wilms' tumor. The most widely quoted studies are those of NWTS and SIOP (23,44,69). A review of the major studies of these two groups follows.

The NWTS and SIOP Strategies

The SIOP studies began with the presumption that treatment with radiation therapy or chemotherapy before surgery would render a Wilms' tumor less vulnerable to intraoperative rupture and surgery-related tumor seeding. Downstaging the tumor was also hoped to reduce treatment-related morbidity by reducing the total amount of treatment (65,66). In accordance with this philosophy, the initial strategy of SIOP was to evaluate the roles of radiotherapy and chemotherapy before definitive surgery based on clinical diagnosis. Subsequently, treatment was assigned according to the extent of disease found at surgery. The advantages attributed to the SIOP were the aforementioned arguments that preoperative treatment may diminish the risk of

operative tumor rupture, seeding, or nonresectability. One disadvantage is the risk of misdiagnosis and mistreatment (i.e., treating a tumor other than Wilms' tumor or treating benign disease). In SIOP 9, the error rate (i.e., the proportion of patients who were found not to have Wilms' tumor) was 6%. In addition, the SIOP approach runs the risk of obscuring important prognostic clues in individual patients (67). Lymph node involvement and histologic subtype may be affected by preoperative therapy. A particular drawback of preoperative therapy is that one may miss diffuse anaplasia. Because prognosis and subsequent therapy are influenced by histology and lymph node involvement, the SIOP approach may render therapy less precise by interfering with histology obtained at the time of definitive surgery. Supporting this contention was a review of data from two SIOP studies indicating that necrotic changes were more frequently seen in patients pretreated with radiotherapy than in those pretreated with chemotherapy. However, an analysis of posttreatment histology in these two SIOP studies and in 83 patients who underwent prenephrectomy chemotherapy in NWTS-3 showed no evidence that prenephrectomy therapy altered the detection of anaplastic histology (63,64,66). It appears that the SIOP presurgical therapy approach does not influence histology.

The disadvantages of preoperative chemoradiotherapy include the possibility that the diagnosis may be in error. Preoperative therapy may obscure the true tumor stage and may lead to more children receiving anthracyclines than necessary. On the other hand, the disadvantage of confining therapy to the postoperative period is that there may be fewer stage I patients. The rate of tumor spillage may be higher, and, ultimately, more radiotherapy may be administered than with preoperative strategies. The general criticism is that preoperative therapy suppresses evidence.

The NWTS strategy is to forgo preoperative therapy in order to obtain the maximum amount of information concerning prognostic factors and tailor therapy accordingly. Therefore, the local extent of the primary tumor, degree of anaplasia, presence of unusual histology, and presence or absence of lymph node involvement are assessed in the absence of the confounding influence of preoperative chemotherapy or radiotherapy in order to select therapy. The benefits of the NWTS approach are the generation of a large body of information about prognostic clues, the avoidance of misdiagnosis, and the customization of therapy. The disadvantages include the need for a hospital providing all clinical services necessary for major pediatric surgery and pathology. In addition, there is the risk that a patient who might benefit from preoperative therapy would be denied it by the insistence upon initial surgery (67). Finally, the complexity of the NWTS prognostic and treatment algorithm may discourage the participation of some physicians and inhibit patient accrual to clinical trials.

We will review the major clinical trials and their outcomes in turn.

The National Wilms' Tumor Studies

NWTS-1 (1969–1974) asked several important treatment questions: Is postoperative radiotherapy necessary in group I disease? Is single-agent chemotherapy with either vincristine or actino-

mycin D equivalent to combining these drugs for group II and III disease? Is preoperative vincristine of value in group IV disease? The study is shown schematically in Fig. 13-7, and the results are summarized in Table 13-6 (15,48,60). Radiotherapy dosages were age adjusted (birth to 18 months of age, 18 to 24 Gy; 18 to 30 months, 24 to 30 Gy; 31 to 40 months, 30 to 35 Gy; 41 months or older, 35 to 40 Gy). Radiotherapy appeared to be unnecessary in group I babies, combined drug therapy was superior in groups II and III, and preoperative vincristine was not helpful in group IV (10,13,42,70).

NWTS-1 generated additional important information. The study demonstrated the significance of the UH versus FH distinction, with a 2-year relapse-free survival of 29% for UH and 89% for FH (41,42). Large tumor size, lymph node involvement, and age older than 2 years were confirmed as poor prognostic factors. No radiation dose–response relationship was discerned in the 10- to 40-Gy range, delays of up to 10 days in initiating postoperative irradiation appeared acceptable, and whole abdomen irradiation was not found to be necessary for tumor spills confined to the flank or for prior tumor

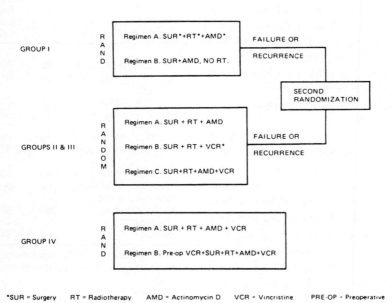

FIG. 13-7. The design of NWTS-1. (From D'Angio GJ. Informational bulletin #19. National Wilms' Tumor Study. Seattle, WA: NWTS Data and Statistical Center, 1991, with permission.)

TABLE 13-6. *NWTS-1 results*

Group and therapy	n	4-Year relapse-free survival (%)	4-Year survival (%)
I. Age <2 yr	38	89	94
A. Radiotherapy	38	89	94
B. No radiotherapy	41	88	90
I. Age ≥2 yr			
A. Radiotherapy	42	76	98
B. No radiotherapy	42	57	81
II and III.			
A. AMD	63	56*	71*
B. VCR	44	57*	71*
C. AMD and VCR	63	79	84
IV.			
A. Immediate surgery	13		83*[a]
B. Preoperative VCR	13		29*[a]

AMD, actinomycin D; VCR, vincristine.
*$p \leq 0.02$.
[a]2-year survival.
From references 17, 42, 54, and 72, with permission.

biopsy (10,13,24,44,61). In these patients, limited radiotherapy fields sufficed.

NWTS-1 showed an advantage for patients older than 2 years with group I tumors treated with irradiation. However, patients with group II tumors receiving actinomycin D with vincristine seemed to do as well as those with group I disease. It was postulated that postoperative vincristine with actinomycin D could substitute for postoperative radiotherapy with actinomycin D. Investigators also were interested in the potential value of adriamycin in the initial treatment of Wilms' tumor because the drug was effective in recurrent disease (70).

NWTS-2 (1974–1979) explored three major questions: Can vincristine and actinomycin D substitute for radiotherapy in older children with group I disease? Are adjuvant vincristine and actinomycin D for protracted periods helpful in group I? Is the addition of adriamycin to actinomycin D and vincristine of value in groups II–IV? The study is shown schematically in Fig. 13-8 (71). Flank irradiation was given in group II–IV disease according to the same age-dependent scale as NWTS-1. Whole abdomen irradiation was reserved for diffuse peritoneal

seeding. Lung metastases were initially treated with 14 Gy of WLI, but when a 10% incidence of pneumonitis occurred the dosage was scaled back to 12 Gy. Study results are summarized in Table 13-7. About 85% of the patients were FH and 15% UH (70). Two-year survival rates were 54% for UH, 90% for FH, 54% for lymph node positive, and 82% for lymph node negative. Excellent survival rates appeared to be achievable without irradiation in group I, and adriamycin added considerable benefit in groups II–III FH and some benefit in groups II–III UH and group IV. The 2-year relapse-free survival for all NWTS-2 patients was 88% for group I, 78% for group II, 70% for group III, and 49% for group IV (17,71–73).

NWTS-3 (1979–1985) incorporated two major changes in treatment planning: Patients were stratified by stages rather than by groups (Tables 13-3 and 13-4), and the distinction between FH and UH was incorporated into the treatment algorithm (Fig. 13-9). Although data from NWTS-1 and NWTS-2 were analyzed by

TABLE 13-7. *NWTS-2 results*

Group and therapy	n	3-Year relapse-free survival (%)	3-Year survival (%)
I.			
E. 6 mo, ADR, VCR	88	89	97
F. 15 mo, ADR, VCR	91	84	92
II and III FH.			
C. VCR, AMD	121	70*	82
D. VCR, AMD, ADR	11	88	92
II and III UH.			
C. VCR, AMD	16	35	38
D. VCR, AMD, ADR	19	42	78
IV.			
C. VCR, AMD	22	43*	44
D. VCR, AMD, ADR	27	60*	60
Lymph node status			
Negative or not examined	383	82[a]	
Positive	84	54	

ADR, adriamycin; AMD, actinomycin D; FH, favorable histology; UH, unfavorable histology; VCR, vincristine.
*$p \leq 0.05$.
[a]2-year survival.
From references 17, 42, 72, and 73, with permission.

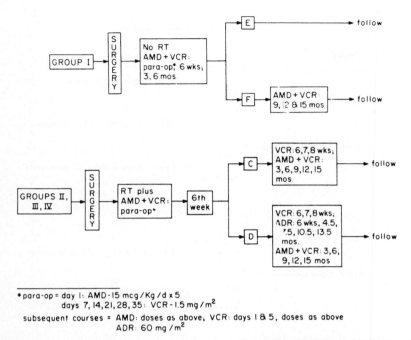

* para-op = day I: AMD-15 mcg/Kg/d x 5
  days 7, 14, 21, 28, 35: VCR-1.5 mg/m²

subsequent courses = AMD: doses as above; VCR: days I & 5, doses as above
ADR: 60 mg/m²

FIG. 13-8. The design of NWTS-2. (From D'Angio GJ, Tefft M, Breslow N, et al. Radiation therapy of Wilms' tumor: results according to dose, field, post-operative timing and histology. *Int J Radiat Oncol Biol Phys* 1978;4:769–780, with permission.)

histology, histology was not used to stratify treatment (10,74).

NWTS-3 considered five major questions: Can the duration of chemotherapy be shortened for stage I FH? Can radiotherapy be eliminated for stage II FH? What is the minimum effective radiotherapy dosage for stage III FH? Is cardiotoxic adriamycin clearly beneficial and therefore necessary in stages II and III FH? Will the addition of cyclophosphamide improve survival in stages I–III UH and in stage IV FH and UH?

NWTS-3 results are summarized in Tables 13-8 and 13-9. Short-course therapy appeared equivalent to long-course therapy in stage I FH. Patients in this group can be treated successfully with a 10-week program of vincristine and actinomycin D without irradiation and can achieve a 4-year relapse-free survival of 89% and overall survival of 96%. Elimination of radiotherapy was acceptable in stage II FH. The 4-year relapse-free and overall survival for the patients not receiving irradiation were 87% and 91%, respectively. In stage III FH, 10 Gy was equivalent

to 20 Gy. There was no statistically significant difference in frequency of intra-abdominal relapse between 10 and 20 Gy, although the trend favored the use of adriamycin or irradiation (intra-abdominal relapse for vincristine, actinomycin D, and 10 Gy, seven out of 61, or 11%; vincristine, actinomycin D, and 20 Gy, three out of 68, or 4%; vincristine, actinomycin D, adriamycin, and 10 Gy, three out of 70, or 4%). In an analysis of patients with stage III, local relapse with doxorubicin occurred in four out of 134 patients, whereas without doxorubicin, it occurred in 11 out of 141 patients, suggesting that chemotherapy played a role in establishing local control. The addition of adriamycin was not clearly beneficial in stage II but seemed to be of benefit in stage III FH. Cyclophosphamide did not benefit stage IV FH. The 4-year survival rate for stage IV FH treated with vincristine, actinomycin D, adriamycin, and abdominal and lung irradiation was 81%. The use of cyclophosphamide seemed to help patients with focal anaplasia. Patients with CCSK did well,

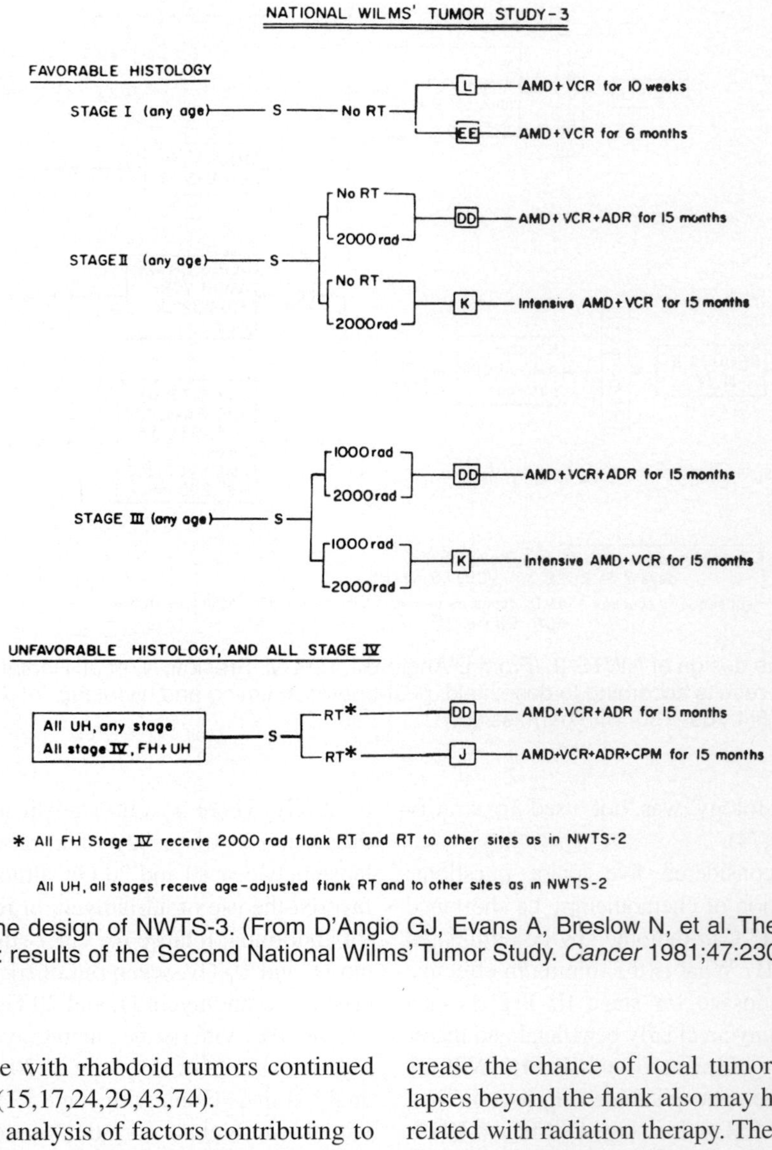

NATIONAL WILMS' TUMOR STUDY-3

FAVORABLE HISTOLOGY

STAGE I (any age)── S ──── No RT ──┬── L ── AMD+VCR for 10 weeks
                                   └── EE ── AMD+VCR for 6 months

STAGE II (any age)── S ──┬── No RT ──┐
                         └── 2000 rad ──┴── DD ── AMD+VCR+ADR for 15 months
                         ┌── No RT ──┐
                         └── 2000 rad ──┴── K ── Intensive AMD+VCR for 15 months

STAGE III (any age)── S ──┬── 1000 rad ──┐
                          └── 2000 rad ──┴── DD ── AMD+VCR+ADR for 15 months
                          ┌── 1000 rad ──┐
                          └── 2000 rad ──┴── K ── Intensive AMD+VCR for 15 months

UNFAVORABLE HISTOLOGY, AND ALL STAGE IV

┌─────────────────────────┐
│ All UH, any stage   │── S ──┬── RT* ──── DD ── AMD+VCR+ADR for 15 months
│ All stage IV, FH+UH   │   └── RT* ──── J ── AMD+VCR+ADR+CPM for 15 months
└─────────────────────────┘

＊ All FH Stage IV receive 2000 rad flank RT and RT to other sites as in NWTS-2

All UH, all stages receive age-adjusted flank RT and to other sites as in NWTS-2

FIG. 13-9. The design of NWTS-3. (From D'Angio GJ, Evans A, Breslow N, et al. The treatment of Wilms' tumor: results of the Second National Wilms' Tumor Study. *Cancer* 1981;47:2302–2311, with permission.)

whereas those with rhabdoid tumors continued to do poorly (15,17,24,29,43,74).

A detailed analysis of factors contributing to flank relapse in NWTS III disclosed some interesting patterns. The 8-year flank relapse rate in patients with stage II disease who had received no radiation was 12.8%, whereas for those who had received 20 Gy of irradiation it was 0%. The relapse rate beyond the flank was 4.6% in the unirradiated patients and 4% in the radiated patients. Similarly, the flank relapse rate in stage II and III disease for patients who received no radiation was 3.2%, whereas it was 1.6% for those who received less than 15 Gy and 0% for those who received more than 15 Gy. Data of this sort indicate that involved-field radiation can in-

crease the chance of local tumor control. Relapses beyond the flank also may have been correlated with radiation therapy. The flank relapse rate in various subgroups of patients who had stage III or IV disease was between 3.5% and 11.8% for those who received 10 to 20 Gy. It fell to 0.18% for those who received 10 Gy and was 0% for those who received 20 Gy (75).

NWTS-4 (1986–1994) addressed issues of minimization of therapy (and, presumably, therapy-related toxicity) and customization of therapy by stage and histology. The trial was the first study of a pediatric population to evaluate the economic impact of two different treatment approaches, one of which entailed fewer clinic visits. By the end of NWTS-3 it had been shown

TABLE 13-8. *NWTS-3 results*

Stage and therapy	*n*	4-Year relapse-free survival (%)	4-Year survival (%)
Stage I FH.			
L. 10 wk ADR, VCR	306	89	96
EE. 6 m ADR, VCR	301	92	97
Stage II FH.			
DD. No radiotherapy; AMD, VCR, ADR	70	88	94
DD2. 20 Gy; AMD, VCR, ADR	71	87	90
K. No radiotherapy; AMD, VCR	67	87	91
K2. 20 Gy; AMD, VCR	70	90	95
Stage III FH.			
DD1. 10 Gy; AMD, VCR, ADR	68	82	91
DD2. 20 Gy; AMD, VCR, ADR	66	86	87
K1. 10 Gy; AMD, VCR	71	71	85
K2. 20 Gy; AMD, VCR	70	77	85
Stage IV FH.[a]			
DD. AMD, VCR, ADR	64	72	78
J. AMD, VCR, ADR, CPM	56	78	87
Stages I–III UH.[a]			
DD. AMD, VCR, ADR	69	67	68
J. AMD, VCR, ADR, CPM	61	62	68
Stage IV UH.[a]			
DD. AMD, VCR, ADR	12	58	58
J. AMD, VCR, ADR, CPM	17	53	52
Anaplastic.[a]			
DD. AMD, VCR, ADR	31	1:80	
II–IV	37	1:78	
II–IV	38*		
J. AMD, VCR, ADR, CPM	17	1:100	
II–IV	83	1:100	
II–IV	82*		
CCSK.[a]			
DD. AMD, VCR, ADR	25	71	75
J. AMD, VCR, ADR, CPM	25	60	76
Rhabdoid.[a]			
DD. AMD, VCR, ADR	13	23	25
J. AMD, VCR, ADR, CPM	18	27	26

ADR, adriamycin; AMD, actinomycin D; CPM, cyclophosphamide; FH, favorable histology; UH, unfavorable histology; VCR, vincristine.
*$p \le 0.05$.
[a]Radiotherapy also given; not a randomized radiotherapy question.
From references 43 and 102, with permission.

TABLE 13-9. *NWTS-3 relapse rates*

Stage and dosage	Flank relapse (8 year)	Beyond flank
0 Gy	3.2%	
<15 Gy	1.6%	
>15 Gy	0%	
II: 0 Gy	12.8%	4.6%
II: 20 Gy	0%	4%
III–IV		
10–20 Gy		3.5–11.8%
10 Gy		0–1.8%
20 Gy		0%

From references 8, 15, 17, 29, 43, and 75.

that 62% of patients with Wilms' tumor (stages I–II, FH) needed neither irradiation nor adriamycin. The study was designed to compare the relapse-free and overall survival rates of patients with stage I and II FH and stage I anaplastic tumors treated with conventional actinomycin D and vincristine and with pulsed, intensive actinomycin D and vincristine. Stages III and IV FH and stage I–IV clear cell sarcoma were treated with conventional actinomycin D, vincristine, and adriamycin, compared with pulsed, intensive actinomycin D, vincristine, and adriamycin; all patients received radiotherapy (for

FH, 10.8 Gy to the abdomen; 12 Gy WLI where appropriate; for stage II–IV anaplastic tumors a sliding scale of radiation dosage was used, as in NWTS-1). Stages II–IV anaplastic Wilms' tumor were treated with appropriate irradiation followed by actinomycin D, vincristine, and adriamycin, compared with these three drugs plus cyclophosphamide. Stages II–IV favorable histology and stages I–IV clear cell sarcoma were treated with 26 weeks or 54 weeks of chemotherapy (Fig. 13-10).

The results of NWTS-4 are shown in Table 13-10. There was no difference in the low-risk or high-risk patients for standard or pulse-intensive therapy. When one breaks down the results based on histology, stage, standard or pulse-

intensive therapy, and, for the more advanced patients, short or long course of therapy, there are, once again, no significant differences between the various treatment groups (76–79). Comparing the results from NWTS-4 with those of the United Kingdom Children's Cancer Study Group Wilms' Tumor Study 2, reported contemporaneously, we see surprisingly similar results (Table 13-11) (78).

Recently there have been detailed analyses of the factors that predict local recurrence in NWTS-4. As seen in Table 13-12, the relative risk of locally recurrent disease was higher in higher-stage disease and with more aggressive histologies. A positive surgical margin and the presence of positive lymph nodes also contributed to the

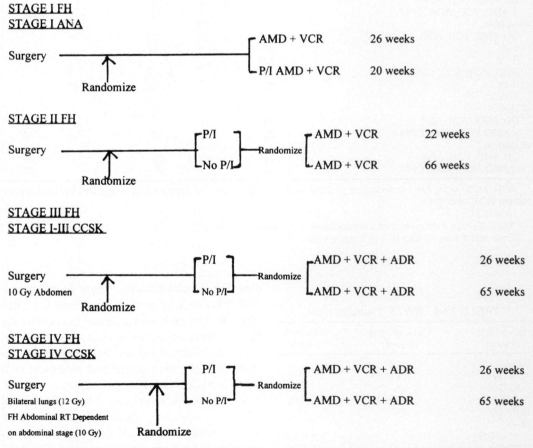

FIG. 13-10. NWTS-4 simplified schema. Stage IV anaplastic tumors continued the randomization of NWTS-3. (From Thomas PRM. Wilms' tumor: changing role of radiation therapy. *Semin Radiat Oncol* 1997;7:204–211, with permission.)

TABLE 13-10. *NWTS-4 results*

4-Year relapse-free survival			
Low risk		High risk	
STD	PI	STD	PI
88%	84%	89%	90%

Stage and treatment	Relapse-free survival (%)
I: FH-STD	93
I: FH-PI	95
I: Ana-STD	93
I: Ana-PI	88
II: FH-STD + Short	82
II: FH-STD + Long	88
II: FH-PI + Short	86
II: FH-PI + Long	89
III: FH-STD + Short	94
III: FH-STD + Long	91
III: FH-PI + Short	92
III: FH-PI + Long	90
IV: FH-STD + Short	82
IV: FH-STD + Long	93
IV: FH-PI + Short	83
IV: FH-PI + Long	78

ANA, anaplastic; FH, favorable histology; Long, long therapy course; PI, pulse intense; Short, short therapy course; STD, standard; UH, unfavorable histology.
From references 24, 44, 79, and 80.

risk of local relapse. Older children and those with incomplete tumor removal were also at higher risk for relapse. Invasion of adjacent organs and tumor spillage placed children at risk for relapse, and when one combines those who had spillage, preoperative tumor rupture, and tu-

TABLE 13-11. *Comparing results: NWTS-4 and UK Children's Cancer Study Group Wilms' Tumor Study 2*

Stage and histology	Relapse-free survival/event-free survival[a]	Survival[b]
Stage I FH	89/87	96/94
Stage II FH	88/82	91/91
Stage III FH	91/82	/84
Stage IV FH	~80/70	80/75

FH, favorable histology.
From references 79, 80, and 84.
[a] The number to the left of the slash is the NWTS-4 relapse-free survival. The number to the right of the slash is the UKCCSG Wilms' Tumor Study 2 event-free survival.
[b] The number to the left of the slash is the NWTS-4 survival. The number to the right of the slash is the UKCCSG Wilms' Tumor Study 2 survival.

TABLE 13-12. *Risk of local recurrence in NWTS-4*

Stage	Relative risk
I	1
II	2.1
III	3.2
Histology	
Favorable histology	1
Diffuse anaplasia	4.7
Clear cell sarcoma of the kidney	2.8
RTK (with other sarcoma)	3.1
Invasion of adjacent organs	
No	1
Yes	1.8
Spillage (local and diffuse)	
No	1
Yes	3.7
Biopsy, spillage, preoperative rupture, and tumor cut across	
No	1
Yes	2.5
Age	
0–23 mo	1
24–47 mo	0.9
48+ mo	2.6
Removal	
Complete	1
Incomplete	2.7
Margin	
−	1
+	2
Nodes	
Negative	1
Hilar	1.1
Aortic	3
None examined	2.6

RTK, Rhabdoid tumor of the kidney.
From Shamberger RC, Guthrie KA, Ritchey ML, et al. Surgery-related factors and local recurrence of Wilms' tumor in National Wilms' Tumor Study 4. *Ann Surg* 1999;229:292–297.

mor cut across, the risk of relapse was elevated. An analysis of relative risks shows that patients with stage II disease and tumor spill were at particularly high risk for local relapse (Tables 13-13 and 13-14). However, the 8-year overall death rate for patients with stage II disease and no spill was 6.1%, compared with 8% for those with spill (not a significant difference). Although the rate of abdominal relapse was higher in those with spill, it did not contribute to an increase in the overall mortality rate (Table 13-15).

The data on the risk of local relapse in stage II disease have prompted a recent debate as to whether any major changes will be implemented in future NWTS chemotherapy programs for FH

TABLE 13-13. *Relative risk of local recurrence in NWTS-4*

	Stage I	Stage II	Stage III
No spill	1	1	1
Spill		4.5	1.9
Negative nodes	1	1	1
Positive nodes	0	0	1.1
Nodes not examined	6	1.4	1.2

From Shamberger RC, Guthrie KA, Ritchey ML, et al. Surgery-related factors and local recurrence of Wilms' tumor in National Wilms' Tumor Study 4. *Ann Surg* 1999;229:292–297.

TABLE 13-15. *NWTS-4 relapse and death rates*

	Abdominal relapse at 8 years	Any relapse
Stage II, no spill	2.7%	14.1%
Stage II, spill	9.3%	23.5%

	8-Year overall death rate
Stage II, no spill	6.1%
Stage II, spill	8%

From Shamberger RC, Guthrie KA, Ritchey ML, et al. Surgery-related factors and local recurrence of Wilms' tumor in National Wilms' Tumor Study 4. *Ann Surg* 1999;229:292–297.

tumors. Some want to reintroduce radiotherapy for patients with stage II disease and a spill, although many oppose this because there is no evidence that the tumor spill affects mortality.

The evidence from NWTS-4 is that pulse-intensive initial chemotherapy is as effective as a longer program. Shorter-course subsequent chemotherapy appears as effective as a longer program. Overall survival rates are excellent, and few patients are irradiated (75).

NWTS-5 (1995 to present) treats stage I favorable and anaplastic histology and stage II FH with 18 weeks of actinomycin D and vincristine. Stage I FH in children younger than 24 months of age and with tumor weight less than 550 g is treated with surgery alone. Stage III–IV FH and stages II–IV focal anaplasia are treated with 24 weeks of actinomycin D, vincristine, adriamycin, and local irradiation and WLI as appropriate (Table 13-16). Stages II–IV diffuse anaplastic sarcoma and stage I–IV CCSK are treated with cyclophosphamide, vincristine, adriamycin, and etoposide along with local irradiation and WLI as appropriate. Stages I–IV

TABLE 13-14. *Local recurrence in patients registered in NWTS-4 before 1994*

I, No spill	2.3%
II, No spill	4.3%
II, Spill	16.4%
III, No spill	4.9%
III, Spill	7.8%

From Shamberger RC, Guthrie KA, Ritchey ML, et al. Surgery-related factors and local recurrence of Wilms' tumor in National Wilms' Tumor Study 4. *Ann Surg* 1999;229:292–297.

rhabdoid tumor of the kidney is treated with carboplatin, etoposide, cyclophosphamide, and radiotherapy. As major objectives, NWTS-5 has an assessment of the importance of loss of heterozygosity for chromosome 1p and 16q markers for prognosis.

SIOP Wilms' Tumor Studies

A classic study by Schweisguth and Bamberger (78), published in 1963, suggested that about one-third of patients with Wilms' tumor could be cured by preoperative radiotherapy and nephrectomy (Table 13-17). The SIOP studies built on this experience.

SIOP Study 1 (1971–1974) registered 397 patients from 42 participating centers: 194 were eligible and randomized, and 203 were excluded from the randomization but were followed. The nonrandomized patients included 44 errors in diagnosis (10%, most commonly neuroblastoma and cysts), 62 children younger than 1 year of age, and 54 with metastases. In patients older than 1 year and younger than 15 years of age at diagnosis, the randomized trial was designed to ascertain whether preoperative plus postoperative primary tumor site irradiation is superior to postoperative irradiation only and whether a single postoperative course of actinomycin D is equal to multiple courses. To answer the first question, 73 children were randomized to receive 20 Gy before surgery, and 64 children underwent immediate surgery. SIOP stage I (Table 13-5) patients randomized

TABLE 13-16. *Simplified scheme of radiation therapy used in NWTS-5*

Stage	FH	Anaplastic tumors	Clear cell sarcoma of the kidney and rhabdoid tumor
I–II	No irradiation.	No irradiation for stage I. For stage II, follow the guidelines for FH, stage III.	Follow the guidelines for FH, stage III.
III	If the tumor involved the renal hilar nodes, gross or microscopic residual disease confined to the flank, or the para-aortic nodes, irradiate the flank, crossing the midline to include the bilateral para-aortic nodes. If there was peritoneal seeding, gross residual abdominal disease, preoperative intraperitoneal tumor rupture, or diffuse abdominal tumor spill, irradiate the whole abdomen. Administer 10.8 Gy in 6 fractions. Boost tumor >3 cm in maximum diameter an additional 10.8 Gy.	Follow the guidelines for FH, stage III.	Follow the guidelines for FH, stage III.
IV	Treat the abdomen per the guidelines for the intra-abdominal stage, i.e., irradiate the abdomen for local stage III but not I–II. Whole lung irradiation to 12 Gy. Boost persistent lung metastases to 19.5 Gy or resect them. In certain circumstances, liver metastases are irradiated.	As for stage IV FH.	As for stage IV FH except that stage I and II abdominal disease is also locally irradiated.

FH, favorable histology.
From references 70 and 147 with permission.

to undergo preoperative irradiation received no additional irradiation, and stage II and III patients were given an additional 15 Gy. Children who were randomized to the postoperative irradiation arm received 20 Gy for stage I and were given 30 Gy for stages II and III, with provision for additional boosts for bulky stage III (Table 13-18). Three of 72 evaluable patients who received preoperative radiotherapy had tumor rupture during surgery (4%), whereas 20 of 60 patients who received no preoperative irradiation suffered from tumor rupture (33%, $p = 0.001$). The 5-year recurrence-free survival was 51% for those without tumor rupture and 27% for those with rupture ($p = 0.01$), with no difference in 8-year overall survival (66% vs. 61%) between the two groups (8). In the randomization between one and seven courses and

TABLE 13-17. *Results of the treatment of new cases of historically confirmed Wilms' Tumor, with more than 2 years of follow-up, as reported by Schweisguth and Bamberger of the Institut Gustave–Roussy in 1963*

Treatment	n	Alive without metastases	Alive with metastases treated	Dead
No nephrectomy	4	0	0	100%
Nephrectomy done	3	0	0	100%
XRT and nephrectomy	15	27%	0	73%
Nephrectomy and XRT	24	33%	0	67%
XRT, nephrectomy, and XRT	50	40%	4%	56%
Laparotomy, XRT, nephrectomy, and XRT	2	0	0	100%
	98	33	2%	65%

Derived from Schweisguth O, Bamberger J. Le nephroblastome de l'enfant. *Ann Chir Enfant Paris* 1963;4:335–354. Translation from French courtesy of Dr. Gustavo Montana.

TABLE 13-18. *SIOP 1 Wilms' tumor treatment protocol*

Randomization	S	Stage	Postoperative treatment	Maintenance	Months
RT (20 Gy)	N	I	A	No treatment	0
		II	RT (15 Gy) + A		
Randomize		III[a]	RT (15 Gy) + A	Randomize	
		I	RT (20 Gy) + A		
Nephrectomy		II	RT (30 Gy) + A		
		III[a]	RT (30 Gy) + A	A (6 courses)	16

A, actinomycin D; N, radical nephrectomy; RT; radiation therapy; S, surgery.
[a]RT whole abdomen: dosage to kidney 12 Gy; dosage to liver 30 Gy.
From references 65, 66, 68, and 70, with additional material supplied by Professor F. Oldenburger.

actinomycin D (15 mg/kg per day $\times$ 5 days), there was no survival difference (Table 13-19) (65,66,68,70).

SIOP Trial 2 (1974–1976) was a nonrandomized study comparing 86 patients receiving 20 Gy of irradiation and 5 days of actinomycin D before surgery with a concurrent group of 52 children treated with primary surgery (Table 13-20). Tumor rupture occurred in 5% of the preoperatively treated patients and in 20% of the other patients ($p = 0.0025$) (53,54,56). The main reason for not giving preoperative therapy was small tumor size. Survival was only 61% in patients with larger tumors who received preoperative and postoperative irradiation. SIOP Trials 1 and 2 demonstrated that presurgical treatment with radiotherapy reduced the number of tumor ruptures. This, in turn, reduced the need for whole abdomen irradiation and its attendant ill effects in young children (Table 13-21) (66,70).

TABLE 13-19. *SIOP 1 results*

Randomization	Outcome
Radiotherapy, surgery, and radiotherapy[a]	4% ruptures 31% stage I
Surgery and radiotherapy[b]	32% ruptures 14% stage I
Actinomycin D, 1 course Actinomycin D, 6 courses	n.s.

From references 65, 66, 68, and 70, with additional material supplied by Professor F. Oldenburger.
[a] vs. [b], $p = 0.001$.

SIOP Trial 5 (1977–1980) was designed to ascertain whether preoperative actinomycin D (two 3-day courses, 15 mg/kg) and vincristine (four weekly injections, 1.5 mg/m^2) were equally effective preoperative therapy when compared with the previously used program of 20 Gy plus actinomycin D. After surgery the preoperatively irradiated patients were given an additional 15 Gy for NWTS group II or III disease, whereas those treated preoperatively only with chemotherapy received 30 Gy for group II or III disease. All patients received postoperative maintenance vincristine and actinomycin (Table 13-22). An analysis of the 172 randomized patients showed no significant difference in the reduction in tumor size, incidence of tumor rupture, stage distribution, mean weight of the tumor specimen, or 3-year recurrence-free survival (89% for preoperative chemotherapy alone vs. 83% for chemotherapy plus radiotherapy). Major histologic changes such as necrosis were significantly less common after preoperative chemotherapy than after preoperative chemoradiotherapy (Tables 13-23 and 13-24) (54,56,58,59).

SIOP Trial 6 (1980–1987) adopted the prenephrectomy chemotherapy used in SIOP Trial 5. All patients received actinomycin D and vincristine. Patients who had stage I disease at the time of surgery were randomized to receive postoperative vincristine and actinomycin D for 17 or 38 weeks. All lymph node–negative stage II patients received 38 weeks of vincristine and actinomycin D and were randomized to receive or not receive 20 Gy of involved-field irradiation. Stage II node-positive patients and stage III patients were randomized to receive vincristine, ac-

TABLE 13-20. *SIOP 2 Wilms' Tumor treatment protocol*

First treatment	Stage	Postoperative treatment	Maintenance
Preoperative RT 20 Gy + S (average tumors)	I II–III	AV AV + RT (15 Gy)	1 or 5 courses A for 6 or 15 mo
A + S (small tumors)	I II–III	AV AV + RT (30 Gy)	1 or 5 courses A for 6 or 15 mo

A, actinomycin D; RT, radiation therapy; S, nephrectomy; V, vincristine.
From references 63, 64, 66, and 70, with additional material supplied by Professor F. Oldenburger.

TABLE 13-21. *SIOP 2 results*

V added to A postoperatively	9 mo vs. 15 mo	Disease-free survival and survival equal
Preoperative RT Surgery (e.g., small tumors)	Ruptures Ruptures	5% } $p = 0.0025$ 20%

A, actinomycin D; RT, radiation therapy; V, vincristine.
From references 63, 64, 66, and 70, with additional material supplied by Professor F. Oldenburger.

TABLE 13-22. *SIOP 5 Wilms' Tumor treatment protocol*

Preoperative treatment	S	Stage	Postoperative treatment	Maintenance	Weeks
VA (4 wk)	S	I II/III	AV AV + RT (30 Gy)		} 43
Randomization				AV (5 courses)	
RT (20 Gy) + A	S	I II/III	AV + RT (15 Gy)		} 45

A, actinomycin D; RT, radiation therapy; S, nephrectomy; V, vincristine.
From references 63, 64, 66, and 70, with additional material supplied by Professor F. Oldenburger.

TABLE 13-23. *SIOP 5 results*

	Relapse-free survival (%)	Survival (%)
Chemotherapy first	77	84
Radiotherapy first	67	83
Overall	71	86

From Lemerle J, Voute PA, Tournade MF, et al. Effectiveness of preoperative chemotherapy in Wilms' tumor: results of an International Society of Pediatric Oncology (SIOP) clinical trial. *J Clin Oncol* 1983;1:604–610, with additional material supplied by Professor F. Oldenburger.

tinomycin D with intensified vincristine, or the two drugs with doxorubicin (Table 13-25). The stage distribution for the 396 SIOP Trial 6 patients was stage I (56%), stage II node negative (27%), and stage II node positive and stage III (17%). Tumor rupture was found in 6% of cases.

In the radiotherapy randomization for stage II node-negative patients in SIOP Trial 6, there were eight relapses among 50 nonirradiated patients. Of these eight, seven had subdiaphragmatic regrowths of tumor, and in six the tumor bed was the site of first relapse. This was in contrast to only one local recurrence of the 58 patients given postoperative irradiation. However, 12 of the 58 children developed lung metastases. Three of the 50 nonirradiated patients died, and five of the 58 irradiated patients died, all of disseminated Wilms' tumor. The overall survival of the two groups at 4 years was not different: 90% of the nonirradiated patients and 85% of the irradiated patients (Table 13-26) (66,68,70).

SIOP Trial 9 (1987–1993) had, as its primary question, the appropriate duration of prene-

TABLE 13-24. *Effect of preoperative treatment: SIOP Trial 5*

Effect	Chemotherapy	Chemotherapy and radiotherapy	p Value
Major clinical reduction in tumor size (%)	84%	88%	n.s.
Mean weight of the specimen (g)	519	473	n.s.
Tumor rupture (%)	9%	6%	n.s.
Stage (% of cases)			
I	43%	52%	n.s.
II	36%	32%	n.s.
III	21%	16%	n.s.
Major change in pathologic pattern (% of cases)	17%	53%	p < .001
3-year recurrence-free survival			
Stage I	43%	52%	
Stage II	36%	32%	
Stage III	21%	16%	
Overall 3-year survival	89%	83%	n.s.

From references 66, 68, and 100, with additional material supplied by Professor F. Oldenburger.

phrectomy chemotherapy. One-half of the patients with disease confined to the abdomen received 4 weeks of actinomycin D and vincristine, and one-half received 8 weeks. After nephrectomy, patients with multicystic, tubular, and nephroblastoma with fibroadenomatous-like structures received no additional therapy. Patients with UH received actinomycin D, epidoxorubicin, vincristine, ifosfamide, and, generally, irradiation. Patients with FH tumors received the following postoperative treatments: stage I, actinomycin D and vincristine; stage II node negative, actinomycin D, vincristine, and epi-

doxorubicin; stage II node positive and stage III, actinomycin D, vincristine, and epidoxorubicin; along with local irradiation (15 Gy to the tumor bed with an optional boost to residual disease up to 30 Gy). Infants younger than 6 months underwent up-front nephrectomy. Children with a preoperative diagnosis of stage IV disease received actinomycin D, vincristine, and epidoxorubicin. This was followed by nephrectomy and possible metastasectomy. Those rendered free of disease continued on actinomycin D, vincristine, and epidoxorubicin. Those with persistent metastatic disease received ifosfamide,

TABLE 13-25. *SIOP 6 Wilms' Tumor treatment protocol*

Preoperative treatment	S	Stage	Postoperative treatment	Maintenance	Weeks
	S	I	AV	AV (2 courses) ↑ Randomization ↓ AV (5 courses)	17 ↓ 38
AV × 4 wk	S	II N0	RT (20 Gy) + AV ↑ Randomization ↓ AV	AV (5 courses) ↓ AV (5 courses)	38 ↓ 38
	S	II N1	IntVCR + RT (30 Gy) ↑ Randomization ↓	AV (5 courses)	40
		III	AdriaAV + RT (30 Gy) (6 courses)	AV (5 courses)	38

A, actinomycin D; Adria, adriamycin; IntVCR, intensified vincristine (2 extra injections during maintenance courses); RT, radiation therapy; S, radical nephrectomy; V, vincristine.
From references 66, 68, and 70.

TABLE 13-26. *SIOP 6 results*

Stage	2-Year disease-free survival (%)	5-year survival (%)	p value
All stages	80	84	
Stage I (trial)	82	89	
Short arm	92	95	} n.s.
Long arm	88	92	
Stage II N0	76	86	
Radiotherapy	72	78	} n.s.
No radiotherapy	88	85	
Stage II N1–III	61	75	
Intensive vincristine	49	74	
Adriamycin	77	80	
Favorable histology	97	97	
Unfavorable histology		58	

From Tournade MF, Com-Nougue C, Coute PA, et al. Results of the Sixth International Society of Pediatric Oncology Wilms' Tumor Trial and Study: a risk-adapted therapeutic approach in Wilms' tumor. *J Clin Oncol* 1993;11:1014–1023.

vincristine, and actinomycin D and irradiation (Tables 13-27–13-29). The study's results show that the duration of prenephrectomy chemotherapy did not influence the stage distribution at the time of surgery. There was also no difference in toxicity between the 4-week and 8-week chemotherapy arms (66,68,70).

SIOP Trial 93-01 opened in 1993. Patients were classified into three histologic groups as shown in Table 13-1. Because the available results show no difference between 4-week and 8-week preoperative chemotherapy, 4 weeks has been adopted as the standard. Patients with stage I low-grade histology received no additional therapy.

Patients with stage I intermediate or high-grade tumors were randomized to a 4-week postoperative program of vincristine and actinomycin D or a 6-week program. All stage II and III

TABLE 13-27. *SIOP 9 Wilms' Tumor treatment protocol*

Preoperative treatment	Eligible for randomization	N	Stage	Histology	Postoperative treatment	Weeks
AV 4 weeks	AV 4 weeks ↑		I	FH	None	0
	Yes → Randomize ↓	S	I	ST	AV × 3	18
	No further preoperative treatment		I	UF	AV × 3	18
	No	S	II N0	ST	AVE × 5	27
			II N1	ST	AVE × 5 + RT 15Gy[a]	27
			III	ST	AVE × 5 + RT 15Gy[a]	27
			II–III	UF	DEVI × 5 + RT 30 Gy[b]	36

A, actinomycin; D, actinomycin D; E, anthracycline; FH, favorable histology; I, ifosfamide; N, radical nephrectomy; RT, radiation therapy; S, surgery; ST, standard; UH, unfavorable histology; V, vincristine.
[a]Stages II N1/III standard histology: RT 15 Gy ± boost 10–15 Gy.
[b]Unfavorable histology: RT 30 Gy ± boost 5–10 Gy.
From references 66, 68, 70, 137, and 138.

TABLE 13-28. *SIOP 9: stage IV protocol*

Preoperative chemotherapy	N ± R	Response of metastases	Abdomen stage	RT lung/boost (Gy)	RT abdomen/boost (Gy)	Postoperative chemotherapy	Weeks
AVE 6 wk	N ± R	M–	I	0	0	A*VE	32
			II N1	0	15/15	A*VE	32
			III	0	15/15	A*VE	32
		M+	I	0	0	A*VI	25
			II N1	17.5/5–10	15/15	A*VI	25
			III	17.5/5–10	15/15	A*VI	25

A, actinomycin D 0.5 mg/m^2 i.v.; A*, actinomycin D 0.9 mg/m^2 i.v.; E, epiadriamycin 50 mg/m^2 i.v. I, ifosfamide 3,000 mg/m^2 i.v.; M, metastases; M–, complete response or completely resected; M+, not a complete response or incompletely resected or multiple inoperable metastases; N, nephrectomy; R, metastasectomy; RT, radiation therapy; V, vincristine 1.5 mg/m^2 i.v.
From references 66, 68, 70, 138, and 139.

TABLE 13-29. *SIOP 9 results*

	2-Year event-free survival (%)	5-Year survival (%)
Tumor rupture, 4 wk	84	92
Tumor rupture, 8 wk	83	87
Tumor volume regression >50%	88	93
Tumor volume regression <50%	82	89
Stage I, favorable histology	100	100
Stage I, standard and anaplastic	86	93
Stage II N0, standard	82	87
Stage II N1, III	77	89
Unfavorable histology	64	79
Entire pre-eligible population		
Stage I–III nonanaplastic	86	92
Stage I, anaplastic	75	92
Randomized patients	84	90
Pre-eligible, nonrandomized patients	81	88

From Tournade MF, Com-Nougue C, de Kraker J., et al. Optimal duration of preoperative therapy in unilateral and nonmetastatic Wilms' tumor in children older than 6 months: results of the ninth International Society of Pediatric Oncology Wilms' tumor trial and study. *J Clin Oncol* 2001;19:488–500.

TABLE 13-30. *SIOP 93-01 Wilms' Tumor treatment: postoperative treatment strategies for unilateral Wilms' Tumor*

Stage	Postoperative	Maintenance
I, low risk	None	None
I, intermediate risk	AV (4 wk)	AV for 2 courses, 18 wk ↑ Randomization ↓ No further treatment
II N0, anaplasia	AVE	AVE for 27 wk
II N1 and III	AVE + RT	AVE for27 wk
High risk (I–III)	E/I/Vp/C	E/I/Vp/C for
	+ RT[a]	34 wk

A, actinomycin; C, carboplatin 600 mg/m^2 i.v.; E, epirubicin 50 mg/m^2 i.v.; I, ifosfamide 3 g/m^2 i.v.; RT, radiation therapy; V, vincristine; Vp, etoposide 100 mg/m^2 i.v.
[a]Stage I high risk, no abdominal RT.
From references 139 and 140.

patients with intermediate-grade tumors received therapy as in SIOP Trial 9. Stage II and III high-grade tumors were treated with ifosfamide, etoposide, and carboplatin (Table 13-31). The survival results are excellent (Tables 13-30–13-33).

A summary of SIOP Trials 1, 2, 5, 6, 9, and 93-01 shows that 4 weeks of prenephrectomy chemotherapy, without irradiation, results in 56% of patients having stage I disease at surgery. In most cases these patients go on to receive postoperative chemotherapy and have a survival rate of more than 90%. Stage II node-positive and stage III patients have approximately a 61% relapse-free survival and a 75% overall survival (37). A diminishing number of patients have received radiotherapy in the sequential SIOP trials. The estimated percentages of patients who received irradiation are as follows: SIOP 1, 90%; SIOP 2, 90%; SIOP 5, 72%; SIOP 6, 34%; SIOP 9, 24% (68). If one excludes patients with metastases, then only about 16% of SIOP patients receive irradiation (66).

The latest SIOP protocol 2001 is summarized in Tables 13-34–13-39.

SELECTION OF THERAPY

Surgery

If one follows the NWTS philosophy, 90–95% of intra-abdominal tumors are resectable at diagnosis, and surgery is the initial definitive treatment. Operative approaches have included a vertical incision or a thoracoabdominal exposure. The current preferred approach is a wide transverse abdominal incision (17,67,81,82). The incision is extended to the thorax when needed for adequate exposure. This is rarely necessary, and the thoracoabdominal incision has been associated with higher complication rates (8). Total resection generally is achievable with the transverse transperitoneal incision. Data regarding the value of adjuvant irradiation and chemotherapy for those with small deposits of residual tumor demonstrate that heroic attempts at tumor removal are not indicated (83). A recent analysis of NWTS-1, NWTS-2, and NWTS-3 shows no significant reduction in survival rates with direct extension or contiguous

TABLE 13-31. *SIOP 93-01 stage IV protocol*

Preoperative chemotherapy	N ± R	Response to metastases	Abdominal stage	RT lung (Gy)	RT abdomen (Gy)	Postoperative chemotherapy	Weeks
AVE 6 wk	N ± R	M−	I	0	0	AVE	27
		M−	II N1	0	15/10	AVE	27
		M−	III	0	15/10	AVE	27
		M+ at	I	15/5–10	0	Vp/C/I/E	34
		Week 11	II+	15/5–10	15/10	Vp/C/I/E	34
		Evaluation	III	15/5–10	15/10	Vp/C/I/E	34
			High risk II/III	15/5–10	25	Vp/C/I/E	34

A, actinomycin; C, carboplatin 600 mg/m^2 i.v.; E, epirubicin 50 mg/m^2 i.v.; I, ifosfamide 3 g/m^2 i.v.; M, metastases; M−, complete response or completely resected; M+, not a complete response or incompletely resected or multiple inoperable metastases; N, nephrectomy; R, metastasectomy; RT, radiation therapy; V, vincristine; Vp, etoposide 100 mg/m^2 i.v.

From references 139–141.

TABLE 13-32. *SIOP 93-01 results*

	Disease-free survival (%)		Survival (%)	
Stage	2 Years	5 Years	2 Years	5 Years
Stage I				
VCR and actinomycin	91	88	98	97
No further treatment	89	87	98	95
Stage II	88	88		
Stage III	78	75		

From references 139–142 with additional material generously supplied by Professor F. Oldenburger.

TABLE 13-33. *SIOP 93-01 results*

Risk group	4-Year event-free survival
Low	100%
Intermediate	~85%
High	~65%

Tumor volume	4-Year event-free survival
≤500 mL	85%
≥500 mL	72%, $p = .0095$

Subtype	Survival
Focal anaplasia	~90%
Blastemal predominant	~75%
Diffuse anaplasia	~55%

From references 139, 140, and 142 with additional material generously supplied by Professor F. Oldenburger.

TABLE 13-34. *SIOP 2001 postoperative treatment strategies for localized tumors*

Risk level	Stage I	Stage II	Stage III
Low risk	No further treatment	AV-2 (27 wk)	AV-2
Intermediate risk	AV-1 (4 wk)	Randomize to either:	Randomize to either:
		Dox + AVD or	RT + Dox + AVD (27 wk) or
		Dox − AV-2	RT + Dox − AV-2
High risk	AVD (27 wk)	High risk + RT (34 wk)	High risk + RT

A, actinomycin; D, adriamycin; Dox, doxorubicin; RT, radiation therapy; V, vincristine; AV-1 is a 4-week program; AV-2 is a 27-week program.

From references 69, 141, and 143 with additional material generously supplied by Professor F. Oldenburger.

TABLE 13-35. *SIOP 2001 protocol for metastatic disease*

Pretreatment: vincristine, actinomycin D, and doxorubicin (6 wk)
Surgery for primary tumor
Evaluation of metastatic sites
Treatment protocol will further be determined by
  Local stage of the tumor
  Histologic type
  Result of evaluation of metastatic sites

From references 69, 141, and 143.

TABLE 13-36. *SIOP 2001 protocol for pulmonary and pulmonary metastases*

Starting points

Metastases absent or completely removed
Metastases incompletely removed or multiple
  inoperable metastases
Patients with high-risk histology of the primary tumor

From references 69, 141, and 143.

TABLE 13-37. *SIOP 2001 stage IV postoperative treatment*

Metastases absent or completely resected, intermediate risk		
Act, Vcr, Dox (27 wk)	Local stage I–II	No RT
	Local stage III	Abdominal RT wk 2–5
Multiple inoperable metastases or incompletely resected metastases		
VP16, Carbo, Cyclo, Dox (34 wk)	Local stage I–II	No abdominal RT
	Local stage III RT	Abdominal RT wk 1–4

Act, actinomycin; Carbo, carboplatin; Cyclo, cyclophosphamide; Dox, doxorubicin; RT, radiation therapy; Vcr, vincristine; VP16, etoposide.
From references 69, 141, and 143 with additional material generously supplied by Professor F. Oldenburger.

involvement of the liver in comparison to other stage III presentations. Survival is diminished with hematogenous intraparenchymal liver metastasis (85).

In NWTS-3, surgeons encountered renal vein involvement in 10% of patients. Extension into the inferior vena cava and atrium occurs in up to 5% more. En bloc removal of the kidney and renal vein tumor thrombus is possible in most children, and separate removal is possible in others. In some cases the thrombus is "milked" from the inferior vena cava to the renal vein before removal. With meticulous surgery, renal vein involvement does not adversely affect prognosis (11,86).

Surgical staging is important in determining treatment and prognosis. Palpation and visual assessment of the opposite kidney and liver are routine (although, as noted earlier in this chapter, some surgeons believe that preoperative imaging studies, particularly MRI, can ex-

TABLE 13-38. *SIOP 2001 stage IV postoperative treatment for a high-risk primary tumor*

VP16, Carbo, Cyclo, Dox (34 wk)
Local stage I: No abdominal RT with pulmonary RT
Local stage II–III: Both abdominal RT and pulmonary RT
    Radiotherapy in wk 1–4
    Pulmonary RT: Start of pulmonary RT is decided by the local radiation oncologist
    Pneumocystis carinii prophylaxis with cotrimoxazole at wk 9

Carbo, carboplatin; Cyclo, cyclophosphamide; Dox, doxorubicin; RT, radiation therapy; VP16, etoposide.
From references 69, 141, and 143.

clude contralateral kidney involvement with tumor). The prognostic importance of lymph node involvement has been established (Table 13-7). Only 56% of patients in whom the surgeon thought that the nodes were involved by tumor in fact had pathologic confirmation of nodal tumor. If the surgeon thought the nodes were negative, 11% proved to be positive. Because the presence of nodal involvement upstages from II to III, it is important to sample the nodes and obtain pathologic confirmation (87).

As previously discussed, the incidence of operative rupture or spill of generally large, often "soft" tumors ranges from 15% to 30% (47,72–73,88). Most cases of operative spill are focal (limited to the operative site) rather than diffuse (contamination of the peritoneal cavity) (61). The risk of abdominal relapse and mortality has been significantly greater after surgical spill (41,47,64). In cases with marginally operable tumors or with large areas of central necrosis, preoperative radiotherapy or chemotherapy may be preferable to attempted resection with spill (89). As noted earlier in this chapter, the SIOP philosophy, using preoperative chemotherapy, has significantly reduced the risk of operative spill and tumor rupture.

Inoperability results primarily from large tumor size with direct involvement of the liver or retroperitoneal structures. Some surgeons recommend preoperative chemotherapy to improve the chance of resectability. Those who subscribe to the viewpoints of the SIOP studies will be predisposed to using preoperative chemotherapy without a biopsy. For those who feel uncomfort-

TABLE 13-39. *SIOP 9, SIOP 93-01, and SIOP 2001 stage IV differences*

Study	Preoperative chemotherapy	N R	Metastases to lungs	Local stage	RT abdomen	RT lungs	Postoperative chemotherapy	Weeks
SIOP 9	AVE	+	M−		II+/III	0	AVE	32
			M+		II+/III	20 Gy	AVI	25
SIOP 93-01	AVE	+	M−	I/II− or II+/III	II+/III		AVE	32
			M+/high-grade	I		15 Gy/wk 11+[a]	E/Ca/I/Epi	34
			primary	II−/III	II+/−/III	15 Gy/wk 11+	E/Ca/I/Epi	34
SIOP 2001	AVD	+	A. M−	I−II−III	III		AVD	27
			B. M+	I−II−III	III	15 Gy/wk 9[b]	E/Ca/Cy/D	34
			C. High-grade primary	I		15 Gy	E/Ca/Cy/D	34
				II−III	II−III	15 Gy	E/Ca/Cy/D	34

A, actinomycin; Ca, carboplatin; CR, complete response; Cy, cyclophosphamide; D, doxorubicin; E etoposide; Epi, epirubicin; I, ifosfamide; M−, complete response or completely resected; M+, not a complete response or incompletely resected or multiple inoperable metastases; N, nephrectomy; R, resection of metastases, RT, radiation therapy, V, vincristine.

[a]Evaluation at wk 11: CR, no RT to lungs; if no CR, RT lungs.
[b]Evaluation at wk 9: CR, no RT to lungs; if no CR, RT lungs.

From references 66, 68, 69, 139, and 144 with additional material generously supplied by Professor F. Oldenburger.

able with a diagnosis made by physical findings and diagnostic imaging, percutaneous biopsy is indicated, and tumor resection is planned after response to preoperative chemotherapy (84). A needle biopsy may entail general anesthesia or heavy sedation with local anesthesia. Ultrasound or contrast-enhanced CT scans may be used to localize the biopsy site. A proper biopsy must provide an adequate, representative specimen (47,72). Subtumor capsular bleeding is a possible biopsy-related complication. For this reason, some clinicians prefer a posterior approach for the biopsy so that bleeding is more locally confined and less likely to spill into the abdominal cavity.

In the 1930s, nephrectomy alone achieved cure in 15% to 30% of children (58,90). Recent experience with the management of highly selected small intrarenal primary Wilms' tumor suggests that one can identify a group of patients at extremely low risk of systemic micrometastasis potentially treatable with surgery alone (82,91). In a pilot study at Children's Hospital in Boston, eight patients younger than 2 years old with unilateral, nonmetastatic, small (less than 550 g total tumor and kidney specimen weight) FH tumors

(stage I) (58,59) underwent nephrectomy with no additional therapy. With mean follow-up of 5 years, all eight children are alive. Seven are continuously disease free; one developed a metachronous bilateral tumor and was treated successfully (83). Other investigators have found that the risk of tumor recurrence in stage I FH is negligible if the following factors are absent: inflammatory pseudocapsule, renal sinus invasion, capsular invasion, and intrarenal vessel invasion (92). A review of children treated on NWTS-1, NWTS-2, and NWTS-3 supports the hypothesis that changes in the NWTS regimens have not improved on the excellent prognosis of children younger than 2 years old at diagnosis with tumors less than 550 g (see also Table 13-33) (53,74). In NWTS-5 this group of children is treated with surgery only.

Radiation Therapy

In 1950 Gross and Neuhauser (93) of Boston Children's Hospital reported that ten of 31 (32%) patients treated for Wilms' tumor from 1931 to 1939 appeared to be cured of their tumors, compared with 18 of 38 (47%) cured when treated between 1940 and 1947. The authors suspected that the difference resulted from the radiotherapy administered to 36 of the 38 patients in the later period. It was customary to irradiate children in the immediate postoperative period (i.e., shortly after they left the operating room). Dosages of 200 roentgen per day were given to a total dosage of 4,000 to 5,000 roentgen.

At present approximately 70–75% of children with Wilms' tumor are treated without radiation therapy. The number rises to 80–85% if metastatic disease is excluded. The NWTS and SIOP trials that have led to this restricted use of radiation therapy are described earlier in this chapter. When irradiation is used, it is successful in limiting the frequency of abdominal relapse to 0–4% of children with FH tumors (73).

There are additional single-institution data concerning the role of radiotherapy for nonmetastatic Wilms' tumor. For example, studies at St. Jude Children's Research Hospital (SJCRH) eliminated radiation therapy for stage II disease after 1979 and began using reduced-dose irradiation for stage III (12 Gy; whole abdomen irradiation until 1985, local field irradiation since 1985 for FH without diffuse peritoneal contamination) (94). Abdominal disease control was obtained in 97% of patients. Under a neoadjuvant chemotherapy protocol at the Hospital for Sick Children, Toronto, 15 of 54 patients with localized disease at presentation needed radiation therapy (27%), nine for stage III or anaplastic disease and six for recurrence (66).

Chemotherapy

In 1966, Sidney Farber (90) reported improved results in the treatment of recurrent and metastatic Wilms' tumor. His series included 16 patients with recurrent disease and 15 with metastatic disease at diagnosis. Patients were treated primarily with actinomycin D and, to a limited degree, vincristine. The 2-year survival rate was 58%.

The addition of effective chemotherapy has substantially improved the overall results in Wilms' tumor in the past two decades. The NWTS and SIOP studies that have substantially established the indications for chemotherapy are discussed earlier in this chapter.

RADIOTHERAPEUTIC MANAGEMENT

The current guidelines for external beam radiation therapy on NWTS-5 are summarized in Table 13-16 (15,67,70,94–96). Indications for radiation therapy in the current SIOP trial are summarized in Tables 13-34 and 13-40–13-42 (69).

The timing of postoperative irradiation is important. Delayed initiation of treatment beyond 10 days after surgery has been related to higher risk of abdominal recurrence in several, but not all, studies (43,61,72,73). Most relapses related to delayed start of therapy have been in patients with UH (73). A recent analysis looked at the influence of delay of radiation therapy on outcome in Wilms' tumor. In NWTS-1 and NWTS-2, a radiotherapy delay of 10 days or more was associated with adverse outcomes. In NWTS-3 and NWTS-4, in patients with stages II–IV FH tumors, approximately 1,200 patients were subjected to analysis. The mean delay in radiotherapy was 10.9 days from surgery, and the median was 9 days; 59% of children were treated 8 to 12 days postoperatively. For children who were treated 0 to 9 days postoperatively and those treated at least 10 days postoperatively, there was no difference in the rate of flank or abdominal recurrence. In NWTS-1 and NWTS-2, 80% of children were treated with radiotherapy during week 1, whereas in NWTS-3 and NWTS-4 24% of children were treated in week 1 but 66% were treated with radiotherapy in week 2 (97). NWTS-5 recommends that postoperative irradiation begin no later than the ninth postoperative day.

Volume

Local-regional irradiation treatment fields include the tumor bed, importantly differentiated from the renal bed to include the entire preoperative tumor extent in the abdomen. The tumor bed is defined as the outline of the kidney and any associated tumor. The tumor volume is established by careful review of the surgical findings, IVP, CT, ultrasound, or MRI. The superior margin of the field is placed at the upper pole of the kidney, with an additional 1-cm margin in a child with a lower pole neoplasm, and the inferior portal margin encompasses the lower margin of the tumor with a 1-cm margin. The field should extend to the dome of the diaphragm only in patients in whom the tumor is known to have extended that far superiorly (98). A variable proportion of the liver is necessarily included to adequately encompass the initial tumor extent for right-sided lesions. Medially, the target volume should encompass the entire width of the vertebral bodies, with adequate contralateral extension to include the entire para-aortic lymph node chain but exclude the remaining kidney. The choice of the medial margin reflects the importance of lymph node radiation therapy. In addition, homogeneous irradiation of the vertebral bodies avoids one mechanism of late scoliosis by equally affecting growth on each side of the vertebral body. Laterally, the treatment field tangentially includes the abdominal wall. Parallel opposed anterior and posterior fields are used.

For patients with preoperative intraperitoneal tumor rupture, intraoperative rupture with diffuse dissemination of tumor, diffuse peritoneal implants, or massive abdominal disease, irradiation must address the entire abdominal cavity. The target volume includes all of the peritoneal surfaces, defined superiorly by the diaphragms and inferiorly through the lower pelvic region, generally at the bottom of the obturator foramen (99). The acetabulum and femoral heads are blocked. Attempts to limit irradiation by blocking the contralateral pelvic region of the peritoneal cavity have been associated with abdominal recurrence when abdominal irradiation was appropriate (100).

WLI must be administered carefully to encompass both apices and the posterior inferior extent of the lungs. The average field extends above the clavicles and down to L1. The shoulders are excluded from the field by blocks. Care should be taken not to irradiate the uninvolved kidney in the whole lung field (101).

Some clinical situations call for WLI plus flank irradiation, such as anaplastic Wilms' tumor (stage II) in the abdomen with lung metastases (overall stage IV). Some patients can be treated with one large field, reducing off the lungs at approximately 12 Gy to continue the flank irradiation. Usually the lungs and flank are irradiated separately. Field matching with appropriate gaps and feathering are important in avoiding excessive liver irradiation in right-sided disease and avoiding irradiation of the remaining kidney in the lower border of the WLI field.

Dosage for Abdominal Disease

Earlier data regarding radiation control of abdominal disease recommended local irradiation to 24 to 30 Gy (58,89,99). The first two NWTS trials incorporated an age-dependent scale of dosages ranging from 18 to 40 Gy (13,67). Review of these trials showed an overall rate of initial abdominal failure of 2–4% with FH in groups II and III (75). Details of radiation therapy showed no apparent dose–response relationship, with equal frequency of abdominal recurrence at dosage levels of 18 to 20 Gy, 20 to 24 Gy, and 24 to 40 Gy (13,75).

NWTS-3 randomly assigned patients with stage III disease to receive 10 or 20 Gy postoperatively, including an option for supplemental dosages up to 10 Gy for regions of gross residual disease (43,44,102). This boost was used in only 2% of the patients with stage III FH tumors (43). As shown in Table 13-8, the NWTS noted no difference in survival or relapse-free survival between the 10- and 20-Gy arms. The current NWTS-5 trial incorporates a boost at the investigator's option from 10.8 Gy to a cumulative dosage of 21.6 Gy for patients with residual disease larger than 3 cm in diameter. SJCRH used 12 Gy postoperatively for patients with stage III disease. Two-year disease-free survival for patients with stage III FH and stage IV FH was 88% and 71%, respectively. Abdominal failure occurred in three of 52 patients (94).

The frequency of abdominal recurrence after protocol-directed therapy has been impressively reduced by the use of radiotherapy with adriamycin, actinomycin D, vincristine, and cyclophosphamide for patients with anaplastic Wilms' tumor (Tables 13-12–13-15). A dose-response relationship for anaplastic Wilms' tumor has not clearly been identified. The frequency of in-field recurrence at low dosages has led some investigators to recommend an age-modulated dosage scheme: younger than 12 months, 12 to 18 Gy; 13 to 18 months, 18 to 24 Gy; 19 to 30 months, 24 to 30 Gy; 31 to 40 months, 30 to 35

TABLE 13-40. *SIOP 2001 indications for radiotherapy*

Flank RT:
  Stage III, intermediate risk
  Stage II, high risk, except blastemal type
  Stage III, high risk
  Stage IV: Abdominal stage III, intermediate risk
             Abdominal stage II–III high risk
Whole abdomen RT: in all risk groups
  Stage III, diffuse spillage, peritoneal metastases
Pulmonary RT: if pulmonary metastases at diagnosis:
  Persistent metastases at wk 9 after chemotherapy
    or surgery
  High-risk primary tumor, independent of pulmonary
    metastases
  Secondary metastases

RT, radiation therapy.
From references 69, 141, and 143, and summarized by Professor F. Oldenburger.

TABLE 13-41. *SIOP 2001 radiation therapy dosage (total dose/dose per fraction)*

Hemiflank:
  Intermediate risk: 14.1/1.8 Gy ± boost: 10.8/1.8 Gy
  High risk, II and III: 25.2/1.8 Gy
Whole abdomen: 14.4 Gy up to a maximum of 21 Gy
  Dosage/fraction 1.25–1.5 Gy
  Children <1 year: 10–12 Gy total
Lungs: 15.0/1.5 Gy, boost 5–10 Gy
Brain: 25.5/1.5 Gy, boost 4.5 Gy
Liver: 20.01/1.5 Gy

From *Nephroblastoma clinical protocol SIOP 2001.* International Society of Pediatric Oncology, Zurich, 2001.

Gy; 41 months or older, 35 to 40 Gy. This is not because of an age-related dose–response relationship but because of a fear of toxicity in the young.

In recent SIOP trials local-regional radiation therapy is given to patients who, after preoperative chemotherapy and nephrectomy, are found to have stage II high-risk tumors or stage III. These categories comprise approximately no more than 25% of patients. The dosage to the tumor bed is 14.4 to 25.2 Gy, with an optional boost to localized areas of tumor as needed (Tables 13-40–13-42) (66,68).

Brachytherapy and Intraoperative Radiation

Three cases of bilateral Wilms' tumor have been reported in which afterloading brachytherapy was used to treat renal disease in the remaining kidney after nephrectomy on one side and to spare surrounding normal tissue as much as possible. Brachytherapy may be of use in selected cases (103,104). Intraoperative radiation, including *ex vivo* bench surgery irradiation, has also been used in selected cases (Fig. 13-11) (62).

Bilateral Wilms' Tumor

Stage V or bilateral Wilms' tumor is found in 4–8% of patients (12,22,44,105). The 2-, 5-, and

TABLE 13-42. *SIOP radiation therapy volumes and dosages*

Study	Volume	Stage	Abdomen dosage (Gy)	Lung[a] dosage (Gy)	Brain dosage (Gy)	Bone dosage (Gy)	Liver dosage (Gy)
SIOP 6	Initial	II N0	±20 Gy				
		II N1/III	30 Gy				
SIOP 9	Initial	II N1/III	15 ± 10–20	15 ± 5–10			
		WA	15 ± 10				
		II/III UH	15/15 + 10				
SIOP 93-01	Preoperative	II N1/III	15 + 10–15	15 ± 5–10			
		WA	15–20 ± 10				
		HR II/III	25				
SIOP 2001	Preoperative	III	14.4 + 10.8	15 ± 5–10	25.2 ± 4.5	30	20
		WA	15–21 ± 10				
		HR II/III	25.2				

Kidney dosage not higher than 12 Gy; liver dose not higher than 20 Gy.
HR, high risk; UH, unfavorable histology; WA, whole abdomen.
[a]With air correction.
From references 69, 141, and 143, and summarized by Professor F. Oldenburger.

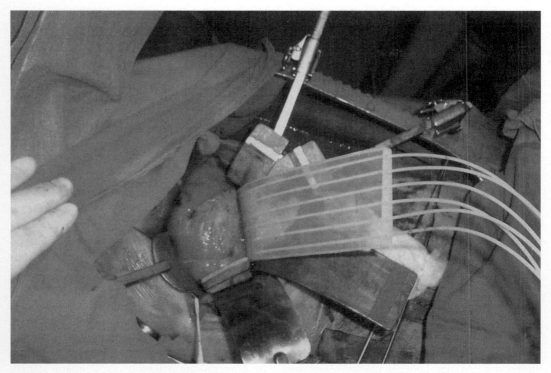

FIG. 13-11. Three weeks before birth, the patient was diagnosed with polyhydramnios. Ultrasound at birth, and periodically thereafter, showed bilateral renal enlargement. At 3 years of age bilateral solid renal masses were seen on abdominal computed tomography. Bilateral Wilms' tumors, favorable histology, were confirmed at exploratory laparotomy. She was treated with vincristine and actinomycin D and right nephrectomy. Biopsies of the left kidney were negative. She then received adriamycin. No radiotherapy was given.

Nine years later, the child, 12 years old, developed abdominal pain. She had a 16 × 9 × 16–cm left renal mass and multiple lung nodules consistent with metastases. Ultrasound-guided renal biopsy confirmed Wilms' tumor. After treatment with etoposide and carboplatin, the pulmonary nodules resolved, and the renal mass was smaller. She received 12 Gy of whole lung irradiation and 12 Gy to the left abdomen, followed by a 3-Gy boost, all at 1.5 Gy per fraction. The residual tumor was resected from the lower pole of the left kidney. Microscopic tumor was at the margin of resection. Intraoperative high–dose rate brachytherapy was administered with a 6-cm-wide applicator to the distal 5 cm of the tumor with [192]Ir. The dosage was 8 Gy at a depth of 0.5 cm in 403 seconds. Uninvolved tissue was shielded with lead sheets. (See color plate)

10-year survival rates are 83%, 73%, and 70%, respectively (12,14,105,106). The majority of bilateral cases present with simultaneous or synchronous involvement in both kidneys. As with bilateral retinoblastoma, the extent of disease in each kidney is often disparate, often including a large unilateral tumor and scattered nodules involving the contralateral kidney. UH is found in 10%, and discordant histology (i.e., UH on one side and FH on the other) is found in some patients (12). Unfavorable histology, older age at

diagnosis, and the most advanced stage of the individual tumors are the most important prognostic factors (14,105–108).

There are a variety of therapeutic approaches to stage V disease. The goal of therapy is cure with preservation of renal function. Radical nephrectomy should almost never be performed as part of the initial surgical procedure. Rather, the initial operation defines the extent of tumor in each kidney, obtains bilateral biopsies to histologically confirm the diagnosis, and biopsies suspicious lymph nodes. Subsequently, the child should be treated with chemotherapy. If NWTS-5 guidelines are followed, the chemotherapy is tailored to the worst histology (favorable or unfavorable) and the stage of the primary tumors (i.e., more aggressive chemotherapy if one of the tumors is intra-abdominal stage III, less aggressive if both tumors are stage I). After this initial chemotherapy, the child is returned to the operating room for second-look surgery. If tumor can be removed with preservation of renal function, it should. If surgery successfully removes the tumors and there is no gross or pathological evidence of persistent or residual disease, chemotherapy is continued appropriate to the surgical stage. If there is gross or microscopic residual intra-abdominal tumor after second-look surgery, the patient is switched to alternative chemotherapy. If abnormalities persist in the kidneys on repeat imaging, a third operation may be attempted to finally excise the tumors. The reader will appreciate the general strategy: alternating between chemotherapy and surgery to achieve sufficient cytoreduction of tumor to achieve successful cancer surgery with preservation of functioning kidneys (12,82,98, 107,108).

Radiation therapy in stage V Wilms' tumor is indicated when definitive surgery has been accomplished and one or both of the primary tumors are found to be stage III FH, stages II–III anaplastic tumors, or stages I–III CCSK or rhabdoid tumor or when preoperative chemotherapy and one or two surgeries have not achieved successful extirpation of cancer. In the latter case, preoperative low-dose irradiation, 12 to 16 Gy, may produce sufficient tumor shrinkage to achieve tumor removal (99,109).

Metachronous or asynchronous bilateral disease has a decidedly less favorable outcome than does synchronous disease. Malcolm et al. (106) reported zero of four survivors with metachronous disease, compared with ten of 16 with simultaneous presentations; speculatively, the less favorable results with metachronous involvement may be interpreted as representing a pattern of relapse rather than independent tumor development. Jones et al. (81) confirmed a less

favorable outcome with metachronous bilateral tumors: 39% 2-year survival in contrast to 87% with simultaneous presentations (111).

Metastatic Disease

The ability to control overt pulmonary metastasis was the major advance consequent to the addition of actinomycin D to irradiation in the management of Wilms' tumor (54,58,89,90). In stage IV with pulmonary metastasis at diagnosis, conventional NWTS management begins with nephrectomy, postoperative chemotherapy, abdominal irradiation if appropriate, and WLI. The indications for infradiaphragmatic irradiation are dictated by the degree of abdominal disease. Abdominal irradiation is given for stage IV patients with in-the-abdomen stage III FH, stages II–III anaplastic histology, and stages I–III CCSK and rhabdoid tumor. For patients with pulmonary metastasis by chest radiograph at diagnosis, the addition of lung radiation therapy is standard (10,16, 74,83,96,112). Although earlier reports documented excellent control at dosage levels of 16 to 18 Gy, the impressive results in recent series using dosages limited to 12 Gy at 1.5 Gy per fraction approach the control rates for abdominal disease with attenuated dosage levels (43,47,94,96). A boost to local sites of residual pulmonary nodules to cumulative levels of 30 Gy is appropriate if permitted by the lung volumes. Stage IV FH with lung metastases had an 80% 4-year survival rate on NWTS-3, whereas survival for those with stage IV UH was about 55% (15,17,113).

In the new SIOP protocol, stage IV disease is treated with preoperative chemotherapy. Nephrectomy is then performed. Radiation therapy is administered according to SIOP guidelines for intra-abdominal disease (discussed earlier in this chapter). WLI is reserved for those who do not have a complete pulmonary tumor response and are not rendered free of disease by metastasectomy (Tables 13-36–13-41) (66,68).

Is WLI necessary in stage IV (pulmonary) Wilms' tumor? In a United Kingdom Children's Cancer Group study, patients with stage

IV FH were spared WLI if they had complete resolution of pulmonary metastases after chemotherapy. Thirty-five of 39 patients were treated without WLI. The 6-year disease-free survival was 50%, overall survival 65% (94). These results appear to be somewhat worse than those of the NWTS and may be used to argue in favor of WLI. In a SIOP study, 36 patients with stage IV FH received chemotherapy, with abdominal irradiation given for stage III or node-positive stage II (46). Chemotherapy eradicated lung disease in 27 of 36 patients. Six additional patients were cleared of lung metastases with surgery. Only seven children ultimately received WLI: seven for recurrent tumor, one immediately after nephrectomy for inoperable multiple metastases, and two after complete tumor clearance by chemotherapy. Five-year actuarial disease-free survival is 83% (10,46,66,68,74).

Radiation therapy was considered fundamental for control of stage IV Wilms' tumor. From the aforementioned data, one may assert that this view might have to be modified for children whose lung metastases completely respond to chemotherapy with supplemental surgery in selected cases and for patients with minimal disease, such as CT-positive, chest radiograph–negative disease (56). One hopes that future studies will help identify patients with stage IV disease who, on the basis of biologic markers, need WLI and those who may be spared it with equivalent survival probabilities (10).

It is important to take account of prior abdominal irradiation in patients who need thoracic irradiation. One must respect liver tolerance when adjoining fields that encompass the hepatic region. One must also respect the upper pole of the remaining kidney in delineating thoracic irradiation fields in a child with previous abdominal irradiation.

Liver metastases may be treated by hepatic irradiation in addition to chemotherapy. Whole liver irradiation is sometimes given for diffuse disease, with supplementary boosts to gross disease (15,67,72). When possible, however, more limited radiotherapy fields are used if the disease is more localized in the liver.

RECURRENT WILMS' TUMOR

A large body of evidence has been developed concerning the important prognostic factors after relapse of Wilms' tumor (99). The major prognostic factors will be considered in turn.

Site of Recurrence

Patients who relapse in the abdomen may be separated into two general groups. The first is those who have recurrences in previously irradiated fields. These patients have resistant disease. In NWTS-3 the 3-year postrelapse survival for such patients was 15%. The second group is those with intra-abdominal recurrences after surgery and chemotherapy only. These patients are amenable to retreatment, and the 3-year postrelapse survival is 77% (100,114–116).

The lung is a common site of recurrence of Wilms' tumor. Relapse confined to the lung has a 44% 3-year postrelapse survival. Relapse in the liver portends a worse prognosis: 14% 4 years after relapse (47,110,115). There are some survivors of solitary metastases to brain or liver (117,118).

Initial Stage of Disease

The prognosis after relapse is related to the initial stage. In both the NWTS trials and the United Kingdom Children's Cancer Study Group Wilms' tumor trials, group I patients had a better ultimate survival after relapse than did groups II or III. In NWTS-2 and NWTS-3 the 3-year postrelapse survival was 57% for initial stage I, 36% for initial stage II and III, and 17% for initial stage IV (10, 115,119).

Histology

The survival after relapse of patients with FH is two to four times greater than that of patients with UH (21,115). The United Kingdom Children's Cancer Study Group has reported only

17 survivors out of 71 patients (24%) who relapsed during or after treatment. Fifteen of 51
(29%) patients with relapsed FH survived,
compared with two of 20 (10%) with UH
(118,120).

Time of Relapse

Relapse after initial therapy is demonstrated
within 1 year of diagnosis in 75% of cases with
ultimate failure. Fewer than 3% of proven relapses have been documented beyond 2 years
after diagnosis (72,73). The longer the time between diagnosis and the development of recurrent disease, the better the ultimate outcome
(10). The 3-year postrelapse survival for patients in NWTS-2 and NWTS-3 who relapsed 0
to 5 months after diagnosis was 18%, 6 to 11
months after diagnosis was 30%, and 12
months or more after diagnosis was 41%
(115,119).

Nature of Prior Therapy

Patients who relapse after initial therapy that included adriamycin or abdominal irradiation fare
worse than those who did not receive such therapy (10,115). Presumably this is because the use
of adriamycin or radiotherapy is a surrogate
marker for initially more advanced disease and
because tumor that recurs after such therapy
may represent more resistant disease.

The rate of success in achieving secondary disease-free survival varies inversely with the intensity of the initial treatment regimen. Data reporting salvage in the NWTS studies demonstrate
lower rates of secondary control that parallel the
selective use of more aggressive treatment in
high-risk patients. Serial reduction in the actual
rate of demonstrated pulmonary metastases has
paralleled reduction in later control of metastatic
disease. Secondary disease-free survival has been
reported in 51% of relapsed cases from NWTS-1,
40% from NWTS-2, and 34% from NWTS-3
(47,121).

When tumor relapses in the lung, a surgical
biopsy or excision is performed to confirm the
diagnosis. However, surgical excision of metastases does not reduce the risk of second relapse

(10). Chemotherapy and WLI are generally
given.

When FH relapses in the abdomen in a child
with initial stage I or II disease who did not receive prior irradiation, the treatment generally
includes preoperative chemotherapy, tumor
excision, and involved-field irradiation (10,73,
104,115). A local relapse of initial stage III disease calls for preoperative chemotherapy, tumor
excision, and reirradiation (115).

TOXICITIES

The late effects of treatment of childhood cancer
and the causes and frequency of treatment-
induced second malignant neoplasms are considered in detail in Chapters 19 and 20. In this
section we will review the late ill effects, including induced neoplasms, particularly associated
with the treatment of Wilms' tumor.

Complications Attributable to Surgery

Small bowel obstruction occurred in 7% of
children who underwent primary nephrectomy
in NWTS-3. Factors contributing to obstruction include tumor rupture, intravascular extension of tumor, the necessity of resecting other
organs at the time of nephrectomy, and the
presence of postoperative residual tumor.
Other complications attributable to surgery include extensive intraoperative hemorrhage
(6%), vascular injuries (1%), injuries to uninvolved organs (1%), and death (0.5%) (11,
122). The operative mortality rate in the United
Kingdom Children's Cancer Wilms' Tumor
Study was 1% (123).

Hematologic Toxicity

Review of the data from NWTS-3 indicates
clinically significant acute hematologic toxicities. Fatal toxicities occur in a small proportion
of patients. Depending on the drugs given, severe hematologic toxicity occurs in 6–64% of
patients over a 6-week course of treatment. Toxicity and infections account for 15% of the
deaths of NWTS children, producing a 1% treatment-related mortality rate (15).

Hepatic Effects

Hepatotoxicity from Wilms' tumor therapy may be indicated by an increase in transaminases or by hyperbilirubinemia. Veno-occlusive disease consists of the clinical triad of hepatomegaly, ascites, and icterus. In unirradiated NWTS-4 patients the frequency of hepatic toxicity related to actinomycin D (serum glutamic-oxaloacetic transaminase, serum glutamic-pyruvic transaminase elevations) rose from 2.8% in patients receiving 15 μg/kg of standard divided-dose therapy to 3.7% in those receiving pulse-intensive 45 μg/kg and 14.3% in those receiving 60 μg/kg pulse-intensive therapy. These data prompted replacement of the 60-μg/kg treatment with the 45-μg/kg dosage (117). A review of cases accrued via the German Pediatric Oncology Hematology Group to SIOP Trial 9 studied 58 patients who received chemotherapy and abdominal irradiation. Eleven of these 58 patients developed signs of hepatotoxicity, four of them with veno-occlusive disease. There was a predominance of children with right-sided tumors in the group with hepatic injury (nine out of 33, 27%, vs. two out of 24, 8%) (124). This probably reflects the larger volume of liver irradiated in right-sided tumors. Plowman from St. Bartholomew's Hospital/The Hospital for Sick Children, London, has described the use of a partial transmission block to reduce the radiation dosage administered to the liver in right-sided Wilms' tumor and thereby reduce the risk of late toxicity (125).

Orthopedic Effects

In long-term follow-up studies of Wilms' tumor survivors, scoliosis and musculoskeletal abnormalities are more common in irradiated patients than in those not irradiated. This may result from irradiation of the vertebral bodies or the paraspinal musculature. Asymmetric irradiation of either produces the deformity. Rate et al. (126) identified 31 children with Wilms' tumor who received abdominal irradiation between 1970 and 1984 and were followed past skeletal maturity. Ten of the children were irradiated with

orthovoltage and 21 with megavoltage. Of the children irradiated with megavoltage, the most common orthopedic abnormalities were lower rib hypoplasia (57%) and mild scoliosis (10 to 20 degrees) (48%). In the patients irradiated with orthovoltage, lower rib hypoplasia occurred in 50%, mild scoliosis in 40%, severe scoliosis (more than 20 degrees) in 40%, and limb length inequality in 20% (126,127). Scoliosis as a late ill effect of abdominal irradiation for Wilms' tumor was confirmed by a report from the University of Helsinki in which 21 of 24 patients (88%) had some degree of scoliosis. Most patients had been irradiated with cobalt-60 (128,129).

Renal Effects

After unilateral nephrectomy in childhood, the remaining kidney generally adjusts its function and size; this is called compensatory hypertrophy of the kidney. One year after nephrectomy for Wilms' tumor the glomerular filtration rate (GFR) and effective renal plasma flow are approximately 90% of normal values for age-matched children with two normal kidneys. Children treated with surgery and chemotherapy also have close to normal values. The addition of radiation to chemotherapy results in a diminished renal function, to approximately 73% of normal GFR (Table 13-43) (130).

Cardiac Effects

Cardiac injury in long-term survivors is associated with the use of doxorubicin or the cardiac irradiation that occurs during WLI (Table 13-44).

TABLE 13-43. *Long-term complications of renal function*

Dosage (Gy)	Impaired creatinine clearance
<12	19%
12–24	32%
>24	73%

From Egeler RM, Wolff JE, Anderson RA, et al. Long-term complications and post-treatment follow-up of patients with Wilms' tumor. *Semin Urol Oncol* 1999; 17:55–61.

TABLE 13-44. *Long-term complications of cardiac function*

Treatment	Congestive heart failure at 15 years
Doxorubicin	1.7%
No whole lung irradiation	1.0%
Whole lung irradiation	5.4%

From Egeler RM, Wolff JE, Anderson RA, et al. Long-term complications and post-treatment follow-up of patients with Wilms' tumor. *Semin Urol Oncol* 1999; 17:55–61.

Pregnancy Outcome

There is now long-term follow-up on pregnancy outcome in irradiated women who were treated, as children, for Wilms' tumor. As Table 13-45 indicates, the risk of early or threatened labor, malposition of the fetus, short gestation, or low birth weight appears directly correlated with the irradiation dosage. The outcome also appears worse for those treated with abdominal–pelvic fields and those treated with higher irradiation dosages (131,132).

Treatment-Induced Neoplasms

Initial reports concerning the risk of second malignant neoplasms after treatment of Wilms' tumor indicated that the cumulative incidence 10 years after diagnosis was 1% (102,132–134). A recent update of long-term survivors indicates a significant increase of second malignancies as assessed by an observed:expected relative risk ratio (8.4). Patients who received both adriamycin and higher-dose irradiation (35 Gy) had the highest relative risk (36.3) (135).

Long-term follow-up indicates that there is a risk of acute myelocytic leukemia in long-term survivors of Wilms' tumor. This may be related to the administration of alkylating agents and abdominal irradiation (136).

Growth Abnormalities

Abdominal irradiation can also produce significant reduction in sitting height and a more modest decrease in standing height. These effects are more pronounced the younger the patient is at the time of radiotherapy (129,132). Long-term analysis of predicted height deficits in children who receive flank radiation for Wilms' tumor indicates, as shown in Table 13-46, that the younger a child is at the time of flank irradiation, the greater the predicted height deficit. Furthermore, the higher dosage of irradiation administered, the greater the predicted height deficit. These effects are related to irradiation of the thoracolumbar vertebral bodies. Abnormalities can also ensue from asymmetric irradiation of the paravertebral musculature, which may, over time, lead to a risk of scoliosis.

FUTURE DEVELOPMENTS

In the future we may begin to assess the risk of local and distant recurrence of Wilms' tumor and select appropriate therapy based on a variety of molecular biologic and related markers. These include assessments of the loss of heterozygosity of certain chromosomes. One may also measure vascular density and telomerase

TABLE 13-45. *Pregnancy outcome*

Flank dosage	Early or threatened labor	Malposition of fetus	Gestation <36 wk	Birthweight <2,500 g
0	13%	3%	82%	11%
0.01–15 Gy	8%	8%	74%	16%
15.01–25 Gy	19%	3%	79%	13%
25.01–35 Gy	23%	19%	68%	26%
>35 Gy	29%	14%	68%	24%
p	*0.03*	0.007	0.0005	0.017

From Green DM, Peabody EM, Nan B, et al. Pregnancy outcome after treatment for Wilms' tumor: a report from the National Wilms' Tumor study Group. *J Clin Oncol* 2002;20:2506–2513.

TABLE 13-46. *Predicted deficit in height at age 18 Years after flank irradiation at selected ages and dosages*

Age at treatment (yr)	Height deficit (cm) after a dosage of:		
	10 Gy	20 Gy	30 Gy
2	2.4	4.8	7.2
4	1.8	3.5	5.3
6	1.2	2.4	3.6
8	0.8	1.5	2.3

From Hogeboom CJ, Grosser SC, Guthrie KA, et al. Stature loss following treatment for Wilms' tumor. *Med Pediatr Oncol* 2001;36:295–304.

activity. The evolving field of proteomics may offer us the opportunity, via initial protein profile and changes in protein profile during the course of therapy, to assess prognosis and therapy. Interstitial pO_2 measurements and noninvasive oxygenation status assessments may prove of value in assessing tumors at risk for local failure and distant metastases. Quantitative positron emission tomography and single-photon emission computed tomography may also be of use.

In the future, we may hope to answer some of the remaining clinical radiotherapy research questions. These include the establishment of the dose–response relationship for the treatment of anaplastic Wilms' tumor and the assessment of the appropriate role of radiotherapy for stage II disease after tumor spill (137).

REFERENCES

References particularly recommended for further reading are indicated by an asterisk.

1. Rance TM. Case of fungus haematodes in kidnies. *Med Phys* 1814;32:19.
2. Gairdner E. Case of fungus haematodes in the kidneys. *Edinburgh Med Surg J* 1828;29:312–315.
3. Osler W. Two cases of striated myosarcoma of the kidney. *J Anat Physiol* 1879;14:229.
4. King SC. Wilms' tumor. *N C Med J* 1991;52:74.
5. Zantinga AR, Coppes MJ. Historical aspects of the identification of the entity Wilms tumor, and its management. *Hematol Oncol Clin North Am* 1995;9:1145–1155.
6. Paterson R. The genital organs. In: *The treatment of malignant disease by radium and X-rays.* London: Edward Arnold, 1948:404–405.
7. Dean AL, Guttman RJ. Radiation therapy in malignant diseases of the genito-urinary tract. In: Pohle EA, ed. *Clinical radiation therapy.* Philadelphia: Lea & Febiger, 1950:491–514.
8. Jacox HW, Cahill GF. Treatment of diseases of the kidney and adrenal gland. In: Portmann UV, ed. *Clinical therapeutic radiology.* New York: Thomas Nelson & Sons, 1950:254–275.
9. Green DM, Breslow N, Li YI, et al. The role of surgical excision in the management of relapsed Wilms' tumor patients with pulmonary metastases. *J Pediatr Surg* 1991;26:728–733.
10. Green DM. Wilms' tumor. *Eur J Cancer* 1997;33:409–418.
11. Haase GM. Current surgical management of Wilms' tumor. *Curr Opin Pediatr* 1996;8:268–275.
12. Blute ML, Kelalis PP, Offord KP, et al. Bilateral Wilms' tumor. *J Urol* 1987;138(2):968–973.
13. D'Angio GJ, Breslow N, Beckwith JB, et al. Treatment of Wilms' tumor: results of the Third National Wilms' Tumor Study. *Cancer* 1989;64:349–360.
14. Montgomery BT, Kelalis PP, Blute MD, et al. Extended follow-up of bilateral Wilms' tumor: results of the National Wilms' Tumor Study. *J Urol* 1991;146:514–518.
15. D'Angio GJ. Informational bulletin #19. National Wilms' Tumor Study. Seattle, WA: NWTS Data and Statistical Center, 1991.
16. Breslow NE, Churchill G, Nesmith B, et al. Clinicopathologic features and prognosis for Wilms' tumor patients with metastases at diagnosis. *Cancer* 1986;58:2501–2511.
17. Green DM, Finkelstein JZ, Breslow NE, et al. Remaining problems in the treatment of patients with Wilms' tumor. *Pediatr Clin North Am* 1991;38:475–488.
18. Hadley GP, Jacobs C. The clinical presentation of Wilms' tumour in black children. *S Afr Med J* 1990;77:565–567.
19. Knudson AG. Hereditary cancer, oncogenes, and antioncogenes. *Cancer Res* 1985;45:1437–1443.
20. Knudson AG, Strong LC. Mutation and cancer: a model for Wilms' tumor of the kidney. *J Natl Cancer Inst* 1972;48:313–324.
21. Grundy P, Coppes M. An overview of the clinical and molecular genetics of Wilms' tumor. *Med Pediatr Oncol* 1996;27:394–397.
22. Grundy P, Coppes MJ, Haber D. Molecular genetics of Wilms' tumor. *Hematol Oncol Clin North Am* 1995;9:1201–1215.
23. Pritchard-Jones K, Grundy PE, Coppes MJ. A report of the 3rd International Conference on the Molecular and Clinical Genetics of Childhood Renal Tumors, together with the Mitchell Ross Symposium on anaplastic and other high risk embryonal tumors of childhood. *Med Pediatr Oncol* 2000;35:126–130.
*24. Blakely ML, Ritchey ML. Controversies in the management of Wilms' tumor. *Semin Pediatr Surg* 2001;10:127–131.
25. Douglass EC, Look AT, Webber B, et al. Hyperdiploidy and chromosomal rearrangements define the anaplastic variant of Wilms' tumor. *J Clin Oncol* 1986;4:975–981.
26. Riccardi VM, Hittner HM, Francke U, et al. The aniridia-Wilms' tumor association: the critical role of chromosome band 11p13. *J Cancer Genet Cytogenet* 1980;2:131–137.
27. Palmer N, Evans AE. The association of aniridia and

Wilms' tumor: methods of surveillance and diagnosis. *Med Pediatr Oncol* 1983;11:73–75.

28. Pendergrass TW. Congenital anomalies in children with Wilms' tumor: a new survey. *Cancer* 1976;37: 403–409.

29. Breslow NE. Epidemiological features of Wilms' tumor: results of the National Wilms' Tumor Study. *J Natl Cancer Inst* 1982;68:429–436.

30. Beckwith JB. Wilms' tumor and other renal tumors of childhood. *Hum Pathol* 1983;14:481–492.

31. Coppes MJ, Ritchey ML, D'Angio GJ. Preface. *Hematol Oncol Clin North Am* 1995;9:xiii–xvii.

32. Ritchey ML. Recent progress in the biology and treatment of Wilms' tumor. *Curr Urol Rep* 2001;2: 127–131.

33. Howell CG, Othersen HB, Kiviat NE, et al. Therapy and outcome in 51 children with mesoblastic nephroma: a report of the National Wilms' Tumor Study. *J Pediatr Surg* 1982;17:826–831.

*34. Dome JS, Coppes MJ. Recent advances in Wilms tumor genetics. *Curr Opin Pediatr* 2002;14:5–11.

35. Puri P, Kalidasan V. Mesoblastic nephroma and Wilms' tumour. In: Puri P, ed. *Neonatal tumours.* London: Springer, 1996:43–48.

*36. Coppes MJ, Pritchard-Jones K. Principles of Wilms' tumor biology. *Urol Clin North Am* 2000;27: 423–433.

37. Walterhouse D. Mesoblastic nephroma. *Med Pediatr Oncol* 1990;18:64–67.

38. Beckwith JB. Wilms' tumor and other renal tumors in childhood. In: Finegold M, ed. *Pathology of neoplasia in children and adolescents.* Philadelphia: WB Saunders, 1986:313–332.

39. Beckwith JB, Palmer NF. Histopathology and prognosis of Wilms' tumor: results from the First National Wilms' Tumor Study. *Cancer* 1978;41:1937–1948.

40. Schmidt D, Beckwith JB. Histopathology of childhood renal tumor. *Hematol Oncol Clin North Am* 1995;9:1179–1200.

41. Breslow NE, Palmer NF, Hill LR, et al. Wilms' tumor: prognostic factors for patients without metastases at diagnosis: results of the National Wilms' Tumor Study. *Cancer* 1978;41:1577–1589.

42. D'Angio GJ, Tefft M, Breslow N, et al. Radiation therapy of Wilms' tumor: results according to dose, field, post-operative timing and histology. *Int J Radiat Oncol Biol Phys* 1978;4:769–780.

43. D'Angio GJ, Evans AE, Breslow N, et al. The treatment of Wilms' tumor: results of the National Wilms' Tumor Study. *Cancer* 1976;38:633–646.

*44. Neville HL, Ritchey ML. Wilms' tumor: overview of National Wilms' Tumor Study Group results. *Urol Clin North Am* 2000;27:435–442.

45. Bonadio JF, Storer B, Norkool P, et al. Anaplastic Wilms' tumor: clinical and pathologic studies. *J Clin Oncol* 1985;3:513–520.

46. de Kraker J, Lemerle J, Voute PA, et al. Wilms' tumor with pulmonary metastases at diagnosis: the significance of primary chemotherapy. *J Clin Oncol* 1990; 8:1187–1190.

47. Breslow N, Churchill G, Beckwith JB, et al. Prognosis for Wilms' tumor patients with nonmetastatic disease at diagnosis: results of the Second National Wilms' Tumor Study. *J Clin Oncol* 1985;3:521–531.

48. Faria P, Beckwith JB, Mishra K, et al. Focal versus diffuse anaplasia in Wilms tumor—new definitions with prognostic significance: a report from the National Wilms' Tumor Study Group. *Am J Surg Pathol* 1996;20:909–920.

49. Haas JE, Bonadio JF, Beckwith JB. Clear cell sarcoma of the kidney with emphasis of ultrastructural studies. *Cancer* 1984;54:2978–2987.

50. Green DM, Thomas PRM, Shochat S. The treatment of Wilms' tumor: results of the National Wilms' Tumor Studies. *Hematol Oncol Clin North Am* 1995;9: 1267–1274.

51. Gutjahr P. Progress and controversies in modern treatment of Wilms' tumor. *World J Urol* 1995;13: 209–212.

52. Leape L, Breslow N, Bishop H. Surgical resection of Wilms' tumor: results of the National Wilms' Tumor Study. *Ann Surg* 1978;181:351–356.

53. Green DM, Jaffe N. Wilms' tumor: model of a curable pediatric malignant solid tumor. *Cancer Treat Rev* 1978;5:143–172.

54. Wilimas JA, Douglass EC, Magill L, et al. Significance of pulmonary computed tomography at diagnosis in Wilms' tumor. *J Clin Oncol* 1988;6: 1144–1146.

55. Flentje M, Weirich A, Potter R, et al. Hepatotoxicity in irradiated nephroblastoma patients during postoperative treatment according to SIOP9/GPOH. *Radiol Oncol* 1994;31:222–228.

56. Feusner JH, Beckwith JB, D'Angio GJ. Clear cell sarcoma of the kidney: accuracy of imaging methods for detecting bone metastases. Report from the National Wilms' Tumor Study. *Med Pediatr Oncol* 1990;18:225–227.

57. Green DM, Breslow NE, Beckwith JB, et al. Treatment with nephrectomy only for small, stage I/favorable histology Wilms' tumor: a report from the National Wilms' Tumor Study Group. *J Clin Oncol* 2001;19:3719–3724.

58. Cassady JR, Tefft M, Filler RM, et al. Considerations in the radiation therapy of Wilms' tumor. *Cancer* 1973;32:598–608.

59. Cassady JR, Jaffe N, Paed D, et al. The increasing importance of radiation therapy in the improved prognosis of children with Wilms' tumor. *Cancer* 1977;39:825–829.

60. Garcia M, Douglass C, Schlosser JV. Classification and prognosis in Wilms' tumor. *Radiology* 1963;80: 574–580.

61. Tefft M, D'Angio GJ, Grant W. Post-operative radiation therapy for residual Wilms' tumor: review of group III patients in the National Wilms' Tumor Study. *Cancer* 1976;37:2768–2772.

62. Jereb B, Tournade MF, Lemerle J, et al. Lymph node invasion and prognosis in nephroblastoma. *Cancer* 1980;45:1632–1636.

63. Lemerle J, Voute PA, Tournade MF, et al. Preoperative versus postoperative radiotherapy, single versus multiple courses of actinomycin D, in the treatment of Wilms' tumor. *Cancer* 1976;38:647–654.

64. Lemerle J, Voute PA, Tournade MF, et al. Effectiveness of preoperative chemotherapy in Wilms' tumor: results of an International Society of Pediatric Oncology (SIOP) clinical trial. *J Clin Oncol* 1983;1:604–610.

65. De Kraker J. Commentary on Wilms' tumor. *Eur J Cancer* 1997;33:419–420.

66. De Kraker J, Weitzman S, Voute PA. Preoperative strategies in the management of Wilms' tumor. *Hematol Oncol Clin North Am* 1995;9:1275–1285.

67. D'Angio GJ. Editorial: SIOP and the management of Wilms' tumor. *J Clin Oncol* 1983;1:595–596.

68. Jereb B, Burgers JMV, Tournade MF, et al. Radiotherapy in the SIOP (International Society of Pediatric Oncology) nephroblastoma studies: a review. *Med Pediatr Oncol* 1994;22:221–227.

69. *Nephroblastoma clinical protocol SIOP 2001.* International Society of Pediatric Oncology, Zurich, 2001.

70. Thomas PRM. Wilms' tumor: changing role of radiation therapy. *Semin Radiat Oncol* 1997;7:204–211.

71. D'Angio GJ, Evans A, Breslow N, et al. The treatment of Wilms' tumor: results of the Second National Wilms' Tumor Study. *Cancer* 1981;47:2302–2311.

72. Tefft M, D'Angio GJ, Beckwith B, et al. Patterns of intra-abdominal relapse in patients with Wilms' tumor who received radiation: analysis by histopathology, a report of National Wilms' Tumor Studies 1 and 2. *Int J Radiat Oncol Biol Phys* 1980;6:663–667.

73. Thomas PR, Tefft M, Farewell VT, et al. Abdominal relapses in irradiated second national Wilms' tumor study patients. *J Clin Oncol* 1984;2:1098–1011.

74. Green DM, Coppes MJ. Future directions in clinical research in Wilms' tumor. *Hematol Oncol Clin North Am* 1995;9:1329–1339.

*75. Shamberger RC, Guthrie KA, Ritchey ML, et al. Surgery-related factors and local recurrence of Wilms tumor in National Wilms' Tumor Study 4. *Ann Surg* 1999;229:292–297.

76. Green DM. Disease committee chair update: Wilms' tumor. *POG Perspectives* 1997;Fall:10–11.

77. Green D, Breslow N, Beckwith J, et al. A comparison between single dose and divided dose administration of dactinomycin and doxorubicin: a report from the National Wilms' Tumor Study Group. *Med Pediatr Oncol* 1998;16:237–245.

78. Schweisguth O, Bamberger J. Le nephroblastome de l'enfant. *Ann Chir Enfant Paris* 1963;4:335–354.

*79. Green DM, Breslow NE, Beckwith JB, et al. Comparison between single-dose and divided-dose administration of dactinomycin and doxorubicin for patients with Wilms' tumor: a report from the National Wilms' Tumor Study Group. *J Clin Oncol* 1998;16:237–245.

80. Green DM, Breslow NE, Evans I, et al. The effect of chemotherapy dose-intensity on the hematological toxicity of the treatment for Wilms' tumor. A report from the National Wilms' Tumor Study. *Am J Pediatr Hematol Oncol* 1994;16:207–212.

81. Jones B, Hrabovsky E, Kiviat N, et al. Metachronous bilateral Wilms' tumor: National Wilms' Tumor Study. *Am J Clin Oncol* 1982;5:545–550.

82. Larsen E, Perez-Atayde A, Green DM, et al. Surgery only for the treatment of patients with stage I (Cassady) Wilms' tumor. *Cancer* 1990;66:264–266.

*83. Green DM, Breslow NE, Beckwith JB, et al. Effect of duration of treatment on treatment outcome and cost of treatment for Wilms' tumor: a report from the National Wilms' Tumor Study Group. *J Clin Oncol* 1998;16:3744–3751.

84. Mitchell C, Jones PM, Kelsey A, et al. The treatment of Wilms' tumour: results of the United Kingdom Children's Cancer Study Group second Wilms' tumour study. *Br J Cancer* 2000;83:602–508.

85. Thomas PR, Sochat SJ, Norkool P, et al. Prognostic implications of extension, invasion or metastases to the liver at diagnosis of Wilms' tumor. *Proc Am Soc Clin Oncol* 1988;7:255.

86. Ritchey ML, Othersen HB Jr, de Lorimier AA, et al. Renal vein involvement with nephroblastoma: a report of the National Wilms' Tumor Study 3. *Eur Urol* 1990;17:139–144.

87. Othersen HB Jr, DeLarimer A, Hrabovsky E, et al. Surgical evaluation of lymph node metastases in Wilms' tumor. *J Pediatr Surg* 1990;25:330–331.

88. Gonzalez-Chirinas P, Aguilar M, Rivera M. Preoperative vincristine in children with Wilms' tumor. *Proc ASCO* 1991;10:314.

89. Burgers JMV, Tournade MF, Bey P, et al. Abdominal recurrences in Wilms' tumours: a report from the SIOP Wilms' tumour trials and studies. *Radiother Oncol* 1986;5:175–182.

90. Farber S. Chemotherapy in the treatment of leukemia and Wilms' tumor. *JAMA* 1966;138:826–836.

91. Hughes E, Klavell L, Cassady JR, et al. Wilms' tumor treated by surgery without chemotherapy. *Proc Am Soc Clin Oncol* 1985;4:241.

92. Weeks DA, Beckwith JB, Luckey DW. Relapse-associated variables in stage I favorable histology Wilms' tumor: a report of the National Wilms' Tumor Study. *Cancer* 1987;60:1202–1204.

93. Gross RE, Neuhauser EBD. Treatment of mixed tumors of the kidney in childhood. *Pediatrics* 1950;6:843–852.

94. Tobin RL, Fantanesi J, Kun LE, et al. Wilms' tumor: reduced-dose radiotherapy in advanced-stage Wilms' tumor with favorable histology. *Int J Radiat Oncol Biol Phys* 1990;19:867–871.

95. Thomas PR, Tefft M, D'Angio GJ, et al. Validation of radiation dose reductions used in the Third National Wilms' Tumor Study. *Proc Am Soc Clin Oncol* 1988;29:227.

96. Wilimas JA, Douglass EC, Lewis S, et al. Reduced therapy for Wilms' tumor: analysis of treatment results from a single institution. *J Clin Oncol* 1988;6:1630–1635.

97. Kalapurakal JA, Li AM, Breslow NE, et al. Influence of radiation therapy delay on abdominal tumor recurrence in patients with favorable histology Wilms' tumor treated on NWTS-3 and NWTS-4: a report from the National Wilms' Tumor Study Group. *Int J Radiat Oncol Biol Phys* 2003;57:495–499.

98. Pediatric Oncology Group. POG 9440/CCG 4941. *National Wilms' Tumor Study 5: therapeutic trial and biology study.* Chicago, IL, August 16, 1995.

99. Paulino AC. Relapsed Wilms tumor: is there a role for radiation therapy? *Am J Clin Oncol* 2001;24:408–413.

100. Jeal P, Jenkins RDT. Abdominal irradiation in the treatment of Wilms' tumor. *Int J Radiat Oncol Biol Phys* 1980;6:655–661.

101. Donaldson SS, Moskowitz PS, Canty EL, et al. Combination radiation–adriamycin therapy: renoprival growth, functional and structural effects in the immature mouse. *Int J Radiat Oncol Biol Phys* 1980;6:851–859.

102. D'Angio GJ. Results of the Third National Wilms' Tumor Study: a preliminary report. *AACR* 1984;723(abst).

103. Duckett CP, Zderic S, Goldwein J, et al. Brachytherapy for residual intra-renal Wilms' tumor. *Med Pediatr Oncol* 1997;28:316–320.

104. Thoms WW Jr, Goldwein JW, D'Angio G. A technique for the use of afterloading [137]brachytherapy in renal-sparing irradiation of bilateral Wilms' tumor. *Int J Radiat Oncol Biol Phys* 997;39:1121–1124.

105. Longaker MT, Harrison MR, Adzick NS, et al. Nephron-sparing approach to bilateral Wilms' tumor: *in situ* or *ex vivo* surgery and radiation therapy. *J Pediatr Surg* 1990;25:411–414.

106. Malcolm AW, Jaffe N, Folkman MJ, et al. Bilateral Wilms' tumor. *Int J Radiat Oncol Biol Phys* 1980;6: 167–174.

107. Laberge JM, Nguyen LT, Homsy YL, et al. Bilateral Wilms' tumors: changing concepts in management. *J Pediatr Surg* 1987;22:730–735.

108. Ritchey ML, Coppes MJ. The management of synchronous bilateral Wilms tumor. *Hematol Oncol Clin North Am* 1995;9:1303–1315.

109. Ritchey ML, Kelalis PP, Haase GM, et al. Preoperative therapy for intracaval and atrial extension of Wilms' tumor. *Cancer* 1993;71:4104–4110.

110. Jereb B, Issac R, Tournade MF, et al. Survival of patients with metastases from Wilms' tumor (SIOP 1, SIOP 2, SIOP 5). *Eur Paediatr Haematol Oncol* 1985;2:71–76.

111. Bishop HC, Tefft M, Evans AE, et al. Survival in bilateral Wilms' tumor: review of 30 national Wilms' tumor study cases. *J Pediatr Surv* 1977;12: 631–638.

112. Sutow WW, Breslow NE, Palmer NF, et al. Prognosis in children with Wilms' tumor metastases prior to or following primary treatment: results from the First National Wilms' Tumor Study (NWTS-1). *Am J Clin Oncol* 1982;5:339–347.

113. Green D, Fernbach D, Narkool P, et al. The treatment of Wilms' tumor patients with pulmonary metastases detected only with computerized tomography. A report from the National Wilms' Tumor Study. *Proc ASCO* 1991;10:309.

114. Green DM, Finkelstein JZ, Tefft ME, et al. Diffuse interstitial pneumonitis after pulmonary irradiation for metastatic Wilms' tumor: a report from the National Wilms' Tumor Study. *Cancer* 1989;63:450–453.

115. Miser JS, Tournade MF. The management of relapsed Wilms tumor. *Hematol Oncol Clin North Am* 1995;9: 1287–1302.

116. Thoms WW Jr, Vega R, Abramowsky C, et al. Multimodal management of recurrent Wilms' tumor: the role of radiation therapy. *Med Pediatr Oncol* 1996; 27:179–184.

117. Green DM, Narkool P, Breslow NE, et al. Severe hepatic toxicity after treatment with vincristine and dactinomycin using single-dose or divided-dose schedules: a report from the National Wilms' Tumor Study. *J Clin Oncol* 1990;8:1525–1530.

118. Groot-Loonen JJ, Pinkerton CR, Morris-Jones PH, et al. How curable is relapsed Wilms' tumor? *Arch Dis Child* 1990;65:968–970.

119. Grundy P, Breslow NE, Green DM, et al. Prognostic factors for children with recurrent Wilms' tumor: results from the second and third Wilms' tumor study. *J Clin Oncol* 1989;7:638–647.

120. Pinkerson CR, Groot-Loonen JJ, Morris-Jones PH, et al. Response rates in relapsed Wilms' tumor: a need for new effective agents. *Cancer* 1991;67:567–571.

121. Larsen E, Griffin GC, Grundy P, et al. *Phase II upfront therapy for recurrent Wilms' tumor.* Concept sheet. St Louis, MO: Pediatric Oncology Group, 1991.

122. Ritchey ML, Kelalis PP, Etzioni R, et al. Small bowel obstruction after nephrectomy for Wilms' tumor: a report of the National Wilms' Tumor Study 3. *Ann Surg* 1993;218:654–659.

123. Pritchard J, Imeson J, Cotterill S, et al. Results of the United Kingdom Children's Cancer Study Group first Wilms' tumor study. *J Clin Oncol* 1995;13:124–133.

*124. Egeler RM, Wolff JE, Anderson RA, et al. Long-term complications and post-treatment follow-up of patients with Wilms' tumor. *Semin Urol Oncol* 1999;17:55–61.

125. Plowman PN. Hepatotoxicity in irradiated nephroblastoma patients. *Radiother Oncol* 1994;31:191.

126. Rate WR, Butler MS, Roibertson WW Jr, et al. Late orthopedic effects in children with Wilms' tumor treated with abdominal irradiation. *Med Pediatr Oncol* 1991;19:265–268.

127. Westerinki HP, Alberts AS. Letter to the editor. *Med Pediatr Oncol* 1992;21:382.

128. Makipernaa A, Heikkila JT, Merikanto J, et al. Spinal deformity induced by radiotherapy for solid tumours of childhood: a long-term follow up study. *Eur J Pediatr* 1993;152:197–200.

129. Wallace WHB, Shalet SM, Morris-Jones PH, et al. Effect of abdominal irradiation on growth in boys treated for a Wilms' tumor. *Med Pediatr Oncol* 1990; 18:441–446.

130. De Graaf SSN, van Gent H, Reitsma-Bierens WCC, et al. Renal function after unilateral nephrectomy for Wilms' tumour: the influence of radiation therapy. *Eur J Cancer* 1996;32A:465–469.

131. Green DM, Peabody EM, Nan B, et al. Pregnancy outcome after treatment for Wilms tumor: a report from the National Wilms' Tumor Study Group. *J Clin Oncol* 2002;20:2506–2513.

132. Paulino AC, Wen B, Brown CK, et al. Late effects in children treated with radiation therapy for Wilms' tumor. *Int J Radiat Oncol Biol Phys* 2000;46:1239–1246.

133. Breslow NE, Norkool PA, Olshan A, et al. Second malignant neoplasms in survivors of Wilms' tumor: a report from the National Wilms' Tumor Study. *J Natl Cancer Inst* 1988;80:592–595.

134. Kovalic JJ, Thomas PRM, Beckwith JB, et al. Hepatocellular carcinoma as second malignant neoplasms in successfully treated Wilms' tumor patients: a National Wilms' Tumor Study report. *Cancer* 1991;67: 342–344.

135. Breslow NE, Takashima JR, Whitton JA, et al. Second malignant neoplasms following treatment for Wilms' tumor: a report from the National Wilms' Tumor Study Group. *J Clin Oncol* 1995;13:1851–1859.

136. Shearer P, Kapoor G, Beckwith JB, et al. Secondary acute myelogenous leukemia in patients previously treated for childhood renal tumors: a report from the National Wilms' Tumor Study Group. *J Pediatr Hematol Oncol* 2001;23:109–111.

*137. Davies-Johns T, Chidel M, Marcklis RM. The role of radiation therapy in the management of Wilms' tumor. *Semin Urol Oncol* 1999;17:46–54.

138. Tournade MF, Com-Nougue C, Coute PA, et al. Results of the Sixth International Society of Pediatric

Oncology Wilms' Tumor Trial and Study: a risk-adapted therapeutic approach in Wilms' tumor. *J Clin Oncol* 1993;11:1014–1023.

139. Godzinski J, Weirich A, Tournade MF, et al. Primary nephrectomy for emergency: a rare event in the International Society of Paediatric Oncology Nephroblastoma Trial and Study no. 9. *Eur J Pediatr Surg* 2001; 11:36–39.

140. Weirich A, Leuschner I, Harms D, et al. Clinical impact of histologic subtypes in localized non-anaplastic nephroblastoma treated according to the trial and study SIOP-9/GPOH. *Ann Oncol* 2001;12:311–319.

141. Trobs RB, Hansel M, Friedrich T, et al. A 23-year experience with malignant renal tumors in infancy and childhood. *Eur J Pediatr Surg* 2001;11:92–98.

142. Suryanarayan K, Marina N. Wilms' tumour. Optimal treatment strategies. *Drugs* 1998;56:598–605.

143. SIOP Web page: http://www.siop.nl.

*144. Ludin A, Macklis RM. Radiotherapy for pediatric genitourinary tumors. *Urol Clin North Am* 2000;27: 553–563.

145. Clinical Trials Web site: http://www.clinicaltrials.gov.

146. Tournade MF, Com-Nougue C, de Kraker J, et al. Optimal duration of preoperative therapy in unilateral and nonmetastatic Wilms' tumor in children older than 6 months: results of the ninth International Society of Pediatric Oncology Wilms' tumor trial and study. *J Clin Oncol* 2001;19:488–500.

147. Hogeboom CJ, Grosser SC, Guthrie KA, et al. Stature loss following treatment for Wilms tumor. *Med Pediatr Oncol* 2001;36:295–304.

148. Vujanic GM, Sandstedt B, Harms D, et al. Revised International Society of Paediatric Oncology (SIOP) working classification of renal tumors of childhood. *Med Pediatr Oncol* 2002;38:79–82.

14

Hepatoblastoma and Hepatocellular Carcinoma

Edward C. Halperin, M.D.

Childhood primary malignant liver tumors (PMLTs) constitute 0.5–2% of pediatric cancer in Europe and the United States. They are more common in Japan, southeast Asia, and sub-Saharan Africa (1,2). A cure is highly dependent on the physician's ability to achieve a surgical extirpation of the tumor. Chemotherapy supports surgery in curative treatment.

CLINICAL PRESENTATION, STAGING, AND WORKUP

Children with PMLTs present with an abdominal mass or generalized abdominal enlargement. The child may have pain localized to the right upper quadrant, fever, anorexia, weight loss, jaundice, or vomiting. The first presentation may, on occasion, be an acute abdominal crisis caused by tumor rupture and hemoperitoneum. Paraneoplastic syndromes have been associated with PMLTs (3). Anemia and thrombocytosis often occur. This is probably related to the ability of hepatoblastoma (HBL) cells to secrete interleukin-1B (IL-1B), which induces IL-6 production in fibroblasts of endothelial cells (4).

HBL is the most common PMLT occurring in the first 20 years of life and accounts for 1% of all pediatric malignancies and about 43–51% of PMLTs in the pediatric age group (3,5,6). The annual incidence is 0.5 to 1.5 diagnoses per million children less than 15 years old in western countries (4). The median age at diagnosis is 1 to 2 years. Most diagnoses are made in children younger than 3 years old. As with all PMLTs, there is a male predominance (2.3, 7–10). HBL has been reported to be associated with a host of other conditions, including Beckwith–Wiedemann syndrome, Wilms' tumor, adrenal cortical tumors, fetal alcohol syndrome, familial adenomatous polyposis, prematurity, low birthweight, precocious puberty in boys caused by human chorionic gonadotropin secretion, and thrombocytosis (6,7,11–15). The cell of origin is thought to be a pluripotent hepatic stem cell.

HBL may be histologically subclassified into six patterns (Table 14-1). Conventional HBLs contain fetal hepatoblasts, embryonal hepatoblasts, or a mixture of the two cell types (Fig. 14-1). Fetal-type hepatoblasts recapitulate the cytoarchitecture of the normal human fetal liver. Cells of the early fetal liver and the cells of fetal HBL are of similar size and configuration. Both proliferate as cuboidal cells with trabeculae one to two cells thick. Both display strong positivity for α-fetoprotein (AFP). Both tissues also display sinusoidal hematopoiesis and a lack of intrahepatic bile ducts (16). Fetal cells are slightly smaller than normal hepatocytes and have a low nuclear-to-cytoplasm ratio. In contrast, embryonal hepatoblasts have a higher nuclear-to-cytoplasm ratio than do fetal cells, and they also have a compact basophilic cytoplasm. This gives a light-microscopic impression of a higher cell density (2,8,17–19). Small-cell undifferentiated or anaplastic HBL contains sheets and nests of medium-sized cells, with little or no evidence of hepatoblastic differentiation. There is scant cytoplasm and a high mitotic rate. Mixed epithelial and mesenchymal HBL is composed of typical areas of fetal epithelial and embryonal type cells mixed with primitive mesenchyme and various mesenchymally derived tissue (Fig. 14-2) (16).

It is debatable whether the recognized histologic subtypes are clearly related to prognosis. The subtypes can occur together in varying amounts, and present definitions do not take this

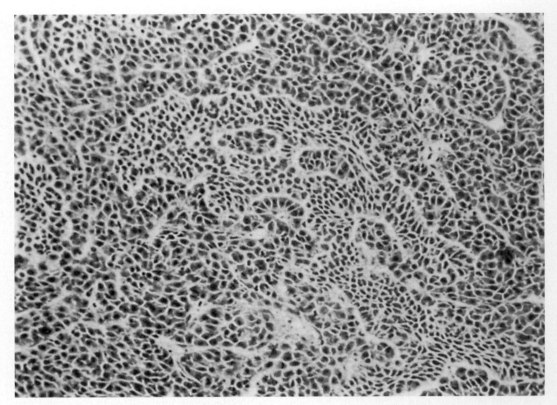

FIG. 14-1. Hepatoblastoma. In this example of a mixed cellular pattern the elongated tumor cells are between nodules of darker-staining larger cells resembling fetal hepatocytes (hematoxylin and eosin; ×365). (From Stringer MD, Hennaye ER, Hoowlad ER, et al. Improved outcome for children with hepatoblastoma. *Br J Surg* 1995;82:336–391, with permission.)

TABLE 14-1. *Histologic classification of hepatoblastoma*

Epithelial type (56%)	Mixed epithelial and mesenchymal type (44%)
Fetal pattern (31%)	Without teratoid features (34%)
Embryonal and fetal pattern (19%)	With treated features (10%)
Macrotrabecular pattern (3%)	
Small-cell undifferentiated pattern (3%)	

Modified from Perilango G, Dall'Igna P, Sainati L. Modern treatment of childhood hepatoblastoma: what do clinicians and pathologists have to say to each other? *Med Pediatr Oncol* 2002;39:474–477, with permission.

into account (20). Some investigators report that in long-term survivors of HBL the most common histology is the conventional type, with a predominantly fetal cell pattern (7). However, there is no uniformly accepted definition of "predominantly" or "pure" fetal histology (21). Although conventional epithelial tumors constitute 60% of all HBLs, they represent 85% of HBLs in children who have undergone complete tumor resection and who are long-term survivors (2,17). Almost no children with anaplastic HBL survive the disease. A Pediatric Oncology Group (POG)–Children's Cancer Study Group (CCSG) trial showed the distinction between fetal HBL and other histologic subtypes to be of prognostic importance in stage I disease (3-year progression-free survival of 79% vs. 56%, $p = 0.11$) (22). However, not all investiga-

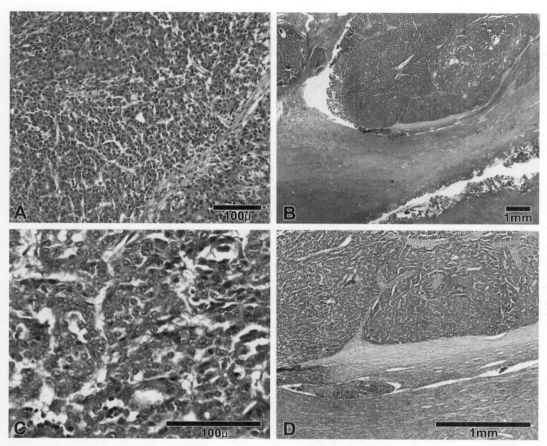

FIG. 14-2. This 10-month-old girl was found to have a right upper quadrant mass. A tumor was resected from the right lobe of the liver. The microscopic sections showed mixed epithelial–mesenchymal hepatoblastoma. The tumor was keratin positive, carcinoembryonic antigen (CEA) positive, and vimentin negative.

tors have confirmed the prognostic importance of histologic subtyping in all stages (8). For example, in a large analysis the Japanese Study Group for Pediatric Liver Tumor found no significant influence of HBL histologic classification on outcome (23).

Hepatocellular carcinoma (HCC), the second most common PMLT in children, accounts for about one-fourth to one-third of pediatric hepatic malignancies (3). HCC is unusual in children younger than 5 years of age (Fig. 14-3). The median age of presentation for pediatric HCC is 10 to 12 years (3,9,10,18). Approximately 25% of cases in children are associated with cirrhosis (7). Causes of this cirrhosis include biliary atresia, Fanconi's anemia, glucose-

6-phosphatase deficiency, and hereditary tyrosinemia. HCC has also been reported in association with hemihypertrophy, anomalies of the abdominal venous drainage system, and the use of oral contraceptives. The tumor occurs in areas with a high prevalence of hepatitis B viral infection (5,24). Hepatitis B carrier status varies by geographic area. Molecular hybridization studies have shown that viral DNA is integrated into the DNA of cellular lines derived from human HCC and into morphologically nonmalignant adjacent liver cells (3).

There is a fibrolamellar (FL) histologic variant of HCC, which occurs in the noncirrhotic livers of older children. This variant is characterized by large polygonal neoplastic hepato-

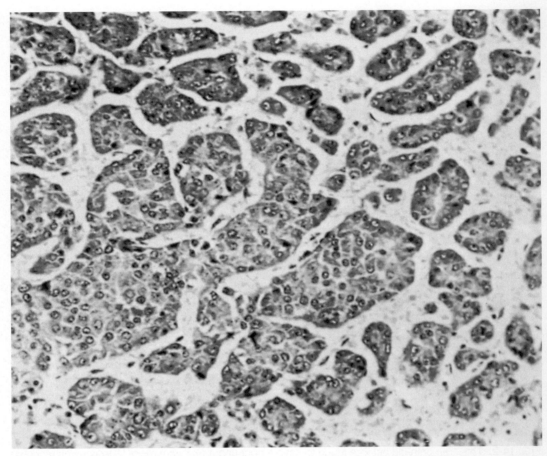

FIG. 14-3. Hepatocellular carcinoma: large cells with abundant cytoplasm in a trabecular configuration (hematoxylin and eosin; ×100). (From Stringer MD, Hennaye ER, Hoowlad ER, et al. Improved outcome for children with hepatoblastoma. *Br J Surg* 1995;82:336–391, with permission.)

cytes and lamellar bundles of collagen. Although patient numbers are small, some think that this tumor is associated with a higher frequency of resectability and a good probability of cure. However, others have failed to demonstrate a favorable effect of the FL variant in children (8,10,11,25,26).

Together, HBLs and HCCs constitute 75–90% of PMLTs of childhood. The remainder include malignant mesenchymoma, undifferentiated embryonal sarcoma, primary hepatic malignant tumor with rhabdoid features, leiomyosarcoma, angiosarcoma, biliary rhabdomyosarcoma (see Chapter 11), hepatic sinusoid tumor simulating neuroblastoma, carcinoid, and primary hepatic and hepatosplenic non-Hodgkin's lymphoma.

Benign tumors account for approximately one-third of all liver tumors of childhood. The benign tumors may be classified by their cell of origin as either mesenchymal (hemangioma, hemangioendothelioma, and hematoma) or epithelial (cysts, focal nodular hyperplasia, and adenoma) (Fig. 14-4).

If a hepatic or biliary tumor produces biliary obstruction, there may be elevations of serum hepatic enzymes or bilirubin (27,28). During the imaging evaluation, an excretory urogram may be performed. This will help to determine that the mass is not of renal origin and that it lies in the peritoneal cavity. An ultrasound examination helps to establish the presence of a hepatic mass and differentiates cystic from

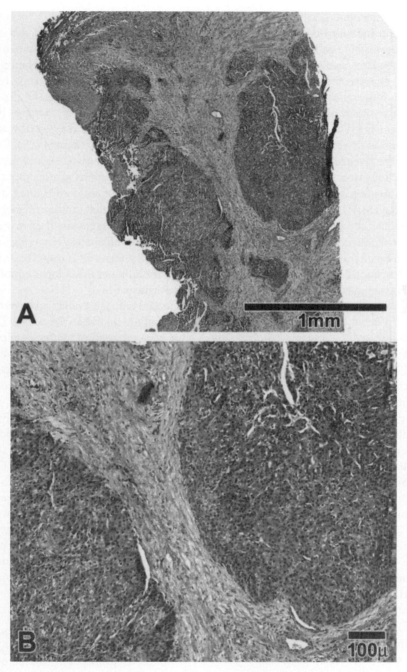

FIG. 14-4. A hepatic mass was identified in a 19-month-old boy. A core biopsy of the tumor showed cells with round nuclei and small, single nucleoli. The tumor was composed of epithelial component. The diagnosis was epithelial hepatoblastoma.

solid lesions. Ultrasound permits evaluation of the adrenals and the kidneys, helps to exclude these organs as possible primary sites of tumor metastatic to the liver, and allows evaluation of the inferior vena cava for tumor thrombus. Color Doppler ultrasound may be performed to demonstrate the relationship of the tumor to hepatic vessels (29). The technetium-90m sulfur colloid scan is of some value in localizing the tumor to the liver and defining its boundaries. It is a sensitive test, but not specific. Computed tomography (CT) and magnetic resonance imaging (MRI) provide superior delineation of the mass and show evidence of multifocality. On nonenhanced CT, epithelial HBL is a homogeneous hypodense mass. The mixed type is heterogenous. Calcifications can be present. Contrast enhancement of the periphery or septa may be seen. On MRI, the epithelial type is homogeneous and hypointense on T1 and hyperintense on T2. The mixed type may be more heterogeneous and hypointense on T1 and T2, and hemorrhage will show high signal intensity on T1 and T2. On CT, HCC will show solitary or multiple masses. Calcification can occur. The tumor rim may enhance with contrast. On MRI the T1 images may be isointense or hyperintense. On T2 images a mosaic pattern (caused by necrosis, hemorrhage, septa, and fatty metaplasia) is common (9). The operating surgeon may request an angiogram to obtain information about the origin and distribution of the right and left hepatic arteries to allow an informed decision about resectability (3). Routine chest radiographs and thoracic CT scans are necessary because 10–20% of patients with HBL and 30% of patients with HCC have lung metastasis at the time of diagnosis (4,15,30–32).

A valuable test in evaluating PMLT is the serum AFP. The clinician should note that AFP, synthesized by the fetal liver, may be detected in pregnant women. AFP levels are high in the normal newborn infant but drop rapidly by 1 month of age. AFP should be barely detectable by 2 years of age (15). Approximately two-thirds of children with HBL and HCC have an elevated AFP (28). However, the clinician should be cautioned that AFP is not always elevated in HBL or HCC and that this protein may be slightly elevated in benign hamartomas. Absence of AFP elevation may be a poor prognostic sign in HBL; it is associated with the small cell (anaplastic) histologic type and responds poorly to therapy. For patients with elevated AFP, it may be of value in monitoring the course of therapy (29). Complete resection of HBL or HCC should result in a normal AFP by 2 months postoperatively (13). No change in an elevated AFP after surgery indicates either residual tumor or regenerating normal liver. The diagnosis of growing tumor depends on confirmatory imaging studies. An elevation in the AFP during the follow-up period generally heralds a local tumor recurrence or metastasis (28).

Limited data are available concerning genetic abnormalities in HBL. Trisomies 2, 8, and 20 have been reported in tumor samples as well as t(1;4)(q12;34). Mutations of the B-catenin gene have been described (20). Loss of heterozygosity of 11p15 is seen in about one-third of cases (4).

There are two major staging systems for PMLT. All are based on resectability and, to a lesser extent, microscopic residual tumor (4,33,34). The staging systems are shown in Tables 14-2 and 14-3 and Fig. 14-5. The clinician must be wary of the pitfalls in the extant staging systems. There are at least two important drawbacks of some of the systems shown. First, the systems are applied at initial diagnosis. If upfront chemotherapy is given and if it produces a substantive tumor response before delayed surgery, then the initial stage may no longer be per-

TABLE 14-2. *Children's Cancer Study Group and Pediatric Oncology Group staging system for primary malignant liver tumors, now generally used*

Stage	Description
I	Complete resection of the tumor
II	Microscopic residual disease
III	Macroscopic residual tumor
IV	Distant metastatic tumor

From references 3, 4, 29, and 44.

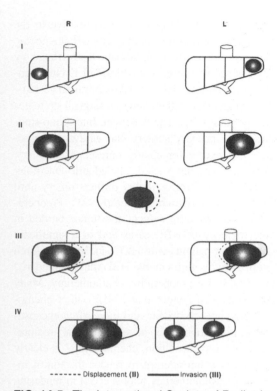

R   L

I

II

III

IV

------- Displacement (II)   ———— Invasion (III)

FIG. 14-5. The International Society of Pediatric Oncology Liver Tumor Study Group Pretreatment Extent of Disease (PRETEXT) grouping system divides the liver into four parts, called sectors. The left lobe of the liver *(L)* is divided into a lateral sector (segments 2 and 3) and a medial sector (segment 4), whereas the right lobe *(R)* is divided into an anterior sector (segments 5 and 8) and a posterior sector (segments 6 and 7). Tumors are classified into one of the four PRETEXT categories, depending on the number of liver sectors affected by the tumor. PRETEXT I, one sector involved; PRETEXT II, two sectors involved, PRETEXT III, two nonadjoining sectors free or three sectors involved; and PRETEXT IV, all four sectors involved. Extrahepatic growth is indicated by adding one or more of the following characters: V, hepatic/caval vein; P, portal vein; E, extrahepatic extension; and M, distant metastases. (From Schnater JM, Aronson DC, Plaschkes J, et al. Surgical view of the treatment of patients with hepatoblastoma: results from the first prospective trial of the International Society of Pediatric Oncology Liver Tumor Study Group (SIOPEL-1). *Cancer* 2002;94: 1111–1120, with permission.)

TABLE 14-3. *TNM staging system*

Primary tumor (T)	
TX	Primary tumor cannot be assessed
T0	No evidence of primary tumor
T1	Solitary tumor without vascular invasion
T2	Solitary tumor with vascular invasion or multiple tumors ≥5 cm
T3	Multiple tumors >5 cm or tumor involving a major branch of the portal or hepatic veins
T4	Tumors with direct invasion of adjacent organs other than the gallbladder or with perforation of visceral peritoneum

Regional lymph nodes (N)	
NX	Regional lymph nodes cannot be assessed
N0	No regional lymph node metastasis
N1	Regional lymph node metastasis

Distant metastasis (M)	
MX	Distant metastasis cannot be assessed
M0	No distant metastasis
M1	Distant metastasis

Stage grouping			
Stage I	T1	N0	M0
Stage II	T2	N0	M0
Stage IIIA	T3	N0	M0
Stage IIIB	T4	N0	M0
Stage IIIC	Any T	N1	M0
Stage IV	Any T	Any N	M1

From Greene FL, Page DL, Fleming, ID, et al., eds. *AJCC cancer staging manual,* 6th ed. New York: Springer-Verlag, 2002, with permission.

tinent. Second, a surgeon's determination of resectability is somewhat subjective and differs among practitioners (35).

In the German HBL Study HB89-94, the following six factors predicted poor prognosis:

- Metastatic disease
- Initial AFP greater than 1×10^6 ng/mL
- Extrahepatic and intrahepatic vascular invasion

- Multifocal disease and involvement of both liver lobes
- Stage (tumor, node, metastasis [TNM])
- Poor epithelial differentiation

In the International Society of Pediatric Oncology Liver Tumor Study Group 1 (SIOPEL-1) study, only metastatic disease and involvement of all four sections of the liver predicted poor outcome (20,36,37).

SELECTION OF THERAPY

Surgery

Localized HBL or HCC is curable with complete surgical excision of the tumor. It is also possible to achieve a cure with a near-complete excision in conjunction with adjuvant therapy that is able to sterilize residual tumor. Tumor resectability is determined by tumor size, the existence of bilobar involvement necessitating more than three liver segments for hepatic resection, vascular invasion, or distant metastases (38).

Some surgeons believe that therapy begins with an attempt at resection rather than biopsy. One-half to two-thirds of patients with HBL have resectable tumors at presentation (39). After chemotherapy the probability of resection rises to about 90%. Only 30–50% of the cases of HCC are amenable to complete resection at presentation because of multilobar involvement or massive tumor size.

Many cases are managed with preoperative chemotherapy. Therefore, the surgeon must first deal with the question of whether to perform a biopsy before chemotherapy is administered in order to histologically confirm the presence of PMLT or accept the diagnosis based on a characteristic clinical presentation, supportive diagnostic imaging, thrombocytosis, and an elevated AFP (2). When chemotherapy is initiated without a histologic diagnosis, there is about a 4% risk that the patient will not have HBL or HCC. Errors in diagnosis include hemangioendothelioma, angiosarcoma, neuroblastoma, and germ cell tumor (21). Most clinicians prefer to have a histologic diagnosis. The classic way to obtain tissue is via an open-wedge biopsy. Some controversy exists over the use of CT or ultrasound-directed needle biopsy as an alternative to the wedge biopsy. Some are concerned that a needle biopsy will cause a significant hemorrhage by disruption of a highly friable PMLT. Other authorities believe that the risk is minimal (2,12).

Broadly stated, there are two surgical strategies for treating HBL. The American Intergroup studies favor primary surgery and adjuvant chemotherapy, except for clearly unresectable tumors. The International Society of Pediatric Oncology (SIOP), after biopsy, defers further surgery until after preoperative chemotherapy (21). Preoperative chemotherapy reduces the tumor burden in the majority of HBL cases and in a significant number of patients with HCC (1). Many children with initially unresectable HBL may be rendered resectable by preoperative chemotherapy. Many surgeons also believe that PMLTs, after chemotherapy, are less friable and more often encapsulated. For patients who have tumors that are unresectable at presentation, chemotherapy is clearly indicated in an attempt to render the tumor resectable. Radiotherapy may succeed in rendering an unresectable tumor resectable if this goal is not achieved by chemotherapy (1).

When the patient comes to definitive surgery, an extensive incision allowing a large area of exposure often is performed (40). A simple tumorectomy with adequate margins is rarely possible. Rather, hepatic lobectomy or extended lobectomy is needed. Perioperative mortality was reported to be as high as 18–33% (7,30,41) in the past but is now on the order of 5–10% in specialized centers (42). Surgical complications include severe bleeding, bile leakage, pleural effusion, rupture of the inferior vena cava, cardiac arrest, convulsions, and subhepatic abscess (35). Improved surgical techniques such as vascular reconstruction, ultrasonic aspiration, and dissection under vascular exclusion and improvements in anesthesia, blood product replacement, and postoperative intensive care have produced the significant reduction in operative and perioperative mortality (1).

In stage IV disease surgical resection of pulmonary metastases can be considered if they persist after preoperative chemotherapy and if the primary tumor has been rendered resectable by drug treatment (42). In patients with stage I disease at initial diagnosis that recurs with isolated pulmonary disease, surgical resection may result in extended survival. Feusner et al. (43) reported six patients with pulmonary relapses of stage I HBL. Three had concurrent relapses in brain, bone, or abdomen and died of metastatic disease. Three of the six, having recurrence only in the lung, were long-term survivors (less than 5 years) after metastasectomy and chemotherapy. Fuchs et al. (36) also reported good results with aggressive excision of pulmonary metastases.

Because it is difficult to resect some PMLTs, there has been interest in the use of total hepatectomy and liver transplantation (28,44). Tagge et al. (45) reported 18 children who underwent laparotomy for a possible hepatectomy and liver transplantation for HBL or HCC. Thirteen were transplanted. Five of the six transplanted patients with HBL are survivors (83%) and three of the seven patients with HCC are survivors (44%). Superina and Billik (46) from the Hospital for Sick Children, Toronto, selected patients suitable for transplant based on absence of lymph node disease and tumor confined to the liver without breech of the capsule. Of three transplanted patients with HBL, two are alive at 2 and 2.5 years. Of five patients with HCC, three are alive at 1, 3, and 5 years of follow-up; for two patients the follow-up is short. Srinivasan et al. (47) from Saudi Arabia recently reported 13 children transplanted for advanced HBL. Of the 12 patients electively transplanted, 11 are alive without evidence of tumor, and 1 has pulmonary metastases (mean follow-up 33 months). One child emergently transplanted died after transplant. In an analysis of 291 liver transplants performed in 265 children from 1984 to 1999 at Baylor University, eight patients were transplanted for HBL (3%). Five are long-term survivors (48). In children who undergo liver transplantation primarily for end-stage nonneoplastic liver disease but who have an incidental PMLT identified, survival is quite good. A living related donor procedure is a new option for some patients.

The therapy of multifocal tumor is one the perplexing clinical problems in the surgical management of HBL. If disease is present diffusely in the liver, and if there is a substantial tumor response to chemotherapy, can one reasonably attempt a partial liver resection? Must one assume microscopic residual tumor is present and perform a hepatectomy and liver transplantation? The answers are unclear (49).

Radiation Therapy

Radiation therapy has been used preoperatively and postoperatively in the curative treatment of HBL and HCC. Its preoperative use has been intended to reduce the tumor burden and increase the probability of resection. Contemporary practice favors using chemotherapy alone for preoperative therapy (7,13,27,33). In children who have unresectable tumors after initial chemotherapy, radiotherapy is warranted (1,11,50). POG 8697, described in the chemotherapy section of this chapter, included five patients treated with radiotherapy because they remained unresectable after chemotherapy. Three became resectable (44,51).

Some evidence exists that postoperative radiotherapy is valuable in children who have residual disease after an attempt at resection. A combined CCSG–POG protocol studied 177 children with HBL or HCC. Patients with microscopic residual disease (stage II) received postoperative chemotherapy and 45 Gy to the tumor bed. Those unable to undergo complete excision after preoperative chemotherapy received 30 Gy whole liver irradiation. The 3-year progression-free survival was 60% for stage II and 22% for stage III (22). The Institut Gustave–Roussy administered preoperative chemotherapy, performed surgical resection, and then gave radiotherapy and additional chemotherapy if there was microscopic or macroscopic persistent tumor at surgery. A dosage of 25 to 45 Gy was given targeted to the area of postoperative disease only. Seven of nine children are disease free at 22 to 98 months of follow-up. One died with a local failure, and one died with a local plus distant failure (1). Habrand et al. (1) described eight cases treated after incomplete resection (four with gross and four with microscopic disease) with combined radiation and chemotherapy. Six are free of disease at 4 to 83 months of follow-up (13). The evidence in favor of the use of irradiation for residual disease is not unequivocal, and we cannot prove that chemotherapy by itself would have failed to control persistent microscopic disease. No dogmatic policy may be adopted based on current evidence (7,12,13).

There is large body of clinical experience concerning the irradiation of adults with unresectable HCC. By definition, these patients have large tumors. Many are also treated with chemotherapy and transcatheter arterial chemoembolization. Three-dimensionally planned radiotherapy or intensity-modulated radiation therapy (IMRT) is used. The initial response rate is generally good (about 60%), but long-term survival is rare (52).

Is whole lung irradiation (WLI) appropriate in metastatic HBL? Data on the subject are sparse. Patients with metastatic disease to the lung only can be cured with surgical resection of the metastatic deposits plus chemotherapy. However, there is a risk of subsequent pulmonary relapse (43). This may be used as an argument in favor of WLI to treat presumed small deposits of well-oxygenated metastatic disease. Reasoning from Wilms' tumor, Ewing's, or osteosarcoma data, for example, a total dosage of 12 to 13 Gy would be sound.

Chemotherapy

Chemotherapy has been used preoperatively in an attempt to improve the probability of resection of HCC and HBL. It has also been used postoperatively, either as adjuvant therapy when there is no apparent residual disease or to treat obvious residual disease. In the presence of metastatic disease, chemotherapy has been used in attempts to prolong survival (7,13,14,53).

Children's Cancer Group (CCG) Trial 831, opened to patient accrual in 1972, gave no adjuvant chemotherapy to patients with stage I disease. Patients with residual tumor in one hepatic lobe received actinomycin D, vincristine, and cyclophosphamide plus involved-field irradiation. Patients with disseminated tumors received only chemotherapy. No patients responded to drug alone. Of 40 patients entered on the study, the only seven long-term survivors were children with stage I disease or with minor residual tumor who had been irradiated (54).

CCG Trial 881 added doxorubicin and 5-fluorouracil to the three drugs used in Trial 831.

Twelve (44%) of 27 patients with measurable disease achieved a response with a median duration of 18 months. Adjuvant chemotherapy was given to 24 patients who did not have measurable disease after surgery. Of these, 83% were disease-free survivors with median follow-up of 30 months (54).

CCG Trial 823F used doxorubicin and cisplatin for four courses after histologic diagnosis but before definitive surgery for disease confined to the liver. Thirty-three children with HBL and 14 with HCC were entered in the study. Of the 26 patients with HBL who completed the prescribed four courses of chemotherapy, 25 achieved a response and were eligible for second-look surgery, 22 were taken to the operating room, and 16 had complete resections. There was no viable tumor in nine of these patients. Of these 16 children, 15 are alive without evidence of disease. Of the 25 children who completed the chemotherapy and were eligible for surgery, 19 (78%) are alive and disease free. The estimated 2-year survival for the initial 33 patients with HBL is 67%. Of the 14 patients with HCC, 12 died of progressive disease, and two remain free of disease. Only 14% of the HCC patients had complete removal of the tumor at second-look laparotomy (54).

The Pediatric Intergroup Hepatoma Study (CCG-8881 and POG 8945) enrolled 173 patients with HBL. Ninety-one patients were randomized to receive cisplatin, vincristine, and 5-fluorouracil, and 82 were randomized to receive cisplatin and doxorubicin. The later program was more toxic; patients had a higher probability of neutropenia, thrombocytopenia, need for parenteral nutrition, and toxic deaths. As shown in Table 14-4, the chemotherapy programs were equally effective in terms of overall and event-free survival (EFS; $p = 0.219$). The results for stage I to III HBL were reasonably good. Patients with more advanced disease did poorly (55,56). For patients with HCC there was also no difference between the two programs for either EFS ($p = 0.88$) or overall survival (OS; $p = 0.68$). All seven stage I patients were event-free survivors (57). Clearly, better therapy is needed for advanced-stage HCC.

Stringer et al. (58) reported 40 children with HBL, treated with the intent to cure, from the

TABLE 14-4. *Results of the Pediatric Intergroup Hepatoma Study (CCG-8881 and POG 8945)*

Stage of hepatoblastoma	Cisplatin, vincristine, 5-fluorouracil			Cisplatin, doxorubicin		
	n	Survival	Event-free survival	*n*	Survival	Event-free survival
I	22	95%	85%	20	95%	95%
II	4	100%	100%	3	100%	100%
III	43	70%	62%	39	65%	61%
IV	23	45%	23%	19	36%	33%

From Ortega JA, Douglas E, Feusner J, et al. Randomized comparison of cisplatin/vincristine/5-fluorouracil and cisplatin/continuous infusion/doxorubicin. Continuous infusion for treatment of pediatric hepatoblastoma: a report from the Children's Cancer Group and Pediatric Oncology Group. *J Clin Oncol* 2000;18:2665–2675, with permission.

Hospital for Sick Children, London. Two received surgery only, 26 received preoperative chemotherapy (most commonly cisplatin and doxorubicin); postoperative chemotherapy (usually cisplatin and doxorubicin also) was given to 12 patients, 11 of whom were suspected of having residual disease. Of the 40 patients, 26 are disease-free survivors after surgery and chemotherapy, one is alive and well after a partial response to chemotherapy and a liver transplant, one died perioperatively, 11 died with tumor, and one is alive with disease at the time of reporting.

The German Cooperative Pediatric Liver Tumor Studies HB89 and HB94 treated 141 patients with HBL. Some patients were treated with total resections alone. Most received ifosfamide, cisplatin, and adriamycin. In cases of insufficient tumor response, high-dose cisplatin and adriamycin were added. With a median follow-up of 6 years, disease-free survival is 98% for stage I, 55% for stage II, 63% for stage III, and 78% for stage IV (35,36,42).

POG 8697 enrolled 60 evaluable patients with HBL. Children with POG stage I favorable histology were followed. Children with stage I unfavorable histology or stage II received cisplatin, vincristine, and 5-fluorouracil. Patients with stage III or IV disease were evaluated for resection after five cycles of chemotherapy. Those who remained unresectable received 33 to 39 Gy of local irradiation plus additional chemotherapy. Disease-free survival is shown in Fig. 14-6. Of the five irradiated patients, three became resectable, achieved a complete resec-

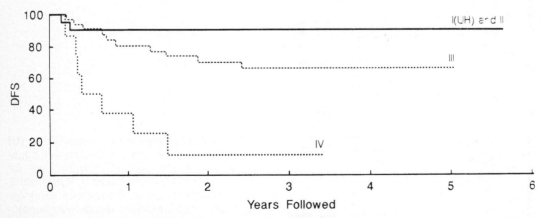

FIG. 14-6. Disease-free survival for children with hepatoblastoma treated with surgery and cisplatin, vincristine, and 5-fluorouracil in Pediatric Oncology Group Study 8697: stage I unfavorable histology (UH) and stage II, 91% ± 9.2% at 3 yr; stage III, 67% ± 10.8%; stage IV, 12.5% ± 11.7%. Staging is described in Table 14-2. (From Pritchard J, Brown J, Shafford E, et al. Cisplatin, doxorubicin, and delayed surgery for childhood hepatoblastoma: a successful approach—results of the first prospective study of the International Society of Pediatric Oncology. *J Clin Oncol* 2000;18:3819–3828, with permission.)

tion, and were alive and well at the time of the study's publication (44,51).

The Japanese Study Group for Pediatric Liver Tumor enrolled 145 patients with HBL from 1991 to 1999. Preoperative and postoperative cisplatin and tetrahydrapyranyl–adriamycin were administered, and 134 patients are evaluable. The complete resection rates by stage were 89% for stage I, 100% for stage II, 84% for stage IIIA, 40% for stage IIIB, and 58% for stage IV. The 6-year survival rate was 100% for stage I, 96% for stage II, 74% for stage IIIA, 50% for stage IIIB, and 39% for stage IV (23).

Guglielmi et al. (41) reported an Italian trial in which six children with stage I HBL were treated with surgery alone. There was one postoperative death. The remaining five patients are alive and well with a follow-up of 19–36 months. Thirteen patients with localized but unresectable HBL received cisplatin and doxorubicin. Ten had partial responses, and eight had radical resections. One patient had minimal change in the tumor but a drop in AFP; this patient also had a radical resection. The nine

resected patients are free of tumor with a median follow-up of 2 years. Two patients with stage I HCC are alive. Two children with HCC had initial chemotherapy. Neither had significant tumor shrinkage. One of the two is disease free.

A SIOP trial followed guidelines similar to those of the Italian study and treated 138 patients with HBL preoperatively with platinum and doxorubicin. Tumor response, defined as "any tumor shrinkage associated with a severe decrease in AFP," occurred in 82% (59).

POG 9345 was open from 1993 to 1995. The study was confined to advanced disease (stage III–IV), and patients were treated with carboplatin, vincristine, fluorouracil, and etoposide according to the plan outlined in Fig. 14-7. A total of 33 patients were entered and eligible for analysis. Twenty-two (67%) had stage III, and 11 (33%) had stage IV. The 5-year OS was 73% in stage III, with an EFS of 59%. In stage IV the 5-year OS was 27% and EFS was also 27% (39). Nineteen of the 33 patients (58%) were completely resected. The EFS of this group was 79%.

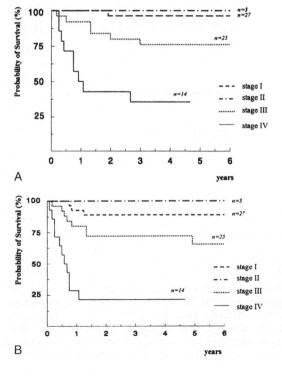

FIG. 14-7. (A) Disease-free survival and **(B)** overall survival, by stage, of children with hepatoblastoma in the German Pediatric Liver Tumor Study HB94. (From Fuchs J, Rydzynski J, Von Schweinitz D, et al. Pretreatment prognostic factors and treatment results with hepatoblastoma: a report from the German Cooperative Pediatric Liver Tumor Study HB94. *Cancer* 2002;95:172–182. Copyright © 2002 American Cancer Society. Reprinted by permission of Wiley-Liss, Inc., a subsidiary of John Wiley & Sons, Inc.)

The treatment results of POG 9345 were comparable to those of other published studies (61).

The German Cooperative Pediatric Liver Tumor study HB94 used a complex treatment algorithm involving surgery, cisplatin, ifosfamide, and doxorubicin, or etoposide and carboplatin (Fig. 14-8). Disease-free and event-free survival are shown in Fig. 14-9 (36,37).

The current intergroup HBL trial (P-9645) compares cisplatin and carboplatin with cisplatin, vincristine, and fluorouracil in patients with advanced-stage disease. Patients on both chemotherapy arms are randomized to receive amifostine (http://www.cancer.gov/search/clinical_trials/results_clinicaltrials.aspx), cisplatin in low-risk HBL, or cisplatin, carboplatin, and doxorubicin in high-risk HBL.

Thirty-nine patients with HCC were registered on the SIOP trial and treated as previously described. Overall survival, by Pretreatment Extent of Disease (PRETEXT) group, was 50% for I–II, 20% for III, and 12% for IV (32). In POG 8945 and CCG-8881, there were 46 patients with HCC, randomized postoperatively to either cisplatin, vincristine, and fluorouracil or cisplatin and doxorubicin. The 5-year event-free survival was 88% for stage I, 8% for stage II, and 0% for stage IV. There was no difference between the two chemotherapy programs (64). In meta-analyses in adults, a clear benefit of adjuvant chemotherapy in HCC cannot be shown (57).

The preponderance of the available data indicates that chemotherapy, most often cisplatin and adriamycin, produces a good response in 70–90% of primary HBL (Table 14-5) (53). In view of these data, and because of the frequent conversion by chemotherapy of unresectable disease to resectability, most authorities now

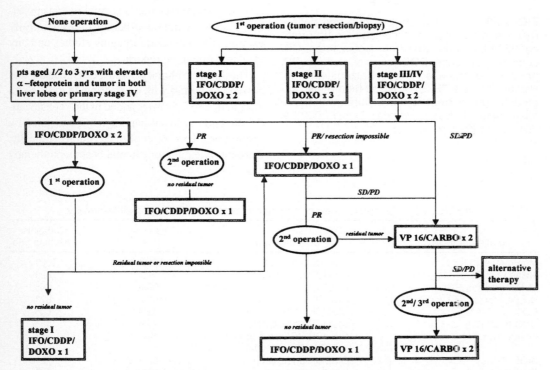

FIG. 14-8. The study design of the German Pediatric Liver Tumor Study HB94. Carbo, carboplatin; CDDP, cisplatin; Doxo, doxorubicin; IFO, ifosfamide; PD, progressive disease; PR, partial response; SD, stable disease; VP16, etoposide. (From Fuchs J, Rydzynski J, Von Schweinitz D, et al. Pretreatment prognostic factors and treatment results with hepatoblastoma: a report from the German Cooperative Pediatric Liver Tumor Study HB94. *Cancer* 2002;95:172–182. Copyright © 2002 American Cancer Society. Reprinted by permission of Wiley-Liss, Inc., a subsidiary of John Wiley & Sons, Inc.)

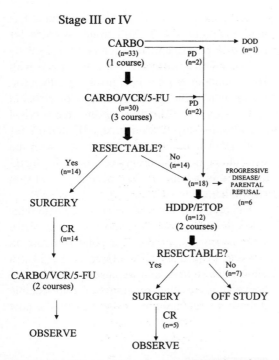

Stage III or IV

FIG. 14-9. The treatment program and patient responses for Pediatric Oncology Group protocol 9345 for stages III–IV hepatoblastoma. CR, complete response; DOD, dead of disease; PD, progressive disease. (From Katzenstein HM, Rigsby C, Shaw PH, et al. Novel therapeutic approaches in the treatment of children with hepatoblastoma. *J Pediatr Hematol Oncol* 2002;24: 751–755, with permission.)

use chemotherapy before definitive resection in all potentially resectable cases of HBL. Postoperatively, at least some chemotherapy is also generally given. There is clearly a need to develop more effective chemotherapy for anaplastic HBL and HCC. At present, the response of these histologies to chemotherapy is poor. HCL, which is often multicentric, can rarely be converted to resectability by up-front chemotherapy. Studies on various combinations of chemotherapy will be hampered by the small number of patients (65). High-dose chemotherapy with autologous stem cell rescue has been attempted with little success (61).

RADIOTHERAPEUTIC MANAGEMENT

If radiotherapy is administered preoperatively before a second-look celiotomy or postoperatively for residual disease, definition of the liver tumor volume is of paramount importance. It is essential to spare as much normal liver as possible. Therefore, the radiotherapist must carefully examine the diagnostic imaging studies and any available operative reports.

The tumor volume should be delineated and covered by portals with a 1- to 2-cm margin. Extra margin (0.5 to 2.5 cm) is added in the cephalocaudal direction to cover diaphragmatic excursion by respiration. This is confirmed fluoroscopically. Respiratory gating for external beam radiotherapy

TABLE 14-5. *Response rates of advanced hepatoblastoma to chemotherapy*

Trial (reference)	Chemotherapy	Response rate	Complete resection rate
Munro et al. (39)	CISDDP and DOXO	100%	100%
Italian Pilot Study (41)	CISDDP and DOXO	77%	62%
M. D. Anderson (76)	CISDDP	100%	86%
Hospital for Sick Children (75)	CISDDP and DOXO	100%	87%
POG 8697 (51)	CISDDP, VCR, and 5FU	92%	64%
CCG 823F (73)	CISDDP and DOXO	76%	48%
Intergroup I (56)	CISDDP, VCR, and 5FU or CISDDP and DOXO	NA	38%
SIOP (58)	CISDDP and DOXO	82%	72%
POG 9345 (59)	See Fig. 14-4	82%	58%
JPLT I (23)	CISDDP and THP	NA	60%

CCG, Children's Cancer Study Group; CISDDP, cisplatin; DOXO, doxorubicin; 5FU, 5-fluorouracil; JPLT, Japan Study Group for Pediatric Liver Tumor; NA, not available; POG, Pediatric Oncology Group; SIOP, International Society of Pediatric Oncology; THP, tetrahydrapyranyl–adriamycin; VCR, vincristine.

may enable a margin reduction on tumor volume. This, in turn, may allow dosage escalation without increasing toxicity (66). In the majority of cases, three-dimensionally planned or intensity-modulated fields from a linear accelerator are used. On occasion, the best treatment plan is anterior and posterior fields. If a fair portion of liver may be spared, then a total dosage of 50 to 60 Gy is appropriate. As we described in the previous section concerning POG 8697, irradiation of an unresectable HBL may convert it to resectability (51).

When postoperative irradiation is given for residual disease after a resection, 45 Gy to a limited area is appropriate for microscopic disease, and 50 to 60 Gy is appropriate for bulkier disease. Full attention must be given to respecting hepatic radiation tolerance. In adults with unresectable HCC, the available retrospective reviews support a dosage of at least 50 Gy (52).

If radiotherapy is to be administered to the whole liver for advanced tumor, then parallel opposed anterior and posterior fields are almost always indicated. The dosage generally is prescribed to the midportion of the liver, and the accepted parameters of liver tolerance to irradiation should not be exceeded. Therefore, with palliative intent for advanced HBL or HCC, 20 to 25 Gy in 2 to 2.5 weeks is reasonable. The treatment of metastasis from HBL or HCC is generally rewarding, and usual palliative dosages of irradiation (based on the surrounding normal tissue tolerance) may be used.

Investigational techniques that may have some promise include intraoperative irradiation, regional hyperthermia in conjunction with intra-arterial yttrium-90 microspheres, intra-arterial iodine-131 lipiodol, and iodine-131 antiferritin administered along with chemotherapy (18,67–69).

COMPLICATIONS

Radiation-induced liver disease (RILD), previously called radiation hepatitis, is a potential risk of radiation therapy for HBL or HCC. RILD is characterized by central liver lobule congestion, sinusoidal congestion, atrophy of the liver plates, and foci of necrosis. RILD can occur weeks to months after radiotherapy. One is particularly concerned about the risk of RILD in patients already compromised by prior hepatic surgery, chronic viral hepatitis, or liver cirrhosis. Recognized laboratory signs of RILD include elevation of the alkaline phosphatase level and elevated transaminases.

The risk of RILD is related to the administered radiation dosage and the treatment volume. In an analysis of dosage–volume histograms in irradiated adults with HCC, Cheng et al. (70,71) found that the mean hepatic dosage was higher in patients who developed RILD (25.0 vs. 19.7 Gy, $p = 0.02$), and the percentage of normal liver with dosage greater than 30 Gy was higher (42% vs. 33%, $p = 0.05$). It appears that IMRT, compared with three-dimensional conformal radiotherapy, can reduce the incidental dosage to the spinal cord, kidneys, and stomach. Because IMRT uses multiple fields, the mean dosage to the liver is higher than with three-dimensional planning (29.2 vs. 25.0 Gy, $p = 0.009$). This increase in whole organ dosage from IMRT is the result of the use of a larger number of fields exposing larger amounts of liver to radiation. The clinical import of this change in dosage distribution from IMRT is unknown.

RESULTS

For stage I–II HBL the survival rate is 70–100%. For stage III–IV the survival rate is 20–60% (3,12–15,20,22,23,72). In CCG-8881

TABLE 14-6. *Five-year survival of 154 children with hepatoblastoma from the first study of the International Society of Pediatric Oncology Liver Tumor Study Group*

Pretreatment extent of disease group	Overall survival	Event-free survival
I	100%	100%
II	91%	83%
III	68%	56%
IV	57%	46%

From Schnater JM, Kohler SE, Lameis WH, et al. Where do we stand with hepatoblastoma?: a review. *Cancer* 2003;98:668–678, with permission.

there was a 70% survival rate for children treated with initially localized and completely excised (stage I) HBL treated with combination chemotherapy. Only 29% of initial stage I patients were alive 3 years after documented recurrence. Results for the SIOP Liver Tumor Study Group are shown in Table 14-6. The survival rate for early stage HCC is about 50% but is 10–20% for stage III–IV disease (6,32,55,62).

REFERENCES

References particularly recommended for further reading are indicated by an asterisk.

*1. Habrand JL, Nehme D, Kalifa C, et al. Is there a place for radiation therapy in the management of hepatoblastoma and hepatocellular carcinomas in children? *Int J Radiat Oncol Biol Phys* 1992;23:525–531.

2. Weinberg AG, Finegold MS. Primary hepatic tumors of childhood. *Hum Pathol* 1983;14(6):512–537.

3. Bellani FF, Massimino M. Liver tumors in childhood: epidemiology and clinics. *J Surg Oncol Suppl* 1993;3:119–121.

*4. Schnater JM, Kohler SE, Lameis WH, et al. Where do we stand with hepatoblastoma?: a review. *Cancer* 2003;98:668–678.

5. Malt RA. Surgery for hepatic neoplasms. *N Engl J Med* 1985;313:1591–1596.

6. Novick DM, Deluca SA. Hepatoblastoma. *Am Fam Physician* 1986;33(2):141–142.

7. Lack EE, Neave C, Vawter GF. Hepatoblastoma: a clinical and pathologic study of 54 cases. *Am J Surg Pathol* 1982;6:693–705.

8. Schmidt D, Harms D, Lang W. Primary malignant hepatic tumors in childhood. *Virchows Arch* 1985;407:387–405.

9. Helmberger TK, Ros PR, Mergo PJ, et al. Pediatric liver neoplasms: a radiologic–pathologic correlation. *Eur Radiol* 1999;9:1339–1347.

10. Czaudema S, Papadiuk S, Korzon M, et al. Multicenter retrospective analysis of various primary pediatric malignant hepatic tumors: management in a series of 47 Polish patients (1985–1999). *Eur J Pediatr Surg* 2001;11:82–85.

11. Clatworth HW Jr, Schiller M, Grosfeld JL. Primary liver tumors in infancy and childhood: 41 cases variously treated. *Arch Surg* 1974;109:143–147.

12. Farhi DC, Shikes RH, Murari PJ, et al. Hepatocellular carcinoma in young people. *Cancer* 1983;52:1516–1525.

13. Gauthier F, Valayer J, Thai BL, et al. Hepatoblastoma and hepatocarcinoma in children: analysis of a series of 29 cases. *J Pediatr Surg* 1986;21:424–429.

14. Quinn JJ, Altman AJ, Robinson HT, et al. Adriamycin and cisplatin for hepatoblastoma. *Cancer* 1985;56:1926–1929.

15. Smith WL, Franken EA, Mitros FA. Liver tumors in children. *Semin Roentgenol* 1983;18:136–148.

16. Stocker JT. Hepatoblastoma. *Semin Diagn Pathol* 1994;11(2):136–143.

17. Finegold MS, Weinberg AC. Hepatoblastoma: histologic classification has important prognostic and therapeutic implications. *Pediatr Res* 1983;17(4):233A.

18. Grady ED, McLaren J, Auda SP, et al. Combination of internal radiation therapy and hyperthermia to treat liver cancer. *South Med J* 1983;76:1101–1105.

19. Manivel C, Wick MR, Abenoza P, et al. Teratoid hepatoblastoma: the nosologic dilemma of solid embryonic neoplasms of childhood. *Cancer* 1986;57:2168–2174.

20. Plaschkes J. Into the year 2000. *Med Pediatr Oncol* 2001;36:380–382.

21. Perilango G, Dall'Igna P, Sainati L. Modern treatment of childhood hepatoblastoma: what do clinicians and pathologists have to say to each other? *Med Pediatr Oncol* 2002;39:474–477.

22. Ablin A, Krailo M, Hass J, et al. Hepatoblastoma and hepatocellular carcinoma in children: a report from the Children's Cancer Study Group (CCG) and the Pediatric Oncology Group (POG). *Med Pediatr Oncol* 1988;16:417.

23. Sasaki F, Matsunaga T, Iwafuchi M, et al. outcome of hepatoblastoma treated with the JPLT-1 (Japanese Study Group for Pediatric Liver Tumor). *J Pediatr Surg* 2002;37:851–856.

24. Exelby PR, Filler RM, Grosfeld JL. Liver tumors in children with particular reference to hepatoblastoma and hepatocellular carcinoma: American Academy of Pediatrics Surgical Section Surgery, 1974. *J Pediatr Surg* 1975;10:329–337.

25. Exelby PR, el-Domeri A, Huvos AG, et al. Primary malignant tumors of the liver in children. *J Pediatr Surg* 1971;6:272–276.

26. Katzenstein HM, Krailo MD, Malogolowkin MH, et al. Fibrolamellar hepatocellular carcinoma in children and adolescents. *Cancer* 2003;97:2006–2012.

27. Mahour GH, Wogo GU, Seigel SE, et al. Improved survival in infants and children with primary liver tumors. *Am J Surg* 1983;146:236–240.

28. Giacomantonio M, Ein SH, Mancer K, et al. 30 years of experience with pediatric primary malignant liver tumors. *J Pediatr Surg* 1984;19:523–526.

29. Cohen MD, Bugaieski EM, Haliloglu M, et al. Visual presentation of the staging of pediatric tumors. *Radiographics* 1996;16(3):523–545.

30. Miller JH, Weinberg K. Liver and spleen. In: Miller JA, ed. *Imaging and pediatric oncology.* Baltimore: Williams & Wilkins, 1985:164–215.

31. Schnater JM, Aronson DC, Plaschkes J, et al. Surgical view of the treatment of patients with hepatoblastoma: results from the first prospective trial of the International Society of Pediatric Oncology Liver Tumor Study Group (SIOPEL-1). *Cancer* 2002;94:1111–1120.

32. Czauderna P, MacKinlay G, Perilango G, et al. Hepatocellular carcinoma in children: results of the first prospective study of the International Society of Pediatric Oncology Group. *J Clin Oncol* 2002;20:2798–2804.

33. Evans AE, Land VJ, Newton WA, et al. Combination chemotherapy (vincristine, adriamycin, cyclophosphamide, and 5-fluorouracil) in the treatment of children with malignant hepatoma. *Cancer* 1982;50:821–826.

34. Morita K, Okabe I, Ochino J, et al. The proposed

Japanese TNM classification of primary liver carcinoma in infants and children. *Jpn J Clin Oncol* 1983;13:361–370.

35. Von Schweinitz D, Burger D, Mildenberger H. Is laparotomy the first step in treatment of childhood liver tumors? The experience from the German Cooperative Pediatric live 89. *Eur J Pediatr Surg* 1994;4:82–86.

*36. Fuchs J, Rydzynski J, Hecker H, et al. The influence of preoperative chemotherapy and surgical technique in the treatment of hepatoblastoma: a report from the German Cooperative Liver Tumour Studies HB89 and HB94. *Eur J Pediatr Surg* 2002;12:255–261.

*37. Fuchs J, Rydzynski J, Von Schweinitz D, et al. Pretreatment prognostic factors and treatment results with hepatoblastoma: a report from the German Cooperative Pediatric Liver Tumor Study HB94. *Cancer* 2002;95:172–182.

38. Reynolds M. Conversion of unresectable to resectable hepatoblastoma and long-term follow-up study. *World J Surg* 1995;19:814–816.

39. Nagasue M, Yakaya H, Chang YC, et al. Active uptake of testosterone by androgen receptors of hepatocellular carcinoma in humans. *Cancer* 1986;57:2162–2167.

40. Munro FD, Azmy AF, Simpson E. Resectability of advanced liver tumours in children after combination chemotherapy. *Ann R Coll Surg Engl* 1994;76:253–256.

41. Filler RM, Tefft M, Vawter GF, et al. Hepatic lobectomy in childhood: effects of x-ray and chemotherapy. *J Pediatr Surg* 1969;17(4 Pt 2):233A.

42. Guglielmi M, Perilongo G, Cecchetto G, et al. Rationale and results of the International Society of Pediatric Oncology (SIOP) Italian pilot study on childhood hepatoma: surgical resection d'emblee or after primary chemotherapy? *J Surg Oncol Suppl* 1993;3:122–126.

43. Feusner JH, Krailo MD, Haas JE, et al. Treatment of pulmonary metastases of initial stage I hepatoblastoma in childhood: report from the Children's Cancer Study Group. *Cancer* 1993;71:859–864.

44. Bowman LC, Riely CA. Management of pediatric liver tumors. *Surg Oncol Clin North Am* 1996;5(2):451–459.

45. Tagge EP, Tagee DU, Reyes J, et al. Resection, including transplantation for hepatoblastoma and hepatocellular carcinoma. Impact on survival. *J Pediatr Surg* 1992;27:292–296.

46. Superina R, Billik R. Results of liver transplantation in children with unresectable liver tumors. *J Pediatr Surg* 1996;31:835–839.

47. Srinivasan P, McCall J, Pritchard J, et al. Orthotopic liver transplantation for unresectable hepatoblastoma. *Transplantation* 2002;74:652–655.

48. Molmenti EP, Nagata D, Raden J, et al. Liver transplantation for hepatoblastoma in the pediatric population. *Am J Transplant* 2002;2:535–538.

*49. Dall'Igna P, Cechetta G, Toffolu HT, et al. Multifocal hepatoblastoma: is there a place for partial hepatectomy? *Med Pediatr Oncol* 2003;40:113–117.

50. Berry CL, Keeling JW. Hepatoblastoma. In: Berry CL, ed. *Pediatric pathology.* Berlin: Springer-Verlag, 1981:660–662.

51. Douglass EC, Reynolds M, Finegold M, et al. Cisplatin, vincristine, and fluorouracil therapy for hepatoblastoma: a Pediatric Oncology Group study. *J Clin Oncol* 1993;11:96–99.

53. Douglass EC, Green AA, Wrenn E, et al. Effect of *cis*-platinum (DDP) based chemotherapy in treatment of hepatoblastoma. *Med Pediatr Oncol* 1985;13:187–190.

54. Pazdur R, Bready B, Cangir A. Pediatric hepatic tumors: clinical trials conducted in the United States. *J Surg Oncol* 1993;3(12):127–130.

55. Douglass E, Ortega J, Feusner J, et al. Hepatocellular carcinoma (HC) in children and adolescents: results from the Pediatric Intergroup Hepatoma Study (CCG 8881/POG 8945). *Proc Am Soc Clin Oncol* 1994;13: A–1439, 420.

56. Ortega JA, Douglas E, Feusner J, et al. Randomized comparison of cisplatin/vincristine/5-fluorouracil and cisplatin/continuous infusion/doxorubicin. Continuous infusion for treatment of pediatric hepatoblastoma: a report from the Children's Cancer Group and Pediatric Oncology Group. *J Clin Oncol* 2000;18: 2665–2675.

57. Schwartz JD, Schwartz M, Mandeli J, et al. Neoadjuvant and adjuvant therapy for resectable hepatocellular carcinoma: review of the randomized clinical trials. *Lancet Oncol* 2002;3:593–603.

58. Stringer MD, Hennaye ER, Hoowlad ER, et al. Improved outcome for children with hepatoblastoma. *Br J Surg* 1995;82:336–391.

59. Pritchard J, Brown J, Shafford E, et al. Cisplatin, doxorubicin, and delayed surgery for childhood hepatoblastoma: a successful approach—results of the first prospective study of the International Society of Pediatric Oncology. *J Clin Oncol* 2000 18:3819–3828.

60. Katzenstein HM, London WB, Douglas EC, et al. Treatment of unresectable and metastatic hepatoblastoma: a Pediatric Oncology Group phase II study. *J Clin Oncol* 2002;20:3438–3444.

61. Katzenstein HM, Rigsby C, Shaw PH, et al. Novel therapeutic approaches in the treatment of children with hepatoblastoma. *J Pediatr Eemctol Oncol* 2002; 24:751–755.

62. Greene FL, Page DL, Fleming ID, et al., eds. *AJCC cancer staging manual,* 6th ed. New York: Springer-Verlag, 2002.

63. Sobin LH, Witlekind CL, eds. *TVM: classification of malignant tumours.* New York: Wiley, 1997.

64. Katzenstein HM, Krailo MD, Malogolowkin MH, et al. Hepatocellular carcinoma in children and adolescents: results from the Pediatric Oncology Group and the Children's Cancer Group Intergroup Study. *J Clin Oncol* 2002;20:2789–2797.

65. Yoo HS, Park CH, Suh JH, et al. Radioiodinated fatty acid esters in the management of hepatocellular carcinoma: preliminary findings. *Cancer Chemother Pharmacol* 1989;23[Suppl]:554–558.

66. Wagman R, Yorke E, Ford E, et al. Respiratory gating for liver tumors: use in dose escalation. *Int J Radiat Oncol Biol Phys* 2003;55:659–668.

67. Tan SB, Chung YFA, Tai BC, et al. Elicitation of prior distributions for a phase III randomization controlled trial of adjuvant therapy with surgery for hepatocellular carcinoma. *Control Clin Trials* 2003;24:110–121.

68. Leichner PK, Yang NC, Franke TL, et al. Dosimetry and treatment planning for ^{90}Y-labeled antiferritin in hepatoma. *Int J Radiat Oncol Biol Phys* 1988;14:1033–1042.

69. Order SE, Stillwagon GB, Klein JL, et al. Iodine 131 antiferritin, a new treatment modality in hepatoma: a

Radiation Therapy Oncology Group study. *J Clin Oncol* 1985;3:1573–1582.

*70. Cheng JCH, Wu JK, Huang CM, et al. Dosimetric analysis and comparison of three-dimensional conformal radiotherapy and intensity-modulated radiation therapy for patients with hepatocellular carcinoma and radiation-induced liver disease. *Int J Radiat Oncol Biol Phys* 2003;56:229–234.

71. Cheng JCH, Wu JK, Huang CM, et al. Radiation-induced liver disease after three-dimensional conformal radiotherapy for patients with hepatocellular carcinoma: dosimetric analysis and implication. *Int J Radiat Oncol Biol Phys* 2002;54:156–162.

72. Goladay ES, Mollitt PK, Osteen NP, et al. Conversion to resectability by intra-arterial infusion chemotherapy after failure of systemic chemotherapy. *J Pediatr Surg* 1985;20:715–717.

73. Ortega JA, Kraila MD, Haas JE, et al. Effective treatment of unresectable or metastatic hepatoblastoma with cisplatin and continuous infusion doxorubicin chemotherapy: a report from the Children's Cancer Study Group. *J Clin Oncol* 1991;9:2167–2176.

74. Ninane J, Perilongo G, Staten JP, et al. Effectiveness and toxicity of cisplatin and doxorubicin in childhood hepatoblastoma and hepatocellular carcinoma. *Med Pediatr Oncol* 1991;19:199–203.

75. Filler RM, Ehrlich PF, Greenberg PL, et al. Preoperative chemotherapy for hepatoblastoma. *Surgery* 1991;110:591–596.

76. Black CT, Cangir A, Choroszy M, et al. Marked response to pre-operative high dose cis-platinum in children with unresectable hepatoblastoma. *J Pediatr Surg* 1991;26:1070–1073.

15

Germ and Stromal Cell Tumors of the Gonads and Extragonadal Germ Cell Tumors

Edward C. Halperin, M.D.

Pediatric germ cell tumors (GCTs) have three important distinguishing features:

- Because the origin is related to abnormal migration of primordial germ cells, the tumor often occurs in extragonadal locations.
- Serum tumor markers allow evaluation of the extent of resection and the development of recurrent tumor.
- Cisplatin, etoposide, and bleomycin (PEB) and cisplatin, vinblastine, and bleomycin (PVB) have significantly improved survival (1).

In the human embryo the primordial germ cells are found in the vicinity of the allantoic stalk. From this position the germ cells migrate into the adjoining mesenchyme at 4 to 5 weeks of gestation. The cells then assume positions in the germinal ridges and migrate along these structures. During this migration the cells are surrounded by the epithelium of the developing gonad and develop into the primitive testis or ovary. GCTs are thought to arise from totipotent primordial germ cells that escape normal organizing influences during development (2). Malignant GCTs account for approximately 3% of childhood cancers (1,3). There are 225 to 300 cases in children younger than 15 years old each year in the United States (4,5). GCTs may occur in the ovary, testes, sacrococcygeal region, vagina, retroperitoneum, pelvis, omentum, and mediastinal areas. Extragonadal and testicular sites predominate in children younger than 3 years old. Gonadal sites are most common during and after puberty (1). The main histologic types are germinoma, embryonal carcinoma, yolk sac tumor (also known as endodermal sinus tumor or Teilum tumor), malignant mixed GCTs, and malignant teratomas (sometimes called immature teratomas) (Fig. 15-1, Table 15-1) (2,6–8). Endodermal sinus tumor typically shows microcytic areas, Shiller–Duval bodies, and periodic acid–Schiff–positive extracellular hyaline droplets. The tumor is often positive, on immunohistochemistry, for α-feto-

TABLE 15-1. *Biological characteristics of pediatric germ cell tumors*

Type	Grade	AFP	HCG	Chemotherapy response	Radiotherapy response
Dysgerminoma	Malignant	−	+/−	+++	+++
Embryonal carcinoma	Malignant	−	−	+++	+
Yolk sac tumor	Malignant	+++	−	+++	+
Choriocarcinoma	Malignant	−	+++	+++	+
Mature and immature teratoma	Benign to potentially malignant	+/−	−	+	+

AFP, α-fetoprotein; HCG, human chorionic gonadotropin.
Derived from Gobel U, Schneider DT, Calaminus G, et al. Germ-cell tumors in childhood and adolescence. *Ann Oncol* 2000;11:263–271.

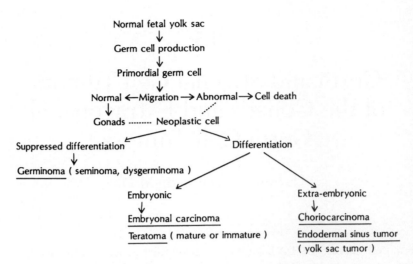

FIG. 15-1. Classification of germ cell tumors.

protein (AFP) and cytokeratin (9). Structural abnormalities of chromosome 1 are frequent (1).

Teratomas (from Greek *teratos,* "monster," and *onkoma,* "swelling") are the most common pediatric GCTs. Malignant teratomas may develop anywhere along the pathway of germinal tissue migration. By definition, teratomas are composed of tissues derived from two or three germinal layers (tridermal ancestry): ectoderm, mesoderm, and endoderm. Malignant teratomas are so named because of foci of endodermal sinus tumor, embryonal carcinoma, germinoma, or choriocarcinoma. There may also be foci of neuroblastoma, nephroblastoma, or hepatoblastoma. In general, frank malignancy is identified in about 20% of teratomas (2). The distinction must be made between immature teratomas with distinct malignant elements, which warrant aggressive adjuvant therapy, and immature teratomas with primitive neuroepithelium, which can be cured with surgery alone. Immature teratomas are graded by the system of Norris, which also predicts relapse (Table 15-2).

GENERAL ASPECTS OF CLINICAL PRESENTATION, STAGING, AND WORKUP

There is a bimodal age distribution for GCTs, with a peak in children younger than 3 years old and a second peak in children older than 12 years old. The male:female ratio is 2:1 (10). Girls predominate in the patient population during the first 3 years of life because of a female predominance in sacrococcygeal tumors. There is an association with intersex disorders (1,11,12). The association between undescended testes and the development of testicular cancer has been established.

The staging workup should include assays for AFP and human chorionic gonadotropin (HCG). AFP is elevated in almost all cases of endodermal sinus tumor and in many other patients with GCTs (13,14). Successful treatment, whether by surgery, chemotherapy, or radiotherapy, is regularly associated with AFP decline consistent with its half-life of 5 days in children 2 months or younger, 33 days in 2- to 4-month-olds, and 5 days in children 8 months or older (1,14,15). AFP falling too

TABLE 15-2. *Grading of immature teratomas*

Grade	Description	Approximate relapse rate
0	Mature	10%
I	Immaturity with PE limited to one lower-magnification field (×40) per slide	14%
II	<4 fields of PE per slide	23%
III	>4 fields of PE per slide	33%

PE, primitive neuroepithelium.
From references 1, 3, and 44.

slowly, failing to normalize after treatment, or rising generally signifies inadequate tumor response and precedes clinical or radiographic evidence of treatment failure. HCG activity is present in some tumors, particularly choriocarcinoma.

Diagnostic imaging of the pelvis and presacral space is best performed with computed tomography (CT), magnetic resonance imaging (MRI), and ultrasound (2). CT scanning is useful to assess the presence of pathologic retroperitoneal lymph nodes and extension of tumor into bone. Chest CT and bone scan should be used to assess the most likely sites of metastatic disease, including the lungs and bone. Imaging may show GCTs to be cystic, solid, or a combination of both. Sacrococcygeal and ovarian lesions that are predominantly cystic are less likely to be malignant, whereas solid lesions are more likely to be malignant. However, the correlation is far from perfect. This is particularly important because it argues strongly against using the term *solid teratoma* as the equivalent of *malignant* or *immature teratoma* (2,8,16,17).

Ovary

Of primary ovarian tumors of childhood, about 71% are GCTs, 17% epithelial, and 12% sex cord stromal tumors (1,16,18). The histologic distribution is approximately as follows: mature teratoma, 47%; immature teratoma, 12%; dysgerminoma, 5%; yolk sac tumor (endodermal sinus), 10%; mixed GCTs, 0–24%; and choriocarcinoma, <1% (1,3,19).

In the series by Germa et al. (19) from Barcelona, 46% of childhood ovarian GCTs presented with pain. The ovary descends from the abdomen to the bony pelvis during puberty. For this reason, in younger children and most adolescents, the pain is abdominal rather than pelvic. The long infundibular pedicle in the child is susceptible to torsion (13,19). Other presenting signs and symptoms included an asymptomatic palpable mass (19%), abdominal distention (36%), and, less commonly, menstrual irregularities, malaise, nausea, vomiting, or vaginal bleeding (10,19–29). The stromal Sertoli–Leydig cell tumors may present with de-feminization or virilization. Ovarian dysgerminomas are rarely hormonally active or productive of tumor markers. If a patient with an ovarian dysgerminoma is found to have an elevated AFP or signs of hormonal imbalance, there should be a meticulous search of the pathology specimen for elements of other tumor types.

Childhood ovarian GCTs are most often staged according to the practice of the Children's Oncology Group (COG; Table 15-3).

Both primary and second-look surgery are used to treat ovarian GCT. The initial surgical procedure should remove as much tumor as possible with a reasonable possibility of retention of fertility. At the time of laparotomy, the entire peritoneal surface should be examined for the presence of metastasis. Particular attention should be paid to the surfaces of the liver and to the inferior surface of the diaphragm (13). The involved ovary should be removed. Dysgerminoma has a 5–10% incidence of bilaterality (18). For childhood ovarian GCT other than dysgerminoma, the probability of bilateral involvement ranges from 0% to 14% (22). Therefore, the contralateral ovary should be biopsied and, if there is no evidence of malignancy, preserved (23). Palpation and biopsy of all suspicious lymph nodes in the pelvic and para-aortic regions

TABLE 15-3. *Children's Oncology Group staging for pediatric ovarian germ cell tumors*

Stage	Extent of disease
I	Limited to ovaries, with no clinical, radiographic, or histologic evidence of disease beyond the ovaries; no malignant cells in ascites or peritoneal washings; omentum grossly normal by visual inspection or pathologically normal if removed; tumor markers normal after appropriate half-life decline (α-fetoprotein = 5 days; β-human chorionic gonadotropin = 16 hr). IA, tumor limited to one ovary; IB, tumor limited to both ovaries.
II	Microscopic residual; tumor markers inappropriately elevated; preoperative or intraoperative rupture.
III	Retroperitoneal lymph node involvement or metastatic nodule; gross residual or biopsy only; contiguous visceral involvement.
IV	Distant metastases, including liver.

should be done. Peritoneal biopsies and washings (or collection of ascites) for cytology are important to complete the surgical staging (24).

The role of second-look laparotomy after chemotherapy for ovarian GCT is controversial. The initial abdominal exploration is used to establish disease status by visual inspection and biopsies. Some authorities favor second-look surgery as a therapeutic guide; that is, patients found free of tumor or with only mature teratoma do not need additional chemotherapy. However, others argue that few patients need second-look surgery. The possibility of a positive second-look operation in the face of a negative physical examination, imaging studies, and negative serum markers is small, and the procedure probably is not necessary in such cases (19).

Ovarian GCTs are lethal malignancies that can kill by early metastasis and rapid invasion of abdominal and pelvic structures. The prognosis of girls with these tumors was poor when they were treated with surgery only or surgery in combination with either radiotherapy or single-agent chemotherapy, except in some cases of dysgerminoma (16). An increasing body of evidence indicates that postoperative chemotherapy has increased the probability of survival (1,3,8,14,16,19,23,25–29). Active drugs include cisplatin (P), vinblastine (V), bleomycin (B), adriamycin (Ad), actinomycin (A), cyclophosphamide (C), etoposide (E), methotrexate (M), and vincristine (O) (10,30–32). Combinations used include VAC, POMB-ACE-PAV, PVB-ACAd, and PEB (2,11,16). PEB or PVB are most commonly used (3,33,34).

The generally accepted standard of care for pediatric ovarian GCT is summarized as follows:

- Benign mature teratomas and immature teratomas: surgery and observation
- Stage I malignant GCT: surgery and observation
- Stages II–IV malignant GCT: surgery and PEB or PVB (1)

AFP and HCG are valuable in patient follow-up.

Radiotherapy appears to be able to maintain local control of ovarian GCT in treated areas for prolonged periods of time. It has never been demonstrated, outside dysgerminoma, that this improved local control leads to an improvement in survival (17,33). In one study, most patients could not complete the planned course of irradiation because of acute toxicities. Intestinal obstruction and sterilization may result from large-field abdominal radiotherapy (11). Contemporary treatment programs do not use radiotherapy if initial surgery and, if used, chemotherapy render the child is disease-free (4). Radiotherapy is reserved for residual disease that cannot be resected at second operation and is not treated with alternative chemotherapy. The persistent tumor volume, generally with progressive shrinking fields, is irradiated to 40 Gy (4,11,14,19).

Historically, special consideration was given to an evaluation of treatment options for ovarian dysgerminoma. Radiation therapy was once considered the treatment of choice, much like adult stage I testicular seminoma. This is no longer the case.

The risk of failure after unilateral oophorectomy for stage I dysgerminoma (no tumor on external surface, capsule intact) had been reported by some to be 17–53%. Most failures that occurred in stage I patients developed in the ipsilateral para-aortic or common iliac lymph nodes and were usually salvaged. However, prophylactic irradiation of these areas almost always prevented such failures. With proper pelvic shielding, the risk of radiation-induced ovarian failure and subsequent sterilization is low.

The two principal treatment options in patients with stage I dysgerminoma are surgery followed by observation, using chemotherapy or radiation only on relapse; and surgery plus prophylactic ipsilateral common iliac plus para-aortic irradiation (15). To avoid irradiating most girls with ovarian dysgerminoma, the following are the criteria for treatment with unilateral salpingo-oophorectomy alone: unilateral encapsulated tumor (stage I); greatest tumor diameter less than 10 cm (although this is not uniformly found to be a prognostic sign); no ascites; no evidence of enlarged or abnormal lymph nodes by palpation, lymphangiogram, biopsy, or CT; well-differentiated pure dysgerminoma; and confidence that the patient will attend regular follow-up appointments. Under these criteria, selected patients may be cured with preservation of fertility (20-21,24,34,35).

If ovarian dysgerminoma is locally extensive (beyond stage I) or bilateral, then chemotherapy should be administered (4,19,31). When chemotherapy is used, PEB as for other ovarian GCT histologies is selected. In a series from Germa et al. (19), chemotherapy-induced amenorrhea was reversed in 14 of 15 patients after chemotherapy. Three patients attempted to become pregnant: Two had uneventful pregnancies and one had a spontaneous abortion. Whether ovarian failure will ultimately develop in chemotherapy-treated patients remains to be seen, although Mann et al. (14) stated that "in ovarian dysgerminoma, chemotherapy is preferable to radiotherapy to preserve fertility."

The few remaining proponents of radiotherapy for ovarian dysgerminoma believe that the indications for radiotherapy are as follows: tumor present on the external surface or tumor rupture, tumor adhesion or extension in the pelvis (stage II or III), and intra-abdominal nodal metastasis detected by biopsy, palpation, lymphangiogram, or CT scan (stage III). However, even the few remaining proponents of radiotherapy agree that mediastinal and supraclavicular disease and ascites are indications for chemotherapy. Brody (36) recommends hemipelvic irradiation if the extension of tumor is strictly within the ipsilateral pelvis. In this way, ovarian function may be preserved. However, ovarian dysgerminoma may spread throughout the abdomen, and a limited hemipelvic field runs the risk of abdominal tumor recurrence. Therefore, Buskirk et al. (18; also see ref. 24) recommended whole abdomen irradiation as initial treatment, with a boost to sites of bulk disease.

If ovarian dysgerminoma is treated with radiotherapy rather than chemotherapy, and if disease extends in a nodal drainage pattern through the pelvis and para-aortic nodes, then large fields are needed. In the absence of extranodal spread the para-aortic nodes and pelvis are irradiated. Whole abdomen irradiation was thought by some to be indicated for bulky abdominal nodes or extracapsular extension. The entire abdomen was irradiated if there was proven abdominal spread or a high risk of abdominal

seeding (positive peritoneal biopsies, tumor rupture). Prophylactic mediastinal irradiation is rarely done in the presence of abdominal disease because it compromises the child's tolerance to chemotherapy (18,20,21). However, the common pattern of practice for ovarian dysgerminoma is to treat stage I with surgery and stages II–IV with surgery plus PVB or PEB, not radiotherapy.

The dosages needed for dysgerminoma are less than those for other GCTs. Sites that are felt to be clinically uninvolved but are being treated prophylactically receive 20 to 25 Gy in 3 to 4 weeks. Areas of bulk disease are boosted with an additional 10 to 15 Gy. If one treats the whole abdomen, then appropriate blocking to the liver and kidneys is needed. When one is reirradiating for recurrent disease, the possibility of cure is significant, and the tolerance of normal tissue to irradiation must be respected (18,20,21,24,37).

For all histologies of ovarian GCTs combined, the reported probability of survival is 60–90%. For the most part, deaths appear to be in stage IV presentations (1,3,4,6,14,19–26,31,34,38,39). The survival of children with ovarian dysgerminoma is 95–100% when disease is confined to the pelvis or has limited abdominal involvement (6,31,36). Tumor rupture or extensive metastasis reduces the probability of survival (36).

Ovarian stromal and epithelial tumors are rare in children. Stromal tumors of the childhood ovary, including juvenile granulosa cell tumors, often are cured by surgical resection alone (40). These stromal tumors usually present with precocious pseudopuberty in prepubertal girls because of estrogen production by the tumor. The roles of surgery and chemotherapy for ovarian epithelial tumors in adolescents (mucinous or serous cystadenocarcinomas) follow the same guidelines as those for adults (1,28,41).

Testis

Testicular GCTs generally present as a palpable painless mass or with signs and symptoms that simulate infection, torsion, or post-traumatic hematoma (42). The diagnostic workup includes testicular ultrasonography, CT of the abdomen and chest, AFP, and HCG. The most common

GCT of the testes in pubertal children is yolk sac tumor (endodermal sinus) (14,16,42). Less common histologies include embryonal carcinoma, mature, immature, and malignant teratoma and mixed tumor. Prepubertal children more often have non–germ cell tumors such as Sertoli or Leydig cell tumors or sarcomas. Testicular GCTs usually are staged by the COG system (Table 15-4). Most cases are stage I at diagnosis. Teenagers may hesitate to discuss the presence of testicular mass and tend to have more advanced disease at diagnosis (10,13,42).

Most testicular tumors are suspected before surgery. A radical orchiectomy should be performed with high ligation of the spermatic cord. Transscrotal procedures should be avoided because they can spread tumor and alter the proportion of lymphatic metastases. If a scrotal biopsy has been done, some authorities advise a hemiscrotectomy (42). Others cite data from adults to argue that there is no increase in the relapse rate in stage I tumors if hemiscrotectomy is not done (43). There is also some support in the literature to treat testicular teratomas with tumor enucleation rather than orchiectomy (44).

The debate concerning the role of retroperitoneal lymph node dissection in early-stage testicular GCT appears to be resolving in favor of a limited role for the procedure. The older literature indicates that 0–33% of children with GCT have involved retroperitoneal lymph nodes (5,10,13,46,47). Proponents of retroperitoneal lymph node dissection suggested that it was important in staging and in the removal of small foci of malignant cells and that it possibly improved the chance of cure. Objections to dissection, based on loss of ejaculatory function, were obviated by the use of the modified retroperitoneal dissection (40). With the widespread availability of serum tumor marker studies and CT screening, however, it is now clear that the staging node dissection is unnecessary in stage I disease. In children with tumor confined to the testes, where AFP levels normalize within 1 month after orchiectomy and where the chest radiograph and retroperitoneal imaging studies are normal, retroperitoneal lymph node dissection is unnecessary. In one study, 28 patients with stage I testicular yolk sac tumors were treated with radical orchiectomy alone; 24 (86%) were cured. The remaining four (14%) relapsed and were rendered free of disease by chemotherapy (47). Both the U.K. Children's Cancer Study Group and the St. Jude Children's Research Hospital (SJCRH) series have almost uniform survival for stage I patients treated with radical orchiectomy alone (15,40). There is no difference in disease-free survival between children with stage I disease who undergo retroperitoneal lymph node dissection and those who do not (13,22,47). Retroperitoneal lymph node dissection may still be appropriate for children with no markers or unknown markers at diagnosis to confirm staging, more aggressive histologies (i.e., embryonal cell), demonstrable moderate-sized nodal metastasis at the time of presentation (i.e., SJCRH stage II), or an elevated AFP after surgery (22,40,45).

The management strategy for testicular GCT is as follows:

- Stage I, surgery alone
- Stages II–IV, surgery followed by PEB

For stage I, chemotherapy is used for documented relapse. The survival for all stages is on the order of 90–100%.

TABLE 15-4. *Children's Oncology Group staging for pediatric testicular germ cell tumor*

Stage	Extent of disease
I	Limited to testes; completely resected by high inguinal orchiectomy; no clinical, radiographic, or histologic evidence of disease beyond the testes; tumor markers normal after appropriate half-life decline (AFP = 5 days; β-HCG = 16 hr); scrotal orchiectomy with negative margin on cord structures.
II	Microscopic residual in scrotum or high in spermatic cord or inappropriately elevated tumor markers after appropriate half-life interval (AFP = 5 days; β-HCG = 16 hr); tumor rupture or scrotal biopsy followed at a later time by a scrotal or inguinal orchiectomy.
III	Retroperitoneal lymph node involvement but no visceral or extra-abdominal involvement.
IV	Distant metastases, including liver.

AFP, α-fetoprotein; β-HCG, β-human chorionic gonadotropin.

Extragonadal

Extragonadal GCTs usually are found in the midline, consistent with embryonic patterns of migration. The most common site is the sacrococcygeal, presacral, and buttock region. This is followed by the mediastinal, vaginal, uterine, and prostatic regions. Other reported sites of origin include the neck and face, retroperitoneum, stomach, orbit, pancreas, heart, and pericardium (1,3,48).

Sacrococcygeal GCTs may develop early in fetal life. Urinary tract obstruction, compression of the umbilical vessels, and chronic hemorrhage into the tumor and amniotic sac may occur. Prenatal ultrasonography may demonstrate the mass, hydronephrosis, fetal hydrops, or prominent polyhydramnios (2). More than one-half of patients with malignant and benign sacrococcygeal teratomas present to medical attention on the first day of life. These children often have other congenital anomalies such as abnormalities of the genitourinary tract or of the lower vertebral bodies (49).

Approximately 60–70% of sacrococcygeal teratomas are unequivocally benign by virtue of the exclusive presence of mature somatic tissue. These lesions in newborns may be cured by surgery. Many are diagnosed by prenatal ultrasonography. Ten percent to 15% of teratomas are composed of a mixture of embryonic or fetal elements in mature structures along with poorly differentiated embryonic tissue. These lesions constitute a category of indeterminate biologic behavior and are called immature benign teratomas. In the surgical treatment of benign and intermediate-grade sacrococcygeal teratomas in infants, every effort must be made to remove the tumor mass. The early, safe, and total extirpation of the tumor and coccyx is necessary. The coccyx should always be removed with the mass because failure to remove the coccyx is associated with a local recurrence rate of 37% (50). Even piecemeal excision of mature and intermediate sacrococcygeal teratomas in infants is rarely associated with local recurrence (25, 27,42–44). Some neonates may benefit from a staged surgical approach with initial ligation of the vascular supply. Only 2–10% of sacrococcygeal region tumors are malignant when removed in infants younger than 4 months old. After 4 months of age, the rate of malignancy rises to 50–90% (2,28,50). Simply put, there are two basic types of sacrococcygeal GCT: large, predominantly benign masses in neonates, and pelvic, primarily malignant masses in older children.

A useful classification system for sacrococcygeal GCT has been developed by the Surgical Section of the American Academy of Pediatrics. Type I tumors are primarily external; type II tumors are dumbbell-shaped, with significant external and intrapelvic components; type III tumors have a small external component, with the majority of the lesion extending into the pelvic and abdominal spaces; and type IV tumors occupy the presacral space and have no appreciable external component. As a general rule, the prevalence of malignancy is lowest in type I tumors and increases as one moves from type II through type IV (2,49). Malignancy rates by type are 8% for type I, 21% for type II, 34% for type III, and 38% for type IV (1). The malignancy rate also rises with age. The COG staging system for malignant extragonadal GCT is shown in Table 15-5.

Preoperative imaging studies help to determine the lesion's type, and they also evaluate whether the lesion is invading adjacent structures rather than displacing them, a suggestion of malignancy. Only a few malignant sacrococcygeal GCTs are resectable *per primum*. In general, the surgeon obtains an initial biopsy, and chemotherapy is administered. There is evidence docu-

TABLE 15-5. *Children's Oncology Group staging for pediatric malignant extragonadal germ cell tumors*

Stage	Extent of disease
I	Complete resection of any site; coccygectomy for sacrococcygeal site; negative tumor margins; in infants >8 mo old tumor markers are normal after appropriate half-life decline. For infants <8 mo, tumor markers return to normal by 8 mo of life.
II	Microscopic residual; lymph nodes negative; tumor markers inappropriately elevated.
III	Gross residual or biopsy only; primarily resected but lymph nodes positive.
IV	Distant metastases, including liver.

menting complete responses of both metastatic and primary disease to chemotherapy with long-term survival (4,14,25,31,51–54). Unresectable tumors have been rendered resectable, with long-term survivorship reported. If there is a satisfactory reduction of tumor volume, the tumor may be deemed resectable at a later date (4,50). If a complete response is achieved with surgery and chemotherapy, the probability of local control and cure is quite good (4,14). In summary, stage I extragonadal mature and immature sacrococcygeal teratomas and completely resected malignant GCTs are resected and observed. Stages II–IV malignant GCTs are treated with PEB or PVB plus surgery. The survival rate of the advanced malignant lesions is about 80% (1).

Mediastinal GCTs may be identified as a result of vascular or pulmonary obstructive symptoms or may be found incidentally on a routine chest radiograph. In young children the histology usually is teratoma. Mediastinal yolk sac (endodermal sinus) tumor almost always occurs in boys and men between the ages of 15 and 35 years. The tumor grows rapidly and metastasizes early via lymphatic and hematogenous pathways (55). An occasional case has been reported in female patients (7). Mature and immature teratomas are treated with surgery. Malignant mediastinal GCTs are treated with surgery and chemotherapy.

In general, the survival rate for extragonadal GCT is not as high as for ovarian and testicular lesions. As previously noted, the survival rate in the United States for sacrococcygeal tumors is 80%, for mediastinum 40–60%, and for other sites 50% (1,4,12,14,22,25,31,51,53–61). In the recent International Society of Pediatric Oncology (SIOP) and German protocols, the 10-year event-free results are as follows: ovarian, 89%; sacrococcygeal, 81%; testicular, 97%; and all others (except brain) 88% (3,43).

Radiotherapy is not necessary for children who have a documented complete response to surgery and chemotherapy (4). The local recurrence rate in this particular set of patients is low. In a study by Flamant et al. (25), the majority of children with nonseminomatous malignant GCT (stages III and IV) did not need radiotherapy when aggressive induction chemotherapy was used as a complement to surgery. In 11 of Flamant et al.'s cases failing initial therapy, nine had a local recurrence as the site of first failure. However, when only a partial response to chemotherapy and surgery is achieved in localized disease, the chance of irradiation achieving local control is only fair. Ablin et al. (4) described 17 children with GCTs of gonadal and extragonadal location who were irradiated for persistent disease after chemotherapy. Radiotherapy failed in the field of treatment in ten of the 17 cases. The primary site of failure in all seven sacrococcygeal GCTs was at the initial site of tumor. Mann et al. (14) reported irradiating eight patients with GCT in a variety of locations. When obvious disease was present, no sustained responses occurred. There were three survivors who had normal AFP levels at the time of irradiation and who may have been already cured before irradiation. Kersh et al. (20) reviewed the results of radiotherapy in adult and pediatric patients with nonseminoma GCTs in the mediastinal, retroperitoneal, and sacrococcygeal regions. Local control was obtained in two of 11 patients with mediastinal lesions, zero of two patients with retroperitoneal tumors, and one of four sacrococcygeal lesions. In summary, the results of radiotherapy for patients with persistent disease after chemotherapy are poor, and the radiotherapy literature derives from older forms of chemotherapy. However, it is also clear that with residual unresected disease after chemotherapy, the risk of tumor regrowth at the primary site is almost a certainty (50). Therefore, we conclude that radiotherapy is worth the effort, albeit with only modest claims for success. There has also been a report of local hyperthermia treatment with platinum chemotherapy for local recurrence (3).

If radiotherapy is used for extragonadal GCT, dosages of 45 to 50 Gy are recommended, as limited by the tolerance of surrounding normal tissue. The radiotherapy portals are dictated by radiographic imaging studies and surgical exploration. Metastatic lesions may necessitate palliative treatment with local field irradiation.

RESULTS

Survival for stages I–II GCTs at gonadal sites approaches 100%. Survival for stages III–IV

GCTs at gonadal sites is about 95%. Extragonadal GCT survival is about 90% for stages I–II and about 75% for stages III–IV (1).

REFERENCES

References particularly recommended for further reading are indicated by an asterisk.

*1. Rescorla FJ, Breitfeld PP. Pediatric germ cell tumors. *Curr Probl Cancer* 1999;23:257–303.

2. Wells RG, Sty JR. Imaging of sacrococcygeal germ cell tumors. *Radiographics* 1990;10:701–713.

*3. Gobel U, Schneider DT, Calaminus G, et al. Germ-cell tumors in childhood and adolescence. *Ann Oncol* 2000; 11:263–271.

4. Ablin AR, Krailo MD, Ramsay NKC, et al. Results of treatment of malignant germ cell tumors in 93 children: a report from the Children's Cancer Study Group. *J Clin Oncol* 1991;9:1782–1792.

5. Dehnard LP. Gonadal and extragonadal germ cell neoplasms: teratomas in childhood. In: Feingold M, ed. *Pathology of neoplasia in children and adolescents.* Philadelphia: WB Saunders, 1986:282–312.

6. Brodeur GM, Howarth CB, Pratt CB, et al. Malignant germ cell tumors in 57 children and adolescents. *Cancer* 1981;48:1890–1898.

7. Hawkins EP, Finegold MJ, Hawkins HK, et al. Nongerminomatous malignant germ cell tumors in children: a review of 89 cases from the Pediatric Oncology Group, 1971–1984. *Cancer* 1986;58:2579–2584.

8. Slayton RE, Park RC, Silverberg SG, et al. Vincristine, dactinomycin, and cyclophosphamide in the treatment of malignant germ cell tumors of the ovary: a Gynecologic Oncology Group study (a final report). *Cancer* 1985;56:243–248.

9. Manavis J, Alexiadis G, Lambropoulou M, et al. Extragonadal retroperitoneal endodermal sinus tumor in an eighth-month-old female infant. *Eur J Gynaecol Oncol* 2001;22:345–346.

10. D'Angio GJ. Yolk sac carcinoma. *Med Pediatr Oncol* 1987;15:96–101.

11. Jereb B, Wollner N, Exelby P. Radiation in multidisciplinary treatment of children with malignant ovarian tumors. *Cancer* 1979;43:1037–1042.

12. Lack EE, Travis WD, Welch KJ. Retroperitoneal germ cell tumors in childhood: a clinical and pathologic study of 11 cases. *Cancer* 1985;56:602–608.

13. Green DM. The diagnosis and treatment of yolk sac tumors in infants and children. *Cancer Treat Rev* 1983; 10:265–288.

14. Mann JR, Pearson D, Barrett A, et al. Results of the United Kingdom Children's Cancer Study Group's malignant germ cell tumor studies. *Cancer* 1989;63:1657–1667.

15. Huddart SN, Mann JR, Gornall P, et al. The UK Children's Cancer Study Group: testicular malignant germ cell tumours 1979–1988. *J Pediatr Surg* 1990;25:406–410.

16. Brammer HM III, Buck JL, Hayes WS, et al. Malignant germ cell tumors of the ovary: radiologic–pathologic correlation. *Radiographics* 1990;10:715–724.

17. Cham WC, Wollner N, Exelby P, et al. Patterns of ex-

tension as a guide to radiation therapy in the management of ovarian neoplasms in children. *Cancer* 1976; 37:1443–1448.

18. Buskirk SJ, Schray MF, Podartz KC, et al. Ovarian dysgerminoma: a retrospective analysis of results of treatment, sites of treatment failure, and radiosensitivity. *Mayo Clin Proc* 1987;62:1149–1157.

19. Germa JR, Izquierdo MA, Segui MA, et al. Malignant ovarian germ cell tumors: the experience at the Hospital de la Santa Creu i Sant Pau. *Gynecol Oncol* 1992;45: 153–159.

20. Kersh CR, Constable WC, Hahn SS, et al. Primary malignant extragonadal germ cell tumors: an analysis of the effect of radiotherapy. *Cancer* 1990;65:2681–2685.

21. Lucraft HH. A review of thirty-three cases of ovarian dysgerminoma emphasizing the role of radiotherapy. *Clin Radiol* 1979;30:585–589.

22. Grosfeld JL, Billmire DF. Teratomas in infancy and childhood. *Curr Probl Cancer* 1985;9:1–53.

23. Red E. Study: save contralateral ovary in girls with ovarian malignancy. *Oncol Times* 1986;8:1–16.

24. Tewfik HH, Tewfik FA, Lataurette HB. A clinical review of seventeen patients with ovarian dysgerminoma. *Int J Radiat Oncol Biol Phys* 1982;8:1705–1709.

25. Flamant F, Schwartz L, Delons E, et al. Nonseminomatous malignant germ cell tumors in children: multi-drug therapy in stages III and IV. *Cancer* 1984;54:1687–1691.

26. Gershenson DM, Kavanaugh JJ, Copeland LJ, et al. Treatment of malignant non-dysgerminomatous germ cell tumors of the ovary with vinblastine, bleomycin, and *cis*-platinum. *Cancer* 1986;57:1731–1737.

27. Nichols CR, Heerema NA, Palmer C, et al. Klinefelter's syndrome associated with mediastinal germ cell neoplasms. *J Clin Oncol* 1987;5:1290–1294.

28. Noseworthy J, Lack EE, Kozakewich HPW, et al. Sacrococcygeal germ cell tumors in childhood: an updated experience with 118 patients. *J Pediatr Surg* 1981;16:358–364.

29. Raney RB, Sinclair L, Uri A, et al. Malignant ovarian tumors in children and adolescents. *Cancer* 1987;59: 1214–1220.

30. Donnellan WA, Swenson O. Benign and malignant sacrococcygeal teratomas. *Surgery* 1968;64 834–846.

31. Etcubanas E, Thompson E, Rao B, et al. Treatment of childhood germ cell tumors (GCT): results of a prospective study. *Proc ASCO* 1985;4:238.

32. Williams SD, Birch R, Einhorn LH, et al. Treatment of disseminated germ-cell tumors with cisplatin, bleomycin, and either vinblastine or etoposide. *N Engl J Med* 1987;315:1435–1440.

33. Gobel G, Calaminus G, Harms D. SIOP teratoma 95, a randomized cooperative protocol for chemotherapy. *Med Pediatr Oncol* 1995;25:319.

34. Creasman WT, Fedder BF, Hammond CB, et al. Germ cell malignancies of the ovary. *Obstet Gynecol* 1979;53:226–230.

35. Kephart G, Smith JP, Rutledge F, et al. The treatment for dysgerminoma of the ovary. *Cancer* 1978;41:986–990.

36. Brody S. Clinical aspects of dysgerminoma of the ovary. *Acta Radiol* 1961;56:209–230.

37. Lawson AP, Adler GF. Radiotherapy in the treatment of ovarian dysgerminoma. *Int J Radiat Oncol Biol Phys* 1988;14:431–434.

38. Wollner N, Exelby PR, Woodruff M, et al. Malignant

ovarian tumors in childhood. Prognosis in relation to initial stage. *Cancer* 1976;37:1953–1964.

39. Norris HJ, Zirkin HJ, Benson WL. Immature (malignant) teratoma of the ovary: a clinical and pathological study of 58 cases. *Cancer* 1976;37:2359–2372.

40. Vassai G, Falmant F, Caillaud JM, et al. Juvenile granulosa cell tumor of the ovary in children: a clinical study of 15 cases. *J Clin Oncol* 1988;6:990–995.

41. Vogelzang NJ, Anderson RW, Kennedy BJ. Successful treatment of mediastinal germ cell/endodermal sinus tumors. *Chest* 1985;88:64–69.

42. Fernandes ET, Etcubanas E, Rao BN, et al. Two decades of experience with testicular tumors in children at St. Jude Children's Research Hospital. *J Pediatr Surg* 1989;24:677–682.

43. Kennedy CL, Hendry, WF, Peckham, MJ. The significance of scrotal interference in stage I testicular cancer managed by orchiectomy and surveillance. *Br J Urol* 1986;58:705–708.

44. Rushton HG, Belman, AB, Sesterhenn, I, et al. Testicular sparing surgery for prepubertal teratoma of the testis: a clinical and pathological study. *J Urol* 1990;144:726–730.

45. Duckett J. Testicular tumors in childhood. In: Hays DM, ed. *Pediatric surgical oncology.* Orlando, FL: Grune & Stratton, 1986:189–204.

46. Ise T, Ohtsuka H, Matsumoto K, et al. Management of malignant testicular tumors in children. *Cancer* 1976;37:1539–1545.

47. Flamant F, Diez P. Cure of testicular Stage I yolk sac tumor (endodermal sinus tumor) in children by conservative treatment. *Proc ASCO* 1985;4:235.

48. Puri A, Chandrasekharam VVSS, Agarwala S, et al. Pediatric extragonadal germ cell tumor of the scalp. *J Pediatr Surg* 2001;36:1602–1603.

49. Altman RP, Randolph JG, Lilly JR. Sacrococcygeal teratoma: American Academy of Pediatric Surgical Section Survey—1973. *J Pediatr Surg* 1974;9:389–398.

50. Ein SH, Mancer K, Adeyemi SD. Malignant sacrococ-

cygeal teratoma—endodermal sinus, yolk sac tumor—in infants and children: a 32 year review. *J Pediatr Surg* 1985;20:473–477.

51. Thomas WJ, Kelleher JF, Duval-Arnould B. Successful treatment of metastatic extragonadal endodermal sinus (yolk sac) tumor in childhood. *Cancer* 1981;48:2371–2374.

52. Valdiserri RO, Yunis EJ. Sacrococcygeal teratomas: review of 68 cases. *Cancer* 1981;48:217–221.

53. Cushing BA, Phillippart AI, Brough AJ, et al. Extragonadal endodermal sinus tumor in early childhood: treatment response and longterm effects. *Proc ASCO* 1985;4:242.

54. Greene FL, Page DL, Fleming, ID, et al., eds. *AJCC cancer staging manual,* 6th ed. New York: Springer-Verlag, 2002.

55. Feun LG, Sampson MK, Stephens RL. Vinblastine, bleomycin, *cis*-platinum, and disseminated extragonadal germ cell tumors: a Southwest Oncology Study. *Cancer* 1980;45:2543–2549.

56. Gooneratne S, Keh P, Streekanth S, et al. Anterior mediastinal endodermal sinus (yolk sac) tumor in a female infant. *Cancer* 1985;56:1430–1433.

57. Anderson WA, Sabio H, Durso N, et al. Endodermal sinus tumor of the vagina: the role of primary chemotherapy. *Cancer* 1985;56:1025–1027.

58. Atkins J. Malignant ovarian and other germ cell tumors. In: Hays DM, ed. *Pediatric surgical oncology.* Orlando, FL: Grune & Stratton, 1986:123–138.

59. Beddis IR, Noblett H, Mott MG. Effective chemotherapy for metastatic malignant sacrococcygeal tumor. *Med Pediatr Oncol* 1984;12:231–232.

60. Israel A, Bosl GJ, Golbey RB, et al. The results of chemotherapy for extragonadal germ-cell tumors in the cisplatin era: the Memorial Sloan–Kettering Cancer Center experience (1975–1982). *J Clin Oncol* 1985;3:1073–1078.

61. Logothetis CJ, Samuels ML, Selig DE, et al. Chemotherapy of extragonadal germ cell tumors. *J Clin Oncol* 1985;3:316–325.

16

Endocrine, Aerodigestive Tract, and Breast Tumors

Edward C. Halperin, M.D.

ENDOCRINE CARCINOMA

Adrenal Cortical Carcinoma

Adrenal cortical carcinoma (ACC) makes up approximately 0.2% of childhood cancer (1–7). There are about 25 cases per year in the United States (8). The tumor is more common in girls than in boys. Tumors may be functional or nonfunctional, depending on whether they produce cortisol, aldosterone, androgens, or estrogens (4).

The molecular pathogenesis of ACC has been explored. In studies of largely adult patients, the cell cycle regulators and molecular markers that are associated with some cases of ACC include the Ki-67 proliferation marker (65% of cases in the Memorial Sloan–Kettering Cancer Center series), p53 (5%), mdm-2 negative (80%), and p21 (70%) (4,5).

In the more than half of ACC cases that are secretory, virilization is the most common sign. There is premature pubic hair, clitoromegaly or phallomegaly, and excessive muscular development. Bone age may be advanced. In Cushing's syndrome there is moon facies, plethora, hypertension, striae, weight gain, acne, hirsutism, and an intracapsular fat pad. Children with ACC rarely have pure Cushing's syndrome; most also have some evidence of virilization. Feminization or aldosterone-secreting tumors are quite rare. A mixed pattern of hormone production is seen in some patients. Hypokalemia may result from aldosterone excess. Urinary 17-keto- and 17-hydroxycorticosteroids may be elevated (2). ACC steroid production generally is not influenced by adrenocorticotropic hormone (ACTH) suppression. Children with non-functioning ACC usually present with pain,

pressure, a palpable mass, weight loss, malaise, hematuria, varicocele, or dyspnea. Ultrasound, computed tomography (CT), and magnetic resonance imaging (MRI) are used to assess the size and extent of the primary tumor and the presence of liver and lymph nodes metastases (9). Most ACCs are more than 6 cm in diameter (4). The primary tumor usually is hypovascular on angiography (5).

Surgical removal of a localized primary ACC is the standard curative treatment (4,10–12). The surgeon attempts a complete excision of the primary tumor and resectable regional metastases. Meticulous attention must be given to perioperative steroid management. Surgery may also be used to treat resectable abdominal recurrences or localized distant metastases (13).

The distinction between benign and malignant ACC is made on cytologic abnormality, tumor weight, and presence of metastases (13,14). Some lesions are frankly malignant on microscopic examination. For those of borderline histologic appearance, one should consider resectability, the extent of capsular invasion, adherence to surrounding structures, the presence of aberrant vessels on angiography, tumor size, and the presence or absence of metastases in distinguishing benign from malignant lesions. Well-encapsulated and easily excised tumors may be cured by surgery alone. In the remaining resected but more locally advanced cases, there is a substantial risk of local relapse and distant metastases (5,11,12,15).

External beam radiation therapy is almost never used after complete resection of ACC. Clinical reports describing a role of adjuvant radiotherapy appeared infrequently in older reports. Stewart et al. (12) recommended 15 to 30 Gy of whole abdomen irradiation, with shielding of the contralateral kidney and adrenal, as adjuvant therapy for resected tumors. They administered whole abdomen irradiation without chemotherapy to four children. There were three survivors, without recurrence of tumor, at 1 to 6 years. One of these children had unresectable tumor invading the inferior vena cava. She was free of tumor at reexploration after irradiation. Percarpio and Knowlton (16) gave preoperative irradiation to two adults with ACC (50 Gy, 45 Gy). Resection was possible in one patient. Four patients (three adults and one child) received postoperative irradiation for unresectable lesions or for tumor spillage. Three patients recurred in field in 2 to 34 months. One failed outside the field 11 years later. Bradley (1) administered adjuvant external beam radiotherapy to four adults (2,300 to 4,500 R). One patient is a long-term survivor 15 years after surgery. Magee et al. (13) described 15 patients, including five children, nine of whom had postoperative irradiation. Three of Magee's patients were girls who presented under the age of 2 years with hormonally active tumors and who survived for more than 10 years after gross total tumor resection and 30 Gy of postoperative irradiation in 4 weeks. Two of the three patients died of second malignancies arising in the irradiated field. Markoe et al. (17) reported 13 patients, including a 9-year-old girl. Local relapse was a common contributor to tumor relapse, and the authors argue that in some cases local irradiation (50 to 60 Gy) may have contributed to improved local control. Kasperlik-Zaluska et al. (18) gave postoperative irradiation to two patients who survived only 5 and 12 months. Zografos et al. (19) briefly mentioned giving radiotherapy to seven patients with inoperable tumors. The results were not explicitly stated. These data may be used to support the use of adjuvant radiotherapy for gross or microscopic residual disease after surgery. Although there is no clear evidence of radiotherapy's usefulness after a gross total tumor resection, an argument may be made for adjuvant irradiation in this situation in view of the poor overall survival

statistics, the lack of other adjuvant treatment options, and the aforementioned older reports (13). The second malignancies in Magee's series are chastening, however. Metastasis can be found in lung, liver, lymph nodes, bone, and brain (20). Palliation of bone pain or soft tissue masses has been achieved with 30 to 45 Gy in 2 to 6 weeks.

It is not clear whether adjuvant chemotherapy is useful after gross total resection of tumor (10,21). Many authorities believe that chemotherapy is clearly indicated for inoperable, recurrent, and metastatic disease (5,11,13,17,21). At one time mitotane was considered to be the drug of choice. The drug, an isomer of the insecticide DDD and a chemical congener of the insecticide DDT, has adrenolytic activity. Pooled data showed approximately a 35% response rate. The median duration of response is 6 to 7 months (4,6,21,22). Responses may be more common when high serum levels of the drug are achieved. The drug has significant toxicity including anorexia, nausea, vomiting, diarrhea, and central nervous system toxicity. There are some long-term survivors of metastatic adrenal cortical carcinoma treated with mitotane (8). Aminoglutethimide blocks adrenocortical hormone synthesis. It has been used to decrease signs and symptoms of Cushing's disease along with mitotane (4). In view of the unimpressive results with mitotane, it is not surprising that a large number of combination chemotherapy programs have been tried as adjuvant therapy and for metastatic disease. Programs that include etoposide, cisplatin, doxorubicin, and mitotane or etoposide, vincristine, doxorubicin, and mitotane have been studied (4,23–25).

The probability of survival of childhood ACC has been reported to range between 10% and 80% (7,11,12,26). The consensus is a 30–50% 5-year survival for patients who undergo complete resection of a localized tumor (22). This wide variation between institutions is certainly the result of case selection, quality of steroid management, and treatment policies. Factors predicting improved survival in resected tumors include resected tumors weighing 160 g or less, fewer than six mitotic figures per ten high-power fields, absence of histologic evidence of intratumor hemorrhage, venous, capsular, or adjacent organ invasion, and tumor necrosis (4,5,7).

Pheochromocytoma

Pheochromocytoma is a rare tumor of childhood. The tumors arise from the chromaffin cells in the sympathetic–adrenal system (27–29). In contrast to adults, children with pheochromocytoma have a higher incidence of bilaterality, a higher incidence of multiple endocrine neoplasia (MEN) syndromes, and a lower incidence of malignant neoplasms (27,30). The tumor is responsible for approximately 1% of cases of childhood nonessential hypertension, and it typically presents between 8 and 14 years of age (31,32). Familial pheochromocytoma is associated with other endocrine tumors in MEN syndromes (33). MEN type II includes familial pheochromocytoma or adrenal medullary hyperplasia, medullary thyroid cancer, and hyperparathyroidism. MEN type III includes pheochromocytoma or adrenal medullary hyperplasia, medullary thyroid cancer, mucosal neuromas, marfanoid habitus, thickened corneal nerves, ganglioneuromata of the alimentary tract, and, rarely, hyperparathyroidism (33).

Almost two-thirds of children with pheochromocytoma are boys. The most common presenting signs and symptoms in childhood include sustained hypertension (in contrast to adults, who usually have paroxysmal hypertension), diaphoresis, fever, nausea, weight loss, fatigue, and headache (27,28,31,34). Convulsions can also occur.

Adrenal medullary pheochromocytomas produce epinephrine and norepinephrine, whereas most extra-adrenal pheochromocytomas (about 10% of cases) produce only norepinephrine. Screening studies include urinary levels of epinephrine, norepinephrine, metanephrine, and vanillylmandelic acid (28,32,34). Preoperative tumor imaging is most often accomplished with ultrasound, CT, or MRI (28). Examination with iodine-131 metaiodobenzylguanidine (MIBG) scans may be of value in assessing tumor location. MIBG is concentrated in catecholamine-producing cells and therefore can be used to image pheochromocytoma and neuroblastoma (1). Children in families known to be at risk for pheochromocytoma can be screened with imaging and plasma or urine catecholamine and metanephrine measurements.

The definitive therapy for pheochromocytoma in childhood is surgical, generally transperitoneal adrenalectomy. There have also been reports of laparoscopic adrenalectomy (29). Preoperative and intraoperative adrenergic receptor blockade of catecholamine-induced receptor stimulation is necessary for successful resection. Phenoxybenzamine is the principal drug used (35,36). Other drugs such as phentolamine, prazosin, metyrosine, nifedipine, labetalol, nitroprusside, propranolol, α-methyl-tyrosine, and lidocaine have been used. During and after tumor resection, blood volume correction (i.e., normal saline, plasma, whole blood) and pressors may be necessary for variable periods of time to maintain the blood pressure (28,36,37).

Total tumor resection usually is curative (37). Recurrences may develop several years after initial surgery, usually are heralded by recurrent hypertension, and are cured by additional surgery (38).

About 10% of pheochromocytomas are malignant. They are characterized by diffuse local infiltration or distant metastases. Surgery remains the primary treatment (39). In some cases disease may be rendered resectable by adriamycin and cisplatin. External beam radiation therapy is effective for palliation of bone, lymph node, brain, and spinal cord metastases (40). High-dose ^{131}I MIBG has been tried for malignant tumors with only modest success (29,35). Palliation may last for years, and long-term survival is possible (30,38,39).

In a series of 14 patients with malignant pheochromocytoma, eight partially or completely responded for a median duration of 21 months to cyclophosphamide, vincristine, and dacarbazine (29,35).

Thyroid Carcinoma

Thyroid carcinoma represents 1–1.5% of childhood cancer (41–51). Sixty-five to 80% of the patients are female (44,45,52).

The types of thyroid cancer in children include the following:

- Papillary carcinoma (65–90% of childhood thyroid cancer). These lesions tend to be infiltrative and multicentric (45). Lymphatic metastases occur in about 60% of childhood cases (41,43). Hematogenous metastases occur, most commonly to the lungs in 10–20% of cases. A mixed papillary–follicular pattern is common in children and is included with the papillary classification (49).
- Follicular carcinoma (10–30%). No papillary elements are present in these tumors. Vascular invasion is common.
- Medullary carcinoma (2% or less). These tumors develop from neural crest parafollicular or C cells. Medullary carcinoma may arise as part of one of the MEN type IIa and IIb syndromes. The tumor is associated with an immunoreactive thyrocalcitonin marker. Missense mutations in the *ret* proto-oncogene on chromosome 10 are associated with MEN IIA and IIB. Medullary thyroid cancer is more aggressive than papillary or follicular cancer and can be fatal. For this reason, some authorities advocate genetic testing to identify children from at-risk families who will develop MEN IIA or IIIB and then perform prophylactic total thyroidectomy before the cancer spreads beyond the thyroid (44,45,53). Medullary thyroid carcinoma surveillance should begin by age 5 years in MEN type 2A and 6 months in type 2B. Unless MEN type 2 has been ruled out by *ret* testing, serum calcium and 24-hour excretion of metanephrine and catecholamines should be measured preoperatively to avoid inadvertently putting a child with hyperparathyroidism and pheochromocytoma under general anesthesia (54).
- Undifferentiated carcinoma (rare). The undifferentiated carcinoma may contain sheets of small cells with large dark nuclei, spindle cells, or giant cells. The prognosis of undifferentiated carcinoma is poor, with death usually occurring within 6 months of diagnosis (55).
- Insular carcinoma (very rare). The insular variant is a type of poorly differentiated cancer intermediate in clinical behavior and morphology between well-differentiated and anaplastic tumors. It is characterized by nests of tumor cells separated from surrounding cells by artifactual clefts. The tumor may behave aggressively (56).

The first sign of thyroid cancer in childhood is either a thyroid nodule or a palpable cervical node (46). If palpable and microscopic lymph node disease is included, then about 60% of children with papillary thyroid cancer have neck node metastases at presentation, a number significantly higher than the incidence in adults (46,49,57–59). Approximately 10–20% have distant metastases at presentation, most commonly lung (60,61). Most children with thyroid carcinoma are euthyroid. Conventional neck radiographs or xeroradiographs may show laminated thyroid calcifications. Such calcifications should raise the suspicion of the psammoma bodies of papillary carcinoma. Imaging with an iodine radionuclide is of greatest value. A cold area in the thyroid is highly suspicious for carcinoma (39,46). However, it is not possible to definitively distinguish malignant from benign thyroid nodules on clinical or imaging grounds. Fine-needle aspiration is being increasingly used in adolescents to evaluate thyroid nodules (44,62).

On April 26, 1986, operators at the Chernobyl Unit 4 Nuclear Power Plant in the Ukraine were doing a low-power engineering test. A succession of human and mechanical errors culminated in a series of explosions and a fire that lasted for 10 days and burned through the roof of the building containing the 1,000-MW water-cooled, graphite-moderated reactor. Approximately 40,000,000 to 50,000,000 Ci of ^{131}I was released into the atmosphere, a staggering number when compared with the 15 to 20 Ci released at the Three Mile Island accident in the United States. Measurements of cesium-137 exceeded 37 KB/qm^2 in Belarus, Ukraine, and areas of the Russian Federation. In addition, large amounts of radioisotopes of xenon, krypton, and strontium were also released (50,50a,63,64).

The incidence of childhood thyroid cancer in Belarus and Ukraine began to rise in 1989. Long-term studies continue to show an increase in childhood cancer. It is almost six times more common among children who received the highest estimated dosages (1 Gy or more) than among those who received the lowest dosage (less than 0.3 Gy) (Fig. 16-1) (50,63–68). Almost all the new cases in children are papillary tumors (94–98%).

Radiation-associated thyroid cancer in children exposed by the Chernobyl accident occurs disproportionately in children less than 5 years old at the time of exposure. The tumors are more aggressive, with a short latency between exposure and disease, and the patients had a lower female:male ratio than sporadic cases (66). Some of the cases of thyroid cancer may be explicable by chronic iodine deficiency in many of the contaminated areas before the accident. A thyroid deficient in iodine would have quickly taken up the radioactive isotopes (63,65).

Surgery is the principal treatment for childhood thyroid cancer (41,43,44,66,67,69–86). However, the extent of surgery for the primary tumor and

potentially involved lymph nodes is hotly debated. Depending on the situation, there are advocates of subtotal lobectomy, lobectomy and isthmusectomy, and total thyroidectomy (Table 16-1). For management of the cervical nodes there are advocates of node picking, advocates of modified and radical neck dissection, and advocates of no node operation. Underlying the surgical controversy is the extent to which subsequent radioactive iodine (RAI) therapy will sterilize residual tumor after surgery (46,57,68). Although we cannot do justice to the breadth of data brought to bear in the argument, we can address the outlines of the controversy. The arguments in favor of total thyroidectomy include the following:

- Papillary foci are in both thyroid lobes in 60–85% of patients.
- 5–10% of recurrences of papillary thyroid carcinoma after unilateral surgery are in the contralateral lobe.

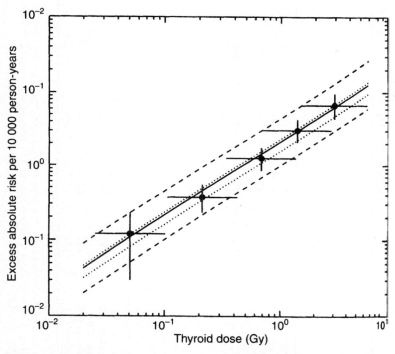

FIG 16-1. Childhood thyroid cancer incidence rates for 1991–1995 from cities and settlements in Belarus and Russia. (From Jacob P, Kenigsberg Y, Zvonova I, et al. Childhood exposure due to the Chernobyl accident and thyroid cancer risk in contaminated areas of Belarus and Russia. *Br J Cancer* 1999;80:1461–1469, with permission.)

TABLE 16-1. *Differentiated thyroid cancer in children from ten pediatric series*

	Jianping et al. (82)	Harness et al. (83)	Samuel and Sharma (314)	Zimmerman et al. (68)	La Quaglia et al. (86)	Ceccarelli et al. (85)	Schlumberger et al. (84)	Newman et al. (76)	Jarzab et al. (43)	Giuffrida et al. (41)
					Clinical Series					
No. of patients	14	89	314	58	100	49	72	329	109	48
Mean age (yr)	NA	12.8	NA	11.9	13.3	14.0	11	15.2	13.6	18.1
Female (%)	NA	81	66	69	71	69	71	76	69	71
Histology (%)										
Papillary	86	93	63	100	87	90	69	90	71	83
Follicular	14	7	32	0	7	8	29	10	29	17
Medullary	0	0	2	0	0	2	0	0	0	0
Other	0	0	3	0	6	0	0	0	0	0
Metastasis (%)	86	88	50	90	71	73	75	74	75	52
Surgical Procedure (%)										
Total thyroidectomy	93	89	83[a]	36	46[a]	0	40	54	74	NA
Subtotal thyroidectomy	7	11		63		100		46	26	NA
Subtotal lobectomy							60			
Other subtotal lymph node procedure		84	NA	84	89	73	83	78	NA	100
Percentage receiving radioactive iodine	NA	82	71	17	22	98	42	43	64	NA
Median follow-up (yr)	6	NA	11	28	20	7.7	13	11.3	5	6.1
Cancer mortality (%)	0	2.2	NA	3.4	0	2.0	17	0.7	0	0

NA, data not available.

[a] In these studies, the children who had a total or near-total thyroidectomy were not subgrouped.

Expanded and modified from a table in Skinner MA. Cancer of the thyroid in infants and children. *Semin Pediatr Surg* 2001;10:119–126.

- RAI is more useful after total thyroidectomy.
- Serum thyroglobulin is a more useful tumor marker with the prior resection of as much thyroid tissue as possible (54).

Arguments for a unilateral procedure include

- Absence of a substantial survival benefit with extensive surgery
- A lower risk of hypoparathyroidism with less extensive surgery
- A lower risk of laryngeal nerve injury after less extensive surgery (41,44,49,54,59,61)

In large-scale retrospective analyses, the 20-year tumor recurrence rate is lower after total thyroidectomy than lobectomy (54). Disease-free survival probably is improved by total thyroidectomy, although overall survival is not (41,43). Several consensus guidelines favor total thyroidectomy. It is appropriate

- If the primary papillary carcinoma is 1 cm in diameter or larger
- If the tumor extends beyond the thyroid
- If there are metastases
- If there is a primary history of exposure to ionizing radiation of the head and neck in view of the increased role of multicentrality and the high rate of tumor recurrence associated with subtotal thyroidectomy (54)

Because there is a high incidence of pulmonary metastases in children, total thyroidectomy allows early detection of occult metastases with RAI scan (44).

Unilateral lobectomy might be sufficient for

- Papillary carcinoma less than 1 cm in diameter
- Tumor confined to one lobe of the gland (54)

For follicular thyroid carcinoma, the absence of multicentric disease is an argument against bilateral thyroidectomy, but most consensus guidelines recommend total thyroidectomy to allow subsequent RAI. In view of the high frequency of multifocal intrathyroidal disease, locoregional spread, and extracervical metastases in children, total thyroidectomy, nodal dissection, adjuvant RAI, and lifelong surveillance are recommended (54).

Most surgeons would support removal of adjacent, grossly involved nodes at the time of surgery for the primary tumor. Opponents of carrying the node surgery to the extent of a radical neck dissection point out that the type of lymphatic dissection does not predict the risk of tumor recurrence and the efficacy of RAI in controlling metastatic disease from well-differentiated thyroid cancer (49).

Well-differentiated thyroid cancers usually are hormone dependent. The suppression of thyroid-stimulating hormone (TSH) by the administration of exogenous thyroid hormone (TH) is indicated because it decreases the probability of tumor recurrence in higher-risk patients (46, 53,62). Exogenous thyroid hormone also ensures that the child remains euthyroid regardless of the extent of the thyroidectomy. Serum TH is maintained in the upper third of normal range, and TSH is suppressed toward the lower range of normal. The risks of properly supervised long-term administration of TH in children are debatable (27). Several studies have suggested that long-term TSH suppression below the lower range of normal may decrease bone mineral density in children (53,62).

RAI is taken up by 50–80% of well-differentiated thyroid tumors but is taken up by few poorly differentiated malignancies. RAI has the potential to deliver extremely high focal dosages of irradiation to ablate thyroid tissue remaining after surgery and to treat neck nodes or distant metastases. RAI also delivers a small dosage of whole-body irradiation. Bone marrow depression is uncommon unless bone metastases are present. Pulmonary fibrosis occurs occasionally when RAI is repeatedly administered for pulmonary metastases. Parotiditis and sialadenitis, nausea, glossalgia, hypogeusia, gastrointestinal discomfort, and thyroiditis rarely occur (41,69, 70). Potential long-term complications of RAI have been alleged, with varying degrees of supporting evidence. These include leukemia, myelosuppression, bladder cancer, salivary cancer, gastric cancer, breast cancer, and infertility. These risks may be attributable to the reported use, in the past, of high, repetitive dosages of RAI.

Controversy also surrounds certain aspects of the use of RAI after surgery for childhood thyroid cancer. There is little question about the necessity of postsurgical ablation of iodine-131 concentrating tissue in the thyroid bed in the presence of nodal or distant metastatic disease. One wants to eliminate thyroid tissue that will concentrate iodine-131 so that, subsequently, one can use iodine-131 therapeutically against the metastases. However, there is much uncertainty over the use of RAI for the routine ablation of remaining thyroid tissue in patients with well-differentiated thyroid cancer who are not thought to have metastatic disease (69,71). In the occasional pediatric patient with a small papillary carcinoma treated by lobectomy, RAI may not be indicated (62). In the more common forms of childhood differentiated thyroid cancer, many argue that RAI is necessary to treat multifocal disease. It is debatable whether RAI will reduce the risk of local tumor failure in postoperative patients treated with TH suppression (49,60,71). Some studies argue it does (43,72). At present, because of the high incidence of nodal and distant metastases in childhood thyroid cancer, many authorities favor routine RAI thyroid ablation, and it is frequently done (41,57,73).

Although most studies show that children with well-differentiated thyroid cancer have, on average, larger tumors, more extensive local invasion, and more nodal and distant metastases than adults, these young patients have an excellent prognosis. Cancer-related deaths, particularly from papillary carcinoma, are rare (41,74). Survival rates for children with thyroid cancer do not differ significantly from those for age-matched population controls at 20, 25, and 30 years (41,44,68). There have been no tumor-induced deaths among 100 children in the Memorial Hospital series (median follow-up 20 years), although 35% had tumor recurrence after initial surgery (49). There is a tumor recurrence rate of 0–39% and a risk of death from disease of 0–17% (Table 16-1, Fig. 16-2) (60,82–85).

There is very little place for external beam radiotherapy to the neck in the local treatment of childhood thyroid cancer. It may be used in the rare instance of locally unresectable tumor that does not take up RAI or is so bulky that RAI would not be able to control it. Neck or mediastinal recurrences of tumors that are bulky or do not take up RAI may also be externally irra-

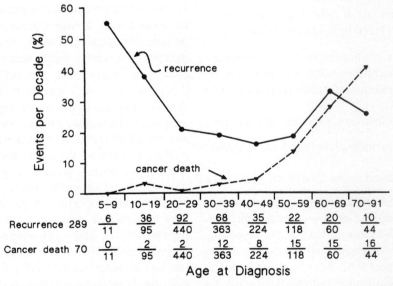

FIG. 16-2. Tumor recurrence and death rates in patients with differentiated thyroid carcinoma as a function of age at diagnosis. It is interesting to note that children and adolescents tend to have more advanced differentiated thyroid carcinoma at presentation than adults, yet they have a higher survival probability. (From Mazzaferri EL, Jhiang SM. Long-term impact of initial surgical and medical therapy on papillary and follicular thyroid cancer. *Am J Med* 1994;97:418–428, with permission.)

diated (48,75–78). Adjuvant external beam radiotherapy might be effective in prevention of locoregional recurrence in patients more than 45 years old with locally invasive papillary carcinoma (54). A retrospective review of 91 patients with locally advanced papillary thyroid cancer, which included some adolescents, found that in T4 disease locoregional control was improved by postoperative external beam irradiation (median dosage 61.2 Gy, spinal cord shielded at 40 Gy). Half of the patients receiving external beam irradiation also were treated with RAI (79). A minimum tumor dosage of 55 Gy is administered with an anterior photon field, anterior photons plus electrons, or weighted anterior and posterior parallel opposed fields with appropriate spinal blocking. The treatment volume encompasses the neck and upper mediastinum. Gross disease in the neck is not hopeless and may be cured by external beam radiotherapy (80). In adults, adjuvant external beam radiation to the neck sometimes is considered in patients with extensive extrathyroid invasion or microscopic residual disease; this view is based on a few retrospective reviews (80). Bone or soft tissue metastases that are not suitable for RAI or do not respond to it may be treated effectively with conventional external beam dosages. In the extremely rare situations in which chemotherapy is considered, adriamycin and paclitaxel have been used (81).

AERODIGESTIVE TRACT

Juvenile Nasopharyngeal Angiofibroma

Juvenile nasopharyngeal angiofibroma (JNA) is a rare tumor that is far more common in boys than in girls (87–95). Various theories have been proposed to explain the origin of these lesions. Because they are most common in male adolescents, a hormonal target has been suggested. Other theories include a desmoplastic response of nasopharyngeal periosteum to an ectopic nidus of vascular tissue, an origin from embryologic chondrocartilage, an origin from nonchromaffin paraganglionic cells, and a proposed role of growth factors including tissue growth factor β-1, platelet-derived growth factor B, and insulin-like growth factor type II (94,96).

The average age at clinical presentation for JNA is 14–16 years (97–99). Arising from the nasopharynx, the lesion may extend to the nasal cavities, the maxillary and sphenoid sinuses, the orbit, the anterior or middle cranial fossae, the infratemporal region, or the pterygopalatine fossa. The lesion is thought to arise from the vascular structures of the basisphenoid region, particularly in the region of the sphenopalatine foramen (99). The histologic appearance of the tumor is characteristic: numerous thin-walled vessels, lined by endothelium and devoid of a complete muscular layer, with interspersed fibroblasts and collagen (Fig. 16-3). Presenting signs and symptoms include recurrent epistaxis, nasal obstruction, cheek swelling, facial deformity, proptosis, hearing loss, dysphagia, headache, mouth breathing, and cranial nerve palsies (94,100,101).

JNAs are firm, red masses. Superimposed infection may produce secondary surface ulcerations. Axial, coronal, and sagittal CT and MRI are invaluable in demonstrating tumor extent (Fig. 16-4) (88,102,103). A typical CT pattern of JNA is a contrast-enhancing nasopharyngeal mass with widening of the pterygopalatine fossa. One can also see erosion of the roof of the medial pterygoid plate or indentation of the posterior wall of the maxillary sinus (Holman–Miller sign) (89). In a series from India, erosion of the sphenoid sinus was detected in 86% of cases by CT, and erosion of the maxillary sinus and extension into the oropharynx was present in 27% (101). The vascular supply may be from the internal maxillary, accessory meningeal, ascending pharyngeal, or ascending palatine arteries. In cases of intracranial extension, blood supply may come from branches of the internal carotid artery including the mandibulovidian and cavernous arteries (99,104–106). During angiography a characteristic reticulated pattern is seen in the arterial phase, with a subsequent dense blush persisting in the venous phase (88).

The definitive therapies for JNA are surgery and external beam radiotherapy. Chemotherapy with doxorubicin and dacarbazine or vincristine, actinomycin, and cyclophosphamide has been used for recurrent lesions that are not amenable to

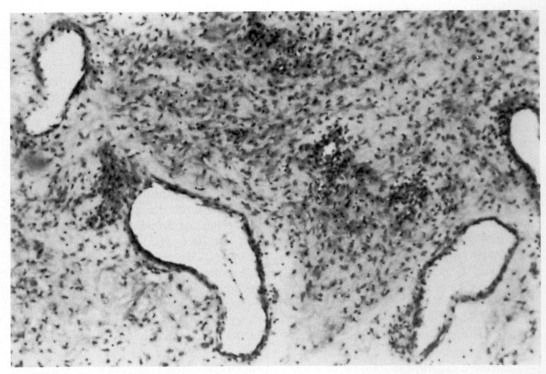

FIG. 16-3. Juvenile nasopharyngeal angiofibroma with vessels devoid of a complete muscle layer. (From Ozkaynak MF, Ortega JA, Laug W, et al. Role of chemotherapy in pediatric pulmonary blastoma. *Med Pediatr Oncol* 1990;18:53–56, with permission.)

additional surgery or irradiation with some success (89,107). Antiangiogenesis agents have been considered, but to date there is no substantial body of published reports. Other treatments include packings until the tumor undergoes spontaneous regression (a rare occurrence), cryotherapy, electrocoagulation, embolization, and implantation of radioisotopes (97,98,102,107–128a). Rather than being competitive, surgery and radiotherapy have complementary roles in the management of JNA. As is often the case, proper patient selection is the key. A wide variety of systems of staging and classification have been proposed by many centers (Table 16-2) (87,106,116,117,128,128a). All systems recognize that local infiltration of JNA, particularly into the infratemporal region or within the cranial vault, makes definitive surgery more difficult and dangerous.

The treatment of smaller JNA is generally accepted to be surgical (120). There are several surgical approaches, including transpalatal, lateral rhinotomy, and craniofacial resection with an infratemporal approach (89,106,129). In recent years several centers have reported endoscopic resection (93,121). Operative blood loss may be as high as 3,000 mL. Preoperative hormone therapy and embolization may be useful preoperative adjuvants to minimize blood loss. The fact that JNAs are far more common in boys than in girls led to the hypothesis that the tumors were related to some imbalance in the pituitary adrenogenital system. Some surgeons believe hormone therapy to be useful in an attempt, preoperatively, to decrease tumor vascularity. However, others have not been impressed (91). Preoperative arterioembolization with particles (i.e., gelatin foam or dura mater) or balloons carried out 1–2 days before surgery has been claimed to significantly reduce operative blood loss (104). However, a recent review from Sweden found no significant

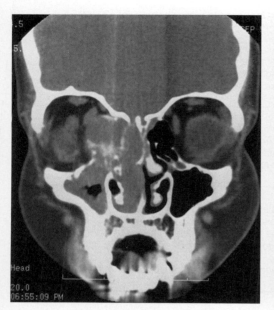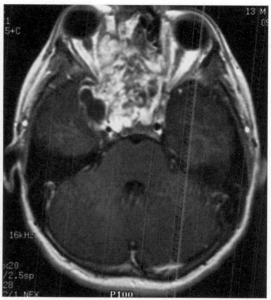

FIG. 16-4. Coronal computed tomography *(left)* and axial magnetic resonance imaging (MRI) *(right)* of a 13-year-old boy with headaches, diplopia, and right proptosis. The mass produced destruction of the ethmoid air cells and superior turbinates, mass effect in the right orbit, compression of the right cavernous sinus, displacement of the right internal carotid artery, and displacement of the pituitary. A biopsy proved the diagnosis of juvenile nasopharyngeal angiofibroma. Three-dimensional treatment planning was used to prepare a four-field noncoplanar external beam radiotherapy treatment technique using rigid head immobilization. A dosage of 36 Gy at 2 Gy per fraction was administered. One and one-half years after irradiation the symptoms had significantly improved and the mass was smaller on physical examination and MRI. Shortly thereafter the symptoms recurred and the MRI demonstrated regrowth of the angiofibroma, within and outside the irradiated field. Interferon was administered as an antiangiogenesis agent.

decrease in blood loss with embolization (122). With adequate operative exposure and resection, 70–100% of patients need no additional treatment beyond surgery (87,89,99,108).

Intracranial, orbital, or pterygopalatine extension of JNA increases the risks of resection (116,120). Some surgeons still favor surgery because of concerns related to the risk of second malignant neoplasms, neuroendocrine dysfunction, bone and soft tissue damage, and cataract formation (91,122). However, many others feel that external beam radiotherapy is best used for the definitive treatment of these advanced cases. This is particularly true for patients in whom disease recurs after surgery (Fig. 16-5). Many of the ill effects attributed to external beam irradiation for JNA occurred in patients treated with higher dosages than are used currently or in patients irra-

diated more than once (95). Parallel opposed lateral field treatment or two lateral fields with an anterior field usually were found to be adequate in the era before three-dimensional treatment planning. In modern practice these patients are immobilized in a head holder and planned with multifield conformal and intensity-modulated techniques. Inadequate treatment fields are a major course of failure of local control of JNA by irradiation (123). If marginal misses are to be avoided, proper mapping of the tumor volume is crucial, including the intracranial extensions. The pertinent studies (CT, MRI, and angiography) must be reviewed with care to establish the treatment volume.

From 30 to 55 Gy of external beam radiation has been used at 1.8–2 Gy per fraction for 3–5 weeks. Economou et al. (109) and McGahan et

TABLE 16-2. *Six proposed staging systems for juvenile nasopharyngeal angiofibroma*

Chandler et al. (160) and Jacobsson et al. (106)	
Stage I	Tumor confined to nasopharynx.
Stage II	Extension into nasal cavity or sphenoid sinus.
Stage III	Extension into one or more of the following: antrum, ethmoid sinuses, pterygomaxillary and infratemporal fossae, orbit, or cheek.
Stage IV	Intracranial extension.
Fields et al. (87)	
Stage I	Tumor confined to nasopharynx or nasal fossae.
Stage II	Extending into the sphenoid sinus or pterygomaxillary fossae.
Stage III	Extending beyond stage II limits into maxillary sinus, ethmoid sinuses, orbits, infratemporal fossae, cheeks, or palate.
Stage IV	Intracranial extension.
Sessions et al. (117)	
Stage IA	Limited to posterior nares or nasopharynx.
Stage IB	Extension into one or more paranasal sinuses.
Stage IIA	Minimal spread into pterygopalatine fossa.
Stage IIB	Occupation of the pterygopalatine fossa displacing posterior maxillary wall; possibly erosion into orbit.
Stage IIC	Extension through pterygopalatine fossa into infratemporal fossa or cheek.
Stage III	Intracranial extension.
Andrews et al. (114)	
Type I	Tumor limited to the nasopharynx and nasal cavity. Bone destruction negligible or limited to the sphenopalatine foramen.
Type II	Tumor invading the pterygopalatine fossa or the maxillary, ethmoid, or sphenoid sinus with bone destruction.
Type IIIa	Tumor invading the infratemporal fossa or orbital region without intracranial involvement.
Type IIIb	Tumor invading the infratemporal fossa or orbit with intracranial extradural (parasellar) involvement.
Type IVa	Intracranial intradural tumor without infiltration of the cavernous sinus, pituitary fossa, or optic chiasm.
Type IVb	Intracranial intradural tumor with infiltration of the cavernous sinus, pituitary fossa, or optic chiasm.
Fisch (118, 129)	
Type I	Tumor limited to the nasopharynx and nasal cavity with no bone destruction.
Type II	Tumor invading the pterygomaxillary fossa, maxillary, ethmoid, and sphenoid sinus with bone destruction.
Type III	Tumors invading the infratemporal fossa, orbit, and parasellar region remaining lateral to the cavernous sinus.
Type IV	Tumor with massive invasion of the cavernous sinus, optic chiasm region, or pituitary fossa.
Radkowski et al. (119)	
Type IA, IB, IIA, IIB	Same as the system of Sessions et al.
Type IIC	As in Sessions et al. or posterior to pterygoid plates.
Type IIIA	As in Sessions et al., erosion of skull base, minimal intracranial.
Type IIIB	As in Sessions et al., erosion of skull base, extensive intracranial with or without cavernous sinus.

al. (128) have argued, based on retrospective data, that dosages of 32–36 Gy are necessary. However, others do not support this view and have achieved good results with 30 Gy. Most of the available data support a total dosage of 30–36 Gy with excellent results (Table 16-3).

An interesting multimodality report by Rao et al. (101) describes 19 boys with JNA. All re-ceived 20–30 Gy of irradiation, estrogen therapy, and then resection with preoperative embolization and temporary external carotid artery ligation. The authors report better regression of the tumor at the time of surgery with 30 Gy than with 20–22.5 Gy.

Intracavitary irradiation has been used rarely (109). Such treatment runs the obvious risks of

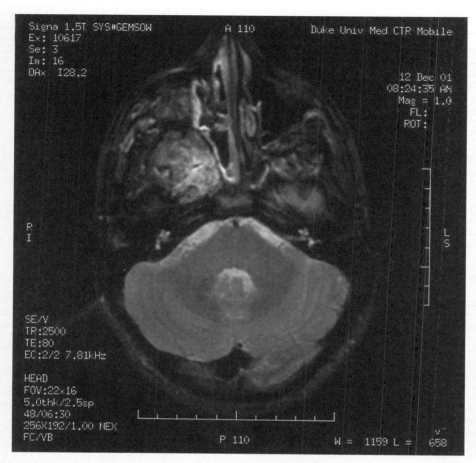

FIG. 16-5. A 14-year-old boy presented to the radiation oncology department after multiple surgical and embolization procedures intended to remove and devascularize a juvenile nasopharyngeal angiofibroma. Detailed three-dimensional mapping of the tumor was performed using magnetic resonance imaging accompanied by careful fiberoptic examination. The mass was treated, with a margin, with a mixture of 6- and 15-MV photons to a cumulative dosage of 40 Gy. Over the subsequent 2 years, striking regression of the mass was seen. Before radiotherapy, the child had been subjected to repeated episodes of bleeding, which ceased after radiotherapy.

major bleeding and inadequate coverage of the treatment volume (123).

Nasopharyngeal Carcinoma

Many of the principles established in adult head and neck oncology apply to childhood nasopharyngeal carcinoma (NPC). However, it would be a mistake to treat children with this tumor by uncritically following the guidelines applicable to adults. Childhood NPC is distinguished from the adult form by certain peculiar features: a close association with Epstein–Barr virus infection, undifferentiated histology, and high incidence of advanced locoregional disease (130).

Two percent to 20% of NPCs occur in people less than 30 years old. In general, NPC represents less than 1% of all childhood malignant tumors but constitutes 20–50% of pediatric malignancies of the nasopharynx (131,132). NPC constitutes a higher proportion of childhood cancer in Asia or Africa than North or South America or Europe. In the United States it may be more common in African Americans than Caucasians (133).

TABLE 16-3. *Radiotherapy for juvenile nasopharyngeal angiofibroma*

Reference	Year of report	Number of cases	Dosage range	Local control	Follow-up
Apostol and Frazell (108)	1965	9	3,000–3,600 rad[a]	6/9 (67%)[b]	1–12 yr
Briant et al. (97)	1970[c]	22	30 Gy	17/22 (77%)[d]	1–<3 yr
Jereb et al. (111)	1970	66	2,000–6,000 rad[a]	>80% ("minimal")	1–<40 yr
Ward et al. (116)	1974	4	3,000 rad[a]	response "left much to be desired"	
		2	45–55 Gy	2/2 (100%)	1–2 yr
Briant et al. (98)	1978[c]	45	30–35 Gy	35/45 (78%)[e]	2–20 yr
Sinha and Aziz (124)	1978	7	30–36 Gy	6/7 (86%)	8–26 yr
Cummings et al. (123)	1984[c]	40	30 Gy	32/40 (80%)[e]	3–26 yr
		15	35 Gy	12/15 (80%)[e]	
Mannai and Schwartz (126)	1986	1	35 Gy	1/1 (100%)	1 yr
Benghait (102)	1986	1	30 Gy	1/1 (100%)	9 mo
Harrison (127)	1987	2	40 Gy	2/2 (100%)	1 yr
Economou et al. (109)	1988	3	<36 Gy	0/3 (0%)	1–25 yr
		11	>36 Gy	11/11 (100%)	
Cuyler (120)	1988	1	36–84 cGy	1/1 (100%)	1 yr
McGahan et al. (128)	1989	4	32 Gy	0/4 (0%)	1–14 yr
		10	36–46 Gy	10/10 (100%)	
Robinson et al. (100)	1989	10	30–40 Gy	9/10 (90%)	8–141 mo
Fields et al. (87)	1990	13[f]	35–52 Gy	11/13 (85%)	29–255 mo
Gullane et al. (125)	1992	7	30–35 Gy	3/7 (42%)	7–10 yr
Kasper et al. (103)	1993	9[f]	30–35 Gy	9/9 (100%)	3–15 yr
Wiatrak et al. (298)	1993	3	36–50.4 Gy	3/3 (100%)	1.7–4.5 yr
Ungkanont et al. (89)	1996	2	35–45 Gy	1/2 (50%)	
Reddy et al. (92)	2001	15	30–35 Gy	13/15 (85%)	2.5–24 yr
Lee et al. (95)	2002	27	30–55 Gy	23/27 (85%)	3–42 yr

[a]It is not clear whether dosages are reported in roentgens or rads. In the Jereb series, some patients received brachytherapy.
[b]Some of the failures may have died of complications while the angiofibroma was controlled.
[c]These series include many of the same patients.
[d]The local control rate is not clear.
[e]Many of the failures were salvaged by additional irradiation or surgery.
[f]Some of these patients had relapses after surgery rather than primary radiotherapy.

The median age of onset in children is 13 years (130). In most series there are more boys than girls (133–141).

It was noted early in this century that the disease is common among Chinese living in China (137). For example, Hong Kong has a very high incidence of NPC (140). Among Chinese living outside China, NPC is less common, although still greater than in a comparable non-Chinese population. These observations suggest that both genetic and environmental factors are important in the development of this neoplasm (141,142). Elevated anti–Epstein–Barr virus (EBV) antibody titers have been found in patients with NPC, and childhood cases of NPC seem to have a closer association with EBV than adults (143). There appears to be a correlation of titer levels with stage at presentation. Measure-

ment of EBV titers during and after treatment is a good indicator of disease activity. Treated patients with no evidence of recurrence have low titers. *In situ* hybridization studies by Hawkins et al. (144) showed EBV in 9 of 11 children; the virus was in the neoplastic epithelial cells but not the lymphocytes. Similar studies by Zubizarieta et al. (145) demonstrated EBV in eight of eight children.

NPC constitutes 20–50% of all primary nasopharyngeal malignant tumors in children. The World Health Organization (WHO) has classified NPC as follows: WHO-1, well to moderately differentiated squamous, including transitional carcinoma with obvious keratin production; WHO-2, nonkeratinizing carcinoma; and WHO-3, undifferentiated carcinoma including lymphoepithelioma with anaplastic, clear

TABLE 16-4. *Staging system for carcinoma of the nasopharynx*

Primary Tumor

Tis	Carcinoma in situ
T1	Tumor confined to the nasopharynx
T2	Tumor extends to soft tissues
T2a	Tumor extends to the oropharynx or nasal cavity without parapharyngeal extension[a]
T2b	Any tumor with parapharyngeal extension[a]
T3	Tumor involves bony structures or paranasal sinuses
T4	Tumor with intracranial extension or involvement of cranial nerves, intratemporal fossa, hypopharynx, orbit, or masticator space

Nodes

N0	No regional lymph node metastases
N1	Unilateral metastasis in lymph node 6 cm or less in greatest dimension, above the supraclavicular fossa
N2	Bilateral metastasis in lymph nodes, 6 cm or less, above the supraclavicular fossa
N3	Metastasis in a lymph nodes >6 cm or to supraclavicular fossa

Distant Metastases

N3a	>6 cm in dimension
N3b	Extension to supraclavicular fossa
MX	Distant metastases cannot be assessed
M0	No distant metastases
M1	Distant metastases

Stage

0	TisN0M0
I	T1N0M0
IA	T2aN0M0
IIB	T1N0IM0, T2NIM0, T2aNIM0, T2bN0M0, T2bNIM0
III	T1N2M0, T2a–2bN2M0, T3N0–1M0
IVA	T4N0–2M0
IVB	T1–4N3M0
IVC	T1–4N0–3MI

[a]Parapharyngeal extension = posterolateral infiltration of tumor beyond the pharyngobasilar fascia.

From Greene FL, Page DL, Fleming ID, et al., eds. *AJCC Cancer Staging Manual*, 6th ed. Heidelberg: Springer, 2002.

cell, and spindle cell variants (Table 16-4) (132,146). Lymphoepithelioma is characterized by a syncytium of malignant epithelial cells with penetration of the tumor mosaic by lymphocytes. The neoplastic element is epithelial, not lymphocytic (142,147). Most cases of childhood NPC are undifferentiated epidermoid carcinoma (147,148).

The most common symptoms in 50 patients less than 16 years old with NPC, evaluated at the University of Istanbul, were neck swelling (70–90%); nasal obstruction, bleeding, or discharge (60–70%); auditory symptoms (40–45%); headache (32%); and neurological symptoms (26%) (Table 16-5). A group of children evaluated in Buenos Aires, Argentina, presented with node swelling (100%), epistaxis (54%), headache (36%), trismus (36%), and otalgia (27%).

The clinical examination discloses cervical lymphadenopathy, a nasopharyngeal mass, or cranial nerve palsies (130,141,145,149). Metastases to the neck nodes often are bilateral. The route of spread is most commonly to the digastric region and to the anterior and middle cervical nodes of the anterior cervical triangle (Fig. 16-6).

The appropriate diagnostic workup includes cranial CT or MRI to assess local tumor extent and base of skull involvement and an evaluation for distant metastases with chest radiograph and bone scan. CT and MRI often demonstrate mucosal thickening of the maxillary antra. This is generally the result of postobstruction inflammation rather than tumor extension (108). In recent years, positron emission tomography scans have been used to assess the primary tumor and questionable neck nodes. The American Joint Committee for Cancer (AJCC) staging system is generally

TABLE 16-5. *Distribution of histologic subtypes in childhood nasopharyngeal carcinoma*

		WHO-1	WHO-2	WHO-3
Well to moderately nonkeratinizing undifferentiated Differentiated squamous including lymphoepithelioma				
Institution	N			
Ibd Rochd Cancer Center Casablanca, Morocco (136)	65	[a]	[a]	81%
Oncology Hospital, Ankara (135)	33	3%	24%	64%
University of Istanbul, Turkey (134)	32	3%	47%	50%
Memorial Sloan–Kettering, New York (152)	33	0%	27%	73%

[a]WHO 1 + 2 = 19%.

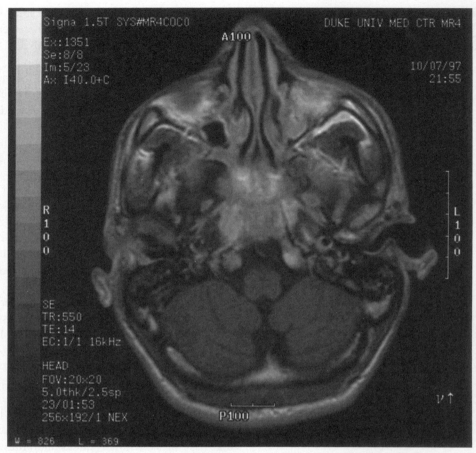

FIG. 16-6. A 17-year-old African American boy presented to medical attention with hearing loss and nasal congestion. He eventually developed headaches and neck swelling. CT and MRI studies showed a large mass involving the nasopharynx. There were bilateral enlarged jugulodigastric lymph nodes. A biopsy made the diagnosis of undifferentiated nasopharyngeal carcinoma. The tumor cells were surrounded by lymphocytic infiltrate, which was consistent with the diagnosis of lymphoepithelioma. Immunostains with keratin were positive in the tumor cells. The patient was treated with a combined program of chemotherapy and twice-daily irradiation. Progressive cone-down techniques were used to treat the primary tumor to 70.8 Gy at 1.2 Gy twice daily. The enlarged lymph nodes were treated to 56.8 Gy and regressed completely. Concurrent 5-fluorouracil and cisplatinum were administered. The patient was without evidence of persistent or recurrent carcinoma 5 years after completion of radiotherapy.

used for NPC (Table 16-4), although some Asian authorities prefer the classification proposed by Ho (101). Almost all children have AJCC stage III or IV disease at presentation, and fewer than 20% have stage I or II: Memorial Sloan–Kettering Cancer Center, 49% stage III, 39% stage IV; Medical College of Georgia, 100% stage IV; Northern Israel Oncology Center, 20% stage III, 80% stage IV; University of Istanbul, 87.5% stage IV (130–131,150–152).

Surgical therapy of the primary tumor is limited to biopsy (153). Tumors of this region are generally regarded as unresectable. The initial diagnostic biopsy may also be obtained from a neck node. Surgical treatment of the neck with a radical neck dissection is appropriate if the primary tumor appears to be controlled and there are persistent neck nodes after neck irradiation, or if tumor recurs in the neck after definitive radiotherapy (153). Many clinicians use planned excision of bulky nodes after an initial treatment with irradiation and chemotherapy. This philosophy is predicated on the view that large aggregates of tumor are unlikely to be controlled by tolerable dosages of cytotoxic therapy alone.

Radiation therapy is the principal management of the primary tumor and neck disease. In preparation for radiotherapy, dental evaluation and a vigorous program of dental prophylaxis are necessary. Because portions of the hypothalamic pituitary axis often are irradiated, baseline neuroendocrine testing is performed. The inclusion of portions of the auditory apparatus in the beam and the common use of cisplatin argue for baseline audiograms.

Precision external beam radiotherapy for childhood NPC calls for a customized face mask stabilization device. A bite block should be considered to move part of the tongue and floor of the mouth away from the beam. The anatomy of the primary tumor volume is established by physical examination and diagnostic imaging studies. At a minimum, the anatomic limits of the nasopharynx are irradiated with a margin. The anatomy of the nasopharynx, pertinent to the design of an external radiotherapy field, is precisely detailed by Wang:

> Anatomically, the nasopharynx is a cubical chamber that has four walls. The superior and posterior walls are bordered by the base of the skull and floor of the sphenoid sinus, sloping downward continuously to the second cervical vertebra at the level of the uvula. The lateral walls are perforated by the cartilaginous portion of the eustachian tube, which enters the nasopharynx through the sinus of Morgagni. The latter is a gap between the uppermost fibers of the superior pharyngeal constrictor muscle and the base of the skull. The gap is closed by a fascia known as the pharyngobasilar fascia, which is attached to the base of the skull superiorly and passes inferiorly deep to the constrictor muscles. The raised anterior portion of the cartilaginous portion of the eustachian tube is termed the torus tubarius, lying posteriorly to the eustachian tube orifice. The lateral nasopharyngeal recess or the fossa of Rosenmüller lies posterosuperiorly to the torus. The inferior wall of the nasopharynx is the dorsal surface of the soft palate and its posterior portion opens into the oropharynx at the isthmus.

The nasopharyngeal structures are supported by the pharyngobasilar fascia, which is continuous with the foramen lacerum and in close proximity with the eustachian tube and foramina in the base of the skull, including the ovale, spinosum, carotid, jugular, and hypoglossal, which provide routes of direct tumor intracranial extension and access to the carotid canal, middle ear, and petro-occipital suture. Other routes of tumor spread may occur into the nasal cavity anteriorly and the oropharynx posteriorly (146).

Conventional simulation is facilitated by the use of radiopaque markers on palpable neck nodes and the fleshy outer canthi of the eyes. Younger children express concern about having lead wires taped to the skin or near the eyes. This is readily dealt with by calm reassurance and demonstration of the technique on a parent or other adult. NPC external beam irradiation is generally thought to be significantly improved by three-dimensional treatment planning for conformal and intensity-modulated irradiation (Fig. 16-7). The tumor volume is mapped out using CT or MRI, and forward or inverse treatment planning is brought to bear in creating multiple beams and blocks. Minimization of dosage to the optic pathway and hypothalamic–pituitary axis is sought. Generally, three to six fields to the primary site are accompanied by neck treatment fields.

The incidence of neck node disease at presentation is 80–90%; 50% of cases have bilateral neck involvement (132). Because node disease is so common, radiotherapy is always directed to the primary tumor site and the neck, even if the neck is clinically free of disease.

The nature of the radiation dose–response relationship for NPC in children is debatable (154), particularly in light of the growing use of chemotherapy. Some retrospective reviews support a dosage to the primary tumor of 60–65 Gy, whereas others have failed to show an association between dosage and improved local control (134,136,152). In general, if conventional 1.8- to 2-Gy per day fractionation is used, 40–50 Gy is delivered to the primary tumor and the upper neck. The clinically uninvolved low anterior neck and paraclavicular region receives 45–50 Gy. The field then excludes the spinal cord, and

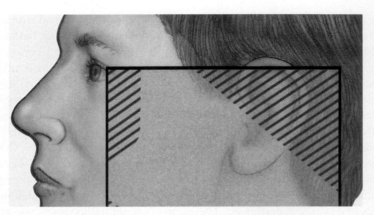

FIG. 16-7. A schematic of a traditional lateral field for irradiation of nasopharyngeal carcinoma in an adolescent. Increasingly, physicians are using three-dimensionally planned conformal fields for all or part of the external beam treatment.

with boost fields, an additional 10 to 25 Gy is given to the primary tumor and palpable nodes (139,155). Some clinicians use a cesium-137 brachytherapy application in an ovoid or a pediatric endotracheal tube for a single application final boost of 5 to 9 Gy to the primary site. Others use a remote afterloading Ir-192 brachytherapy machine and fractionate the boost (134). Bulky neck nodes are boosted with photons or electrons. The final total dosage to the primary tumor is 50 to 72 Gy (143). The spinal cord dosage is limited to 50 Gy or less, the brainstem to 55 Gy or less, and the optic chiasm to 55 Gy or less. Involved neck nodes receive a similar dosage to the primary tumor, although, as previously noted, many physicians prefer surgical resection to high-dose boosting of neck nodes (137,149,156–159). With dosages of this size, local tumor control of childhood NPC is excellent (140,143). However, the radiotherapist is well advised not to be complacent. Inadequate attention to tumor volume mapping and insufficient attention to field and block design in this complex anatomic area can lead to tumor relapse caused by a marginal miss (143). On occasion, the patient with local relapse can be salvaged with reirradiation.

In an attempt to capitalize on the apparent benefits of multiple-fraction-per-day (MFD) irradiation, some clinicians treat adults with advanced NPC with two or three fractions per day irradiation. Many authorities on adult radiother-

apy consider MFD irradiation the standard of care for advanced NPC, and growing body of prospective clinical trials supports this view (160). In the twice-daily technique, 1.2 to 1.6 Gy per fraction is used. The possibility must be considered that MFD irradiation may provide good local control for childhood NPC with diminution in undesirable late effects. This hypothesis may warrant testing in pilot studies in children.

In Table 16-6, we summarize the results of treatment of NPC in children. Prognosis appears to be related directly to T stage (136,155). The N stage is not a significant influence on survival independent of T stage. This is undoubtedly because of the high incidence of neck disease (143). Survival in modern series is 50–80%; many of the treatment failures are in distant sites, particularly bone (135). The incidence of distant failures increases with increasing N stage (143,161).

Prolongation of radiotherapy treatment may adversely affect prognosis (134). Exceptionally good results with chemotherapy plus irradiation in children suggest that chemotherapy is indicated in T3 or T4 disease (130,131,143,148, 150–152,155,155a,162). A randomized prospective trial conducted jointly by several adult oncology cooperative groups found that progression-free survival achieved with radiotherapy (70 Gy in 35 fractions over 7 weeks) plus concomitant cisplatin and 5-fluorouracil was superior to that achieved with radiotherapy alone. Two-year survival was 80% for radiation plus chemotherapy, compared with 55% for radiation alone ($p = 0.0007$) (163). Chemotherapy appears to be more effective when it is given concurrently with radiotherapy (163–165).

Radiotherapy fields for NPC may include a portion of the hypothalamic–pituitary axis. Radiotherapy for NPC is associated with decreases, at long-term follow-up, in serum values of growth, follicle-stimulating, and leuteinizing hormones and prolactin and cortisol levels. The serum TSH level may rise. These changes in serum hormone levels are of clinical significance is about one-third of cases (130,137,143). Xerostomia, hearing loss, neck atrophy, chronic sinusitis, second malignancies, trismus, optic neuropathy, and dental caries are other potential late effects (130,134–136,152,166). In adults amifostine is often used with the goal of reducing xerostomia related to head and neck irradiation (167). The drug has not been tested adequately in children.

Other Nasopharyngeal Neoplasms

A wide variety of neoplasms can arise in or project into the nasopharynx. These include germ cell tumors such as teratomas and, rarely, endodermal sinus tumors (167–169). In addition, there are gliomas, hemangiomas, congenital rhabdomyomas, and hematomas. The radiotherapist may be asked to participate in the management of nasopharyngeal rhabdomyosarcoma, Hodgkin's disease, or non-Hodgkin's lymphoma (171). In addition, nasopharyngeal projections of chordoma or craniopharyngioma may necessitate irradiation. These latter neoplasms are considered in their respective chapters.

Esthesioneuroblastoma or Olfactory Neuroblastoma

Esthesioneuroblastoma (ENB) is a rare tumor of neural crest origin arising from the olfactory epithelium of the superior nasal cavity close to the cribriform plate (172–174). It was first described in the French literature in 1924 as "l'esthesioneuroepitheliome olfactif" (175). The origin

is unclear. Chemical and viral carcinogenesis theories have been advanced (176). The histologic features of the tumor include neuroepithelial cells arranged in pseudorosettes (called olfactory rosettes by some), a surrounding stroma of undifferentiated nuclei and fibrillary cords, palisading of neuroepithelial cells around blood vessels, few miotic figures, and interstitial calcification (172,173,177). The tumor may stain positive for neuron-specific enolase S-100 protein, neurofilament protein, or neural cell adhesion molecule (176,178). Tumors may be separated into grades, a distinction that may be important in predicting survival. There is a low-versus-high grade system and a Hyman's grade 1–4 system (178,179). Many centers find histologic grading of no use. The clinical presentation may include nasal obstruction, facial pain, recurrent epistaxis, loss of smell, sinus pain, neck mass, facial numbness, proptosis, diplopia, lethargy, or syncope (180,181). There is a slight male predominance in all age groups, including adolescents (172,173,177).

ENB presents as an intranasal nasopharyngeal, or paranasal soft tissue mass. The ethmoid and maxillary sinuses are most commonly involved. Bone destruction is common. Intracranial extension of the tumor can occur. Neck node involvement has been reported as ranging from 10% to 50% (173,174,177,179,181). There are several staging systems. The most commonly used is by Kadish et al. (146,177,181,182): Group A patients have a tumor confined to the nasal cavity, group B patients have a tumor involving the nasal cavity and paranasal sinuses, and group C patients exhibit tumor spread beyond the nasal cavity and paranasal sinuses. About half of patients are in group C and one-third in group B. Radiotherapy retrospective reviews consist largely of group B and C patients.

The mainstays of therapy are surgery and radiotherapy (Table 16-7). Groups A and B have been treated by resection alone. However, the local recurrence rate is 45–100% (177,179). Therefore, most authorities recommend a combination of surgery and radiotherapy for group A disease (except for small low-grade lesions) and, even more strongly, for groups B and C (179).

TABLE 16-6. *Survival in childhood nasopharyngeal carcinomas*

Year of report (reference)	Number of cases	Treatment	Survival		
			T1–T2	Combined	T3–T4
1973 (312)	7	R + Cy	7/7		
1974 (301)	1	R or R-RND	1/1		
1974 (147)	9	R or R + Cy	5/9		
1974 (302)	1	R or R + Ch	0/1		
1976 (149)	10	R or R + Ch	2/2		4/8
1975, 1977 (113, 142)	7	R or R + RND		4/7	
1977 (186)	22	R	11/22		
1978 (303)	83	R	8/15		20/63
1980 (137)	39	R or R + Ch		45% at 3 yr	
1980 (304)	16	R	2/6		0/10
1980 (299)	25	R	8/12		5/13
1981 (159)	103	R ± Ch	30/41		23/62
1987 (156)	10	R ± Ch	2/2		2/8
1982 (305)	20	R ± CAV	7/8		1/12
1983 (306)	27	R	8/11		6/16
1984 (307)	17	R	3/9		0/8
1985 (308)	21	R + Ch		10/21	
1986 (309)	10	R ± Ch		4/10	
	12	R ± Ch		10/12	
1986 (310)	18	R ± Ch		7/18	
1987, 1988 (155, 162)	15 (T3–T4)	R + Ch		20% 5-yr RFS	
	12 (T3–T4)	R + Ch		75% 5-yr RFS	
1988 (139)	67	R		43 (64%) 5 yr	
1989 (143)	27	R ± Ch	9/10		6/17
1989 (148)	7	R + CAV + 5FU			7/7
1990 (161)	57	R ± Ch	61%	49%	
1994 (150)	10	R or R + cisDDP + 5FU		8/10	

Year (Ref.)	N (stage)	Treatment	Outcome	Outcome
1994 (151)	1 (T1–T2) 9 (T3–T4)	R R + CAV or R + cisDDP + 5FU or R + ABVD or R + cisDDP + 5FU + ABVD or R + Bleo + 5FU		63% 5-yr DFS 54% 10-yr DFS	69% n_{0-1} 28% n_{2-3}
1996 (131)	13 (T1–T2) 35 (T3–T4)	R R + cisDDP/5FU R + Bleo + cisDDP + Epi R + cisDDP + 5FU or R + Cy + cisDDP		R: 47% 10-yr FFS R then Ch: 54% 5-yr FFS Ch then R: 72% 3-yr FFS	
1996 (132)	6 stage IV			83% 5 yr a	
1997 (154)	1 (T1–T2) 4 (T3–T4)	R R + BACON R + UICC2 or R + UICC2 + V		4/5	
1999 (136)	65	R (34) R + Cy	58%		
2000 (152)	33	R + Epi + Bleo + cisDDP R (13) or R + T6		58%	
2000 (145)	11 (all stage IV)	R (4) or cisDDP R + CAV Ch or 5FU	91% at 75 mo		
2001 (135)	33			63%	
2001 (134)	32	R + 5FU + cisDDP R (10) or R + 5FU + cisDDP (6) or R + Epi + Bleo + cisDDP (3) or R + MTX + Bleo + cisDDP (3)	73%		

5FU, 5-fluorouracil; ABVD, adriamycin, bleomycin, vinblastine, and dacarbazine; BACON, bleomycin, doxorubicin, lomustine, vincristine; Bleo, bleomycin; CAV, cyclophosphamide, doxorubicin, and vincristine; Ch, chemotherapy, not otherwise specified; cisDDP, cisplatin; Cy, cyclophosphamide; DFS, disease-free survival; Epi, epirubicin; FFS, failure-free survival; MTX, methotrexate; OS, overall survival; R, radiotherapy; RFS, relapse-free survival; R-RND, radical neck dissection for relapse; T6, actinomycin, cyclophosphamide, bleomycin, vincristine, methotrexate, and oidiomycin; UICC2, bleomycin, methotrexate, cisplatin, and vinblastine; V, vincristine.

TABLE 16-7. *Local recurrence rates in retrospective series of the treatment of esthesioneuroblastoma: combined adult and pediatric series*

Author (reference)	Surgery alone	Surgery and preoperative or post operative radiotherapy
Argiris et al. (182)	40%	63%
Dulguerov and Calcaterra (186)	86%	40%
Eich et al. (176)	—	17%
Elkon et al. (180)	44%	0%
Foote et al. (179)	59%	8%
Gruber et al. (185)	—	46%
Kadish et al. (177)	50%	0%
O'Connor et al. (188)	75%	29%
Resto et al. (181)	33%	11%
Crude average[a]	**55%**	**24%**

[a]Does not account for variations in age, stage, number of patients, or details of therapy between retrospective series. The "surgery alone" patients generally have lower-stage disease. In view of the higher relapse rate in these more favorable patients, the role of radiotherapy is reinforced.

The surgical procedure usually begins with a lateral rhinotomy followed, as necessary, by maxillectomy, ethmoidectomy, and sphenoidectomy for tumor excision. Often, a combined otorhinolaryngology and neurosurgical procedure of craniofacial resection is necessary for adequate tumor excision (174,183). In a craniofacial resection a frontal craniotomy is combined with a lateral rhinotomy or midfacial degloving for an en bloc resection, which may include tumor, cribriform plate, olfactory bulbs, medial maxillae, septum, fovea ethmoidalis, ethmoid air cells, and anterior cranial fossa dura. A defect engendered by a dural resection can be repaired with a pericranial flap or fascia grafts. The nasal defect may be repaired with a split-thickness skin graft.

Unequivocal complete surgical extirpation of ENB is rarely achieved in advanced cases, and local tumor control with surgery alone is poor. Therefore, one often combines surgery with irradiation (179). Some authorities favor using radiation postoperatively to allow assessment of surgical margins unimpeded by prior therapy, establishment of sinus drainage, and intraoperative evaluation of tumor anatomy before radio-

therapy (177). Proponents of postbiopsy but pre–definitive surgery irradiation argue that the tumor is best treated before extensive manipulation to improve the resection and that preoperative radiation may decrease wound seeding by tumor (174). Some physicians also favor preoperative chemotherapy. Patients who respond well to chemotherapy receive high-dose irradiation, potentially avoiding extensive surgery (184). Both approaches are defensible, but the sparse data do not support substituting chemotherapy for radiotherapy.

Establishing local control of ENB appears to entail dosages of 50–65 Gy at 1.8–2 Gy per fraction, in combination with surgery. (146,174, 179,191). As with other nasal, nasopharyngeal, and paranasal sinus tumors, treatment planning based on sophisticated imaging, computerized dosimetry, and rigid head immobilization is crucial to successful intensity-modulated radiation therapy or conformal treatment. Early evidence supports a higher local control rate with conformal therapy (151). The anterior cranial fossa and cribriform plate are included in the field. Careful attention is necessary to protect the pituitary, optic chiasm, and globes if the tumor position allows.

Several centers believe there is a role for chemotherapy in ENB. Popular programs include cyclophosphamide, doxorubicin, and vincristine (CAV); these drugs plus etoposide (CAV-E); intra-arterial adriamycin; vincristine and cyclophosphamide; cisplatin and 5-fluorouracil; and cisplatin and etoposide. They have been given before or after surgery and radiotherapy. Tumor responses have been seen, and some retrospective data have been brought to bear, arguing that survival has been favorably influenced (178, 181,182,184,185). Some patients with relapsed ENB have been successfully treated with high-dose chemotherapy and autologous bone marrow transplantation (183).

It is generally stated that with a low but variable risk of cervical nodal disease, prophylactic neck dissection or irradiation is not indicated (177). This proposition may be arguable in children who appear to have more advanced and aggressive disease than their elders. Relapse in cervical lymph nodes is common (179,183). The role of elective neck dissection or radiation to the neck in advanced cases has been discussed. Some institutions use 50 Gy of prophylactic irradiation to the clinically negative neck (181). At the very least, radiotherapy fields should be generous, and the threshold for biopsy of suspicious neck nodes should be low. Modern combined adult and pediatric series report a survival of 45–69% (176,178,181,182,185,186–191).

Malignancies of the Oral Cavity, Oropharynx, Hypopharynx, and Larynx; Salivary Gland Tumors

Squamous cell carcinoma of the head and neck rarely occurs in children (191,192). Epidermoid cancers constituted only 2.5% of the 388 head and neck cancers in children seen at the Institut Gustave–Roussy from 1975 to 1987 (193). They constituted 5.8% of head and neck tumors seen at Saint Sofia Children's Hospital in Athens (194). Some pediatric cases may be related to smoking, tobacco chewing, or passive smoking. Chronic irritation by dental caries or poor oral hygiene may contribute to a malignant change. Other proposed causal factors include oral viral infections, xeroderma pigmentosa (particularly for lip cancer), and a genetic predisposition (i.e., a history of hereditary retinoblastoma) (195).

Children have been reported to develop squamous cell carcinoma of the lip, floor of the mouth, buccal mucosa, tongue, tonsil, palate, hypopharynx, and larynx (196,197). There is nothing to suggest that the clinical presentation or routes of spread of childhood head and neck cancer differs substantially from that of adults.

Therapeutic guidelines mimic those for adults. One seeks to control the primary site and the routes of tumor spread in the neck with surgery or radiotherapy. Cosmetic considerations, preservation of swallowing, vocal quality, and the long-term consequences of radiation play a role in the selection of therapy (195–198).

Salivary gland tumors in children have been reported (Table 16-8). In adults, 15–25% of salivary gland tumors are malignant. In children, nearly 50% are malignant. These lesions usually present with a mass. These tumors are more common in girls. The dominant location is the

TABLE 16-8. *Epithelial salivary gland neoplasms in children and adolescents*

Pleomorphic adenoma	~45%
Mucoepidermoid carcinoma	~30%
Acinic cell carcinoma	~7%
Adenocarcinoma	~6%
Undifferentiated carcinoma	~4%
Adenoid cystic carcinoma	~3%

From de Cassia Broga Ribeiro R, Kowalski LP, Saba LMB, et al. Epithelial salivary gland neoplasm in children and adolescents: a forty-four-year experience. *Med Pediatr Oncol* 2002;39:594–600. Also see references 203, 312, and 313.

parotid gland. Surgery is the preferred option for the initial treatment of pediatric salivary gland neoplasms. In parotid tumors special attention is directed to preserving the facial nerve. In children, the facial nerve is proportionally longer than in adults and generally more superficial in location (199). Facial nerve involvement can occur with parotid neoplasms. In some cases, resection of some branches or the main trunk of the facial nerve may be necessary. Facial nerve grafting may be used to restore deficits. Occult nodal metastases in the neck are rare, and neither elective neck dissection nor irradiation is routinely indicated (200,201). Local tumor control is highly associated with the absence of aggressive features such as nodal metastases, local extraglandular tumor extension, and perineural, perivascular, or perilymphatic invasion.

In general, postoperative radiotherapy is indicated for high-grade malignancies, microscopic residual tumor, perineural invasion, soft tissue extension, cervical lymph node involvement, or local relapse. The indications for radiotherapy include high-grade primary malignancy, cervical metastases, positive margins, gross postoperative residual tumor, aggressive histologic findings such as the perineural invasion typical of adenoid cystic carcinoma, vascular or lymphatic invasion, local extraglandular soft tissue extension, or inoperability (200). Potential but rare complications of radiotherapy are trismus and osteoradionecrosis. Careful treatment planning and postradiotherapy dental care reduce the risk of dental caries. In young children facial deformity is also a risk. In a series from Brazil, the 5-year survival rate for children with mucoepidermoid carcinoma was 100% for clinical stages I–II and 50% for clinical stages III–IV (199). Fast neutron radiotherapy appears effective in treating malignant salivary gland tumors and recurrent pleomorphic adenomas, particularly for gross disease. Because of the high RBE of neutrons, typical fraction sizes are 1.1–1.2 neutron Gy four times per week to 17–22 neutron Gy. There are recognized risks of neutron therapy including osteoradionecrosis, vascular injury, and hearing loss (202).

Rhabdomyosarcoma of the larynx may occur in childhood. Its management is discussed in Chapter 11. Involvement of the mucosal surfaces of the upper respiratory tract by acquired immune deficiency syndrome–associated Kaposi's sarcoma may cause pain, hemorrhage, or airway obstruction (204). Dosages of 20 to 25 Gy, in 2–2.5 weeks, often produce a satisfactory response.

Infantile Subglottic Hemangiomas

Infantile subglottic hemangiomas are rare lesions. There is a 2:1 female to male predominance, and 80–90% of patients present before the age of 6 months. The most common symptoms are respiratory distress (inspiratory stridor), a hoarse cry, cough, dysphagia, cyanosis, emesis, and hemoptysis. Cutaneous hemangiomas occur in 44–51% of these patients. The diagnosis usually is made by direct laryngoscopy (205–210). Therapy aims to maintain a patient airway, shorten the natural course of the tumor, and avoid serious side effects such as subglottic stenosis, a delay in speech, and induction of second malignant neoplasms.

Spontaneous regressions have occurred but are uncommon. The low rate of spontaneous regression is the impetus for more definitive therapy. Many forms of treatment have been proposed: CO_2 laser, intralesional steroid injection, cryotherapy, systemic steroids, injection of sclerosants, tracheostomy alone or in combination with other treatments, surgical excision, external beam irradiation, and ^{198}Au or ^{32}P have been used alone or in combination (205–207,211–216).

Many consider tracheostomy and observation for involution of the hemangioma to be the standard of care. A drawback of this therapy is that it may affect speech and language development. Some clinicians advocate the use of the CO_2 laser to remove subglottic hemangiomas. However, subglottic stenosis is a recognized possible complication of this approach. Small, circumscribed lesions can be treated by surgical excision. Intralesional steroid therapy is advocated by some.

Because of concerns about the development of secondary malignancy (particularly thyroid) and deleterious effects of radiation on growth and development of the larynx, radiotherapy is almost never used in modern practice (197,208). In 1919, New and Clark (217) applied radium outside the larynx for infantile subglottic hemangioma and reported that radium "is specific for all true vascular growths of the larynx, as well as other parts of the body." There are reports of treatment with brachytherapy that are of historical interest (211–213). Using endolaryngeal microsurgical technique, a ^{198}Au seed was inserted into a submucosal pocket below and medial to the edge of the true vocal cord. Seed position was checked by a postoperative radiograph or xeroradiogram. Responses occur over 1 to 2 months. Beta ray brachytherapy with ^{32}P was also tried (215).

The cure rate with external radiotherapy used alone or in combination with tracheostomy is approximately 80%. Between 3.5 and 5 Gy at 0.5 to 1.5 Gy per fraction is used. Advocates of irradiation point out its generally satisfactory and reliable results and raise concerns of late scarring with laser surgery. When dealing with a life-threatening situation, one should be prepared to use irradiation if other treatment modalities are either inapplicable or unsuccessful. However, radiotherapy is rarely used.

Esophagus

Esophageal carcinoma may develop in children; it may arise spontaneously, years after chemical burns in the setting of Barrett's esophagus, and, in one reported case, in association with Cornelia de Lange syndrome (218–224). Both squamous cell carcinoma and adenocarcinomas have been reported. They are managed similarly to those in adults (225). The rare case of esophageal sarcoma (leiomyosarcoma, carcinosarcoma, malignant schwannoma) may be treated with preoperative or postoperative irradiation (226). Palliative radiotherapy is occasionally necessary for leukemia or secondary or primary lymphomatous infiltration of the esophagus (227,228). Other rare esophageal neoplasms include leiomyoma, desmoid, and teratoma (229–231).

Lung

Primary lung and pleural tumors rarely occur in children. In 1983 Hartman and Shochat (232) reviewed 241 well-documented cases of primary pediatric pulmonary neoplasms. Of the total group, 67% were malignant and 33% benign. Of the malignancies, 49% were carcinoids, 29% were bronchogenic carcinoma, and 9% were pulmonary blastomas. Other reported tumors are mucoepidermoid tumors, mesothelioma, mesenchymal sarcoma, bronchioalveolar carcinoma, and lymphoepithelioma (60,233–241).

The pleuropulmonary blastoma is thought to originate from pluripotent primitive blastemal cells. The tumor contains mesenchymal and epithelial cellular components. It morphologically mimics the embryonal structure of the lung (242–245). It was originally called fetal embryoma because it resembles fetal lung. Mean age of onset is 2.5 years, with a male predominance (236). Most cases are managed initially with surgery. Total resection is associated with better outcomes (236). The tumors often are large and locally extensive, making complete surgical excision uncommon (243–246). Local recurrence and distant metastases (brain, liver, and bone) are common, particularly among patients with tumors more than 5 cm in diameter (237,245). Thoracic irradiation has been used for the postoperative treatment of patients with large tumors or positive margins (30 to 55 Gy) (246). One should also consider radiotherapy for the treatment of local tumor recurrence, where the situation is grim but not hopeless (245,246). The use

of intraoperative irradiation has been reported (247). Chemotherapy has shown some promise as adjuvant therapy postoperatively and for preoperative tumor reduction. Drugs used include various combinations of actinomycin D, adriamycin, cyclophosphamide, cisplatin, etoposide, and vincristine, but there are too few cases to claim that a particular drug combination is indicated (248). The overall survival at 2 years is 63%. A case has been reported in which high-dose chemotherapy with autologous blood stem cell transplantation failed to prevent local recurrence of tumor and death (249).

Endobronchial adenomas usually are slow-growing but possess a low-grade malignant potential. The tumors fill and invade the bronchus and produce obstructive symptoms. The mucoepidermoid, carcinoid, and cylindroid adenomas are increasingly malignant, in that order. Cures are possible with complete resection (249,250). Malignant mesotheliomas rarely occur in childhood. There is rarely a history of asbestos exposure in children (251). Radiotherapy may be used for palliative treatment or after an attempted resection with close or positive margins.

Bronchogenic carcinoma occurs in children, arising *de novo* or associated with cigarette smoking (240,251,253,254).

Stomach

Non-Hodgkin's lymphoma is the most common malignancy of the stomach in childhood (255). Its management is discussed in Chapter 8. As a group, leiomyosarcoma and leiomyoblastoma are the second most common gastric malignancies in children (256–259). The average size of a gastric leiomyosarcoma in childhood is 6–7 cm in diameter. Infiltration of tumor to adjacent structures, including the liver or nodal metastasis, may occur (258). Therapy of gastric leiomyosarcoma begins with surgery. The operative bed and the upper abdomen are common sites of tumor recurrence. Postoperative external beam irradiation is justifiable when there is a particularly high risk of local recurrence created by positive surgical margins or posterior penetration. However, the efficacy of adjuvant radiotherapy in this setting is not proven.

Gastric adenocarcinoma is rare in children (228,259,259a). It may occur *de novo* or in association with Peutz–Jeghers syndromes (249, 260). There is epidemiologic evidence that longstanding *Helicobacter pylori* infection and chronic gastritis are involved in the development of a variety of gastric malignancies including adenocarcinomas, lymphomas, and mucosa-associated lymphoid tissue lymphomas. Acquisition of infection in childhood appears to be a risk factor for development of neoplasia as an adult. However, there is no evidence at present that the treatment of all *H. pylori*–infected children would influence the risk of gastric malignancy decades later (261). Rhabdomyosarcoma, Hodgkin's disease, malignant teratoma, gastrointestinal stromal tumor, and nerve sheath tumors also may occur in the stomach (262). (See Chapters 7, 11, and 12.)

Pancreas

Primary neoplasms of the pancreas are rare in childhood. The most common malignant forms are listed in Table 16-9. Pancreatoblastoma is characterized by well-formed acinar areas along with squamoid corpuscles and zymogen-like granules. Because these organoid structures are similar to the pancreatic anlage, pancreoblas-

toma is thought to originate from pancreatic multipotential primordial cells (263). Positive staining by periodic acid–Schiff, α-trypsin, and α-keratin are common (264). About two-thirds of cases have been associated with a high level of α-fetoprotein (263–266).

Pancreatoblastoma generally is slow growing. Localized, nonmetastatic tumor that can be completely resected is generally cured (267). In some cases, unfortunately, the tumor is clearly malignant, with local invasion, recurrence, and metastasis. About 35% of patients present with metastases, and 50% die of tumor (264,268).

A resectable tumor without metastases can be treated with surgery alone. If the tumor secretes α-fetoprotein, this marker can be used along with CT and ultrasound for follow-up. The role of radiation therapy in managing pancreatoblastoma is not clearly defined. Griffin et al. (269) reported a case of locally recurrent pancreatoblastoma treated with 46.2 Gy. Six weeks after irradiation, exploratory laparotomy was performed. Multiple biopsies showed no evidence of tumor. Therefore, is possible to infer that some cases of pancreatoblastoma may be curable by radiation. However, in most cases in which radiotherapy is considered it is because of tumor spillage at the time of surgery or positive surgical margins. Radiation therapy has been used to render unresectable tumors resectable, to treat local regional recurrent tumor, and as postoperative therapy for microscopic disease and tumor spillage. A dosage of 40 to 50 Gy seems appropriate (263,266,267). We are aware of patients successfully treated for recurrent tumor with intraoperative radiation (20 Gy) (266,270).

A variety of chemotherapy programs have been used to shrink unresectable tumors, to treat metastatic disease, or as adjuvant therapy. There have been some notable successes in rendering unresectable tumors resectable. Cyclophosphamide, vincristine, 5-fluorouracil, adriamycin, mitomycin-C, cisplatin, etoposide, ifosfamide, actinomycin D, bleomycin, vinblastine, and epirubicin have been used. Cases are so rare that firm statements regarding the indications and specifics of chemotherapy treatment policy are inappropri-

TABLE 16-9. *Malignant pancreatic tumors in childhood and adolescence seen at Memorial Sloan–Kettering Cancer Center, 1967–2002 (exclusive of patients with multiple endocrine neoplasia syndromes)*

	n
Solid papillary tumors	7
Pancreatoblastoma	5
Pancreatic endocrine neoplasm	2
Primitive neuroectodermal tumor	2
Total	16

From Shorter NA, Glick RD, Klimstra DS, et al. Malignant pancreatic tumors in childhood and adolescence: the Memorial Sloan–Kettering experience, 1967 to present. *J Pediatr Surg* 2002;37:887–892.

ate (265–267,268,271–273). Childhood pancreatic carcinoma has been reported (274).

Appendix

Carcinoids are the most common neoplasm of the appendix in children. Almost all appendiceal carcinoids are incidental findings, usually 2 cm in diameter or less, and are found in specimens removed because of appendicitis or during abdominal surgery. Metastasis to lymph nodes occurs in less than 5% of pediatric cases. Some assert that the risk of metastases is related to tumor size and local invasion.

Surgical excision is the treatment of choice. For the typical small tumor, appendectomy is curative. Some authors favor hemicolectomy in tumors larger than 2 cm, for invasive lesions, or for nodal metastases. Others advocate a resection restricted to the cecum as an alternative. The overall prognosis of appendiceal carcinoid tumors is excellent. Radiotherapy is almost never used (275–277).

Small Bowel

Non-Hodgkin's lymphoma is the most common malignancy of the small intestine in children (see Chapter 8) (168,255). Small intestine adenocarcinoma develops *de novo* or in association with Peutz–Jeghers syndrome (249). Surgery is the initial treatment. Nonfixed jejunal and ileal lesions usually are treated with surgery alone. As a general rule, radiation therapy should not be used for routine adjuvant treatment of small bowel carcinoma when the primary tumor is in a mobile part of the small bowel. In the retroperitoneal fixed portions of the duodenum, where local recurrence after surgery is a risk, an argument may be made for postoperative irradiation. Unresectable tumors may be treated with palliative irradiation for pain and bleeding. The survival rate for small bowel adenocarcinoma is poor.

Sarcomas of the small bowel are treated with surgery. Adjuvant radiation therapy is appropriate when there are close or positive surgical margins (278). Small intestinal carcinoids are

treated surgically (277). Palliative radiation therapy may be used for liver metastases.

Large Bowel

Carcinomas of the colon and rectum in childhood present with pain, vomiting, anemia, a palpable mass, hematochezia, diarrhea, or constipation (279,279a,280). Because of the lack of specificity of the symptoms and the rarity of the disease (about one case per million children per year), the possibility of a child having colorectal carcinoma is rarely considered, and the interval between clinical complaints and diagnosis often is long (228,280–283). In Japan, for example, one to three pediatric colon carcinomas are identified annually (279,279a). These tumors may arise *de novo* or may be associated with one of the polyposis syndromes such as Gardner's syndrome, Turcot's syndrome, and Peutz–Jeghers syndrome. They also may occur as second malignant neoplasms after treatment of childhood leukemia, rhabdomyosarcoma, Wilms' tumor, or Hodgkin's disease (284). Carcinoma may also arise in the chronically irritated colon of ulcerative colitis (285). It is generally felt that when a carcinoma arises in ulcerative colitis, a total colectomy should be performed. Unfortunately, involvement of regional lymph nodes, distant metastases, and inoperability are common in children (280).

Clinical management of colon cancer in children is the same as in adults. However, the prognosis for young patients is worse. In a review of the Japanese literature concerning children less than 15 years old, 48% of the patients were disease-free survivors (279). This is attributed to a delay in diagnosis resulting in more advanced disease (286,287).

Leiomyosarcoma of the colon has been reported in children. It is curable by surgical resection (288).

BREAST

Adenocarcinoma of the breast rarely occurs in children and adolescents. The most common form of breast cancer occurring in young girls is juvenile secretory carcinoma. The malignant cells are characterized by abundant secretion of mucin and mucopolysaccharide-containing materials (289–293). A unique pathological feature is the presence of a thick-walled capsule that is thought to be caused by a desmoplastic reaction around the tumor. This may be responsible for its cystic appearance on ultrasound (294). Estrogen and progesterone receptors are generally negative (226). Some surgeons believe that local tumor excision alone may be adequate therapy in juvenile secretory carcinoma. Others favor simple, modified radical, and radical mastectomies (225,226,228,229). The prognosis is excellent in this benign tumor, and no radiotherapy or chemotherapy is generally necessary. There is minimal experience with lumpectomy and radiotherapy.

Infiltrating ductal, lobular, medullary, and inflammatory carcinoma have been reported in young girls. With almost no data available in children, we would be cautious about varying from the principles of clinical management set by adult oncology (225,227,231,294).

There have been case reports of primary non-Hodgkin's lymphoma, rhabdomyosarcoma, adenoid cystic carcinoma, radiation-induced spindle cell sarcoma, and cystosarcoma phyllodes of the breast in children (290–296). Reported breast metastases in children include hepatocarcinoma, non-Hodgkin's lymphoma, rhabdomyosarcoma, Hodgkin's disease, neuroblastoma, and adenocarcinoma (297).

REFERENCES

References particularly recommended for further reading are indicated by an asterisk.

1. Bradley EL III. Primary and adjunctive therapy in carcinoma of the adrenal cortex. *Surg Gynecol Obstet* 1975;141:507–511.
2. Honour JW, Price DA, Grant DB. Virilizing adrenocortical tumors in childhood. *Pediatrics* 1986;78:547.
3. Jones GS, Shah KJ, Mann JR. Adreno-cortical carcinoma in infancy and childhood: a radiological report of ten cases. *Clin Radiol* 1985;36:257–262.
4. Dackiw APB, Lee JE, Gagel RF, et al. Adrenal cortical carcinoma. *World J Surg* 2001;25:914–926.
5. Stajadinovic A, Ghassein RA, Haas A, et al. Adrenocortical carcinoma: clinical, morphologic, and molecular characterization. *J Clin Oncol* 2002;20:941–950.
6. Icard P, Goudet P, Charpenay C, et al. Adrenocortical carcinomas: surgical trends and results of a 253-patient series from the French Association of Endocrine Surgeons study group. *World J Surg* 2001;25:891–897.
7. Michalkiewicz EL, Sandrini R, Bugg MF, et al. Clinical characteristics of small functioning adrenocortical tumors in children. *Med Pediatr Oncol* 1997;28; 175–178.
8. De Leon DD, Lage BJ, Walterhouse D, et al. Long-term (15 years) outcome in an infant with metastatic adrenocortical carcinoma. *J Clin Endocrinol Metab* 2002;87:4452–4456.
9. Petrus LV, Hall RT, Boechat MI, et al. The pediatric patient with suspected adrenal neoplasm: which radiologic test to use? *Med Pediatr Oncol* 1992;20:53–57.
10. Neblett NW, Frexes-Steed M, Scott HW Jr. Experience with adrenocortical neoplasms in childhood. *Am Surg* 1987;53:117–125.
11. Vierhapper H. Adrenocortical tumors: clinical symptoms and biochemical diagnosis. *Eur J Radiol* 2001;41:88–94.
12. Stewart DR, Morris-Jones PH, Jolleys A. Carcinoma of the adrenal gland in children. *J Pediatr Surg* 1974;9:59–67.
13. Magee BJ, Gattameneni HR, Pearson D. Adrenal cortical carcinoma: survival after radiotherapy. *Clin Radiol* 1987;38:587–588.
14. Page DL, DeLellis RA, Hough AJ Jr. *Atlas of tumor pathology, second series, fascicle 23. Tumors of the adrenal.* Washington, DC: Armed Forces Institute of Pathology, 1985:203–207.
15. Daneman A, Chan HSL, Martin DJ. Adrenal carcinoma and adenoma in children: a review of 17 patients. *Pediatr Radiol* 1983;13:11–18.
16. Percarpio B, Knowlton AH. Radiation therapy for adrenal cortical carcinoma. *Acta Radiol Ther Phys Biol* 1976;15:288–292.
17. Markoe AM, Serber W, Micaily B, et al. Radiation therapy for adjunctive treatment of adrenal cortical carcinoma. *Am J Clin Oncol* 1991;14:170–174.
18. Kasperlik-Zaluska AA, Migdalska BM, Zgliczyinski S, et al. Adrenocortical carcinoma: a clinical study and treatment results of 52 patients. *Cancer* 1995;75: 2587–2591.
19. Zografos GC, Driscoll DL, Karakousis CP, et al. Adrenal adenocarcinoma: a review of 53 cases. *J Surg Oncol* 1994;56:160–164.
20. Romaguera RL, Minagar A, Bruce JH, et al. Adrenocortical carcinoma with cerebral metastasis in a child: case report and review of the literature. *Clin Neurol Neurosurg* 2001;103:46–50.
21. Haak HR, Hermans J, van de Velde CJH, et al. Optimal treatment of adrenocortical carcinoma with mitotane: results in a consecutive series of 96 patients. *Br J Cancer* 1994;69:947–951.
22. Wooten MD, King DK. Adrenal cortical carcinoma: epidemiology and treatment with mitotane and a review of the literature. *Cancer* 1993;72:3145–3155.
23. Sloan DA, Schwartz ARW, McGrath PC, et al. Diagnosis and management of adrenal tumors. *Curr Opin Oncol* 1996;8:30–36.
24. Ahlman H, Khorram-Manesh A, Jansson S, et al. Cytotoxic treatment of adrenocortical carcinoma *World J Surg* 2001;25:927–933.
25. Abraham J, Bakke S, Ruff A, et al. A phase II trial of

combination chemotherapy and surgical resection for the treatment of metastatic adrenocortical carcinoma. *Cancer* 2002;94:2333–2343.

26. Bartley GB, Campbell RJ, Salomao DR, et al. Adrenocortical carcinoma metastatic to the orbit. *Ophthal Plast Reconstr Surg* 2001;17:215–220.

27. Newman KD, Ponsky T. The diagnosis and management of endocrine tumors causing hypertension in children. *Ann NY Acad Sci* 2002;970:155–158.

28. Caty MG, Coran AG, Geagen M, et al. Current diagnosis and treatment of pheochromocytoma in children: experience with 22 consecutive tumors in 14 patients. *Arch Surg* 1990;125:978–981.

29. Miller KA, Albanese C, Harrison M, et al. Experience with laparoscopic adrenalectomy in pediatric patients. *J Pediatr Surg* 2002;37:979–982.

30. Misra AK, Agarwal G, Mishra A, et al. Pheochromocytoma in children and adolescents: an institutional experience. *Indian Pediatr* 2002;39:51–57.

30a. American Joint Committee on Cancer. *AJCC cancer staging manual*, 6th ed. New York: Springer, 2002.

31. Fonkalsrud EW. Pheochromocytoma in childhood. *Prog Pediatr Surg* 1991;26:103–111.

32. Januszewicz P, Wieteska-Klimczak A, Wyszynska T. Pheochromocytoma in children: difficulties in diagnosis and localization. *Clin Exp Hypertens* 1990; A12(4):571–579.

33. Gagel RF, Tashijian AH Jr, Cummings T, et al. The clinical outcome of prospective screening for multiple endocrine neoplasia type 2a: an 18-year experience. *N Engl J Med* 1988;318:478–484.

34. Gakce O, Gakce C, Gunel S, et al. Pheochromocytoma presenting with headache, panic attacks and jaundice in a child. *Headache* 1991;31:473–475.

35. Raum WJ. Pheochromocytoma. *Curr Ther Endocrinol Metab* 1994;5:172–178.

36. Matsota P, Avgerinopaulou-Vlahou A, Velegrakis D. Anaesthesia for phaeochromocytoma removal in a 5-year-old boy. *Paediatr Anaesth* 2002;12:176–180.

37. Loh KC, Shlossberg AH, Abbott EC, et al. Phaeochromocytoma: a ten-year survey. *QJM* 1997;90:51–60.

38. Ein SH, Shandling B, Wesson D, et al. Recurrent pheochromocytomas in children. *J Pediatr Surg* 1990;25:1063–1065.

39. Ein SH, Weitzman S, Thorner P, et al. Pediatric malignant pheochromocytoma. *J Pediatr Surg* 1994;29:1197–1201.

40. Yu L, Fleckman AM, Chadha M, et al. Radiation therapy of metastatic pheochromocytoma: case report and review of the literature. *Am J Clin Oncol* 1996;19:389–393.

41. Giuffrida D, Scollo C, Pellegriti G, et al. Differentiated thyroid cancer in children and adolescents. *J Endocrinol Invest* 2002;25:18–24.

42. Brink JS, van Heerden JA, McIver B, et al. Papillary thyroid cancer with pulmonary metastases in children: long-term prognosis. *Surgery* 2000;128:881–887.

43. Jarzab B, Junak DH, Wloch J, et al. Multivariate analysis of prognostic factors for differentiated thyroid cancer in children. *Eur J Nucl Med* 2000;27:833–841.

*44. Skinner MA. Cancer of the thyroid in infants and children. *Semin Pediatr Surg* 2001;10:119–126.

45. Geiger JD, Thompson NW. Thyroid tumors in children *Otolaryngol Clin North Am* 1996;29:711–719.

46. Desjardins JG, Bass J, Leboeuf G, et al. A twenty-year experience with thyroid carcinoma in children. *J Pediatr Surg* 1988;23:709–713.

47. Fjalling M, Tisell L, Carlsson S, et al. Benign and malignant thyroid nodules after neck irradiation. *Cancer* 1986;58:1219–1224.

48. Klopp CT, Rosvoll RV, Winship T. Is destructive surgery ever necessary for treatment of thyroid cancer in children? *Ann Surg* 1967;165:745–750.

49. LaQuaglia MP, Corbally MT, Heller G, et al. Recurrence and morbidity in differentiated thyroid carcinoma in children. *Surgery* 1988;104:1149–1156.

50. Jacob P, Kenigsberg Y, Zvonova I, et al. Childhood exposure due to the Chernobyl accident and thyroid cancer risk in contaminated areas of Belarus and Russia. *Br J Cancer* 1999;80:1461–1469.

50a. Maysich KB, Menezes RJ, Michalek AM. Chernobyl related ionising radiation exposure and cancer risk: an epidemiological review. *Lancet Oncol* 2002;3:269–279.

51. Winship T, Rosvoll RV. Childhood thyroid carcinoma. *Cancer* 1961;14:734–743.

52. Wiersinga WM, Thyroid cancer in children and adolescents: consequences in later life. *J Pediatr Endocrinol Metab* 2001;14:1289–1296.

53. McClellan DR, Francis GL. Thyroid cancer in children, pregnant women, and patients with Graves' disease. *Endocrinol Metab Clin North Am* 1996;25:27–49.

54. Sherman SI. Thyroid carcinoma. *Lancet* 2003;361:501–511.

55. Shvero J, Gal R, Avidor I, et al. Anaplastic thyroid carcinoma: a clinical histologic and immunohistochemical study. *Cancer* 1988;62:319–325.

56. Flynn SD, Forman BH, Stewart AF, et al. Poorly differentiated ("insular") carcinoma of the thyroid gland: an aggressive subset of differentiated thyroid neoplasms. *Surgery* 1988;104:963–970.

57. Ceccarelli C, Pacini F, Lippi F, et al. Thyroid cancer in children and adolescents. *Surgery* 1988;104:1143–1148.

58. Duffy BJ Jr, Fitzgerald PJ. Thyroid cancer in childhood and adolescence: report of 28 cases. *J Clin Endocrinol* 1950;10:1296–1308.

59. LoGerfo P, Chabot J, Gazetas P. The intraoperative incidence of detectable bilateral and multicentric disease in papillary cancer of the thyroid. *Surgery* 1990;108:958–963.

60. McCann MP, Fu Y, Kay S. Pulmonary blastoma: a light and electron microscopic study. *Cancer* 1976;38:789–797.

61. Webb AJ, Brewster S, Newington D. Problems in diagnosis and management of goitre in childhood and adolescence. *Br J Surg* 1996;83:1586–1590.

62. Hanna CE, LaFranchi SH. Adolescent thyroid disorders. *Adolesc Med* 2002;13:13–35.

63. Balter M. Children become the first victims of fallout. *Science* 1996;272:357–360.

64. Becker DV, Robbins J, Beebe GW, et al. Childhood thyroid cancer following the Chernobyl accident. *Endocrinol Metab Clin North Am* 1996 25:197–211.

65. Antonelli A, Miccoli P, Derzhitski VE, et al. Epidemiologic and clinical evaluation of thyroid cancer in children from the Gomel Region (Belarus). *World J Surg* 1996;20:867–871.

66. Deodhar SD, Joshi S, Khubchandani S. Cystosarcoma phyllodes. *J Postgrad Med* 1989;35:98–103.
67. Ontai S, Straehley CJ. The surgical treatment of well-differentiated carcinoma of the thyroid. *Am Surg* 1985;51:653–657.
68. Zimmerman D, Hay ID, Gough IR, et al. Papillary thyroid carcinoma in children and adults: long-term follow-up of 1039 patients conservatively treated at one institution during three decades. *Surgery* 1988; 104:1157–1166.
69. Beirwaites WH. Controversies in the treatment of thyroid cancer: the University of Michigan approach. *Thyroid Today* 1983;6:1–5.
70. Harbert JC. Radioiodine therapy of differentiated thyroid cancer. In: *Nuclear medicine therapy.* New York: Thieme Medical Publishers, 1987:37–89.
71. Leeper R. Controversies in the treatment of thyroid cancer: the New York Memorial Hospital Approach. *Thyroid Today* 1982;5:1–4.
72. Mazzaferri EL, Jhiang SM. Long-term impact of initial surgical and medical therapy on papillary and follicular thyroid cancer. *Am J Med* 1994;97:418–428.
73. Mazzaferi EL. Treating differentiated thyroid carcinoma: where do we draw the line? *Mayo Clin Proc* 1991;66:105–111.
74. Buckwalter JA, Thomas CG, Freeman JB. Is childhood thyroid cancer a lethal disease? *Ann Surg* 1975; 181:632–639.
75. Sheline GE, Galante M, Lindsay S. Radiation therapy in the control of persistent thyroid cancer. *AJR* 1966;97:923–930.
76. Newman KD, Black T, Heller G, et al. Differentiated thyroid cancer: determinants of disease progression in patients less than 21 years of age at diagnosis—a report of the Surgical Discipline Committee of the Children's Cancer Group, 1998;227:533–541.
77. Smedal MI, Meissner WA. Results of x-ray treatment in undifferentiated carcinoma of the thyroid. *Radiology* 1961;76:927–935.
78. Tubiana M, Locour J, Mannier JP, et al. External radiotherapy and radio-iodine in the treatment of 359 thyroid cancers. *Br J Radiol* 1975;48:894–907.
79. Kim TH, Yang DS, Jung KY, et al. Value of external irradiation for locally advanced papillary thyroid cancer. *Int J Radiat Oncol Biol Phys* 2003;55:1006–1012.
80. Brierley JD, Tsang RW. External-beam radiation therapy in the treatment of differentiated thyroid cancer. *Semin Surg Oncol* 1999;16:42–49.
81. Ain KB, Egarin MJ, DeSimone PA. Treatment of anaplastic thyroid cancer with paclitaxel: phase 2 trial using ninety-six–hour infusion. *Thyroid* 2000; 10:588–594.
82. Jianping G, Renxi Z, Huanqiu C. Childhood thyroid cancer: an analysis of 14 cases. *Chin J Oncol* 2000; 22:324–326.
83. Harness JA, Thompson NW, McLeod MK, et al. Differentiated thyroid carcinoma in children and adolescents. *World J Surg* 1992;16:547–554.
84. Schlumberger M, De Vathaire F, Travagli JP, et al. Differentiated thyroid carcinoma in childhood: long term follow-up in 72 patients. *J Clin Endocrinol Metab* 1987;65:1088–1094.
85. Ceccarelli C, Pacini F, Lippi F, et al. Thyroid cancer in children and adolescents. *Surgery* 1988;104:1143–1148.
86. La Quaglia MP, Corbally MT, Heller G, et al. Recurrence and morbidity in differentiated thyroid carcinoma in children. *Surgery* 1988;104:1157–1163.
87. Fields JN, Halverson KJ, Devinein VR, et al. Juvenile nasopharyngeal angiofibroma: efficacy of radiation therapy. *Radiology* 1990;176:263–265.
88. Palmer FJ. Preoperative embolisation in the management of juvenile nasopharyngeal angiofibroma. *Australas Radiol* 1989;33:348–350.
89. Ungkanont K, Byers RM, Weber RS, et al. Juvenile nasopharyngeal angiofibroma: an update of therapeutic management. *Head Neck* 1996;Jan/Feb:60–66.
*90. Paris J, Guelfucci B, Moulin G, et al. Diagnosis and treatment of juvenile nasopharyngeal angiofibroma. *Eur Arch Otorhinolaryngol* 2001;258:120–124.
*91. Scholtz AW, Appenroth E, Kammen-Jolly K, et al. Juvenile nasopharyngeal angiofibroma: management and therapy. *Laryngoscope* 2002;111:681–687.
*92. Reddy KA, Mendenhall WM, Amdur RJ, et al. Long-term results of radiation therapy for juvenile nasopharyngeal angiofibroma. *Am J Otolaryngol* 2001; 22:172–175.
93. Roger G, Tran Ba Huy P, Fraehlich P, et al. Exclusively endoscopic removal of juvenile nasopharyngeal angiofibroma. *Arch Otolaryngol Head Neck Surg* 2002;128:928–935.
94. Tewfik TL, Tan AK, Alnoviy K, et al. Juvenile nasopharyngeal angiofibroma. *J Otolaryngol* 1999;28: 145–151.
*95. Lee JT, Chen P, Safa A, et al. The role of radiation in the treatment of advanced juvenile angiofibroma. *Laryngoscope* 2002;112:1213–1220.
96. Zito J, Fitzpatrick P, Amedee R. Juvenile nasopharyngeal angiofibroma. *J La State Med Soc* 2001;153: 395–398.
97. Briant TDR, Fitzpatrick PJ, Book H. The radiological treatment of juvenile nasopharyngeal angiofibromas. *Ann Otolaryngol* 1970;79:1108–1113.
98. Briant TDR, Fitzpatrick PJ, Berman J. Nasopharyngeal angiofibroma: a twenty year study. *Laryngoscope* 1978;88:1247–1251.
99. Iannetti G, Belli E, DePonte F, et al. The surgical approaches to nasopharyngeal angiofibroma. *J Craniomaxillofac Surg* 1994;22:311–316.
100. Robinson ACR, Khoury GG, Ash DV, et al. Evaluation of response following irradiation of juvenile angiofibromas. *Br J Radiol* 1989;62:245–247.
101. Rao BN, Shewalkar BK. Clinical profile and multimodality approach in the management of juvenile nasopharyngeal angiofibroma. *Indian J Cancer* 2000; 37:133–139.
102. Benghait A. Juvenile nasopharyngeal angiofibroma treated by radiotherapy. *J Laryngol Otol* 1986;100: 351–356.
103. Kasper ME, Parsons JT, Mancuso AA, et al. Radiation therapy for juvenile angiofibroma: evaluation by CT and MRI, analysis of tumor regression, and selection of patients. *Int J Radiat Oncol Biol Phys* 1993;25:689–694.
104. Garcia-Cervigan E, Bien S, Rufenacht D, et al. Preoperative embolization of nasopharyngeal angiofibromas: report of 58 cases. *Neuroradiology* 1988;30: 556–560.
105. Bales C, Katapka M, Loevner LA, et al. Craniofacial resection of advanced nasopharyngeal angiofibroma.

Arch Otolaryngol Head Neck Surg 2002;128:1071–1078.

106. Jacobsson M, Petruson B, Svendsen P, et al. Juvenile nasopharyngeal angiofibroma: a report of eighteen cases. *Acta Otolaryngol* 1988;105:132–139.

107. Goepfert H, Cangir A, Lee YY. chemotherapy for aggressive juvenile nasopharyngeal angiofibroma. *Arch Otolaryngol* 1985;111:285–289.

108. Apostol JV, Frazell EL. Juvenile nasopharyngeal angiofibroma: a clinical study. *Cancer* 1965;18:869–878.

*109. Economou TS, Abemayor E, Ward P. Juvenile nasopharyngeal angiofibroma: an update of the UCLA experience, 1960–1985. *Laryngoscope* 1988;98:170–178.

110. Gross M, Gutjahr P. Therapy of rhabdomyosarcoma of the larynx. *Int J Pediatr Otorhinolaryngol* 1988;15:93–97.

111. Jereb B, Anggard A, Baryd I. Juvenile nasopharyngeal angiofibroma: a clinical study of 69 cases. *Acta Radiol (Ther)* 1970;9:302–310.

112. Makek MS, Andrews JC, Fisch U. Malignant transformation of a nasopharyngeal angiofibroma. *Laryngoscope* 1989;99:1088–1092.

113. Snow JB Jr. Neoplasms of the nasopharynx in children. *Otolaryngol Clin North Am* 1977;10:11–24.

114. Andrews C, Fish U, Valavanis A, et al. The surgical management of extensive nasopharyngeal angiofibromas with infratemporal fossa approach. *Laryngoscope* 1989;99:429–437.

115. Hedlund GL, Bisset GS III, Bove KE. Malignant neoplasms arising in cystic hamartomas of the lung in childhood. *Radiology* 1989;173:77–79.

116. Ward PH, Thompson R, Calcaterra T, et al. Juvenile angiofibroma: a more rational therapeutic approach based upon clinical and experimental evidence. *Laryngoscope* 1974;84:2181–2194.

117. Sessions RB, Bryan R, Naclerio R, et al. Radiographic staging of juvenile angiofibroma. *Head Neck Surg* 1981;3:279–183.

118. Fisch U. The infratemporal fossa approach for nasopharyngeal tumors. *Laryngoscope* 1983;93:36–44.

119. Radkowski D, McGill T, Healy GB, et al. Angiofibroma: changes in staging and treatment. *Arch Otolaryngol Head Neck Surg* 1996;122:122–129.

120. Cuyler JP. Treatment options for angiofibroma. *J Otolaryngol* 1988;17:214–218.

121. Kamel RH. Transnasal endoscopic surgery in juvenile nasopharyngeal angiofibroma. *J Laryngol Otol* 1996;110:962–968.

122. Petruson K, Rodriguez-Catarina M, Petruson B, et al. Juvenile nasopharyngeal angiofibroma: long-term results in preoperative embolized and non-embolized patients. *Acta Otolaryngol* 2002;122:96–100.

123. Cummings BJ, Blend R, Keane T, et al. Primary radiation therapy for juvenile nasopharyngeal angiofibroma. *Laryngoscope* 1984;94:1599–1605.

124. Sinha PP, Aziz HI. Juvenile nasopharyngeal angiofibroma: a report of seven cases. *Radiology* 1978;178:501–505.

125. Gullane PJ, Davidson J, O'Dwyer T, et al. Juvenile angiofibroma: a review of the literature and a case series report. *Laryngoscope* 1992;102:928–933.

126. Mannai C, Schwartz HC. Juvenile nasopharyngeal angiofibroma presenting as a facial swelling. *J Maxillofac Surg* 1986;14:329–331.

127. Harrison DF. The natural history, pathogenesis, and treatment of juvenile angiofibroma: personal experience with 44 patients. *Arch Otolaryngol Head Neck Surg* 1987;113:936–942.

128. McGahan RA, Durrance FY, Parke RB Jr, et al. The treatment of advanced juvenile nasopharyngeal angiofibroma. *Int J Radiat Oncol Biol Phys* 1989;17:1067–1072.

128a. Radkowski D, McGill T, Healy GB, et al. Angiofibroma: changes in staging and treatment. *Arch Otolaryngol Head Neck Surg* 1996;122:122–129.

129. Fisch U. The infratemporal fossa approach for nasopharyngeal tumors. *Laryngoscope* 1983;93:36–44.

130. Ayan I, Kaytan E, Ayan N. Childhood nasopharyngeal carcinoma: from biology to treatment. *Lancet Oncol* 2003;39:51–57.

131. Ayan I, Altun M. Nasopharyngeal carcinoma in children: retrospective review of 50 patients. *Int J Radiat Oncol Biol Phys* 1996;35:485–492.

132. Werner-Wasik M, Winkler P, Uri A, et al Nasopharyngeal carcinoma in children. *Med Pediatr Oncol* 1996;26:352–358.

133. Ong YK, Tan KK. Case report: nasopharyngeal carcinoma in children. *Int J Pediatr Otorhinolaryngol* 2000;55:149–154.

*134. Uzel O, Yoruk SO, Sahinler I, et al. Nasopharyngeal carcinoma in childhood: long-term results of 32 patients. *Radiother Oncol* 2001;58:137–141.

*135. Berberoglu S, Illhan I, Cetindag F, et al. Nasopharyngeal carcinoma in Turkish children: review of 33 cases. *Pediatr Hematol Oncol* 2001;18:305–315.

136. Sahraoui S, Acharki A, Benider A, et al. Nasopharyngeal carcinoma in children under 15 years of age: a retrospective review of 65 patients. *Ann Oncol* 1999;10:1499–1502.

137. Counter RT, Linares L, Shaw HJ, et al. Cancer of the nasopharynx in under 21-year-olds: a review. *Clin Oncol* 1980;6:213–220.

138. Farrow JH, Ashikari H. Breast cancer in young girls. *Surg Clin North Am* 1969;49:261–269.

139. Gin D, Hu Y, Yan J, et al. Analysis of 1379 patients with nasopharyngeal carcinoma treated by radiation. *Cancer* 1988;61:1117–1124.

140. Papvasiliou C, Pavaltou M, Pappas J. Nasopharyngeal cancer in patients under the age of thirty years. *Cancer* 1977;40:2312–2316.

141. Tsao SY, Shiu WCT. Radiotherapy and chemotherapy for nasopharyngeal carcinoma. *Ear Nose Throat J* 1990;69:272–278.

142. Snow JB Jr. Carcinoma of the nasopharynx in children. *Ann Otol* 1975;84:817–826.

143. Pao WJ, Hustu OH, Douglass EC, et al. Pediatric nasopharyngeal carcinoma: long term follow-up of 29 patients. *Int J Radiat Oncol Biol Phys* 1989;17:299–305.

144. Hawkins EP, Krischer JP, Smith BE, et al. Nasopharyngeal carcinoma in children—a retrospective review and demonstration of Epstein–Barr viral genomes in tumor cell cytoplasm: a report of the Pediatric Oncology Group. *Hum Pathol* 1990;21:805–810.

145. Zubizarreta PA, D'Antonio G, Raslawski E, et al. Nasopharyngeal carcinoma in childhood and adolescence: a single-institution experience with combined therapy. *Cancer* 2000;89:690–695.

146. Wang CC. *Radiation therapy for head and neck neoplasms,* 3rd ed. Chicago: Wiley-Liss, 1997.

147. Pick T, Maurer HM, McWilliams NB. Lymphoepithelioma in childhood. *J Pediatr* 1974;84:96–100.

148. Kim TH, McLaren J, Alvardo CS, et al. Adjuvant chemotherapy for advanced nasopharyngeal carcinoma in childhood. *Cancer* 1989;63:1922–1926.

149. Fernandez CH, Camgir A, Samaan N, et al. Nasopharyngeal carcinoma in children. *Cancer* 1976;37:2787–2791.

150. Arush MB, Stein ME, Rosenblatt E, et al. Advanced nasopharyngeal carcinoma in the young: the Northern Israel Oncology Center experience, 1973–1991. *Pediatr Hematol Oncol* 1995;12:271–276.

151. Zabel A, Thilmann C, Milker-Zabel S, et al. The role of stereotactically guided conformal radiotherapy for local control of esthesioneuroblastoma. *Strahlenther Onkol* 2002;178:187–191.

*152. Wolden SL, Steinherz PG, Kraus DH, et al. Improved long-term survival with combined modality therapy for pediatric nasopharynx cancer. *Int J Radiat Oncol Biol Phys* 2002;46:859–864.

153. Burkey B, Koopman CF, Brunberg J. The use of biopsy in the evaluation of pediatric nasopharyngeal masses. *Int J Pediatr Otorhinolaryngol* 1990;20:169–179.

154. Strojan P, Benedik MD, Kragelj B, et al. Combined radiation and chemotherapy for advanced undifferentiated nasopharyngeal carcinoma in children. *Med Pediatr Oncol* 1997;28:366–369.

*155. Gasparini M, Lombardi F, Rottoli L, et al. Improved relapse free survival with combined radiotherapy and chemotherapy in stage T3–T4 nasopharyngeal carcinoma. *J Clin Oncol* 1988;6:491–494.

155a. Palmer RE, Hustu HO. Combined radiotherapy and chemotherapy of lymphoepithelioma in children. *Proc Am Assoc Cancer Res* 1973;421:106.

156. Baker SR, McClathey KD. Carcinoma of the nasopharynx in childhood. *Otolaryngol Head Neck Surg* 1987;89:555–559.

157. Martin WD, Shah KJ. Carcinoma of the nasopharynx in young patients. *Int J Radiat Oncol Biol Phys* 1994;28:991–999.

158. Haghbin M, Kramer S, Patchefsky AS, et al. Carcinoma of the nasopharynx: a 25-year study. *Am J Clin Oncol* 1985;8:334–392.

159. Jenkin RDT, Anderson JR, Jereb B, et al. Nasopharyngeal carcinoma—a retrospective review of patients less than thirty years of age: a report from Children's Cancer Study Group. *Cancer* 1981;47:360–366.

160. Chandler JR, Goulding R, Moskowitz L, et al. Nasopharyngeal angiofibromas: staging and management. *Ann Otol Rhinol Laryngol* 1984;93:322–329.

160a. Nguyen LN, Ang KK. radiotherapy for cancer of the head and neck: altered fractionation regimens. *Lancet Oncol* 2002;3:693–701.

161. Ingersoll L, Woo SY, Donaldson S, et al. Nasopharyngeal carcinoma in the young: a combined M. D. Anderson and Stanford experience. *Int J Radiat Oncol Biol Phys* 1990;19:881–887.

162. Gasparini M, Rottoli L, Ballerini E, et al. Improved RFS in stage T3–T4 nasopharyngeal carcinoma of children with radiotherapy and ADM + VCR + CTX. *Proc Am Soc Clin Oncol* 1987;6:A864.

163. Al Sarraf M, LeBlanc M, Gin M, et al. Chemoradiotherapy versus radiotherapy in patients with advanced nasopharyngeal cancer: phase III randomized intergroup study 0099. *J Clin Oncol* 1998;16:1310–1317.

164. Chua DT, Sham JS, Choy D, et al. Preliminary report of Asian–Oceanian Clinical Oncology Association randomized trial comparing cisplatin and epirubicin followed by radiotherapy versus radiotherapy alone in the treatment of patients with locally advanced nasopharyngeal carcinoma. *Cancer* 1998;83:2270–2283.

165. International Nasopharynx Cancer Study Group. VUMCA trial I: preliminary results of randomized trial comparing neoadjuvant chemotherapy (cisplatin, epirubicin, bleomycin) plus radiotherapy vs. radiotherapy alone stage IV (>N2, Mo) undifferentiated nasopharyngeal carcinoma: a positive effect on progression-free survival. *Int J Radiat Oncol Biol Phys* 1996;35:463–469.

166. Chatani M, Teshima T, Inoue T, et al. Radiation therapy for nasopharyngeal carcinoma: retrospective review of 105 patients based on a survey of Kansai Cancer Therapist Group. *Cancer* 1986;57:2267–2271.

167. Brizel DM, Overgaard J. Does amifostine have a role in chemoradiation treatment? *Lancet Oncol* 2003;4:378–381.

168. Aughton DJ, Sloan CT, Milad MP, et al. Nasopharyngeal teratoma ("hairy polyp"), Dandy–Walker malformation, diaphragmatic hernia, and other anomalies in a female infant. *J Med Genet* 1990;27:788–790.

169. Har-El G, Zirkin HY, Tovi F, et al. Congenital pleomorphic adenoma of the nasopharynx: report of a case. *J Laryngol Otol* 1985;99:1281–1287.

170. Tischer W, Reddemann H, Herzog P, et al. Experience in surgical treatment of pulmonary and bronchial tumors in childhood. *Prog Pediatr Surg* 1987;21:118–135.

171. Mallouh A. Nasopharyngeal Hodgkin's disease with intracranial extension in a child. *Med Pediatr Oncol* 1989;17:174–177.

172. Silva EG, Butler JJ, MacKay B, et al. Neuroblastomas and neuroendocrine carcinomas of the nasal cavity: a proposed new classification. *Cancer* 1982;50:2388–2405.

*173. Slevin NJ, Irwin CJR, Banerjee SS, et al. Olfactory neural tumours: the role of external beam radiotherapy. *J Laryngol Otol* 1996;110:1012–1016.

174. Spaulding CA, Kranyak MS, Constable WC, et al. Esthesioneuroblastoma: a comparison of two treatment eras. *Int J Radiat Oncol Biol Phys* 1988;15:581–590.

175. Berger L, Lue G, Richard D. L'esthesioneuroepitheliome olfactif. *Bull Assoc Fr Etude Cancer* 1924;13:410–421.

*176. Eich HT, Staar S, Micke O, et al. Radiotherapy of esthesioneuroblastoma. *Int J Radiat Oncol Biol Phys* 2001;49:155–160.

177. Kadish S, Goodman M, Wang CC. Olfactory neuroblastoma: a clinical analysis of 17 cases. *Cancer* 1976;37:1571–1576.

178. Eriksen JG, Basthold L, Kroshal AS, et al. Esthesioneuroblastoma: what is the optimal treatment? *Acta Oncol* 2000;39:231–235.

179. Foote RL, Morita A, Ebersold MJ, et al. Esthesioneuroblastoma: the role of adjuvant radiotherapy. *Int J Radiat Oncol Biol Phys* 1993;27:835–842.

180. Elkon D, Hightower SI, Lim ML, et al. Esthesioneuroblastoma. *Cancer* 1979;44:1087–1094.

181. Resto VA, Eisele DW, Forastiere A, et al. Esthe-

sioneuroblastoma: the Johns Hopkins experience. *Head Neck* 2000;22:550–558.

182. Argiris A, Dutra J, Tseke P, et al. Esthesioneuroblastoma: the Northwestern experience. *Laryngoscope* 2003;113:155–160.

*183. Eden BV, Debo RF, Larner JM, et al. Esthesioneuroblastoma. *Cancer* 1994;73:10:2556–2562.

184. Bhattacharyya N, Thornton AF, Joseph MP, et al. Successful treatment of esthesioneuroblastoma and neuroendocrine carcinoma with combined chemotherapy and proton radiation. *Arch Otolaryngol Head Neck Surg* 1997;123:34–40.

185. Gruber G, Laedrach K, Baumeit B, et al. Esthesioneuroblastoma: irradiation alone and surgery alone are not enough. *Int J Radiat Oncol Biol Phys* 2002;54:486–491.

186. Dulguerov P, Calcaterra T. Esthesioneuroblastoma: the UCLA experience 1979–1990. *Laryngoscope* 1992;102:843–848.

187. Elkon D, Hightower SI, Lin ML, et al. Esthesioneuroblastoma *Cancer* 1979;44:1087–1094.

188. O'Connor TA, McLean P, Julliard GJF, et al. Olfactory neuroblastoma. *Cancer* 1989;63:2426–2428.

189. de Campora E, Radici M, de Campora L. Neurogenic tumors of the head and neck in children. *Int J Pediatr Otorhinolaryng* 1999;49[Suppl 1]:S231–S233.

190. Ang KK, Garden AS, Morrison WH. Sinonasal cancer. In: Gunderson LL, Tepper JE (eds). Clinical radiation oncology. New York: Churchill Livingstone, 2000:504–518.

191. Gudea F, Van Limbergen E, Van Den Bogaert W. High dose level radiation therapy for local tumour control in esthesioneuroblastoma. *Eur J Cancer* 1994;12;1757–1760.

192. Mendez P Jr, Maves MD, Panje WR. Squamous cell carcinoma of the head and neck in patients under 40 years of age. *Arch Otolaryngol* 1985;111:762–764.

193. Schwaab G, Bouzouita K, Janot F, et al. Les cancers oral de l'enfant repartition histologique et topographique. Indications therapeutiques (a propos de 380 cas IGR 1975–1987). *Bull Cancer* 1989;76:757–762.

194. Rapidis AD, Economidis J, Goumas PD, et al. Tumours of the head and neck in children: a clinicopathological analysis of 1007 cases. *J Craniomaxillofac Surg* 1988;16:279–286.

195. Usenius T, Karja J, Collan Y. Squamous cell carcinoma of the tongue in children. *Cancer* 1987;60:236–239.

196. Moore C. Visceral squamous cancer in children. *Pediatrics* 1958;21:573–581.

197. New GB, Hertz CS. Malignant disease of the face, mouth, pharynx, and larynx in the first three decades of life. *Surg Gynecol Obstet* 1940;70:163–169.

198. Patel DD, Dave RI. Carcinoma of the anterior tongue in adolescence. *Cancer* 1976;37:917–921.

199. Wysocki J. Minimal distances between temporal bone structures and their mutual correlations. *Med Sci Monit* 2002;8:BR80–BR83.

200. Callender DL, Frankenthaler RA, Luna MA, et al. Salivary neck neoplasms in children. *Arch Otolaryngol Head Neck Surg* 1992;118:474–476.

201. Castro EB, Huvos AG, Strong EW, et al. Tumors of the major salivary glands in children. *Cancer* 1972;29:312–317.

202. Douglas JG, Einck J, Austin-Seymour M, et al. Neutron radiotherapy for recurrent pleomorphic adenomas of major salivary glands. *Head Neck* 2001;23:1037–1042.

203. Gustafson H, Dahlquist A, Anniko M, et al. Mucoepidermoid carcinoma in a minor salivary gland in childhood. *J Laryngol Otol* 1987;101:1320–1323.

204. Roy TM, Dow FT, Puthuff DL. Upper airway obstruction from AIDS-related Kaposi's sarcoma. *J Emerg Med* 1991;9:23–25.

205. Meeuwis J, Bas CE, Hoeve LJ, et al. Subglottic hemangiomas in infants: treatment with intralesional corticosteroid injections and intubation. *Int J Pediatr Otorhinolaryngol* 1990;19:145–150.

206. Remacle M, Declaye X, Mayne A. Subglottic hemangioma in the infant: contribution of CO_2 laser. *J Laryngol Otol* 1989;103:930–934.

207. Shikhani AH, Marsh BR, Jones MM, et al. Infantile subglottic hemangiomas: an update. *Ann Otol Rhinol Laryngol* 1986;95:336–347.

208. Phipps CD, Gibson WS, Wood WE. Infantile subglottic hemangioma: a review and presentation of two cases of surgical excision. *Int J Pediatr Otorhinolaryngol* 1997; 41:71–79.

209. Gregg CM, Wiatrak BJ, Koopmann Jr CF. Management options for infantile subglottic hemangioma. *Am J Otolaryngol* 1995;16:409–414.

210. Hoeve LJ, Kuppeis GLE, Verwoerd CDA. Management of infantile subglottic hemangioma: laser vaporization, submucous resection, intubation, or intralesional steroids? *Int J Pediatr Otorhinolaryngol* 1997;42:179–186.

211. Holborow CA, Mott TJ. Subglottic haemangioma in infancy. *J Laryngol Otol* 1973;87:1013–1017.

212. Benjamin B. Treatment of infantile subglottic hemangioma with radioactive gold grain. *Ann Otol* 1978;87:18–21.

213. Benjamin B, Carter P. Congenital laryngeal hemangioma. *Ann Otol Rhinol Laryngol* 1983;92:448–455.

214. Hertzanu Y. Mendelsohn DB, Davidge-Pitts K, et al. Preoperative embolization in paediatric maxillofacial haemangiomas. *J Laryngol Otol* 1985;99:1089–1095.

215. Mouzard A, Damalain MN, Chassagne D. Intubation tracheale des angiomas sous-glottiques due nourisson brachytherapie locale du ^{32}P. *Intensive Care Med* 1977;3:186.

216. Seid AB, Pransky SM, Kearns DB. The open surgical approach to subglottic hemangioma. *Int J Pediatr Otorhinolaryngol* 1991;22:85–90.

217. New GB, Clark CM. Angiomas of the larynx. Report of three cases. *Ann Otol Rhinol Laryngol* 1919;28:1025–1037.

218. DuVall GA, Walden DT. Adenocarcinoma of the esophagus complicating Cornelia de Lange syndrome. *J Clin Gastroenterol* 1996;22(2):131–133.

219. Hassoun AAK, Hay ID, Goellner JR, et al. Insular thyroid carcinoma in adolescents. *Cancer* 1997;79:1044–1048.

220. Hassall E. Barrett's esophagus: new definitions and approaches in children. *J Pediatr Gastroenterol Nutr* 1993;16:345–364.

221. Isolauri J, Markkula H. Lye ingestion and carcinoma of the esophagus. *Acta Chir Scand* 1989;155:269–271.

222. Wahrendorf J, Chang-Claude J, Liang QS, et al. Precursor lesions of oesophageal cancer in young people

in a high-risk population in China. *Lancet* 1989;2: 1239–1241.

223. Schettini ST, Ganc A, Saba L. Esophageal carcinoma secondary to a chemical injury in a child. *Pediatr Surg Int* 1983;13:519–520.

224. Hoeffel JC. Letter to the editor. *Eur J Pediatr Surg* 2001;11:143.

225. Shahi UP, Sundersan D, DaHagupta S, et al. Carcinoma oesophagus in a 14 year old child: report of a case and review of literature. *Trop Gastroenterol* 1989;10:225–228.

226. Perch SJ, Saffen EM, Whittington R, et al. Esophageal sarcomas. *J Surg Oncol* 1991;48:194–198.

227. Bolandi L, DeGiorgia R, Santi V, et al. Primary non-Hodgkin's T-cell lymphoma of the esophagus: a case with peculiar endoscopic ultrasonographic pattern. *Dig Dis Sci* 1990;35:1426–1430.

228. Goldthorn JF, Canizaro PC. Gastrointestinal malignancies in infancy, childhood, and adolescence. *Surg Clin North Am* 1986;66:845–861.

229. Bourque MD, Spigland N, Bensoussan AL, et al. Esophageal leiomyoma in children: two case reports and reviews of the literature. *J Pediatr Surg* 1989;24: 1103–1107.

230. Vade A, Nolan J. Posterior mediastinal teratoma involving the esophagus. *Gastrointest Radiol* 1989;14: 106–108.

231. Wolf Y, Katz S, Lax E, et al. Dysphagia in a child with aggressive fibromatosis of the esophagus. *J Pediatr Surg* 1989;24:1137–1139.

232. Hartman GE, Shochat SJ. Primary pulmonary neoplasms of childhood: a review. *Am J Thorac Surg* 1983;36:108–119.

233. Curcio LD, Cohen JS, Grannis FW, et al. Primary lymphoepithelioma-like carcinoma of the lung in a child. *Chest* 1996;111:250–251.

234. Kern WH, Stiles QR. Pulmonary blastoma. *J Thorac Cardiovasc Surg* 1976;72:801–808.

235. Kantar M, Getingul N, Veral A, et al. Rare tumors of the lung in children. *Pediatr Hematol Oncol* 2002;19: 421–428.

236. Granata C, Gambini C, Carlini C, et al. Pleuropulmonary blastoma. *Eur J Pediatr Surg* 2001;11: 271–273.

237. Jimenez JF. Pulmonary blastoma in childhood. *J Surg Oncol* 1987;34:87–93.

238. Kowalski P, Rodziewicz B, Pejcz J. Bilateral bronchioalveolar carcinoma of the lungs in a 7 year old girl treated for Hodgkin's disease. *Tumor* 1989;75: 449–451.

239. Lodge JPA, Hamilton JRL, Walker DR, et al. Surgical management of thoracic malignancy in childhood: eight years' experience in Leeds. *Ann R Coll Surg Engl* 1988;70:109–112.

240. Niitu Y, Kubota H, Hasegawa S, et al. Lung cancer (squamous cell carcinoma) in adolescence. *Am J Dis Child* 1974;127:108–111.

241. Pettinato G, Manivel JC, Saldana MJ, et al. Primary bronchopulmonary fibrosarcoma of childhood and adolescence: reassessment of a low grade malignancy. *Hum Pathol* 1989;20:463–471.

242. Barnard WG. Embryoma of lung. *Thorax* 1952; 7:299–301.

243. Koss MN, Hochholzer L, O'Leary T. Pulmonary blastomas. *Cancer* 1991;67:2368–2381.

244. Merriman TE, Beasley SW, Chow CW, et al. A rare tumor masquerading as an empyema: pleuropulmonary blastoma. *Pediatr Pulmonol* 1996;28:408–411.

245. Senac MO Jr, Wood BP, Isaacs H, et al. Pulmonary blastoma: a rare childhood malignancy. *Radiology* 1991;179:743–746.

246. Manivel JC, Priest JR, Walterson J, et al. Pleuropulmonary blastoma: the so-called pulmonary blastoma of childhood. *Cancer* 1988;62:1516–1526.

247. Nag S, Tippin D, Ruymann FB. Intraoperative high–dose-rate brachytherapy for the treatment of pediatric tumors: the Ohio State University experience. *Int J Radiat Oncol Biol Phys* 2001;51:729–735.

248. Ozkaynak MF, Ortega JA, Laug W, et al. Role of chemotherapy in pediatric pulmonary blastoma. *Med Pediatr Oncol* 1990;18:53–56.

249. Schmaltz C, Sauter S, Opitz O, et al. Pleuropulmonary blastoma: a case report and review of the literature. *Med Pediatr Oncol* 1995;25:479–484.

250. Tovar JA, Eizaguirre I, Albert A, et al. Peutz–Jeghers syndrome in children: report of two cases and review of the literature. *J Pediatr Surg* 1983;18:1–6.

251. deParedes CG, Pierce WS, Groff DB, et al. Bronchogenic tumors in children. *Arch Surg* 1970;100: 574–576.

252. Fraire AE, Cooper S, Greenberg SD, et al. Mesothelioma of childhood. *Cancer* 1988;62:838–847.

253. Sawyer KC, Sawyer RB, Lubchenco AE, et al. Fatal primary cancer of the lung in a teenage smoker. *Cancer* 1967;20:451–457.

254. DeCaro L, Benfield JR. Lung cancer in young persons. *J Thorac Cardiovasc Surg* 1982;83:372–376.

255. Azab MB, Henry-Amar M, Rougier P, et al. Prognostic factors in primary gastrointestinal non-Hodgkin's lymphoma: a multivariate analysis, report of 106 cases, and review of the literature. *Cancer* 1989;64: 1208–1217.

256. Lavin P, Hajdu SI, Foote FW Jr. Gastric and extragastric leiomyosarcomas: clinicopathologic study of 44 cases. *Cancer* 1972;29:305–311.

257. Mahour GH, Isaacs H Jr, Change L. Primary malignant tumors of the stomach in children. *J Pediatr Surg* 1980;15:603–608.

258. Jaeger HJ, Schmitz-Stolbrink A, Albrecht M, et al. Gastric leiomyosarcoma in a child. *Eur J Radiol* 1996;23:111–114.

259. Wright JR Jr, Kyriakos M, DeSchryver-Keeskemeti K. Malignant fibrous histiocytomas of the stomach. *Arch Pathol Lab Med* 1988;112:251–258.

259a. Siegel SE, Hays DM, Romansky S, et al. Carcinoma of the stomach in childhood. *Cancer* 1976;38:1781–1784.

260. Chatura KR, Nadar S, Pulimood S, et al. Gastric carcinoma as a complication of dyskeratosis congenita in an adolescent boy. *Dig Dis Sci* 1996;41:2340–2342.

261. Kuragoglu S, Mihmanli I, Gelken T, et al. Radiological features in paediatric primary gastric MALT lymphoma and association with *Helicobacter pylori*. *Pediatr Radiol* 2002;32:82–87.

262. Li P, Wei J, West AB, et al. Epithelioid gastrointestinal stromal tumor of the stomach with liver metastases in a 12-year-old girl: aspiration cytology and molecular study. *Pediatr Dev Pathol* 2002;5:386–394.

263. Defachelles AS, de Lassalle EM, Boutard P, et al. Pancreatoblastoma in childhood: clinical course and

therapeutic management of seven patients. *Med Pediatr Oncol* 2001;37:47–52.

264. Klimstra DS, Wenig BM, Adair CF, et al. Pancreatoblastoma: a clinicopathologic study and review of the literature. *Am J Surg Pathol* 1995;19:1371–1389.

265. Ogawa T, Okinaga K, Nakumare K, et al. Pancreatoblastoma treated by delayed operation after effective chemotherapy. *J Pediatr Surg* 2000;35:1663–1665.

266. Murakami T, Ueki K, Kawakami H, et al. Pancreatoblastoma: case report and review of treatment in the literature. *Med Pediatr Oncol* 1996;27:193–197.

267. Willnow U, Willberg B, Schwamborn D, et al. Pancreatoblastoma in children case report and review of the literature. *Eur J Pediatr Surg* 1996;6:369–372.

*268. Shorter NA, Glick RD, Klimstra DS, et al. Malignant pancreatic tumors in childhood and adolescence: the Memorial Sloan–Kettering experience, 1967 to present. *J Pediatr Surg* 2002;37:887–892.

269. Griffin BR, Wisbeck WM, Schaller RT, et al. Radiotherapy for locally recurrent infantile pancreatic carcinoma (pancreatoblastoma). *Cancer* 1987; 15:1734–1736.

270. Kaushal V, Goel A, Rattan KN, et al. Pancreatoblastoma. *Indian J Pediatr* 2001;68:1075–1077.

271. Horie A, Yano Y, Kotoo Y, et al. Morphogenesis of pancreatoblastoma, infantile carcinoma of the pancreas: report of two cases. *Cancer* 1977;39:247–254.

272. Luttges J, Stigge C, Pacena M, et al. Rare ductal adenocarcinoma of the pancreas in patients younger than age 40 years. *Cancer* 2004;100:173–182.

273. Rich RH, Dehner LP, Okinaga K, et al. Surgical management of islet–cell adenoma in infancy. *Surgery* 1978;84:519–526.

274. Vejcho S. Carcinoma of the pancreas in childhood: a case report of long term survival. *J Med Assoc Thai* 1993;76:177–183.

275. Pelizza G, La Riccia A, Bouvier R, et al. Carcinoid tumors of the appendix in children. *Pediatr Surg Int* 2001;17:399–402.

276. Assadi M, Kubiak R, Kaiser G. Appendiceal carcinoid tumors in children: does size matter? *Med Pediatr Oncol* 2002;38:65–66.

277. Spunt SL, Pratt CB, Rao BN, et al. Childhood carcinoid tumors: the St. Jude Children's Research Hospital experience. *J Pediatr Surg* 2000;35:1282–1286.

278. Freeman J. Leiomyosarcoma of small bowel: a case report. *J Pediatr Surg* 1979;14:477–478.

279. Yamamoto K, Tanaka T, Kuno K, et al. Carcinoma of the colon in children: case report and review of the Japanese literature. *J Gastroenterol* 1994;29:647–652.

279a.Taguchi T, Suita S, Hirata Y, et al. Carcinoma of the colon in children: a case report and review of 41 Japanese cases. *J Pediatr Gastroenterol Nutr* 1991;12:394–399.

280. Lamego CMB, Tarlani H. Colorectal adenocarcinoma in childhood and adolescence: report of 11 cases and review of the literature. *Pediatr Radiol* 1989;19:504–508.

281. Ko WS, Lin LH, Chen DF. Carcinoma of the colon in a child. *Acta Paediatr Sin* 1994;36:227–230.

282. Hwang EH, Chung WH. Adenocarcinoma of the transverse colon in a child with survival: a case report. *Kyoemi Med J* 1993;34:287–292.

283. Takahoshi H, Hansmann ML. Primary gastrointestinal lymphoma in childhood (up to 18 years of age). *J Cancer Res Clin Oncol* 1990;116:190–196.

284. Deutsch M, Wollman R, Ramanathan R, et al. Rectal cancer twenty-one years after treatment of childhood Hodgkin's disease. *Med Pediatr Oncol* 2002;38:280–281.

285. Pratt CB, Rivera G, Shanks E, et al. Colorectal carcinoma in adolescents: implications regarding etiology. *Cancer* 1977;40:2464–2472.

286. Rose RH, Axelrod DM, Aldea PA, et al. Colorectal carcinoma in the young: a case report and review of the literature. *Clin Pediatr* 1988;27:105–108.

287. Umpleby HC, Williamson RC. Large bowel cancer in the young. *Ann Acad Med Singapore* 1987;16:456–461.

288. Nagaya M, Tsuda M, Ishiguro Y. Leiomyosarcoma of the transverse colon in a neonate: a rare case of meconium peritonitis. *J Pediatr Surg* 1989 24:1177–1180.

289. Dugue G, Back G, Molho L, et al. Breast cancer in the young. *J Natl Med Assoc* 1989;81:1184–1187.

290. Eskelinen M, Vainio J, Tuominen L, et al. Carcinoma of the breast in children. *Z Kinderchir* 1990;45:52–55.

291. Bower R, Bell MJ, Ternberg JL. Management of breast lesions in children and adolescents. *J Surg* 1976;11:337–346.

292. Sears JB, Schlesinger MJ. Carcinoma of the breast in a ten-year old girl: report of a case. *N Engl J Med* 1940;223:760–761.

293. Templeman C, Hertweck SP. Breast disorder in the pediatric and adolescent patient. *Obstet Gynecol Clin North Am* 2000;27:19–34.

294. Murphy JJ, Marzaria S, Gowk W, et al. Breast cancer in a 6-year-old child. *J Pediatr Surg* 2000;35:765–767.

295. Hildreth NG, Shore RE, Dvoretsky PM. The risk of breast cancer after irradiation of the thymus in infancy. *N Engl J Med* 1989;321:1281–1284

296. Miliauskas JR, Leong ASY. Adenoid cystic carcinoma in a juvenile male breast. *Pathology* 1991;23:298–301.

297. Rogers DA, Lobe TE, Rao BN, et al. Breast malignancy in children. *J Pediatr Surg* 1994;24:48–51.

298. Wiatrak BJ, Koopmann CF, Turrisi AT. Radiation therapy as an alternative to surgery in the management of intracranial juvenile nasopharyngeal angiofibroma. *Int J Pediatr Otorhinolaryngol* 1993;28:51–61.

299. Berry MP, Smith CR, Brown TC, et al. Nasopharyngeal carcinoma in the young. *Int J Radiat Oncol Biol Phys* 1980;6:415–421.

300. Greene FL, Page DL, Fleming, ID, et al., eds. *AJCC cancer staging manual,* 6th ed. Heidelberg: Springer, 2002.

301. Stier J, Huh C, Lapidot A. Squamous carcinoma of nasopharynx in a child. *Bull N Y Acad Med* 1974;49:610–612.

302. LaNasa JJ, Putney FJ. Nasopharyngeal malignancy in childhood. *South Med J* 1974;67:1363–1364.

303. Ellouz R, Cammoun M, Attia RB, et al. Nasopharyngeal carcinoma in children and adolescents in Tunisia: clinical aspects and the paraneoplastic syndrome. In: de The G, ed. *NPC etiology and control.* WHO-IARC science publication no. 20. WHO–IARC. Lyon: International Agency for Research on Cancer, 1978:115–130.

304. Jereb B, Huvos AG, Steinherz P, et al. Nasopharyngeal carcinoma in children. Review of 16 cases. *Int J Radiat Oncol Biol Phys* 1980;6:415–421.
305. Lombardi F, Gasparini M, Gianni C, et al. Nasopharyngeal carcinoma in childhood. *Med Pediatr Oncol* 1982;10:243–250.
306. Castro-Vita, Mendiondo O, Shaw E, et al. Nasopharyngeal carcinoma in second decade of life. *Radiology* 1983;148:253–256.
307. Morales P, Bosch A, Salaverry S, et al. Cancer of nasopharynx in young patients. *J Surg Oncol* 1984;27: 181–185.
308. Sarrazin D, Schwaab G, Fontaine F, et al. La radiotherapie des carcinomes nasopharynx chez l'enfant après chimotherapie primable. Resultants preliminaires sur 21 cas traites a l'institut Gustave–Roussy entre 1978 et 1981. *Ann Otolaryngol* 1985;175–178.
309. Lobo-Sanahuja F, Garcia I, Carranza A, et al. Treatment and outcome of undifferentiated carcinoma of the nasopharynx in childhood: a 13-year experience. *Med Pediatr Oncol* 1986;14:6–11.
310. Roper RH, Essex-Cater A, Marsen HB, et al. Nasopharyngeal carcinoma in children. *Pediatr Hematol Oncol* 1986;3:143–152.
311. de Cassia Broga Ribeiro R, Kowalski LP, Saba LMB, et al. Epithelial salivary gland neoplasm in children and adolescents: a forty-four-year experience. *Med Pediatr Oncol* 2002;39:594–600.
312. Hicks J, Flaitz C. Mucoepidermoid carcinoma of salivary glands in children and adolescents: assessment of proliferation markers. *Oral Oncol* 2000;36:454–460.
313. Luna MA, Batsakis JG, El-Naggar AK. Salivary gland tumors in children. *Ann Otol Rhinol Laryngol* 1991;100:869–871.
314. Samuel AM, Sharma SM. Differentiated thyroid carcinoma in children and adolescents. *Cancer* 1981:67: 2186–2190.

17

Langerhans Cell Histiocytosis

Edward C. Halperin, M.D.

HISTORICAL BACKGROUND

Paul Wilhelm Heinrich Langerhans (1847–1888) was born in Berlin. His father and his two brothers were physicians. While still an undergraduate student, Langerhans used Cohnheim's gold chloride staining technique to identify a novel non-pigmentary dendritic cell in the epidermis. When he was 21 years old, he described this finding in an 1868 paper titled "Uber die Nerven der menschlichen Haut [On the nerves of the human skin]" (2). Langerhans initially regarded these cells as intraepidermal receptors for extracutaneous signals of the nervous system. He later changed his mind and in 1882 wrote that "my cells are in no way essential for nerve endings" (3). Langerhans studied medicine with Heckel and Virchow. He defended his thesis in 1869, titled "Contributions to the Microscopic Anatomy of the Pancreas." He identified a cell in the human pancreas, now called Langerhans islets. After his thesis defense, Langerhans demonstrated that cinnabar was taken up by white blood corpuscles but never by the red. This opened the door for Aschoff's concept of the reticuloendothelial system.

In 1874 Langerhans became Professor Extraordinarius in Freiburg. Unfortunately, one week later he was diagnosed with renal tuberculosis. After a leave of absence he was released from his duties at the university and left for Madeira. He continued to do research on the flora and fauna of the Atlantic Islands and Madeira in particular. His contributions were of such high quality that in 1909 a polychaete worm was named after him. Langerhans practiced medicine whenever his health allowed. The majority of his patients were German and British citizens who lived on the island for health reasons, usually tuberculosis. Langerhans died of progressive renal degeneration caused by tuberculosis on July 20, 1888, in Madeira. He published two papers on tuberculosis, undoubtedly influenced by his own condition and by the fact that his mother had died of tuberculosis and his half brother had also contracted the disease (4,5).

In 1893, Dr. Alfred Hand, Jr., a 25-year-old resident at the Children's Hospital of Philadelphia, reported the case of a 3-year-old boy with "a history of great thirst and polyuria . . . undersized and puny." At autopsy, he found a lesion in the skull (6):

> A yellow spot about the size of a five-cent piece was noticed near the right parietal eminence. When the skull-cap was removed, this spot was seen on the inner side as well, and the entire thickness of the bone there was soft and movable. . . . The lymphatic glands . . . all through the body were greatly enlarged. . . . The liver and spleen were enlarged and firm, and the former had minute gray nodules in its substance. . . . Microscopial sections showed nodular masses of small, round-celled infiltration in the liver, spleen, kidneys.

Hand suspected that he was dealing with a case of tuberculosis. In 1921, he noted the similarity of his original case to ones subsequently reported by Schuller, Christian, and Kay. Eventually, the term *Hand–Schuller–Christian disease* or *triad* was used to describe a disease occurring in children more than 2 years old. It was characterized by exophthalmos, lesions in the bones of the skull, and diabetes insipidus. The full triad was rarely seen, and the prognosis was good (1,7–9).

In 1924 and 1933, pathologist Letterer and pediatrician Siwe described what they perceived to be an entity distinct from Hand–Schuller–Christian disease. Letterer–Siwe disease generally occurred in children less than 2 years old.

The diagnostic criteria included splenomegaly, hepatomegaly, lymphadenopathy, anemia, and a hemorrhagic diathesis. The prognosis was poor (6–9).

In 1940, Otani and Ehrlich (10) described a granuloma of bone simulating a primary neoplasm. Eventually, the solitary eosinophilic granuloma was described as occurring in children more than 2 years old and characterized by a solitary, usually bony site of involvement. The prognosis was excellent (8,9).

In 1953, pathologist Lichtenstein argued that eosinophilic granuloma of bone, Letterer–Siwe disease, and Hand–Schuller–Christian disease were related manifestations of a single nosologic entity (6,9). He used the name *histiocytosis X* to refer to a spectrum of diseases of the mononuclear phagocyte (histiocyte). The *X* referred to the unknown etiology and pathogenesis of the disease or diseases. The diseases formerly grouped under the heading *histiocytosis X* are now called *Langerhans cell histiocytosis* (LCH) (1).

DEFINITION, PATHOGENESIS, AND PATHOLOGY

LCH was reclassified by the writing group of the Histiocyte Society as class I histiocytosis. The current definition of the disease is an accumulation or proliferation of a clonal population of cells bearing the phenotype of a Langerhans cell that has been arrested in early stage of activation and is functionally deficient. LCH can affect multiple different organs including the skin, bone, lymph nodes, ear, gums, lungs, and gastrointestinal tract including the liver. They can affect the central nervous system by causing diabetes insipidus (Table 17-1).

The Langerhans cells are a family of related cells characterized by their dendritic morphology and multiple thin membrane projections. Dendritic cells are scarce. They constitute 0.2% of white blood cells in the blood and are present in even smaller proportions in tissues such as the skin. Because of their rarity, their true function eluded scientists for nearly a century after Langerhans first identified them in 1868. In 1973, Ralph M. Steinman of Rocke-

TABLE 17-1. *Organ system involvement in Langerhans cell histiocytosis*

Organ	Percentage of cases
Bone	80%
Skin	60%
Liver, spleen, and lymph nodes	33%
Bone marrow	30%
Lungs	25%
Orbits	25%
Oral cavity and teeth	20%
Ears	20%
Endocrine system	
Diabetes insipidus	15%
Growth failure	<1%

From Usami GN, Westra SJ, Younes S. Case 13-2003: a 14-month-old boy with hepatomegaly, perianal lesions, and a bony lump on the forehead. *N Engl J Med* 2003;348:1692–1702, with permission.

feller University rediscovered the cells in mouse spleens and recognized that they are part of the immune system (11). The cells were unusually potent in stimulating immunity in experimental animals. He renamed the cells *dendritic* because of their spiky arms, or dendrites. The subset of dendritic cells that occur in the epidermis of the skin are commonly still called Langerhans cells. In normal anatomy, Langerhans cells are found in the epidermis and skin appendages, in squamous mucosal epithelium such as the buccal mucosa, vagina, cervix, and esophagus, and in the spleen and lymphatic system. Dendritic cells attack invading bacteria, digest them, and display their antigens on the surface. Antigen-bearing dendritic cells travel to lymph nodes or the spleen, where they interact with other cells of the immune system, including B cells, which make antibodies, and killer T cells, which attract microbes and ingest them. This is all part of the immune defense against bacterial invasion.

LCH cells cause tissue damage by infiltration and excessive production of cytokines and prostaglandins. Cells produce interleukin-1 (IL-1) and prostaglandin E2, which can cause bone resorption through osteoclast activation. IL-1 may cause release of IL-2 and gamma interferon from helper-inducer T lymphocytes, leading to the stimulation of other lymphocytes and histiocytes. Tissue injury results from the local immune response as the collection of immune cells impairs normal tissue structure and function (12). On microscopic evaluation, the lesions of LCH are found to be consistent with Hand's original description: a pleomorphic infiltrate of lymphocytes, eosinophils, polymorphonuclear leukocytes, and Langerhans cells (Fig. 17–1). A more definitive diagnosis is made when electron microscopy shows Birbeck granules or when light microscopy shows that the Langerhans cells are ATPase-positive; stain for S-100 protein, CD11 and CD14, anti-CD1 marker (also called the T6 surface marker), and α-D-mannosidase; and bind peanut lectin (Table 17-2) (13,14). Bierbeck granules are membranous cytoplasmic structures, 200–400 mm wide and shaped like tennis rackets (Fig. 17-2) (15). The function of Bierbeck granules is unknown. Bone is the most common site of disease, although skin, lymph node, lung, and other sites may be involved.

TABLE 17-2. *Immunophenotype of Langerhans cell histiocytosis*

Marker	Percentage of cases positive
CD1a	~100%
S-100	~100%
CD21	~0%
CD35	~0%
CD68	<50%
Lysozyme	~0%

From Usami GN, Westra SJ, Younes S. Case 13-2003: a 14-month-old boy with hepatomegaly, perianal lesions, and a bony lump on the forehead. *N Engl J Med* 2003;348:1692–1702.

Lesional cells of LCH may represent Langerhans cells arrested in early stage of activation. Therefore, immunohistochemical expression of fascin, a protein that is a marker for dendritic cells, is likely. Immunoreactivity for fascin is observed in many cases of LCH. This immunoreac-

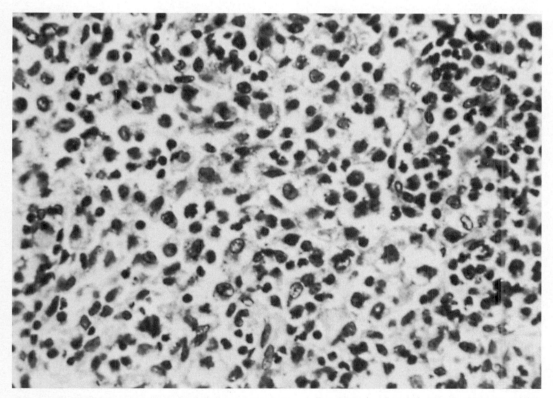

FIG. 17-1. This pleomorphic infiltrate of Langerhans cell histiocytosis in a lymph node includes eosinophils, large mononuclear lymphocytes, and polymorphonuclear leukocytes (hematoxylin and eosin, (180). (From Berry CL, ed. *Paediatric pathology.* Berlin: Springer-Verlag, 1991, with permission.)

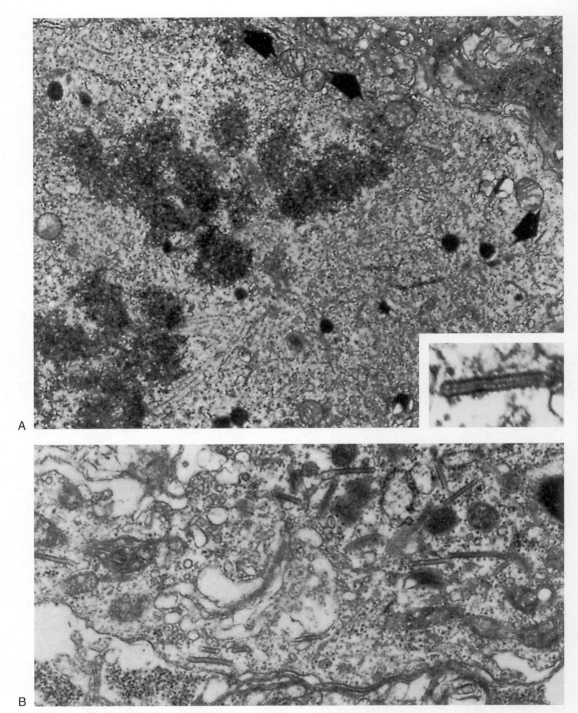

FIG. 17-2. (A) The Birbeck granule is a small rod- or tennis racket–shaped cytoplasmic organelle found in Langerhans cells. It is diagnostic for Langerhans cell histiocytosis. In this transmission electron micrograph (×11,500; inset ×70,100) a granule is shown in the inset and marked by arrows in the larger picture. (From Ceci A, DeTerlizzi M, Calella R, et al. Etoposide in recurrent childhood Langerhans' cell histiocytosis: an Italian cooperative study. *Cancer* 1988;62:2528–2531, with permission.) **(B)** A group of Birbeck granules are seen in the cytoplasm of a normal Langerhans cell of human epidermis. Some of the granules have a drumstick configuration (×41,600). (From Berry CL, ed. *Paediatric pathology.* Berlin: Springer-Verlag, 1991, with permission.)

tivity for fascin supports LCH's pathogenesis from cells of the dendritic system and provides another marker that may be detected for these cells in paraffin section (16).

LCH has been traditionally treated by oncologists (7,17). Until recently, the disease generally was not thought to be monoclonal in origin. It was argued that the individual cells do not show atypia and that the disease lacked the usual histologic criteria for malignancy. Therefore, LCH was generally considered to fall within the realm of reactive immunologic disorders or perhaps to be of infectious origin. However, viral and immune causation theories generally have lacked supporting evidence. In 1994, Williman et al. (18) provided evidence that LCH is a clonal proliferative disorder. These investigators studied ten lesions from patients with LCH and found that they all contained clonal populations of cells. The proportion of clonal cells corresponded to the proportion of lesional Langerhans-like cells, whether from solitary lesions or extensive multisystem disease (19). Yu et al. (20) reported similar findings by flow-sorting CD1a-positive cells from three patients. The hypothesis that LCH arises from somatic mutation of DNA in a normal Langerhans or precursor cell must be considered (21). The evidence of a genetic mutation or mutations leading to LCH is circumstantial. On average, patients with multiorgan LCH are younger than those with single-bone disease. In the rare instances of familial LCH, all the affected members have multiorgan disease. These two observations, reminiscent of the pattern of heritable versus nonheritable retinoblastoma, suggested to Egeler the possibility that LCH's behavior was explicable by Knudson's two-hit hypothesis and a tumor suppressor gene (22,23). (The two-hit hypothesis is discussed in detail in Chapter 5.)

The distinction between calling LCH malignant and considering it a reactive immunologic disorder is important. Classification has significant consequences for how the clinician thinks about and manages the disease. If one believes that LCH is primarily a malignancy, then radiation therapy, cytotoxic chemotherapy, and even bone marrow ablation and transplantation seem to be acceptable primary therapies. However, if one thinks about LCH primarily as a reactive disorder, then at least initially one would be likely to use more conservative and less toxic therapies, in many cases including nothing more than expectant observation. For the clinician, the truth lies between these two classifications. Most cases of LCH are not life-threatening and can be managed with minimal therapy. There are a few instances of the disease running a fulminant and fatal course, a situation that calls for an aggressive response.

CLINICAL PRESENTATION, DIAGNOSTIC EVALUATION, AND STAGING

The annual incidence of LCH is approximately 0.5 to 2.0 cases per 100,000 children per year. There is a male predominance, with 56–66% of patients male (13,16,24–26).

The Writing Group of the Histiocyte Society has identified three levels of confidence in the diagnosis of LCH:

- *Presumptive diagnosis:* The disease is clinically consistent with LCH, and histology is consistent with the diagnosis.
- *Diagnosis:* Histology is consistent with LCH, and lesional cells are shown to express S100 or α-D-mannosidase activity.
- *Definitive diagnosis:* Histology is consistent with a diagnosis of LCH, and the lesional cells are shown to express CD1a or to have cytoplasmic Bierbeck granules on electron microscopy (27).

The form of clinical presentation is related to the child's age (24,27–40). In children less than 2 years old, there may be a widespread seborrheic rash (Fig. 17-3). The rash is often most pronounced on the scalp and in the groin. Petechial hemorrhages in the involved skin are characteristic. Erosive intertrigo in the groin, axilla, and perianal region is a common feature. Ulceration and secondary skin infection may occur. Involvement of the mastoid and middle ear may present as a chronic draining otitis. The child's parents may have noted the infant to be irritable, with a diminished appetite and failure to thrive. Palpable lymphadenopathy may be

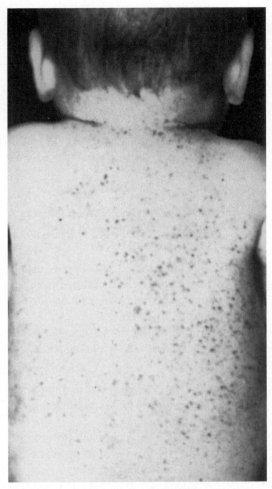

FIG. 17-3. Truncal rash and hepatosplenomegaly in an infant with Langerhans cell histiocytosis. (From Berry CL, ed. *Paediatric pathology.* Berlin: Springer-Verlag, 1991, with permission.)

seen secondary to LCH infiltration. Liver involvement is common in disseminated LCH. Hepatomegaly, elevation of liver enzymes, increased conjugated bilirubin, ascites, edema, and failure to thrive may be attributable to liver disease or involvement of the gastrointestinal tract. Diarrhea may be the result of abnormal bile acid metabolism or malabsorption (14). Splenomegaly may be accompanied by anemia, leukopenia, or thrombocytopenia (39). In children more than 2 years old, the most common presenting symptoms are related to bone involvement (Table 17-3). The most commonly involved bones, in order of frequency, are the skull (including the mandible), ribs, pelvis, vertebrae, upper extremity, and lower extremity (31,41,42). There is localized pain, with or without an associated soft tissue mass. Involvement of the orbital bones may cause exophthalmos. LCH may produce premature eruption of the teeth or tooth loss because of gum and mandibular disease (39). Back pain and loss of vertebral height may be seen. Spinal cord compression is rare.

Diabetes insipidus (DI) is the most common complication of central nervous system (CNS) involvement in LCH. The incidence varies, in different reports, from 11% to 50%. Magnetic resonance imaging (MRI) may show lesions in the posterior pituitary or the pituitary stalk (42). The mechanism of injury is thought to be either infiltration of the meninges adjacent to the posterior hypothalamic–pituitary axis or direct involvement of the brain. DI often is associated

TABLE 17-3. *Sites of bone involvement in Langerhans cell histiocytosis: a summary from the published literature*

Author (Ref.) Number of patients	Slater (123) 639	Kilpatrick (77) 263	Sessa (122) 40
Bone(s) Involved			
Skull, including mandible	51%	73%	80%
Ribs	14%	16%	38%
Pelvis	13%	18%	20%
Vertebrae	10%	16%	50%
Upper extremity	7%	12%	5%
Lower extremity	18%	33%	30%
Other	9%	20%	15%

The percentages shown represent patients with this/these bone(s) involved/total number of patients in series *not* patients with this/these bone(s) involved/total number of bony sites involved.

with skull lesions, which may be seen before the DI (27,43–45). This may be important because if the index of suspicion for DI is high, and it is diagnosed early, then some authors believe prompt irradiation may reverse or ameliorate the DI. Lung and oral mucous membrane involvement with LCH often occurs in patients in whom DI develops (44). In a Dutch–German–Austrian study, 3 of 93 patients (3%) with primary localized disease and 16 of 106 patients (15%) with dissemination of LCH at diagnosis had DI (42). In a series of patients from London's Hospital for Sick Children, DI was more common among children with multisystem disease (12 of 32) than among those with disease apparently confined to bone (3 of 20). Fourteen of the 15 children with DI had bone disease involving the skull. The cumulative risk of developing DI during the first 4 years after presentation with LCH was 42% (46). In a series from San Francisco, 25% of patients developed DI (28).

Pulmonary LCH has been reported in infants and older adults. However, it affects primarily adults in their twenties and thirties. Chest CT demonstrates multiple nodules with a predominance in the upper lobes. If bronchioalveolar lavage yields more than 5% LCH cells, then the procedure is diagnostic. The cells are CD1A positive. In adults, the natural history of LCH is variable. It is often associated with cigarette smoking, and patients who continue to smoke progress to end-stage fibrotic disease or develop extrapulmonary complications. Smoking cessation is the most effective therapy in adults (46).

Skull lesions often are the first sign of LCH. They may be single or multiple and can occur without other bony involvement. They are often very slow growing. Although they have a predilection for the temple area, they can be found anywhere on the skull. On plain radiographs they will appear as punched-out lesions. With time they can develop a sclerotic border (47). Calvarial lesions can have epidural extension. They may extend beneath the dura into the brain parenchyma. In disseminated LCH cerebral involvement may occur (22). CNS involvement with LCH can take several forms. There can be meningeal involvement with formation of large plaques of subdural tumor. There can also be in-

traparenchymal lesions. The most common sites for intraparenchymal disease are the hypothalamus and cerebellum. Less common locations are the frontal and temporal lobes (48). Occasionally, LCH can first present to medical attention as an isolated, unifocal lesion of the CNS. The hypothalamus is the most common site for this rare situation. In such cases, the diagnosis is made after surgical exploration and biopsy (49,50). It is clear that LCH has a wide clinical spectrum and can affect many different organs. The frequency of presenting symptoms seen by a practitioner results from the intrinsic nature of LCH but is also likely to be influenced by referral patterns. A diagnostic radiograph skeletal survey should be performed to assess the extent of bony involvement (Fig. 17-4). LCH is one of the few conditions in which conventional skeletal surveys are of more value than isotopic bone scans (51,52). In skeletal radiographs, LCH produces a focal area of rarefaction (53,54). The lucent area begins with the medullary cavity and extends to involve the inner table of the cortical bone. MRI may show that the area of bone abnormality is larger than suspected from other studies.

Some clinicians have urged that the term *staging* be abandoned in reference to LCH and replaced with *scoring the extent of disease*. This view reflects a concern that by invoking the notion of staging we are reinforcing the view that LCH is a malignancy (55,56). This concern does not seem to us to be warranted. LCH has a variable prognosis, and a system of grouping patients by predicted outcome is a valuable guide for the clinician (57–59). The two clinical extremes of LCH are well defined. At one extreme is the good-risk group, characterized by a unifocal lesion in bone that responds to minimal therapy. At the other extreme is the poor-risk group, less than 2 years old, with organ dysfunction. Lahey and co-workers (33,34,60,61) found a striking difference in survival between patients with and without organ dysfunction. Of the 50 patients without organ dysfunction, 33 (66%) responded to chemotherapy and 2 (4%) died. In 33 patients with dysfunction of one or more of the three organ systems, only 11 (33%) responded to chemotherapy, and 22 (67%) died.

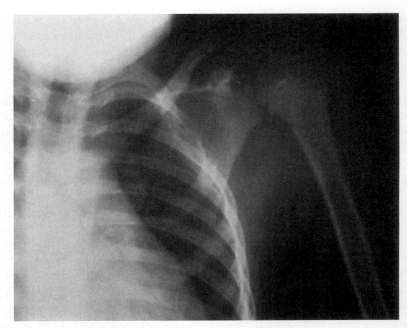

FIG. 17-4. Langerhans cell histiocytosis (LCH) involving the left second rib in a 5-year-old girl. The lesion was painful. The involved portion of the rib was subtotally resected and was diagnostic of LCH. This localized, unifocal bone lesion was adequately treated with surgery alone. There was no recurrence of LCH.

The stage distribution of LCH at presentation is almost certainly influenced by referral patterns. A children's hospital is likely to see a higher proportion of advanced disease than a community hospital. In the Children's Hospital of Philadelphia series, 33 of 64 patients (52%) had localized disease at presentation, 22 (34%) had multifocal disease without organ dysfunction, and 9 (14%) had multifocal disease with evidence of organ dysfunction (25). In a series by McLelland et al. (17) of 58 children, 14 (24%) had single-system disease, 22 (38%) had multisystem disease without organ dysfunction, and 22 (38%) had multisystem disease with organ dysfunction (17).

SELECTION OF THERAPY

In many cases LCH can take an indolent course or spontaneously remit. If there is no organ dysfunction or systemic effects threatening the child, it may be possible to use minimal or no therapy. Asymptomatic lesions in older patients with disease confined to one organ system often are best managed by observation (52,55,62,63). One should carefully balance the risks of treatment against the apparent course of the disease. The potentially toxic effects of therapy should not be engendered unless absolutely necessary (63). In Table 17-4 the authors outline a conservative management strategy for LCH. A detailed discussion of the particulars of therapy follows.

Surgery

Regression of an isolated LCH orbital bone lesion with no further treatment after the initial fine needle aspiration biopsy has been reported. It is possible that a small amount of mechanical perturbation of an LCH lesion is sufficient to initiate its regression without further treatment (64). Pediatric Oncology Group (POG) Study 8047 evaluated the response rate of LCH bone lesions to incisional or excisional biopsy. The study was open to patients less than 21 years old with no more than two bone lesions and no systemic involvement by LCH. Open biopsy was recommended, with curettage when possible.

TABLE 17-4. *Management strategy for Langerhans cell histiocytosis*

Stage of involvement	Anatomic site	Symptoms	Recommended options for therapy
Localized disease without organ dysfunction	Bone or soft tissue	None	If the diagnosis is not established, then excisional biopsy (or biopsy and curettage) is diagnostic and therapeutic. If the diagnosis is already established, then expectant observation is appropriate.
Localized disease without organ dysfunction	Bone, soft tissue, or skin	Pain or disruption of function	Disease in noncrucial bone and soft tissue sites can be managed by biopsy, excision, curettage, or steroid injection. At some sites, such as adjacent to the eye, ear, or spine or in critical weight-bearing bones with the potential to fracture, consider systemic steroids or local irradiation. Symptomatic skin disease may be treated with topical nitrogen mustard, although some authorities prefer systemic therapy.
Multifocal, no organ dysfunction	Any sites	None	Complete absence of symptoms in this situation is rare, but if the child is truly asymptomatic, then expectant observation is felt to be appropriate by some authorities; others begin chemotherapy.
Multifocal, with organ dysfunction	Any sites	Fever, weight loss, failure to thrive, local symptoms from bone and soft tissue lesions	Patients may be stratified into a high-risk group based on young age (<3 years) and organ dysfunction. Older children without organ dysfunction are low risk. Chemotherapy is given in accordance with the results of cooperative group trials as described in the text. If this fails and the situation is life-threatening, consider bone marrow transplantation.

Needle biopsy was performed for vertebral lesions, and excision was performed for expendable bone. Surgery proved highly effective, because 20 of 23 lesions (87%) were controlled without local LCH relapse (65).

POG study 8047, in conjunction with other literature, strongly supports the notion that solitary bone lesions may be treated surgically. There is an equal probability of local control with biopsy, curettage, or excision (66,67). A wide excision may be considered in an expendable bone such as the clavicle, ribs, or tip of the scapula. In nonexpendable bone locations, a small, mill-like biopsy instrument allows a tissue diagnosis and access to the medullary cavity for a curettage. Relative contraindications to curettage are situations in which the procedure would result in loss of function, severe orthopedic deformity, or poor cosmetic result. A curettage should not be performed at the axis, atlas,

or femoral neck because of the risk of bone instability. Gingival curettage may be useful for gum disease.

Direct Injection of Steroids

Methylprednisolone (40–80 mg) or depomedrone may be injected into some bone lesions under fluoroscopic guidance. Because the transient expansion of the medullary cavity causes extreme pain, the procedure should be performed under general anesthesia (Table 17-5). One cannot be certain whether responses are obtained from the steroids or from the disruption of the microenvironment caused by the needle (27).

Radiation Therapy

The use of radiation therapy to manage localized bone or soft tissue LCH is decreasing. This

TABLE 17-5. *Treatment of localized Langerhans cell histiocytosis of bone with intralesional corticosteroid injection*

Reference	Anesthesia needed: general/ local	Speed of pain relief (wk)	Speed of resolution of bone disease (mo)	Complete responders/ total number of patients	Complications
Cohen et al. (115)	8/1	1	2–4	8/9	None
Scaglietti et al. (116)	9/0	<1	2	9/9	None
Nauert et al. (117)	10/2	1–2	NS	12/12	None
Ruff et al. (118)	1/0	NS	NS	1/1	None
Capana et al. (78)	11/0	2	3	11/11	None
Fradia et al. (119)	3/0	NS	NS	3/3	None
Wirtschafter et al. (120)	1/0	NS	NS	1/1	None
Jones et al. (121)	1/0	NS	NS	1/1	Abscess
Kindy-Degnan et al. (122)	NS	1	12	1/1	None
Egeler et al. (123)	8/0	1–2	3–6	8/8	Osteomyelitis

NS, not stated.
Modified from Egeler RM, Thompson RC Jr, Voute PA, et al. Interlesional infiltration of corticosteroids in localized Langerhans cell histiocytosis. *J Pediatr Orthop* 1992;12:811–814; and Egeler RM, Nesbit ME. Langerhans cell histiocytosis and other disorders of monocyte–histiocyte lineage. *Crit Rev Oncol Hematol* 1995;18(1):9–35.

trend is attributable to a better understanding of the prognostic factors predicting the behavior of LCH, an appreciation of the frequency of disease remission after minimally toxic therapy, and concern about the long-term ill effects of radiation, albeit at low dosages (14). The complete response rate of solitary LCH in bone to curettage or excision is 70–90% (65,66). There is no evidence that immediate postoperative irradiation improves these results. Therefore, postoperative irradiation should be reserved for patients who have no clinical or radiographic signs of local healing. In addition, radiotherapy may be indicated in the following situations: for local relapse after surgery when the relapsed bone is the sole site of recurrent disease, where curettage is not appropriate because of the risk of fracture (i.e., a lytic lesion of the femoral neck; mandibular involvement producing a loose, painful tooth and reluctance to eat) or poor cosmesis (i.e., the orbital bones) (67–70), when the potential compromise of critical structures from expansile bone lesions (spinal cord compression, pressure on the globe or optic nerve) demands a reliable and rapid response, or for pain relief (65).

Selch and Parker (30) obtained local control with radiotherapy in 15 of 15 LCH lesions in pediatric patients, compared with 29 of 41 (71%) in adults. Bone pain resolved within 4 months in all 40 treated sites. Radiographic healing occurred in 37 of 40 lesions (93%), with long-term control documented in 35 (88%). El-Sayed and Brewin (71) found that radiation relieved bone pain symptoms in 14 of 15 cases (93%). Willis et al. (28) achieved uniform in-field control of lesions with radiotherapy in 37 patients.

Asymptomatic bone lesions with sclerotic margins often resolve spontaneously (72). Radiotherapy usually is not necessary in these situations. If the clinician obtains follow-up radiographs of the child with bony LCH, evidence of healing is common. Meyer et al. (73) described radiographic lesion improvement in 14 out of 15 patients with multifocal LCH (93%) and 7 out of 8 patients with unifocal LCH (88%). A change from a nontrabecular to a trabecular pattern, evolution of sclerosis in a nonsclerotic lesion, and loss of distinct margins indicate healing (74). Minimum time from diagnosis to evidence of mild healing was 3 months, although complete resolution often takes longer (67).

Vertebral lesions should be considered a special situation. Partial or complete collapse (vertebra plana) of a vertebral body may be asymptomatic (Fig. 17-5). These asymptomatic lesions generally do not warrant therapy because partial regrowth usually occurs irrespective of treatment. However, if a vertebral lesion is painful, it may be irradiated (75).

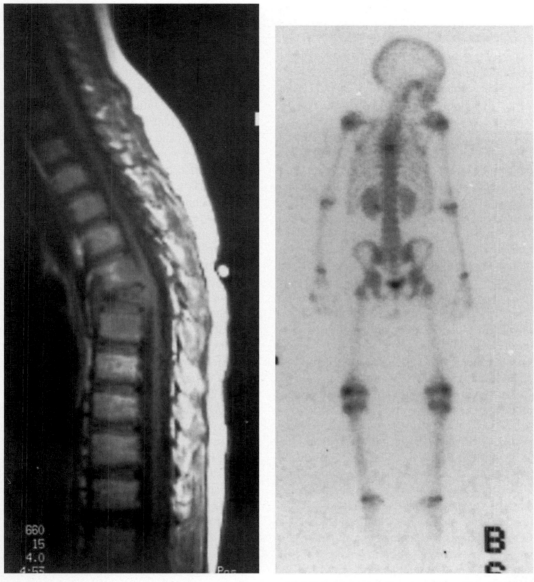

FIG. 17-5. (A) Magnetic resonance imaging scan and **(B)** bone scan showing complete vertebral collapse (vertebra plana) secondary to Langerhans cell histiocytosis (LCH) in 1992. No therapy was given beyond a needle biopsy to establish the diagnosis. Pain resolved over a month. Typically, healing includes fusion to adjacent vertebrae. The child remains without evidence of recurrent LCH.

In patients with multifocal LCH or with organ dysfunction, local irradiation may have a place. Lesions that are painful despite chemotherapy should be considered for local irradiation (76). Disfiguring bone or soft tissue lesions or bones at substantial immediate risk for fracture may also be appropriate for local radiation therapy.

Recalcitrant skin lesions may be treated with electron beam or orthovoltage photon therapy, but this should rarely be necessary in view of the other available agents (46,70).

The value of irradiation for LCH-associated DI is controversial. Greenberger et al. (68) reported 21 patients irradiated for DI. They noted a complete reversal of symptoms in four patients with discontinuation of pitressin for 2, 5, 5, and 25 years. A complete response to irradiation was observed in three of four patients treated within 1 week of the onset of symptoms. Only 1 of 15 patients responded when the duration of symptoms before radiotherapy exceeded 2 weeks. However, Smith et al. (77) reported no response in seven patients irradiated for DI. Broadbent and Chu (79) have reported six patients with DI who failed to respond to irradiation. Selch and Parker (30) irradiated two patients with DI 3 months after the onset of symptoms. Neither of these patients responded. There were no responses among 7 patients treated with chemotherapy with or without irradiation by Willis et al. (28). El-Sayed and Brewin (71) reported successful radiotherapy of two patients with DI. Grois et al. (42) found that none of five patients treated with 10 Gy of radiotherapy to the pituitary within 1 month of the occurrence of DI was able to decrease the necessary desmopressin dosage. Some have discounted the value of radiation therapy for DI without contributing additional supporting data to the literature (22,43).

The largest series of DI in LCH has been reported by Minehan et al. (44) and Kilpatrick et al. (31) from the Mayo Clinic. In 45 evaluable patients, the principal findings were as follows: 10 of the 28 (36%) irradiated patients had a complete or partial improvement in their DI, as opposed to none of the 17 nonirradiated patients; 6 patients were complete responders, 5 of whom were irradiated within 14 days of the diagnosis of DI; 77% of all patients with LCH and DI had a non-CNS head and neck site involved with LCH; computed tomography (CT) or MRI improvement in a pituitary–hypothalamic mass did not correlate well with improvement in DI; and in 12 of the 28 patients (43%) irradiated for DI, growth hormone deficiency or parahypopituitarism developed. Minehan et al. (44) did a literature review, to which we can add published patients they did not include, to generate an overall response rate of less than 25% of DI to radiation (30,31,43–45,78). We believe that radiotherapy is worth a trial in DI if symptoms are of recent onset (approximately 1 week). Others recommend radiotherapy even for long-standing DI in the hope of preventing local disease progression and additional neuroendocrine dysfunction.

Focal LCH involving the brain can be treated successfully with radiotherapy. On rare occasions, LCH may diffusely involve the parenchyma of the brain (50). The true incidence of this event is not known. Brain involvement of this sort occurs in the most aggressive form of the disease. On MRI, cerebral LCH may demonstrate parenchymal masses that intensively enhance after gadolinium is administered. Other patients may show diffuse infiltration of brain structures without tumor formation.

Treatment strategies for cerebral LCH are not well defined. A retrospective review by Hund et al. (50) identified 36 histologically evaluated cases of cerebral LCH with an extrahypothalamic localization. Sixteen of the patients had cerebral involvement during the course of the previously diagnosed LCH, whereas 20 patients had cerebral LCH without a history or symptoms of systemic disease before the neurologic presentation. Solitary brain lesions were treated by surgery in 13 patients. Six remained free of disease for up to 2 years of follow-up. In another 6 follow-up was not reported. One patient died 4 weeks after resection of a posterior fossa mass. In an additional 6 patients, surgery was followed by radiation therapy (10–41 Gy) because of recurrence of a lesion or incomplete resection. In 5 of the 6 patients, the lesions disappeared and did not recur for up to 2 years of follow-up. In 3 patients with multiple lesions, the disease was controlled by radiation or chemotherapy for up to 3 years. In others, regression, relapse, or new lesions occurred despite various treatment. Eight of the 36 patients died; 4 had multiple intracranial lesions, and the remaining 4 had localized lesions. Although it is difficult to draw firm conclusions from the available literature, some suggestions may be made concerning the management of cerebral LCH. Dural and choroid plexus lesions probably are best treated by resection. Solitary interparenchymal lesions may also be resected. Radiation after biopsy (if necessary for diagnosis) is a reasonable alternative to surgery. Although there are reports concerning the use of chemotherapy, its role has not been well defined.

A single patient with systemic LCH is reported in the literature as having been treated with hemibody irradiation, vincristine, and prednisone. The patient died of a peripheral neuropathy, and an autopsy revealed no evidence of LCH in irradiated tissues but extensive involvement of unirradiated tissues (80). A multi-institution trial of hemibody irradiation for LCH was closed after only six patients were accrued. In these patients, hemibody irradiation appeared to be more effective in those without sclerotic pulmonary nodules than in those with long-standing pulmonary involvement (T.W. Griffin, personal communication, 1987). Later in this chapter, we will consider the use of total body irradiation before bone marrow transplantation for LCH.

Chemotherapy

We have previously emphasized that children with solitary LCH of bone or multifocal but single-system disease (usually bone, skin, or lymph nodes) have a good prognosis. Expectant observation or local therapy (surgery, local irradiation, or topical chemotherapy) is appropriate and generally results in a favorable outcome (17,78). In the first three editions of this book, we stated that in multifocal LCH the indications for systemic therapy are controversial. Because there was no agreement on the important prognostic factors in LCH, the selection of patients needing chemotherapy was difficult (81–82). The lack of a uniformly applied staging system made comparison of specific chemotherapy programs difficult. Many clinicians were reluctant to use chemotherapy in multisystem disease because of the study of McLelland et al. (17).

Forty-four children with multisystem disease, including 22 with organ dysfunction, were treated conservatively. Five had no treatment, 1 received topical nitrogen mustard only, 2 received radiotherapy alone, and 36 were treated with prednisone. Of these 36, 21 later were given cytotoxic drugs when disease progressed despite prednisone. The 2-year mortality rate of the patients in the study by McLelland et al. (17) (36% with organ dysfunction, 0% without) was no different

from that of historical studies using aggressive upfront systemic cytotoxic chemotherapy. The rate of development of DI in the group of McLelland et al. was 36%, which is higher than that in some but not all other series of the era (17,78).

From the 1970s to the 1990s, the reported complete and partial response rates of advanced LCH to prednisone, indomethacin, and a wide variety of single-agent cytotoxic chemotherapeutic agents (chlorambucil, cyclophosphamide, etoposide, vinblastine, and vincristine) was between 50% and 100% (17,28,44,82–89). (These data are reviewed in Table 6 of Chapter 17 in the third edition of this book.) Relapse after initial therapy was common (69). By the early 1990s, if systemic therapy was elected for LCH, then the consensus view was to begin with high-dose steroids, usually prednisone. If that failed, then most clinicians opted for either etoposide or vinblastine as a single agent. Because of the immune system abnormalities detected in patients with LCH, calf thymus extract (thymosin), interleukin-2, and cyclosporine were also proposed as treatments. Experience with these agents was limited, response rates varied, and responses often were short-lived (12,58,90–93).

There are now several large cooperative group studies that offer guidance in selecting appropriate patients for chemotherapy. In these studies, patients were stratified into prognostic groups according to the extent of disease and the presence or absence of organ dysfunction.

A prospective multicenter trial that included 12 different Italian institutions was undertaken to evaluate therapy for disseminated LCH (87). The trial is abbreviated as AIEOP-CNR-H.X*83. The objectives of the study were to determine the outcome of patients therapeutically stratified according to the presence or absence of organ dysfunction, to test the efficacy of different single-agent chemotherapy approaches in patients with a good prognosis, and to determine the incidence of disease-related disabilities before and after treatment.

Ninety eligible patients were evaluated. In children with a single lesion, treatment was variable and consisted of either incisional biopsy, curettage, or total excision, radiation therapy, or chemotherapy. The initial therapeutic approach in this good-prognosis group consisted of immunotherapy with crude calf thymic extract and then sequential single-agent chemotherapy. First-line treatment was with vinblastine. Poor responders then went to doxorubicin, and patients in whom doxorubicin failed were placed on etoposide. The poor prognostic group, consisting of patients with organ dysfunction, were treated with vincristine, cyclophosphamide, and prednisone.

Of the 90 eligible patients, 84 were evaluable for results of therapy. The 16 patients with mono-ostotic LCH or a paravertebral intradural mass are alive. All had initial complete responses, and 15 were recurrence free 3–6 months after diagnosis. Fifty-four patients with systemic disease but without organ dysfunction received good-prognosis chemotherapy. Thirty-four achieved a complete response with vinblastine. The multiagent program for the poor prognosis group was given to 11 patients. Only 2 achieved complete response and were recurrence free at 36 and 66 months, respectively.

The overall survival for the 84 evaluable children was 93% at 48 months. Survival at 48 months was 100% for the 60 children more than 2 years old and 79% for the 24 children less than 2 years old. All 73 children without organ dysfunction were long-term survivors, and the 11 patients with organ dysfunction had a 46% survival rate at 12 months. Of the total 90 eligible patients, 18 developed DI. One patient developed acute nonlymphocytic leukemia 2 years after diagnosis and treatment with vinblastine and etoposide.

The DAL-HX83 trial accrued patients from institutions in Austria, Germany, and the Netherlands from June 1983 to December 1989 (62,89). One hundred six patients with disseminated LCH were studied. Disseminated disease was defined as the presence of multiple LCH lesions of any type or combination, with the exception of multiple skin lesions. Group A patients were those with multifocal bone disease: lesions in multiple bones or more than two lesions in one bone. Group B patients had soft tissue involvement with or without bone lesions and without signs of organ dysfunction. Group B also included patients with a single bone lesion and a biopsy-proven contiguous soft tissue mass, regional lymph node involvement, or endocrinological disabilities. Group C patients had dysfunction of liver, lung, or the hematopoietic system.

All patients with disseminated disease received chemotherapy immediately after diagnosis with prednisone, vinblastine, and etoposide. Thereafter, all patients received continuous oral 6-mercaptopurine for 46 weeks. Patients in group A received prednisone and vinblastine. Patients in group B received continuation treatment with prednisone, vinblastine, and etoposide. Patients in group C received continuation therapy with those three agents plus methotrexate.

Complete resolution was achieved in 86% of all patients at 4 months. In group A 25 of 28 patients (89%) achieved initial complete resolution of LCH. Recurrence occurred in only 3 children (12%). In group B, 52 of 57 patients (91%) achieved resolution of disease. Twelve patients (23%) had recurrent disease. In group C, 14 of 21 patients, (67%) achieved resolution of disease. Of these 14 patients, 6 (42%) developed a recurrence. Disease-free survival was 88% in group A, 73% in group B, and 64% in group C ($p < 0.05$). DI developed in 15% of patients.

The Histiocyte Society's LCH trial 1 was the first LCH randomized trial (88). All patients with disseminated LCH received high-dose methylprednisolone. Patients were then randomized to receive either etoposide or vinblastine. One hundred forty-three patients with multisystem disease were randomized. Vinblastine and etoposide were equivalent in response at week 6 of therapy, response at the last evaluation, toxicity, probability of survival, frequency of disease reactivation, and risk of diabetes insipidus. In general the results of the LCH1 trial compared unfavorably with those of the DAL-HX83/90 studies. The response rate was lower, and the activation rate was higher.

The results of the LCH1 and the DAL-HX studies formed the basis of the Histiocyte Society's LCH2 study, which opened in 1996. This is a randomized trial to compare the effect of oral prednisolone combined with vinblastine with or without the addition of etoposide in high-risk patients, defined as those with multisystem disease with at least one of the organ systems involved. Low-risk patients are more than 2 years old without involvement of the hematopoietic system, liver, lungs, or spleen (94).

The LCH1S study was established to study salvage therapy for patients who did not respond to initial chemotherapy. In this trial, a combination of cyclosporine A, antithymus globulin, and prednisolone was proposed as therapy for patients who did not respond to chemotherapy and were not appropriate for a bone marrow transplantation because of the absence of a donor. Very few patients have been accrued to this study (52,86).

It is interesting that the incidence of DI in conservatively treated patients with multisystem disease, for whom treatment was reserved only for exacerbations, was 36% compared with a 15% incidence in the DAL series and 20% in the Italian trial, both of which used intensive chemotherapy. However, the McLelland series is from a single institution, and referral may have accounted for the difference (95).

Skin involvement is a common component of multisystem LCH in younger children. Skin symptoms may include pruritus, ulceration, purulent exudation, odor, and painful defecation caused by anogenital involvement (27,96). Sheehan et al. (97) treated 16 patients with symptomatic cutaneous LCH with a topical nitrogen mustard solution made by adding tap water to nitrogen mustard powder and applying it to the skin with a watercolor brush. A complete or partial response was obtained in all cases. The nitrogen mustard is made up of at a concentration of 20 mg per 100 mg tap water and applied on a daily basis. In patients who do not respond to topical nitrogen mustard or become very sensitive to it, oral psoralen with ultraviolet A (PUVA) is a very useful treatment. LCH cells are very sensitive to ultraviolet, and PUVA and can be effective in controlling skin disease. Mayou et al. (98) successfully treated a case of cutaneous LCH in an adult with oral etoposide. Concerned about the mutagenicity of nitrogen mustard, these authors labeled the topical use of that compound for LCH as "retrogressive." Systemic cor-

ticosteroids have been advocated for the treatment of children with persistent or recalcitrant skin disease (27).

2-Chlorodeoxyadenosine (2-CdA) is a purine analog resistant to the enzyme adenosine deaminase (ADA) but not to the enzyme deoxycytidine kinase (DCK). ADA has an essential role in the intracellular degradation of purine nucleosides derived from DNA breakdown. Normal mature lymphocytes and monocytes express high levels of DCK. In vitro studies have shown that 2-CdA is a highly selective antimonocyte agent that causes decreased monocyte function and viability and decreased IL-6 secretion. Because tissue histiocytes are derived from the same stem cells as circulating monocytes, 2-CdA may be a rational agent for treating patients with histiocytic disorders. In a report by Rodriguez-Galindo et al. (94), five out of six patients with multisystem LCH achieved remission with 2-CdA. Although the efficacy of 2-CdA in treating LCH probably results from its direct effects on histiocytes, the drug also may interfere with the immune abnormalities that are part of the pathogenesis of LCH.

Liver and Bone Marrow Transplantation

Liver involvement is common in young children with multisystem LCH. The cause of liver damage in LCH is not well understood. Several mechanisms have been postulated, including histiocytic and immunocyte proliferation in the portal tracts, which produces biliary damage, fibrosis, and chronic cholestasis; extrahepatic biliary obstruction by lymphadenopathy in the porta hepatis; primary sclerosing cholangitis; and iatrogenic injury from chemotherapy, transfusion-related hepatitis, or total parenteral nutrition. In some children, liver failure is the immediate cause of death from LCH. There are a few case reports of successful orthotopic liver transplantations for LCH. These patients did not appear to have active LCH at the time of the transplant. It is tantalizing to speculate that the cyclosporine used for immunosuppression after the transplant may also have an effect against recrudescence of the LCH (12,76,99).

There have been a small number of children with refractory LCH, despite chemotherapy, who have been successfully treated with autologous bone marrow rescue, unrelated cord blood, stem cells, or other forms of allogeneic bone marrow transplantation. A variety of conditioning programs have been used, including the treatment of many patients with programs that include total body irradiation (TBI, e.g., 2–2.25 Gy per fraction daily or twice daily to 12–15.75 Gy or some combination of cyclophosphamide, busulfan, and carmustine). However, because many of the children who will receive bone marrow transplantation for chemotherapy-resistant LCH are young at the time of transplantation, TBI-containing conditioning programs should be used only with great caution. From the available literature, about 60% of patients treated with bone marrow transplantation may be expected to be long-term survivors (7,24,55,63,100–105).

be exercised in interpreting retrospective dose–response data. The bone dosage obviously would be higher from kilovoltage irradiation than from megavoltage treatment. Dosages may have been modified based on the extent of disease.

Greenberger et al. (68) described 89 patients receiving radiotherapy to 380 fields for control of bone lesions. Between 100 and 2,000 cGy, local control was obtained in 75% of courses (Fig. 17-6). In a study of 56 irradiated sites, Selch and Parker (30) found no difference in median dosage between controlled and relapsed bony sites (9 vs. 10 Gy) or soft tissue sites (median dosage 15 Gy for either controlled or relapsed sites). Overall local control was 82% (Fig. 17-7). Reviews describe the use of total dosages of 5–35 Gy, with 5–10 Gy in three to five fractions being the favored range (Fig. 17-8) (46,76,81). Cassady (107) advised using a total dosage of 15–20 Gy in patients older than 18 years because

RADIOTHERAPEUTIC MANAGEMENT

Dosage

There is no clear relationship between the dosage of irradiation and local control of LCH. Childs and Kennedy (53) reported 12 patients treated with radiotherapy. Their series began with an infant treated in 1927–1928 with a radium source. They thought that a dosage of approximately 600 roentgens was necessary to control individual lesions. Smith et al. (77) reported on 89 courses of irradiation administered with 250-kV X-rays or cobalt-60. Less than 1,000 cGy was administered in 92% of the cases, and the local success rate was 87%. Three of five sites treated with less than 450 cGy had a local failure but were salvaged with additional irradiation. Dosages greater than 1,000 cGy did not appear to be more effective than dosages of 450–1,000 cGy. Ochsner (54) reported that radiotherapy was effective for bony sites at dosages of 600–1,000 cGy. Similarly, in a report confined to solitary lesions of the skull, Rawlings and Wilkins (106) noted almost uniformly successful results with dosages of 600–2,500 cGy. McGaran and Spady (66) had good results with 300–3,500 cGy. Caution should

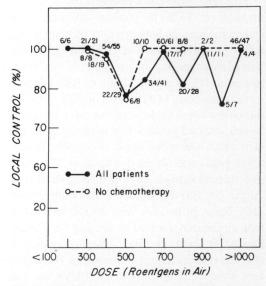

FIG. 17-6. Local control of bone lesions as a function of dosage delivered. (From Greenberger JS, Cassady JR, Jaffe N, et al. Radiation therapy in patients with histiocytosis: management of diabetes insipidus and bone lesions. *Int J Radiat Oncol Biol Phys* 1979;5:1749–1755, with permission.)

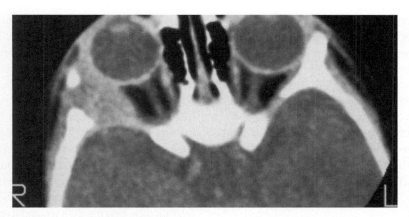

FIG. 17-7. A 4-month-old boy developed a seborrheic skin rash with focal areas of ulceration. Skin biopsy showed Langerhans cell histiocytosis (LCH). No other organ systems were involved. At 6 months of age, proptosis was noted, and orbital computed tomography scan demonstrated erosion of the lateral wall of the right orbit by a destructive lesion. Surgery was felt to be ill-advised because of concern over damage to the lateral rectus muscle and an unacceptable cosmetic result. Vinblastine and prednisone were administered. Proptosis improved but then subsequently worsened. A total dosage of 6 Gy in four fractions was administered with a right anterior oblique half-beam–blocked 4-MV photon field with shielding of the lens and two-thirds of the globe in 1984. Vinblastine was continued for 15 months after radiotherapy. The bone lesion healed within 2 months after irradiation. There is no evidence of LCH 18 years after the initial diagnosis. The young man is now being treated for attention deficit disorder.

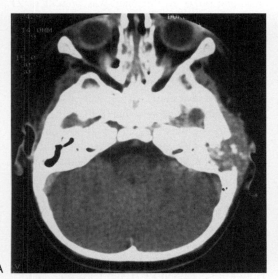
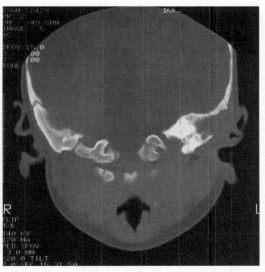

A   B

FIG. 17-8. An 11-month-old boy presented to medical attention with protrusion of the superior aspect of the left ear. Computed tomographic scan showed a left mastoid soft tissue mass with erosion into the temporal bone. Open biopsy made the diagnosis of Langerhans cell histiocytosis (LCH). In 1987, the child received local irradiation with 12-MeV electrons to a total dosage of 6 Gy in three fractions. After irradiation he was treated with vinblastine and prednisone. He remains without evidence of persistent or recurrent LCH.

of a perceived higher risk of local failure and a lower risk of bone damage by radiation.

For DI, Smith et al. (77) reported no relief in seven patients treated with 500–1,830 cGy. Greenberger et al. (68) administered 345–1,600 cGy to 21 patients and, as discussed previously, observed a complete response in 4 patients and a partial response in another 4. Minehan et al. (44) reported three of five patients (60%) with DI responding when treated with more than 15 Gy, compared with 7 of 23 (30%) treated with less than 15 Gy.

Volume

To treat DI, one uses a 5 × 5- to 7 × 7-cm set of parallel opposed fields, arcs, a three-field technique, or conformally planned fields to cover the hypothalamic–pituitary axis. Bone lesions should be treated with a field designed to cover the radiographic abnormality with a small margin. In the treatment of skull lesions, we attempt to minimize the dosage to the underlying brain by treating with electrons or orthovoltage equipment. If electrons are used, an adjustment for attenuation by compact bone infiltrated by LCH should be made. This is best done by taking density measurements of the involved bone with a cranial CT scan.

LONG-TERM SEQUELAE OF LCH AND ITS TREATMENT

Because of the low dosage of irradiation used, acute side effects of radiotherapy for LCH are rare. However, it is common to see late sequelae of LCH, most of which may be attributable to the disease and some of which may be attributable to the treatment (95,108).

Long-term disabilities are common in survivors of LCH. The French Langerhans Cell Histiocytosis Group reported 320 living patients followed for a median of 39.5 months. The most common sequelae were DI (18%), growth hormone deficiency and short stature (5%), hypothyroidism (2.5%), deafness (2.5%), and vertebra plana and orthopedic sequelae (2.5%) (24). The most common sequelae in the University of California, San Francisco, series were DI (26%),

growth failure (20%), sex hormone deficiency (16%), and hearing loss (16%) (28). The 90 children followed by the Italian Cooperative Group had an overall incidence of disease-related disabilities of approximately 48%. These included DI, orthopedic abnormalities, growth defects, tooth loss, chronic hepatitis, exophthalmus, and hearing loss (87,109). The Southwest Oncology Group has described a significant incidence of neurologic symptoms, intellectual problems, and growth failure (107). McLelland et al. (17,56) described orthopedic abnormalities, endocrine dysfunction, hearing deficits, and liver fibrosis as well as DI. In a study of 15 long-term survivors of LCH, Ransom et al. (110) found that 7 had an IQ lower than 89. In a large study of the Histiocyte Society, DI (24%), orthopedic abnormalities (20%), hearing loss (13%), and neurological consequences (11%) were most frequent (111).

Growth and endocrine disorders are common in multisystem LCH. A detailed study of 144 patients with multisystem LCH evaluated at the Great Ormond Street Hospital for Sick Children in London showed that of the 144 patients, 50 had endocrinopathy, 49 of whom had DI. Growth hormone (GH) insufficiency was present in 21 patients. GH therapy was able to significantly improve growth in these patients. It was not clear that radiotherapy to the head increased the incidence of GH insufficiency. It is clear that children with LCH should be investigated for hormone insufficiency, especially those who have DI or growth failure. It appears that GH insufficiency is secondary to direct hypothalamic–pituitary involvement by the disease. Thickening of the pituitary stalk on MRI scan provides additional evidence of GH insufficiency (95).

The frequency of secondary malignancy after therapy for LCH is uncertain (8,59,107). In a report describing the association between LCH and other malignancies (91 patients), 39 had LCH and lymphoma (Hodgkin's or non-Hodgkin's), 22 had LCH and leukemia, and 30 had LCH and a solid tumor, most commonly lung cancer. Although the leukemias and non-lung solid tumors most commonly occurred years after LCH, most of the lymphomas and lung cancers preceded LCH or were diagnosed concurrently, in an unexplained association

(111). Affected patients had initially received irradiation and chemotherapy, irradiation only, or chlorambucil only for LCH (45,61,112). One case of leukemia was seen among 90 patients followed in the Italian Cooperative Group Study (87). One case of leukemia was seen in 51 patients followed more than 3 years at the University of California, San Francisco (28). There were no second malignancies in 106 patients with LCH treated in the Dutch–German–Austrian DAL-HX83 Trial (52,89).

Haupt et al. (113) evaluated children with LCH enrolled in three protocols of the Italian Association of Pediatric Hematology/Oncology. These patients received a variety of chemotherapy programs including vinblastine, adriamycin, etoposide, vincristine, cyclophosphamide, and prednisone. The median follow-up after entry into the study cohort was 5 years and 5 months. There were three cases of acute nonlymphocytic leukemia (ANLL), all in children who had received etoposide. Two had received etoposide alone, and one had received etoposide in combination with alkylating agent chemotherapy and other chemotherapy or irradiation. Although the absolute number of patients in this study is small, the occurrence of three episodes of ANLL results in a high simple incidence rate of secondary leukemia.

RESULTS

In patients presenting with solitary LCH of bone, close to 100% survival has been reported (26,43,66,67,113). In the presence of organ dysfunction with multisystem disease, survival ranges from 33% to 54%. In its absence, survival ranges from 82% to 96% (25,33,34, 36,61,78). In the 348 patients reported from 32 French centers treated from 1983 to 1993, the 6-year actuarial survival according to the DAL-HX staging system was as follows: localized disease, isolated unifocal or bifocal bone involvement, 100%; soft tissue involvement with or without bone involvement, no organ dysfunction, 90%; liver, lung, or bone marrow dysfunction, 49% (24). In the DAL-HX83 Trial the probability of survival, using the DAL-HX83 staging system for disseminated disease described earlier in this chapter, was 100% for group A, 96% for group B, and 62% for group C. The 15-year survival rates in the series of Willis et al., by type of initial presentation, were skin disease only, 83%; monostotic disease, 100%; polyostotic disease, 100%; and multisystem disease, 76% (52,89).

REFERENCES

References particularly recommended for further reading are indicated by an asterisk

1. D'Angio GJ, Favara BE, Ladisch S. Editorial: toward an understanding of the childhood histiocytoses. *Med Pediatr Oncol* 1986;14:104.
2. Langerhans P. Uber die nerven der menschlichen haut. *Arch Pathol Anat* 1868;44:325–327.
3. Langerhans P. Berichtigungen (u.a. zu den nervenenden der haut, und nervenfasern im rete). *Arch Mikrosk Anat* 1882;20:641–643.
4. Egeler RM, Zantinga AR, Coppes MJ. Paul Langerhans Jr. (1847–1888): a short life, yet two eponymic legacies. *Med Pediatr Oncol* 1994;22:129–132
5. Egeler RM. The Langerhans cell histiocytosis X files revealed. *Br J Hematol* 2002;116:3–9.
6. Hand A. Polyuria and tuberculosis. *Arch Pediatr* 1893;10:673–675.
7. Komp DM. Concepts in staging and clinical studies for treatment of Langerhans' cell histiocytosis. *Semin Oncol* 1991;18:18–23.
8. Lieberman PH, Jones CR, Dargeon HWK, et al. A reappraisal of eosinophilic granuloma of bone, Hand–Schuller–Christian syndrome and Letterer–Siwe syndrome. *Medicine* 1969;48:375–400.
9. Lichtenstein L. Histiocytosis X: integration of eosinophilic granuloma of bone, "Letterer–Siwe disease," and "Schuller–Christian disease" as related manifestations of a single nosologic entity. *Arch Pathol* 1953;56:84–102.
10. Otani E, Ehrlich J. Solitary eosinophilic granuloma of bone simulating primary neoplasm. *Am J Pathol* 1940;16:479–490.
*11. Banchereau J. The long arm of the immune system. *Sci Am* 2002;287:52–59.
12. Mahmoud HH, Wang WC, Murphy SB. Cyclosporine therapy for advanced Langerhans cell histiocytosis. *Blood* 1991;77:721–725.
13. Castleman B, McNeely BU. Case records of the Massachusetts General Hospital, case 17-1970. *N Engl J Med* 1970;282:917–925.
14. Velez-Yanguas MC, Warrier RP. Langerhans' cell histiocytosis. *Orthop Clin North Am* 1996;27:615–623.
15. Hurwitz CA, Faquin WC. A 15-year-old boy with a retro-orbital mass and impaired vision. *N Engl J Med* 2002;146:513–520.
16. Pinkkus GS, Lones MA, Matsumara F, et al. Langerhans cell histiocytosis: immunohistochemical expression of fascin, a dendritic cell marker *Am J Clin Pathol* 2002;118:335–343.
*17. McLelland DJ, Broadbent V, Yeomans E, et al.

Langerhans cell histiocytosis: the case for conservative treatment. *Arch Dis Child* 1990;65:301–303.

*18. Willman CL, Busque L, Griffith BB, et al. Langerhans cell histiocytosis (histiocytosis X): a clonal proliferative disease. *N Engl J Med* 1994;331:154–160.

19. Cotter FE, Pritchard J. Clonality in Langerhans cell histiocytosis. *BMJ* 1995;310:74–75.

20. Yu RC, Chu C, Buluwela L, et al. Clonal proliferation of Langerhans cells in Langerhans cell histiocytosis. *Lancet* 1994;343:767–768.

*21. Cotter FE, Pritchard J. Clonality in Langerhans' cell histiocytosis. *BMJ* 1995;310:74–75.

22. Egeler RM, Nesbit ME. Langerhans cell histiocytosis and other disorders of monocyte-histiocyte lineage. *Crit Rev Oncol Hematol* 1995;18:9–35.

23. Knudson AG. Mutation and cancer: statistical study of retinoblastoma. *Proc Natl Acad Sci USA* 1971;68:620–623.

*24. French Langerhans' Cell Histiocytosis Study Group. A multicentre retrospective survey of Langerhans' cell histiocytosis. 348 cases observed between 1983 and 1993. *Arch Dis Child* 1996;75:17–24.

25. Raney RB Jr, D'Angio GJ. Langerhans' cell histiocytosis (histiocytosis X): experience at the Children's Hospital of Philadelphia, 1970–1984. *Med Pediatr Oncol* 1989;17:20–28.

26. Starling KA, Donaldson MH, Haggard ME, et al. Therapy of histiocytosis X with vincristine, vinblastine, and cyclophosphamide. *Am J Dis Child* 1972;123:105–110.

27. Chu T. Langerhans cell histiocytosis. *Aust J Dermatol* 2001;42:237–242.

28. Willis B, Ablin A, Weinberg V, et al. Disease course and late sequelae of Langerhans' cell histiocytosis: 25-year experience at the University of California, San Francisco. *J Clin Oncol* 1996;14:2073–2082.

29. Gadner H, Heitger A, Grois N, et al. Treatment strategy for disseminated Langerhans cell histiocytosis. *Med Pediatr Oncol* 1994;23:72–80.

30. Selch MT, Parker RG. Radiation therapy in the management of Langerhans cell histiocytosis. *Med Pediatr Oncol* 1990;18:97–102.

31. Kilpatrick SE, Wenger DE, Gilchrist GS, et al. Langerhans' cell histiocytosis (histiocytosis X) of bone. *Cancer* 1995;76:2471–2484.

32. Broadbent V, Heaf D, Pritchard J, et al. Occult multisystem involvement in histiocytosis X (HX). *Med Pediatr Oncol* 1986;14:113.

33. Lahey ME. Histiocytosis X: comparison of three treatment regimens. *J Pediatr* 1975;87:179–183.

*34. Lahey ME. Prognostic factors in histiocytosis X. *Am J Pediatr Hematol Oncol* 1981;3:57–60.

35. Lechner W, Ortner A, Thoni A, et al. Histiocytosis X in gynecology. *Gynecol Oncol* 1983;15:253–260.

36. Lipton J. The pathogenesis, diagnosis, and treatment of histiocytosis syndromes. *Pediatr Dermatol* 1983;1:112–120.

37. Starling KA. Chemotherapy of histiocytosis. *Am J Pediatr Hematol Oncol* 1981;3:157–160.

38. Dagenais M, Pharoah MJ, Sikorski PA. The radiographic characteristics of histiocytosis X. *Oral Surg Oral Med Oral Pathol* 1992;74:230–236.

39. Filcoma D, Weedleman H, Arceci R, et al. Pediatric histiocytomas: characterization, prognosis and oral

management. *Am J Pediatr Hematol Oncol* 1993;15:226–230.

40. Sessa S, Sommelet D, Lascombes P, et al. Treatment of Langerhans-cell histiocytosis in children. Experience at the Children's Hospital of Nancy. *J Bone Joint Surg Am* 1994;76(10):1513–1525.

41. Slater JM, Swarm OJ. Eosinophilic granuloma of bone. *Med Pediatr Oncol* 1980;8(2):151–164.

42. Grois N, Flucher-Wolfram B, Heitger A, et al. Diabetes insipidus in Langerhans cell histiocytosis: results from the DAL-HX 83 study. *Med Pediatr Oncol* 1995;24:248–256.

43. Angeli SI, Hoffman HT, Alcalde J, et al. Langerhans cell histiocytosis of the head and neck in children. *Ann Otol Rhinol Laryngol* 1995;104:173–180.

44. Minehan KJ, Chen MG, Zimmerman D, et al. Radiation therapy for diabetes insipidus caused by Langerhans cell histiocytosis. *Int J Radiat Oncol Biol Phys* 1992;23:519–524.

45. Dunger DB, Broadbent V, Yeoman E, et al. The frequency and natural history of diabetes insipidus in children with Langerhans' cell histiocytosis. *N Engl J Med* 1989;321:1157–1162.

46. Seo P. Cases from the Osler medical service of Johns Hopkins University. *Am J Med* 2002;112:667–669.

47. Pittman T, Grant J, Darling C, et al. An eight-month-old boy with a skull mass. *Pediatr Neurosurg* 2002;37:100–104.

48. Hayward J, Packer R, Finlay J. Central nervous system and Langerhans' cell histiocytosis. *Med Pediatr Oncol* 1990;18:325–328.

49. Rube J, Para SDL, Pickren JW. Histiocytosis X with involvement of brain. *Cancer* 1967;20:486–492.

50. Hund E, Steiner HH, Jansen O, et al. Treatment of cerebral Langerhans cell histiocytosis. *J Neurol Sci* 1999;171:145–152.

51. Gerrard MP, Hendry MM, Eden OB. Comparison of radiographic and scintigraphic assessment of skeletal lesions in histiocytosis X. *Med Pediatr Oncol* 1986;14:113.

*52. Broadbent V, Gadner H. Current therapy for Langerhans cell histiocytosis. *Hematol Oncol Clin North Am* 1998;12:327–338.

53. Childs DS Jr, Kennedy RLJ. Reticuloendotheliosis of children: treatment with roentgen rays. *Radiology* 1951;57:653–661.

54. Ochsner SF. Eosinophilic granuloma of bone. Experience with twenty cases. *AJR* 1966;97:719–726.

55. Komp DM. Therapeutic strategies for Langerhans cell histiocytosis. *J Pediatr* 1991;119:274–275.

56. McLelland J, Pritchard J, Chu AC. Current controversies. *Hematol Oncol Clin North Am* 1987;1:147–162.

57. Chu A, D'Angio GJ, Favara BE, et al. Report and recommendations of the workshop on the childhood histiocytosis: comments and controversies. *Med Pediatr Oncol* 1968;14:116.

58. Osband ME, Lipton JM, Lavin P, et al. Histiocytosis X: demonstration of abnormal immunity, T-cell histamine H2-receptor deficiency, and successful treatment with thymic extract. *N Engl J Med* 1981;304:146–153.

*59. Greenberger JS, Crocker AC, Vawter G, et al. Results of treatment of 127 patients with systemic histiocytosis (Letterer–Siwe syndrome, Schuller–Christian syndrome and multifocal eosinophilic granuloma). *Medicine* 1981;60:311–338.

60. Lahey ME. Histiocytosis X: comparison of three treatment regimens. *J Pediatr* 1975;87:179–183.

61. Lahey ME, Heyn RM, Newton WA Jr, et al. Histiocytosis X: clinical trial of chlorambucil: a report from Children's Cancer Study Group. *Med Pediatr Oncol* 1979;7:197–203.

62. Gadner H, Heitger A, Ritter J, et al. Langerhanszell-histiozytose im kindesalter-ergebnisse der DAL-HX 83 studies. *Klin Padiatr* 1987;199:173–182.

63. Komp DM. Langerhans cell histiocytosis. *N Engl J Med* 1987;316:747–748.

64. Smith JH, Fulton L, O'Brien JM. Spontaneous regression of orbital Langerhans cell granulomatosis in a three-year-old girl. *Am J Ophthalmol* 1999;128: 119–121.

65. Berry DH, Gresik M, Maybee D, et al. Histiocytosis in bone only. *Med Pediatr Oncol* 1990;18:292–294.

66. McGaran MH, Spady HA. Eosinophilic granuloma of bone. A study of 28 cases. *J Bone Joint Surg* 1960;42A:979–992.

67. Womer RB, Rainey RB, D'Angio GJ. Healing rates of treated and untreated bone lesions in histiocytosis X. *Pediatrics* 1985;76:286–288.

68. Greenberger JS, Cassady JR, Jaffe N, et al. Radiation therapy in patients with histiocytosis: management of diabetes insipidus and bone lesions. *Int J Radiat Oncol Biol Phys* 1979;5:1749–1755.

69. Matus-Ridley M, Raney RB Jr, Thawerani H, et al. Histiocytosis X in children: patterns of disease and results of treatment. *Med Pediatr Oncol* 1983;11: 99–105.

70. Richter MP, D'Angio GJ. The role of radiation therapy in the management of children with histiocytosis X. *Am J Pediatr Hematol Oncol* 1981;3:161–163.

71. El-Sayed S, Brewin TB. Histiocytosis X: does radiotherapy still have a role? *Clin Oncol* 1992;4:27–31.

*72. Sartoris DJ, Parker BR. Histiocytosis X: rate and pattern of resolution of osseous lesions. *Radiology* 1984;152:679–684.

73. Meyer JS, Harty MP, Mahboudi S, et al. Langerhans cell histiocytosis: presentation and evolution of radiologic findings with clinical correlation. *Radiographics* 1995;15:1135–1146.

74. Alexander JE, Seibert JJ, Berry DH, et al. Prognostic factors for healing of bone lesions in histiocytosis X. *Pediatr Radiol* 1988;18:326–332.

*75. Kieffer SA, Nesbit ME, D'Angio GJ. Vertebra plane due to histiocytosis X: serial studies. *Acta Radiol* 1969;8:241–250.

76. Concepcion W, Esquivel CO, Terry A, et al. Liver transplantation in Langerhans' cell histiocytosis (histiocytosis X). *Semin Oncol* 1991;8:24–28.

*77. Smith DG, Nesbit ME Jr, D'Angio GJ, et al. Histiocytosis X: role of radiation therapy in management with special reference to dose levels employed. *Radiology* 1973;106:419–422.

78. Capana R, Springfield DS, Ruggieri P, et al. Direct cortisone injection in eosinophilic granuloma of bone. *Radiology* 1980;136:289–293.

79. Broadbent V, Chu AC. Langerhans cell histiocytosis. In: Plowman PN, Pinkerson CR, eds. *Paediatric oncology: clinical practices and controversies, second*

edition. London: Chapman & Hall, 1997:547–560.

80. Griffin TW. The treatment of advanced histiocytosis X with sequential hemibody irradiation. *Cancer* 1977;39:2435–2436.

81. Nezelof C, Barbey S, Gane P, et al. Histiocytosis X: a proliferation disorder of the Langerhans' cell system. *Med Pediatr Oncol* 1986;14:108–109.

82. Berry DH, Gresik MV, Humphrey GB, et al. Natural history of histiocytosis X: a Pediatric Oncology Group study. *Med Pediatr Oncol* 1986;14:1–5.

83. Raney RB Jr. Chemotherapy for children with aggressive fibromatosis and Langerhans' cell histiocytosis. *Clin Orthop* 1991;262:58–63.

84. Savinas A, Rageliene L. Role of chemotherapy in disseminated Langerhans cell histiocytosis. *Med Pediatr Oncol* 1992;20:452.

85. West WO. Velban as treatment for disseminated eosinophilic granuloma of bone: follow-up note after seventeen years. *J Bone Joint Surg Am* 1984;66.1128.

86. Katz BZ. Treatment for multisystem Langerhans' cell histiocytosis. *J Pediatr* 2002;140:280.

87. Ceci A, DeTerlizzi M, Colella R, et al. Langerhans cell histiocytosis in childhood: results from the Italian Cooperative AIEOP-CNR-H.X. 1983 study. *Med Pediatr Oncol* 1993;21:259–264.

*88. Gadner H, Grois N, Arico M, et al. A randomized trial of treatment for multisystem Langerhans cell histiocytosis. *J Pediatr* 2001;138:728–734.

89. Gadner H, Heitger A, Grois N, et al. Treatment strategy for disseminated Langerhans cell histiocytosis. *Med Pediatr Oncol* 1994;23:72–80

90. Arico M. Cyclosporine therapy for refractory Langerhans' cell histiocytosis. *Blood* 1991;78: 3107.

91. Davies EG, Levinsky RJ, Butler M, et al. Thymic hormone therapy for histiocytosis X? *N Engl J Med* 1983;309:493–494.

92. Hirose M, Saito S, Yoshimoto T, et al. Interleukin-2 therapy of Langerhans cell histiocytosis. *Acta Paediatr* 1995;84:1204–1206.

93. Osband ME, Cohen EB, Shipman DL. Treatment of histiocytosis X with suppression. In: Byrom NA, Hobbs JR, eds. *Thymic factor therapy* New York: Raven Press, 1984:391–398.

94. Rodriguez-Galindo C, Kelly P, Jeng M, et al. Treatment of children with Langerhans cell histiocytosis with 2-chlorodeoxyadenosine. *Am J Hematol* 2002; 69:179–184.

95. Nandurf VR, Barelile P, Pritchard J, et al. Growth and endocrine disorders in multisystem Langerhans' cell histiocytosis. *Clin Endocrinol* 2000;53:509–515.

96. Iwatsuki K, Tsugiki M, Yoshizawa N, et al. The effect of phototherapies on cutaneous lesions of histiocytosis X in the elderly. *Cancer* 1986;57:1931–1936.

97. Sheehan MP, Atherton DJ, Broadbent V. et al. Topical nitrogen mustard: an effective treatment for cutaneous Langerhans cell histiocytosis. *J Pediatr* 1991;119:317–321.

98. Mayou SC, Chu AC, Munro DD, et al. Langerhans cell histiocytosis: excellent response to etoposide. *Clin Exp Dermatol* 1991;16:292–294.

99. Mahmoud H, Gaber O, Wang W, et al. Successful orthotopic liver transplantation in a child with Langerhans' cell histiocytosis. *Transplantation* 1991;51: 278–280.

100. Arceci RJ. Treatment options: commentary. *Br J Cancer* 1994;23[Suppl]:558–560.

101. Conter V, Reciputo A, Arrigo C, et al. Bone marrow transplantation for refractory Langerhans' cell histiocytosis. *Haematologica* 1996;81:468–471.

102. Greinix HT, Storb R, Sanders JE, et al. Marrow transplantation for treatment of multisystem progressive Langerhans' cell histiocytosis. *Bone Marrow Transplant* 1992;10:39–44.

103. Morgan G. Myeloablative therapy and bone marrow transplantation for Langerhans' cell histiocytosis. *Br J Cancer* 1994;23[Suppl]:552–553.

104. Suminoe A, Matsuzaki A, Hattari H, et al. Unrelated cord blood transplantation for an infant with chemotherapy-resistant progressive Langerhans cell histiocytosis. *J Pediatr Hematol Oncol* 2001;23:633–636.

105. Nagarajan R, Neglia J, Ramsay N, et al. Successful treatment of refractory Langerhans cell histiocytosis with unrelated cord blood transplantation. *J Pediatr Hematol Oncol* 2001;23:629–632.

106. Rawlings CE III, Wilkins RH. Solitary eosinophilic granuloma of the skull. *Neurosurgery* 1984;15:155–161.

107. Cassady JR. Current role of radiation therapy in the management of histiocytosis X. *Hematol Oncol Clin North Am* 1987;1:123–130.

108. Komp DM. Long-term sequelae of histiocytosis X. *Am J Pediatr Hematol Oncol* 1981;5:165–168.

109. Ceci A, DeTerlizzi M, Calella R, et al. Etoposide in recurrent childhood Langerhans' cell histiocytosis: an Italian cooperative study. *Cancer* 1988;62:2528–2531.

110. Ransom JL, Morris P, John RG, et al. Neuropsychological late sequelae of histiocytosis X. *Pediatr Res* 1978;12:47(abst).

111. Haupt R, Nanduri V, Calevo MG, et al. Permanent consequences in Langerhans cell histiocytosis patients: a pilot study from the Histiocyte Society—Late Effects Study Group. *Pediatr Blood Cancer* 2004;42:483–484.

112. Egeler RM, Neglia JP, Puccetti DM, et al. The association of Langerhans' cell histiocytosis with malignant neoplasms. *Cancer* 1993;71:865–874.

113. Haupt R, Fears TR, Rosso P, et al. Increased risk of secondary leukemia after single-agent treatment with etoposide for Langerhans' cell histiocytosis. *Pediatr Hematol Oncol* 1994;11:499–507.

114. Berry CL, ed. *Paediatric pathology*. Berlin: Springer-Verlag, 1991.

115. Cohen M, Fornoza J, Cangir A, et al. Direct injection of methylprednisolone sodium succinate in the treatment of solitary eosinophilic granuloma of bone. *Radiology* 1980;136:289–293.

116. Scaglietti O, Marchetti PG, Bartolozzi P. Final results obtained in the treatment of bone cysts with methylprednisolone acetate (Depo-Medrol) and a discussion of results achieved in other bone lesions. *Clin Orthop* 1982;165:33–42.

117. Nauert C, Zornoza J, Ayala A, et al. Eosinophilic granuloma of bone: diagnosis and management. *Skeletal Radiol* 1983;10:227–235.

118. Ruff S, Chapman GK, Taylor TKF, et al. The evolution of eosinophilic granuloma of bone: a case report. *Skeletal Radiol* 1983;10:37–39.

119. Fradia M, Podoshin L, Ben-Davie J, et al. Eosinophilic granuloma of the temporal bone. *J Laryngol Otol* 1985;99:475–479.

120. Wirtschafter JD, Nesbit ME, Anderson P, et al. Intralesional methylprednisolone for Langerhans cell histiocytosis of the orbit and cranium. *J Pediatr Ophthalmol Strabismus* 1987;24:194–197.

121. Jones LR, Toth BB, Cangir A. Treatment for solitary eosinophilic granuloma of the mandible by steroid injection: report of a case. *J Oral Maxillofac Surg* 1989;47:306–309.

122. Kindy-Degnan NA, Laflamme P, Duprat G, et al. Intralesional steroid in the treatment of an orbital eosinophilic granuloma [Letter]. *Arch Ophthalmol* 1991;109:617–628.

*123. Egeler RM, Thompson RC Jr, Voute PA, et al. Interlesional infiltration of corticosteroids in localized Langerhans cell histiocytosis. *J Pediatr Orthop* 1992;12:811–814.

18

Hemangioma, Lymphangioma, and Skin Cancer

Edward C. Halperin, M.D., and John P. Kirkpatrick, M.D., Ph.D.

HEMANGIOMAS

Hemangiomas are common developmental vascular abnormalities. These benign blood vessel tumors may be encountered in any portion of the body (1–7). In this chapter, we consider cutaneous, ocular, and vertebral body hemangiomas. Subglottic hemangiomas are discussed in Chapter 16.

Historically, hemangiomas were divided into three clinical types. Nevus flammeus (port-wine stains) usually is located on the head and neck, varying in size and color. Facial nevus flammeus in the cutaneous distribution of cranial nerve V, in association with leptomeningeal angiomas, is called the Sturge–Weber syndrome (8). Nevus vasculosus (strawberry mark) is red and elevated. Angiocavernosum (cavernous hemangioma) was considered a lesion of the deep vasculature, especially the veins (9,10). Cavernous hemangioma may be complicated by life-threatening thrombocytopenia, hemolytic anemia, and consumptive coagulopathy caused by platelet sequestration and high shear stresses within the lesion (Kasabach–Merritt syndrome) (11–13).

Modern classification divides vascular birthmarks into two broad categories—vascular tumors and vascular malformations—based on vasculogenesis, histopathology, and clinical features (1,14–18). Vascular tumors are dynamic lesions characterized by a growth phase, marked by endothelial proliferation and hypercellularity, followed by involution (1,14–18). This category includes the common hemangioma of infancy and rarer entities such as Kaposiform hemangioendothelioma, which is associated with Kasabach–Merritt syndrome (19,20). In contrast, vascular malformations are essentially stable, demonstrating little or no growth over time. These structural malformations include capillary (port-wine stain), venous, lymphatic, and arteriovenous malformations (Table 18-1).

Hemangiomas often can be diagnosed by a thorough history and physical examination. If the natural history or appearance suggests a more aggressive neoplasm, imaging studies may prove useful in establishing a diagnosis. Doppler ultrasonography offers a rapid and inexpensive method of differentiating hemangiomas from vascular malformations (21). However, contrasted computed tomography or magnetic resonance imaging scans provide detailed anatomic information of greater utility in planning therapy (22–24). The choice of imaging modality depends on the specific anatomic location of the lesion. For example, contrasted T1-weighted and T2-weighted magnetic resonance imaging are particularly effective at distinguishing vascular tumors of the head and neck from other soft tissue structures.

Only 20% of hemangiomas are present at birth. The other 80% arise within the first 8 weeks of life. The natural history of the common hemangioma of infancy is one of rapid growth during the first 6–9 months of life and then a period of more slowly increasing size that parallels the infant's growth. Involution generally follows at a rate of about 10% per year, with complete disappearance of 50% of the lesions by 4 or 5 years of age and 90% by 9 years (1,25–27). In most cases, hemangiomas of infancy are best managed by observation. There are some indications for treatment, including rapid progression of the lesion producing unacceptable symptoms

TABLE 18-1. *Classification of congenital vascular abnormalities*

Vascular tumors	Vascular malformations
Types	
Hemangioma of infancy	Simple
Kaposiform hemangio-endothelioma	Capillary (port-wine stain)
Tufted angioma	Venous
Pyogenic granuloma	Arterial
Hemangiopericytoma	Lymphatic
	Complex
	Arterial–venous, capillary–venous, capillary–arterial–venous etc.
Characteristics	
Usually absent at birth	Present at birth
Appear during first weeks of life	
Dynamic: Proliferation ↓	Adynamic, stable
Stabilization ↓	
Slow, spontaneous involution	

Adapted from references 2, 14, and 18.

(e.g., an eyelid hemangioma, obstructing vision and producing deprivation amblyopia); progressive ulceration and infection (perineal lesions are at particular risk); progression of a lesion causing unacceptable deformity from compression, or overgrowth of an extremity from increased blood flow in a hemangioma (hemangiomatous gigantism); growth of a lesion in an intertriginous area, where it is subject to trauma and secondary infection; facial lesions producing severe cosmetic deformity; high-output cardiac failure; and life-threatening Kasabach–Merritt syndrome (1,4–7,28–31).

When the decision is made to treat a hemangioma, options available include steroids, embolization, vasoligation, surgical excision, laser therapy, interferon, and cyclophosphamide (1, 28–40). In the treatment of hemangiomas, 30–80% of lesions respond to steroids (1,4,33). Interferon is often effective, although there have been reports of severe neurotoxicity, including spastic diplegia (36,37). Whereas some physicians use it primarily in cases that have failed to respond to steroids, others consider it first-line therapy. Resection or arterial ligation is indicated for small lesions for which excision would produce significant cosmetic deformity. Surgery is also appropriate for treatment of uncontrolled ulceration, bleeding, or infection, arteriovenous shunts with high-output cardiac failure, or visual obstruction (1,4–7).

Radiotherapy should be considered only for lesions that have failed to respond to steroids or interferon and are not appropriate for treatment with other modalities. Significant late effects have been attributed to irradiation of hemangiomas, including scarring, bone growth abnormalities, and secondary neoplasms (10,28,41–47). The incidence of cancer after radiotherapy for skin hemangiomas has been studied extensively in a series of articles from Sweden. These reports describe a total of 14,633 children less than 18 months old irradiated at the Radiumhemmet in Stockholm from 1909 to 1959 and 12,055 treated at Sahlrenska Hospital, Goteborg, from 1930 to 1965 (41–47). At the Radiumhemmet, treatment was most commonly by ^{226}Ra applicators (81%) or contact X-ray therapy (60 kVp or less, 16%). At Goteborg ^{226}Ra was used for 99% of the treatments. The median age of treatment was 6 months at Radiumhemmet and 5 months at Goteborg. There is a higher-than-expected incidence of cancer in these irradiated children. Significantly higher levels of breast cancer were detected in the pooled studies (hazard ratio 1.2, 95% confidence interval 1.06–1.36), and there was an approximate twofold increase in the expected incidence thyroid cancer. Recalculation of the dosages from the ^{226}Ra applicators suggests a linear dose–response relationship. Conceivably, the use of electron therapy in lieu of ^{226}Ra might mitigate the long-term effects of radiotherapy in these patients. However, these studies strongly argue against the routine use of radiotherapy to treat hemangiomas of infancy and indicate that irradiation of the thyroid, breast buds, and gonads should be avoided (41–47).

The response of cutaneous hemangiomas of infancy to irradiation can be dramatic. In 1946, MacKee and Cipallaro (10) reported that the "results of beta-ray therapy in nevus vasculosus are so striking, so perfect, that they may be placed among the most notable achievements of radiation therapy in the treatment of cutaneous diseases." Furst et al. (39) reported good results in 88% of treated cases. In treatment of hemangiomas in 13 patients with Kasabach–Merritt syndrome, Ogino et al. (40) demonstrated regression of the lesion and an increase in platelet count to more than $10^5/mm^3$ within 40 days of radiotherapy. When radiotherapy is used, the clinical treatment volume should include the visible and palpable lesion with a small margin. The dosage per fraction should be 150–300 cGy. The majority of lesions respond to two or three fractions, for a total dosage of 300–750 cGy. Occasionally, higher dosages may be indicated, but the total dosage should not exceed 10 Gy (10,40,48). If these guidelines are observed, regressions generally will occur rapidly, and scarring should be minimal.

On rare occasions, the radiation oncologist is consulted on cases of hemangiomas that began in infancy and continued to enlarge slowly rather than regress. These older children or young adults present with severe deformity and, rarely, hemodynamic compromise, anemia, or coagulopathy (49). A host of other treatments fail before radiotherapy is considered for these patients. The response of these large, symptomatic lesions often is substantial (29,30, 50). Before treatment, the lesion should be evaluated by careful physical examination and by imaging, preferably by magnetic resonance imaging, as described earlier. The lesion is irradiated with tight margins using fractionated radiotherapy in 150- to 200-cGy daily fractions, typically to a total dosage of 30–40 Gy (Fig. 18-1) (50).

Orbital hemangiomas are another special treatment case (48,51,52). When irradiation of the lid is needed, the eye is protected by a lead shield placed behind the lid and over the lens of the eye. Superficial X-rays or electrons are then used for treatment. Posterior orbit hemangiomas may be successfully treated to a total dosage of 12–18 Gy using techniques similar to the commonly used lateral beam approach for retinoblastoma (see Chapter 5) (30,51).

Hemangiomas of the bone are benign, slow-growing tumors that can exhibit cavernous or capillary architecture. The majority of these lesions are asymptomatic and are detected on routine radiographs. The hemangioma produces replacement of the normal cancellous bone with thick bony trabeculae. On plain radiographs and computed tomography scan a honeycomb or polka-dot appearance is characteristic (53,54). The incidence increases with age, and less than 10% occur in the first two decades of life (55). Hemangiomas of the vertebrae may give rise to neurologic signs and symptoms ranging from pain to severe spinal cord compression. The pathophysiology of these lesions includes ballooning of the vertebrae with narrowing and deformation of the spinal canal, extension of the hemangioma into the epidural space, and, rarely, vertebral body compression fracture. Although asymptomatic vertebral bodies do not warrant treatment, intervention is needed for paresis, paraplegia, or severe pain. Laminectomy is recommended by some in the setting of rapid-onset cord compression but is hazardous because of the chance of severe hemorrhage. Catheter embolization of feeder vessels has been successful but runs the risk of vascular catastrophe (54).

Rades et al. (56) analyzed the results from University Hospital Eppendorf and published reports on the outcome after radiation therapy in the treatment of symptomatic vertebral hemangiomas (54–62). A total of 117 patients were evaluable, ranging in age from 12 to 78 years (median age 47 years). To identify a dose–effect relationship, patients were divided into two groups based on the total radiation dosage of 20–34 Gy ($n = 62$, median total dosage = 30 Gy) or 36–44 Gy ($n = 55$, median 40 Gy). Total radiation dosages were calculated based on a 2 Gy per fraction equivalent dosage using an α/β ratio of 3 Gy. Complete pain relief was achieved in 82% of the higher-dose group and 39% of the lower-dose group ($p = 0.003$). Complete or partial pain relief was obtained in 100% and 87% of the higher- and lower-dose patients, respectively. This analysis suggests that a total of 40 Gy delivered in 2 Gy per fraction can provide

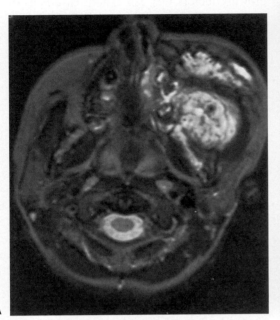

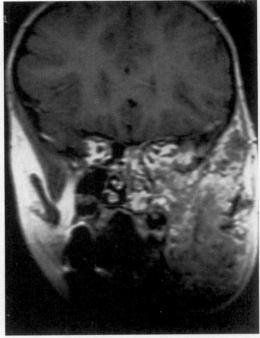

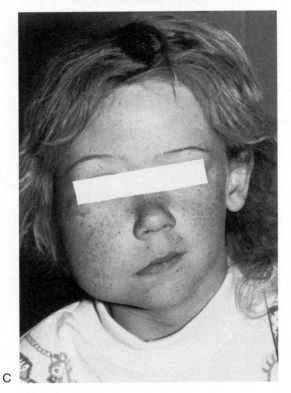

FIG. 18-1. (A, B) This hemangioma grew from birth until, when the child was 8 years old, there was significant facial deformity and bleeding from the intraoral component of the lesion. There was a moderate response after a split course of irradiation to a total dosage of 45 Gy. **(C)** Disease remains stable 11 years after irradiation. At last follow-up contact, the patient was 3 months pregnant.

effective palliation of symptomatic vertebral hemangiomas (56).

LYMPHANGIOMAS

Lymphangiomas usually are first noted in the neonate and can produce symptoms at any age. They can occur throughout the body but predominate in the neck. They may infiltrate the tongue or the floor of the mouth, causing deformity, pain associated with frequent infections, and obstruction of the aerodigestive passages. Spontaneous regression of these lesions is rare (63,64).

Lymphangiomas are composed of dilated lymph vessels, the walls of which consist of endothelial cells and connective tissues (65). Four distinct forms have been described. These include capillary lymphangiomas, an uncommon lesion that may have the appearance of an ordinary wart or group of small vesicles. These lesions consist of a network of lymphatic spaces formed by small- and medium-sized vessels. Cavernous lymphangiomas occur in the skin and subcutaneous tissue, salivary glands, and lips. These are diffuse spongy masses, often with indistinct margins. They consist of multiple dilated lymph channels that are lined with either single or multiple layers of endothelial cells. Cystic hygromas are the most common lymphangiomas. They are composed of cysts ranging from a few millimeters to several centimeters in diameter. The cysts compress surrounding tissues, and small vessels course over their walls. Finally, lymphangial hemangiomas consist of a combination of blood- and lymph-containing channels. Although these lesions are quite similar to cavernous lymphangiomas, some spaces in these lesions also contain erythrocytes and are therefore presumed to be in direct communication with blood vessels (63,65,66).

Surgical excision is the preferred therapy for lymphangiomas, although this may be difficult in certain situations and entail repeated operations (66–68). Sclerosing agents have been used, but the results have been problematic because of poor cosmetic outcome and fistula formation. Bleomycin fat emulsions and, more recently, OK-432, an immunostimulant composed of group A *Streptococcus pyogenes* and benzylpenicillin, have been advocated for the treatment of unresectable lymphangiomas (66,69–74). However, the availability of the latter drug is limited, and the efficacy of this agent in treating large lesions has been questioned (75).

Radiation therapy is rarely used. Dosage inhomogeneity and the risk of infection have discouraged radiation oncologists from using interstitial brachytherapy. Some dramatic responses of neck, chest, and mesenteric lymphangiomas to external beam radiotherapy have been reported in the literature (76–80). However, one must be cautious because physicians are more likely to report their therapeutic successes than their failures (65).

Fractionated radiotherapy to a total dosage of 15–30 Gy has been used to treat lymphangiomas of the head and neck. However, the known risks of radiation to this region, including inhibition of bone growth and soft tissue development and the increased risk of thyroid cancer, should be considered in the decision to treat.

BASAL AND SQUAMOUS CELL CARCINOMAS

Basal and squamous cell skin cancers are rarely diagnosed in children (81–84). When they do occur in childhood, there is usually a predisposition to skin cancer, that is, basal cell nevus syndrome (BCNS) or xeroderma pigmentosa. They have also been reported as arising in a nevus sebaceous (85), after cranial irradiation for acute lymphoblastic leukemia (86), and after thorium X treatment of a hemangioma (87). BCNS (also known as nevoid basal cell carcinoma syndrome or Gorlin's syndrome) is characterized by the occurrence of multiple basal cell epitheliomas, a positive family history for the syndrome, keratocysts of the jaw, epidermal cyst and hamartoma formation, palmar and plantar pits, skeletal abnormalities, and oculoneurologic abnormalities (88,89). The basal cell epitheliomas that warrant treatment develop on the face, neck, and trunk. Patients may be treated with chemotherapy, immunotherapy, electrodesiccation, cryotherapy, Mohs' chemosurgery, or primary surgery with reconstruction of the defect. Some children have been treated with radiotherapy, although this treatment is generally reserved for adults.

BCNS may provide a unique example of the genetic–environmental interaction in the production of malignancies. Several patients have been reported with BCNS who have also developed medulloblastoma in early childhood (90). In many survivors, multiple basal cell epitheliomas have developed within 6 months to 3 years of craniospinal irradiation. These skin cancers develop at an age distinctly earlier and in a distribution unlike that of family members with BCNS. The distribution of basal cell epitheliomas corresponds to the radiotherapy ports. The development of multiple cutaneous skin cancers has not been generally reported in the general population of long-term survivors in medulloblastoma (91). This unusual illustration of multihit mutagenesis may suggest that radiotherapy for skin epitheliomas is relatively contraindicated in young children with BCNS.

Xeroderma pigmentosa (XP) is an autosomally dominant inherited disease. The clinical manifestations occur primarily on sun-exposed skin that develops abnormal pigmentation and multiple malignant tumors. Areflexia, mental retardation, and other neurologic abnormalities are associated with XP. The biochemical defect appears to be a poor ability to repair ultraviolet-induced DNA damage. Basal cell and squamous cell carcinomas of the skin may develop in patients with XP. These carcinomas usually are treated with the standard techniques of electrodesiccation, curettage, surgery, cryosurgery, or chemosurgery. Because ionizing radiation damage to XP cells is repaired normally, there is no theoretical objection to radiotherapy treatment of tumors if indicated. However, situations in which radiotherapy is appropriate are quite rare (92).

At St. Jude Children's Research Hospital (SJCRH), eight children with skin carcinomas were seen from 1962 to 1986. In four patients, basal cell epitheliomas developed in previously irradiated fields (acute lymphoblastic leukemia, Hodgkin's disease, neuroblastoma). There was a fifth patient with BCNS. The three patients treated for squamous cell carcinoma had a prior diagnosis of XP (93). From 1971 to 1991, seven cases of basal cell carcinoma and three cases of squamous cell carcinoma were encountered at the National Institute of Pediatrics in Mexico City (81). Five of the seven children with basal cell carcinoma had XP, one had BCNS, and one developed in a previous radiotherapy field. One of the three patients with squamous cell carcinoma also had XP.

MALIGNANT MELANOMA

The incidence of malignant melanoma before the age of 15 years is estimated at 1–2 per million population in the United States and United Kingdom and approximately 4 per million in Australia. Fewer than 2% of malignant melanomas are seen in children and adolescents (84,94). Childhood melanoma in Australia is higher than that reported in other series, accounting for 3.3% of all pediatric neoplasms. This high incidence is attributed to excessive exposure to sunlight (84,95). In the United States, the reported incidence of cutaneous melanoma rose approximately twofold between 1974 and 1994, with the increase observed across all age groups (96–98).

At least seven factors should be considered in the etiology of childhood malignant melanoma: large congenital nevocytic nevi (LCNN), the total number of melanocytic nevi, dysplastic nevus syndrome, immunosuppression, transplacental malignant melanoma (i.e., mother-to-child transmission), XP, and cumulative sun exposure. LCNN are defined as congenital nevi 20 cm in diameter or larger. They may occur anywhere on the body and include the so-called "bathing trunks" nevi. There is controversy in the literature regarding the relative risk of malignant melanoma arising in LCNN, with lifetime risks ranging from 2% to 31% (99–102). The total number of melanocytic nevi strongly influences the risk of developing melanoma later in life (103–108). In turn, the number of melanocytic nevi in children is closely associated with the degree of sun exposure and the nevus counts in the parents (108).

Familial dysplastic nevus syndrome is an autosomal dominant trait characterized by unusual nevi at risk for developing melanoma. Patients with XP are at significant risk for developing melanoma, as described earlier. The risk of malignant melanoma is higher in congenital immunodeficiency syndromes and iatrogenic immunosuppression, suggesting that immunoincompetence adversely influences melanoma development. There are rare reports of transplacental transmission of metastatic melanoma from mother to child (99). The infant usually has disseminated disease at birth, and the prognosis is poor.

Sun exposure is a critical epidemiological factor in the development of malignant melanoma (94,108–112). Although there is debate about the timing of sun exposure, particularly severe sunburns, and the eventual development of malignant melanoma, the data strongly support the concept that the lifetime total exposure to sunlight is directly related to the incidence of malignant melanoma. Thus, medical practitioners, including radiation oncologists, should counsel parents to protect children from excessive sun exposure.

Childhood melanoma may be staged with the following system: stage I, localized disease; stage II, regional lymph node involvement; stage III, distant metastatic disease (113). Three important factors should be considered in evaluating stage I patient: the presence of local ulceration, Clark's level of invasion, and Breslow's depth of invasion (Table 18-2). All three have been shown to be important prognostic indicators in childhood melanoma (114). In children, metastatic disease is rare in lesions less than 1.5 mm thick (113). In the SJCRH series of 33 children treated from 1967 to 1988, there were no tumor-related deaths in children with thin melanomas (Clark's level I–II, Breslow thickness less than 1.5 mm). Twenty-four patients 16 years of age or younger with malignant melanoma were reviewed at St. Thomas' Hospital, London, from 1981 to 1993. Three of three patients with tumors 1.2 mm or smaller were alive without tumor. In contrast, of the 19 children with tumors 1.6 mm or larger, 15 were disease-free, 3 were alive but suffered locoregional relapse, and 1 died of disease (102). As in adult patients, brain metastases often occur and convey a poor prognosis (115).

It is important to distinguish malignant melanoma from juvenile melanoma or nevi of large spindle or epithelioid cells or Spitz nevi. In 1948, Sophie Spitz, a pathologist at New York's Memorial Hospital, described 12 of 13 children who were long-term survivors of this peculiar "benign" childhood melanoma (116). Spitz nevi

TABLE 18-2. *Classification of the primary lesion in malignant melanoma*

Clark et al.'s "levels" (147)	Breslow's "thickness" (148)	American Joint Committee on Cancer T category (149)
Level I: All tumor cells above the basement membrane	Using an ocular micrometer, measure maximal thickness of lesion from granular cell layer to deepest point of lesion. If the lesion is ulcerated, measure from the ulcer base over the deepest point of the lesion (i.e., <0.76 mm, 0.76–1.50 mm, >1.50 mm).	T_0 No evidence of primary tumor
Level II: Tumor cells into the papillary but not reticular dermis		T_{is} Melanoma in situ
Level III: Tumor of the papillary–reticular dermis interface		T_1 Melanoma ≤1.0 mm thick with or without ulceration
Level IV: Neoplastic cells into the collagen bundles of the reticular dermis		T_2 Melanoma 1.01–2 mm thick, with or without ulceration
Level V: Invasion of subcutaneous tissue		T_3 Melanoma 2.01–4 mm thick, with or without ulceration
		T_4 Melanoma >4 mm thick, with or without ulceration

usually are symmetric and small, exhibit epithelial hyperplasia, contain clefts between nests of melanocytes and epidermis, exhibit mature melanocytes, and contain dull, pink epidermal globules called Kamino bodies (117–119). The histologic differentiation of Spitz nevi and malignant melanoma is difficult, even among expert dermatopathologists (120).

The inclusion of benign Spitz nevi cases in pediatric malignant melanoma series results in an overdiagnosis of malignant melanoma and an underestimate of mortality rate (121–123). Analysis of pediatric malignant melanoma series that exclude the benign Spitz tumors indicates that survival rates in children are similar to those of adults. Among the 8,635 patients registered with the Duke Melanoma Clinic, only 85 (less than 1%) were under age 18 (99,124). Fifty-nine percent of the patients had the superficial spreading histologic type, and 20% of the remaining patients were Clark's level III or IV. There was no difference in the actuarial survival rates between adult and juvenile stage I patients (Fig. 18-2).

Overall, on a stage-by-stage basis, survival in children and adults appears comparable (121).

The standard treatment for localized malignant melanoma is wide local excision (125–127). In certain situations, a skin graft may be used to close the resulting defect. The role of elective node dissection of clinically uninvolved regional lymph nodes has been a subject of debate. It is clear that not all patients are candidates for elective lymph node dissection. However, for patients with melanoma more than 0.75 mm thick, the proper initial extent of surgery is debatable. The arguments in favor of elective node dissection include staging, detecting microscopic disease, and treating occult metastatic disease if present, thereby reducing tumor burden and removing a potential source of future metastases (126,127).

Sentinel lymph node biopsy is emerging as the standard method of staging metastasis to regional lymph nodes. To identify the sentinel node (i.e., the first node draining an anatomical site), a colloidal dye or radioactive isotope is in-

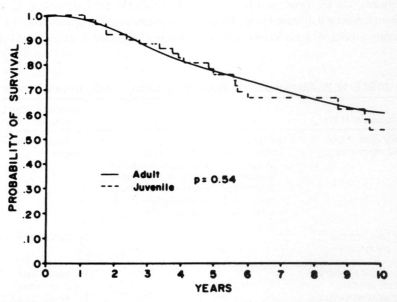

FIG. 18-2. Actuarial survival rates of the adult and juvenile stage I patients registered at the Duke University Melanoma Clinic. Of 18 pediatric patients who were disease-free for more than 7 years, 12 (67%) ultimately developed recurrent disease, including 5 patients whose disease recurred more than 13 years after the initial diagnosis. Late recurrences indicate that patients must be followed for life. (From Reintgen DS, Vollmer R, Seigler HF. Juvenile malignant melanoma. *Surg Gynecol Obstet* 1989;168:249–253, with permission).

jected at the tumor bed. During surgery, the sentinel node is identified by visual inspection or by a handheld gamma probe, and the node is excised for sectioning and immunohistochemical staining. In adults, this low-morbidity procedure offers an accurate and sensitive method of determining nodal involvement (128). In turn, the regional lymph node status has been found to be the strongest prognostic factor in early-stage melanoma (128–131). Although data on the utility of sentinel lymph node biopsy in malignant melanoma for the pediatric population are limited because of the rarity of this disease, the similarities between malignant melanoma in the adult and child suggest that sentinel lymph node biopsy should be considered in staging pediatric patients (132–135).

Patients with positive sentinel nodes usually undergo completion lymphadenectomy and may be candidates for clinical trials. There is some published evidence supporting the use of chemotherapy or immunotherapy to treat metastatic or relapsed disease. SJCRH has reported a complete or partial response in 8 of 18 patients (44%) receiving cyclophosphamide, vincristine, and dacarbazine (136). Responses have also been observed with single-agent dacarbazine and melphalan with hyperthermic isolated limb perfusion (137,138). In Eastern Cooperative Oncology Group (ECOG) 1684, the use of high-dose interferon α–2b in adults with high-risk melanoma appeared to improve survival at the cost of significant toxicity (139). However, a subsequent larger intergroup study (ECOG 1690) failed to confirm significant benefit of this approach (140). In an adult population, interleukin-2 has also shown activity in the treatment of metastatic melanoma (141).

Radiotherapy is reasonably effective for the symptomatic palliation of metastases. Radiobiologic interest had been focused on the possibility that at a cellular level, malignant melanoma is truly radioresistant (142). A survey of D_q values (width of the shoulder of the cell survival curve in response to ionizing radiation) of various mammalian cell lines suggests that a typical value for D_q is about 90 cGy. However, observations from several investigators suggest that malignant melanoma *in vitro* has a particularly

broad-shouldered survival curve, with a D_q greater than 200 cGy. These data reinforced the belief that malignant melanoma, though intrinsically radioresistant, might be more responsive to high dosages per fraction. A review of several retrospective studies of the effect of fraction size on disease response in malignant melanoma in adults suggested that the probability of a complete response was 34% for dosages less than 400 cGy but 59% for dosages 400 cGy or greater (143). This analysis excluded bone metastases, which showed equal responses for small and large fractions (144).

Subsequently, a prospective clinical trial of patients at least 15 years old, with measurable melanoma lesions, randomized 126 patients to either 4 weekly fractions of 8 Gy per fraction or 20 fractions of 2.5 Gy per fraction 5 days per week (145). In both the large and conventional fraction arms, equivalent complete and partial clinical responses were observed. Stratification by tumor size (greater than or less than 5 cm) or tumor site (soft tissue or skin, nodal, other) also failed to show any difference between the 8- and 2.5-Gy fractionation schemes (127). Based on the retrospective results, it seems reasonable to use high-dose-per-fraction radiotherapy for palliation of metastatic melanoma when late effects are not an issue. The prospective trial suggests that conventional fraction is equally reasonable when there is a significant probability of long-term survival.

REFERENCES

References particularly recommended for further reading are indicated by an asterisk.

*1. Drolet BA, Esterly NB, Freiden IJ. Hemangiomas in children. *N Engl J Med* 1999;341:173–181.
 2. Powell J. Update on hemangiomas and vascular malformations. *Curr Opin Pediatr* 1999;11:456–463.
 3. Garzon M. Hemangiomas: update on classification, clinical presentation, and associated aromalies. *Cutis* 2000;66:325–328.
 4. Metry DW, Hebert AA. Benign cutaneous vascular tumors of infancy: when to worry, what to do. *Arch Dermatol* 2000;136:905–914.
 5. Garzon MC, Frieden IJ. Hemangiomas: when to worry. *Pediatr Ann* 2000;29:58–57.
 6. Donald PJ. Vascular anomalies of the head and neck. *Facial Plast Surg Clin North Am* 2001;9:77–92.
 7. Gampper TJ, Morgan RF. Vascular abnormalities:

hemangiomas. *Plast Reconstr Surg* 2002;110:572–585.

8. Paller AS. The Sturge–Weber syndrome. *Pediatr Dermatol* 1987;4:300–304.

9. Braun-Falco O, Goldschmidt H, Lukacs S. *Dermatologic radiotherapy.* New York: Springer-Verlag, 1976.

10. MacKee GM, Cipallaro AC. *X-rays and radium in the treatment of disease of the skin.* Philadelphia: Lea & Febiger, 1946:513–521.

11. Kasabach HH, Merritt KK. Capillary hemangioma with extensive purpura: report of a case. *Am J Dis Child* 1940;59:1063–1070.

12. Shim WKT. Hemangiomas of infancy complicated by thrombocytopenia. *Am J Surg* 1968;116:896–906.

13. Esterly NB. Kasabach–Merritt syndrome in infants. *J Am Acad Dermatol* 1983;8:504–513.

14. Mulliken JB, Glowacki J. Hemangiomas and vascular malformations in infants and children: a classification based on endothelial characteristics. *Plast Reconstr Surg* 1982;69:412–422.

15. Mulliken JB. Classification of vascular birthmarks. In: Mulliken JB, Young AE, eds. *Vascular birthmarks: hemangiomas and malformations.* Philadelphia: Saunders, 1988:24–40.

16. Enjolras O, Mulliken JB. Vascular tumors and vascular malformations (new issues). *Adv Dermatol* 1998;13:375–422.

17. Pasyk KA. Classification and clinical and histopathological features of hemangiomas and other vascular malformations. In: Ryan TJ, Cherry GW, eds. *Vascular birthmarks: pathogenesis and management.* Oxford: Oxford University Press, 1987:1–55.

*18. Hand JL, Frieden IJ. Vascular birthmarks of infancy: resolving nosologic confusion. *Am J Med Genet* 2002;108:257–264.

19. Vin-Christian K, McCalmont T, Frieden IJ. Kaposiform hemangioendothelioma: an aggressive, locally invasive vascular tumor that can mimic hemangioma of infancy. *Arch Dermatol* 1997;133:1573–1578.

20. Sarkar M, Mulliken JB, Kozakewich HP, et al. Thrombocytopenic coagulopathy (Kasabach–Merritt phenomenon) is associated with Kaposiform hemangioendothelioma and not with common infantile hemangioma. *Plast Reconstr Surg* 1997;100:1377–1386.

21. Dubois J, Patriquin HB, Garel L, et al. Soft-tissue hemangiomas in infants and children: diagnosis using Doppler sonography. *AJR* 1998;171:247–252.

22. Kern S, Niemeyer C, Darge K, et al. Differentiation of vascular birthmarks by MR imaging. *Acta Radiol* 2000;41:453–457.

23. Dubois J, Garel L, Grignon A, et al. Imaging of hemangiomas and vascular malformations in children. *Acad Radiol* 1998;5–390–400.

24. Burrows PE, Laor T, Paltiel H, et al. Diagnostic imaging in the evaluation of vascular birthmarks. *Dermatol Clin* 1998;16:455–488.

25. Mulliken JB. Diagnosis and natural history of hemangiomas. In: Mulliken JB, Young AE, eds. *Vascular birthmarks: hemangiomas and malformations.* Philadelphia: Saunders, 1988:41–62.

26. Lister WA. The natural history of strawberry nevi. *Lancet* 1938;1:1429–1434.

27. Nakayama H. Clinical and histological studies of the classification and natural history of the strawberry birthmark. *J Dermatol* 1981;2:277–291.

28. Enjolras O, Richie MC, Merland JJ, et al. Management of alarming hemangiomas in infancy: a review of 25 cases. *Pediatrics* 1990;85:491–498.

29. Schild SE, Buskirk SJ, Frick LM, et al. Radiotherapy for large symptomatic hemangiomas. *Int J Radiat Biol Phys* 1991;21:729–735.

30. Dutton SC, Plowman PN. Paediatric hemangiomas: the role of radiotherapy. *Br J Radiol* 1991;64:261–269.

31. Dinehart SM, Kincannon J, Geronemus R. Hemangiomas: evaluation and treatment. *Dermatol Surg* 2001;27:475–485.

32. Armstrong DC, ter Brugge K. Selected interventional procedures for pediatric head and neck vascular lesions. *Neuroimaging Clin N Am* 2000;10:271–292.

33. Akyüz C, Yaris N, Kutluk NT, et al. Management of cutaneous hemangiomas: a retrospective analysis of 1109 cases and comparison of conventional dose prednisolone with high-dose methylprednisolone therapy. *Pediatr Hematol Oncol* 2001;18:47–55.

34. Ezekowitz RA, Mulliken JB, Folkman J. Interferon alfa-2a therapy for life-threatening hemangiomas of infancy. *N Engl J Med* 1992;326:1456–1463.

35. Ricketts RR, Hatley RM, Corden BJ, et al. Interferon-alpha-2a for the treatment of complex hemangiomas of infancy and childhood. *Ann Surg* 1994;219:605–614.

36. Barlow CF, Priebe CJ, Mulliken JB, et al. Spastic diplegia as a complication of interferon alfa-2a treatment of hemangiomas of infancy. *J Pediatr* 1998;132:527–530.

37. Greinwald JH Jr, Burke DK, Bonthius DJ, et al. An update on the treatment of hemangiomas in children with interferon-alpha-2a. *Arch Otolaryngol Head Neck Surg* 1999;125:21–27.

38. Hurvitz CH, Alkalay AL, Sloninsky L, et al. Cyclophosphamide therapy in life-threatening vascular tumors. *J Pediatr* 1986;109:360–363.

*39. Furst CJ, Lundell M, Holm LE. Radiation therapy of hemangiomas, 1909–1959. A report based on 50 years of clinical practice at Radiumhemmet, Stockholm. *Acta Oncol* 1987;26:33–36.

40. Ogino I, Torikai K, Kobayasi S, et al. Radiation therapy for life- or function-threatening infant hemangioma. *Radiology* 2001;218:834–839.

*41. Furst CJ, Lundell M, Holm LE, et al. Cancer incidence after radiotherapy for skin hemangioma: a retrospective cohort study in Sweden. *Natl Cancer Inst* 1988;80:1387–1392.

*42. Furst CJ, Silfversward C, Holm LE. Mortality in a cohort of radiation treated childhood skin hemangiomas. *Acta Oncol* 1989;28(6):789–794.

*43. Lindberg S, Karlsson P, Arvidsson B, et al. Cancer incidence after radiotherapy for skin hemangioma during infancy. *Acta Oncol* 1995;34:735–740.

*44. Lundel M, Haulinen T, Holm LE. Thyroid cancer after radiotherapy for skin hemangioma in infancy. *Radiat Res* 1994;140:334–339.

*45. Lundel M, Holm LE. Risk of solid cancers after irradiation in infancy. *Acta Oncol* 1995;34:727–734.

*46. Lundel M, Mattson A, Haulinen T, et al. Breast cancer after radiotherapy for skin hemangioma in infancy. *Radiat Res* 1996;145:225–230.

47. Lundberg S. Radiotherapy of childhood haeman-

giomas: from active treatment to radiation risk estimates. *Radiat Environ Biophys* 2001;40:179–189.

48. Freire JE, Brady LW, Shields JA, et al. Eye and orbit. In: Perez CA, Brady LW, Halperin EC, et al., eds. *Principles & practice of radiation oncology.* Philadelphia: Lippincott Williams & Wilkins, 2003:876–892.

49. Morelli JG. Hemangiomas and vascular malformations. *Pediatr Ann* 1996;25:91–96.

50. Sealy B, Barry L, Buret E, et al. Cavernous hemangioma of the head and neck in the adult. *J R Soc Med* 1989;82:198–202.

51. Plowman PN, Harnett AN. Radiotherapy in benign orbital disease. I. Complicated ocular angiomas. *Br J Ophthalmol* 1988;72:286–288.

52. Garza G, Fay A, Rubin PAD. Treatment of pediatric vascular lesions of the eyelid and orbit. *Int Ophthalmol Clin* 2001;41:43–55.

53. Jeleniewski-Rudyk A. Treatment of vertebral hemangiomas. *Pol Rev Radiol Nucl Med* 1967;31:155–160.

54. Raco A, Ciapetta P, Artico M, et al. Vertebral hemangiomas with cord compression: the role of embolization in five cases. *Surg Neurol* 1990;34:164–168.

55. Unni KK, Irvius JC, Beabul JW. Hemangioma, hemangiopericytoma, and hemangioendothelioma (angiosarcoma) of bone. *Cancer* 1971;27:1403–141.

*56. Rades D, Bajrovic A, Alberti W, et al. Is there a dose-effect relationship for the treatment of symptomatic vertebral hemangioma? *Int J Radiat Oncol Biol Phys* 2003;55:178–181.

57. Glanzmann C, Rust M, Horst W. Radiotherapie bei Angiomen der Wirbelelsäule: Ergebnisse bei 62 Patienten aus dem Zeitraum. 1939–1975. *Strahlenther Onkol* 1990;2:159–1975.

58. Asthana AK, Tandon SC, Pant GC, et al. Radiation therapy for symptomatic vertebral hemangioma. *Clin Oncol* 1990;2:159–162.

59. Winkler C, Dornfeld S, Baumannn, et al. Effizienz der Strahlentherapie bei Wirbelhämangiomen. *Strahlenther Onkol* 1996;172:681–684.

60. Guedea F, Majo J, Guardia E, et al. The role of radiation therapy in vertebral body hemangiomas without neurological signs. *Int Orthop* 1994;18:77–79.

61. Sakata K, Hareyama M, Oouchi A, et al. Radiotherapy of vertebral hemangiomas. *Acta Oncol* 1997;36:719–724.

62. Miszczyk L, Ficek K, Trela K, et al. The efficacy of radiotherapy for vertebral hemangiomas. *Neoplasma* 2001;48:82–84.

63. Gordon RF, Parkin JL. Lymphangioma of the head and neck. *Ear Nose Throat J* 1982;61:338–342.

64. Saija M, Munro JR, Mancer K. Lymphangioma: a long-term follow-up study. *Plast Reconstr Surg* 1975;56:642–651.

65. Holmes GW, Hawes LE. Radiation treatment of lymphangioma. *AJR* 1943;49:799–802.

66. Tanigawa N, Shimayatsu T, Takahashi K, et al. Treatment of cystic hygroma and lymphangioma with the use of bleomycin fat emulsions. *Cancer* 1987;60:741–749.

67. Alqahtani A, Nguyen LT, Flageole H, et al. 25 years' experience with lymphangiomas in children. *J Pediatr Surg* 1999;34:1164–1168.

68. Fliegelman LJ, Friedland D, Brandwein M, et al. Lymphatic malformation: predictive factors for recurrence. *Otolaryngol Head Neck Surg* 2000;123:706–710.

69. Orford J, Barker A, Thonell S, et al. Bleomycin therapy for cystic hygroma. *J Pediatr Surg* 1995;30:1282–1287.

70. Sanlialp I, Karnak I, Tanyel FC, et al. Sclerotherapy for lymphangioma in children. *Int J Pediatr Otorhinolaryngol* 2003;67:795–800.

71. Ogita S, Tsuto T, Nakamura K, et al. OK-432 therapy in 64 patients with lymphangioma. *J Pediatr Surg* 1994;29:784–785.

72. Claesson G, Kuylenstierna R. OK-432 therapy for lymphatic malformation in 32 patients (28 children). *Int J Pediatr Otorhinolaryngol* 2002;65:1–6.

73. Laranne J, Keski-Nisula L, Rautio R, et al. OK-432 (Picibanil) therapy for lymphangiomas in children. *Eur Arch Otorhinolaryngol* 2002;259:274–278.

74. Giguère CM, Bauman NM, Sato Y, et al. Treatment of lymphangiomas with OK-432 (Picibanil) sclerotherapy. *Arch Otolaryngol Head Neck Surg* 2002;128:1137–1144.

75. Hall N, Ade-Ajayi N, Brewis C, et al. Is intralesional injection of OK-432 effective in the treatment of lymphangiomas in children? *Surgery* 2003;133:238–242.

76. Johnson DW, Klazynski PT, Gordon WH, et al. Mediastinal lymphangioma and chylothorax: the role of radiotherapy. *Ann Thorac Surg* 1986;41:325–328.

77. Ikemura K, Hidaka H, Fujiwara T, et al. A case of cystic lymphangioma extending from the neck to the tongue. *J Craniomaxillofac Surg* 1987;15:369–371.

78. Dajee H, Woodhouse R. Lymphangiomas of the mediastinum with chylothorax and chylopericardium: role of radiation treatment. *J Thorac Cardiovasc Surg* 1994;108:594–595.

79. Tai PTH, Jewell LF. Case report: mesenteric mixed haemangioma and lymphangioma; a report of a case with 10-year follow-up after radiation treatment. *Br J Radiol* 1995;68:657–661.

80. Kandil A, Rostom AY, Mourad WA, et al. Successful control of extensive thoracic lymphangiomatosis by irradiation. *Clin Oncol* 1997;6:309–411.

81. de la Luz Orozco-Cavarrubias M, Tamoyc-Sanchez L, Duran-McKinster C, et al. Malignant cutaneous tumors in children: twenty years of experience in at a large pediatric hospital. *J AM Acad Dermctol* 1994;30:243–249.

82. Hay WE. Nonmelanoma skin cancer in Albuquerque, New Mexico: experience of a major health care provider. *Cancer* 1996;77:2849–2495.

83. Wyatt AJ, Hansen RC. Pediatric skin tumors. *Pediatr Clin North Am* 2000;47:937–963.

84. Pearce MS, Parker L, Cotterill SJ, et al. Skin cancer in children and young adults: 28 years' experience from the Northern Region Young Person's Malignant Disease Registry, UK. *Melanoma Res* 2003;13:421–426.

85. Hughes JR, O'Donnell PJ, Pembroke AC. Basal cell carcinoma arising in a naevus sebaceous in a 5-year old girl. *Clin Exp Dermatol* 1995;20:177.

86. Yoshihara T, Ikuta H, Hibi S, et al. Second cutaneous neoplasms after acute lymphoblastic leukemia in childhood. *Int J Hematol* 1993;59:67–71.

87. Scerri L, Navaratnam AE. Basal cell carcinoma presenting as a delayed complication of thorium X used for treating congenital hemangioma. *J Am Acad Dermatol* 1994;31:796–797.

88. Southwick GJ, Schwartz RA. The basal cell nevus

syndrome: disasters occurring among a series of 36 patients. *Cancer* 1979;44:2294–2305.

89. Kimonis VE, Goldstein AM, Pastakia B, et al. Clinical manifestations in 105 persons with nevoid basal cell carcinoma syndrome. *Am J Med Genet* 1997;69: 299–308.

90. Amlashi SF, Riffaud L, Brassier G, et al. Nevoid basal cell carcinoma syndrome: relation with desmoplastic medulloblastoma in infancy. A population-based study and review of the literature. *Cancer* 2003;98: 618–624.

91. Strong LC. Genetic and environmental interactions. *Cancer* 1977;40:1861–1866.

92. Robbins JH, Kraemer KH, Latzner MA, et al. Xeroderma pigmentosum: an inherited disease with sun sensitivity, multiple cutaneous neoplasms, and abnormal DNA repair. *Ann Intern Med* 1974;80:221–248.

93. Pratt CB, George SL, Green AA, et al. Carcinomas in children. Clinical and demographic characteristics. *Cancer* 1988;61:1046–1050.

*94. Hamre MR, Chuba P, Bakshi S, et al. Cutaneous melanoma in childhood and adolescence. *Pediatr Hematol Oncol* 2002;19:309–317.

95. Swetter SM. Dermatological perspectives of malignant melanoma. *Surg Clin North Am* 2003;83:77–95.

96. McWhirter WR, Dobson C, Ring I. Childhood cancer incidence in Australia, 1982–1991. *Int J Cancer* 1996;65:34–38.

97. Dennis LK. Analysis of the melanoma epidemic, both apparent and real: data from the 1973 through 1994 surveillance, epidemiology, and end results program registry. *Arch Dermatol* 1999;135:275–280.

98. Hall HI, Miller DR, Rogers JD, et al. Update on the incidence and mortality from melanoma in the United States. *J Am Acad Dermatol* 1999;40:35–42.

99. Reintgen DS, Vollmer R, Seigler HF. Juvenile malignant melanoma. *Surg Gynecol Obstet* 1989;168: 249–253.

100. Gari LM, Rivers JK, Kopf AW. Melanomas arising in large congenital nevocytic nevi: a prospective study. *Pediatr Dermatol* 1988;5:151–158.

101. Marghoob AA, Schoenbach SP, Kopf AW, et al. Large congenital melanocytic nevi and the risk for the development of malignant melanoma. A prospective study. *Arch Dermatol* 1996;132:170–175.

102. Handerfeld-Jones SE, Smith NP. Malignant melanoma in childhood. *Br J Dermatol* 1996;134: 607–616.

103. Swerdlow AJ, English J, MacKie RM, et al. Benign melanocytic naevi as a risk factor for malignant melanoma. *Br Med J Clin Res Ed* 1986;292:1555–1559.

104. Grob JJ, Gouvernet J, Aymar D, et al. Count of benign melanomocytic nevi as a major indicator of risk for nonfamilial nodular and superficial spreading melanoma. *Cancer* 1990;66:387–395.

105. Bauer J, Garbe C. Acquired melanocytic nevi as a risk factor for melanoma development. A comprehensive review of epidemiological data. *Pigment Cell Res* 2003;16:297–306.

106. Garbe C, Buttner P, Weiss J, et al. Risk factors for developing cutaneous melanoma and criteria for identifying persons at risk: multicenter case-control study of the Central Melanoma Registry of the German Dermatological Society. *J Invest Dermatol* 1994;102:695–696.

107. Makkar HS, Frieden IJ. Congenital melanocytic nevi: an update for the pediatrician. *Curr Opin Pediatr* 2002;14:397–403.

108. Wiecker TS, Luther H, Buettner P, et al. Moderate sun exposure and nevus counts in parents are associated with development of melanocytic nevi in childhood. A risk factor study in 1812 kindergarten children. *Cancer* 2003;97:628–638.

109. Whiteman DC, Whiteman CA, Green A. Childhood sun exposure as a risk factor for melanoma: a systematic review of epidemiologic studies. *Cancer Causes Control* 2001;12:69–82.

110. Elwood JM, Jopson J. Melanoma and sun exposure: an overview of published studies. *Int J Cancer* 1997;73:198–203.

111. Siskind V, Aitken J, Green A, et al. Sun exposure and interaction with family history in risk of melanoma, Queensland, Australia. *Int J Cancer* 2002;97: 90–95.

112. Pfahlberg A, Kölmel KF, Gefeller O, et al. Timing of excessive ultraviolet radiation and melanoma: epidemiology does not support the existence of a critical period of high susceptibility to solar ultraviolet radiation-induced melanoma. *Br J Dermatol* 2001;144: 471–475.

113. Pratt CB, Palmer MK, Thatcher N, et al. Malignant melanoma in children and adolescents. *Cancer* 1981; 47:392–397.

114. Rao BN, Hayes FA, Prah CB, et al. Malignant melanoma in children: its management and prognosis. *J Pediatr Surg* 1990;25:198–203.

115. Rodriguez-Gaindo C, Pappo AS, Kaste SC, et al. Brain metastases in children with melanoma. *Cancer* 1997;79:2440–2245.

116. Spitz S. Melanomas of childhood. *Am J Pathol* 1948;24:591–609.

117. Barnhill RL, Flotte TJ, Fleischli M, et al. Cutaneous melanoma and atypical Spitz tumors in childhood. *Cancer* 1995;76:1833–1845.

118. Helm KF, Schwartz RA, Janniger CK. Juvenile melanoma (Spitz nevus). *Cutis* 1996;57:35–39.

119. Barnhill RL. Childhood melanoma. *Semin Diagn Pathol* 1998;15:189–194.

120. Wechsler J, Bastuji-Garin S, Spatz A, et al. Reliability of the histopathologic diagnosis of malignant melanoma in childhood. *Arch Dermatol* 2002;138:625–628.

121. Saenz NC, Saenz-Bandilllos J, Busam K, et al. Childhood melanoma survival. *Cancer* 1999;85:750–754.

122. Jemal A, Devesa SS, Fears TR, et al. Cancer surveillance series: changing patterns of cutaneous malignant melanoma mortality rates among whites in the United States. *J Natl Cancer Inst* 2000;92:811–818.

123. Conti EMS, Cercato MC, Gata G, et al. Childhood melanoma in Europe since 1978: a population-based survival study. *Eur J Cancer* 2001;37:780–784.

124. Davidoff AM, Cirrincione C, Seigler HF. Malignant melanoma in children. *Ann Surg Oncol* 1994;1: 278–282.

125. Schmid-Wendtner MH, Berking C, Baumert J, et al. Cutaneous melanoma in childhood and adolescence: an analysis of 36 patients. *J Am Acad Dermatol* 2002;46:874–879.

126. Wagner JD, Gordon MS, Chuang TY, et al. Current therapy for cutaneous melanoma. *Plast Reconstr Surg* 2000;105:1774–1799.

127. Essner R. Surgical treatment of cutaneous melanoma. *Surg Clin North Am* 2003;83:109–156.

128. Morton DL, Thompson JF, Essner R, et al. Validation of the accuracy of intraoperative lymphatic mapping and sentinel lymphadenectomy for early-stage melanoma. A multicenter trial. *Ann Surg* 1999;230: 453–465.

129. Balch CM, Soong SJ, Gershenwald JE, et al. Prognostic factors analysis of 17,600 melanoma patients: validation of the American Joint Committee on Cancer melanoma staging system. *J Clin Oncol* 2001; 19:3622–3634.

130. Essner R, Chung MH, Bleicher R, et al. Prognostic implications of thick (≥4-mm) melanoma in the era of intraoperative lymphatic mapping and sentinel lymphadenectomy. *Ann Surg Oncol* 2002;9:754–761.

131. Bleicher RJ, Essner R, Foshag LJ, et al. Role of sentinel lymphadenectomy in thin invasive cutaneous melanomas. *J Clin Oncol* 2003;21:1326–1331.

132. Gibbs P, Moore A, Robinson W, et al. Pediatric melanoma: are recent advances in the management of adult melanoma relevant to the pediatric population? *J Pediatr Hematol Oncol* 2000;22:428–432.

133. Zuckerman R, Maier JP, Huntsman WT, et al. Pediatric melanomas: confirming the diagnosis with sentinel node biopsy. *Ann Plast Surg* 2001;46:394–399.

134. Toro J, Ranieri JM, Havlik RJ, et al. Sentinel lymph node biopsy in children and adolescents with malignant melanoma. *J Pediatr Surg* 2003;38:1063–1065.

135. Bisseck M, Shen P, Pranikoff T. Sentinel lymph node biopsy in a young child with thick cutaneous melanoma. *Oncology* 2003;17:1003–1005.

136. Hayes FA, Green AA. Malignant melanoma in childhood: clinical course and response to chemotherapy. *J Clin Oncol* 1984;2:1229–1238.

137. Boddie AW Jr, Cangir A. Adjuvant and neoadjuvant chemotherapy with dacarbazine in high-risk childhood melanoma. *Cancer* 1987;60:1720–1723.

138. Baas PC, Hoekstra HJ, Koops HS, et al. Hyperthermic isolated regional perfusion in the treatment of extremity melanoma in children and adolescents. *Cancer* 1989;63:199–203.

139. Kirkwood JM, Strawderman MH, Ernstoff MS, et al. Interferon alfa-2b adjuvant therapy of high-risk resected cutaneous melanoma: the Eastern Cooperative Oncology Group Trial EST 1684. *J Clin Oncol* 1996;14:7–17.

140. Kirkwood JM, Ibrahim J, Sondak V, et al. Role of high-dose IFN in high-risk melanoma: preliminary results of the E1690/S9111/C9190 US intergroup trial of high and low-dose IFN2b (HDI and LDI) in high-risk primary or lymph node metastatic melanoma. *Proc Am Soc Clin Oncol* 1999;35:2072A.

141. Atkins MB, Lotze MT, Dutcher JP, et al. High-dose recombinant interleukin 2 therapy for patients with metastatic melanoma: analysis of 270 patients treated between 1985 and 1993. *J Clin Oncol* 1999;17: 2105–2116.

142. Dewey DL. The radiosensitivity of melanoma cells in culture. *Br J Radiol* 1971;44:816–817.

143. Geara FB, Ang KK. Radiation therapy for malignant melanoma. *Surg Clin North Am* 1996;76:1383–1398.

144. Overgaard J. The role of radiotherapy in recurrent and metastatic malignant melanoma: a clinical radiobiological study. *Int J Radiat Oncol Biol Phys* 1986;12:867–872.

145. Konefal JB, Emami B, Pilepich MV. Analysis of dose fractionation in the palliation of metastases from malignant melanoma. *Cancer* 1988;61:243–246.

*146. Sause WT, Cooper JS, Rush S, et al. Fraction size in external beam radiation therapy and the treatment of melanoma. *Int J Radiat Oncol Biol Phys* 1990;20: 429–432.

147. Clark WH Jr, Fram L, Bernardino EA, et al. The histogenesis and biologic behavior of primary human malignant melanomas of the skin. *Cancer Res* 1969; 29:705–726.

148. Breslow A. Tumor thickness, level of invasion and node dissection in stage I cutaneous melanoma. *Ann Surg* 1975;182:572–575.

149. American Joint Committee on Cancer. Green FL, Balch CM, Page DL, et al. eds. *Cancer staging manual*, 6th ed. Philadelphia: Lippincott Raven, 2002: 209–217.

19

Late Effects of Cancer Treatment

Debra L. Friedman, M.D., and Louis S. Constine, M.D.

The use of radiation and chemotherapy to manage childhood cancer must be determined, in part, by knowledge of the late effects of these modalities on normal tissues. As more children with cancer survive after therapy, the obligation grows for the oncologist to critically assess the adverse effects of therapy on the physical, intellectual, and emotional development of children.

The integration of radiation, chemotherapy, and surgery for childhood cancer has resulted in markedly improved survival. For the period of 1985–1997, the 5-year survival rate for childhood cancer reported by the National Cancer Institute Surveillance and End Results (SEER) section is 75% (1). Both radiotherapy (RT) and chemotherapy can result in adverse long-term health-related outcomes that manifest months to years after completion of cancer treatment and are commonly called *late effects*. Late effects include organ dysfunction, second malignant neoplasms, and adverse psychosocial sequelae. The impact of death due to treatment complications on overall survival and the increase in its relative importance with the increasing survival of children with cancer is demonstrated by data from St. Jude Children's Research Hospital (Fig. 19-1) (2) and from the Childhood Cancer Survivor Study (3).

Clearly, the potential to ameliorate or prevent such normal tissue damage, or to manage and rehabilitate affected patients, requires an understanding of tissue tolerance to therapy. Because late effects can manifest months or years after cessation of treatment, therapeutic decisions intended to prevent such effects can be based only on the probability, not the certainty, that such effects will develop. Risk factors for late effects may be tumor, treatment, or host related. RT factors include the total and fractional dosage of ir-

radiation, dosage rate, overall treatment time, machine energy, treatment volume (4), and dosage distribution. Chemotherapy factors include the specific agent used, the dosage, route, and rate of administration. Both modalities are affected by interactions with each other and with chemical protectors, sensitizers, and biologic therapy. Host factors include the child's developmental status, genetic predisposition (e.g., ataxia-telangiectasia), inherent tissue sensitivities and capacity for normal tissue repair, underlying disease (e.g., collagen vascular disease) or other abnormalities (structural and functional), and compensating mechanisms (e.g., the presence of a nonirradiated second kidney). Tumor factors include direct tissue effects (such as extent of organ invasion), systemic effects of tumor-induced organ dysfunction or chemical secretion, and indirect mechanical effects (e.g., renal obstruction).

Determining the prevalence, cumulative incidence, spectrum, and pathogenesis of late effects is difficult for several reasons: The patient must be a long-term survivor to manifest late effects; the numbers of affected and unaffected patients must be known in order to assign a probability risk; dramatic late effects are recognized by most physicians, whereas more subtle or subclinical damage receives little attention; the use of combined-modality therapy and the latent period resulting in the development of late effects make it difficult to unequivocally define the contribution of any single therapy; and the influence of modifying factors, such as other health behaviors, illnesses, or genetic contributions, is difficult to identify.

In rapidly proliferating tissues, cell kill is expressed clinically as an acute injury. Tissues in which cells are postmitotic and fully differenti-

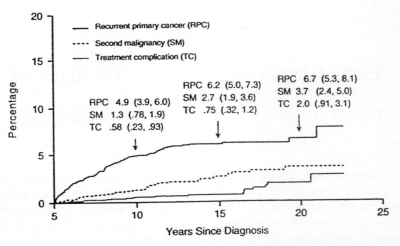

FIG. 19-1. Cumulative incidence functions for mortality from recurrence, second malignancy, and nonneoplastic treatment complication for patients treated between 1971 and 1983. (From Hudson M, Jones D, Boyett J, et al. Late mortality of long-term survivors of childhood cancer. *J Clin Oncol* 1997;15:2205–2213, with permission.)

ated were previously thought to be resistant to chemotherapy. It is now known that drug action is so diverse that such assessments are inaccurate. For example, doxorubicin affects mature cardiac myocytes by cell membrane or DNA binding, producing cell damage even when cell replication is not occurring (5). It is clear that cell injury may occur, depending on the chemotherapeutic agent, at different levels of cell cycle activity or cell differentiation. The effect of chemotherapeutic insult may not necessarily be expressed as frank cell injury. It may be expressed as a depletion of stem cell reserve or as loss of the normal mitotic potential of reserve stem cells.

Radiation damage is produced by some combination of parenchymal cell loss and injury to the underlying vasculature (6,7). Initial tissue recovery results mainly from parenchymal cell repopulation. The progressive component of damage is the arteriocapillary fibrosis, which predominates in the late irreparable injury and accentuates the cellular depletion of the parenchyma. It is the vascular changes that follow irradiation, but not chemotherapy, that partially account for the differences in late effects of the two modes of treatment. The distribution of late radiation damage reflects primarily vascular injury and cannot be explained simply as an indirect effect of parenchymal cell loss. Devastating late effects of

RT or of RT and chemotherapy can occur in both rapidly and slowly proliferating normal tissues without a clinically recognizable acute phase because of this vascular injury.

Advances in molecular biophysiology have provided insights into the responses of normal tissues to chemotherapeutic and radiation injury. The classic concept of a single target cell that can explain the dynamic sequence of events leading to organ damage is supplanted by that of multiple cell systems interacting. Moreover, the acute and late phases of adverse effects are actually manifestations of an ongoing sequence of events caused by autocrine, paracrine, and endocrine messages that occur immediately after injury to a variety of cells: epithelial, endothelial, fibroblastic, and inflammatory. A variety of growth and inhibitory factors are released, specific cell receptors are altered, and the resulting signals received by these receptors are translated into postreceptor cytoplasmic, nuclear, and interstitial events. Thus a combination of cell death, the production of reactive oxygen species, alterations in gene expression, and the expression of both proinflammatory and profibrotic cytokines are viewed as integral in the pathogenesis of late effects. The importance of this view is that interventions are possible that can upregulate or downregulate cytokine responses, leading to a modulation of the toxic reaction (8).

EFFECTS OF CHEMOTHERAPY AND RADIOTHERAPY ON NORMAL TISSUE

Late effects have been reported in patients who received dosages of chemotherapy and RT below the generally accepted threshold levels for either of the two when used alone. Therefore, one must be circumspect in accepting "tolerance dosages" for normal tissues and organs in the combined–treatment modality era. Untoward reactions can occur at unexpected times and in unpredictable ways. Chemotherapy acts predominantly on the cellular parenchymal component, whereas radiation acts on the microcirculatory

system and the parenchymal cells. In rapid renewal systems, the same stem cell population is affected, and one can usually reduce the increase in acute toxicity of both modes by applying them sequentially. In slow renewal tissues, the additive ill effects of drugs and radiation often are related to entirely different target cell populations in the same organ system. Late effects may not be avoidable because chemotherapy, whenever applied, can result in additional stem cell kill and lead to expression of subclinical radiation effects. Therefore, the tolerance dosages of fractionated RT, listed in Table 19-1 (8), might be lower in the setting of chemotherapy and in younger children. Table 19-2 lists some of the common adverse effects of chemotherapy, which may act synergistically with RT.

TABLE 19-1. *Tolerance dosages, $TD_5–TD_{50}$ (fractionated dosage, whole or partial organ)*

Target cell	Complication endpoint	Dosage range (Gy), $TD_5–TD_{50}$
Range: 2–10 Gy		
Lymphoid and lymphocytes	Lymphopenia	2–10
Testes spermatogonia	Sterility	1–2
Ovarian oocytes	Sterility	6–10
Diseased bone marrow (CLL or multiple myeloma)	Severe leukopenia and thrombocytopenia	3–5
Range: 10–20 Gy		
Lens	Cataract	6–12
Bone marrow stem cell	Acute aplasia	15–20
Range: 20–30 Gy		
Kidney: renal glomeruli	Arterionephrosclerosis	23–28
Lung: type II vasculoconnective tissue systems	Pneumonitis or fibrosis	20–30
Range: 30–40 Gy		
Liver central veins	Hepatopathy	35–40
Bone marrow	Hypoplasia	25–35
Range: 40–50 Gy		
Heart, whole organ	Pericarditis and pancarditis	40–45
Bone marrow microenvironments, sinusitis	Permanent aplasia	45–50
Range: 50–75 Gy		
Gastrointestinal	Infarction necrosis	50–55
Heart, partial organ	Cardiomyopathy	50–55
Spinal cord	Myelopathy	50–60
Brain	Encephalopathy	54–70
Mucosa (upper aerodigestive tract)	Ulcer	65–75
Rectum	Ulcer	65–75
Bladder	Ulcer	65–75
Mature bones	Fracture	65–70
Pancreas	Pancreatitis	

CLL, Chronic lymphoblastic leukemia.

Modified from Rubin P, Constine L, Williams J. Late effects of cancer treatment: radiation and drug toxicity. In: Perez C, Brady L, eds. *Principles and practice of radiation oncology.* Philadelphia: Lippincott-Raven, 1998: 155–211, with permission.

TABLE 19-2. *Common chemotherapy late effects*

System	Agents	Potential effects	Monitoring guidelines
Central nervous system	Intrathecal chemotherapy High-dose methotrexate Cytarabine	Cognitive dysfunction Leukoencephalopathy (risk increases with increased dosage) Cerebellar dysfunction	Neurocognitive evaluation Neurologic evaluation
Cardiac	Doxorubicin Daunomycin Idarubicin Epirubicin	Cardiomyopathy Arrhythmias	Electrocardiogram, echo-cardiogram, Holter, or cardiac stress dependent on dosage, age at time of treatment, symptoms, or radiation exposure
Hearing	Cisplatin Carboplatin	Hearing loss	Audiology evaluation
Vision	Corticosteroids	Cataracts	Ophthalmologic evaluation
Dentition	Vincristine	Dental enamel, bone, and root abnormalities	Dental evaluation
Pulmonary	Bleomycin Lomustine Carmustine Busulfan	Pulmonary fibrosis Abnormal pulmonary diffusion Restrictive or obstructive disease	Pulmonary function tests
Urologic	Cyclophosphamide Ifosfamide	Chronic hemorrhagic cystitis Second bladder cancers	Urinalysis
Hepatic	Methotrexate Thioguanine Mercaptopurine Dactinomycin Busulfan	Hepatic dysfunction Veno-occlusive disease (Dactinomycin D, busulfan, thioguanine)	Liver function tests Doppler ultrasound
Renal	Cisplatin > carboplatin High-dose methotrexate Ifosfamide	Renal insufficiency or failure Renal electrolyte wasting or insufficiency	Urinalysis Renal function tests Creatinine clearance
Gonadal	Mechlorethamine Cyclophosphamide Procarbazine Dacarbazine Ifosfamide Busulfan Melphalan Lomustine Carmustine	Ovarian failure, early menopause Testicular failure, Leydig cell dysfunction	Leuteinizing hormone, follicle-stimulating hormone Estradiol or testosterone Reproductive counseling or endocrinology evaluation Gynecologic evaluation Sperm analysis Tanner staging Menstrual history
Second malig-nancies	Mechlorethamine > other alkylating agents Etoposide Doxorubicin Cisplatin Cyclophosphamide	Leukemia Transitional bladder carcinoma	Complete blood count Urinalysis

INFLUENCE OF THE DEVELOPMENTAL STAGE OF THE TARGET ORGAN ON ITS SENSITIVITY TO THERAPY

The potential for the development of debilitating effects in normal tissues is related to the cellular activity and maturation in the tissue under consideration. In children, a mosaic of different tissues are developing at different rates and in different temporal sequences. The vulnerability of tissues to adverse effects is increased during the periods of rapid proliferation, whereas in adults the same tissues are in a mature steady state with slow cell renewal kinetics (9,10). Immature pediatric tissue contains cells that are initially totipotent, then multipotent, and eventually unipotent. At this final stage they are either resting or actively proliferating, with or without differentiation, into specialized tissues or organs. Inherent in this development sequence are critical time points of exquisite vulnerability to therapy. Adding to the complexity is the fact that some slow renewal systems can become active if challenged or stimulated. Therefore, recognition of the various stages of cellular development in pediatric tissues is vital to determining the potential for late effects. Traditionally, radiation dosages in children are modified by age, but without specific recognition of the periods of active proliferation, differentiation, and eventual maturation of one organ or tissue as it differs from another. When does a pediatric tissue or organ become similar to an adult tissue or organ? This is a major question that must be addressed in order to predict the sensitivity to late effects (9,10).

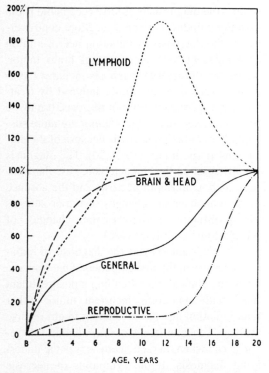

FIG. 19-2. Growth curves of different tissues. (From Tanner JM. *Growth at adolescence.* Oxford: Blackwell Scientific, 1962; and Harris JM, Jackson CM, Patterson DG. *The measurement of man.* Minneapolis: University of Minnesota Press, 1930, with permission.)

The growth of any given tissue follows one of four general developmental patterns (Fig. 19-2) (11,12). The first is commonly recognized skeletal pattern with peak growth rates in the early postnatal period and during puberty. The organs of circulation and digestion also follow this pattern. The second is the neural type, characterized by a rapid postnatal growth that slows in late infancy and ceases in adolescence. The respiratory and renal organs tend to follow this pattern. The third is the genital pattern, which shows little change during early life but shows rapid development just before and coincident with puberty. The sequence is followed by breast tissue, testes, and ovaries. The fourth pattern is the lymphoid type, characterized by a gradual evolution and involution to the time of puberty. Identifying these different rates and ages at which each tissue matures is necessary for determining its radiosensitivity. In addition, recognizing the mechanism of organ growth— that is, an increase in the size of cells (hypertrophy) as opposed to the number of cells (proliferation)—allows better identification of relative radiosensitivity because organs that only hypertrophy are less vulnerable to functional disturbance by irradiation.

LATE EFFECTS BY ORGAN SYSTEM

Central Nervous System

Pathophysiology

The brain develops rapidly in the first 3 years of life and very little after age 6. This growth is caused by an increase in the size but not the number of neurons. Axonal growth, dendritic arborization, and synaptogenesis are most active at this time (13). If maturation is judged by the degree of myelinization, then most regions are well developed by the second year but are not complete until puberty (14). Radiation injury would be expected to be profound during the early years. The essential radiation insult in radiation injury to the central nervous system (CNS) is a demyelinating lesion with focal or diffuse areas of white matter necrosis (15–17). In the first weeks after irradiation, early demyelinating changes are generally limited to scattered astrocytic or microglial reactions with occasional perivascular collections of mononuclear cells. Subsequently, neural tissue begins to break down with the appearance of regions of myelin destruction, proliferative and degenerative changes in glial cells, and vascular changes including endothelial cell loss, proliferation, capillary occlusion, degeneration, and hemorrhagic exudates. When a critical mass of capillary endothelial cells fails, then vasogenic edema develops in response to the loss of essential support of dependent neurons, reflecting cerebral cortical atrophy. Intracerebral calcifications sometimes are present and presumably represent lesions of mineralizing microangiopathy.

The basic mechanisms underlying the pathologic changes are not precisely known for any particular syndrome of irradiation damage. The three most commonly proposed mechanisms may act alone or in combination. The vascular mechanism acknowledges that the endothelial cell is essential for patency of the microcirculation. This cell is radiosensitive, and damage is expressed as cell death or endothelial hyperplasia. Because endothelial cell turnover is slow, injury based on these cells occurs over a prolonged time interval. The evolution of hyalin degeneration and obliterating sclerosis of the arterioles produces areas of complete and incomplete necrosis (18). The clonogenic death of glial cells mechanism postulates a radiation-induced reproductive death of the slowly reproducing oligodendrocyte. The oligodendrocyte maintains myelin. These cells show a decrease in numbers within weeks after irradiation. Damage in individual nerve fibers can be demonstrated quantitatively by electron microscopy as early as 2 weeks after irradiation and before vascular damage (19). Effects on myelin synthesis and maintenance may be especially important in childhood because myelogenesis is most active in the first year of life. The ultimate result is demyelination. Radiation-induced endothelial cell death followed by vascular occlusion also promotes necrosis (20). The allergic mechanism of pathologic change in the brain after irradiation argues that the lesions of delayed radiation necrosis sometimes consist of disseminated plaques of demyelination with central necrosis and occasional petechial hemorrhage. In the patent blood vessels that remain, there may be perivascular cuffing with lymphocytes and plasma cells. The postulated autoimmune mechanism is that an antigen is produced by the reaction of ionizing irradiation with the oligodendromyelin complex. This antigen would stimulate the accumulation of inflammatory cells (18). One cannot prove that a single hypothesis explains delayed radiation necrosis, and it is possible that the pathophysiology is explicable by some combination of the three mechanisms.

The classic findings of radiation-induced necrosis of the CNS are large areas of confluent, coagulative necrosis of the white matter and deep layers of the cortex; the vascular changes of fibrinoid necrosis or fibrin incontinence; atypia or absence of endothelial cells; vascular thickening; telangiectasis; and vascular proliferation (15,18,20). When radiation necrosis occurs at a distance from the neoplasm—as might occur, for example, after large dosages of radiation to extracranial lesions such as one on the scalp—the diagnosis is readily acceptable if the histologic findings are present. More controversial is the diagnosis of radiation necrosis in an area adjacent to a parenchymal brain tumor, where the differential diagnosis includes therapeutic necrosis of the tumor induced by treatment and spontaneous tumor necrosis. It may be true that areas adjacent to a tumor are more susceptible to radiation necrosis because of the preexisting tissue injury (15,18,20). The diagnosis usually rests on the characteristic vascular findings such as fibrinoid necrosis and the absence of the characteristic changes of tumor such as the proliferative microvascular changes of glioblastoma multiforme (20).

It is important to make the diagnosis of radiation necrosis in the treated patient. One wants to avoid the clinical trap of calling a posttreatment mass with symptoms recurrent tumor rather than radiation necrosis. A patient might receive "salvage" chemotherapy or reirradiation for "recurrence" when, in fact, necrosis was the underlying diagnosis. If the symptoms of necrosis spontaneously improved, as they sometimes do, then a patient might be erroneously scored as a chemotherapy responder.

Pediatric radiation oncologists have a variety of imaging tools at their disposal to aid in the diagnosis of radiation necrosis. Computed tomography (CT) of the brain shows regions of low density without mass effect or contrast enhancement, a localized low-density contrast-enhancing mass, or diffuse lesions of varying density without mass effect but with occasional enhancement. Such lesions develop months to years after therapy. Magnetic resonance imaging (MRI) shows prolonged T1 and T2 relaxation times (21). Positron emission tomography (PET) is particularly promising. Hypermetabolic areas, using glucose, are more likely to represent proliferating tumor. Hypometabolic areas, which do not use glucose, are more likely to represent radiation necrosis. However, no imaging modality is infallible, and the clinician can only rely on biopsy to make the diagnosis, with the caution that even biopsy can be misleading because of the possibility of sampling error (20,22).

Clinical Manifestations

Necrosis

The incidence of radiation necrosis after therapeutic dosages is uncertain. Quoted incidence data range from 0.1% to 5% after dosages of 50–60 Gy fractionated over 5–6 weeks (16–18, 23). The variability in the data is the result of the uncertainty, in some studies, concerning the denominator; the long time delay until the occurrence of necrosis; the lack of histologic confirmation in many surviving patients; and the absence of postmortem data in patients who succumb. The clinical signs and symptoms of radiation necrosis are headache and mass effect. Surgical debulking is performed when possible and is often therapeutic (23–25). Corticosteroids may offer transient relief (26). Anecdotal reports exist of the benefits of anticoagulation with heparin or warfarin compounds (18,22,25, 27,28).

Necrotizing Leukoencephalopathy and Mineralizing Microangiopathy

Leukoencephalopathy is a late complication of cranial irradiation and chemotherapy, particularly intravenous (IV) and intrathecal (IT) meth-

otrexate (MTX). The histologic appearance is of multifocal white matter destruction, especially in the centrum semiovale and periventricular regions, with loss of myelin and oligodendrocytes. Hypodense areas emerge in the white matter, and there is cerebral atrophy, an increase in the sulcal width, and enlargement of the ventricles. Mineralizing microangiopathy can occur and is visualized on CT scanning as intracerebral calcification (21,22,25,27). The clinical features include lethargy, seizures, spasticity, paresis, and ataxia. The multifactorial origin and risk of leukoencephalopathy have been studied in acute lymphoblastic leukemia (ALL) survivors. As shown in Fig. 19-3, radiation and MTX appear to be contributing factors (29). Of interest is a report from the German Late Effects Working Group, which documented CT and MRI evidence of atrophy, leukoencephalopathy, calcification, or gray matter changes in approximately 50% of children treated for ALL (30). The frequency and severity of abnormalities were greater in children treated with cranial RT and MTX than in those treated with MTX alone. It is worth emphasizing that the situation is decidedly worse in children who have CNS involvement with ALL. In these cases, the pres-

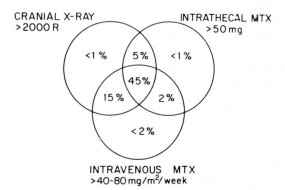

FIG. 19-3. Approximate risks of leukoencephalopathy. (From Griffin TW. White matter necrosis, microangiopathy and intellectual abilities in survivors of childhood leukemia. Association with central nervous system irradiation and methotrexate therapy. In: Gilbert HA, Kagan AR, eds. *Radiation damage to the nervous system.* New York: Raven Press, 1980:155–174, with permission.)

ence of leukemia can alter the cerebrospinal clearance of MTX and increase the risk of injury.

Neuropsychologic and Intellectual Deficits

Cranial irradiation of children may have significant adverse effects on intelligence, learning, and social and emotional adjustment (25,27,28, 31,32). Neurocognitive late effects most commonly follow treatment of malignancies that necessitate CNS-directed therapies, such as cranial radiation or intraventricular or IT chemotherapy. Thus, children with CNS tumors, head and neck sarcomas, and ALL are most commonly affected. Studies of patients with brain tumors must account for the confounding variables of CNS injury by the tumor, seizures and their therapy, elevated intracranial pressure, and surgery. In patients with leukemia and brain tumors, the use of chemotherapy and the impact of the illness on body image and school attendance may complicate the issue.

Deficits occur in a variety of areas, which include general intelligence, age-appropriate developmental progress, academic achievement (especially in reading language and mathematics), visual and perceptual motor skills, nonverbal and verbal memory, receptive and expressive language, and attention (13,27,28,33–35). Younger age at time of treatment is associated with a greater neurocognitive deficit (36–40).

The effects of cranial radiotherapy on subsequent intellectual function have been studied in detail, most comprehensively in survivors of CNS tumors and leukemia. However, the effects of radiation on the brain are difficult to define, especially when cranial radiation is often routinely a part of multimodality therapy that may also include surgery and systemic or IT chemotherapy. Moreover, tumor-related deficits caused by direct invasion of the brain, seizures, and hydrocephalus must be recognized. The review of the literature that follows is selective, concentrating on the findings that are clinically important and are supported by most of the data. We measure intelligence using various tools. The intelligence scale or intelligence quotient (IQ) generally is reported as three values. The verbal

IQ (VIQ) measures performance on vocabulary, general fund of information, and reasoning. The performance IQ (PIQ) assesses visuospatial tasks such as puzzle assembly, block construction, visual memory, and nonverbal reasoning. The full-scale IQ (FSIQ) combines verbal and performance scores (41). We may also evaluate children with achievement tests of skills such as spelling or arithmetic and with questionnaires designed to ascertain social and emotional functioning (31,32). School performance and the need for special schooling are another indicator of intellectual performance. All of these tools have been used to assess the effects of radiation, chemotherapy, and surgery on children.

Older studies that reported a high functional level in most (70–80%) children after cranial RT for brain tumors used simple clinician-scored performance scales (32,42). More detailed assessment of IQ, achievement tests, learning ability, and school performance suggests a far less favorable outcome. The results of a variety of studies are summarized in Table 19-3. It is worth emphasizing several important points concerning these studies: Ill effects are more severe the younger the age at the time of treatment; undesirable effects may be more likely with higher dosages of RT and whole brain, as opposed to limited-field, treatment; particularly in the very young (under age 5); IQ loss may worsen as the time interval from treatment increases; the practical implications of lowered IQs include an increased demand for special schooling and educational resources; the presence of hydrocephalus at diagnosis does not correlate with intellectual outcome; and tumor location may help predict outcome, such that patients with hemispheric and hypothalamic tumors have worse sequelae than patients with infratentorial tumors (13,22, 23,27,28,31,32,43,44).

With changes in the dosage, fields, and volumes of cranial and craniospinal RT, changes in the incidence and spectrum of these adverse effects of therapy are expected. More recent studies using lower dosages and more targeted volumes have demonstrated better results (45–47). Ris et al. (45) evaluated the intellectual outcome of 43 children treated on Children's Cancer Group study 9892 for posterior fossa medul-

TABLE 19-3. *Neurocognitive effects of cranial radiotherapy for brain tumors*

Reference	Year	Number of patients	Outcome
Hirsh et al. (505)	1979	28	12% had IQs >90, 31% had IQs <70, 93% had behavior disturbances.
Raimondi and Tomita (506)	1979	18	46% had IQs <70.
Spunberg et al. (507)	1981	14	42% were retarded.
Danoff et al. (508)	1982	38	17% had IQs <70, 56% had IQs >90, 37% had emotional difficulties.
Duffner et al. (509)	1983	10	50% had IQs <80, 20% had IQs >90, 4 of 5 with IQs >80 were learning disabled.
Kun et al. (32)	1983	30	The number with IQs <90 was greater than the distribution normally expected; 53% with supratentorial tumors or posterior fossa tumors necessitating whole brain RT had test results significantly below normal.
Ellenberg et al. (510)	1987	73	Ages at the time of treatment and whole brain RT were associated with increased cognitive deficits.
Packer et al. (511)	1988	28	Mean IQ was 96 (range 50–120).
Packer et al. (512)	1989	18[a]	Children ≤7 years of age at diagnosis had a mean decline in IQ of 25 points at 2 years.
Packer et al. (513)	1992	17	No significant IQ drop in older children.
Ris et al. (45)	2001	43	Decline in full-scale IQ of 17.4 points.

[a]Full-scale IQ and academic performance were worse in the irradiated group than in 14 children with brain tumors in similar sites who were not irradiated.

loblastoma or primitive neuroectodermal tumor (PNET). The study used a reduced craniospinal RT regimen of 23.4 Gy to the neuraxis and 32.4-Gy boost to the posterior fossa with adjuvant chemotherapy. The mean age at time of treatment was 6 years, with a range of 3–15 years. The estimated rate of change of FSIQ was −4.3 points/year, for VIQ −4.2 points/year, and for nonverbal IQ (NVIQ) −4.0 points/year. In examining host-related factors, a more significant decline was seen for girls (–8 points/year) than boys (–3 points/year) for VIQ and for children less than 7 years old (–5.2 points/year) as opposed to children 7 years and older (–0.8) for NVIQ. This latter observation was noteworthy in that the older children's baseline was lower, with little decline over time, as compared with the younger children, who had a much higher baseline followed by a steep decline. The effect of baseline intelligence was examined for the whole group, and the same phenomenon was seen. Children who had a baseline IQ of 100 or higher had a much steeper decline in FSIQ, VIQ, and NVIQ than children who had a baseline under 100. The effect on FSIQ is shown in Fig. 19-4.

Another recent study supports the hypothesis that patients with medulloblastoma demonstrate a decline in IQ values because of an inability to acquire new skills and information at a rate comparable to that of their healthy same-age peers rather than a loss of previously acquired information and skills (48). In a recent Danish study of 133 children treated for brain tumors, younger age at diagnosis, tumor site in the cerebral hemisphere, hydrocephalus treatment with shunt, and radiation therapy predicted lower cognitive functions (49). Finally, a reduction in the volume of normal-appearing white matter has been observed in some survivors of childhood brain tumors, and this was associated with decreased attentional abilities, which led to an IQ deficit and impaired academic achievement (50).

For ALL, older studies again show significant neurocognitive impairment (51). Even when combined with IT chemotherapy, reduction in the cranial radiation dosage has resulted in less neurocognitive impairment (40,52–55).

Studies on CNS prophylaxis for ALL comparing craniospinal RT with cranial RT combined with IT MTX showed that children who were less than 5 years old at time of treatment

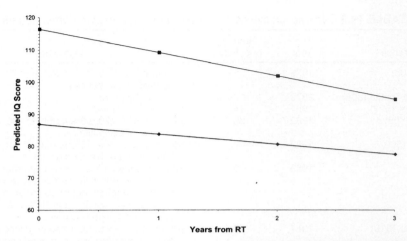

FIG. 19-4. Full-scale IQ change by baseline intelligence. *Diamond,* baseline IQ < 100; *square,* baseline IQ > 100. (From Ris MD, Packer R, Goldwein J, et al. Intellectual outcome after reduced-dose radiation therapy plus adjuvant chemotherapy for medulloblastoma: a Children's Cancer Group study. *J Clin Oncol* 2001;19:3470–3476, with permission.)

and had received RT and IT chemotherapy had lower IQ scores than those who received craniospinal RT alone (56). Similarly, Meadows et al. (51) found a significant IQ deficit in children treated with 24 Gy cranial RT combined with IT MTX, as compared with childhood cancer survivors who received no CNS-directed therapy, with the effect greatest among those less than 5 years old. A similar effect on cognition with the addition of IT MTX has been found in children treated for medulloblastoma (57).

Systemic MTX, in high dosages and when combined with RT, can lead to a well-described leukoencephalopathy, described earlier, in which severe neurocognitive deficits are obvious (22,28, 58). Leukemic involvement of the CNS, intracranial bleeding, or solid tumor obstruction of cerebrospinal fluid (CSF) outflow may affect the clearance of IT MTX. Transependymal flow of the drug into the surrounding brain parenchyma may produce a greater chance of leukoencephalopathy. MTX also appears to be more injurious when administered after irradiation rather than before (23,27,28). Because of its penetrance into the CNS, systemic MTX has been used in a variety of low- and high-dose regimens for leukemia CNS prophylaxis. The deleterious effects of systemic MTX, especially at dosages greater than

1 g/m^2, may be no different from those of 18 Gy cranial RT (59,60). At lower MTX dosages, there does not appear to be a consistent pattern of neurocognitive deficits (61). A recent long-term study of infants who received high-dose systemic MTX combined with IT cytarabine and MTX for CNS leukemia prophylaxis and were tested 3–9 years after treatment showed that cognitive function was in the average range (62).

In a recent small study from Italy, cognitive outcome was evaluated in 21 children who received both cranial RT and IT MTX. Mean total IQ was within normal limits, but there was a large discrepancy between the VIQ and PIQ, with the former being significantly higher than the latter. In addition, intracerebral calcifications on MRI were associated with the number of intrathecal MTX dosages and with low scores on IQ, attention, and visual integration tests. Age at treatment and RT dosage were not associated with neuropsychiatric outcomes (63).

Chemotherapy without RT for ALL may result in cognitive dysfunction. Brown et al. (59) examined 48 children treated for leukemia without cranial RT and found impairment in tasks of higher-order cognitive functioning and learning disabilities in the area of mathematics. Waber et al. (54) showed that children, particularly girls, treated with systemic and IT MTX for CNS leukemia prophylaxis showed impairment of verbal memory and coding. Hill et al. (64) reported mild visual and verbal short-term memory deficits in leukemia survivors treated with intrathecal chemotherapy. More recently, the substitution of dexamethasone for prednisone in the treatment of ALL has been implicated in increasing cognitive dysfunction (55,62). Treatment intensity and duration can also adversely affect cognitive performance by causing absences from school and interruption of studies (65). It is appropriate to point out that the combination of IT MTX and high-dose IV MTX, without irradiation, may produce memory impairment (66).

Children who suffer a CNS relapse of ALL and receive IT chemotherapy and cerebrospinal irradiation (CSI) are at risk for leukemia-, radiation-, and drug-associated cognitive impairment. Kumar et al. (67) prospectively studied 11 long-term survivors of a CNS relapse of ALL treated with CSI (24 Gy cranium, 15 Gy spine) and systemic and IT chemotherapy. FSIQ did not fall significantly in children 4 years of age or older. The combination of young age at diagnosis and low initial IQ predicted a low IQ after treatment.

Controversy regarding the role of RT in impairing neurocognition will continue, largely because of differences in the radiation dosages and drugs used in various protocols and different endpoints. For example, in contrast to the aforementioned data is a multi-institutional report on 110 survivors of childhood ALL in which patients were treated with chest radiotherapy (CRT; 24 Gy) and IT MTX, or intermediate-dose MTX and IT-MTX (Cancer and Leukemic Groups B [CALGB] protocol); the former group had significantly poorer academic achievement, poorer self-images, and greater psychological stress (43). In summary, prophylactic cranial irradiation of 24 Gy at 2 Gy per fraction in the treatment of ALL can lower IQ and achievement test scores. IQ loss may be on the order of 8–10 points (i.e., median of normals of 100 down to 90–92). A drop of this magnitude results in children being at the lower end of the normal range (41). Learning disabilities most commonly manifested are memory (especially short-term) deficits, difficulty in acquiring new knowledge, and decreased speed of mental processing and attention span (37). Some studies suggest that the undesirable consequences of 18 Gy are less than 24 Gy, but the data on this point are not definitive (41,51,66,68).

Somnolence Syndrome

Irradiation of the brain of children can result in the somnolence syndrome. This syndrome was first described by Druckmann (69) in 1929 in children who were irradiated for ringworm of the scalp. The syndrome has its onset 4–8 weeks after irradiation and is characterized by drowsiness, nausea, irritability, anorexia, apathy, and dizziness. The majority of children reported to have developed this syndrome were irradiated for ALL, although it can occur after treatment of a brain tumor. The incidence may be as high as 60% of cases (18,25,70). Rarely, a previously resolved neurologic deficit may reappear for a short time. This should not be confused with recurrent malignancy. The somnolence syndrome resolves spontaneously, but corticosteroids hasten recovery.

Arterial vasculopathy is an uncommon occurrence, almost always described after irradiation to the parasellar region, primarily in children. Single- or multiple-vessel narrowing or obliteration results in typical stroke deficits (71).

Myelopathy

The spectrum of radiation injuries to the spinal cord includes transient and irreversible syndromes (18). A rare, rapidly evolving permanent paralysis is presumed to result from an acute infarction of the cord. A more common form of radiation injury to the cord was first described by French neurologist Lhermitte as a sign of multiple sclerosis. The so-called Lhermitte's sign or Lhermitte's symptom consists of an electric shock–like sensation that radiates down the spine and often into the limbs (72). The location of the sensation can change with time. The symptoms may be precipitated by flexion of the neck, walking on a hard surface, sitting on a hard surface, or other forms of physical exertion. The syndrome generally occurs a few months after spinal irradiation. The incidence after full-dose mantle irradiation for Hodgkin's disease (HD) may be 10–15% (73). The mechanism is thought to be transient demyelinization, although detailed human pathologic studies are lacking. There are no known CT or MRI correlations. It is also reported in association with cisplatin administration, where the results may be long-lasting (74).

Chronic progressive radiation myelitis (CPRM) is rare. Intramedullary vascular damage that progresses to hemorrhagic necrosis or infarction is the likely mechanism, although extensive demyelination, which progresses to white matter necrosis, is an alternative explanation. The initial symptoms, generally subtle, are usually paresthesias and sensory changes (including diminished temperature sensation or proprioception), which start 9–15 months after therapy and progress over the subsequent year (75). Much longer intervals to initial symptoms are seen occasionally. Because a definitive diagnosis of myelitis includes pathology, which cannot be obtained except at autopsy, the diagnosis rests on supportive information. The neurologic lesion must be within the irradiated volume. Recurrent or metastatic tumor must be ruled out. CSF protein may be elevated, and myelography can demonstrate cord swelling or atrophy. MRI and CT provide additional supportive information.

The incidence of CPRM and the radiation dosage causing this event are poorly defined because of the diagnostic difficulties and the variety of radiation techniques (with uncertain dosimetries). A review by Wara et al. (76) suggests that 42 Gy in 25 fractions carries a 1% risk, 45 Gy a 5% risk, and 61 Gy a 50% risk. Cohen and Creditor's (4) data indicate a 5% risk at 49 Gy. Data from Marcus and William (77) suggest that the cervical cord may be more tolerant to radiation than previously presumed when 1.8- to 1.9-Gy fractional doses are used; in 324 patients treated to dosages of 55 Gy or less,

no cases of myelitis were seen. A review by Schultheiss et al. (75) supports this and suggests that the 5% incidence of myelopathy, at least in adults, probably occurs at total dosages of 57–61 Gy. However, tolerance in children might be lower.

A higher risk of myelopathy is associated with higher individual fraction sizes, shorter overall treatment time, higher total dosages, and long lengths of the cord treated (especially more than 10 cm) (78). Children may be more susceptible to CPRM, developing it after lower radiation dosages and with shorter latency periods (75). Actinomycin D may decrease the dosage threshold (79).

Table 19-4 reviews several CNS late effects with respect to causative treatments, signs and symptoms, screening and diagnostic tests, and management and intervention (80).

Psychosocial

Psychological Effects

Psychological effects of childhood cancer and its treatment were first described by Koocher and O'Malley (81), who used the term *Damocles syndrome* to refer to the uncertainty of future health faced by families of childhood cancer survivors. In a group of 117 survivors, they found a higher risk of maladjustment, poor self-esteem, lower self-satisfaction, anxiety, and depression than in controls who had chronic nonmalignant conditions. Shorter and less intensive treatment courses with fewer and less severe side effects were associated with a better outcome. They also described a similar syndrome in parents of these patients, more severe in those with lower socioeconomic status and income.

Studies in the early 1990s described childhood cancer survivors as generally well-adjusted, although a subset had psychological difficulties that resulted in functional impairment (82–84). Further in-depth analyses have led to the description of posttraumatic stress disorder (PTSD) in some childhood cancer survivors and their mothers. The core features include experiencing an event perceived as life-threatening, with an accompanying reaction of intense fear, horror, or helplessness; persistent reexperiencing of the event; avoidance of things, events, or people surrounding the event or decreased responsiveness to same; and persistent symptoms of sleep disturbance, irritability, hypervigilance, and difficulty concentrating (85). PTSD has been reported in mothers of childhood cancer survivors and in adolescent and young adult survivors. There are common features in presentation and risk factors for the syndrome. There is intense anxiety and psychological distress. Because avoidance of places and people associated with the cancer is part of PTSD, the syndrome may interfere with appropriate access to health care. Those with PTSD perceived greater current threats to their or their children's lives and greater treatment intensity. Other risk factors include poor family functioning, decreased social support, and noncancer stressors (86–91). Among 78 young adult survivors of childhood cancer, Hobbie et al. (86) found 21% to meet criteria for PTSD. In contrast, only 5% of younger children met the criteria for the syndrome. In several studies performed by the same group of investigators, 9–10% of parents of childhood cancer survivors met criteria for PTSD (90,92).

A combined analysis of symptoms of somatic distress and depression has been completed from the Childhood Cancer Survivor Study (CCSS) cohort. This included 1,834 survivors of HD who were compared with sibling controls. Eighty-seven had scores on the Brief Symptom Index symptomatic for depression and 237 for somatic distress. Risk factors included female sex, low socioeconomic status, lack of a complete high school education, lack of employment, intensive chemotherapy, and elapsed time since therapy (93). In a subsequent analysis of the entire CCSS cohort, Mulrooney et al. (94) evaluated risk factors for fatigue or sleep impairment. In univariate analysis, compared with other diagnostic groups, a diagnosis of HD or sarcoma was associated with higher risks of fatigue, depression, and sleep impairment. In multivariate analysis of the fatigue risk factors, hypothyroidism and depres-

sion were independent risk factors, and radiation therapy had a marginal association (OR = 1.10, 95% CI 0.98–1.28).

This is a rapidly emerging area of research that is still limited by sample size and selection bias. It is unclear what the extent of the true problem is and how many childhood cancer survivors have lower quality of life or other adverse psychological outcomes. The role that therapy, specifically radiotherapy, plays in these adverse psychological outcomes is not clear. A recent review of behavioral, emotional, and social adjustment among survivors of childhood brain tumors illustrates this point, where rates of psychological adjustment range from 25% to 93% (95).

Neuroendocrine

Hypothalamic–pituitary (HP) irradiation may produce a spectrum of neuroendocrine abnormalities.

Growth Hormone

The effects of cranial irradiation on growth hormone (GH) production and release are most common and worthy of detailed consideration. GH is secreted episodically by the anterior pituitary gland. Growth hormone–releasing hormone (GHRH), produced in the hypothalamus, stimulates GH production, whereas the hypothalamic neuropeptide somatostatin excretes an inhibitory effect. In the liver and other tissues, circulating GH stimulates the production of insulin-like growth factor 1 (IGF-1, also called somatomedin-C), which promotes cell proliferation and protein synthesis. GH is secreted in bursts throughout the day and night. A simple and reliable test for GH reserve is not yet available. Current technology relies on a variety of provocative agents capable of stimulating GH release to assess GH reserve. These agents include insulin-induced hypoglycemia, IV arginine hydrochloride, oral levodopa, and oral clonidine (96,97). The anatomic site of the radiation injury that produces GH deficiency probably is the hypothalamus. Both Lannering and

TABLE 19-4. *Evaluation of patients at risk for late effects: central nervous system*

Late effects	Causative treatment			Signs and symptoms	Screening and diagnostic tests	Management and intervention
	Chemotherapy	Radiation	Surgery			
Neurocognitive deficit	High-dose IV MTX, IT MTX	>18 Gy	Resection of central nervous system tumor	Difficulty with reading, language, verbal and nonverbal memory, arithmetic, receptive and expressive language, decreased speed of mental processing, attention deficit, decreased IQ, behavior problems, poor school attendance, poor hand-eye coordination	Neurocognitive testing: Psychoeducational Neuropsychologic	Psychoeducation assistance
Leukoencephalopathy	IT or IV MTX IT cytosine arabinoside	>18 Gy (with MTX)		Seizures, neurologic impairment; compare with premorbid status	CT and MRI for baseline and symptoms	Symptom management: muscle relaxants, anticonvulsants, physical therapy, occupational therapy

Focal necrosis	IT or high-dose IV MTX Carmustine, cisplatin	>50 Gy (especially with >2 Gy daily fraction)	Tumor resection	Headaches; nausea; seizures; papilledema; hemiparesis or other focal findings; speech, learning, and memory deficits	CT and MRI for baseline, PRN Positron emission tomography or single-photon emission computed tomography	Steroid therapy Debulking of necrotic tissue
Large-vessel stroke		>60 Gy		Headache, seizures, hemiparesis, aphasia, focal neurologic findings	CT and MRI Arteriogram	Determined by specific neurologic impairment
Vision loss	Intra-arterial carmustine, cisplatin	>50 Gy (optic nerve chiasm, occipital lobe)	Tumor resection	Progressive visual loss	Ophthalmic evaluation Visual-evoked response	Visual aids
Ototoxicity	cisplatin, carboplatin	>35 Gy (middle and inner ear)	Surgery, CSF shunting	Abnormal speech development Hearing	Audiogram for baseline, PRN	Speech therapy Hearing aid
Myelitis		45–50 Gy	Spinal cord surgery	Paresis, spasticity, altered sensation, loss of sphincter control	MRI	Steroids Physical therapy Occupational therapy

CSF, cerebrospinal fluid; CT, computed tomography; IT, intrathecal; IV, intravenous; MRI, magnetic resonance imaging; MTX, methotrexate; PRN, as needed.

From Constine LS, Hobbie W, Schwartz C. Facilitated assessment of chronic treatment by symptom and organ systems. In: Schwartz C, Hobbie W, Constine L, et al., eds. *Survivors of childhood cancer: assessment and management.* St Louis: Mosby, 1994:21–80, with permission.

Albertsson-Wikland (98) and Blacklay et al. (99) have studied children who are GH deficient after irradiation to the HP axis. Most demonstrate a prompt rise in GH after administration of GHRH. This implies that GH deficiency in the irradiated patient may be the result of disturbances in the hypothalamic production of GHRH. This finding is supported by a study of GH-deficient patients with brain tumors who received irradiation to the posterior fossa. Although the pituitary gland was excluded from the treatment field, the ventromedian nucleus of the hypothalamus, which is thought to be the site of GHRH production, was included (23,25).

Clinical Manifestations

Having considered the anatomic site of radiation's damage to GH production, we may turn our attention to the frequency of the ill effect, the dose–response relationship, and the time interval between therapy and the onset of the deficiency.

The potential for neuroendocrine damage is likely to decrease with the use of more focused RT and a decrease in dosage in some settings such as medulloblastoma. Approximately 60–80% of irradiated pediatric brain tumor patients who have received dosages greater than 30 Gy have impaired serum GH response to provocative stimulation. This usually occurs within 5 years of treatment. The dose–response relationship has a threshold of 18–20 Gy, and the higher the radiation dosage, the earlier the GH deficiency will occur after treatment. A recent study of conformal radiotherapy in children with CNS tumors indicates that GH insufficiency usually can be demonstrated within 12 months of radiotherapy depending on hypothalamic dose–volume effects (100). Children treated with CNS irradiation for leukemia are also at greater risk of GH deficiency. Sklar et al. (101) evaluated 127 patients with ALL treated with 24 Gy, 18 Gy, or no cranial irradiation. The change in height standard deviation score (SDS) was significant for all three groups, with a dose–response relationship noted: -0.49 ± 0.14 for no RT group, -0.65 ± 0.15 for the 18 Gy RT group, and -1.38 ± 0.16 for the 24 Gy group. Schriock et al. (102) found similar results in 118 ALL survivors treated with 24 Gy cranial irradiation, where 74% had an SDS of at least -1 and the remainder at least -2.

Children who receive bone marrow transplantation (BMT) with total body irradiation (TBI) have a significant risk of GH deficiency. Risk is higher with single-dose as opposed to fractionated radiation, pretransplant cranial irradiation, female sex, and posttreatment complications such as graft-versus-host disease (103–106). Regimens with busulfan and cyclophosphamide also increase risk (106). Hyperfractionation of the TBI dosage markedly reduces risk in the absence of pretransplant cranial radiation (107). In a recent review of late effects after BMT, Socie et al. (108) discuss this risk at length. The mean loss of height is estimated to be approximately 1 SDS (6 cm) compared with the mean height at time of stem cell transplantation and mean genetic height. In a report from the European Group for Blood and Marrow Transplantation, among 181 patients with aplastic anemia, leukemias, and lymphomas who underwent stem cell transplantation before puberty, an overall decrease in final height SDS value was found compared with the height at transplant and with the genetic height. The type of transplantation, graft-versus-host disease, GH, or steroid treatment did not influence final height. TBI (single greater than fractionated dosage), male sex, and young age at transplant were found to be major factors for long-term height loss. The majority of patients (140 of 181) reached adult height within the normal range of the general population. Data from this study demonstrating the changes in SDS by type of radiotherapy are shown in Fig. 19-5 (109).

GH deficiency should be treated with replacement therapy. There has been some controversy surrounding this therapy, with a concern over increased risk of recurrence and second malignant neoplasms (SMNs). However, most studies are limited by selection bias and small sample size. Leung et al. (110) at St. Jude Children's Research Hospital evaluated final height of 47 patients

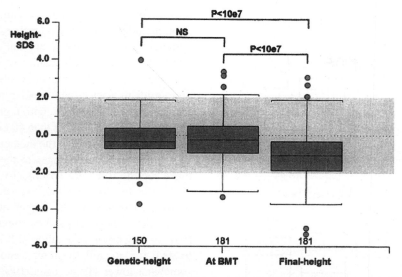

FIG. 19-5. Correlation between the genetic height, height standard deviation score (SDS) at bone marrow transplantation, and final height SDS. Numerals indicate the number of cases studied in each group. The dotted area indicates the height SDS distribution for the normal general population. The lower line in the box plot indicates the 25th percentile, the upper line indicates the 75th percentile, and the horizontal lines above and below the boxes represent the 3rd and the 97th percentile, respectively. Statistical analyses: paired Student's *t* test. (From Cohen A, Rovelli A, Bakker B, et al. Final height of patients who underwent bone marrow transplantation for hematological disorders during childhood: a study by the Working Party for Late Effects–EBMT. *Blood* 1999;93:4109–4115, with permission.)

treated for GH deficiency from a larger group of 910 patients treated for ALL. They also compared risk of leukemia relapse and SMN with those who had not been treated with GH. After a median duration of 4.5 years, the adult height SDSs approached height SDSs at the time of diagnosis. The median adult height for men was 173.2 cm (157–191.9 cm) and for women, 158.1 (141–168 cm). Height SDSs of survivors treated with GH from this study are shown in Fig. 19-6. There was no difference in leukemia recurrence or SMN in those treated with GH and the 544 control subjects who did not receive GH therapy. Among the GH-treated group, there were no recurrences and 2 SMNs, compared with 8 relapses and 16 SMNs among the control subjects (110). Sklar et al. (111) studied 361 GH-treated cancer survivors enrolled in the CCSS and compared risk of recurrence, risk of SMN, and risk of death between survivors who did and did not receive treatment with GH. The relative risk of disease recurrence was

0.83 (95% CI 0.37–1.86) for GH-treated survivors. GH-treated subjects were diagnosed with 15 SMNs, all solid tumors, for an overall relative risk of 3.21 (95% CI 1.88–5.46), mainly because of a small excess number of SMNs observed in survivors of acute leukemia. The data surrounding SMNs must be interpreted with caution given the small number of events.

Non–Growth Hormone Trophins

Pubertal growth can also be adversely affected by cranial radiation. Dosages greater than 50 Gy may result in gonadotrophin deficiency, and dosages of 18–47 Gy can result in precocious puberty. Precocious puberty has occurred mostly in girls who received dosages of at least 24 Gy cranial radiation. However, earlier puberty and earlier peak height velocity are seen in girls treated with 18 Gy cranial radiation (112,113). Shalet and et al. (114) showed that the age of pu-

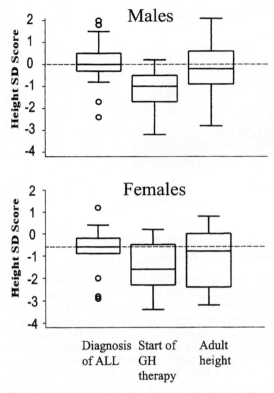

FIG. 19-6. Box plot of height standard deviation scores of survivors who received GH. The solid line in the middle of box represents 50th percentile, the box extends from 25th to 75th percentile, and whiskers extend to the upper and lower adjacent values that are no more than 1.5 times the interquartile range. More extreme values, if any, are individually plotted *(open circles).* (From Leung W, Rose SR, Zhou Y, et al. Outcomes of growth hormone replacement therapy in survivors of childhood acute lymphoblastic leukemia. *J Clin Oncol* 2002;20:2959–2964, with permission.)

bertal onset is positively correlated with the age at the time of cranial irradiation (Fig. 19-7). The impact of early puberty in a child with radiation-associated GH deficiency is significant, and the timing of GH is especially important for GH-deficient girls also at risk of precocious puberty. With higher dosages of cranial irradiation (more than 35 Gy), deficiencies in the gonadotropins can be seen, with a cumulative incidence of 10–20% at 5–10 years (115).

Constine et al. (116) documented non-GH abnormalities in 20 children treated with irradia-

tion for brain tumors not involving the HP region, including low free T4 levels caused by hypothalamic or pituitary injury and low luteinizing hormone (LH) and estradiol with oligomenorrhea. The frequency of central hypothyroidism after cranial irradiation relates to the dosage to the HP axis, with a greater likelihood after dosages greater than 40 Gy. Although some reports suggest that the incidence is as low as 6%, the radiation dosages to the HP axis in those reports were not specifically determined (117,118). In Constine et al.'s series (119), 65% of patients treated in the higher dosage range had evidence of subclinical or clinical hypothyroidism. In a report by Paulino (120) on children treated for medulloblastoma, and thus with somewhat lower HP dosages, 19% of children developed central hypothyroidism.

Adrenocorticotropin deficiencies and hyperprolactinemia are rare in children because dosages greater than 50 Gy are needed for their development (116,121). Samaan et al. (122) described 110 patients treated for nasopharyngeal or paranasal sinus carcinoma, in whom more than 60 Gy was typically administered. They found deficiencies in 83%. Twenty-seven percent had thyroid abnormalities, attributed to hypothalamic injury in one-third of the patients and pituitary injury in the remainder. Cortisol deficiency attributable to hypothalamic injury also occurred in 27% of patients. Abnormalities of prolactin and LH were noted in 39% and 30%, respectively. A summary of neuroendocrine complications of therapy, the relationship to dosage, diagnostic studies, and interventions are provided in Table 19-5 (80).

Thyroid

Radiation-induced thyroid neoplasms are considered in Chapter 20. In this section, we will review the effects of therapeutic irradiation on the endocrine function of the thyroid. The thyroid may be directly irradiated in the treatment of childhood head and neck cancers such as rhabdomyosarcoma, nasopharyngeal lymphoepithelioma, and squamous cell carcinoma, a variety of other aerodigestive tract tumors, and HD. A photon spinal field used during craniospinal ir-

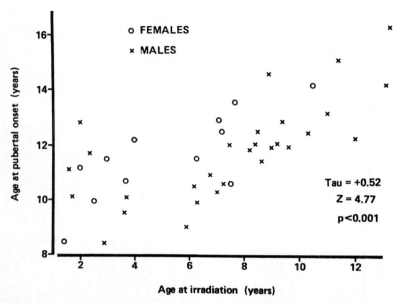

FIG. 19-7. The relationship between age at the time of cranial or craniospinal irradiation and age of pubertal onset. (From Shalet SM, Ogilvy-Stuart AL, Crowne EC, et al. Indications for human growth hormone treatment of radiation-induced growth hormone deficiency. In: Green DM, D'Angio GJ, eds. *Late effects of treatment for childhood cancer.* New York: Wiley-Liss, 1992:71–79, with permission.)

radiation for brain and spinal tumors and for leukemia will deliver radiation to the thyroid.

Pathophysiology

The thyroid gland is the largest pure endocrine gland and is located between the thyroid cartilage and third or fourth tracheal cartilages. It consists of follicles filled with colloid and lined by follicular cells, which trap iodide. The glycoprotein thyroglobulin is a major component of the colloid and participates in the formation and storage of thyroid hormones. The primary, hormonally active iodothyronines, triiodothyronine (T3) and thyroxine (T4), are largely bound to plasma proteins when released by the gland. Thyroxine-binding globulin is the major transport protein, and only a small percentage of unbound T3 and T4 is available for activity. The pituitary hormone thyroid-stimulating hormone (TSH) regulates synthesis and release of T3 and T4. TSH secretion is stimulated by the hypothalamic hormone thyrotropin-releasing hormone (TRH) and inhibited by the circulating free thyroid hormones (123, 124). The pathophysiology of radiation-induced

thyroid dysfunction is not precisely defined. Direct radiation damage to the thyroid follicular cells, the thyroid vasculature, or the supporting stroma may occur. Less likely mechanisms that could contribute include the induction by RT of an immunologic reaction or damage from the iodine load administered for lymphangiography. Support for the latter is based on the observation that radioiodine induces hypothyroidism in patients with autoimmune thyroiditis (125). Histopathologic changes in an irradiated thyroid gland include progressive obliteration of the fine vasculature, degeneration of follicular cells and follicles, atrophy of the stroma, and, less commonly, lymphocytic infiltration (8,126,127). Because radiation damage depends on the degree of mitotic activity and the thyroid of a developing child grows in parallel with body growth, this gland might be expected to show an age-related degree of injury and repair.

Hypothyroidism

The legion of symptoms include cold intolerance, constipation, inordinate weight gain, dry

TABLE 19-5. *Evaluation of patients at risk for late effects: neuroendocrine*

Late effects	Causative treatment			Signs and symptoms	Screening and diagnostic tests	Management and intervention
	Chemotherapy	Radiation	Surgery			
GH deficiency		>18 Gy to HP axis	Tumor in region of HP axis	Falling off of growth curve Inadequate growth velocity Inadequate pubertal growth spurt	Annual stadiometer height (q 6 mo at age 9–12 yr) Growth curve Bone age at 9 yr, then q yr to puberty Insulin stimulation test and pulsatile GH analysis	GH therapy Delay puberty with GnRH agonist
Adrenocorticotropic hormone deficiency		>40 Gy to HP axis	Tumor in region of HP axis	Muscular weakness, anorexia, nausea, weight loss, dehydration, hypotension, abdominal pain, increased pigmentation (skin, buccal mucosa)	Cortisol (a.m.) for baseline, PRN Insulin–hypoglycemia; metapyrone stimulation tests	Hydrocortisone
Thyrotropin-releasing hormone deficiency		>40 Gy HP axis	Tumor in region of HP axis	Hoarseness, fatigue, weight gain, dry skin, cold intolerance, dry brittle hair, alopecia, constipation, lethargy, poor linear growth, menstrual irregularities; pubertal delay, bradycardia, hypotension	Free T4, T3, thyroid-stimulating hormone baseline, q 3–5 yr	Hormone replacement with thyroxine Anticipatory guidance regarding symptoms of hypothyroidism
Precocious puberty (especially girls)		>20 Gy to HP axis	Tumor in region of HP axis	Early growth spurt False catch-up Premature sexual maturation: Female: Breast development and pubic hair before 8 yr and menses before 9 yr Male: Testicular and penile growth and pubic hair before 9.5 yr	Height, growth curve q yr Bone age q 2 yr until mature LH, FSH, estradiol, or testosterone Pelvic ultrasound, GnRH stimulation testing	GnRH agonist

Late effect	Predisposing treatment		Highest risk factor	Signs and symptoms	Screening/diagnosis	Management
Male gonadotropin deficiency	>40 Gy to hypothalamic region		Tumor in region of hypothalamus	Delayed, arrested, or absent pubertal development: Lack of or diminished pubic and axillary hair, penile and testicular enlargement, voice change, body odor, acne; Testicular atrophy (softer and smaller); Failure to impregnate	LH, testosterone q 3–5 yr; GnRH testing	Testosterone replacement
Female gonadotropin deficiency	>40 Gy to hypothalamic region		Tumor in region of hypothalamus	Delayed, arrested, or absent pubertal development, including breasts, female escutcheon, female habitus, vaginal estrogen effect, body odor; Acne; Changes in duration, frequency, and character of menstruation (less cramping); Estrogen deficiency: hot flashes, vaginal dryness, dyspareunia, low libido; Infertility *If not on birth control pills	Tanner stage; LH, FSH, estradiol q 3–5 yr; GnRH stimulation tests	Anticipatory guidance regarding symptoms of estrogen deficiency; Hormone replacement; Early intervention may prevent osteoporosis, atherosclerosis
Hyperprolactinemia	>40 Gy HP axis		Tumor in region of hypothalamus	Female: menstrual irregularities, loss of libido, infertility, galactorrhea, hot flashes, osteopenia; Male: loss of libido, impotence, infertility	Prolactin level baseline, then PRN	Dopamine agonist (bromocriptine)
Metabolic syndrome	Steroids	? ≥18 Gy (dosage not well established)		Obesity, hypertension, hyperlipidemia, hyperglycemia, insulin resistance with hyperinsulinemia	Fasting lipids, glucose, insulin levels, body mass index evaluation	Refer to endocrinology

FSH, follicle-stimulating hormone; GH, growth hormone; GnRH, gonadotropin-releasing hormone; HP, hypothalamic–pituitary; LH, leuteinizing hormone; PRN, as needed.
From Constine LS, Hobbie W, Schwartz C. Facilitated assessment of chronic treatment by symptom and organ systems. In: Schwartz C, Hobbie W, Constine L, et al., eds. *Survivors of childhood cancer: assessment and management.* St Louis: Mosby, 1994:21–80, with permission.

skin, brittle hair, menorrhagia or spotting, muscle cramps or generalized muscle weakness, and slowed mentation. Signs include a round, puffy face, slow speech, hoarseness, hypokinesia, delayed relaxation of deep tendon reflexes, periorbital or peripheral edema, and pleural or pericardial effusions (128,129). In addition to the classic signs and symptoms of hypothyroidism or hyperthyroidism, patients who present with pleural or pericardial effusions, cardiac arrhythmias, or hypercholesterolemia after cervical or mantle irradiation should also be evaluated for thyroid dysfunction (124).

The incidence of radiation-induced hypothyroidism may be significantly influenced by a variety of methodological factors. Clinical hypothyroidism may be defined as the clinical symptoms of hypothyroidism associated with an elevation in basal TSH levels, elevated TSH response to TRH, and depressed levels of T4 and T3 parameters. Subclinical hypothyroidism may be defined as an elevation of the basal TSH level and of TSH response to TRH, but with normal T3 and T4 parameters and no clinical symptoms of hypothyroidism (78). One can readily see that the reported clinical incidence of hypothyroidism after irradiation of the gland may be affected by the laboratory tests the investigator used (i.e., T3 and T4 alone vs. these parameters plus a TSH assessment), by how carefully the clinical symptoms of thyroid dysfunction are pursued (i.e., the degree to which the nonspecific complaint of "being tired" is evaluated by the physician or reported by the patient), and by the frequency with which the patient is evaluated after treatment. It is also possible that the frequency of hypothyroidism after irradiation is affected by the interval since the RT was given, the dosage administered, the nature of the underlying malignant disease, and the age of the patient at the time of RT (24,78,119,121,130–136).

Patients with HD constitute the larger part of the population for the late effects of RT on thyroid function (137). A variable incidence of hypothyroidism after RT has been reported. Most of the available clinical studies are retrospective. Few patients have been subject to detailed baseline thyroid function testing followed by prospective evaluation of the endocrine outcome of treatment (78,135,136). Consequently, if an elevated serum TSH concentration is the determinant, then 4–79% of patients become affected (78,119,126,128,131,135–141).

In a study of 1,677 children and adults with HD who were treated with RT between 1961 and 1989, the actuarial risk at 26 years for overt or subclinical hypothyroidism was 47%, with a peak incidence at 2–3 years after treatment (137). In a study of patients with HD treated between 1962 and 1979, hypothyroidism occurred in 4 of 24 patients who received mantle dosages less than 26 Gy but in 74 of 95 who received more than 26 Gy. The peak incidence occurred at 3–5 years after treatment, with a median of 4.6 years (119). A more recent cohort of childhood HD survivors treated between 1970 and 1986 was evaluated for thyroid disease by use of a self-report questionnaire in the CCSS. Among 1,791 survivors, 34% reported that they had been diagnosed with at least one thyroid abnormality. For hypothyroidism, there was a clear dose–response relationship, with a 20-year risk of 20% for those who received less than 35 Gy, 30% for those who received 35–44.9 Gy, and 50% for those who received more than 45 Gy to the thyroid gland (Fig. 19-8). Compared with that of siblings, the relative risk for hypothyroidism was 17.1. Elapsed time since diagnosis was a risk factor for hypothyroidism, where the risk increased in the first 3–5 years after diagnosis. Of note, female patients were at greater risk (142). A similar dose–response relationship is noted in a report by Bhatia et al. (138), where the relative risk of hypothyroidism increased significantly by 1.02 per gray.

Other groups of childhood cancer survivors are at greater risk of primary hypothyroidism, including survivors of ALL, those with CNS tumors treated with craniospinal RT, and those who received TBI. The frequency of primary hypothyroidism after RT to the spinal axis in the course of treating CNS tumors has not been as well studied. Ogilvy-Stuart et al. (143) evaluated 85 children and found a 32% incidence of compensated hypothyroidism. Constine et al. (116,121) evaluated eight children treated with 4- to 10-MV photon irradiation to the spinal axis (mean dosage 30 Gy). Three demonstrated primary thyroid injury with low free T4 and an exaggerated TSH re-

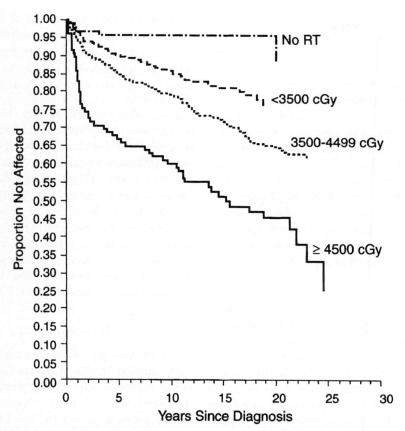

FIG. 19-8. Probability of developing an underactive thyroid after diagnosis of Hodgkin's disease. Patients are grouped according to dosage of thyroid irradiation. RT, radiotherapy. (From Sklar C, Whitton J, Mertens A, et al. Abnormalities of the thyroid in survivors of Hodgkin's disease: data from the Childhood Cancer Survivor Study. *J Clin Endocrinol Metab* 2000;85:3227–3232, with permission.)

sponse to TRH. Oberfield et al. (144) studied 36 patients after craniospinal irradiation for medulloblastoma. Many of the patients also received chemotherapy. Abnormal thyroid function as ascertained by TRH stimulation testing or TSH, T3, and T4 levels was identified in 21 cases (58%). The definition of thyroid dysfunction apparently was broad. Schmiegelow et al. (117) compared the effects of craniospinal irradiation (CSI) and cranial irradiation (CIR) only with or without chemotherapy on the HP thyroid axis in a population-based study of patients treated for childhood brain tumors in Denmark. Thyroid function was evaluated. Primary hypothyroidism was found in 24%, as opposed to central hypothyroidism, seen in 6%. Of those with primary hypothyroidism, 71% had been treated with CSI and 29% with CIR only. When thyroid functions were assessed

in all survivors, both clinical (overt) and subclinical (compensated) hypothyroidism prevalence were 27% and 73%, respectively. The CIR-only group had significantly higher median basal TSH levels than control subjects, and the CSI group had significantly higher median basal TSH levels than the CIR and control groups. Therefore, the authors speculated that this probably resulted from scattered irradiation from both cranial and spinal fields to the thyroid gland.

Survivors of pediatric bone marrow transplantation are at higher risk of thyroid dysfunction, with the risk being much lower (15–16%) after fractionated TBI, as opposed to single-dose TBI (46–48%). Non-TBI regimens do not appear to increase risk. Although mildly elevated TSH is common, it is usually accompanied by normal thyroxine concentration (145–147).

Thyroid abnormalities have been observed among long-term survivors of ALL. Robison et al. (148) collected data on 175 survivors first evaluated 7 years after diagnosis. Seventeen (10%) had thyroid function abnormalities, including 5 with primary hypothyroidism and 11 with compensated hypothyroidism. No significant association was observed between hypothyroidism and the radiation fields (cranial vs. craniospinal), dosage (18 Gy vs. 24 Gy), duration of chemotherapy (3 vs. 5 years), or age at the time of irradiation. At St. Jude, Leung et al. (149) evaluated survivors of infant leukemia. Among those treated with chemotherapy and CNS-directed RT, with or without subsequent bone marrow transplantation, hypothyroidism was seen in 15%.

Some patients may demonstrate a spontaneous recovery of thyroid function, as indicated by a report by Constine et al. (119) in which 20 of 75 (27%) affected patients normalized. Data from St. Jude Children's Research Hospital are supportive. Twenty-nine of 85 children developed abnormal thyroid function tests (34%), and 8 of these patients spontaneously recovered (28%) (150). In the series reported by Robison (148), of 11 ALL survivors with compensated hypothyroidism, 8 later became euthyroid without replacement therapy.

Although radiation dosage is the most relevant parameter in predicting the likelihood of hypothyroidism, as is evidenced by the data just presented, radiation technique must be considered. A differential anterior versus posterior field weighting may have been used, cervical blocks may have been introduced during treatment, specific thyroid blocks may have been used, and anterior beam spoilers to increase the superficial dosage from high-energy linear accelerators may have been in place. All these factors may affect the actual dosage the thyroid received and may have not been reflected in the midplane central axis dosage reported (135,136, 151).

Other factors may affect risk for radiation-induced hypothyroidism. The influence of young age at the time of RT is unclear because most young children are treated with lower-dose radiation in combination with chemotherapy (119,131,137,138). Hancock et al. (137) found that the incidence of hypothyroidism rose from 15% for patients treated before 5 years of age (usually with reduced RT dosages) to 39% for those irradiated between 15 and 20 years of age. The incidence declined gradually during advancing adulthood. Before age 16 years, RT dosage was the predominant determinant of risk, whereas female sex and chemotherapy were additional risk factors in older patients. In Constine et al.'s (119) study age did not affect the incidence of hypothyroidism but was weakly correlated with the degree of abnormality, as suggested by higher serum TSH concentrations in adolescents than in younger children. Such an age effect could reflect the greater sensitivity of the thyroid gland in rapidly growing pubertal children than in preadolescents (10,152).

Hyperthyroidism

Thyrotoxicosis may occur after mantle or cervical irradiation for HD. In Hancock et al.'s report (137), approximately 2% of patients ($n = 34$) developed Graves's disease. Almost all had a diffuse goiter, high free T4, low TSH, and elevated thyroid uptake of radioiodine. One-half of these patients developed infiltrative ophthalmopathy, as did an additional four patients who did not have overt hyperthyroidism. The relative risk for Graves's disease was 7.2–20.4. Six patients developed silent thyroiditis characterized by transient mild symptoms of thyrotoxicosis, elevated serum free T4 and low TSH, no thyroid enlargement or tenderness, and low thyroid uptake of radioiodine (153). All of these patients subsequently developed hypothyroidism.

In the CCSS study of HD survivors by Sklar et al. (142), the relative risk for hyperthyroidism compared with sibling control subjects was 8.0, with cases becoming manifest 3–5 years after diagnosis.

Detection and Screening

Laboratory screening evaluations for asymptomatic patients should include serum concentrations of TSH and thyroxine (usually free T4) tests. The measurement of free T4 rather than other tests (usually total T4 by radioimmunoassay) is recommended because the former is not affected by changes in binding proteins. Because the latent interval to the development of abnormality can be prolonged, systematic clinical and laboratory evaluation should be performed yearly. Although some patients with normal serum free T4 and TSH concentrations might show an exaggerated TSH response to provocative testing with TRH, the clinical significance of this finding is unclear. In patients with clinical and laboratory findings suggestive of thyrotoxicosis, radioiodine uptake aids in distinguishing Graves's disease (increased uptake) from silent thyroiditis (diminished uptake) (124,129). Measurements of serum antimicrosomal, antithyroglobulin, and thyroid-stimulating antibodies can assist in confirming Graves's disease; abnormalities in asymptomatic patients are of uncertain clinical significance.

Management

Patients with uncompensated hypothyroidism (low serum concentration of thyroxine) clearly need thyroid replacement therapy. Patients with elevated serum concentrations of TSH but normal thyroxine are treated with thyroid replacement therapy in most institutions. The rationale for this approach is that subclinical hypothyroidism may evolve into overt hypothyroidism, and prolonged TSH stimulation of an irradiated thyroid gland may increase the risk of carcinoma (119,129,135,137,154). In support of this approach is that thyroid hormone replacement reduces the risk of recurrent cancer after thyroidectomy or an irradiated gland (155). For patients with overt hypothyroidism, thyroxine replacement should be gradual to avoid the rare occurrence of cardiovascular overload (124). Approaches to decrease the risk of thyroid injury in the setting of RT for HD have included shielding the gland from irradiation (151) and administering thyroxine before irradiation (156). The former approach places patients at risk for shielding of involved cervical lymph nodes, and the latter did not prevent subsequent hypothyroidism. Therefore, these approaches are not recommended.

Table 19-6 reviews several thyroid late effects with respect to causative treatments, signs and symptoms, screening and diagnostic tests, and management and intervention (80).

Bone and Body Composition

It has long been established that bone growth can be impaired by radiation. As in so many other areas of scientific inquiry, we are indebted to animal research for developing the foundation of our understanding of radiation's effects on bone growth. In 1903, Perthes (157) reported that chickens irradiated to one wing had slower growth of that wing than in the unirradiated side. In 1906, Forsterling (158) noted gross impairment of growth after irradiation of one-half the body of a rabbit. Studies in the albino rat and dog conducted between 1940 and 1947 by a variety of investigators showed that some epiphyseal growth retardation could be produced at a threshold dosage of 400–600 R. Complete growth inhibition occurred at 1,200 R or more (24,159,160). Highly instructive experiments were reported by Arkin and Simon (161) in 1950. The rabbit vertebral column was exposed to an inhomogeneous radiation dosage by unilateral implantation of radon seeds and by external beam treatment. When the animals were sacrificed, the vertebral bodies were wedge-shaped. There was an absence of cartilaginous columns on the irradiated side. The zones of temporary calcification were acellular (162).

Pathophysiology

The pathophysiology of radiation injury to growing bone probably is attributable to damage to the chondroblasts (159,163,164). Single doses of 2–20 Gy inhibit proliferation of cartilage cells, thereby decreasing cellularity and causing disarray of the cellular columns within the growth plate (165). The resulting retarded bone growth is attributed to this loss of proliferating cells in the growth plate, the decreased ability of surviving cells to synthesize matrix, or the production of an abnormal matrix that fails to calcify.

The effects of radiation on growing bone have been summarized by Rubin et al. (9,10,152):

TABLE 19-6. *Evaluation of patients at risk for late effects: thyroid*

Late effects	Causative treatment			Signs and symptoms	Screening and diagnostic tests	Management and intervention
	Chemotherapy	Radiation	Surgery			
Overt hypothyroidism (elevated TSH, decreased T4)		>20 Gy to the neck, cervical spine; >7.5 Gy total body irradiation	Partial or complete thyroidectomy	Hoarseness, fatigue, weight gain, dry skin, cold intolerance, dry brittle hair, alopecia, constipation, lethargy, poor linear growth, menstrual irregularities, pubertal delay, bradycardia, hypotension	Free T4, TSH annually up to 10 yr postradiation or if symptomatic; Plot on growth chart	Refer to endocrinologist; Thyroxine replacement; Anticipatory guidance regarding symptoms of hyperthyroidism and hypothyroidism
Compensated hypothyroidism (elevated TSH, normal T4)		Same as for overt hypothyroidism	Same as for overt hypothyroidism	Asymptomatic	Same as for overt hypothyroidism	Refer to endocrinologist; Thyroxine to suppress gland activity
Thyroid nodules		Any dosage		Same as for overt hypothyroidism	Same as for overt hypothyroidism; Physical exam; Ultrasound for technetium-99m scan for baseline and then PRN	Refer to endocrinologist; Thyroid scan; Biopsy or resection
Hyperthyroidism (low TSH, elevated T4)		Same as for overt hypothyroidism		Nervousness, tremors, heat intolerance, weight loss, insomnia, increased appetite, diarrhea, moist skin, tachycardia, exophthalmus, goiter	Same as for thyroid nodules; T3, antithyroglobulin, antimicrosomal antibody baseline, then PRN	Refer to endocrinologist; PTU, propranolol; ^{131}I Thyroidectomy

PRN, as needed; PTU, propothiouracil; TSH, thyroid-stimulating hormone.

From Constine LS, Hobbie W, Schwartz C. Facilitated assessment of chronic treatment by symptom and organ systems. In: Schwartz C, Hobbie W, Constine L, et al., eds. *Survivors of childhood cancer: assessment and management.* St Louis: Mosby, 1994:21–80, with permission.

Epiphyseal irradiation, to a sufficient dosage, causes an arrest of chondrogenesis; metaphyseal irradiation results in a failure of absorptive processes in calcified bone and cartilage; and diaphyseal irradiation produces an alteration in periosteal activity, which causes abnormal bone modeling. Therefore, the location of a radiotherapy field on a long bone can significantly influence the nature and severity of the subsequent deformity.

By identifying the location of the most rapidly growing epiphyseal plate of a given bone, we may infer the extent of growth stunting produced by placement of a radiotherapy field. In the femur, approximately 30% of growth comes from the proximal epiphysis and 70% from the distal. In the tibia, 60% of growth is from the proximal epiphysis and 40% is from the distal, whereas in the humerus, 80% is derived from the proximal and 20% is derived from the distal (10,159,163).

Clinical Manifestations

Bone Growth Retardation

Chondroblasts and chondrocytes are affected by radiation therapy in growing children, and this can result in soft tissue hypoplasia and diminution of bone growth. These effects are associated with the total and fractional radiation dosage and the inclusion of the epiphyses in the radiation field (166–169).

Clinically, radiation's effects on growing bone may be most simply characterized as shortening of long bones (i.e., femur, tibia, humerus) or hypoplasia of flat bones (i.e., ilium). The crucial factors influencing the ultimate height of the patient may be inferred from the data previously presented: the radiation total dosage and dosage per fraction; the energy, dosage distribution, and absorptive properties of the beams; the bones that are irradiated and the epiphyseal plates that are encompassed; the age at the time of irradiation (implying that the amount of growth already obtained is important in judging ultimate outcome); the influence of other toxins on growth, such as exogenous steroids and cytotoxic chemotherapy; and the patient's genetic constitution (159,160,163).

A large body of knowledge has been developed concerning loss of height after childhood irradiation. Much of the data published in the 1970s and 1980s reflects treatment with higher dosages of radiotherapy than those currently used. However, several recent reports indicate that stature loss must still be considered in the late effects of RT. For children treated with craniospinal RT for ALL or CNS tumors, the cranial dosage can result in decreased growth by causing growth hormone deficiency, and the spinal dosage can result in stature loss through its effect on the vertebral bodies (102,114, 169–171).

The pediatric radiation oncologist will counsel the young patient's parents about decreased sitting or standing height or limb length discrepancy after radiotherapy. Parents often respond, "But how short will my child be?" An answer couched in terms of standard deviations from the mean usually is unsatisfactory. Silber et al. (168) have attempted to address this problem with a mathematical model to predict adult stature after treatment of cancer in childhood. An estimate of ideal adult stature in the absence of cancer treatment is made based on anthropomorphic data from a normal population. By using the subject's sex, age, stature, weight, and the statures of the subject's mother and father, a prediction can be made of the ultimate ideal adult stature. Silber et al. (168) found that a model that included the irradiation dosage, the vertical distance of the spine irradiated, whether or not the femoral heads or acetabula were irradiated, and sex was highly predictive of the ultimate adult height ($R^2 = 0.74$, multiple correlation coefficient). However, the model was based on data from only 49 patients. Donaldson (164) was unable to confirm the model's efficacy in two of three cases.

Patients who receive radiation therapy for Wilms' tumor are an ideal population for study of the effect of RT and age at time of treatment on stature. As a result of earlier studies showing a higher risk of spinal curvature with asymmetric radiation to the vertebral bodies, standard flank radiation now includes the affected side and extends across the spinal column but excludes the contralateral kidney. Radiation dosages have decreased over successive National Wilms Tumor Study Group (NWTS) protocols. Hogeboom et al. (167) evaluated stature loss in 2,778 children treated on NWTS 1–4. Repeated height measurements were collected during long-term follow-up. The effects of radiation dosage, age at treatment, and chemotherapy on stature were analyzed using statistical models that accounted for the normal variation in height with sex and advancing age. Predictions from the model were validated by descriptive analysis of heights measured at age 17–18 years for 205 patients. For those under 12 months of age at diagnosis who received more than 10 Gy, the estimated adult height deficit was 7.7 cm when contrasted with the nonradiation group. For those who received 10 Gy the estimated trunk shortening was 2.8 cm or less. Among those whose height measurements in the teenage years were available, patients who received more than 15 Gy of RT were 4–7 cm shorter on average than their nonirradiated counterparts, with a dose–response relationship evident. Chemotherapy did not confer additional risk.

Scoliosis and Kyphosis

Scoliosis and kyphosis are common consequences of spinal or flank irradiation. Asymmetric spinal growth has most been seen most often after irradiation for Wilms' tumor and neuroblastoma, where there has been flank surgery (e.g., nephrectomy) and radiation (161,172). The types of deformities observed included a lateral flexion curve, concave to the side of the primary tumor, and a rotary scoliosis (162). However, with current dosages and fields of RT used to treat Wilms' tumor, scoliosis and kyphosis are less common. In a series by Paulino et al. (173), in a group of 42 children treated for Wilms' tumor from 1968 to 1994, 7 developed muscular hypoplasia, 5 were found to have limb length inequality, 3 had kyphosis, and another 3 had iliac wing hypoplasia. Scoliosis was seen in 18, with only one patient needing orthopedic intervention. Median time to development of scoliosis was 102 months, with a range of 16–146

months. The actuarial incidence of scoliosis at 5, 10, and 15 years after RT was 4.8% ± 3.3%, 51.8% ± 9.0%, and 56.7% ± 9.3%, respectively. A clear dose–response relationship was seen, with children treated with lower dosages (less than 24 Gy) having a significantly lower incidence of scoliosis than those who received more than 24 Gy. There was also a suggestion that the incidence was lower in patients who received 10–12 Gy, the dosages currently used for Wilms' tumor, although the sample size was small.

Asymmetric irradiation of the vertebrae seemed to promote the development of rotary scoliosis and lateral flexion curvature. These late effects in humans seemed to recapitulate the early studies in animal models: An inhomogeneous dosage across a growth plate may lead to curvature of bone growth (162). Some clinicians believe that it is better to arrest a growth plate than partially irradiate it and cause a curvature. Neuhauser et al. (160) stated it well: "If the spine is to be included in the field of irradiation in a growing child, as it must in the paraspinal neuroblastomas, the fields should be so arranged that the spine receives uniform intensity of irradiation throughout the course of therapy." It is for this reason that some clinicians prefer true anteroposterior portals. Lateral and tangential ports may give sufficient variation in intensity of radiation to the epiphyseal plates of the spine to produce scoliosis by the irregular advance of the epiphyses. This led to the change in radiotherapy fields now used to treat unilateral intra-abdominal tumors of childhood. If therapy is limited to one-half of the abdomen, it is advisable to bring the ports slightly beyond the midline so that the entire transverse diameter of the spine is included, receiving irradiation of fairly uniform intensity. If the entire abdomen needs treatment and it must be subdivided into quadrants, caution should be exercised in avoiding quadruple cross-firing of the spine, producing a "hot spot" in the region of the first or second lumbar vertebrae.

Slipped Femoral Capital Epiphysis

Slipped femoral capital epiphysis is a clinically significant adverse effect observed in patients after irradiation of the femoral head (174–177). There is a threshold dosage of 25 Gy for this complication. It occurred in about 50% of children irradiated before 4 years of age (7 of 15), compared with only 1 of 21 5- to 15-year-olds (Fig. 19-9). A similar age effect is seen with TBI for hematopoietic stem cell transplantation (HSCT). Fletcher et al. (178) examined 10 children with skeletal surveys 7–9 years after transplant with TBI and found more significant metaphyseal and epiphyseal abnormalities in those treated before 8 years of age than in those treated between 12 and 19 years, supporting the effect of radiation on growing tissue. The mechanism of femoral capital epiphyseal plate slippage is postulated to be a radiation-induced delay in maturation of the epiphyseal plate with disruption of normal calcification and bone matrix deposition. This renders the plate weak and prone to slippage through shearing stress at the tilted femoral line (159). When the femoral heads are shielded during irradiation, the frequency of this complication is small.

Avascular Necrosis

Avascular necrosis of the femoral or humeral heads can occur 2–3 years after irradiation (175). Libshitz and Edeikin (179) reported necrosis in 16 of 44 children receiving 30–60 Gy to the femoral heads. This complication was bilateral in 4 of 5 patients who received irradiation to both hips. This debilitating injury is rare when the femoral and humeral heads are shielded and when lower radiation dosages are used (159,163). Corticosteroids also increase risk of avascular necrosis. In a series from St. Jude Children's Research Hospital, avascular femoral head necrosis was identified in 15 patients treated from 1974 to 1991, most often in survivors of leukemia. Patients ranged from 7 to 27 years of age at diagnosis of this complication, with a median interval of 25 months (range, 0–11 years) from primary diagnosis. Both steroids and RT appear to be implicated in the pathogenesis of avascular necrosis: 9 patients had received high cumulative dosages of

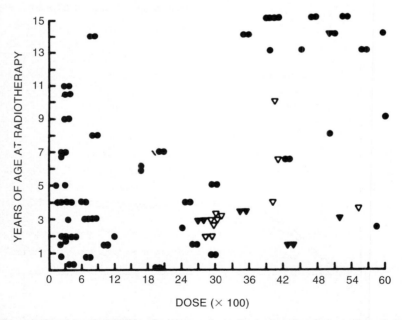

FIG. 19-9. The relationship of radiation dosage and age in the production of slipped capital femoral plates *(closed triangles)*. The open triangles are other reported cases. Refer to Fig. 2. of ref. 176 for references from which data were obtained. Normal epiphyseal plates are represented by closed circles. (From Silverman CL, Thomas PR, McAlister WH, et al. Slipped femoral capital epiphysis in irradiated children: dose, volume, and age relationships. *Int J Radiat Oncol Biol Phys* 1981;7:1357–1363, with permission.)

prednisone (3.4–14 g/m^2), 4 had received 35–64.8 Gy local irradiation involving the femoral head, and 1 underwent TBI (12 Gy) (180). The origin of this complication is unclear but may be related to the combined use of steroids and irradiation.

Of interest is the increasing information on the occurrence of osteonecrosis in children treated for ALL without RT. Corticosteroids are a significant risk factor (178,181–185). Strauss et al. (185) evaluated the incidence of osteonecrosis and fractures among 176 children treated for ALL between 1987 and 1995. With a median follow-up of 7.6 years, the cumulative incidence of any bony morbidity was 30% ± 4%, with a 5-year cumulative incidence of fractures of 28% ± 3% and of osteonecrosis of 7% ± 2% (Fig. 19-10). In multivariate analysis, age 9–18 years at time of treatment, male sex, and use of dexamethasone were associated with bony morbidity. Dexamethasone use was compared with prednisone use in these protocols, and dexamethasone was associated with a higher risk of fractures but not osteonecrosis.

Other Skeletal Abnormalities

A variety of other skeletal abnormalities can be seen after irradiation. These include sternal deformity (hypoplasia, asymmetry, pectus excavatum, pectus carinatum) (186); hypoplasia of the iliac bones or lower ribs; cartilaginous exostoses (187); osteochondromata (162); hypoplasia of the mandible; deformity of orbital, maxillary, nasal, or temporal bone (162,188); and lower extremity abnormalities such as acetabular dysplasia, coxa vara, hip dislocation, and leg shortening (189,190).

Table 19-7 reviews several musculoskeletal late effects with respect to causative treatments, signs and symptoms, screening and diagnostic tests, and management and intervention (80).

Osteopenia

Bone mineral density in childhood cancer survivors may be reduced, especially in children treated for ALL, or with HSCT, where it has been best studied. Risk factors include increased age at time of exposure, estrogen defi-

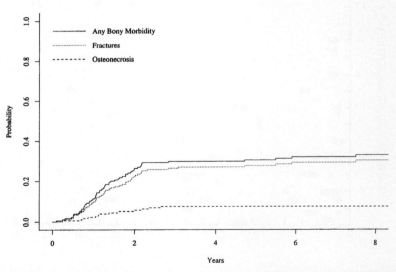

FIG. 19-10. Cumulative incidence (CI) of bony morbidity for 176 children treated for ALL between 1987 and 1991. With 7.6 years of median follow-up, the overall 5-year CI (± *SE*) was 30% ± 4%. The 5-year CI of fracture was 28% ± 3%, and of osteonecrosis, 7% ± 2%. (From Strauss AJ, Su JT, Dalton VM, et al. Bony morbidity in children treated for acute lymphoblastic leukemia. *J Clin Oncol* 2001;19:3066–3072, with permission.)

ciency, female sex, corticosteroid use and type, GH deficiency, and cranial radiation. Prevalence, chronicity, and severity are not consistent across studies, so the risk remains poorly defined (191–202). Further research into the pathophysiology, the contribution of the various risk factors, the type and frequency of screening, the populations at highest risk, and interventions are clearly indicated.

Similarly of concern, but not yet rigorously studied, is abnormal body composition, which is reported in survivors of pediatric ALL. Oeffinger (203) evaluated obesity in 1,764 ALL survivors followed in the CCSS and compared them with a cohort of 2,565 siblings. The odds ratio for being obese was 2.6 for female survivors and 1.9 for male survivors who received dosages greater than 20 Gy. The highest risk was for girls treated at 0–4 years of age and with cranial radiation dosages greater than 20 Gy (Fig. 19-11). Risk of

obesity was not higher among ALL survivors treated with chemotherapy alone or with cranial radiation dosages of 10–19 Gy. Similar findings were reported by Warner et al. (204), where body mass index Z-score, skinfold thickness, percentage fat by dual-energy X-ray absorptiometry, and ratio of central to peripheral fat was higher in girls treated for ALL than in siblings or patients treated for other malignancies. Reilly et al. (205,206) found higher obesity rates in survivors of childhood ALL, with higher risk in younger children and those thinner at time of diagnosis, and associated with premature adiposity. A number of endocrinologic and metabolic findings, which include increased body mass index, can be summarized as the metabolic syndrome. This includes insulin resistance, hyperglycemia, hyperinsulinemia, hypertension, hyperlipidemia, and obesity. In some cancer survivors, the metabolic syndrome is at least in part attributable to en-

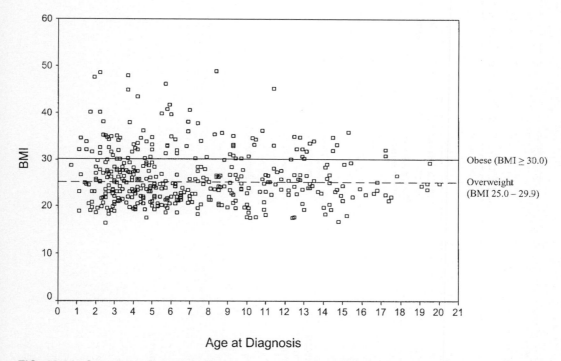

FIG. 19-11. Scatterplot for unadjusted body-mass index (BMI) by age at diagnosis of acute lymphoblastic leukemia for females treated with ≥20 Gy cranial radiotherapy. (From Oeffinger KC, Mertens AC, Sklar CA, et al. Obesity in adult survivors of childhood acute lymphoblastic leukemia: a report from the Childhood Cancer Survivor Study. *J Clin Oncol* 2003;21:1359–1365.)

TABLE 19-7. *Evaluation of patients at risk for late effects: musculoskeletal*

| Late effects | Causative treatment | | | Signs and symptoms | Screening and diagnostic tests | Management and intervention |
	Chemotherapy	Radiation	Surgery			
Muscular hypoplasia		>20 Gy (growing child) Younger children more sensitive	Muscle loss or resection	Asymmetry of muscle mass when compared with untreated area Decreased range of motion Stiffness and pain in affected area (uncommon)	Careful comparison and measurement of irradiated and unirradiated areas Range of motion	Prevention: good exercise program, range of motion, muscle strengthening
Spinal abnormalities: scoliosis, kyphosis, lordosis Decreased sitting height		For young children, RT to hemiabdomen or spine (especially hemivertebral) 10 Gy (minimal effect) >20 Gy (clinically notable defect)	Laminectomy	Back pain Hip pain Uneven shoulder height Rib humps or flares Deviation from vertical curve Gait abnormalities	Standing and sitting height at each visit and plot on chart (stadiometer). During puberty examine spine q 3–6 mo until growth is completed and then q 1–2 yr Spinal films for baseline during puberty, then PRN curvature (Lippman-Cobb technique to measure curvature)	Refer to orthopedist if any curvature is noted, especially during a period of rapid growth
Length discrepancy		>20 Gy		Lower back pain, limp, hip pain, discrepancy in muscle mass and length when compared with untreated extremity, scoliosis	Annual measurement of treated and untreated limb (completely undressed patient to ensure accurate measurements) Radiograph baseline to assess remaining epiphyseal growth Radiographs annually during periods of rapid growth	Contralateral epiphysiodesis Limb-shortening procedures

Pathological fracture	>40 Gy	Biopsy	Pain, edema, ecchymosis	Baseline radiograph of treated area to assess bone integrity, then PRN	Prevention: consider limitation of activities (e.g., contact sports) Surgical repair of fracture; may need internal fixation
Osteonecrosis	Steroids		Pain in affected joint, limp	Radiograph, CT scan PRN	Symptomatic care Joint replacement
Osteocartilaginous exostoses	40–50 Gy (more common in adults) RT		Painless lump or mass noted in the field of radiation	Radiograph for baseline and PRN with growth of lesion	Resection for cosmetic or functional reasons, counsel regarding 10% incidence of malignant degeneration
Osteopenia and osteoporosis	Steroids >18 Gy cranial radiotherapy		Fractures, pain	Dual-energy x-ray absorptiometry: intervals of testing unclear. Pediatric norms not well established. Best data are in adults	Calcium supplementation Increase weight-bearing exercise Refer to endocrinology for possible bisphosphonate therapy
Slipped capitofemoral epiphysis	High-dose steroids >25 Gy (at young age)		Pain in effected hip, limp, abnormal gait	Radiograph baseline to assess integrity of the treated joints, then PRN	Refer to orthopedist for surgical intervention

CT, computed tomography; PRN, as needed; RT, radiotherapy.
From Constine LS, Hobbie W, Schwartz C. Facilitated assessment of chronic treatment by symptom and organ systems. In: Schwartz C, Hobbie W, Constine L, et al., eds. *Survivors of childhood cancer: assessment and management.* St Louis: Mosby, 1994:21–80, with permission.

docrine dysfunction that occurs as a consequence of cancer therapies, such as corticosteroids and cranial radiation. For example, body composition is altered, with decreased fat free mass, in people with untreated GH deficiency or hypogonadism (207–214). Childhood survivors of ALL have been reported to have a 45–62% incidence of the metabolic syndrome (215–217). It results at least in part from disturbances of the HP axis, but much more research is needed to better understand all of the pathogenesis, the specific presentations of the syndrome, and its incidence and prevalence in survivors of childhood cancer.

Cardiac

The functional and structural complexity of the heart places it at risk for a spectrum of RT and chemotherapy injuries that can occur. The radiation-associated sequelae include acute pericarditis during radiation (rare and associated with juxtapericardial cancer); delayed pericarditis, which can present abruptly or as chronic pericardial effusion; pancarditis, which includes pericardial and myocardial fibrosis with or without endocardial fibroelastosis (only after large dosages); myopathy in the absence of significant pericardial disease; coronary artery disease (uncommon), usually involving the left anterior descending artery; functionally valvular injury; and conduction defects (Table 19-8) (218–220). The hallmark of these injuries histologically is fibrosis in the interstitium with normal-appearing myocytes and capillary and arterial narrowing (221).

Several parameters must be considered in the evaluation of these radiation-associated injuries, including the relative weighting of the radiation portals and, therefore, the amount of radiation delivered to different depths of the heart; the presence of juxtapericardial tumor; the volume and specific areas of the heart irradiated; the total and fractional irradiation dosage; the presence of other risk factors in each patient such as age, weight, blood pressure, family history, lipoprotein levels, and habits such as smoking; and the use of specific chemotherapeutic agents.

TABLE 19-8. *Nonfatal cardiac diagnosis among 635 patients treated for Hodgkin's disease (HD) during childhood and adolescence*

Diagnosis	Number (%)	Interval from radiation (yr)	
		Mean	Range
Acute myocardial infarction[a]	3 (0.5)	12	6.2–19.8
Coronary artery disease necessitating revascularization[a]	3 (0.5)	21	18.0–23.8
Pericardiectomy for constrictive pericarditis	12 (1.9)	7	0.8–16.8
Acute pericarditis during HD therapy	8 (1.3)	—	—
Acute pericarditis after HD therapy	30 (4.7)	6	0.3–18.0
Pericarditis after corticosteroid withdrawal	2 (0.3)	11	6.7–14.8
Valvular heart surgery[b]	3 (0.5)	18	15.0–21.3
Heart murmur	26 (4.1)	14	1.1–27.5
Mitral valve prolapse	3 (0.5)	6	4.0–9.3
Valvular disease before HD	6 (0.9)	—	—
Recurrent congestive heart failure or cardiomyopathy	3 (0.5)	13	5.3–22.3
Electrocardiographic abnormalities or arrhythmia[c]	4 (0.6)	15	1.5–23.8
Persistent tachycardia from vagus injury	3 (0.5)	—	—
Total	106 (16.7)	—	—

[a]One underwent cardiac transplantation for ischemic cardiomyopathy; one underwent left ventricular aneurysmectomy and left anterior descending artery bypass.
[b]Coronary revascularization performed with aortic valve replacement in two patients.
[c]Includes two patients with bundle branch block: one patient with pacemaker for complete heart block, one patient with paroxysmal atrial tachycardia.
From Rubin P, Van Houtte P, Constine L. Radiation sensitivity and organ tolerances in pediatric oncology: a new hypothesis. *Front Radiat Ther Oncol* 1982;16:62–82, with permission.

The effects of thoracic RT are difficult to separate from those of anthracyclines because few children are exposed to thoracic RT in the absence of anthracyclines. The pathogenesis of injury differs, however, with radiation affecting primarily the fine vasculature of the heart and anthracyclines directly damaging myocytes (222). However, with current techniques and reduced dosages of RT, these effects are unlikely after treatment for childhood cancer. In a study of 635 patients treated for childhood HD, the actuarial risk of pericarditis necessitating pericardiectomy was 4% at 17 years (occurring only in children treated with higher radiation dosages). Only 12 patients died of cardiac disease, including seven deaths from acute myocardial infarction, but these deaths occurred only in children treated with 42–45 Gy. Among children treated with 15–26 Gy, none developed radiation-associated cardiac problems (218).

Pericarditis

Delayed acute pericarditis can be symptomatically occult or present suddenly with fever, dyspnea, pleuritic chest pain, friction rub, ST and T wave changes, and decreased QRS voltage (223, 224). Up to 30% of patients treated for HD with a mean midplane heart dosage of 46 Gy are affected (225,226). With equally weighted anterior and posterior fields and the use of subcarinal blocking, the frequency decreases to 2.5% (227). The onset of delayed acute pericarditis averages 6 months, and 92% of effusions occur within 12 months. Although the effusion usually resolves in 1–10 months, it may persist for years. Up to 50% of patients develop some degree of tamponade (paradoxical pulse, Kussmaul's sign) occasionally necessitating a pericardiocentesis. Chronic effusive–constrictive pericarditis develops in 10–15% of patients and may necessitate pericardectomy. Pericardectomy is a high-risk procedure in this setting because of the coexistence of other types of radiation-induced damage such as fibrosis of the myocardium and lung, coronary artery and valvular disease, impaired chest wall healing, and the patient's general condition (228). However, Hancock et al. (229) noted a 4% (at 17 years) actuarial risk of pericardiectomy (occurring only in children treated with higher radiation dosages), and most patients improved after surgery. It is noteworthy that constriction may present 5–50 years after irradiation with no antecedent acute disease (223,230,231). Diuretics are sometimes necessary to control peripheral edema or ascites.

Myocardiopathy

Myocardiopathy is highly potentiated by doxorubicin and other anthracyclines (idarubicin, epirubicin, daunomycin) but occurs in its absence (227,232). An autopsy study of patients who were treated with at least 35 Gy, many with anterior-only portals (mean dosage of 56 Gy to anterior heart surface), showed myocardial fibrosis in 50%, fibrous thickening of the mural endocardium in 75%, and pericardial thickening in more than 90% (5,228). Right ventricular end-diastolic function may also be reduced by up to 25% in asymptomatic patients (233,234). Ejection fractions may be decreased in up to 33%. However, with modern radiation techniques and appropriate cardiac blocking, measures of cardiac function including left ventricular ejection fraction (LVEF) and peak filling rate (PFR) in patients irradiated to portions of the heart are commonly preserved. This was demonstrated by Constine et al. (235), who assessed 50 asymptomatic survivors of HD treated with mean central cardiac RT dosages of 35.1 Gy (range 18.5–47.5 Gy). The mean LVEF and PFR were normal, and 2 (4%) and 8 (16%) of patients, respectively, had low test results.

Although an in-depth discussion of the late cardiotoxic effects of anthracycline administration will not be presented, its importance and frequency must be emphasized. This is especially important because more contemporary HD treatment protocols are using lower dosages of radiotherapy but continue to use doxorubicin in the 200- 300-mg/m^2 range. Doxorubicin has been most extensively studied of the anthracyclines, and its cardiotoxicity often is progressive and disabling. Increased risk of doxorubicin-related cardiomyopathy is associated with female sex, cumulative dosages greater than 200–300 mg/m^2, younger age at time of exposure, and increased time from exposure (Fig. 19-12) (236–249). Route of administration of doxorubicin may influence risk of cardiomyopathy. Lipshultz et al. (243) studied the effect of continuous (48 hours) versus bolus (1 hour) infusions of doxorubicin in 121 children who received a cumulative dosage of 360 mg/m^2 for treatment of ALL and found no difference in the degree or spectrum of cardiotoxicity in the two groups. Because the follow-up time in this study was short, it is not yet clear whether the frequency of progressive cardiomyopathy will differ between the two groups over time. Ewer et al. (236) compared cardiac dysfunction in 113 children who received doxorubicin by single-dose infusion or by a consecutive divided daily dose schedule. The divided-dose patients received one-third of the total cycle dosage over 20 minutes for 3 consecutive days. Patients treated according to a single-dose schedule received the cycle dosage as a 20-minute infusion. There was no significant difference in the incidence of car-

diac dysfunction between the divided- and single-dose infusion groups. Earlier studies in adults have shown lower cardiotoxicity with prolonged infusion, so further evaluation of this question is warranted (250–253).

Prevention or amelioration of anthracycline-induced cardiomyopathy is of utmost importance as we continue to use anthracyclines in cancer therapy. Dexrazoxane (DZR) is a bis-dioxopiperazine compound that readily enters cells and is subsequently hydrolyzed to form a chelating agent. DZR has been shown to prevent cardiac toxicity in adults and children treated with anthracyclines (254–258). In two recently closed Pediatric Oncology Group (POG) therapeutic phase III studies for HD (259,260), myocardial toxicity is being measured clinically and sequentially over time by echocardiography, electrocardiography, and the determination of levels of cardiac troponin T (cTnT), a protein that is elevated after myocardial damage (254, 261–265).

The angiotensin-converting enzyme inhibitor enalapril has been used in the attempt to ameliorate doxorubicin-induced left ventricular

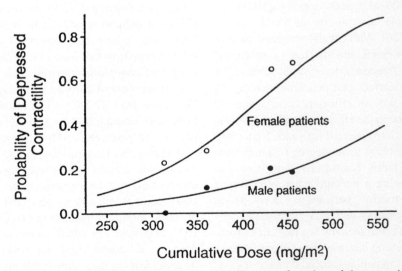

FIG. 19-12. Probability of depressed cardiac contractility as a function of the cumulative dosage of doxorubicin in female and male patients. (From Lipshultz S, Lipsitz S, Sallan S. Chronic progressive left ventricular systolic dysfunction and afterload excess years after doxorubicin therapy for childhood acute lymphoblastic leukemia. *Proc Am Soc Clin Oncol* 2000; 19:580a, with permission.)

(LV) dysfunction. Although a transient improvement in LV function and structure was noted in 18 children, LV wall thinning continued to deteriorate, so the intervention with enalapril was not considered to be successful (243).

Older data from the POG are still relevant and point to the prevalence of the problem. The incidence of clinical cardiotoxicity was determined in 6,493 children who had received anthracycline on POG protocols (239). Types of cardiotoxicity and their frequency were as follows: congestive heart failure not from other causes, 58 patients; abnormal measurements of cardiac function that prompted discontinuation of therapy, 43 patients; and sudden death from presumed cardiac causes, 5 patients. Relative risks (RRs) included cumulative dosage greater than or equal to 550 mg/m^2 (RR = 5.2), maximal individual dosage greater than 50 mg/m^2 (RR = 2.8), female sex (RR = 1.9), black race (RR = 1.7), presence of trisomy 21 (RR = 3.4), and exposure to amsacrine (RR = 2.6). Cardiotoxicity within 1 year after the completion of anthracycline treatment represented 89.5% of cases. The relationship of several other chemotherapeutic agents, such as cyclophosphamide, busulfan, 5-fluorouracil, and paclitaxel, has been reviewed (266).

Children who need HSCT are at especially high risk of cardiac toxicity. They may have received anthracyclines or RT with the heart in the field as part of their initial cancer therapy, and they are subsequently exposed to conditioning regimens that may include high-dose cyclophosphamide and TBI (267–271). Assessment of the cardiovascular complications of bone marrow transplantation will assume greater importance with the increasing number of children undergoing this therapy. In a report from the University of Minnesota on 63 transplanted children, 74% of children old enough to undergo treadmill exercise testing had a borderline or abnormal response to exercise, and 12.7% of patients had symptomatic cardiovascular abnormalities (268). The preparative regimen included TBI in slightly more than half of the patients, but this was independently associated with outcome.

Valvular Disease

Fibrous valvular endocardial thickening occurs in 80% of autopsied patients treated with high radiation dosages. The mitral, aortic, and tricuspid valves are most often affected (272) Although such valvular lesions are common, they rarely evolve into symptomatic valvular disease. In addition, they have not been reported in patients treated with the more commonly used low dosages of RT. In some patients, the radiation-induced cellular injury to the valvular endocardium, combined with chronic pressure-related trauma, may eventually lead to valvular deformity, resulting in stenosis or insufficiency. In a report by Hancock et al. (229) on 635 children treated for HD, 2 patients died of valvular disease, and 3 others have undergone aortic (2 patients) or mitral (1 patient) valve replacement. A contribution of mediastinal irradiation to significant or accelerated valvular disease could not be clearly determined. Unfortunately, in another report, valve replacement in such patients was infrequently successful and operative mortality was high (66%) (273).

Arrhythmia

High-degree atrioventricular (AV) conduction abnormalities are rarely seen and have been attributed to fibrosis of the AV node conducting branches (274). In one series, all patients with radiation-associated AV block had received more than 40 Gy to the chest, with a median time to development of the block of 14 years (275).

Again, as with myocardiopathy, the effect of doxorubicin should be considered. A number of studies have examined cardiac function after RT and anthracycline exposure using cardiopulmonary exercise stress tests and have found abnormalities in exercise endurance, cardiac output, aerobic capacity, echocardiography during exercise testing, and ectopic rhythms (270,271, 273,276–279). However, it remains unclear whether these abnormalities will have clinical impact, and further follow-up of these findings is needed.

Coronary Artery Disease

As the population of cured childhood cancer patients ages and becomes exposed to the risk factors for coronary artery disease (CAD) such as smoking, obesity, hypertension, diabetes, and elevated cholesterol, it is possible that excess morbidity and mortality from ischemic heart disease may occur if RT or chemotherapy accelerates atherosclerosis (280). RT can lead to ischemic heart disease via endothelial damage and obliteration of the microvasculature and via accelerated atherosclerosis of large vessels.

The manner in which thoracic irradiation is administered may significantly affect the incidence of radiation-associated CAD. Mantle irradiation using only a single anterior beam or an anteriorly weighted pair of opposed beams, or treating only one field per day, may significantly increase the cardiac dosage. The cardiac dosage and the risk of CAD may also be influenced by the extent of cardiac blocking via left ventricle and subcarinal blocks, the radiation dosage per fraction, and the total dosage. However, it is important to note that the proximal coronary arteries, which are commonly the site of obstruction, are not shielded with routine cardiac blocking (Fig. 19-13) (219). Data from the University of Rochester demonstrated that the site of coronary artery stenosis in patients irradiated for HD was most commonly in

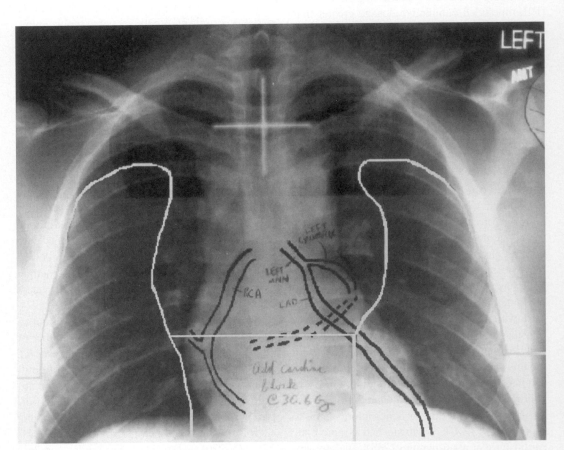

FIG. 19-13. Location of the coronary vessels *(dark lines)* on a standard mantle field is illustrated. The blocks are outlined in white. (From King V, Constine LS, Clark D, et al. Symptomatic coronary artery disease after mantle irradiation for Hodgkin's disease. *Int J Radiat Oncol Biol Phys* 1996;36: 881–889, with permission.)

the proximal coronary arteries, and this was no different than that which would be found in the general population. More specifically, the left main and the proximal portions of the left anterior descending and right coronary arteries are most commonly involved (219). Retrospective reviews that indicate an association between chest irradiation and CAD may reflect the dangers of older forms of radiotherapy and therefore be of only historical interest to the modern pediatric radiation oncologist (223,281).

The risk of myocardial infarction (MI), cardiac failure, and death from same are clearly related to RT dosage and field, although host factors may modify this risk. The Institut Gustave–Roussy reported 13 MIs in 499 mantle-irradiated patients (10-year cumulative incidence of 30%) but observed no MIs in 138 patients who received no irradiation ($p < 0.05$). Among the retrospective series evaluating the incidence of CAD after heart irradiation of adults and adolescents, one can readily find data indicating that moderate- to low-dose irradiation does not increase the risk of MI or cardiac death. Hancock et al. (226) at Stanford found that in patients with HD irradiated with more modern radiotherapeutic techniques, there was no significant difference in MI mortality when compared with that in age- and sex-matched control subjects. Mauch et al. (282) at the Harvard–Joint Center for Radiation Therapy also found no increase in the incidence of MIs in irradiated patients with HD when compared with matched control subjects. Of interest is data from the University of Rochester that assessed the risk of CAD in survivors of HD and also the prevalence of cardiac risk factors. Although the risk of cardiac death was elevated at 2.8 (3.1 for males and 1.8 for females), other risk factors were more common than in the general population; among patients with HD, 72% smoked, 72% were male, 78% had hypercholesterolemia, 61% were obese, 28% had a positive family history, 33% had hypertension, and 6% had diabetes (219). This suggests that RT is one of several risk factors for CAD in patients treated for HD. Data are accumulating on radiation-associated CAD specific to children. Among 635 children treated (less than 21 years old) at Stanford for HD, 12 patients have

died of cardiac disease (RR = 29.6), including seven deaths from acute MI (RR = 41.5). Deaths occurred only in children treated with 42–45 Gy (fraction size 1.5–2.75 Gy to anterior and posterior fields on alternate days). Among children treated with 15–26 Gy, none developed carditis (229,283). Another series of 28 children treated with 30 Gy (average dosage) showed pericardial thickening in 43% but no functional abnormalities (225).

Using a battery of tests, one may detect and quantitate cardiopulmonary abnormalities in children. Among 12 patients treated at the Mayo Clinic with 19.5–55 Gy (median dosage 35 Gy) for HD, 33% had abnormal echocardiograms and 50% had abnormal exercise studies (275). A team at the Children's Hospital of Helsinki (284) studied 21 patients who had received, as children, thoracic irradiation for a variety of malignancies. Many also received chemotherapy. The testing battery included electrocardiography, chest radiograph, echocardiography, auscultation, stress testing, and pulmonary function studies. Fourteen of the 21 patients (67%), followed up 11–27 years after RT, had at least one abnormal test, but in only one case did these abnormalities appear to have clinical impact. It seems safe to conclude that cardiac radiation using sophisticated treatment planning and careful blocking to dosages of up to 25 Gy is generally safe, and 40 Gy may be administered to small cardiac regions. However, we cannot exclude the possibility that longer follow-up of patients treated in the modern era will reveal an unexpected frequency of cardiac-related difficulties.

Although much of the data on doxorubicin and radiation-associated cardiac dysfunction is from survivors of HD and ALL, survivors of other childhood cancers are also at risk. Children who undergo spinal radiation to treat CNS tumors have a low maximal cardiac index on exercise testing, pathologic Q waves in inferior leads on electrocardiography, and higher posterior wall stress (273). A study of self-reported late effects among 1,607 survivors of childhood brain tumors in the CCSS revealed that 18% had cardiovascular conditions. Compared with siblings, risk was elevated for stroke, blood clots, and angina-like symptoms (118). A recent follow-up study of Wilms' tumor survivors reported a cumulative risk of congestive heart failure of 4.4% at 20 years for those who received doxorubicin as part of their initial therapy and 17.4% at 20 years where doxorubicin was received as part of therapy for relapsed disease. Risk factors for congestive heart failure in this cohort included female sex, lung irradiation with dosages 20 Gy or higher, left-sided abdominal irradiation, and doxorubicin dosage of 300 mg/m^2 or more (238). Finally, cardiac complications after bone marrow transplantation may occur, with arrhythmias, pericarditis, and myopathies predominating. High-dose cyclophosphamide clearly is a causative agent. TBI is a secondary contributing factor (285,286).

Table 19-9 reviews several cardiac late effects with respect to causative treatments, signs and symptoms, screening and diagnostic tests, and management and intervention (80).

Lungs

The target cells for pulmonary injury are type I and II pneumocytes, fibrocytes, endothelial cells, and macrophages (9,10,287). Several pulmonary radiation syndromes occur in the child. Acute pneumonitis and chronic fibrosis result from injury to the type II pneumocytes and endothelial cells. Chronic respiratory limitations result from impairment in the development of new alveoli or from growth impairment of established ones. Limitations of a different character result from a reduction in growth of the muscle, cartilage, and bone that form the thoracic cage.

Pathophysiology

The acute reactions of radiation pulmonary injury, known as the exudative phase, can be detected within 24 hours of irradiation. It is signified by intra-alveolar edema and exudation of proteinaceous material into the alveoli, impairing gas exchange. Infiltration by inflammatory cells and desquamation of epithelial cells from the alveolar walls occur. A proliferative phase occurs between 2 and 6 months with accumulation of type II alveolar cells and protein leakage into the alveolar spaces. Interstitial edema organizes into collagen fibrils, leading to the thickening of the alveolar septa and a clinical pneumonitis. Injury to the type II pneumocyte, with resultant changes in the surfactant system (and thus alveolar surface tension and compliance) and in the endothelial cell and capillary permeability, causes these changes (288,289). After 6 months the fibrotic phase occurs. Alveolar septa become fibrotic and thickened by bundles of elastic fibers, forming the basis for chronic respiratory injury. Eventually, the alveoli collapse and are obliterated by connective tissue. Capillaries are lost, replaced, and then recanalized. The target cells that trigger this process are less clearly established but include the septal fibrocyte and endothelial cell (290).

Clinical Manifestations

Acute pneumonitis usually occurs 3–6 months after the start of irradiation. The symptoms include fever, congestion, a hacking but eventually productive cough, dyspnea, chest tightness, and pleuritic pain. Signs are initially absent, but consolidation and pleural fluid or a friction rub may be detected. If a large enough volume (greater than 75%) of lung is treated at dosages greater than 45 Gy, then cor pulmonale and death can occur. Surviving patients experience a protracted phase that slowly resolves. Lung function abnormalities are generally not detected for 4–8 weeks after completion of irradiation. Restrictive changes with volume loss occur, accompanied by a fall in diffusion capacity with mild arterial hypoxemia. Hypoperfusion of the irradiated area and decreased lung compliance can be demonstrated. The earliest radiographic changes (1–3 months after therapy) are a diffuse infiltrate corresponding to the radiation field with volume loss.

Chronic fibrosis is seen months to years after therapy, but most changes are apparent by 1–2 years. Most patients are asymptomatic, but chronic respiratory impairment with dyspnea, orthopnea, cyanosis, or cor pulmonale may oc-

TABLE 19-9. *Evaluation of patients at risk for late effects: cardiac*

Late effects	Causative treatment			Signs and symptoms	Screening and diagnostic tests	Management and intervention
	Chemotherapy	Radiation				
Cardiomyopathy	Anthracycline >300 mg/m^2 >200 mg/m^2 and radiotherapy to mediastinum High-dose CTX Bone marrow transplantation Possibly ifosfamide	>35 Gy >25 Gy and anthracyclines		Fatigue, cough, dyspnea on exertion, peripheral edema, hypertension, tachypnea and rales, tachycardia, cardiomegaly (S3/S4), hepatomegaly, syncope, palpitations, arrhythmias	ECG, ECHO and radionuclide angiogram, and CXR baselines, q 1–5 yr (depending on risk factors) Holter monitor and exercise testing for baseline, PRN, and after high cumulative anthracycline dosage (>300 mg/m^2)	Diuretics, digoxin, afterload reduction, antiarrhythmics, cardiac transplant, education regarding risks of: isometric exercises, alcohol consumption, drug use, smoking, pregnancy, anesthesia
Valvular damage (mitral and tricuspid aortic)		>35 Gy		Weakness, cough, dyspnea on exertion, new murmur, pulsating liver	ECHO and CXR (baseline), q 3–5 yr then PRN	
Pericardial damage		>35 Gy		Fatigue, dyspnea on exertion, chest pain, cyanosis, ascites, peripheral edema, hypotension, friction rub, muffled heart sounds, venous distension, pulsus paradoxus	ECG (ST–T changes, decreased voltage), ECHO, CXR baseline, q 3–5 yr	Penicillin prophylaxis for surgery or dental procedures Pericardial stripping
Coronary artery disease		>30 Gy		Chest pain on exertion (radiates to arm and neck), dyspnea, diaphoresis, pallor, hypotension, arrhythmias	ECG q 3 yr Stress test (consider thallium scintigraphy) baseline, q 3–5 yr or PRN	Diuretics, cardiac medications Low-sodium, low-fat diet, conditioning regimens

CXR, chest radiograph; ECG, electrocardiogram; ECHO, echocardiogram; PRN, as needed.
From Mertens AC, Yasui Y, Neglia JP, et al. Late mortality experience in five-year survivors of childhood and adolescent cancer: the Childhood Cancer Survivor Study. *J Clin Oncol* 2001;19:3163–3172, with permission.

cur. Maximum breathing capacity and tidal volume decrease. Chest radiographs show linear streaking that may extend outside the irradiated field. Regional contraction, pleural thickening, and tenting of the diaphragm occur. The hilum may retract, with resulting compensatory hyperinflation of adjacent lung. CT and perfusion scans have been used to demonstrate and quantitate these changes (291–293).

Radiation Dosage and Volume Parameters

In the modern management of pediatric malignancies, RT often is given in combination with chemotherapy. It is important to recognize that many chemotherapeutic agents either induce lung damage on their own or potentiate the damaging effects of radiation on the lung. Bleomycin, cyclophosphamide, and, to a lesser extent, vincristine also enhance the damaging effects of thoracic irradiation (293).

Changes in lung function in children treated to the whole lung for metastatic Wilms' tumor have been reported. A dosage of 12–14 Gy reduced total lung capacity and vital capacity to about 70% of predicted values, and even lower if the patient had undergone thoracotomy. Fractionation of dosage decreases this risk (293–295). Bleomycin alone can produce pulmonary toxicity and, when combined with radiation therapy, can heighten radiation reactions. Chemotherapeutic agents such as doxorubicin, dactinomycin, and busulfan are radiomimetic agents and can reactivate latent radiation damage (293,294,296).

The development of bleomycin-associated pulmonary fibrosis with permanent restrictive disease is dose dependent, usually occurring at dosages greater than 200 U/m^2, higher than those used in pediatric malignancies (296–298). Mefferd et al. (299) evaluated lung function in 20 children with HD treated with mechlorethamine, vincristine, procarbazine, prednisone/doxorubicin, bleomycin, vinblastine, dacarbazine (MOPP/ABVD) and 1,500- to 2,500-cGy mantle radiation and found 55% to have abnormal diffusing capacity. Marina et al. (300) evaluated serial pulmonary function in children treated with cyclophosphamide, vincristine, procarbazine (COP)/ABVD and mantle radiotherapy and found 65–73% to have only

mildly decreased or normal diffusing capacity. Nysom et al. (301,302) reviewed pulmonary toxicity in survivors of childhood ALL, HD, and non-Hodgkin's lymphoma and found some abnormalities as measured by pulmonary function testing. Of note, clinical symptoms were uncommon and generally not correlated with pulmonary function test results in these studies. After 35- to 40-Gy mantle irradiation for HD, pneumonitis has been documented in 5% of patients. Lowering the radiation dosage to 15–25 Gy essentially eliminates this complication. Therapy with corticosteroids decreases symptoms but must be withdrawn slowly (303). This should be specifically remembered in the unusual instance in which a patient receives full-dose thoracic RT as part of conditioning and then goes on to HSCT for recurrent HD.

Patients who are treated with HSCT are at greater risk of pulmonary toxicity, related to preexisting pulmonary dysfunction (e.g., asthma, pretransplant therapy); to the preparative regimen, which may include cyclophosphamide, busulfan, carmustine, and TBI; and to the presence of graft-versus-host disease (304–309). Although most transplant survivors are not clinically compromised, restrictive lung disease may occur. Obstructive disease is less common, as is the recently described late-onset pulmonary syndrome, which includes the spectrum of restrictive and obstructive disease. Bronchiolitis obliterans, with or without organizing pneumonia, diffuse alveolar damage, and interstitial pneumonia may occur as a component of this syndrome, generally 6–12 months after transplant. Cough, dyspnea, or wheezing may occur with either normal chest radiograph or diffuse or patchy infiltrates; however, most patients are symptom free (308,309).

Cerveri et al. (304) evaluated pulmonary function tests in survivors of pediatric HSCT at baseline, and at 3–6, 12, and 24 months after transplant. Before transplant, at 3–6 months after transplant, and at 24 months after transplant, 44%, 85%, and 62% of children, respectively, had abnormal pulmonary function tests. A restrictive abnormality was most common at 3–6 months after transplant. Data on type of abnormality by follow-up period are shown in Fig. 19-14 (304).

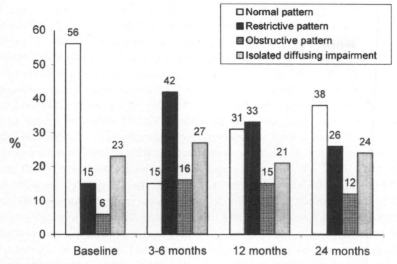

FIG. 19-14. Distribution of different respiratory function patterns in patients before bone marrow transplant and 3–6 months, 12 months, and 24 months after transplant. (From Cerveri I, Fulgoni P, Giorgiani G. Lung function abnormalities after bone marrow transplantation in children: has the trend recently changed? *Chest* 2001;120:1900–1906, with permission.)

Fryer et al. (288) and Keane et al. (310) analyzed the relationship between single doses of irradiation to the whole lung and resulting fatal pneumonitis. After correction for an increased lung transmission of 15–20%, a dose–response relationship was generated. Lethal pneumonitis was seen in 5% of patients after 8.2 Gy, 50% after 9.3 Gy, and 90% after 11 Gy. Thus, a difference of 2 Gy could change mortality from 0% to 50%, which emphasizes the importance of correcting for lung density. Increasing the dose rate from 0.1 to 0.5 Gy per minute increased the frequency of injury from 50% to 90%. TBI for BMT is associated with acute and sometimes fatal pneumonitis and with chronic pulmonary compromise (311). The risk of acute pneumonitis increases from 5% after autologous transplantation to 20% after allogeneic. The use of fractionated and low-dose rate regimens may decrease the risk.

The true overall prevalence or incidence of pulmonary dysfunction in childhood cancer survivors is unknown. No large cohort studies have been performed with clinical evaluations coupled with functional and quality-of-life assessments. A recent analysis of self-reported pulmonary complications of 12,390 survivors of common childhood malignancies has been re-

ported by the CCSS. This cohort includes children treated with both conventional and myeloablative therapies. Compared with siblings, survivors had a higher relative risk of lung fibrosis, recurrent pneumonia, chronic cough, pleurisy, use of supplemental oxygen therapy, abnormal chest wall, exercise-induced shortness of breath, and bronchitis, with relative risks ranging from 1.2 to 13.0, highest for lung fibrosis and lowest for bronchitis. The 25-year cumulative incidence of lung fibrosis was 5% for those who received CRT and less than 1% for those who received pulmonary toxic chemotherapy (PTC). For more subjective complaints, the 25-year cumulative incidences were higher as follows: chronic cough, 15% for combined CRT and PTC, 12% CRT alone, 6% PTC alone; exercise-induced shortness of breath, 20% CRT and PTC, 15% CRT alone, 6% PTC alone. Treatment-related risk factors included chest radiation for lung fibrosis, supplemental oxygen therapy, recurrent pneumonia, exercise-induced shortness of breath, and chronic cough. Cyclophosphamide increased the risk of exercise-induced shortness of breath, supplemental oxygen therapy, chronic cough, bronchitis, and recurrent pneumonia. Bleomycin increased risk of supplemental oxygen therapy, bronchitis, and chronic cough. Busulfan increased the risk of chronic cough and pleurisy. Doxorubicin was associated with a higher risk of emphysema, supplemental oxygen therapy, chronic cough, and shortness of breath. Nitrosoureas were associated with a greater risk of supplemental oxygen therapy. Three survivors had undergone a lung transplant, and another three survivors developed adenocarcinoma of the lung as a second malignancy. Risk continues to increase with time since diagnosis (312). With changes and dosages in RT used since the late 1980s, the incidence of these abnormalities is likely to decrease. However, longer follow-up is needed to confirm this hypothesis.

Table 19-10 reviews several pulmonary late effects with respect to causative treatments, signs and symptoms, screening and diagnostic tests, and management and intervention (80).

Ovary

Radiation and chemotherapy can cause transitory or permanent effects on reproductive capacity, endocrine integrity, and sexual function. The concerns of survivors range from their functional status to consequences on the health of their offspring. The complexity of defining these sequelae stems from the dose-dependent effects caused by different chemotherapy agents, RT, and their combination. Injury to the ovaries can cause both sterilization and suppressed hormone production because of the relationship of the latter to the presence of ova and maturation of the primary follicle (313). Therefore, affected patients can have impaired development of secondary sexual characteristics, menstrual irregularities including amenorrhea, and symptoms associated with menopause such as hot flashes, loss of libido, and osteoporosis (314–317).

Pathophysiology

The ovary produces oocytes and secretes steroid hormones. Active mitosis of oogonia occurs during fetal life, reaching a peak of 6 million at 5 months after conception, dropping to 2 million at birth, with only 100,000 present at puberty (318,319). The cortices of the ovaries harbor the follicles within connective tissue. The follicles arise from the germinal epithelium, which covers the free surface of the ovary. Through involution, atresia, and, to a much lesser extent, ovulation, the follicles disappear entirely at menopause. Hypothalamic gonadotropin-releasing hormone (GnRH) surges in late childhood to initiate puberty. GnRH stimulates release of the pituitary gonadotrophs, which orchestrate follicular maturation (follicle-stimulating hormone, FSH) and ovarian luteinization (LH). With sexual maturity comes the 28-day cycle with an estrogen-dependent midcycle surge of FSH and LH. After ovulation, the corpus luteum forms and produces progesterone, estradiol, and 17-hydroxyprogesterone, and the resultant endometrial changes. Without chorionic gonadotropin from a conceptus, the corpus luteum is exhausted and progesterone and estrogen fall. As FSH increases, the endometrium sloughs (menstruation). The normal premenopausal ovary, $4 \times 3 \times 2$ cm in size, contains degenerating ova and follicles in varying stages of maturity. Ovarian hormones have critical physiologic effects on other organs, including maturation and maintenance of the breasts and vagina, bone mineralization, integrity of the cardiovascular system, and libido. With depletion of oocytes by radiation, chemotherapy, or aging, the ovaries undergo atresia, and menstruation and estrogen production cease.

Radiation causes a decrease in the number of small follicles, impaired follicular maturation, cortical fibrosis and atrophy, generalized hypoplasia, and hyalinization of the capsule. These effects are more direct and indirect through vascular sclerosis (127). Alkylating chemotherapeutic agents affect the resting oocyte in a dose-dependent, cell cycle–independent manner. Thecal cells and ova are depleted, as are the primordial follicles, resulting in arrest of follicular maturation and decreased estrogen secretion. Because girls treated before puberty have a greater complement of ova than do older women, ovarian function is more resistant to RT in younger girls.

Clinical Manifestations

The dosage of radiation that will ablate ovarian function depends on the patient's stage of devel-

TABLE 19-10. *Evaluation of patients at risk for late effects: pulmonary*

Late effects	Causative treatment		Signs and symptoms	Screening and diagnostic tests	Management and intervention
	Chemotherapy	Radiation			
Pulmonary fibrosis	Bleomycin, lomustine, carmustine, CPM, methotrexate, mitomycin, vinca alkaloids	Pulmonary RT 15–20 Gy Risk increases with dosage, larger volume irradiated, and younger age	Fatigue, cough, dyspnea on exertion, reduced exercise tolerance, orthopnea, cyanosis, finger clubbing, rales, cor pulmonale	Baseline chest radiograph and O_2 saturation, pulmonary function test including diffusing capacity of lung for carbon monoxide, then q 3–5 yr or as needed	Consider pulmonary evaluation, steroid therapy Prevention: avoidance of smoking Avoidance of infections: influenza vaccine, Pneumovax After bleomycin: avoid $Fio_2 > 30\%$ intraoperatively and postoperatively Avoid excessive hydration

CPM, cyclophosphamide.
From Constine LS, Hobbie W, Schwartz C. Facilitated assessment of chronic treatment by symptom and organ systems. In: Schwartz C, Hobbie W, Constine L, et al., eds. *Survivors of childhood cancer: assessment and management.* St Louis: Mosby, 1994:21–80, with permission.

opment and whether the dosage is fractionated. Data from Ash (320) summarized the effect of fractionated RT on ovarian function in women of reproductive age (Table 19-11). Ovaries in younger girls are more resistant to the effects of RT than those of adolescents. When one considers dosages to the ovary, after single fractions, temporary sterility can occur with ovarian dosages of 1.7–6.4 Gy and permanent sterility after 3.2–10 Gy (321). Wallace et al. (322) reviewed data to estimate an LD_{50} of 600 cGy for the oocyte. Whole abdomen dosages of 20–30 Gy are associated with primary or premature secondary ovarian failure (322,323).

Stillman et al. (324) studied girls less than 17 years old who were treated with 12–15 Gy, and they confirmed the relationship between ovarian failure and radiation dosage. Ovarian failure occurred in 17 of 25 girls (68%) whose ovaries received the full irradiation dosage. Five of 35 girls (14%) with at least one ovary at the edge of the abdominal treatment volume (estimated dosage 0.9–10 Gy with a mean of 2.9 Gy) experienced ovarian failure. None of 34 girls who received an estimated ovarian dosage of 0.5–1.5 Gy (mean 0.54 Gy), by having at least one ovary outside the treatment volume, had ovarian failure. It is possible that direct or scattered irradiation from the spinal component of craniospinal irradiation may produce ovarian damage (322,325).

To shield the ovaries from direct irradiation during, for example, pelvic irradiation from HD, an oophoropexy may be performed. Typically, the ovaries are moved to a midline position in front of or behind the uterus. Alternately, they may be moved laterally to the iliac wings, which is particularly helpful for young girls or adolescents undergoing irradiation to the midline central pelvis. The ovaries should be marked by the surgeon with clips that can later be identified by a simulator film. Central pelvic blocking at the time of "inverted Y" field will prevent direct irradiation, although scatter dose and transmitted dose will be inevitable. Medial or lateral transposition of the ovaries results in ovarian dosages of 8–10% and 4–5%, respectively, of the pelvic dosage (326–328). For most patients this is compatible with preservation of fertility, although there may be temporary amenorrhea. In a review of HD treated at Stanford University Medical Center, 11 of 11 girls less than 13 years old treated with upper abdominal radiation and 7 of 7 treated to the pelvis with midline ovarian blocking retained ovarian function (283).

Sklar et al. (329) documented amenorrhea and the failure to develop secondary sexual characteristics in prepubertal girls who received 10 Gy TBI and ovarian failure in all pubertal women, of whom 50% had menopausal symptoms. Sanders et al. (330) evaluated gonadal function in HSCT survivors 1–11 years after marrow transplantation. All 15 women less than 26 years old and 3 of 9 more than 26 years old who were treated with 200 mg/kg cyclophosphamide recovered normal gonadotropin levels and menstruation. Three of 38 women who were prepared with 120 mg/kg cyclophosphamide and 920–1,200 cGy TBI had normal gonadotropin levels and menstruation.

Because radiotherapy is no longer used as a single modality to treat most forms of childhood

TABLE 19-11. *Effect of fractionated irradiation on ovarian function in women of reproductive age*

Minimum ovarian dosage (Gy)[a]	Effect
0.6	No deleterious effect.
1.5	No deleterious effect in most young women. Some risk of sterilization especially in women age >40.
2.5–5.0	Variable. Age 15–40 yr: about 60% sterilized permanently. Aged >40: 100% sterilized permanently.
5–8	Variable. Age 15–40 yr: about 70% sterilized permanently, temporary amenorrhea in some of remainder.
>8	100% permanently sterilized.

[a]No attempt has been made to allow for variation in mode of fractionation.
Modified from Ash P. The influence of radiation on fertility in man. *Br J Radiol* 1980;53:271–278, with permission.

cancer, the effects of chemotherapy must also be considered. Cyclophosphamide, nitrogen mustard (mechlorethamine), busulfan, and other alkylating agents and nitrosoureas are capable of causing ovarian dysfunction (313,331,332). Risk of menstrual irregularity, ovarian failure, and infertility increase with age at treatment (333–338). Ovarian function apparently is more resistant to large cumulative dosages of cyclophosphamide in prepubertal girls than in adults (339). Chapman et al. (315) documented chemotherapy-induced ovarian failure in 84% of women older than 30 years, compared with 31% in women under that age, at the time of therapy. Therefore, amenorrhea and premature ovarian failure occur more commonly in adult women treated with cyclophosphamide and other alkylating agents than with adolescents, with prepubertal girls tolerating cumulative dosages as high as 25 g/m^2 (334,340). However two large studies of survivors treated through the 1980s have shown elevated relative risks for infertility and early menopause in female survivors of childhood cancer (323,341). In a study of 2,498 survivors and 3,509 siblings treated between 1945 and 1975, there was a 7% fertility deficit among female survivors as compared with their siblings. Forty-two percent of those with alkylating agent exposure and abdominal radiation experienced menopause by age 31 years (323). In another study of 719 survivors treated between 1964 and 1988, there was a 15.5% failure to conceive (341). Mechlorethamine and procarbazine together are perhaps the most damaging of the agents. Substitution of cyclophosphamide for mechlorethamine appears to have significantly reduced the risk of ovarian dysfunction, which is further lessened by reduction in total dosage of both agents (342). More time must elapse before the effect on premature menopause can be evaluated.

Table 19-12 reviews several ovarian late effects with respect to causative treatments, signs and symptoms, screening and diagnostic tests, and management and intervention (80).

Testes

Germ cell integrity, Leydig and Sertoli cell functioning, and the neuromuscular control of ejaculation are vulnerable to cancer therapy. Although fertility and hormone production are closely related in the ovary because of their dependence on the ova and primary follicle, these functions differ in the testes because of the differing sensitivity of the spermatogonia and Leydig cells to cytotoxic therapy. Therefore, the effects of surgery, radiation, and chemotherapy must be considered in the context of various specific functions.

Pathophysiology

Spermatogenesis, or the formation of spermatozoa from immature germ cells, takes place in the seminiferous epithelium in the tubules The least differentiated germ cells, the spermatogonia, divide to form spermatocytes. Immediately after formation, these cells undergo meiosis to form spermatids, which then metamorphose into motile spermatozoa. This process may take up to 74 days (343). A constant supply of germ cell precursors is essential to the continuous production of spermatozoa, which are then transported through the lumen of the seminiferous tubules into the epididymis, where they are stored. Leydig cells are the primary androgen-secreting cells and account for at least 75% of the total testosterone produced by the normal man (344). Normal secretion of LH by the pituitary gland is essential for Leydig cell function; LH levels rise if inadequate androgen is produced. The physiologic role of FSH in spermatogenesis is to trigger an event in the immature testis that is essential for the completion of spermiogenesis. FSH levels rise if such spermatid differentiation is compromised. Once the process of spermatogenesis is established, it proceeds continuously as long as the supply of testosterone is available. Testosterone also stimulates the development of male secondary sex characteristics and, through negative feedback, pituitary LH secretion. Measurement of testosterone production by the testis therefore is of major significance in the evaluation of testicular function. However, because intact Leydig cell function is necessary for normal spermatogenesis, these measurements may not be necessary when sperm production is determined to be normal (343).

TABLE 19-12. *Evaluation of patients at risk for late effects: ovarian*

Late effects	Causative treatment				Screening and diagnostic tests	Management and intervention
	Chemotherapy	Radiation	Surgery	Signs and symptoms		
Ovarian failure	Nitrogen mustard, cyclophosphamide, procarbazine, busulfan, melphalan, dacarbazine, carmustine, lomustine, ifosfamide	4–12 Gy Tolerance decreases with increasing age	Oophorectomy or oophoropexy	Delayed, arrested, or absent pubertal development, including breasts, female escutcheon, female habitus, vaginal estrogen effect, development of body odor and acne Changes in duration, frequency, and character of menses (cramping) Estrogen deficiency: hot flashes, vaginal dryness, dyspareunia, low libido, infertility	Tanner stage Leutinizing hormone, follicle-stimulating hormone, estradiol: 1) Age 12 yr 2) Failure of pubertal development 3) Baseline when fully mature 4) As needed Assess basal body temperature (midcycle elevation suggests ovulation) Dehydroepiandrosterone for failure of development	Hormone replacement (estrogen), anticipatory guidance regarding symptoms of estrogen deficiency and early menopause Referral to reproductive endocrinology Alternative strategies for parenting, early intervention (hormone replacement may prevent osteoporosis, atherosclerosis)

From Constine LS, Hobbie W, Schwartz C. Facilitated assessment of chronic treatment by symptom and organ systems. In: Schwartz C, Hobbie W, Constine L, et al., eds. *Survivors of childhood cancer: assessment and management.* St Louis: Mosby, 1994:21–80, with permission.

Clinical Manifestations

There can be no question that RT can cause infertility. The testes can be irradiated directly, by scattered irradiation, or by radiation transmitted through shielding blocks. Because the spermatogonia are exquisitely sensitive to radiation, even small dosages can produce measurable damage. Depression of sperm counts is discernible at dosages as low as 15 cGy. This decrease in sperm counts may evolve 3–6 weeks after irradiation, and, depending on the dosage, recovery may take 1–3 years. The germinal epithelium is damaged by much lower dosages (less than 1 Gy) of RT than are Leydig cells (20–30 Gy) (338). Complete sterilization may occur with fractionated irradiation to a dosage of 1–2 Gy (345). Spermatocytes generally fail to complete maturation division at dosages of 2–3 Gy and are visibly damaged after 4–6 Gy with resulting azoospermia. Higher dosages are necessary to damage spermatids than will damage the more sensitive spermatocytes. This sensitivity is convincingly demonstrated by Heller (346), who documented changes in sperm counts in men after various single doses of irradiation. Oligospermia occurred after a dosage as low as 0.5 Gy. Recovery to normal cell counts took 9–18 months after dosages lower than 1 Gy, 30 months after 2–3 Gy, and 5 or more years after 4–6 Gy. At the highest dosages, permanent sterility is common. At lower dosages, this reduced sperm count is seen 60–80 days after exposure, which is the time at which maturation would otherwise be complete (346).

A variety of studies have shown that multiple small fractions of radiation are more toxic to spermatogenesis than a large, single fraction. This has been called the reverse fractionation effect. It is the result of the extreme radiosensitivity of the testicular germinal epithelium, the small number of stem cells, and rapid cell turnover (345,346). Table 19-13 summarizes the fractionated dose-related effect on spermatogenesis and Leydig cell function (320).

For abdominal RT, the effect of the testes results from scatter. Sklar et al. (347) evaluated the effect of 12 Gy radiation to the abdomen on testicular function of long-term ALL survivors and found 55% to have evidence of germ cell dys-

function. Scatter from abdominal radiation with dosages greater than 20 Gy for HD can cause transient elevation in FSH and oligospermia but there is no effect with lower dosages (348). Shalet et al. (349) evaluated 10 men treated for Wilms' tumor as a child. After scattered irradiation dosages of 2.7–9.8 Gy in 20 fractions, 8 (80%) had oligospermia or azoospermia and 7 (70%) had an elevated FSH. When patients are treated for HD, the scattered dosage to the testes from a mantle or para-aortic field is negligible. However, when the pelvis is treated, the calculated dosage depends on the relative location of the testes to the inguinal field, with dosages ranging from 3% to 10% without a specially designed testes shield and less than 1% with such a shield. Therefore, less than 2 Gy is delivered or scattered with well-designed shielding, and this dosage can be reduced further with use of multileaf collimation. That is, the transmitted dosage through the leaves is less than through cut blocks. The available data on males treated for HD suggest that fertility is either maintained or only transiently depressed.

The effects of RT often are combined with those of chemotherapy, particularly alkylating agents. In a study of patients treated at Stanford for pediatric HD, with median follow-up of 9 years, data on gonadal function were available on 15 postpubertal males. Among the eight boys treated with radiation alone, four were able to father a child (three after 40–45 Gy pelvic radiation dosage, one without pelvic radiation) 3–19 years after treatment. Three others who received 30–44 Gy pelvic radiation were oligospermic when tested at 10–15 years after treatment. Semen analyses in 10 of 12 (83%) boys who had been treated with six cycles of mechlorethamine, Oncovin (vincristine), procarbazine, and prednisone (MOPP) with or without pelvic radiation revealed absolute azoospermia with no evidence of recovery up to 11 years later. Age at time of MOPP administration did not ameliorate effect. After prolonged azoospermia, 2 of the 12 boys (17%) had recovery of fertility, with normalization of sperm count or ability to procreate at 12 and 15 years after treatment (328).

A retrospective study was conducted of gonadal and sexual function of 77 adult male sur-

TABLE 19-13. *Effect of fractionated testicular irradiation on spermatogenesis and Leydig cell function*

Testicular dosage (Gy)	Effect on spermatogenesis	Effect on Leydig cell function
<0.1	No effect.	No effect
0.1–0.3	Temporary oligospermia. Complete recovery by 12 mo.	No effect
0.3–0.5	Temporary azoospermia at 4–12 mo after RT. 100% recovery by 48 mo.	Variable
0.5–1.0	100% temporary azoospermia for 3–17 mo after RT. Recovery beginning at 8–26 mo.	Transient rise in FSH with eventual normalization
1–2	100% azoospermia from 2 mo to at least 9 mo. Recovery beginning at 11–20 mo, with return of sperm counts at 30 mo.	Transient rise in FSH and LH
2–3	100% azoospermia beginning at 1–2 mo. Some suffer permanent azoospermia; others show recovery starting at 12–14 mo. Reduced testicular volume.	Prolonged rise in FSH with some recovery. Slight increase in LH. No change in testosterone
3–4	100% azoospermia. No recovery observed up to 40 mo. All have reduced testicular volume.	Permanent elevation in FSH. Transient rise in LH. Reduced testosterone response to HCG stimulation
12	Permanent azoospermia. Reduced testicular volume.	Elevated FSH and LH. Low testosterone. Decreased or absent testosterone response to HCG stimulation. Testosterone replacement may be needed to ensure pubertal changes
>24	Permanent azoospermia. Reduced testicular volume.	Effects more severe and profound than at 12 Gy. Prepubertal testes appear more sensitive to the effects of radiation. Replacement hormone treatment probably needed in all prepubertal cases

FSH, follicle-stimulating hormone; HCG, human chorionic gonadotropin; LH, luteinizing hormone; RT, radiotherapy. Modified from Green DM. Fertility and pregnancy outcome after treatment for cancer in childhood or adolescence. *Oncologist* 1997;2:171–179, with permission.

vivors of childhood malignancies treated at a single center from 1970 to 1989 and followed for a median of 13 years. One-third of the patients were treated for hematologic malignancies, one-third for CNS tumors, and one-third for other malignancies. Eleven patients needed androgen substitution after treatment for tumors of the HP region or acute lymphoblastic leukemia, including testicular irradiation or orchiectomy. In three patients the testicles were removed. The other eight had small testicles, those providing sperm samples had azoospermia, and sexual function was disturbed in most of them. Most of the remaining 66 patients had small testicles. Normozoospermia was found in 63%, oligozoospermia in 20%, and azoospermia

in 17%. Although there was a highly significant correlation between testicular volume and sperm test, 25% of patients with testicles of less than 10 mL had normozoospermia. Sexual function was normal in 46 patients. Twenty-one patients had no signs of gonadal dysfunction (350).

The limited data available indicate that chemical changes in Leydig cell function are observable after direct testicular irradiation. Shalet et al. (351) studied 11 boys irradiated with 24 Gy in 12–16 fractions for a testicular relapse of ALL. Abnormalities of gonadotropin secretion consistent with testicular damage were seen in 9 (82%) of the boys. The mechanism for the increase in FSH is not entirely clear, but it is inversely proportional to the loss of germ cells in the seminiferous tubules. A study of boys who had received 24 Gy of testicular irradiation and who were followed up, on average, 3.8 years after irradiation found that basal testosterone levels were normal in the 12 prepubertal boys. Basal LH levels were normal in 9 and elevated in 3. Plasma testosterone response to human chorionic gonadotropin (HCG) was diminished in 10 and normal in 2. There were 9 pubertal patients. Basal testosterone levels were normal in 3 and diminished in 6. Response of testosterone to HCG was normal in 2 and diminished in 7. There was a correlation between age and response to HCG stimulation ($r = 0.46$) (352). Figure 19.15 depicts the relationship of radiation dosage to testosterone production as gleaned from several reports (344).

Gonadal function was studied in 33 male childhood cancer survivors 2–18 years after treatment to analyze different diagnostic methods and were compared with the results of equivalent tests in 23 age-matched normal controls. These survivors had elevated levels of LH and FSH before ($p < 0.05$; $p < 0.001$) and after ($p < 0.01$; $p < 0.001$) stimulation with GnRH. They also exhibited lower testicular volumes than normal control subjects, as measured with a Prader orchidometer

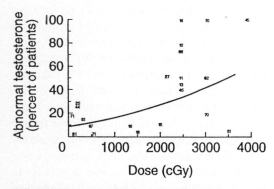

FIG. 19-15. Percentage of patients with an abnormal testosterone value plotted against the stated radiation dosage to the testicles. The curve shows the best fit (extrapolated from the values by logistic regression). (From Izard M. Leydig cell function and radiation: a review of the literature. *Radiother Oncol* 1995;34:1–8, with permission; see Fig. 3 for references from which data were obtained.)

($p < 0.01$) or by ultrasonography ($p < 0.001$). Whereas all spermiograms of normal control subjects ($n = 8$) showed a normal sperm cell density (SCD), only 2 of 14 male survivors exhibited a normal SCD ($p < 0.001$). Treatment with alkylating agents and higher dosages of abdominal radiotherapy increased risk. All male long-term survivors with testicular volumes below the normal range (less than 13 mL) and basal FSH levels above the normal range (more than 10 IU/L) exhibited azoospermia, whereas survivors with normal values for testicular volume and basal FSH had a normal SCD (353).

The germinal epithelium of prepubertal testes is susceptible to damage produced by several chemotherapeutic agents including cyclophosphamide, nitrogen mustard, and procarbazine. Testicular biopsies after chemotherapy have demonstrated aplasia of the germinal epithelium. Spermatogenesis is highly sensitive to cyclophosphamide, with a dose–response relationship and an effect exacerbated by coadministration of other alkylating agents, such as procarbazine (335,354–359). This was illustrated in a study by Bokemeyer et al. (360) in which long-term gonadal toxicity was compared among survivors of HD and non-Hodgkin's lymphoma (NHL). Both groups had received comparable median cumulative dosages of cyclophosphamide, but only the patients with HD received procarbazine. The incidence of gonadal toxicity was more than three times higher in the men in the HD group. The only men in the NHL group who had FSH elevation had received far higher dosages of cyclophosphamide than the mean (360). With the common use of multiagent therapy that includes cyclophosphamide, patients with sarcoma are also at greater risk of infertility, again with a dose–response effect (361–363). Although boys who are younger at the time of treatment demonstrate less of an effect on germinal epithelium, prepubertal boys are not spared because there is less reserve of stem spermatogonia with higher proliferative potential (355). Reduction of alkylating agent therapy in multiagent protocols has reduced the risk of male infertility (335,350, 357,358,364). Review of the available studies has led to the consensus that boys who receive less than 4 g/m^2 of cyclophosphamide without any other alkylating agents and without testicular or cranial radiation are likely to retain their fertility. Dosages greater than 9 g/m² are unlikely to result in any conservation of fertility.

More recently, ifosfamide has been used as part of multimodality therapy for a variety of childhood cancers, often in combination with cyclophosphamide or abdominopelvic radiotherapy. Little is known about its long-term gonadal toxicity. A recent study was performed to evaluate fertility in 96 male patients treated with ifosfamide and no other alkylating agents for osteosarcoma. Eleven patients were prepubertal and 85 were postpubertal at the time of chemotherapy. Of the 96 patients, 26 underwent sperm analysis, and 20 showed oligospermia or azoospermia. Patients who received high-dose ifosfamide showed a higher incidence of azoospermia. Six patients were normospermic and received no ifosfamide or lower dosages of ifosfamide. Eight patients fathered a total of 12 children (365).

With the growing use of bone marrow transplantation to treat malignant and nonmalignant diseases, the effects of the transplantation preoperative regimen on reproduction is of interest. High dosages of alkylating agents often are used in the treatment program. After 200 mg/kg of cyclophosphamide and marrow transplantation for aplastic anemia, 18 prepubertal boys who were 2–13 years old at the time of transplantation were evaluated, on average, 9 years after transplant. All boys over 13 years of age have shown normal progression through puberty and have demonstrated normal LH, FSH, and testosterone levels. In 8 patients who underwent semen analysis, 2 are azoospermic and 6 are normal. Another population of prepubertal boys who received either TBI or TBI plus testicular irradiation have been studied. All boys who received TBI plus additional testicular irradiation of 18–24 Gy had delayed development and elevated FSH and LH levels with diminished testosterone levels. The majority of those who received TBI alone had normal LH levels with elevated FSH (366–368).

Current efforts to protect patients from chemotherapy- or radiation-induced damage to spermatogenesis involve eliminating agents known to damage spermatogenesis and optimizing testicular shielding from irradiation.

Table 19-14 reviews several testicular late effects with respect to causative treatments, signs and symptoms, screening and diagnostic tests, and management and intervention (80).

Reproduction and Offspring

Many survivors of childhood cancer previously treated with cytotoxic therapy remain fertile, so pregnancy outcomes and the risk of cancer or genetic disease in offspring must be addressed. Young women who have been exposed to RT below the diaphragm are also at risk of impaired development of the uterus, which can result in adverse pregnancy outcomes. The magnitude of the risk is related to the radiation field, total dosage, and fractionation schedule. This can lead to premature labor and low-birthweight infants. Female long-term survivors treated with TBI and marrow transplantation are also at risk of ovarian follicular depletion, impaired uterine growth and blood flow, and early pregnancy loss and premature labor if pregnancy is achieved. Despite standard hormone replacement, the uterus of these young girls is often reduced to 40% of normal adult size. Uterine volume correlates with the age at which radiation was received (369).

With more childhood cancer survivors retaining their fertility, pregnancy outcome data are now available. In a study of 4,029 pregnancies among 1,915 women followed in the CCSS, there were 63% live births, 1% stillbirths, 15% miscarriages, 17% abortions, and 4% unknown or in gestation. Risk of miscarriage was 3.6 times higher in women treated with craniospinal radiation and 1.7 times higher in those treated with pelvic radiation. Chemotherapy exposure alone did not increase risk of miscarriage. Compared with siblings, survivors were less likely to have live births, more likely to have medical abortions, and more likely to have low-birthweight babies (370). In the same cohort, Green et al. (371) evaluated pregnancy outcomes of partners of male survivors. Among 4,106 sexually active men, 1,227 reported that they sired 2,323 pregnancies, which resulted in 69% live births, 13% miscarriages, 13% abortions, and

TABLE 19-14. *Evaluation of patients at risk for late effects: testicular*

| Late effects | Causative treatment | | | Signs and symptoms | Screening and diagnostic tests | Management and intervention |
	Chemotherapy	Radiation	Surgery			
Germ cell damage: oligospermia and azoospermia	Cyclophosphamide, nitrogen mustard, lomustine and carmustine, procarbazine, ifosfamide, busulfan, melphalan, dacarbazine	1–6 Gy	Orchiectomy or surgical manipulation	Testicular atrophy (softer and smaller), failure to impregnate	Tanner stage, inquire regarding previous sperm banking, determine testicular size and consistency. LH, FSH, testosterone for failure of pubertal development, for baseline when sexually mature, and for failure to impregnate (repeat q 3 yr for possible recovery). Analysis of sperm at maturity or for failure to impregnate (repeat q 3–5 yr to assess recovery)	Instruct on testicular self-examination. Anticipatory guidance regarding germ cell damage. Referral to reproductive endocrinology. Infertility counseling. Alternative strategies for fathering
Leydig cell damage: testosterone deficiency	Cyclophosphamide Etoposide	>24 Gy to the testes (direct or scattered from pelvis)	Orchiectomy	Delayed, arrested, or absent pubertal development, pubic and axillary hair (female hair pattern), lack of penile and testicular enlargement, voice change, body odor and acne, testicular atrophy (softer and smaller)	LH and testosterone at age 13 yr, failure of pubertal development, baseline if sexually mature, changes in libido or sexual performance	Testosterone replacement. Anticipatory guidance regarding testosterone deficiency

FSH, follicle-stimulating hormone; LH, leuteinizing hormone.
From Constine LS, Hobbie W, Schwartz C. Facilitated assessment of chronic treatment by symptom and organ systems. In: Schwartz C, Hobbie W, Constine L, et al., eds. *Survivors of childhood cancer: assessment and management.* St Louis: Mosby, 1994:21–80, with permission.

5% unknown or in gestation at the time of analysis. Compared with partners of male siblings, there a lower chance of live births (RR = 0.77) but no significant differences of pregnancy outcome by treatment. The rate of miscarriage was higher for the partners of male survivors treated with more than 5,000 mg/m^2 of procarbazine, which includes HD survivors treated with more than six cycles of MOPP or cyclophosphamide, vincristine, procarbazine, prednisone (COPP) chemotherapy (RR = 2.44, 95% CI 1.28–4.67).

In the National Wilms Tumor Study, records were obtained for 427 pregnancies of more than 20 weeks' duration. In this group, there were 409 single and 12 twin live births. Early or threatened labor, malposition of the fetus, lower birthweight (less than 2,500 g) and premature delivery (less than 36 weeks) were more common among women who had received flank radiation, in a dose-dependent manner (See Table 13.45 in Chapter 13). Congenital anomalies in the offspring were also more common in this group (372).

Preservation of fertility and successful pregnancies may occur after BMT, although the conditioning regimens, which include TBI, cyclophosphamide, and busulfan, are highly gonadally toxic. In a group of 21 female patients who had received a bone marrow transplant in the prepubertal years, 12 (57%) were found to have ovarian failure when examined between age 11 and 21 years, and the association with busulfan was significant (373). Sanders et al. (374) evaluated pregnancy outcomes in a group of women treated with bone marrow transplant. Among 708 women who were postpubertal at the time of transplant, 116 regained normal ovarian function and 32 became pregnant. Among 82 women who were prepubertal at the time of transplant, 23 had normal ovarian function and 9 became pregnant. Of the 72 pregnancies in these 41 women, 16 occurred in those treated with TBI, and 50% resulted in early termination. Among the 56 pregnancies in women treated with cyclophosphamide without TBI or busulfan, 21% resulted in early termination. There were no pregnancies among the 73 women treated with busulfan and cyclophosphamide, and only 1 retained ovarian function.

Progress in reproductive endocrinology has resulted in the availability of several options for preserving or permitting fertility in patients about to receive potentially toxic chemotherapy or radiotherapy (333,338). For males, cryopreservation of spermatozoa before treatment is an effective method to circumvent the sterilizing effect of therapy. Although pretreatment semen quality in patients with cancer has been shown to be less than that noted in healthy donors, the percentage decline in semen quality and the effect of cryodamage to spermatozoa from patients with cancer is similar to that of normal donors (375–378). For those unable to sperm bank, newer technologies such as testis sperm extraction may be an option, as recently demonstrated for male survivors of germ cell tumors who had postchemotherapy nonobstructive azoospermia (379). Further micromanipulative technologic advances such as intracytoplasmic sperm injection may be able to render sperm extracted surgically, or even poor-quality cryopreserved spermatozoa from cancer patients, capable of successful fertilization (379,380). In prepubertal and postpubertal females, cryopreservation of ovarian cortical tissue or enzymatically extracted follicles and the *in vitro* maturation of prenatal follicles are of potential clinical use. To date, most of this technology has been performed in laboratory animals (381–383). Another option available to the postpubertal female is the stimulation of ovaries with exogenous gonadotropins and retrieval of mature oocytes for cryopreservation. However, only a few oocytes can be harvested after stimulation of the ovaries (382). *In vitro* fertilization and subsequent embryo cryopreservation has also been successful. These options may not be readily available to the pediatric and adolescent patient, and the necessary delay in cancer therapy for ovarian stimulation or *in vitro* fertilization cycles often renders these interventions impractical (383). Furthermore, all these approaches harbor the risk that malignant cells will be present in the specimen and reintroduced in the patient at a later date. Those with hematologic or gonadal tumors would be at greatest risk for this eventuality (382,383).

For childhood cancer survivors who have offspring, there is the concern about congenital anomalies, generic disease, or risk of cancer in the offspring. In the report from the National Wilms Tumor Group, the rate of congenital anomalies was marginally higher in offspring of women who had received flank radiotherapy (372). In a report of 2,198 offspring of adult survivors treated for childhood cancer between 1945 and 1975 compared with 4,544 offspring of sibling control subjects, there were no differences in the proportion of offspring with cytogenetic syndromes, single-gene defects, or simple malformations. There was similarly no effect of type of childhood cancer treatment on the occurrence of genetic disease in the offspring. Survivors treated with abdominal radiotherapy or alkylating agents did not have a higher risk of offspring with genetic disease than did survivors not exposed to these agents (384). Similar results were reported in a single-institution study of 247 offspring of 148 cancer survivors (385).

With increased use of assisted fertility techniques in survivors of childhood cancer, the risk of congenital anomalies must be followed closely due to reports of increased anomalies in offspring born by *in vitro* fertilization or intracytoplasmic sperm injection (386–390).

In a study of 5,847 offspring of survivors of childhood cancers treated in five Scandinavian countries, in the absence of a hereditary cancer syndrome (such as hereditary retinoblastoma), there was no increased risk of cancer (391). Preliminary data from the CCSS indicate that the risk of cancer in offspring was not significantly elevated (standardized independence ratio [SIR] = 1.67; 95% CI 0.80–3.50), but this was based on a small number of offspring ($n = 11$). However, among survivors who themselves had second neoplasms or SMNs, risk of cancer in offspring was significantly elevated (SIR = 15.08; 95% CI 5.29–43.02) and much higher than for offspring of CCSS non-SMN cases (SIR = 1.0; 95% CI 0.38–2.67) ($p < 0.001$) (392). Further follow-up of offspring is needed to see whether patterns of cancer in offspring change with elapsed time.

Kidney

Pathophysiology

The progression of renal dysfunction after irradiation is grouped into three periods (9). The acute period (up to 6 months) is rarely symptomatic, and the glomerular filtration rate may be low. In the subacute period (6–12 months) the signs and symptoms include dyspnea on exertion, headaches, ankle edema, lassitude, anemia, hypertension, albuminuria, papilledema, elevated blood urea, and urinary abnormalities (granular and hyalin casts, red blood cells). Death might result from chronic uremia or left ventricular failure, pulmonary edema, pleural effusion, and hepatic congestion. In the chronic period (generally after 18 months) either benign or malignant hypertension is seen, depending on the severity of the renal insult. Chronic radiation nephropathy in its mildest forms may not be diagnosed until 14 years after therapy. Abnormalities may include only proteinuria and azotemia with urinary casts and mild or no hypertension. A contracted renal size (mild atrophy) is seen on intravenous pyelogram. When chronic nephropathy is severe, death may result.

The pathologic process is a progressive arteriolonephrosclerosis. The lesion involves the microvasculature with injury to the intercellular connections between the renal capillary and arterioles. There is degeneration and sclerosis of these arterioles, with narrowing or occlusion of the lumen and secondary degeneration of dependent structures (glomeruli, tubules). Associated changes in connective tissue include a thickened basement membrane, increased interstitial connective tissue, hyalinization and fibrosis. Decreased perfusion of the kidney can occur with capillary and venous thrombosis and, eventually, necrosis. Withers et al. (393) used animal data to argue for a different pathogenesis, with the essential lesion involving the tubules and with secondary loss of nephrons and parenchymal cell depletion (394).

Clinical Manifestations

Radiation nephropathy is dose-related. Dosages of more than 25 Gy to both kidneys can cause renal failure at delayed intervals of more than 6 months (395,396). The effect of RT on the kidney has best been examined in survivors of pediatric Wilms' tumor, where unilateral nephrectomy is also common. Unilateral irradiation at dosages of 14–20 Gy may reduce the ability of the contralateral (untreated) kidney to undergo compensatory hypertrophy (397). Ritchey et al. (398) examined the spectrum of renal failure in 55 patients among 5,823 patients treated for Wilms' tumor. The incidence of renal failure at 16 years was 0.6% for patients with unilateral disease and 13% for patients with bilateral disease. The most common causes of renal failure were bilateral nephrectomy for persistent or recurrent tumor, progressive tumor in the remaining kidney without nephrectomy, Denys–Drash syndrome, and radiation nephritis. Long-term renal function was subsequently evaluated in 81 children with synchronous bilateral Wilms' tumor who received treatment. With a median follow-up of 27 months, 28 patients had elevated blood urea nitrogen or serum creatinine levels. Of those, 18 had moderate and 10 had marked renal insufficiency. There was no dose–response relationship for chemotherapy, and tumor recurrence necessitating additional surgery increased the risk of renal dysfunction. Those with less than one kidney remaining had more marked dysfunction (399). In another study from the National Wilms' Tumor Group, of children treated from 1969–1995, 58 of 5,976 children developed renal failure at a median follow-up of 11 years. Patients with bilateral disease and unilateral disease had a 20-year renal failure incidence of 5.5% and 1.0%, respectively (See Table 13.43 in Chapter 13). In a recent study

of 40 Wilms' tumor survivors treated in England with combined surgery and chemotherapy, with and without radiation therapy, no significant nephrotoxicity was seen (400). Patients with predisposition syndromes such as Denys–Drash syndrome; Wilms' tumor, aniridia, genitourinary retardation syndrome; or male genitourinary anomalies had a much higher incidence of renal failure at 20 years of 62.4%, 38.3%, and 10.9%, respectively. Presence of intralobar nephrogenic rests in the unilateral disease group without a defined syndrome resulted in an elevated cumulative risk of renal failure at 20 years of 3.3%, compared with 0.7% without this pathologic finding (401).

Dose–volume histograms of renal radiation correlated with various renal function endpoints will be necessary for accurate determination of functional tolerance levels. In a review of several reports, Cassady (395) determined a threshold dosage of approximately 15 Gy delivered with conventional fractionation (in the absence of interactive drugs and underlying renal disease) as a reasonable estimate, and dosages of more than 25 Gy to the total renal mass are likely to eliminate useful renal function in patients followed for sufficiently long periods of time (Fig. 19-16).

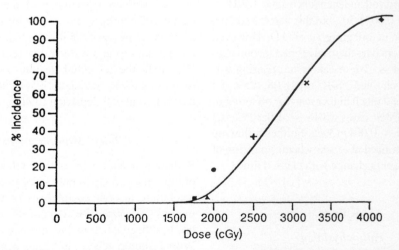

FIG. 19-16. Radiation dose–response curve for the occurrence of symptomatic radiation nephropathy generated from data presented in several reports. An approximate threshold dosage of 15 Gy (conventional fractionation) is seen, and a plateau is noted beyond dosages of 30 Gy. (Modified from Cassady JR. Clinical radiation nephropathy. *Int J Radiat Oncol Biol Phys* 1995;31:1249–1256, with permission.)

Late renal dysfunction has been documented after TBI before BMT for childhood malignancies. Tarbell et al. (402) reported a 35% incidence in children with ALL and a 71% incidence in children with neuroblastoma who received fractionated TBI (12–14 Gy over 3–4 days). All patients had anemia, hematuria, and elevated blood urea nitrogen and creatinine levels. Renal biopsies in two patients showed changes consistent with radiation nephropathy or hemolytic uremic syndrome. The onset of renal dysfunction after TBI is 3–6 months. Therefore, the time course is similar to that of classically described radiation nephritis. Whereas Tarbell et al. (402) found that renal injury occurs at a young age, Lonnerholm et al. (403) found an 18% incidence of renal dysfunction in autografted children without an apparent age effect. With more modern techniques and longer interfraction intervals for TBI, less than 15% of children will develop chronic renal insufficiency or hypertension, and the risk is related both to the nephrotoxic agents used and the TBI fractionation scheme and interfraction interval (308,404). Of interest is that proximal tubular dysfunction is more commonly abnormal than distal tubular function.

Chemotherapy can also adversely affect renal function. Cisplatin at dosages greater than 200 mg/m^2 can result in glomerular or tubular injury and renal insufficiency. Other nephrotoxic agents such as aminoglycosides, amphotericin, and ifosfamide may further increase risk. Effects can be seen acutely and may progress after completion of therapy (405–408). Studies in the early 1990s showed that carboplatin has less acute nephrotoxicity than cisplatin (409–411). However, only a few small studies examining children treated with carboplatin have evaluated short- and long-term nephrotoxicity, finding none significant to date (412,413).

Ifosfamide can also cause glomerular and tubular toxicity, with renal tubular acidosis, or Fanconi's syndrome. Dosages greater than 60 g/m^2, age less than 5 years at time of treatment, and combination with cisplatin and carboplatin increase risk. Abnormalities in glomerular filtration are less common and when found are not clinically significant. More common are abnormalities with proximal greater than distal tubular function, although the prevalence of these findings is uncertain, and further study of larger cohorts with longer follow-up is needed (414–418).

Table 19-15 reviews several renal late effects with respect to causative treatments, signs and symptoms, screening and diagnostic tests, and management and intervention (80).

Digestive Tract

The esophagus, stomach, and small and large intestines are irradiated in a variety of pediatric malignancies. Although primary tumors of these organs are rare in childhood, they may be incidentally irradiated in the treatment of HD and non-Hodgkin's lymphoma, Wilms tumor, neuroblastoma, soft tissue sarcomas, and bone tumors.

The direct effect of digestive tract irradiation is loss of regenerating cells lining the gut. Radiation damage of the fine vasculature of the digestive tract may progress to obliterative vasculitis, with the ultimate development of ischemia (419,420). Acute radiation injury results from the depletion of normally proliferating cell, mucosal sloughing, villus shortening, and subsequent inflammatory infiltration and edema. The patient may suffer from odynophagia, dysphagia, abdominal pain, or diarrhea, depending on the site irradiated. Malabsorption of nutrients and decreased bile salt reabsorption can produce a nutritional wasting state (420). Such nutritional compromise must be treated with the utmost seriousness because it can lead to life-threatening risks of organ failure and, in the long run, severely impair the ability to administer adequate anticancer treatment. The clinician's threshold for the use of vigorous enteral or parenteral nutrition should be low.

Late radiation injury to the digestive tract is attributable to vascular injury. As the radiation vasculopathy progresses to obliteration, necrosis, ulceration, stenosis, or perforation may result (420,421). Late radiation enteropathy is characterized by malabsorption, pain, and recurrent episodes of bowel obstruction, as well as perforation, infection, and death. The onset is generally 6–24 months after the conclusion of radiotherapy. Donaldson et al. (422) evaluated 44 children who

TABLE 19-15. *Evaluation of patients at risk for late effects: genitourinary*

Late effects	Causative treatment			Signs and symptoms	Screening and diagnostic tests	Management and intervention
	Chemotherapy	Radiation	Surgery			
Glomerular dysfunction	Cisplatin, carboplatin			Asymptomatic or with fatigue, poor linear growth, anemia, oliguria	Annual: blood pressure, height, weight, hemoglobin and hematocrit, urinalysis, creatinine, BUN, creatinine clearance baseline and q 3 yr	Low-protein diet, dialysis, renal transplant
Hypoplastic kidney and renal arteriosclerosis		20–30 Gy 10–15 Gy with chemotherapy		Fatigue, poor linear growth, hypertension, headache, edema (ankle, pulmonary), albuminuria, urinary casts, hepatomegaly	Same as for glomerular dysfunction	Same as for glomerular dysfunction
Tubular dysfunction	Cisplatin, carboplatin, ifosfamide			Seizures ($\downarrow$Mg), weakness ($\downarrow$PO$_4$), glycosuria, poor linear growth	Same as for glomerular dysfunction, and Mg, PO$_4$ (24-hr urine for Ca, PO$_4$)	Mg supplement PO$_4$ supplement
Nephrotic syndrome		20–30 Gy		Proteinuria Edema	Urinalysis q yr, blood pressure q yr Serum protein, albumin, Cr, BUN 24-hr urine for protein, Cr	Low-salt diet Diuretics
Bladder: fibrosis or hypoplasia (reduced bladder capacity)	Cyclophosphamide Ifosfamide	>30 Gy prepubertal >50 Gy postpubertal		Urgency, frequency, dysuria, incontinence (nocturia), pelvic hypoplasia	Urinalysis q yr (cystoscopy, intravenous pyelogram, ultrasound: volumetrics)	Exercises to increase bladder capacity Surgical referral

Hemorrhagic cystitis	Cyclophosphamide Ifosfamide	RT enhances chemotherapy effect	Hematuria, frequency, urgency, dysuria, bladder tenderness	Urinalysis q yr to rule out UTI, renal calculi; Cystoscopy if hematuria on 2 exams	Transfusion, antispasmodics, formalin, counsel regarding risk of bladder cancer
Prostate		40–60 Gy (lower dosages inhibit development; higher dosages cause atrophy)	Decreased volume of seminal fluid; Hypoplastic or atrophied prostate	Examination of prostate gland; Semen analysis × 1 (ultrasound)	Counsel regarding possible infertility caused by inadequate seminal fluid; Monitor prostate (exam, ? prostate-specific antigen)
Vagina: fibrosis, diminished growth	Actinomycin D, doxorubicin enhance RT effect	>40 Gy	Painful intercourse, vaginal bleeding, small vaginal vault	Pelvic exam (possibly under anesthesia) for baseline, during puberty, and as needed	Dilations; Reconstructive surgery; Potential need for cesarean section
Uterus: fibrosis, decreased growth		>20 Gy (prepubertal) 40–50 Gy (postpubertal)	Multiple spontaneous abortions; Low birthweight infants; Small uterus	Pelvic exam for baseline, at puberty, then annually	? Endometrial biopsy; Counsel regarding pregnancy
Ureter: fibrosis		50–60 Gy	Frequent UTIs, pelvic hypoplasia, hydronephrosis	Urinalysis q yr; Urethrogram	UTI prophylaxis
Urethra: strictures	GU	>50 Gy	Frequent UTIs, dysuria, stream abnormalities	Urinalysis q yr; Voiding cystogram	UTI prophylaxis; Surgical intervention

BUN, blood urea nitrogen; GU, genitourinary; RT, radiotherapy; UTI, urinary tract infection.
From Constine LS, Hobbie W, Schwartz C. Facilitated assessment of chronic treatment by symptom and organ systems. In: Schwartz C, Hobbie W, Constine L, et al., eds. *Survivors of childhood cancer: assessment and management.* St Louis: Mosby, 1994:21–80, with permission.

received abdominal irradiation for lymphoma, Wilms' tumor, or other malignancies. Eleven percent of the entire population and 36% of the long-term survivors developed bowel obstruction. Contributing factors included prior abdominal surgery, the use of concurrent actinomycin D, and very young age. Late radiation injury to the digestive tract is attributable to vascular injury. Necrosis, ulceration, stenosis, and perforation can occur and are characterized by malabsorption, pain, recurrent episodes of bowel obstruction, perforation, and infection (420,421). In general, fractionated dosages of 20–30 Gy can be delivered to the small bowel without significant long-term morbidity. Dosages greater than 40 Gy are needed to cause bowel obstruction or chronic enterocolitis (423). Sensitizing chemotherapeutic agents such as actinomycin D and anthracyclines can increase this risk. In a report of 42 survivors of Wilms' tumor treated from 1968 to 1994 with megavoltage radiotherapy, actinomycin D, and vincristine with or without doxorubicin, the actuarial incidence of bowel obstruction at 5, 10, and 15 years was $9.5\% \pm 4.5\%$, $13.0\% \pm 5.6\%$, and $17.0\% \pm 6.5\%$. Of 23 patients, 5 irradiated within 10 days of surgery and 1 of 19 irradiated after 10 days developed bowel obstruction (173). In a report from the Intergroup Rhabdomyosarcoma Study Committee, extended follow-up of 86 children and adolescents who were treated for paratesticular rhabdomyosarcoma on the Intergroup Rhabdomyosarcoma Studies I and II (IRS I–II) revealed that four patients who underwent abdominal radiotherapy had chronic diarrhea (361).

The prevention and management of radiation digestive tract injury relies primarily on the exclusion of normal tissues from the treatment beam whenever possible. For the esophagus, stomach, and large bowel, this usually relies on beam direction planning and patient positioning. For the mobile portions of the small bowel, the clinician also evaluates the prone versus supine position; the use of compression, tilt tables, and false table tops; surgical placement of omental slings and absorbable mesh; and other techniques. The patient with acute radiation enteropathy may be helped by symptomatic interventions such as topical anesthetics for esophagitis, antidiarrheal agents, antispasmod-

ics, antiemetics, bile salt–binding agents, and an elemental or lactose-free diet (422). Medical therapy for late-onset radiation enteritis is unsatisfactory and has relied on intermittent steroids, sulfasalazine, parenteral nutrition, and other supportive care. Surgical resection of damaged or obstructed bowel may be used, but there is a high incidence of anastomotic dehiscence, operative mortality, and reobstruction (420).

Liver

The clinical signs and symptoms of radiation hepatitis include abdominal pain, increased girth, ascites, weight gain, jaundice, and elevation of liver enzymes, especially alkaline phosphatase (424,425). Severe thrombocytopenia can be seen, most commonly in children who have also been treated with actinomycin D (426). The clinical and laboratory expression of hepatic injury in terms of its time to expression and association with irradiation with or without chemotherapy is outlined in Table 19-16 (427).

In the acute phase of radiation injury (less than 3 months after irradiation), the liver is hyperemic and enlarged in the treated area (426,428). Dilatation and sinusoidal congestion accompanied by atrophy around the central vein of the lobule may be seen. As the chronic phase evolves (more than 3 months after treatment), characteristic central vein lesions develop. The lumen narrows progressively with fibrotic changes involving the intima, leading to increasing sinusoidal congestion and liver cell atrophy. Inflammatory exudate is uniformly absent. After 6 months and up to 6 years after irradiation, the distance between the central vein and portal space decreases, indicating the atrophy of hepatocytes. Nodules of regeneration are rare. Central veins become small and inconspicuous, and lobules are distorted or collapsed. Concentric fibrosis in the portal spaces around the portal veins occurs. This pathologic picture has been classified as veno-occlusive disease, a process that is accelerated after bone marrow transplantation and can be seen with weeks of conditioning with TBI; with modern chemotherapy and radiotherapy, it is the most critical hepatic toxic-

TABLE 19-16. *Comparison of radiation-induced liver disease and combined modality-induced liver disease*

Clinical feature	Radiation-induced liver disease	Combined-modality liver disease
Time to presentation after treatment	2–16 wk (typically 4–8 wk)	1–4 wk (typically 1–2 wk)
Signs and symptoms		
Jaundice	+	++++
Weight gain	+++	++++
Right upper quadrant pain	+	+++
Hepatomegaly	++	+++
Ascites	++++	++
Encephalopathy	+/−	++
Laboratory findings		
Elevated bilirubin	+	++++
Elevated aspartate aminotransferase	++	++++
Elevated alkaline phosphatase	++++	+++
Outcome	10–20% mortality	30–50% mortality

From Lawrence T, Robertson J, Ansher M, et al. Hepatic toxicity resulting from cancer treatment. *Int J Padiat Oncol Biol Phys* 1995;31:1237–1248, with permission.

ity. It is characterized by occlusion and obliteration of the central veins of the hepatic lobules, with retrograde congestion and secondary necrosis of hepatocytes. Although there may be a dose effect of RT, this complication is also reported after conditioning regimens with cyclophosphamide and busulfan alone. Preexisting hepatic disease, including infection, and GVHD may increase the risk (429–431). Of particular interest is a report from the IRS on the occurrence of veno-occlusive disease in children treated with vincristine, actinomycin D, and cyclophosphamide. Ten patients, or 1.2% of 821 patients, treated according to IRS-IV had evidence of veno-occlusive disease. This incidence was greater than in previous studies and considered to be associated with an escalation of the cyclophosphamide dosage in IRS-IV (432).

The cumulative dosage, volume of liver irradiated, and additional treatment with chemotherapy are important risk factors for hepatic fibrosis. Radiation hepatopathy can occur with dosages of 30–40 Gy to the entire liver, but significantly higher dosages to focal volumes can be given with few clinical complications (433). Lower dosages can be associated with hepatopathy if the child is also receiving sensitizing chemotherapy. This is evident in a series of children treated for Wilms' tumor, neuroblastoma, or hepatoma with radiotherapy to the liver and chemotherapy. Fractionated dosages to 12–25 Gy caused abnormal liver function tests and ra-

dionuclide scans in 50% of patients, 25–35 Gy caused abnormalities in 63%, and more than 35 Gy was toxic in 86% (434). In the National Wilms' Tumor Study, 16 out of 303 patients (5.3%) had liver toxicity. The dosages of radiation to portions of the liver ranged from less than 15 Gy to more than 30 Gy, with right flank or whole abdomen radiation increasing risk significantly more than isolated left flank radiation. The injury was manifest as thrombocytopenia, hepatomegaly, ascites, and, in four cases, hepatic failure. It was interesting to note that 8.6% of patients receiving right flank or whole abdomen irradiation exhibited toxicity, as opposed to 2% of patients receiving left flank irradiation ($p = 0.01$). All patients received chemotherapy, including vincristine, actinomycin D, and, in some patients, doxorubicin (435). In a series by Ingold et al. (426), no cases of radiation-induced liver disease occurred below a dosage of 25 Gy, whereas 21% and 42% of patients had abnormalities after 30–36 Gy and 38–42 Gy, respectively.

The volume of liver irradiated influences tolerance to dosage. The regenerating liver (e.g., after partial hepatectomy) appears to be even less tolerant to irradiation. New developments in three-dimensional organ imaging, in combination with the available clinical data, allow reasonable predictions of the probability of liver injury as a function of radiation dosage. In the absence of chemotherapy, 30 Gy of whole liver irradiation involves a significant risk of radiation hepatitis. In the presence of chemotherapy used to treat childhood malignancy, most authorities are hesitant to treat the whole organ to more than 12 Gy, except perhaps in desperate situations such as that produced by marginally resectable primary hepatic tumors (see Chapter 14). The changes induced in the liver by radiation may be imaged by scintillation nuclear medicine scanning (which will show a cold area), CT, or MRI (425,436).

Table 19-17 reviews several gastrointestinal and hepatic effects with respect to causative treatments, signs and symptoms, screening and diagnostic tests, and management and intervention (80).

Eye

The eye is composed of several tissues that vary greatly in their radiosensitivity. Acute reactions include iridocyclitis, keratitis, conjunctivitis, and blepharitis. Delayed reactions, which generally occur after 6 months, include retinopathy, optic neuropathy, lacrimal gland atrophy or duct stenosis, glaucoma resulting from iridocyclitis, cataract, corneal vascularization and scarring, conjunctival telangiectasia, and eyelid atrophy with entropion or ectropion.

Retina

Radiation retinopathy is characterized by a slowly progressive microangiopathy, which may result in macular edema, capillary nonperfusion, retinal and disk neovascularization, vitreous hemorrhage, and traction retinal detachment. The microangiopathic changes may appear 6 months to 3 years after therapy (437). Visual loss is painless unless neovascular glaucoma develops. Using 1.8–2 Gy per fraction, the threshold for injury is 46 Gy, although the frequency is rare below dosages of 60 Gy. As fraction size increases beyond 2.5 Gy, the frequency of injury increases (438). It is important to note that certain chemotherapeutic agents can cause retinal toxicity, and the risk is higher in children with impaired renal function who thereby accumulate drugs (439).

Lacrimal Apparatus

Radiation may cause scarring of the canaliculi and puncta, ectropion of one punctum, failure of the lacrimal pump secondary to decreased eyelid mobility, and reflex lacrimation associated with ectropion, entropion, or conjunctival keratinization (437). Secondary symptoms can develop within months and be fully developed by 1 year. The patient may suffer from excess tearing, a foreign body sensation, and photophobia secondary to corneal epithelial damage. When injury is severe, corneal ulceration, opacification, and vascularization sufficient to cause visual loss occur. Injury is rare at dosages less than 45 Gy and common above 60 Gy (440).

Lens

Whereas retinitis and lacrimal duct abnormalities are caused only by high RT dosages, low-dose irradiation damages the germinal zone of the epithelium on the equator of the lens (441–446). The radiation-induced cataract is a central, posterior subcapsular opacity that appears as a dot at the posterior pole of the lens. As the cataract enlarges, small vacuoles and granules appear around it. With continued enlargement, the opacity develops a clear center, giving it a doughnut-shaped appearance (437). This progresses to the anterior pole, and the cortex then becomes opaque. Merriam and Focht (447) reported an evaluation of the dose–response relationship in 1957. After single doses of 200 R, abnormalities were detected but were not clinically significant until dosages exceeded 400 R. With fractionated irradiation, a 60% frequency (progressive in one-half) was seen after 750–950 R, whereas 100% was seen after 1,150 R. Other investigators have suggested a threshold for damage of about 2,000 R (448). Reevaluation of atomic bomb survivor data suggests a 20–40% incidence of radiation cataract after a single eye dosage of 5 Gy mixed photons and neutrons (449). The interval to abnormality in various studies is 2–3 years but ranges from 6 months to 35 years depending on dosage.

Patients treated with TBI are also at greater risk of cataracts. Risk ranges from approximately 10% to 60% at 10 years depending on the total dosage and fractionation, with a shorter latency period and more severe cataracts noted after single fraction and higher-dose or higher–dose rate TBI. Deeg et al. (450) reported that 80% of patients were affected after a single dose of 10 Gy but only 19% after fractionated regimens to 12–15 Gy. In a report from France on 494 patients undergoing TBI, high instantaneous dose rate (more than 9 cGy/minute) was identified as the main risk factor for cataractogenesis (451).

Corticosteroids and GVHD may further increase risk. Young children may actually be at a lower risk than adolescents and adults (452–457). Belkacemi et al. (455) reported on cataracts after TBI in a group of 1,063 survivors of leukemia treated with HSCT from the European Group for Blood and Marrow Transplantation. The overall 10-year cataract incidence was 50%: 60% in those who were treated with single-fraction TBI, 43% in those treated with 6 fractions or less, and only 7% in those treated with more than 6 fractions of TBI. In those who received lower–dose rate RT (0.04 Gy/minute or less), the 10-year incidence was 30%, compared with 59% in those treated with more than 0.04 Gy/minute. These data are shown in Fig. 19-17. Independent risk

factors for cataracts in multivariate analysis were age greater than 23 years, higher–dose rate RT (more than 0.04 Gy/minute), allogeneic transplantation, and corticosteroid exposure of more than 100 days.

Radiation-induced cataracts are one of the reported complications of retinoblastoma treatment. Based on first principles, one might think that an unblocked anterior beam for all or part of the treatment, as opposed to an angled lateral lens-sparing setup, would have a higher incidence of cataract formation. However, these data are equivocal, and cataracts may occur after either technique (458,459). This is almost certainly because variations in daily setup make complete lens sparing unlikely with most lateral approaches. If a radiation-induced cataract causes visual impairment in the patient with retinoblastoma, it may be removed. Persistent tumor is a contraindication to cataract removal. Final visual acuity after cataract removal depends on the presence or absence of macular tumor, the existence of radiation-induced keratopathy or retinopathy, severe amblyopia, a history of rhegmatogenous retinal detachment, and tumor control. In the absence of negative factors, visual acuity after cataract removal would be expected to be in the 20/20 to 20/50 range (460).

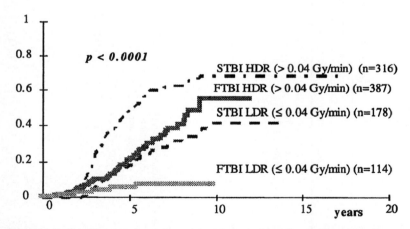

FIG. 19-17. Product-limit estimates for cataract incidence according to fractionation and dose rate. FTBI, fractionated total body irradiation; HDR, high dose rate (>0.04 Gy/min); LDR, low dose rate (≤0.04 Gy/min); STBI, single-dose total body irradiation. (From Belkacemi Y, Labopin M, Vernant JP, et al. Cataracts after total body irradiation and bone marrow transplantation in patients with acute leukemia in complete remission: a study of the European Group for Blood and Marrow Transplantation. *Int J Radiat Biol Oncol Phys* 1998;41(3):659–668, with permission.)

TABLE 19-17. *Evaluation of patients at risk for late effects: gastrointestinal*

Late effects	Causative treatment			Signs and symptoms	Screening and diagnostic tests	Management and intervention
	Chemotherapy	Radiation	Surgery			
Enteritis	Actinomycin D, doxorubicin enhance RT effect	>30 Gy	Abdominal surgery enhances RT effect	Abdominal pain, diarrhea, decreased stool bulk, emesis, weight loss, poor linear growth	Height and weight q yr, Stool guaiac q yr, CBC with MCV q yr, total protein and albumin q 3–5 yr, absorption tests, vitamin B$_{12}$ level, and contrast studies	Dietary management, refer to gastroenterologist
Adhesions		RT enhances effect	Laparotomy	Abdominal pain, bilious vomiting, hyperactive bowel sounds	Abdominal radiograph	NPO, gastric suction, adhesion lysis
Fibrosis: esophagus (stricture)	Actinomycin D, doxorubicin (RT enhancers)	40–50 Gy	Abdomen	Dysphagia, weight loss, poor linear growth	Height and weight q yr, CBC q yr, barium swallow and endoscopy as needed	Esophageal dilation Antireflux surgery
Fibrosis: small intestines		>40 Gy	Abdomen	Abdominal pain, constipation, diarrhea, weight loss, obstruction	Height and weight q yr, CBC with MCV q yr, serum protein and albumin q 3–5 yr, upper GI, small bowel biopsy	High-fiber diet, decompression, resection, balloon dilation
Fibrosis: large intestine, colon		>40 Gy	Abdomen	Abdominal colic, rectal pain, constipation, melena, weight loss, obstruction	Height and weight q yr, rectal exam, stool guaiac q yr, lower GI, colonoscopy, sigmoidoscopy	Stool softeners, high-fiber diet

Evaluation of patients at risk for late effects: hepatic

| Late effects | Causative treatment | | | Signs and symptoms | Screening and diagnostic tests | Management and intervention |
	Chemotherapy	Radiation	Surgery			
Hepatic fibrosis and cirrhosis	Methotrexate, actinomycin D, 6MP 6TG	>30 Gy	Massive resection	Itching, jaundice, spider nevi, bruising Portal hypertension: esophageal varices, hemorrhoids, hematemesis Encephalopathy	Height and weight q yr, CBC, reticulocyte count, platelets q yr, liver function tests q 2–5 yr Hepatic screen Liver biopsy Endoscopy	Hepatitis screen (hepatitis A, B, C/CMV), diuretics, liver transplant Varices: sclerosis, vascular shunting

6MP, 6-mercaptopurine; 6TG, 6-thiguanine; CBC, complete blood cell count; GI, gastrointestinal; MCV, mean cell volume; RT, radiotherapy.
From Constine LS, Hobbie W, Schwartz C. Facilitated assessment of chronic treatment by symptom and organ systems. In: Schwartz C, Hobbie W, Constine L, et al., eds. *Survivors of childhood cancer: assessment and management.* St Louis: Mosby, 1994:21–80, with permission.

Optic Nerve

Injury to the distal nerve end produces ischemic optic neuropathy, whereas more proximal injury produces retrobulbar optic neuropathy. These are potentially blinding complications. The peak onset is 1–2 years, manifested by visual field deficits or central scotoma (461).

Lid

Rounding of the lid margins is not seen below 40 Gy, and ectropion is uncommon below 60 Gy. The eyelash usually is spared by anterior megavoltage beams so that it may remain partially intact (437).

Orbit

For survivors of retinoblastoma, a small orbital volume may result after either enucleation or radiotherapy. Age less than 1 year may increase risk, but this is not consistent across studies (462,463). Better management of prosthetic implants and newer methods of delivering RT are likely to reduce risk (462,464). Newer strategies for treating retinoblastoma use chemotherapy to reduce tumor size, combined with local ophthalmic therapies that include thermotherapy, cryotherapy, and plaque radiation. These strategies may be associated with local complications that can affect vision. Because they are new, further follow-up is needed to determine their long-term effects. Treatment for tumors located near the macula and fovea increases the risk of complications leading to visual loss (464–469).

One group of patients at risk for all of the aforementioned complications are survivors of orbital rhabdomyosarcoma, who are at risk of dry eye, cataract, orbital hypoplasia, ptosis, retinopathy, keratoconjunctivitis, optic neuropathy, lid epithelioma, and impairment of vision after RT dosages of 30–65 Gy. The higher dosages (more than 50 Gy) are associated with lid epitheliomas, keratoconjunctivitis, lacrimal duct atrophy, and severe dry eye. Retinitis and optic neuropathy may also occur after dosages of 50–65 Gy, and even at lower total dosages if the individual fraction size is greater than 2 Gy

(461). Cataracts are reported after lower dosages of 10–18 Gy (441–446).

Table 19-18 reviews several late effects involving the eye with respect to causative treatments, signs and symptoms, screening and diagnostic tests, and management and intervention (80).

Hearing

The auditory apparatus may be irradiated during the treatment of brain tumors, aerodigestive tract malignancies, soft tissue sarcomas, and lymphoma. Fractionated dosages of more than 50 Gy can produce permanent changes in the temporal bone and adjacent soft tissues, including empty lacunae in the bone, resorption, absent marrow, and replacement by fibrous tissue. Temporal bone osteoradionecrosis is extremely rare with modern pediatric RT technique. Radiation changes in the external auditory canal may include thickening of the epithelium overlying the tympanic membrane, atrophic ceruminous glands, and absent hair follicles. On occasion, the combination of abnormal epithelium of the external auditory canal and bacterial overgrowth can produce a persistent otitis externa necessitating the use of wicks, otic antibiotics, and otic steroid preparations (470).

Cranial irradiation alone rarely has a significant effect on hearing. RT can result in cochlear damage, with sensorineural hearing loss (SNHL) occurring in about 25% of patients treated with dosages approaching 60 Gy, but SNHL has been considered rare at lower RT dosages in the absence of cisplatin. Recent data suggest that cochlear dosages of 30–50 Gy can cause intermediate-frequency SNHL and that CSF shunting procedures increase the risk (443,445,471,472). At dosages as low as 270 mg/m^2, cisplatin can result in hearing loss when combined with cranial radiotherapy dosages of 40–50 Gy (445, 473). The sequence of chemoradiotherapy appears to influence risk. Risk and severity of ototoxicity are greater when cisplatin is administered after cranial radiation (Fig. 19-18) (474).

Hearing loss in the speech range (0.5–3 kHz), which may compromise language reception and expression, is reported with cumulative cisplatin dosages of at least 360 mg/m^2, and a 25% inci-

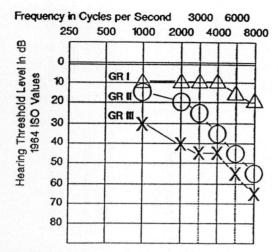

Frequency in Cycles per Second   3000 6000

FIG. 19-18. Mean hearing thresholds for three groups of patients with brain tumors. Group I (GRI; *triangles*) received cranial irradiation only, group II (GRII; *circles*) received cisplatin, and group III (GRIII, *Xs*) received cranial irradiation, then cisplatin. (From McHaney V, Kavnar E, Meyer W, et al. Effects of radiation therapy and chemotherapy on hearing. In: Green DM, D'Angio GJ, eds. *Late effects of treatment for childhood cancer.* New York: Wiley-Liss, 1992:7–10, with permission.)

dence of hearing loss is reported with dosages greater than 720 mg/m^2 in the absence of any radiotherapy. Fifty percent of children treated with cisplatin dosages greater than 450 mg/m^2 have SNHL in the high-frequency range (6–8 kHz). Younger age at time of administration increases risk (408,445,473–475). Carboplatin may be less ototoxic, but further follow-up in patients treated with high cumulative dosages is necessary before a clear dose threshold can be established (475). A recent German study of children treated for neuroblastoma demonstrated the influence of both cisplatin and carboplatin on hearing, again in the absence of radiotherapy. For cisplatin, there was 12% hearing impairment at dosages of 1–200 mg/m^2, 13% at dosages of 201–400 mg/m^2, 26% at dosages of 401–600 mg/m^2, and 22% at 601–800 mg/m^2. There was an additional effect of carboplatin when given as high-dose therapy with autologous stem cell infusion, where 40% of patients developed hearing loss after a dosage of 1,500 mg/m^2 (476).

Hearing loss in the child with cancer merits detailed attention because it may lead to additional difficulties with communication, speech and language acquisition, and development of learning skills. The judicious use of amplification and other hearing aids is well advised, but many survivors report that they are not helpful.

Table 19-19 reviews several late effects involving the ear with respect to causative treatments, signs and symptoms, screening and diagnostic tests, and management and intervention (30).

Teeth and Salivary Glands

Radiation-induced damage to developing teeth causes cosmetic and functional difficulties throughout life. The age of the child at the time of therapy and the radiation dosage determine the consequences. Teeth begin to develop from the dental lamina 6 weeks after conception. The crowns of deciduous incisors are fully formed at birth. Calcification begins 3–5 months after birth in the central incisors, canines, and first molars; by 1 year in the maxillary lateral incisors; and by 2.5 years in premolars. By the end of the third year, the whole deciduous dentition is developed (477).

Developing teeth are irradiated in the course of treating head and neck sarcomas, HD, neuroblastoma, retinoblastoma, and potential or established CNS leukemia and during TBI for bone marrow transplantation. The defects that occur include destruction of the tooth germ causing tooth agenesis, stunted growth of the whole tooth or its root, impaction, incomplete calcification, premature closures of apices, premature eruption, tapering roots with apical constriction, delayed development, and caries (477,478). Maxillofacial abnormalities include trismus, abnormal occlusal relationships, and facial deformities. Tooth defects are most severe before histodifferentiation and incremental calcification of the tooth buds, and the extent of damage is not apparent until the teeth erupt.

Dosages of 20–40 Gy can cause root shortening or abnormal curvature, dwarfism, and hypocalcification. More than 85% of survivors of head and neck rhabdomyosarcoma who receive radiation dosages of more than 40 Gy may

TABLE 19-18. *Evaluation of patients at risk for late effects: eye*

Late effects	Causative treatment			Signs and symptoms	Screening and diagnostic tests	Management and intervention
	Chemotherapy	Radiation	Surgery			
Lacrimal glands: decreased tear production	5FU	>40 Gy		Dry, irritated red eye, foreign body sensation, positive fluorescein staining	Penlight or slit lamp exam, fluorescein staining	Tear replacement, occlude lacrimal puncta, education regarding avoiding rubbing lids when puncta plug is intact
Lacrimal duct: fibrosis	5FU	>50 Gy		Tearing	Ophthalmic exam	Dilation of duct
Eyelids: Ulceration Telangiectasia		>50 Gy >50 Gy		Blepharitis, bleeding and crusted lesion, previous infections Enlarged, tortuous blood vessels Pigmentary changes	Physical exam Slit lamp or penlight exam Open and closed eyelid exam	Topical and oral steroids, skin balm Teach: lid hygiene, radiosensitizing drugs, UV protection Avoid trauma, harsh soaps and lotions
Conjunctiva: Necrosis Scarring Subconjunctival hemorrhage		Radioactive plaque therapy >45 Gy		Dry, irritated eye, foreign body sensation, irregular rough conjunctival surface, telangiectasia Irritated eye, foreign body sensation, dry, irregular conjunctival surface	Slit lamp or penlight exam Fluorescein stain	Steroids and antibiotic drops Tear replacement (resolves spontaneously) Patching Tear replacement
Sclera: thinning		>50 Gy		May be asymptomatic, dry eyes, foreign body sensation, gray, charred, blue sclera	Slit lamp or penlight exam	Antibiotic drops Avoid trauma Protective glasses
Cornea: ulceration		>45 Gy		Pain, foreign body sensation, decreased VA, photosensitivity	Slit lamp or penlight exam Fluorescein staining	Tear replacement, antibiotics, soft bandages, soft contact lens, surgery, ophthalmology
Neovascularization		>50 Gy		Increased tearing, increased vessels surrounding edge of cornea	Slit lamp exam	Same as ulceration

Site/Effect	Dose/Etiology	Clinical manifestations	Evaluation	Management
Keratinization	>50 Gy	Decreased corneal sensation, photosensitivity, fluorescein staining	Slit lamp exam; Fluorescein staining	
Edema	>40 Gy	Decreased visual acuity, hazy cornea	Penlight or slit lamp exam: white, opaque cornea	Prevention by shielding during treatment; Surgical removal; Educate regarding UV protection
Lens: cataract	Steroids (incidence varies with dosage); >8 Gy (single dose); 10–15 Gy (fractionated)	Decreased visual acuity; Opaque lens	Direct ophthalmoscopic exam, decreased red reflex, slit lamp or penlight exam: opaque lens	Steroid drops
Iris: Neovascularization	>50 Gy	May be asymptomatic, new blood vessels in iris (rubeosis)	Slit lamp or penlight exam	Beta-blocker drops, atropine, Diamox
Secondary glaucoma	>50 Gy	blood in anterior chamber, different-colored irises; Eye pain, headache, nausea or vomiting, decreased peripheral vision, increased intraocular pressure	Measure ocular pressure	Photocoagulation
Atrophy		Decreased iris stroma at pupillary margin	Slit lamp or penlight exam	
Retina: Infarction	>50 Gy	Blanched white cotton specs, decreased visual acuity, decreased visual field, blurred vision (central or peripheral)	Visual acuity	Steroids
Exudates	>50 Gy		Visual field (confrontation computerized or Amsler grid)	Photocoagulation
Hemorrhage	>50 Gy	Blood vessels: yellow fluid, bleeding, thin, incompetent vessels, tortuous, enlarged vessels	Direct and indirect ophthalmoscope exam	Education regarding avoiding ASA and bleeding precautions
Telangiectasia	>50 Gy		Fundus photography	
Neovascularization	>50 Gy			
Macular edema (VA and VF)	>50 Gy	Blister of fluid in the macula		
Optic neuropathy	Tumor resection; >50 Gy	Pale optic disc, abnormal pupillary responses	Visual evaluation	Visual aids

5FU, 5 fluoroucil; ASA, aspirin; UV, ultraviolet; VA, visual acuity; VF, visual field.
From Constine LS, Hobbie W, Schwartz C. Facilitated assessment of chronic treatment by symptom and organ systems. In: Schwartz C, Hobbie W, Constine L, et al., eds. *Survivors of childhood cancer: assessment and management.* St Louis: Mosby, 1994:21–80, with permission.

TABLE 19-19. *Evaluation of patients at risk for late effects: ear*

| Late effects | Causative treatment | | Signs and symptoms | Screening and diagnostic tests | Management and intervention |
	Chemotherapy	Radiation			
Chronic otitis		>35 Gy	Dryness and thickening of canal and tympanic membrane Conductive hearing loss Perforation of tympanic membrane	Otoscopic exam Audiometry	Antibiotic therapy, decongestants, myringotomy, PE tubes, preferential seating in school, amplification Preferential seating in school Amplification
Sensorineural hearing loss	Cisplatin, carboplatin	35–50 Gy Cranial RT enhances the platinum effect	High frequency hearing loss (bilateral) Tinnitus Vertigo	Conventional pure tone audiogram baseline and then q 2–3 yr Bilateral, symmetric, irreversible	
Decreased cerumen production		30–40 Gy	Hard and encrusted cerumen in canal Hearing impairment Otitis externa	Examination of canal	Periodic cleaning ear canal, cerumen-loosening agents, otitic drops for otitis externa Keep ear dry: ear plugs, drying solution
Chondritis Chondronecrosis		50 Gy 60 Gy	Cauliflower ear	Inspection of auricle	Antibiotics, surgical repair (reconstruction may be hampered by poor blood supply)

PE, pressure equalization.

have significant dental abnormalities, including mandibular or maxillary hypoplasia, increased caries, hypodontia, microdontia, root stunting, and xerostomia (442,443). In a study of 68 long-term survivors of childhood cancer, Jaffe et al. (188) found that 82% of patients receiving max-illofacial radiation exhibited dental abnormalities. Children treated with 18–30 Gy for leukemia are less frequently affected, with about 40% showing root or crown abnormalities of the maxillary first molars. Children who undergo BMT for high-risk neuroblastoma are clearly at high risk for microdontia, impaired tooth development, and compromised occlusion. These abnormalities are greater if TBI is a component of the conditioning regimen, but they occur even without TBI (479).

Chemotherapy for the treatment of leukemia can cause shortening and thinning of the premolar roots and enamel abnormalities (480–482). This could result from direct inhibiting effects of chemotherapy, altered marrow milieu caused by leukemic involvement, or systemic factors altering growth. Radiographic abnormalities are common after radiotherapy for leukemia and sarcoma (188,481,483).

When 10 Gy of TBI is administered for BMT, impaired root development resulting in short, V-shaped roots is found in all patients, whereas microdontia, enamel hypoplasia, and premature apical closure are found in 30–50% (484). These effects seem to result from irradiation, not chemotherapy.

Salivary gland irradiation causes a qualitative and quantitative change in salivary flow. When salivary glands are irradiated, acinar cells are destroyed and replaced by ductal remnants and loose connective tissue (485,486). Such damage is evident after 20 Gy of fractionated irradiation. Salivary flow rate drops rapidly during a course of fractionated irradiation. Postradiotherapy xerostomia is irreversible if all major salivary glands are treated with dosages of 50–60 Gy (485,486). Stimulated and nonstimulated salivary flow are primarily from the parotid and submandibular glands. In Fromm's study of children treated for head and neck sarcomas, about 40% of parotid glands had absent secretions, and these patients received the highest radiation dosage (mean 51 Gy) (483). Patients treated with less than 40 Gy were not affected. Among patients treated for HD with 40 Gy to regions including the submandibular glands, flow rate reductions of about 55% have been documented (487). The radiation dose–response relationship in the effect of radiation on parotid salivary flow is seen in Fig. 19-19 (488). In normal saliva, car-

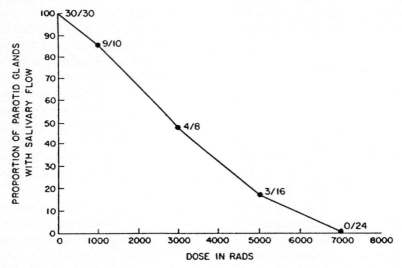

FIG. 19-19. Proportion of unirradiated and irradiated parotid gland with measurable salivary flow as a function of radiation dosage. (From Marks J, Davis C, Gottsman V, et al. The effects of radiation on parotid salivary function. *Int J Radiat Oncol Biol Phys* 1981;7:1013–1019, with permission.)

iogenesis is diminished by salivary antimicrobial substances. Radiation-induced changes in salivary pH and quantity produce a highly cariogenic microflora along with a decrease in protective salivary electrolytes and immunoproteins (485,486). In addition, the pediatric cancer patient often is on a high-carbohydrate diet because of parental indulgence or to maintain adequate calorie intake (478). These circumstances render the patient highly susceptible to radiation-induced caries.

Excellent oral hygiene and attentive dental care are the keys to dealing with radiation's effects on teeth and salivation in children, so these findings give further impetus to routine dental and dental hygiene evaluations for survivors of childhood treatment. Before radiation and chemotherapy a dental evaluation is indicated. As possible foci of infection, loose exfoliating primary teeth and orthodontic appliances should be removed (478). The daily use of topical fluoride can dramatically reduce the frequency of radiation caries in the treated patient (486,489). Xerostomia is palliatively treated with saliva substitutes and sialagogues (485). Data support the efficacy of pilocarpine in improving saliva production and relieving symptoms of xerostomia, with minor risks that are limited predominantly to sweating (490).

Table 19-20 reviews several dental and salivary late effects with respect to causative treatments, signs and symptoms, screening and diagnostic tests, and management and intervention (80).

Bone Marrow

The hematopoietic progenitor cells and their offspring are cradled on a stroma of endothelial cells, adventitial cells, fibroblasts, macrophages, and fat cells. Mechanisms of marrow-induced failure include direct killing of hematopoietic progenitor cells, accessory cells (e.g., lymphocytes and monocytes), damage to the stroma and microcirculation, and disturbance of hematopoietic growth and regulatory factors (491,492).

The bone marrow is extremely sensitive to irradiation, to the degree that some injury is produced by any fractional dosage. Irradiated bone marrow becomes hypocellular. There is destruction of fine vasculature followed by fatty marrow replacement of the normal hematopoietic marrow (493–495). If the radiation dosage is sufficiently high, destruction of the sinusoidal circulation precludes migration of hematopoietic cells from distant nonirradiated sites. The radiation dosage causing permanent local marrow aplasia has been assessed by several investigators using techniques of bone marrow aspiration, scanning with ^{99m}Tc-S, ^{52}Fe, or ^{111}In as tracers, or MRI (493,494,496,497). After 40 Gy fractionated irradiation, 85% of irradiated sites show a return of activity in 2 years; in 55% of those areas, recovery becomes complete. Conversely, single doses of 20 Gy to localized regions can produce permanent aplasia. Radiation-induced changes in bone marrow may be detected by increased signal intensity on MRI because of the decreased T1 relaxation time of the increased fatty marrow content. MRI findings support those of nuclear medicine scanning and bone marrow aspiration studies, namely that dosages of up to 40 Gy, to limited areas, do not preclude repopulation of the irradiated marrow in the years after treatment (495). Dosages greater than 50 Gy seem to produce irreversible depletion of myeloid tissue (498).

The regenerative capacity of the bone marrow depends on the volume irradiated (499). After irradiation to less than 25% of the bone marrow, the unexposed portion is stimulated and successful in compensating for hematopoietic demands, and the treated portion may never regenerate. When larger volumes (more than 50%) are irradiated, the unexposed bone marrow is not adequate to meet the body's demands. Consequently, the paradoxical phenomenon of infield regeneration is seen 2–5 years later, and extension of bone marrow activity into previously quiescent long bones is seen within 1–2 years.

Differences between children and adults in the response of the bone marrow to irradiation relate primarily to the differing extent of active bone marrow at different ages (500). In the immediate postnatal period, conversion from active red to fatty yellow marrow begins and is

TABLE 19-20. *Evaluation of patients at risk for late effects: teeth*

| Late effects | Causative treatment | | Signs and symptoms | Screening and diagnostic tests | Management and intervention |
	Chemotherapy	Radiation			
Xerostomia (decreased salivary gland function)		>40 Gy, and >50% of gland must be radiated	Decreased salivary flow, dry mouth, altered taste perception, dental decay, *Candida* (thrush)	Dental examination, salivary flow studies, attention to early caries, periodontal disease	Encourage meticulous oral hygiene, saliva substitution, prophylactic fluoride, dietary counseling regarding avoiding fermentable carbohydrates, nystatin for oral candidiasis, pilocarpine
Abnormal tooth and root development	Vincristine, cyclophosphamide, actinomycin D, 6MP, procarbazine, nitrogen mustard	Generally 10 Gy can destroy developing roots	Enamel appears pale, teeth appear small, uneven, malocclusion	Dental exam q 6 mo with attention to early caries, periodontal disease, and gingivitis Panorex and bite-wing radiographs for baseline (age 5–6)	Careful evaluation before tooth extraction, endodontics, and orthodontics Fluoride Antibiotics as needed to reduce risk of infection (e.g., with trauma)

6MP, 6 mercaptopurine.

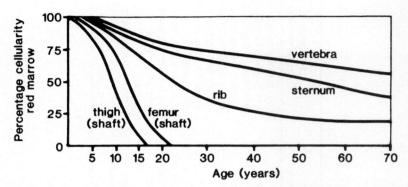

FIG. 19-20. The relative amount of red and yellow bone marrow in different anatomic sites as a function of age. (From Kricun ME. Red–yellow marrow conversion: its effect on the location of some solitary bone lesions. *Skeletal Radiol* 1985;14:10–19, with permission.)

first evident in the extremities. This conversion progresses from peripheral (appendicular) toward the central (axial) skeleton and from diaphyseal to metaphyseal in individual long bones (Fig. 19-20). Beyond these changes in active bone marrow volume, some investigators have suggested that younger people have a greater regenerative capacity for as yet unexplained reasons (497,499). The self-renewal capacity or numbers of stem cells might simply be greater in youth.

The acute and chronic effects of chemotherapeutic agents on the hematopoietic compartment have been reviewed (492) and will not be detailed in this section. However, radiation oncologists must be familiar with the acute myelosuppressive effects of various drugs, and they are summarized in Table 19-21.

TABLE 19-21. *Antineoplastic drug category and agent with their relative degree and duration of myelosuppression*

Drug or drug class	Degree of suppression[a]	Myelosuppression nadir (days)	Time to marrow recovery (days)
Anthracycline	III	6–13	21–24
Vinca alkaloids	I–II	4–9	7–21
Mustard alkylator	III	7–14	28
Antifolates	III	7–14	14–21
Antipyrimidines	III	7–14	22–24
Antipurines	II	7–14	14–21
Podophyllotoxins	II	5–14	22–28
Alkylators	II	10–21	18–40
Nitrosoureas	III	26–60	35–85
Miscellaneous[b]			
Busulphan	III	11–30	24–54
Cisplatin	I	14	21
Dacarbazine	III	21–28	28–35
Hydroxyurea	II	7	14–21
Mithramycin	I	5–10	10–18
Mitomycin	II	28–42	42–56
Procarbazine	II	25–36	35–50
Bispiperazinedione	II	11–16	12–25

[a]I, mild; II, moderate; III, severe (based on common dosing schedules).
[b]Agents differing from their class of compounds.
From Mauch P, Constine L, Greenberger J, et al. Hematopoietic stem cell compartment: acute and late effects of radiation therapy and chemotherapy. *Int J Radiat Oncol Biol Phys* 1995;31:1319–1339, with permission.

CONCLUSIONS AND FUTURE DIRECTIONS

Radiotherapy and chemotherapy can result in adverse long-term physiologic sequelae for survivors of childhood cancer. However, these treatment modalities have resulted in a markedly increased survival rate for almost all pediatric malignancies. Therefore, it is essential to balance the benefits against risks. Both length of survival and the impact of physiologic late effects on the quality of that survival must be considered in therapy selection.

The pathophysiologic mechanisms of damage from RT and chemotherapy to normal tissues are well described. However, what is unclear is the interindividual variation in responses to the same therapeutic exposures. Although many children and adolescents are treated with the same RT dosages, fields, and volumes, there is a significant degree of variability in the proportion that develops radiation-related toxicities. For some, the cytotoxicity of chemotherapy may enhance the RT effects. However, little is known about host-related factors, such as genetic susceptibility. This may include inherited differences in radiation sensitivity to normal tissue or genes of xenobiotic metabolism, nucleotide provision, or DNA repair. In addition, morbidity and premature mortality have been examined with respect to treatment exposures but not yet in association with other factors such as diet, sun, tobacco, and alcohol exposure that are etiologically related to the major problems in an aging population. New patterns of late morbidity and mortality may emerge as survivors continue to age, and it is only through continued study that such patterns will be identified and interventions for treatment and prevention designed.

REFERENCES

References particularly recommended for further reading are indicated by an asterisk.

1. Ries LAG, Smith MA, Gurney JG, et al. Cancer incidence and survival among children and adolescents: United States SEER Program 1975-1995, National Cancer Institute, SEER Program. NIH Pub. No. 99-4649, Bethesda, MD, 1999:1–15.

2. Hudson M, Jones D, Boyett J, et al. Late mortality of long-term survivors of childhood cancer. *J Clin Oncol* 1997;15:2205–2213.

*3. Mertens AC, Yasui Y, Neglia JP, et al. Late mortality experience in five-year survivors of childhood and adolescent cancer: the Childhood Cancer Survivor Study. *J Clin Oncol* 2001;19:3163–3172.

4. Cohen L, Creditor M. Iso-effect tables for tolerance of irradiated normal human tissues. *Int J Radiat Oncol Biol Phys* 1983;9:233–241.

5. Bristow MR, Mason JW, Billingham ME, et al. Doxorubicin cardiomyopathy: evaluations by phonocardiology, endomyocardial biopsy, and cardiac catheterization. *Ann Intern Med* 1978;88:168–175.

6. Casarett GW. Aging. In: Vaeth JM, ed. *Frontiers of radiation therapy and oncology,* Vol. 6. New York: S Karger, 1972:479–485.

7. Casarett GW. Similarities and contrasts between radiation and time pathology. In: Strehler B, ed. *Advances in gerontological research.* New York: Academic Press, 1964:109–163.

8. Rubin P, Constine L, Williams J. Late effects of cancer treatment: radiation and drug toxicity. In Perez C, Brady L, eds. *Principles and practice of radiation oncology.* Philadelphia: Lippincott-Raven, 1998:155–211.

*9. Rubin P, Cassarett GW. *Clinical radiation pathology,* Vols. I and II. Philadelphia: WB Saunders, 1968.

10. Rubin P, Van Houtte P, Constine L. Radiation sensitivity and organ tolerances in pediatric oncology: a new hypothesis. *Front Radiat Ther Oncol* 1982; 16:62–82.

11. Tanner JM. *Growth at adolescence.* Oxford: Blackwell Scientific, 1962.

12. Tanner JM. Physical growth and development. In: Forfar JO, Arneil GCY, eds. *Textbook for pediatrics.* Edinburgh: Churchill Livingston, 1978:249–304.

13. Packer RJ, Meadows AT, Rocke LB, et al. Long-term sequelae of cancer treatment of the central nervous system in childhood. *Med Pediatr Oncol* 1987;15: 241–253.

14. Dobbing J, Sands J. The quantitative growth and development of the human brain. *Arch Dis Child* 1963; 48:757–767.

15. Halperin EC, Burger PC. Conventional external beam radiotherapy for central nervous system malignancies. *Neurol Clin* 1985;3:867–882.

16. Marks JE, Wong J. The risk of cerebral radionecrosis in relation to dose, time, and fractionation. A follow-up study. *Prog Exp Tumor Res* 1985;29:210–218.

17. Martins AN, Johnston JS, Henry MJ, et al. Delayed radiation necrosis of the brain. *J Neurosurg* 1977; 47:336–345.

18. Anscher MS, Green DM, Kneece SM, et al. Radiation injury of the brain and spinal cord. In: Wilkins RH, Rengaaachary SS, eds. *Neurosurgery update II: vascular, spinal, pediatric and function neurosurgery.* New York: McGraw-Hill, 1991:42–49.

19. Van der Kogel A. Mechanisms of late radiation injury in the spinal cord. In: Meyh RE, Withers HR, eds. *Radiation biology in cancer research.* New York: Raven Press, 1980:461.

20. Burger PC, Scheithauer B, Vogel FS. *Surgical pathology of the nervous system and its coverings.* New York: Churchill Livingstone, 1991:229–236.

21. Constine LS, Konski A, Ekholm S, et al. Adverse effects of brain irradiation correlated with MR and CT imaging. *Int J Radiat Oncol Biol Phys* 1988;15: 319–330.

22. Cohen ME, Duffner PK. Long-term consequences of CNS treatment for childhood cancer, Part I: pathologic consequences and potential for oncogenesis. *Pediatr Neurol* 1991;7:157–163.

23. Danoff BF, Cowchock S, Marquette C, et al. Assessment of the long-term effects of primary radiation therapy for brain tumors in children. *Cancer* 1982;49: 1580–1586.

24. D'Angio GJ. An overview and historical perspective of late effects of treatment of childhood cancer. In: Green DM, D'Angio GJ, eds. *Late effects of treatment for childhood cancer.* New York: Wiley-Liss, 1992:1–6.

25. Dropcha EJ. Central nervous system injury by therapeutic irradiation. *Neurol Clin* 1991;9:969–988.

26. Woo E, Lam K, Yu Y, et al. Cerebral radionecrosis: is surgery necessary? *J Neurol Neurosurg Psychiatry* 1982;50:1407–1414.

27. Duffner PK, Cohen ME. Long-term consequences of CNS treatment for childhood cancer. Part II: clinical consequences. *Pediatr Neurol* 1991;7:237–242.

28. Duffner PK, Cohen ME. The long-term effects of central nervous system therapy on children with brain tumors. *Neurol Clin* 1991;9:479–495.

29. Griffin TW. White matter necrosis, microangiopathy and intellectual abilities in survivors of childhood leukemia. Association with central nervous system irradiation and methotrexate therapy. In: Gilbert HA, Kagan AR, eds. *Radiation damage to the nervous system.* New York: Raven Press, 1980:155–174.

30. Hertzberg H, Huk W, Ueberall M, et al. CNS late effects after ALL therapy in childhood. Part I: neuroradiological findings in long-term survivors of childhood ALL. *Med Pediatr Oncol* 1997;28:387–400.

31. Jannoun L. Are cognitive and educational development affected by the age at which prophylactic therapy is given in acute lymphoblastic leukemia? *Arch Dis Child* 1983;58:955–958.

32. Kun LE, Mulhern RK, Crisco JJ. Quality of life in children treated for brain tumors, Intellectual, emotional and academic function. *J Neurosurg* 1983;58:1–6.

33. Glauser TA, Packer RJ. Cognitive deficits in long-term survivors of childhood brain tumors. *Childs Nerv Syst* 1991;7:2–12.

34. Rodgers J, Britton PG, Morris RG, et al. Memory after treatment for acute lymphoblastic leukaemia. *Arch Dis Child* 1992;67:266–268.

35. Stehbens JA, Kaleita TA, Noll RB, et al. CNS prophylaxis of childhood leukemia: what are the longterm neurological, neuropsychological, and behavioral effects? *Neuropsychol Rev* 1991;2:147–177.

36. Cohen BH, Packer RJ, Siegel KR, et al. Brain tumors in children under 2 years: treatment, survival and longterm prognosis. *Pediatr Neurosurg* 1993;19:171–179.

37. Mulhern R, Hancock J, Fairclough D. Neuropsychological status of children treated with brain tumors: a critical review and integrated analysis. *Med Pediatr Oncol* 1992;20:181–191.

38. Radcliffe J, Bunin GR, Sutton LN, et al. Cognitive deficits in long-term survivors of childhood medulloblastoma and other noncortical tumors: age-dependent effects of whole brain radiation. *Int J Dev Neurosci* 1994;12:327–334.

39. Roman DD, Sperduto PW. Neuropsychological effects of cranial radiation: current knowledge and future directions. *Int J Radiat Oncol Biol Phys* 1995; 31:983–998.

*40. Silber JH, Radcliffe J, Peckham V, et al. Whole-brain irradiation and decline in intelligence: the influence of dose and age on IQ score. *J Clin Oncol* 1992;10: 1390–1396.

41. Halberg FE, Kramer JH, Moore IM, et al. Prophylactic cranial irradiation dose effects on late cognitive function in children treated for acute lymphoblastic leukemia. *Int J Radiat Oncol Biol Phys* 1991;22:13–16.

42. Bloom HJC, Wallace ENJ, Henk JM. The treatment and prognosis of medulloblastoma in children: a study of 82 verified cases. *AJR* 1969;105:43–62.

43. Syndikus I, Tait D, Ashley S, et al. Long-term followup of young children with brain tumors after irradiation. *Int J Radiat Oncol Biol Phys* 1994;30:781–787.

44. Packer RJ, Sutton LA, Atkins TE, et al. A prospective study of cognitive function in children receiving whole-brain radiotherapy and chemotherapy: 2-year results. *J Neurosurg* 1989;70:707–713.

45. Ris MD, Packer R, Goldwein J, et al. Intellectual outcome after reduced-dose radiation therapy plus adjuvant chemotherapy for medulloblastoma: a Children's Cancer Group study. *J Clin Oncol* 2001;19:3470–3476.

*46. Mulhern RK, Kepner JL, Thomas PR, et al. Neuropsychologic functioning of survivors of childhood medulloblastoma randomized to receive conventional or reduced-dose craniospinal irradiation: a Pediatric Oncology Group study. *J Clin Oncol* 1998;16: 1723–1728.

47. Packer RJ, Goldwein J, Nicholson HS, et al. Treatment of children with medulloblastomas with reduced-dose craniospinal radiation therapy and adjuvant chemotherapy: a Children's Cancer Group study. *J Clin Oncol* 1999;17:2127–2136.

48. Palmer SL, Goloubeva O, Reddick WE, et al. Patterns of intellectual development among survivors of pediatric medulloblastoma: a longitudinal analysis. *J Clin Oncol* 2001;19:2302–2308.

49. Reimers TS, Ehrenfels S, Mortensen EL, et al. Cognitive deficits in long-term survivors of childhood brain tumors: identification of predictive factors. *Med Pediatr Oncol* 2003;40:26–34.

50. Reddick W, White H, Glass J, et al. Developmental model relating white matter volume to neurocognitive deficits in pediatric brain tumor survivors. *Cancer* 2003;97:2523–2529.

51. Meadows AT, Gordon J, Massari DJ. Declines in IQ scores and cognitive dysfunctions in children with acute lymphocytic leukemia treated with cranial irradiation. *Lancet* 1981;2:1015–1018.

52. Haupt R, Fears TR, Robison LL, et al. Educational attainment in long-term survivors of childhood acute lymphoblastic leukemia. *JAMA* 1994;272:1427–1432.

53. Kingma A, Van Dommelen RI, Mooyaart EL, et al. No major cognitive impairment in young children with acute lymphoblastic leukemia using chemotherapy only: a prospective longitudinal study. *J Pediatr Hematol Oncol* 2002;24:106–114.

54. Waber D, Tarbell N, Fairclough D, et al. Cognitive sequelae of treatment in childhood acute lymphoblas-

tic leukemia: cranial radiation requires an accomplice. *J Clin Oncol* 1995;13:2490–2496.

55. Waber DP, Shapiro BL, Carpentieri SC, et al. Excellent therapeutic efficacy and minimal late neurotoxicity in children treated with 18 gray of cranial radiation therapy for high-risk acute lymphoblastic leukemia: a 7-year follow-up study of the Dana–Farber Cancer Institute Consortium protocol 87-01. *Cancer* 2001;92:15–22.

56. Bleyer A, Robinson L, Fallovollita J, et al. Influence of age, sex and concurrent intrathecal methotrexate therapy on intellectual function after cranial irradiation during childhood. *Pediatr Hematol Oncol* 1990;7:329–338.

57. Riva D, Giorgi C, Nichelli F, et al. Intrathecal methotrexate affects cognitive function in children with medulloblastoma. *Neurology* 2002;59:48–53.

58. Bleyer WA. Neurologic sequelae of methotrexate and ionizing radiation: a new classification. *Cancer Treat Rep* 1981;65[Suppl 1]:89–98.

59. Brown RT, Madan-Swain A, Pais R, et al. Chemotherapy for acute lymphocytic leukemia: cognitive and academic sequelae. *J Pediatr* 1992;121(6):885–889.

60. Ochs J, Mulhern R, Fairclough D, et al. Comparison of neuropsychologic functioning and clinical indicators of neurotoxicity in long-term survivors of childhood leukemia given cranial radiation or parenteral methotrexate: a prospective study. *J Clin Oncol* 1991;9:145–151.

61. Butler RW, Hill JM, Steinherz PG, et al. Neuropsychologic effects of cranial irradiation, intrathecal methotrexate, and systemic methotrexate in childhood cancer. *J Clin Oncol* 1994;12(12):2621–2629.

62. Kaleita TA, Reaman GH, MacLean WE, et al. Neurodevelopmental outcome of infants with acute lymphoblastic leukemia: a Children's Cancer Group report. *Cancer* 1999;85:1859–1865.

63. Iuvone L, Mariotti P, Colosimo C, et al. Long-term cognitive outcome, brain computed tomography scan, and magnetic resonance imaging in children cured for acute lymphoblastic leukemia. *Cancer* 2002;95: 2562–2570.

64. Hill DE, Ciesielski KT, Sethre-Hofstad L, et al. Visual and verbal short-term memory deficits in childhood leukemia survivors after intrathecal chemotherapy. *J Pediatr Psychol* 1997;22:861–870.

65. Williams KS, Ochs J, Williams JM, et al. Parental report of everyday cognitive abilities among children treated for acute lymphoblastic leukemia. *J Pediatr Psychol* 1991;16:13–26.

66. Mulhern R, Wasserman A, Fairclough D, et al. Memory function in disease-free survivors of childhood acute lymphocytic leukemia given CNS prophylaxis with or without 1800 cGy cranial irradiation. *J Clin Oncol* 1988;6:315–320.

67. Kumar P, Kun LE, Rivera GK, et al. A prospective neuropsychological evaluation of children treated with additional chemotherapy and craniospinal irradiation following isolated central nervous system relapse in acute lymphoblastic leukemia. *Int J Radiat Oncol Biol Phys* 1993;27:134(abst).

68. Waber DP, Tarbell NJ, Kahn CM, et al. The relationship of sex and treatment modality to neuropsychologic outcome in childhood acute lymphoblastic leukemia. *J Clin Oncol* 1992;10:810–817.

69. Druckmann A. Schlafsucht als folge der rontgenbestrahlung: beitrag zur strahlenempfindlichkeit des genirns. *Strahlenther Onkol* 1929;33:382–384.

70. Eiser C. Intellectual abilities among survivors of childhood leukemia as a function of CNS irradiation. *Arch Dis Child* 1978;53:391–395.

71. Mitchell WG, Fishman LS, Miller JH, et al. Stroke as a late sequela of cranial irradiation for childhood brain tumors. *J Child Neurol* 1991;6:128–133.

72. Jones AM. Transient radiation myelopathy (with reference to Lhermitte's sign of electrical paresthesia). *Br J Radiol* 1964;37:727–744.

73. Kaplan HS. *Hodgkin's disease.* Cambridge, MA: Harvard University Press, 1980:689.

74. Inbar M, Merimsky O, Wigler N, et al. Cisplatin-related Lhermitte's sign. *Anticancer Drugs* 1992;3: 375–377.

75. Schultheiss TE, Higgins EM, El-Mahdi HM. The latent period in radiation myelopathy. *Int J Radiat Oncol Biol Phys* 1984;10:1109–1115.

*76. Wara W, Phillips T, Sheline G, et al. Radiation tolerance of the spinal cord. *Cancer* 1975;35:1558–1562.

*77. Marcus R, William R. The incidence of myelitis after irradiation of the cervical spinal cord. *Int J Radiat Oncol Biol Phys* 1990;19:3–8.

78. Feyerabend T, Kapp B, Richter E, et al. Incidence of hypothyroidism after irradiation of the neck with special reference to lymphoma patients: a retrospective and prospective analysis. *Acta Oncol* 1990;29:597–602.

79. Littman P, Rosenstock J, Bailey C. Radiation myelitis following craniospinal irradiation with concurrent actinomycin D therapy. *Med Pediatr Oncol* 1978;5: 145–151.

80. Constine LS, Hobbie W, Schwartz C. Facilitated assessment of chronic treatment by symptom and organ systems. In: Schwartz C, Hobbie W, Constine L, et al., eds. *Survivors of childhood cancer: assessment and management.* St Louis: Mosby, 1994:21–30.

81. Koocher GP, O'Malley JE. The Damocles syndrome: psychologic consequences of surviving childhood cancer. New York: McGraw-Hill, 1981.

82. Gray RE, Doan BD, Shermer P, et al. Psychologic adaptation of survivors of childhood cancer. *Cancer* 1992;70:2713–2721.

83. Zeltzer LK. Cancer in adolescents and young adults psychosocial aspects. Long-term survivors. *Cancer* 1993;71:3463–3468.

84. Kazak AE. Implication of survival: pediatric oncology patients and their families. In *Pediatric psychooncology: psychological perspectives on children with cancer.* New York: Oxford University Press, 1994:171–192.

85. Association AP. *Diagnostic and statistical manual (DSM) IV.* Washington, DC: American Psychiatric Press, 1994.

86. Hobbie WL, Stuber M, Meeske K, et al. Symptoms of posttraumatic stress in young adult survivors of childhood cancer. *J Clin Oncol* 2000;18:4060–4066.

87. Kazak AE, Barakat LP, Meeske K, et al. Posttraumatic stress, family functioning, and social support in survivors of childhood leukemia and their mothers and fathers. *J Consult Clin Psychol* 1997;65:120–129.

88. Kazak AE, Simms S, Barakat L, et al. Surviving Cancer Competently Intervention Program (SCCIP): a

cognitive–behavioral and family therapy intervention for adolescent survivors of childhood cancer and their families. *Family Process* 1999;38:175–191.

89. Rourke MT, Stuber ML, Hobbie WL, et al. Posttraumatic stress disorder: understanding the psychosocial impact of surviving childhood cancer into young adulthood. *J Pediatr Oncol Nurs* 1999;16:126–135.

90. Stuber ML, Kazak AE, Meeske K, et al. Predictors of posttraumatic stress symptoms in childhood cancer survivors. *Pediatrics* 1997;100:958–964.

91. Meeske KA, Ruccione K, Globe DR, et al. Posttraumatic stress, quality of life, and psychological distress in young adult survivors of childhood cancer. *Oncol Nurs Forum* 2001;28:481–489.

92. Kazak AE, Stuber ML, Barakat LP, et al. Predicting posttraumatic stress symptoms in mothers and fathers of survivors of childhood cancers. *J Am Acad Child Adolesc Psychiatry* 1998;37:823–831.

93. Zebrack BJ, Zeltzer LK, Whitton J, et al. Psychological outcomes in long-term survivors of childhood leukemia, Hodgkin's disease, and non-Hodgkin's lymphoma: a report from the Childhood Cancer Survivor Study. *Pediatrics* 2002;110:42–52.

94. Mulrooney DA, Mertens AC, Neglia JP, et al. Fatigue and sleep disturbance in survivors of childhood cancer: a report from the Childhood Cancer Survivor Study. *Proc Annu Meet Am Soc Clin Oncol* 2003;22:761.

95. Fuemmeler BF, Elkin TD, Mullins LL. Survivors of childhood brain tumors: behavioral, emotional, and social adjustment. *Clin Psychol Rev* 2002;22:547–585.

*96. Shalet SM, Ogilvy-Stuart AL, Crowne EC, et al. Indications for human growth hormone treatment of radiation-induced growth hormone deficiency. In: Green DM, D'Angio GJ, eds. *Late effects of treatment for childhood cancer.* New York: Wiley-Liss, 1992:71–79.

*97. Sklar CA. Physiology of growth hormone production and release. In: Green DM, D'Angio GJ, eds. *Late effects of treatment for childhood cancer.* New York: Wiley-Liss, 1992:49–54.

98. Lannering B, Albertsson-Wikland K. Growth hormone release in children after cranial irradiation. *Hormone Res* 1987;27:13–22.

99. Blacklay A, Grossman A, Ross RJM, et al. Cranial irradiation for cerebral and nasopharyngeal tumours in children: evidence for the production of a hypothalamic defect in growth hormone release. *J Endocrinol* 1986;108:25–29.

*100. Merchant TE, Goloubeva O, Pritchard DL, et al. Radiation dose-volume effects on growth hormone secretion. *Int J Radiat Oncol Biol Phys* 2002;52:1264–1270.

101. Sklar C, Mertens A, Walter A, et al. Final height after treatment for childhood acute lymphoblastic leukemia: comparison of no cranial irradiation with 1800 and 2499 centigrays of cranial irradiation. *J Pediatr* 1993;123:59–64.

102. Schriock EA, Schell MJ, Carter M, et al. Abnormal growth patterns and adult short stature in 115 long-term survivors of childhood leukemia. *J Clin Oncol* 1991;9:400–405.

103. Sanders JE. Endocrine problems in children after bone marrow transplant for hematologic malignancies. *Bone Marrow Transplant* 1991;8:2–4.

104. Ogilvy-Stuart AL, Clark DJ, Wallace WH, et al. Endocrine deficits after fractionated total body irradiation. *Arch Dis Child* 1992;67:1107–1110.

105. Willi SM, Cooke K, Goldwein J, et al. Growth in children after bone marrow transplantation for advanced neuroblastoma compared with growth after transplantation for leukemia or aplastic anemia. *J Pediatr* 1992;120:726–732.

106. Wingard JR, Plotnick LP, Freemer CS, et al. Growth in children after bone marrow transplantation: busulfan plus cyclophosphamide versus cyclophosphamide plus total body irradiation. *Blood* 1992;79:1068–1073.

107. Huma Z, Boulad F, Black P, et al. Growth in children after bone marrow transplantation for acute leukemia. *Blood* 1995;86:819–824.

108. Socie G, Salooja N, Cohen A, et al. Nonmalignant late effects after allogeneic stem cell transplantation. *Blood* 2003;101:3373–3385.

109. Cohen A, Rovelli A, Bakker B, et al. Final height of patients who underwent bone marrow transplantation for hematological disorders during childhood: a study by the Working Party for Late Effects—EBMT. *Blood* 1999;93:4109–4115.

110. Leung W, Rose SR, Zhou Y, et al. Outcomes of growth hormone replacement therapy in survivors of childhood acute lymphoblastic leukemia. *J Clin Oncol* 2002;20:2959–2964.

*111. Sklar CA, Mertens AC, Mitby P, et al. Risk of disease recurrence and second neoplasms in survivors of childhood cancer treated with growth hormone: a report from the Childhood Cancer Survivor Study. *J Clin Endocrinol Metab* 2002;87:3136–3141.

112. Didcock E, Davies HA, Didi M, et al. Pubertal growth in young adult survivors of childhood leukemia. *J Clin Oncol* 1995;13:2503–2507.

113. Shalet SM, Brennan BM. Puberty in children with cancer. *Horm Res* 2002;57:39–42.

114. Shalet SM, Crowne EC, Didi MA, et al. Irradiation-induced growth failure. *Baillieres Clin Endocrinol Metab* 1992;6:513–526.

115. Rappaport R, Brauner R, Czernichow P, et al. Effect of hypothalamic and pituitary irradiation on pubertal development in children with cranial tumors. *J Clin Endocrinol Metab* 1982;54:1164–1168.

*116. Constine LS, Woolf PD, Cann D, et al. Hypothalamic–pituitary dysfunction after radiation for brain tumors. *N Engl J Med* 1993;328:87–94.

117. Schmiegelow M, Feldt-Rasmussen U, Rasmussen AK, et al. A population-based study of thyroid function after radiotherapy and chemotherapy for a childhood brain tumor. *J Clin Endocrinol Metab* 2003;88:136–140.

118. Gurney JG, Kadan-Lottick NS, Packer RJ. Endocrine and cardiovascular late effects among adult survivors of childhood brain tumors: Childhood Cancer Survivor Study. *Cancer* 2003;97:663–673.

*119. Constine LS, Donaldson SS, McDougall IR, et al. Thyroid dysfunction after radiotherapy in children with Hodgkin's disease. *Cancer* 1984;53:878–883.

120. Paulino AC. Hypothyroidism in children with medulloblastoma: a comparison of 3600 and 2340 cGy craniospinal radiotherapy. *Int J Radiat Oncol Biol Phys* 2002;53:543–547.

*121. Constine LS, Rubin P, Woolf PD, et al. Hyperprolactinemia and hypothyroidism following cytotoxic therapy for central nervous system malignancies. *J Clin Oncol* 1987;5:1841–1851.

122. Samaan NA, Vieto R, Schultz PN, et al. Hypothalamic pituitary and thyroid dysfunction after radiotherapy to the head and neck. *Int J Radiat Oncol Biol Phys* 1982;8:1857–1867.

123. Capen CC. Anatomy, comparative anatomy, and histology of the thyroid. In: Braverman LE, Utiger RD, eds. *Werner and Ingbar's the thyroid.* Philadelphia: Lippincott, 1991:22–40.

*124. Hancock S, McDougall I, Constine L. Thyroid abnormalities after therapeutic external radiation. *Int J Radiat Oncol Biol Phys* 1995;31:1165–1170.

125. Braverman LE, Ingbar SH, Vagenakis AG, et al. Enhanced susceptibility to iodide myxedema in patients with Hashimoto's disease. *J Clin Endocrinol Metab* 1971;32:515–521.

126. Carr RF, LiValsi VA. Morphologic changes in the thyroid after irradiation for Hodgkin's and non-Hodgkin's lymphoma. *Cancer* 1989;64:825–829.

*127. Fajardo LF. *Pathology of radiation injury.* New York: Masson, 1982:205–212.

128. Glatstein E, McHardy-Young S, Brast N, et al. Alterations in serum thyrotropin (TSH) and thyroid function following radiotherapy in patients with malignant lymphoma. *J Clin Endocrinol Metab* 1971;32:833–841.

129. McDougall IR. *Thyroid disease in clinical practice.* London: Chapman & Hall Medical, 1992:304–324.

130. D'Angio G, ed. Delayed consequences of cancer therapy: proven and potential. *Cancer* 1976;37:999–1013.

131. Devney RB, Sklar CA, Nesbit ME Jr, et al. Serial thyroid function measurements in children with Hodgkin's disease. *J Pediatr* 1984;105:223–229.

132. Fjalling M, Tisell LE, Carlsson S, et al. Benign and malignant thyroid nodules after neck irradiation. *Cancer* 1986;58:1219–1224.

133. Fleming ID, Black TL, Thompson EI, et al. Thyroid dysfunction and neoplasia in children receiving neck irradiation for cancer. *Cancer* 1985;55:1190–1194.

134. Liening DA, Duncan NO, Blackeslee DB, et al. Hypothyroidism following radiotherapy for head and neck cancer. *Otolaryngol Head Neck Surg* 1990;103:10–13.

135. Schimpff SC, Diggs CH, Wiswell JG. Radiation-related thyroid dysfunction: implications for the treatment of Hodgkin's disease. *JAMA* 1980;245:48–49.

136. Schimpff SC, Diggs CH, Wiswell JG, et al. Radiation-related thyroid dysfunction: implications for the treatment of Hodgkin's disease. *Ann Intern Med* 1980;92:91–98.

*137. Hancock SL, Cox RS, McDougall IR. Thyroid diseases after treatment of Hodgkin's disease. *N Engl J Med* 1991;325:599–605.

138. Bhatia S, Ramsay N, Bantle J, et al. Thyroid abnormalities after therapy for Hodgkin's disease in childhood. *Oncologist* 1996;1:62–67.

139. Constine L, Schwartz C. The thyroid gland. In: Schwartz C, Hobbie W, Constine L, et al., eds. *Survivors of childhood cancer: assessment and management.* St Louis: Mosby, 1994:151–158.

140. Fuks Z, Glatsten E, Marsa GW, et al. Long-term effects of external radiation on the pituitary and thyroid glands. *Cancer* 1976;37:1152–1161.

141. Nelson DF, Reddy KV, O'Mara RE, et al. Thyroid abnormalities following neck irradiation for Hodgkin's disease. *Cancer* 1978;42:2553–2562.

142. Sklar C, Whitton J, Mertens A, et al. Abnormalities of the thyroid in survivors of Hodgkin's disease: data from the Childhood Cancer Survivor Study. *J Clin Endocrinol Metab* 2000;85:3227–3232.

143. Ogilvy-Stuart A, Shalet S, Gattamamenti H. Thyroid function after treatment of brain tumors in children. *J Pediatr* 1991;119:733–737.

144. Oberfield SE, Sklar C, Allen J, et al. Thyroid and gonadal function and growth of long-term survivors of medulloblastoma/PNET. In Green DM, D'Angio GJ, eds. *Late effects of treatment for childhood cancer.* New York: Wiley-Liss, 1992:55–62.

145. Sanders JE. The impact of marrow transplant preparative regimens on subsequent growth and development. *Semin Hematol* 1991;28:244–249.

146. Borgstrom B, Bolme P. Thyroid function in children after allogeneic bone marrow transplantation. *Bone Marrow Transplant* 1994;13(1):59–64.

147. Leung W, Hudson MM, Strickland DK, et al. Late effects of treatment in survivors of childhood acute myeloid leukemia. *J Clin Oncol* 2000;18:3273–3279.

148. Robison LL, Nesbit ME, Sathes HN, et al. Thyroid abnormalities in long-term survivors of childhood acute lymphoblastic leukemia. *Pediatr Res* 1985;19:266A(abst).

149. Leung W, Hudson M, Zhu Y, et al. Late effects in survivors of infant leukemia. *Leukemia* 2000;14:1185–1190.

150. Hudson M, Greenwald C, Thompson E. Efficacy and toxicity of multiagent chemotherapy and low-dose involved-field radiotherapy in children and adolescents with Hodgkin's disease. *J Clin Oncol* 1993;11:100–108.

151. Marcial-Vega VA, Order SE, Lastner G, et al. Prevention of hypothyroidism related to mantle irradiation for Hodgkin's disease: preoperative photon study. *Int J Radiat Oncol Biol Phys* 1990;18:613–618.

152. Rubin P. The Franz Buschke lecture: late effects of chemotherapy and radiation therapy. A new hypothesis. *Int J Radiat Oncol Biol Phys* 1984;10:5–34.

153. Petersen M, Keeling CA, McDougall IR. Hyperthyroidism with low radioiodine uptake after head and neck irradiation for Hodgkin's disease. *J Nucl Med* 1989;30:255–257.

154. DeGroot LJ. Clinical review 2: diagnostic approach and management of patients exposed to irradiation to the thyroid. *J Clin Endocrinol Metab* 1989;69:925–928.

155. Schneider AB, Recant W, Pinsky SM, et al. Radiation-induced thyroid carcinoma: clinical course and results of therapy in 296 patients. *Ann Intern Med* 1986;105:405–412.

156. Bantle JP, Lee CKK, Levitt SH. Thyroxine administration during radiation therapy to the neck does not prevent subsequent thyroid dysfunction. *Int J Radiat Oncol Biol Phys* 1985;11:1999–2002.

157. Perthes G. Uber den einfluss der roentgenstrahlen auf epitheliale gewebe. Insbesondere aus des carcinom. *Arch Klin Chir* 1903;51:955–1000.

158. Forsterling K. Uber allgemeine und partielle washstums storungen nach kurz davenden rontgen bestrahlungen von saugethieren. *Arch Klin Chir* 1906;81:506.

159. Dalinka MK, Mazzea V. Complications of radiation therapy. *Crit Rev Diagn Imaging* 1984;23:236–267.

*160. Neuhauser EBD, Wittenborg MH, Berman CZ, et al. Irradiation effects of roentgen therapy on the growing spine. *Radiology* 1952;59:637–650.

161. Arkin AM, Simon N. Radiation scoliosis: an experimental study. *J Bone Joint Surg* 1950;32A:396–401.

162. Rutherford H, Dodd GD. Complications of radiation therapy: growing bone. *Semin Roentgenol* 1974;9:15–27.

163. Dawson WB. Growth impairment following radiotherapy in childhood. *Clin Radiol* 1968;19:241–256.

*164. Donaldson SS. Effects of irradiation on skeletal growth and development. In: Green DM, D'Angio GJ, eds. *Late effects of treatment for childhood cancer.* New York: Wiley-Liss, 1992:63–70.

165. Blackburn J, Wells AB. Radiation damage to growing bone: the effect of x-ray doses of 100–1000 rads on mouse tibiae and knee joints. *Br J Radiol* 1963;36:505–513.

166. Willman K, Cox R, Donaldson S. Radiation induced height impairment in pediatric Hodgkin's disease. *Int J Radiat Oncol Biol Phys* 1994;28:85–92.

167. Hogeboom CJ, Grosser SC, Guthrie KA, et al. Stature loss following treatment for Wilms tumor. *Med Pediatr Oncol* 2001;36:295–304.

168. Silber JH, Littman PS, Meadows AT. Stature loss following irradiation for childhood cancer. *J Clin Oncol* 1990;8:304–312.

169. Sklar CA. Growth following therapy for childhood cancer. *Cancer Invest* 1995;13:511–516.

170. Sklar CA. Growth and neuroendocrine dysfunction following therapy for childhood cancer. *Pediatr Clin North Am* 1997;44:489–503.

171. Shalet SM, Brennan BM. Growth and growth hormone status following treatment for childhood leukaemia. *Horm Res* 1998;50:1–10.

172. Riseborough EJ, Grabias SL, Burton RI, et al. Skeletal alterations following irradiation for Wilms' tumor. *J Bone Joint Surg* 1976;58A:526–536.

173. Paulino AC, Wen BC, Brown CK, et al. Late effects in children treated with radiation therapy for Wilms' tumor. *Int J Radiat Oncol Biol Phys* 2000;46:1239–1246.

174. Chapman JA, Deakin DP, Green JH. Slipped upper femoral epiphysis after radiotherapy. *J Bone Joint Surg* 1980;62B:337–339.

175. Prosnitz LR, Lawson JP, Friedlaender GE, et al. Avascular necrosis of bone in Hodgkin's disease patients with combined modality therapy. *Cancer* 1981;47:2793–2797.

*176. Silverman CL, Thomas PR, McAlister WH, et al. Slipped femoral capital epiphysis in irradiated children: dose, volume, and age relationships. *Int J Radiat Oncol Biol Phys* 1981;7:1357–1363.

177. Wolf EL, Berdon WE, Cassady JR, et al. Slipped capital femoral epiphysis as a sequela to childhood irradiation for malignant tumors. *Radiology* 1977;125:781–784.

178. Fletcher BD, Crom DB, Krance RA, et al. Radiation-induced bone abnormalities after bone marrow transplantation for childhood leukemia. *Radiology* 1994;191:231–235.

179. Libshitz A, Edeikin BS. Radiotherapy changes of the pediatric hip. *AJR* 1981;137:585–588.

180. Hanif I, Mahmoud H, Pui CH. Avascular femoral head necrosis in pediatric cancer patients. *Med Pediatr Oncol* 1993;21:655–660.

181. Hoelzer D, Gokbuget N, Ottmann O, et al. Acute lymphoblastic leukemia. *Hematology* 2002;162–192.

182. Gaynon PS, Carrel AL. Glucocorticosteroid therapy in childhood acute lymphoblastic leukemia. *Adv Exp Med Biol* 1999;457:593–605.

183. Shusterman S, Meadows AT. Long term survivors of childhood leukemia. *Curr Opin Hematol* 2000;7:217–222.

184. Gaynon PS, Lustig RH. The use of glucocorticoids in acute lymphoblastic leukemia of childhood. Molecular, cellular, and clinical considerations. *J Pediatr Hematol Oncol* 1995;17:1–12.

185. Strauss AJ, Su JT, Dalton VM, et al. Bony morbidity in children treated for acute lymphoblastic leukemia. *J Clin Oncol* 2001;19:3066–3072.

186. Morris LL, Cassady JR, Jaffe N. Sternal changes following mediastinal irradiation for childhood Hodgkin's disease. *Radiology* 1975;115:701–705.

187. Murphys FD, Blount WP. Cartilaginous exostoses following irradiation. *J Bone Joint Surg* 1981;44:662–668.

188. Jaffe N, Toth BB, Hoar RE, et al. Dental and maxillofacial abnormalities in long-term survivors of childhood cancer: effects of treatment with chemotherapy and radiation to the head and neck. *Pediatrics* 1984;73:816–823.

189. Goldwein JW. Effects of radiation therapy on skeleton growth in childhood. *Clin Orthop* 1991;262:101–107.

190. Katzman H, Waugh T, Berdon W. Skeletal changes following irradiation of childhood tumors. *J Bone Joint Surg* 1969;51:825–842.

191. Kaste SC, Jones-Wallace D, Rose SR, et al. Bone mineral decrements in survivors of childhood acute lymphoblastic leukemia: frequency of occurrence and risk factors for their development. *Leukemia* 2001;15:728–734.

192. Brennan B, Shalet SM. Reduced bone mineral density at completion of chemotherapy for a malignancy [Letter]. *Arch Dis Child* 1999;81(4):372.

193. Arikoski P, Komulainen J, Voutilainen R, et al. Reduced bone mineral density in long-term survivors of childhood acute lymphoblastic leukemia. *J Pediatr Hematol Oncol* 1998;20(3):234–240.

194. Kadan-Lottick N, Marshall JA, Baron AE, et al. Normal bone mineral density after treatment for childhood acute lymphoblastic leukemia diagnosed between 1991 and 1998. *J Pediatr* 2001;138:898–904.

195. Aisenberg J, Hsieh K, Kalaitzoglou G, et al. Bone mineral density in young adult survivors of childhood cancer. *J Pediatr Hematol Oncol* 1998;20(3):241–245.

196. Vassilopoulou-Sellin R, Brosnan P, Delpassand A, et al. Osteopenia in young adult survivors of childhood cancer. *Med Pediatr Oncol* 1999;32:272–278.

197. van Leeuwen BL, Kamps WA, Jansen HW, et al. The effect of chemotherapy on the growing skeleton. *Cancer Treat Rev* 2000;26:363–376.

198. van der Sluis IM, van den Heuvel-Eibrink MM, Hahlen K, et al. Altered bone mineral density and body composition, and increased fracture risk in childhood acute lymphoblastic leukemia. *J Pediatr* 2002;141:204–210.

199. Valimaki MJ, Kinnunen K, Volin L, et al. A prospective study of bone loss and turnover after allogeneic bone marrow transplantation: effect of calcium sup-

plementation with or without calcitonin. *Bone Marrow Transplant* 1999;23:355–361.

200. Kauppila M, Irjala K, Koskinen P, et al. Bone mineral density after allogeneic bone marrow transplantation. *Bone Marrow Transplant* 1999;24:885–889.

201. Bhatia S, Ramsay NK, Weisdorf D, et al. Bone mineral density in patients undergoing bone marrow transplantation for myeloid malignancies. *Bone Marrow Transplant* 1998;22(1):87–90.

202. Nysom K, Holm K, Michaelsen KF, et al. Bone mass after allogeneic BMT for childhood leukaemia or lymphoma. *Bone Marrow Transplant* 2000;25:191–196.

203. Oeffinger KC Mertens AC, Sklar CA, et al. Obesity in adult survivors of childhood acute lymphoblastic leukemia: a report from the Childhood Cancer Survivor Study. *J Clin Oncol* 2003;21:1359–1365.

204. Warner JT, Evans WD, Webb DK, et al. Body composition of long-term survivors of acute lymphoblastic leukaemia. *Med Pediatr Oncol* 2002;38:165–172.

205. Reilly JJ, Ventham JC, Newell J, et al. Risk factors for excess weight gain in children treated for acute lymphoblastic leukaemia. *Int J Obes Relat Metab Disord* 2000;24:1537–1541.

206. Reilly JJ, Kelly A, Ness P, et al. Premature adiposity rebound in children treated for acute lymphoblastic leukemia. *J Clin Endocrinol Metab* 2001;86:2775–2778.

207. American Diabetes Association. Type 2 diabetes in children and adolescents. *Pediatrics* 2000;105:671–680.

208. Arslanian S, Suprasongsin C. Insulin sensitivity, lipids, and body composition in childhood: is "syndrome X" present? *J Clin Endocrinol Metab* 1996;81:1058–1062.

209. Jiang X, Srinivasa SR, Bao W, et al. Association of fasting insulin with longitudinal changes in blood pressure in children and adolescents. *Am J Hypertens* 1993;6:564–569.

210. Manolio TA, Savage PJ, Burke GL, et al. Association of fasting insulin with blood pressure and lipids in young adults. *Arteriosclerosis* 1990;10:430–436.

211. Nysom K, Holm K, Michaelsen KF, et al. Degree of fatness after treatment of malignant lymphoma in childhood. *Med Pediatr Oncol* 2003;40:239–243.

212. Sinaiko AR, Jacobs DR Jr, Steinberger J, et al. Insulin resistance syndrome in childhood: associations of the euglycemic insulin clamp and fasting insulin with fatness and other risk factors. *J Pediatr* 2001;139:700–707.

213. Steinberger J, Daniels SR, et al. Obesity, insulin resistance, diabetes, and cardiovascular risk in children: an American Heart Association scientific statement from the Atherosclerosis, Hypertension, and Obesity in the Young Committee (Council on Cardiovascular Disease in the Young) and the Diabetes Committee (Council on Nutrition, Physical Activity, and Metabolism). *Circulation* 2003;107:1448–1453.

214. Steinberger J, Moran A, Hong CP, et al. Adiposity in childhood predicts obesity and insulin resistance in young adulthood. *J Pediatr* 2001;138:469–473.

215. Didi M, Didcock E, Davies HA, et al. High incidence of obesity in young adults after treatment of acute lymphoblastic leukemia in childhood. *J Pediatr* 1995;127:63–67.

216. Oeffinger KC, Mertens AC, Sklar CA, et al. Obesity in adult survivors of childhood acute lymphoblastic

leukemia: a report from the Childhood Cancer Survivor Study. *J Clin Oncol* 2003;21:1359–1365.

217. Talvensaari KK, Lanning M, Tapanainen P, et al. Long-term survivors of childhood cancer have an increased risk of manifesting the metabolic syndrome. *J Clin Endocrinol Metab* 1996;81:3051–3055.

*218. Hancock SL, Tucker MA, Hoppe RT. Factors affecting late mortality from heart disease after treatment of Hodgkin's disease. *JAMA* 1993;270:1949–1955.

*219. King V, Constine LS, Clark D, et al. Symptomatic coronary artery disease after mantle irradiation for Hodgkin's disease. *Int J Radiat Oncol Biol Phys* 1996;36:881–889.

220. Adams MJ, Lipshultz S, Schwartz C, et al. Radiation associated cardiovascular disease: manifestations and management. *Semin Radiat Oncol* 2003;13:346–356.

221. Fajardo L, Stewart J. Human and experimental observations. In: Bristow M, ed. *Drug-induced heart disease.* Amsterdam: Elsevier/North-Holland, 1980:241–260.

222. Fajardo LF, Eltringham JR, Steward JR. Combined cardiotoxicity of adriamycin and x-radiation. *Lab Invest* 1976;34:86–96.

223. Applefeld MM. The late appearance of chronic pericardial disease in patients treated by radiotherapy for Hodgkin's disease. *Ann Intern Med* 1981;94:338–441.

224. Stewart J, Cohen K, Fajardo L, et al. Radiation-induced heart disease: a study of twenty-five patients. *Radiol* 1967;89:302–310.

225. Green DM, Gingell RL, Pearce J, et al. The effect of mediastinal irradiation on cardiac function of patients treated during childhood and adolescence for Hodgkin's disease. *J Clin Oncol* 1987;5:239–245.

226. Hancock SL, Hoppe RT, Horning SJ, et al. Intercurrent death after Hodgkin's disease therapy in radiotherapy and adjuvant MOPP trials. *Ann Intern Med* 1988;109:183–189.

227. Mauch PM, Weinstein H, Botnick L, et al. An evaluation of long-term survival and treatment complications in children with Hodgkin's disease. *Cancer* 1983;51:925–932.

228. Ni Y, von Segesser LK, Turina M. Futility of pericardiectomy for post-irradiation constrictive pericarditis? *Ann Thorac Surg* 1990;49:445–448.

229. Hancock S, Donaldson S, Hoppe R. Cardiac disease following treatment of Hodgkin's disease in children and adolescents. *J Clin Oncol* 1993;11:1208–1215.

230. Stewart JR, Fajardo LF. Radiation-induced heart disease: an update. *Prog Cardiovasc Dis* 1984;27:173–194.

231. Byhardt R, Brace K, Ruckdeschel J. Dose and treatment factors in radiation-related pericardial effusion associated with the mantle technique for Hodgkin's disease. *Cancer* 1975;35:795–802.

232. LaMonte CS, Yeh S, Straus D. Long-term follow-up of cardiac function in patients with Hodgkin's disease treated with mediastinal irradiation and combination chemotherapy including doxorubicin. *Cancer Treat Rep* 1986;70:439–444.

233. Brosius FCI, Waller BF, Roberts WC. Radiation heart disease. Analysis of 16 young (aged 15–33 years) necropsy patients who received over 3.500 rads to the heart. *Am J Med* 1981;70:519–530.

234. Burns RJ, Bar-Shlomo B, Druck M. Detection of ra-

diation cardiomyopathy by gated radionuclide angiography. *Am J Med* 1983;74:297–302.

*235. Constine L, Schwartz R, Savage D, et al. Cardiac function, perfusion, and morbidity in irradiated long-term survivors of Hodgkin's disease. *Int J Radiat Oncol Biol Phys* 1997;39:897–906.

236. Ewer MS, Jaffe N, Ried H, et al. Doxorubicin cardiotoxicity in children: comparison of a consecutive divided daily dose administration schedule with single dose (rapid) infusion administration. *Med Pediatr Oncol* 1998;31:512–515.

237. Giantris A, Abdurrahman L, Hinkle A, et al. Anthracycline-induced cardiotoxicity in children and young adults. *Crit Rev Oncol Hematol* 1998;27:53–68.

238. Green DM, Grigoriev YA, Nan B, et al. Congestive heart failure after treatment for Wilms' tumor: a report from the National Wilms' Tumor Study Group. *J Clin Oncol* 2001;19:1926–1934.

239. Krischer J, Epstein S, Cuthbertson D, et al. Clinical cardiotoxicity following anthracycline treatment for childhood cancer: the Pediatric Oncology Group experience. *J Clin Oncol* 1997;15:1544–1552.

240. Lipshultz SE, Sanders SP, Goorin AM, et al. Monitoring for anthracycline cardiotoxicity. *Pediatrics* 1994;93:433–437.

241. Lipshultz SE, Lipsitz SR, Mone SM, et al. Female sex and higher drug dose as risk factors for late cardiotoxic effects of doxorubicin therapy for childhood cancer. *N Engl J Med* 1995;332:1738–1743.

242. Lipshultz S, Lipsitz S, Sallan S. Chronic progressive left ventricular systolic dysfunction and afterload excess years after doxorubicin therapy for childhood acute lymphoblastic leukemia. *Proc Am Soc Clin Oncol* 2000;19:580a.

243. Lipshultz SE, Giantris AL, Lipsitz SR, et al. Doxorubicin administration by continuous infusion is not cardioprotective: the Dana–Farber 91-01 Acute Lymphoblastic Leukemia protocol. *J Clin Oncol* 2002; 20:1677–1682.

244. Nysom K, Holm K, Lipsitz SR, et al. Relationship between cumulative anthracycline dose and late cardiotoxicity in childhood acute lymphoblastic leukemia. *J Clin Oncol* 1998;16:545–550.

245. Silber JH, Jakacki RI, Larsen RL, et al. Increased risk of cardiac dysfunction after anthracyclines in girls. *Med Pediatr Oncol* 1993;21:477–479.

246. Steinherz LJ, Graham T, Hurwitz R, et al. Guidelines for cardiac monitoring of children during and after anthracycline therapy: report of the Cardiology Committee of the Children's Cancer Study Group. *Pediatrics* 1992;89:942–949.

247. Steinherz LJ, Steinherz PG, Tan C. Cardiac failure and dysrhythmias 6–19 years after anthracycline therapy: a series of 15 patients. *Med Pediatr Oncol* 1995;24:352–361.

248. Grenier MA, Lipshultz SE. Epidemiology of anthracycline cardiotoxicity in children and adults. *Semin Oncol* 1998;25:72–85.

249. Zinzani PL, Gherlinzoni F, Piovaccari G, et al. Cardiac injury as late toxicity of mediastinal radiation therapy for Hodgkin's disease patients. *Haematologica* 1996;81:132–137.

250. de Valeriola D. Dose optimization of anthracyclines. *Anticancer Res* 1994;14:2307–2313.

251. Shapira J, Gotfried M, Lishner M. Reduced cardiotoxicity of doxorubicin by a 6-hour infusion regimen. A prospective randomized evaluation. *Cancer* 1990;65:870–873.

252. Storm G, van Hoesel QG, de Groot G, et al. A comparative study on the antitumor effect, cardiotoxicity and nephrotoxicity of doxorubicin given as a bolus, continuous infusion or entrapped in liposomes in the Lou/M Wsl rat. *Cancer Chemother Pharmacol* 1989; 24:341–348.

253. Legha SS, Benjamin RS, Mackay B, et al. Reduction of doxorubicin cardiotoxicity by prolonged continuous intravenous infusion. *Ann Intern Med* 1982;96: 133–139.

254. Herman EH, Zhang J, Rifai N, et al. The use of serum levels of cardiac troponin T to compare the protective activity of dexrazoxane against doxorubicin- and mitoxantrone-induced cardiotoxicity. *Cancer Chemother Pharmacol* 2001;48:297–304.

255. Lipshultz SE. Dexrazoxane for protection against cardiotoxic effects of anthracyclines in children. *J Clin Oncol* 1996;14:328–331.

256. Swain SM, Whaley F, Gerber M. Cardioprotection with dexrazoxane for doxorubicin-containing therapy in advanced breast cancer. *J Clin Oncol* 1997;15: 1318–1332.

257. Venturini M, Michelotti A, Del Mastro L, et al. Multicenter randomized controlled clinical trial to evaluate cardioprotection of dexrazoxane versus no cardioprotection in women receiving epirubicin chemotherapy for advanced breast cancer. *J Clin Oncol* 1996;14: 3112–3120.

258. Wexler LH. Ameliorating anthracycline cardiotoxicity in children with cancer: clinical trials with dexrazoxane. *Semin Oncol* 1998;25:86–92.

259. Schwartz C, Tebbi C, London W, et al. Response based therapy for pediatric Hodgkin's disease: Pediatric Oncology Group Protocols 9425/9426. *Med Pediatr Oncol* 2001;37:263(abstr).

260. Tebbi C, Mendenhall N, Schwartz C. Response dependent treatment of stages IA, IIA and IIIA1 micro Hodgkin's disease with DBVE and low dose involved field irradiation with or without dexrazoxane. Fifth International Symposium on Hodgkin's Lymphoma. Harwood Academic, September 22–25, 2001.

261. Hamm CW. Cardiac biomarkers for rapid evaluation of chest pain. *Circulation* 2001;104:1454–1456.

262. Heeschen C, Goldmann BU, Terres W, et al. Cardiovascular risk and therapeutic benefit of coronary interventions for patients with unstable angina according to the troponin T status. *Eur Heart J* 2000;21: 1159–1166.

263. Herman EH, Zhang J, Lipshultz SE, et al. Correlation between serum levels of cardiac troponin-T and the severity of the chronic cardiomyopathy induced by doxorubicin. *J Clin Oncol* 1999;17:2237–2243.

264. Lipshultz SE, Rifai N, Sallan S. Predictive value of cardiac troponin T in pediatric patients at risk for myocardial injury. *Circulation* 1997;96:2641–2648.

265. Mathew P, Suarez W, Kip K, et al. Is there a potential role for serum cardiac troponin I as a marker for myocardial dysfunction in pediatric patients receiving anthracycline-based therapy? A pilot study. *Cancer Invest* 2001;19:352–359.

266. Fishman W, Yee H, Keefe D, et al. Cardiovascular

toxicity with cancer chemotherapy. *Curr Probl Cancer* 1997;21:301–360.

267. Carlson K, Smedmyr B, Backlund L, et al. Subclinical disturbances in cardiac function at rest and in gas exchange during exercise are common findings after autologous bone marrow transplantation. *Bone Marrow Transplant* 1994;14:949–954.

268. Eames G, Crosson J, Steinberger J, et al. Cardiovascular function in children following bone marrow transplant: a cross-sectional study. *Bone Marrow Transplant* 1997;19:61–66.

269. Hertenstein B, Stefanic M, Schmeiser T. Cardiac toxicity of bone marrow transplantation: predictive value of cardiologic evaluation before transplant. *J Clin Oncol* 1994;12:998–1004.

270. Hogarty AN, Leahey A, Zhao H, et al. Longitudinal evaluation of cardiopulmonary performance during exercise after bone marrow transplantation in children. *J Pediatr* 2000;136:311–317.

271. Pihkala J, Happonen JM, Virtanen K, et al. Cardiopulmonary evaluation of exercise tolerance after chest irradiation and anticancer chemotherapy in children and adolescents. *Pediatrics* 1995;95:722–726.

272. Carlson RG, Mayfield WR, Norman S, et al. Radiation-associated valvular disease. *Chest* 1991;99:538–545.

273. Jakacki R, Goldwein J, Larsen R, et al. Cardiac dysfunction following spinal irradiation during childhood. *J Clin Oncol* 1993;11:1033–1038.

274. Cohen SI, Bharati S, Glass J, et al. Radiotherapy as a cause of complete atrioventricular block as Hodgkin's disease: an electrophysiological–pathological correlation. *Arch Intern Med* 1981;141:676–679.

275. Kadota R, Burgert E, Driscoll D, et al. Cardiopulmonary function in long-term survivors of childhood Hodgkin's lymphoma: a pilot study. *Mayo Clin Proc* 1988;63:362–367.

276. De Wolf D, Suys D, Matthys D, et al. Stress echocardiography in the evaluation of late cardiac toxicity after moderate dose of anthracycline therapy in childhood. *Int J Pediatr Hematol Oncol* 1994;1: 399–401.

277. Jenney ME, Faragher EB, Jones PH, et al. Lung function and exercise capacity in survivors of childhood leukaemia. *Med Pediatr Oncol* 1995;24:222–230.

278. Turner-Gomes SO, Lands LC, Halton J. Cardiorespiratory status after treatment for acute lymphoblastic leukemia. *Med Pediatr Oncol* 1996;26:160–165.

279. Schwartz CL, Hobbie WL, Truesdell S. Corrected QT interval prolongation in anthracycline-treated survivors of childhood cancer. *J Clin Oncol* 1993;11:1906–1910.

280. Corn BW, Tract BJ, Goodman RL. Irradiation-related ischemic heart disease. *J Clin Oncol* 1990;8:741–750.

281. Cosset JM, Henry-Amar M, Meerwaldt JH. Long-term toxicity of early stages of Hodgkin's disease therapy: the EORTC experience. *Ann Oncol* 1991;2:77–82.

282. Mauch P, Tarbell N, Weinstein H, et al. Stage IA and IIA supradiaphragmatic Hodgkin's disease: prognostic factors in surgically staged patients treated with mantle and para-aortic irradiation. *J Clin Oncol* 1988;6:1576–1583.

283. Donaldson SS, Kaplan HS. Complications of treatment of Hodgkin's disease in children. *Cancer Treat Rep* 1982;66:977–989.

284. Makinen L, Makipernaa A, Rautanen J, et al. Long-term cardiac sequelae after treatment of malignant tumors with radiotherapy or cytostatics in childhood. *Cancer* 1990;65:1913–1917.

285. Cazin B, Gorin N, Laporte J, et al. Cardiac complications after bone marrow transplantation. *Cancer* 1986;57:2061–2069.

286. Constine L, Rubin P. Morbidity of combined chemotherapy and radiotherapy. In: Plowman DN, McElwain T, Meadows A, eds. *Complications of cancer management survey.* London: Butterworth Heinemann, 1991:13–26.

287. Rubin P, Finkelstein JN, Siemann DW, et al. Predictive biochemical assays for late radiation effects. *Int J Radiat Oncol Biol Phys* 1986;12:469–476.

288. Fryer CJH, Fitzpatrick PJ, Rider WD, et al. Radiation pneumonitis: experience following a large single dose of radiation. *Int J Radiat Oncol Biol Phys* 1978; 4:931–936.

289. Gross NJ. Experimental radiation pneumonitis. IV: Leakage of circulatory proteins onto the alveolar surface. *J Lab Clin Med* 1980;95:19–31.

290. Rosenkrans WA, Penny DP. Cell-cell matrix interactions in induced lung injury: III. Long term effects of X-irradiation on basal laminar proteoglycans. *Anat Rec* 1986;215:127–133.

291. Littman P, Meadows AT, Polgar G, et al. Pulmonary function in survivors of Wilms' tumor. *Cancer* 1976; 37:2773–2776.

292. Mah K, van Dyke J. Quantitative measurements of changes on human lung density following irradiation. *Radiother Oncol* 1988;11:169–179.

293. McDonald S, Rubin P, Maasilta P. Response of normal lung to irradiation tolerance doses/tolerance volumes in pulmonary radiation syndromes. *Front Radiat Ther Oncol* 1989;23:255–276.

294. McDonald S, Rubin P, Phillips T, et al. Injury to the lung from cancer therapy: clinical syndromes, measurable endpoints, and potential scoring systems. *Int J Radiat Oncol Biol Phys* 1995;31:1187–1203.

295. Bradley JI, Zoberi I, Wasserman TH. Thoracic radiotherapy: complications and injury to normal tissue. *Prin Prac Radiat Oncol Updates* 2002;3(1):1–16.

296. Kreisman H, Wolkove N. Pulmonary toxicity of antineoplastic therapy. *Semin Oncol* 1992;19:508–520.

297. Bossi G, Cerveri I, Volpini E, et al. Long-term pulmonary sequelae after treatment of childhood Hodgkin's disease. *Ann Oncol* 1997;8[Suppl 1]: 19–24.

298. Fryer C, Hutchinson RJ, Krailo M, et al. Efficacy and toxicity of 12 courses of ABVD chemotherapy followed by low-dose regional radiation in advanced Hodgkin's disease in children: a report from the Children's Cancer Study Group. *J Clin Oncol* 1990;8: 1971–1980.

299. Mefferd JM, Donaldson SS, Link MP. Pediatric Hodgkin's disease: pulmonary, cardiac, and thyroid function following combined modality therapy. *Int J Radiat Oncol Biol Phys* 1989;16:679–685.

300. Marina NM, Greenwald CA, Fairclough DL, et al. Serial pulmonary function studies in children treated for newly diagnosed Hodgkin's disease with mantle radiotherapy plus cycles of cyclophosphamide, vincristine, and procarbazine alternating with cycles of doxorubicin, bleomycin, vinblastine, and dacarbazine. *Cancer* 1995;75:1706–1711.

301. Nysom K, Holm K, Olsen JH. Pulmonary function

after treatment for acute lymphoblastic leukaemia in childhood. *Br J Cancer* 1998;78:21–27.

302. Nysom K, Holm K, Hertz H, et al. Risk factors for reduced pulmonary function after malignant lymphoma in childhood. *Med Pediatr Oncol* 1998;30:240–248.

303. Castellino R, Glatstein E, Turbow M, et al. Latent radiation injury of lungs or heart activated by steroid withdrawal. *Ann Intern Med* 1974;80:593–599.

304. Cerveri I, Fulgoni P, Giorgiani G. Lung function abnormalities after bone marrow transplantation in children: has the trend recently changed? *Chest* 2001;120:1900–1906.

305. Kaplan EB, Wodell RA, Wilmott RW. Late effects of bone marrow transplantation on pulmonary function in children. *Bone Marrow Transplant* 1994;14:613–621.

306. Nenadov Beck M, Meresse V, Hartmann O, et al. Long-term pulmonary sequelae after autologous bone marrow transplantation in children without total body irradiation. *Bone Marrow Transplant* 1995;16:771–775.

307. Nysom K, Holm K, Hesse B, et al. Lung function after allogeneic bone marrow transplantation for leukaemia or lymphoma. *Arch Dis Child* 1996;74:432–436.

308. Leiper AD. Non-endocrine late complications of bone marrow transplantation in childhood: part II. *Br J Haematol* 2002;118:23–43.

309. Schultz KR, Green GJ, Wensley D, et al. Obstructive lung disease in children after allogeneic bone marrow transplantation. *Blood* 1994;84:3212–3220.

310. Keane T, van Dyke J, Rider W. Idiopathic interstitial pneumonia following bone marrow transplantation: the relationship with total body irradiation. *Int J Radiat Oncol Biol Phys* 1981;7:1365–1370.

311. Champlin R, Gale R. The early complications of bone marrow transplantation. *Semin Hematol* 1984;12:101–108.

312. Mertens AC, Yasui Y, Liu Y. Pulmonary complications in survivors of childhood and adolescent cancer. *Cancer* 2002;95:2431–2441.

313. Green DM. Fertility and pregnancy outcome after treatment for cancer in childhood or adolescence. *Oncologist* 1997;2:171–179.

314. Chapman RM, Sutcliffe SB. Protection of ovarian function by oral contraceptives in women receiving chemotherapy for Hodgkin's disease. *Blood* 1981;58:849–851.

315. Chapman RM, Sutcliffe SB, Malpas JS. Cytotoxic-induced ovarian failure in women with Hodgkin's disease. I. Hormone function. *JAMA* 1979;242:1877–1881.

316. Chapman RM, Sutcliffe SB, Malpas JS. Cytotoxic-induced ovarian failure in women with Hodgkin's disease. II. Effects on sexual function. *JAMA* 1979;242:1882–1884.

317. Shalet SM, Beardwell CG, Jacobs HS, et al. Ovarian failure following abdominal irradiation in childhood. *Br J Cancer* 1976;33:655–658.

318. Jones WH III. Cyclic histology and cytology of the genital tract. In: Jones HWI, Wentz AC, Burnett LS, eds. *Novak's textbook of gynecology.* Baltimore: Williams & Wilkins, 1988.

319. Torano A, Halperin E, Leventhal B. The ovary. In: Schwartz C, Hobbie W, Constine L, et al., eds. *Survivors of childhood cancer, assessment and management.* St Louis: Mosby, 1994:213–224.

320. Ash P. The influence of radiation on fertility in man. *Br J Radiol* 1980;53:271–278.

321. Lushbaugh CC, Casarett GW. The effects of gonadal irradiation in clinical radiation therapy: a review. *Cancer* 1976;37:1111–1120.

322. Wallace WHB, Shalet SM, Crowne EC, et al. Ovarian failure following abdominal irradiation in childhood: natural history and prognosis. *Clin Oncol* 1989;1:75–79.

*323. Byrne J, Mulvihill JJ, Myers MH, et al. Effects of treatment on fertility in long-term survivors of childhood or adolescent cancer. *N Engl J Med* 1987;317:1315–1321.

324. Stillman RJ, Schinfeld JS, Schiff I, et al. Ovarian failure in long-term survivors of childhood malignancy. *Am J Obstet Gynecol* 1981;139:62–66.

325. Halperin EC. Concerning the spinal component of the craniospinal irradiation field for central nervous system malignancies. *Int J Radiat Oncol Biol Phys* 1993;26:357–362.

326. Haie-Meder C, Mlika-Cabanne N, Michel G, et al. Radiotherapy after ovarian transposition: ovarian function and fertility preservation. *Int J Radiat Oncol Biol Phys* 1993;25:419–424.

327. LeFloch O, Donaldson SS, Kaplan HS. Pregnancy following oophoropexy and total nodal irradiation in women with Hodgkin's disease. *Cancer* 1976;38:2263–2268.

328. Ortin TT, Shostak CA, Donaldson SS. Gonadal status and reproductive function following treatment for Hodgkin's disease in childhood: the Stanford experience. *Int J Radiat Oncol Biol Phys* 1990;19:873–880.

329. Sklar CA, Kim TH, Williamson JF, et al. Ovarian function after successful bone marrow transplantation in post-menarchal females. *Med Pediatr Oncol* 1983;11:361–364.

330. Sanders JE, Buckner CD, Leonard JM, et al. Late effects on gonadal function of cyclophosphamide, total-body irradiation, and marrow transplantation. *Transplantation* 1983;36:252–255.

331. Horning SJ, Hoppe RT, Kaplan HS, et al. Female reproductive potential after treatment for Hodgkin's disease. *N Engl J Med* 1981;304:1377–1382.

332. Mackie E, Radford M, Shalet S. Gonadal function following chemotherapy for childhood Hodgkin's disease. *Med Pediatr Oncol* 1996;27:74–78.

333. Bath LE, Hamish W, Wallace B, et al. Late effects of the treatment of childhood cancer on the female reproductive system and the potential for fertility preservation. *Int J Obstet Gynaecol* 2002;109(2):107–114.

334. Damewood MD, Grochow LB. Prospects for fertility after chemotherapy or radiation for neoplastic disease. *Fertil Steril* 1986;45:443–459.

335. Hill M, Milan S, Cunningham D. Evaluation of the efficacy of the VEEP regimen in adult Hodgkin's disease with assessment of gonadal and cardiac toxicity. *J Clin Oncol* 1995;13:1283–1284.

336. Mayer EI, Dopfer RE, Klingebiel T. Longitudinal gonadal function after bone marrow transplantation for acute lymphoblastic leukemia during childhood. *Pediatr Transplant* 1999;3:38–44.

337. Nicosia SV, Matus-Ridley M, Meadows AT. Gonadal effects of cancer therapy in girls. *Cancer* 1985;55:2364–2372.

338. Thomson AB, Critchley HO, Kelnar CJ, et al. Late re-

productive sequelae following treatment of childhood cancer and options for fertility preservation. *Best Pract Res Clin Endocrinol Metab* 2002;16:311–334.

339. Lange B, Littman P. Management of Hodgkin's disease in children and adolescents. *Cancer* 1983;51:1371–1377.

340. Kreuser ED, Felsenberg D, Behles C. Long-term gonadal dysfunction and its impact on bone mineralization in patients following COPP/ABVD chemotherapy for Hodgkin's disease. *Ann Oncol* 1992;3:105–110.

341. Chiarelli AM, Marrett LD, Darlington G. Early menopause and infertility in females after treatment for childhood cancer diagnosed in 1964–1988 in Ontario, Canada. *Am J Epidemiol* 1999;150:245–254.

342. Santoro A, Valagussa P. Advances in the treatment of Hodgkin's disease. *Curr Opin Oncol* 1992;4:821–828.

343. Leventhal B, Halperin E, Torano A. The testes. In: Schwartz C, Hobbie W, Constine L, et al., eds. *Survivors of childhood cancer, assessment and management.* St Louis: Mosby, 1994:225–244.

344. Izard M. Leydig cell function and radiation: a review of the literature. *Radiother Oncol* 1995;34:1–8.

345. Griffin JE, Wilson JD. Disorders of the testes and the male reproductive tract. In: Wilson JD, Foster DW, eds. *Williams textbook of endocrinology.* Philadelphia: WB Saunders, 1992:799–852.

346. Heller GC. Effects on the germinal epithelium in radiobiological factors in manned space flight. In: Langham WH, ed. *NRC Publication 1487.* Washington, DC: National Academy of Sciences, National Research Council, 1967:124–133.

*347. Sklar CA, Robison LL, Nesbit ME, et al. Effects of radiation on testicular function in long-term survivors of childhood acute lymphoblastic leukemia: a report from the Children's Cancer Study Group. *J Clin Oncol* 1990;8:1981–1987.

348. Kinsella T, Fraass B, Glatstein E. Late effects of radiation therapy in the treatment of Hodgkin's disease. *Cancer* 1982;69:1241–1247.

349. Shalet SM, Beardwell CG, Pearson D, et al. The effects of varying doses of cerebral irradiation on growth hormone production in childhood. *Clin Endocrinol* 1976;5:287–290.

350. Relander T, Cavallin-Stahl E, Garwicz S. Gonadal and sexual function in men treated for childhood cancer. *Med Pediatr Oncol* 2000;35:52–63.

351. Shalet SM, Horner A, Akrned SR, et al. Leydig cell damage after testicular irradiation for acute lymphoblastic leukemia. *Med Pediatr Oncol* 1985;13:65–68.

352. Brauner R, Catlabiano P, Rappaport R, et al. Leydig cell insufficiency after testicular irradiation for acute lymphoblastic leukemia. *Horm Res* 1988;30:111–114.

353. Muller H, Klinkhammer-Schalke M, Seelbach-Gobel B, et al. Gonadal function of young adults after therapy of malignancies during childhood or adolescence. *Eur J Pediatr* 1996;155:763–769.

354. Ben Arush MW, Solt I, Lightman A, et al. Male gonadal function in survivors of childhood Hodgkin and non-Hodgkin lymphoma. *Pediat Hematol Oncol* 2000;17(3):239–245.

355. Dhabhar BN, Malhotra H, Joseph R. Gonadal function in prepubertal boys following treatment for Hodgkin's disease. *Am J Pediatr Hematol Oncol* 1993;15:306–310.

356. Gerres L, Bramswig JH, Schlegel W, et al. The effects of etoposide on testicular function in boys treated for Hodgkin's disease. *Cancer* 1998;83:2217–2222.

357. Kulkarni S, Sastry P, Saikia T, et al. Gonadal function following ABVD therapy for Hodgkin's disease. *Am J Clin Oncol* 1997;20:354–357.

358. Muller U, Stahel R. Gonadal function after MACOP-B or VACOP-B with or without dose intensification and ABMT in young patients with aggressive non-Hodgkin's lymphoma. *Ann Oncol* 1993;4:399–402.

359. Pryzant RM, Meistrich ML, Wilson G, et al. Long-term reduction in sperm count after chemotherapy with and without radiation therapy for non-Hodgkin's lymphomas. *J Clin Oncol* 1993;11:239–247.

360. Bokemeyer C, Schmoll HJ, van Rhee J, et al. Long-term gonadal toxicity after therapy for Hodgkin's and non-Hodgkin's lymphoma. *Ann Hematol* 1994;68(3):105–110.

361. Heyn R, Raney RB Jr, Hays DM. Late effects of therapy in patients with paratesticular rhabdomyosarcoma. Intergroup Rhabdomyosarcoma Study Committee. *J Clin Oncol* 1992;10:614–623.

362. Kenney LB, Laufer MR, Grant FD, et al. High risk of infertility and long term gonadal damage in males treated with high dose cyclophosphamide for sarcoma during childhood. *Cancer* 2001;91:613–621.

363. Meistrich ML, Wilson G, Brown BW, et al. Impact of cyclophosphamide on long-term reduction in sperm count in men treated with combination chemotherapy for Ewing and soft tissue sarcomas. *Cancer* 1992;70:2703–2712.

364. Schellong G, Potter R, Bramswig J, et al. High cure rates and reduced long-term toxicity in pediatric Hodgkin's disease: the German–Austrian multicenter trial DAL-HD-90. *J Clin Oncol* 1999;17:3736–3744.

365. Longhi A, Macchiagodena M, Vitali G, et al. Fertility in male patients treated with neoadjuvant chemotherapy for osteosarcoma. *J Pediatr Hematol Oncol* 2003;25:292–296.

366. Blatt J, Sherins RJ, Niebrugge D, et al. Leydig cell function in boys following treatment for testicular relapse of acute lymphoblastic leukemia. *J Clin Oncol* 1985;3:1227–1231.

367. Sanders JE. Effects of bone marrow transplantation on reproductive function. In: Green DM, D'Angio GJ, eds. *Late effects of treatment for childhood cancer.* New York: Wiley-Liss, 1992:95–102

368. Blatt J, Mulvihill JJ, Ziegler JL, et al. Pregnancy outcome following cancer chemotherapy. *Am J Med* 1980;69:828–832.

369. Critchley HO, Bath LE, Wallace WH. Radiation damage to the uterus: review of the effects of treatment of childhood cancer. *Hum Fertil* 2002;5:61–66.

370. Green DM, Whitton JA, Stovall M. Pregnancy outcome of female survivors of childhood cancer: a report from the Childhood Cancer Survivor Study. *Am J Obstet Gynecol* 2002;187:1070–1080.

371. Green DM, Whitton JA, Stovall M. Pregnancy outcome of partners of male survivors of childhood cancer: a report from the Childhood Cancer Survivor Study. *J Clin Oncol* 2003;21:716–721.

*372. Green DM, Peabody EM, Nan B. Pregnancy outcome after treatment for Wilms tumor: a report from the National Wilms Tumor Study Group. *J Clin Oncol* 2002;20:2506–2513.

373. Teinturier C, Hartmann O, Valteau-Couanet D, et al. Ovarian function after autologous bone marrow transplantation in childhood: high-dose busulfan is a major cause of ovarian failure. *Bone Marrow Transplant* 1998;22:989–994.

374. Sanders JE, Hawley J, Levy W. Pregnancies following high-dose cyclophosphamide with or without high-dose busulfan or total-body irradiation and bone marrow transplantation. *Blood* 1996;87:3045–3052.

375. Agarwal A. Semen banking in patients with cancer: 20-year experience. *Int J Androl* 2000;23 [Suppl 2]:16–19.

376. Hallak J, Hendin B, Thomas A, et al. Investigation of fertilizing capacity of cryopreserved spermatogonia from patients with cancer. *J Urol* 1998;159:1217–1220.

377. Khalifa E, Oehninger S, Acosta A. Successful fertilization and pregnancy outcome in in-vitro fertilization using cryopreserved/thawed spermatozoa from patients with malignant diseases. *Hum Reprod* 1992;7:105–108.

378. Muller J, Sonksen J, Sommer P, et al. Cryopreservation of semen from pubertal boys with cancer. *Med Pediatr Oncol* 2000;34:191–194.

379. Damani MN, Master V, Meng MV. Postchemotherapy ejaculatory azoospermia: fatherhood with sperm from testis tissue with intracytoplasmic sperm injection. *J Clin Oncol* 2002;20:930–936.

380. Pfeifer S, Coutifaris C. Reproductive technologies 1998: options available for the cancer patient. *Med Pediatr Oncol* 1999;33:34–40.

381. Bahadur G, Steele S. Ovarian tissue cryopreservation for patients. *Hum Reprod* 1996;11:2215–2216.

382. Donnez J, Godin P, Qu J, et al. Gonadal cryopreservation in the young patient with gynaecological malignancy. *Curr Opin Obstet Gynecol* 2000;12:1–9.

383. Newton H. The cryopreservation of ovarian tissue as a strategy for preserving the fertility of cancer patients. *Hum Reprod Update* 1998;4:237–247.

384. Byrne J, Rasmussen SA, Steinhorn SC. Genetic disease in offspring of long-term survivors of childhood and adolescent cancer. *Am J Hum Genet* 1998;62:45–52.

385. Green DM, Fiorello A, Zevon MA, et al. Birth defects and childhood cancer in offspring of survivors of childhood cancer. *Arch Pediatr Adolesc Med* 1997;15:379–383.

386. Hansen M, Kurinczuk JJ, Bower C, et al. The risk of major birth defects after intracytoplasmic sperm injection and in vitro fertilization. *N Engl J Med* 2002;346:725–730.

387. Bonduelle M, Liebaers I, Deketelaere V, et al. Neonatal data on a cohort of 2889 infants born after ICSI (1991–1999) and of 2995 infants born after IVF (1983–1999). *Hum Reprod* 2002;17(3):671–694.

388. Simpson JL, Lamb DJ. Genetic effects of intracytoplasmic sperm injection. *Semin Reprod Med* 2001;19:239–249.

389. Serafini P. Outcome and follow-up of children born after IVF-surrogacy. *Hum Reprod Update* 2001;7:23–27.

390. Ericson A, Kallen B. Congenital malformations in infants born after IVF: a population-based study. *Hum Reprod* 2001;16:504–509.

391. Sankila R, Olsen JH, Anderson H, et al. Risk of cancer among offspring of childhood-cancer survivors. *N Engl J Med* 1998;338:1339–1344.

392. Friedman DL, Kadan-Lottick N, Liu Y, et al. History of cancer among first-degree relatives of childhood cancer survivors: a report from the Childhood Cancer Survivor Study. *Proc Annu Meet Am Soc Clin Oncol* 2001:433a.

393. Withers R, Mason K, Thames H. Late radiation response of kidney assayed by tubule-cell survival. *Br J Radiol* 1986;59:587–595.

394. McGill CW, Holder TM, Smith TH, et al. Postradiation renovascular hypertension. *J Pediatr Surg* 1979;14:831–833.

395. Cassady JR. Clinical radiation nephropathy. *Int J Radiat Oncol Biol Phys* 1995;31:1249–1256.

396. Irwin C, Fyles A, Wong CS, et al. Late renal function following whole abdominal irradiation. *Radiother Oncol* 1996;38:257–261.

397. Cassady JR, Lebowitz RL, Jaffe N, et al. Effect of low dose irradiation on renal enlargement in children following nephrectomy for Wilms' tumor. *Acta Radiol Oncol* 1981;20:5–8.

*398. Ritchey M, Green D, Thomas P, et al. Renal failure in Wilms' tumor patients: a report from the National Wilms' Tumor Study Group. *Med Pediatr Oncol* 1996;26:75–80.

399. Smith GR, Thomas PR, Ritchey M, et al. Long-term renal function in patients with irradiated bilateral Wilms tumor. National Wilms' Tumor Study Group. *Am J Clin Oncol* 1998;21:58–63.

400. Bailey S, Roberts A, Brock C, et al. Nephrotoxicity in survivors of Wilms' tumours in the North of England. *Br J Cancer* 2002;87(10):1092–1098.

401. Breslow NE, Takashima JR, Ritchey ML, et al. Renal failure in the Denys–Drash and Wilms' tumor–aniridia syndromes. *Cancer Res* 2000;60(15):4030–4032.

402. Tarbell N, Guinan E, Neimeyer C, et al. Late onset of renal dysfunction in survivors of bone marrow transplantation. *Int J Radiat Oncol Biol Phys* 1988;15:99–104.

403. Lonnerholm G, Carlson K, Bratteby LE, et al. Renal function after autologous bone marrow transplantation. *Bone Marrow Transplant* 1991;8:129–134.

404. Patzer L, Hempel L, Ringelmann F, et al. Renal function after conditioning therapy for bone marrow transplantation in childhood. *Med Pediatr Oncol* 1997;28:274–283.

405. Bianchetti MG, Kanaka C, Ridolfi-Luthy A, et al. Persisting renotubular sequelae after cisplatin in children and adolescents. *Am J Nephrol* 1991;11(2):127–130.

406. Cvitkovic E. Cumulative toxicities from cisplatin therapy and current cytoprotective measures. *Cancer Treat Rev* 1998;24:265–281.

407. Hutchison FN, Perez EA, Gandara DR, et al. Renal salt wasting in patients treated with cisplatin. *Ann Intern Med* 1988;108:21–25.

408. McKeage MJ. Comparative adverse effect profiles of platinum drugs. *Drug Saf* 1995;13:228–244.

409. Ettinger LJ, Krailo MD, Gaynon PS, et al. A phase I study of carboplatin in children with acute leukemia in bone marrow relapse. *Cancer* 1993;72:917–922.

410. Ettinger LJ, Gaynon PS, Krailo MD. A phase II study of carboplatin in children with recurrent or progressive solid tumors. *Cancer* 1994;73:1297–1301.

411. Gaynon PS, Ettinger LJ, Baum ES, et al. Carboplatin

in childhood brain tumors. A Children's Cancer Study Group Phase II trial. *Cancer* 1990;66:2465–2469.

412. Meyer WH, Pratt CB, Poquette CA. Carboplatin/ifosfamide window therapy for osteosarcoma: results of the St Jude Children's Research Hospital OS-91 trial. *J Clin Oncol* 2001;19:171–182.

413. Stern JW, Bunin N. Prospective study of carboplatin-based chemotherapy for pediatric germ cell tumors. *Med Pediatr Oncol* 2002;39:163–167.

414. Arndt C, Morgenstern B, Wilson D, et al. Renal function in children and adolescents following 72 g/m² of ifosfamide. *Cancer Chemother Pharmacol* 1994; 34(5):431–433.

415. Arndt C, Morgenstern B, Hawkins D, et al. Renal function following combination chemotherapy with ifosfamide and cisplatin in patients with osteogenic sarcoma. *Med Pediatr Oncol* 1999;32(2):93–96.

416. Loebstein R, Koren G. Ifosfamide-induced nephrotoxicity in children: critical review of predictive risk factors. *Pediatrics* 1998;10:E8.

417. Prasad VK, Lewis IJ, Aparicio SR. Progressive glomerular toxicity of ifosfamide in children. *Med Pediatr Oncol* 1996;27:149–155.

418. Skinner R, Pearson AD, English MW, et al. Risk factors for ifosfamide nephrotoxicity in children. *Lancet* 1996;348:578–580.

419. Chowhan NM. Injurious effects of radiation on the esophagus. *Am J Gastroenterol* 1990;85:115–120.

420. Sher ME, Bauer J. Radiation induced enteropathy. *Am J Gastroenterol* 1990;85:121–128.

421. Churnratanakul S, Wirzba G, Lam T, et al. Radiation and the small intestine. Future perspectives for preventive therapy. *Dig Dis* 1990;8:45–60.

422. Donaldson SS, Jundt S, Ricour C, et al. Radiation enteritis in children. *Cancer* 1975;35:1167–1178.

423. Emami B, Lyman J, Brown A, et al. Tolerance of normal tissue to therapeutic irradiation. *Int J Radiat Oncol Biol Phys* 1991;21:109–122.

424. Woods W, Dehner L, Nesbit M, et al. Fetal venoocclusive disease of the liver following high dose chemotherapy, irradiation and bone marrow transplantation. *Am J Med* 1998;60:285–290.

425. Yankelevitz DF, Knapp PH, Henschke CI, et al. MR appearance of radiation hepatitis. *Clin Imaging* 1992;16:89–92.

*426. Ingold JA, Reed GB, Kaplan HS, et al. Radiation hepatitis. *AJR* 1963;93:200–208.

427. Lawrence T, Robertson J, Ansher M, et al. Hepatic toxicity resulting from cancer treatment. *Int J Radiat Oncol Biol Phys* 1995;31:1237–1248.

428. Fajardo L, Colby T. Pathogenesis of veno-occlusive liver disease after irradiation. *Arch Pathol Lab Med* 1980;104:584–588.

429. Bearman SI. The syndrome of hepatic veno-occlusive disease after marrow transplantation. *Blood* 1995; 85(11):3005–3020.

430. Carreras E, Bertz H, Arcese W, et al. Incidence and outcome of hepatic veno-occlusive disease after blood or marrow transplantation: a prospective cohort study of the European Group for Blood and Marrow Transplantation. *Blood* 1998;92:3599–3604.

431. Hasegawa S, Horibe K, Kawabe T, et al. Veno-occlusive disease of the liver after allogeneic bone marrow transplantation in children with hematologic

malignancies: incidence, onset time and risk factors. *Bone Marrow Transplant* 1998;22:1191–1197.

432. Ortega J, Donaldson S, Percy S, et al. Venoocclusive disease of the liver after chemotherapy with vincristine, actinomycin D, and cyclophosphamide for the treatment of rhabdomyosarcoma. A report of the Intergroup Rhabdomyosarcoma Study Group. *Cancer* 1997;79:2435–2439.

433. Dawson LA, Ten Haken RK, Lawrence TS. Partial irradiation of the liver. *Semin Radiat Oncol* 2001;11: 240–246.

*434. Tefft M, Mitus A, Das L, et al. Irradiation of the liver in children: review of experience in the acute and chronic phases, and in the intact normal and partially resected. *AJR* 1990;108:365–385.

*435. Thomas PRM, Tefft M, D'Angio GJ, et al. Acute toxicities associated with radiation in the second National Wilms' Tumor Study. *J Clin Oncol* 1988;6:1694–1698.

436. Lawrence TS, Ten Haken RK, Kessler ML, et al. The use of 3-D dose volume analysis to predict radiation hepatitis. *Int J Radiat Oncol Biol Phys* 1992;23: 781–788.

437. Nanda SK, Schachat AP. Ocular complications following radiation therapy to the orbit. In: Green DM, D'Angio GJ, eds. *Late effects of treatment for childhood cancer.* New York: Wiley-Liss, 1992:11–22.

438. Wara W, Irvine A, Neger R, et al. Radiation retinopathy. *Int J Radiat Oncol Biol Phys* 1979;5:31–83.

439. Hilliard L, Berkow R, Watterson J, et al. Retinal toxicity associated with cisplatin and etoposide in pediatric patients. *Med Pediatr Oncol* 1997;28:310–313.

440. Parsons J, Fitzgerald C, Hood C, et al. The effects of irradiation of the eye and optic nerve. *Int J Radiat Oncol Biol Phys* 1983;9:609–622.

441. Parsons JT, Bova FJ, Mendenhall WM, et al. Response of the normal eye to high dose radiotherapy. *Oncology (Huntingt)* 1996;10:837–847.

442. Paulino AC. Role of radiation therapy in parameningeal rhabdomyosarcoma. *Cancer Invest* 1999;17:223–230.

443. Paulino AC, Simon JH, Zhen W, et al. Long-term effects in children treated with radiotherapy for head and neck rhabdomyosarcoma. *Int J Radiat Oncol Biol Phys* 2000;48:1489–1495.

444. Oberlin O, Rey A, Anderson J, et al. Treatment of orbital rhabdomyosarcoma: survival and late effects of treatment—results of an international workshop. *J Clin Oncol* 2001;19:197–204.

445. Raney RB, Asmar L, Vassilopoulou-Sellin R. Late complications of therapy in 213 children with localized, nonorbital soft-tissue sarcoma of the head and neck: a descriptive report from the Intergroup Rhabdomyosarcoma Studies (IRS)-II and -III. IRS Group of the Children's Cancer Group and the Pediatric Oncology Group. *Med Pediatr Oncol* 1999;33: 362–371.

446. Raney RB, Anderson JR, Kollath J. Late effects of therapy in 94 patients with localized rhabdomyosarcoma of the orbit: report from the Intergroup Rhabdomyosarcoma Study (IRS)-III, 1984–1991. *Med Pediatr Oncol* 2000;34:413–420.

*447. Merriam G, Focht E. Radiation dose to the lens in treatment of tumors of the eye and adjacent structures: possibilities of cataract formation. *Radiology* 1958;71:357–369.

448. Britten M, Halman K, Meredith W. Radiation

cataract: new evidence on radiation dosage to the lens. *Br J Radiol* 1966;39:612–617.

449. Otake M, Schull WJ. A review of forty-five years study of Hiroshima and Nagasaki atomic bomb survivors radiation cataract. *J Radiat Res* 1991;32:283–293.

450. Deeg H, Flournoy N, Sullivan K, et al. Cataracts after total body irradiation and marrow transplantation: a sparing effect of dose fractionation. *Int J Radiat Oncol Biol Phys* 1984;10:957–964.

451. Belkacemi Y, Ozsahin M, Pene F, et al. Cataractogenesis after total body irradiation. *Int J Radiat Oncol Biol Phys* 1996;35:53–60.

452. van Kempen-Harteveld ML, Struikmans H, Kal HB. Cataract-free interval and severity of cataract after total body irradiation and bone marrow transplantation: influence of treatment parameters. *Int J Radiat Oncol Biol Phys* 2000;48:807–815.

453. van Kempen-Harteveld ML, Belkacemi Y, Kal HB, et al. Dose–effect relationship for cataract induction after single-dose total body irradiation and bone marrow transplantation for acute leukemia. *Int J Radiat Oncol Biol Phys* 2002;52:1367–1374.

454. van Kempen-Harteveld ML, Struikmans H, Kal HB. Cataract after total body irradiation and bone marrow transplantation: degree of visual impairment. *Int J Radiat Oncol Biol Phys* 2002;52:1375–1380.

455. Belkacemi Y, Labopin M, Vernant JP, et al. Cataracts after total body irradiation and bone marrow transplantation in patients with acute leukemia in complete remission: a study of the European Group for Blood and Marrow Transplantation. *Int J Radiat Biol Oncol Phys* 1998;41(3):659–668.

456. Holmstrom G, Borgstrom B, Calissendorff B. Cataract in children after bone marrow transplantation: relation to conditioning regimen. *Acta Ophthalmol Scand* 2002;80:211–215.

457. Zierhut D, Lohr F, Schraube P. Cataract incidence after total-body irradiation. *Int J Radiat Oncol Biol Phys* 2000;46:131–135.

458. Foote RL, Garretson BR, Schomberg PJ, et al. External beam irradiation for retinoblastoma: patterns of failure and dose–response analysis. *Int J Radiat Oncol Biol Phys* 1989;16:823–830.

459. McCormick B, Ellsworth R, Abramson D, et al. Results of external beam radiation for children with retinoblastoma: a comparison of two techniques. *J Pediatr Ophthalmol Strabismus* 1989;26:239–243.

460. Brooks HL Jr, Meyer D, Shields JA, et al. Removal of radiation-induced cataracts in patients treated for retinoblastoma. *Arch Ophthalmol* 1990;108:1701–1708.

461. Kline L, Kim J, Ceballos R. Radiation optic neuropathy. *Ophthalmology* 1985;92:1118–1126.

462. Kaste S, Chen G, Fontanesi J, et al. Orbital development in long-term survivors of retinoblastoma. *J Clin Oncol* 1997;15:1183–1189.

463. Peylan-Ramu N, Bin-Nun A, Skleir-Levy M. Orbital growth retardation in retinoblastoma survivors: work in progress. *Med Pediatr Oncol* 2001;37:465–470.

464. Shields CL, Shields JA. Recent developments in the management of retinoblastoma. *J Pediatr Ophthalmol Strabismus* 1999;36:8–18.

465. Shields CL, Shields JA, Cater J, et al. Plaque radio-

therapy for retinoblastoma: long-term tumor control and treatment complications in 208 tumors. *Ophthalmology* 2001;108:2116–2121.

466. Weiss AH, Karr DJ, Kalina RE, et al. Visual outcomes of macular retinoblastoma after external beam radiation therapy. *Ophthalmology* 1994;101:1244–1249.

467. Buckley EG, Heath H. Visual acuity after successful treatment of large macular retinoblastoma. *J Pediatr Ophthalmol Strabis* 1992;29(2):103–106.

468. Fontanesi J, Pratt CB, Kun LE. Treatment outcome and dose-response relationship in infants younger than 1 year treated for retinoblastoma with primary irradiation. *Med Pediatr Oncol* 1996;26:297–304.

469. Shields JA, Shields CL. Pediatric ocular and periocular tumors. *Pediatr Ann* 2001;30:491–501.

470. Adler M, Hawke M, Bergern G, et al. Radiation effects on the external auditory canal. *J Otolaryngol* 1985;14:226.

471. Huang E, The BS, Strother DR. Intensity-modulated radiation therapy for pediatric medulloblastoma: early report on the reduction of ototoxicity. *Int J Radiat Oncol Biol Phys* 2002;52:599–605.

472. Merchant TE, Gould CJ, Xiong X. Early neuro-otologic effects of three-dimensional irradiation in children with primary brain tumors. *Int J Radiat Oncol Biol Phys* 2002;54:201–202.

473. Schell MJ, McHaney VA, Green AA. Hearing loss in children and young adults receiving cisplatin with or without prior cranial irradiation. *J Clin Oncol* 1989;7:754–760.

474. McHaney VA, Thibadoux G, Hayes FA, et al. Hearing loss in children receiving cisplatin chemotherapy. *J Pediatr* 1983;10:314–317.

475. Landier W. Hearing loss related to ototoxicity in children with cancer. *J Pediatr Oncol Nurs* 1998;15:195–206.

476. Simon T, Hero B, Dupuis W, et al. The incidence of hearing impairment after successful treatment of neuroblastoma. *Klin Padiatr* 2002;214:149–152.

477. Maguire A, Craft A, Evans R, et al. The long-term effects of treatment on the dental condition of children surviving malignant disease. *Cancer* 1987;60:2570–2575.

478. Best JD. The dentist and the pediatric oncology patient. *N Y State Dent J* 1990;56:29–30.

479. Holtta P, Alahuusua S, Saarinen-Pihkala UM, et al. Long-term adverse effects on dentition in children with poor-risk neuroblastoma treated with high-dose chemotherapy and autologous stem cell transplantation with or without total body irradiation. *Bone Marrow Transplant* 2002;29:121–127.

480. Alpaslan G, Alpaslan C, Gogen HA. Disturbances in oral and dental structures in patients with pediatric lymphoma after chemotherapy: a preliminary report. *Oral Surg Oral Med Oral Pathol Oral Radiol Endod* 1999;87:317–321.

481. Kaste S, Hopkins K, Crom D, et al. Dental abnormalities in children treated for acute lymphoblastic leukemia. *Leukemia* 1997;11:792–796.

482. O'Sullivan EA, Duggal MS, Bailey CC. Changes in the oral health of children during treatment for acute lymphoblastic leukaemia. *Int J Paediatr Dentistry* 1994;4:31–34.

483. Fromm M, Littman P, Raney B, et al. Late effects after treatment of twenty children with soft tissue sarcomas of the head and neck. *Cancer* 1986;57: 2070–2076.

484. Dahllof G, Barr M, Balme P, et al. Disturbances in dental development after total body irradiation in bone marrow transplant recipients. *Oral Surg Oral Med Oral Pathol* 1988;65:41–44.

485. Makkonen T, Nordman E. Estimation of long-term salivary gland damage induced before the onset of treatment. *Cancer* 1987;57:1986–1987.

486. Maxymiw WG, Wood RE. The role of dentistry in head and neck radiation therapy. *Can Dent Assoc J* 1988;55:193–198.

487. Bucker J, Fleming T, Fuller L, et al. Preliminary observations on the effect of mantle field radiotherapy on salivary flow rates in patients with Hodgkin's disease. *J Dent Res* 1988;6:518–521.

488. Marks J, Davis C, Gottsman V, et al. The effects of radiation on parotid salivary function. *Int J Radiat Oncol Biol Phys* 1981;7:1013–1019.

489. Myers RE, Mitchell DL. Fluoride for the head and neck radiation patient. *Milit Med* 1988;153:411–413.

490. Johnson J, Ferretti G, Nethery J, et al. Oral pilocarpine for post-irradiation xerostomia in patients with head and neck cancer. *N Engl J Med* 1993;329:390–395.

491. Hendry J. The cellular basis of long-term marrow injury after irradiation. *Radiother Oncol* 1985;3:331–338.

492. Mauch P, Constine L, Greenberger J, et al. Hematopoietic stem cell compartment: acute and late effects of radiation therapy and chemotherapy. *Int J Radiat Oncol Biol Phys* 1995;31:1319–1339.

493. Storb R, Deeg HJ, Applebaum FR, et al. Total-body irradiation in bone marrow transplantation. In: Browne D, ed. *Treatment of radiation injuries.* New York: Plenum Press, 1990:29–33.

494. Sykes M, Chu F, Savel H, et al. The effects of varying dosages of irradiation upon sternal marrow regeneration. *Radiology* 1964;83:1084–1087.

495. Yankelevitz DF, Henschke CI, Knapp PH, et al. Effect of radiation therapy on thoracic and lumbar bone marrow: evaluation with MR imaging. *AJR* 1992; 157:87–92.

496. Parmentier C, Morardet N, Tubiana M. Late effects of human bone marrow after extended field radiotherapy. *Int J Radiat Oncol Biol Phys* 1983;9:1301–1311.

497. Rubin P, Scarantino C. The bone marrow organ: the critical structure in radiation–drug interaction. *Int J Radiat Oncol Biol Phys* 1978;4:3–23.

498. Casamassima F, Ruggkiero C, Carmaella D, et al. Hematopoietic bone marrow recovery after radiation therapy: MRI evaluation. *Blood* 1989;73:1677–1681.

499. Sachs E, Goris M, Glatstein E, et al. Bone marrow regeneration following large field irradiation. Influence of volume, age, dose and time. *Cancer* 1978;42: 1057–1065.

500. Cristy M. Active bone marrow distribution as a function of age in humans. *Phys Med Biol* 1981;26: 389–400.

501. McHaney V, Kavnar E, Meyer W, et al. Effects of radiation therapy and chemotherapy on hearing. In: Green DM, D'Angio GJ, eds. *Late effects of treatment for childhood cancer.* New York: Wiley-Liss, 1992:7–10.

502. Custer RP, Ahlfedt FE. Studies on the structure and function of bone marrow. *J Lab Clin Med* 1932; 17:960–962.

503. Kricun ME. Red–yellow marrow conversion: its effect on the location of some solitary bone lesions. *Skeletal Radiol* 1985;14:10–19.

504. Harris JM, Jackson CM, Patterson DG. *The measurement of man.* Minneapolis: University of Minnesota Press, 1930.

505. Hirsh J, Renier D, Czernechow P. Medulloblastoma in childhood: survival and functional results. *Acta Neurochir* 1979;48:1–15.

506. Raimondi AJ, Tomita T. Advantages of total resection of medulloblastoma and disadvantages of full head postoperative radiation therapy. *Childs Brain* 1979; 5:50–59.

507. Spunberg JJ, Chang CH, Goldman M, et al. Quality of long term survival following irradiation for intracranial tumors in children under the age of two. *Int J Radiat Oncol Biol Phys* 1981;7:727–736.

508. Danoff BF, Cowchock S, Marquette C, et al. Assessment of the long-term effects of primary radiation therapy for brain tumors in children. *Cancer* 1982; 49:1580–1586.

509. Duffner PK, Cohen ME, Thomas PRM. Late effects of treatment on the intelligence of children with posterior fossa tumors. *Cancer* 1983;51:233–237.

510. Ellenberg L, McComb JG, Siegel SE, et al. Factors affecting intellectual outcome in pediatric brain tumor patients. *Neurosurgery* 1987;21:638–644.

511. Packer RJ, Sposto R, Atkins TE, et al. Quality of life for children with primitive neuroectodermal tumors: medulloblastoma of the posterior fossa. *Pediatr Neurosci* 1988;13:169–175.

512. Packer RJ, Sutton LA, Atkins TE, et al. A prospective study of cognitive function in children receiving whole-brain radiotherapy and chemotherapy: 2-year results. *J Neurosurg* 1989;70:707–713.

513. Packer RJ, Radcliffe J, Glauser TA. Prospective evaluation of neuropsychological function in children treated for medulloblastoma. In: Green DM, D'Angio GJ, eds. *Late effects of treatment for childhood cancer.* New York: Wiley-Liss, 1992:41–48.

20

Second Malignant Neoplasms

Smita Bhatia, M.D., M.P.H., and Louis S. Constine, M.D.

With current risk-based multimodality therapeutic approaches, more than 75% of children with cancer can be expected to be long-term survivors (1). As a result of their cancer or therapy, 60–70% of young adult survivors of childhood cancer are reported to develop at least one health-related complication, and second primary cancers (SPCs) might be considered the most emotionally and physically devastating of these complications (2). A spectrum of questions can be raised regarding these events, including their relationship to the primary cancer, chemotherapy, and radiation therapy; innate genetic predispositions; age at diagnosis of the primary malignancies; the risk interval for development of the SPC; patient sex; and environmental influences.

THE INCIDENCE OF SPCS: THE SCOPE OF THE PROBLEM

SPCs After First Primary Cancers in Adults

An SPC is a histologically distinct second neoplasm that develops after the first neoplasm. Several large epidemiologic studies have demonstrated that the risk of second cancers after primary cancers diagnosed and treated in adulthood is modest at best, ranging from no difference from the general population to a two-fold greater incidence (3–5).

SPCs After First Primary Cancers in Childhood

There are several reports describing the risk of SPCs after the first primary cancer in childhood, with the estimated cumulative probability of approximately 3%. This is three to six times higher than the incidence in the general population (6,7).

Data from the Surveillance, Epidemiology, and End Results (SEER) program were used to calculate the influence of subsequent neoplasms on overall incidence trends in childhood cancer (8). Higher annual incidence rates were found for all childhood cancers combined, specifically for acute lymphoblastic leukemia (ALL) and brain tumors but not for other cancer types because of their rarity. However, excluding subsequent neoplasms from the analysis had a negligible effect on the observed trends. The Childhood Cancer Survivor Study Cohort reported the absolute excess risk of SPCs after a first primary cancer diagnosed and treated during childhood to be 1.9 per 1,000 patient-years of follow-up (7). These two analyses demonstrate that the high relative risk of SPC after a primary cancer in childhood does not translate into a high absolute risk. However, the morbidity and mortality associated with SPCs are substantial, validating the need to characterize this complication and identify associated risk factors.

CONTEMPORARY UNDERSTANDING OF CARCINOGENESIS

In the past decade, progress in discerning carcinogenesis has focused on the cumulative mutations that alter specific loci in DNA, leading to downstream alterations in the encoded proteins. Two general types of genes have been the target of interest for unraveling neoplastic transformation. The first is the proto-oncogene, which codes for cellular signaling components that play a role in controlling normal growth and differentiation (9). The ability of proto-oncogenes to participate in neoplastic transformation arises from the fact that the protein products of these genes are crucial relays in the elaborate biochemical circuitry that governs vertebrate cells (10).

There are several general categories of proto-oncogenes. These include growth factor receptors acting via a tyrosine-specific protein kinase pathway, glutamine triphosphate (GTP) binding proteins, membrane- and cytoskeletal-associated tyrosine-specific kinases, extracellular growth factors, serine- and threonine-specific protein kinases, and steroid-type growth factor receptors (Fig. 20-1). Therefore, products of the proto-oncogene may include polypeptide hormones acting on the cell surface, receptors for these hormones, proteins that convey signals from the cell surface to its depths, and chemicals that affect nuclear functions.

The second category of genes involved in carcinogenesis is called tumor suppressor genes (11). These genes restrain cell growth. Carcino-genesis could be the result of inactivation of a tumor suppressor gene, eliminating its growth-suppressing function. This could allow unbridled cell growth and neoplastic transformation.

There has been much interest in tumor suppressor genes in childhood cancer. This interest initially focused on the RB1 gene and its relationship to retinoblastoma and osteogenic sarcoma and is now expanding to a variety of other malignancies (12,13). In late G1 or early S phase the RB1 protein (pRB) becomes progressively more phosphorylated at multiple sites. The enzymes that carry out these phosphorylation reactions are cyclin-dependent kinases, which are activated by complex formation with cyclins A, D, and E and regulate cell cycle events. The level of pRB phosphorylation re-

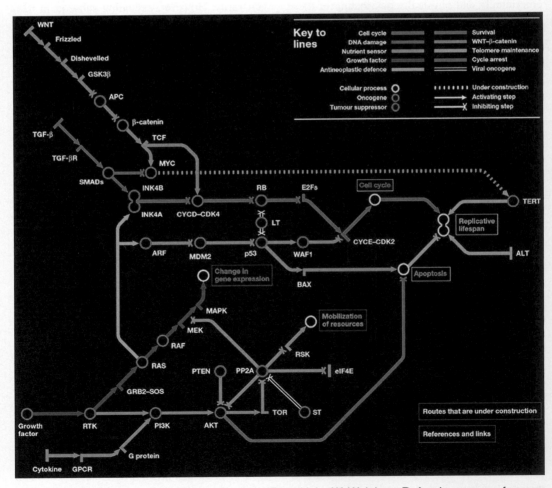

FIG. 20-1. A subway map of cancer pathways. (From Hahn W, Weinberg R. A subway map of cancer pathways. *Nat Rev Cancer* May 2002, with permission.) (See color plate)

mains high until late in M phase, when a phosphatase removes these posttranslational modifications. The pRB is again underphosphorylated in Go/G1. These periodic phosphorylation and dephosphorylation reactions are believed to modulate pRB's physical and functional interaction with a variety of cellular targets.

In resting cells (G0) or cells in early G1, pRB can be found in a complex with a cellular transcription factor called E2F. In general, transcription factors are proteins that, by binding to a specific DNA sequence adjacent to the genes they regulate, promote the expression of particular genes. E2F contributes to the activation of a constellation of genes encoding S-phase functions needed for DNA synthesis. When E2F is complexed to pRB, E2F gene-mediated transcriptional activation does not occur. Therefore, RB1 functions in part by its sequestration of E2F in G1 (14,15).

The p53 gene is another tumor suppressor gene that has provoked interest among those studying childhood cancer. p53 has been shown to be mutated in many histologic types of cancer (11,12,14,15). In various cell lines p53 has been shown to inhibit proliferation, promote differentiation, enable cells to arrest their growth after exposure to certain DNA damaging agents, and mediate apoptosis (14,15).

The mechanism through which p53 exerts its growth suppressive function is under vigorous investigation. Much of the available evidence suggests that p53 acts as a transcriptional activator or a transcription factor (14,15). Some sequence-specific DNA binding has shown that p53 may also function as a transcription factor by interacting with other DNA-bound proteins, thereby affecting their activity. Several transcriptional target genes for p53 have now been identified, with the assumption that such genes are likely to mediate the growth suppressive properties attributed to p53 (14,15).

p21 is one of the most important mediators of p53's actions. The suppression of cell growth by p53 may be related to activation of p21 expression. As a transcription factor, p53 induces p21, which in turn inhibits cyclin-dependent kinases. As an inhibitor of cyclin-dependent kinases, p21 prevents phosphorylation of pRB and hence the expression of genes needed for replication.

Apoptosis, or programmed cell death, is an important biological consequence of exposure to ionizing radiation and other DNA-damaging agents. Initial reports of radiation-induced apoptosis emphasized the importance of p53 in this cellular response. Cell cycle arrest after irradiation at the G1 checkpoint requires the expression of p53 in some cell lines. In tumor cells that undergo p53-dependent apoptosis, it seems that one of the functions of p53 is to screen for damaged DNA. In the presence of damaged DNA, wild-type p53 facilitates cell cycle arrest and DNA repair. Therefore, it prevents the proliferation of cells with damaged DNA (16). One might speculate that p53-negative cells that sustain radiochemotherapeutic damage would exhibit a diminished capacity to detect and respond to such damage. Consequently, the damaged DNA could be duplicated. If a lethal mutation had occurred from radiochemotherapeutic damage, then the cell would die. However, if a sublethal mutation had occurred, it is possible that a lack of p53 might allow amplification of the injured DNA and result in a cancer (14,15).

A pervasive dogma in cancer research is that carcinogenesis is a multistage process. The classic description of this process involved the concepts of initiation, promotion, and progression. More recent models involve multiple chromosomal changes in a variety of genes as growth-stimulating oncogenes are activated and tumor suppressor genes inactivated. How is it possible that exposure to a course of therapeutic radiation can result in mutations at the multiplicity of genetic loci necessary to produce a secondary cancer?

One possibility is that a protracted course of radiation will induce sufficient mutations to produce all or most of the steps necessary to produce a second cancer. For this to be true, ionizing radiation would have to be capable of producing point mutations to activate proto-oncogenes and point mutations and deletions to inactivate tumor suppressor genes. Radiation would produce cancer by the instantaneous creation of initiated cells (17). Because radiation is ineffective at causing point mutations but extremely effective at causing large deletions, inactivation of tumor suppressor genes such as p53 is likely to be an important mechanism of radiation carcinogenesis (18,19). Cell lines derived from primary thyroid tumors, rendered capable of tumor formation in athymic nude mice by radiation, express p53 mutations (20). The cell initiated by radiation may undergo clonal expansion with subsequent promotion. Once a malignant cell is generated, it gives rise to a tumor after some lag period.

It is also possible that in addition to inactivating tumor suppressor genes, radiation may generate a malignant diathesis by other subtle mechanisms. For example, a mutation in the genes responsible for DNA mismatch repair could lead to defective repair phenotype. In this way, multiple mutations may derive from a radiation-induced mutation in a repair system (18,19). In this postulated mechanism, radiation causes persistent genomic instability, resulting in a high rate of spontaneous mutations including those associated with a malignant phenotype (21).

Despite the support for the aforementioned mechanisms of carcinogenesis, accumulating evidence has challenged some of these theories and provoked alternate hypotheses. These include theories hypothesizing that a breakdown in DNA duplication or repair leads to many thousands of random mutations in cells, that damage to a few "master" genes corrupts the genome, leading to deregulation, and that abnormal numbers of chromosomes may lead to the ensuing carcinogenic events (22–26).

RISK FACTORS FOR SECOND CANCERS

Known genetic predisposition to malignancy and exposure to radiation therapy or to specific chemotherapeutic agents have been shown to increase the risk of SPCs in certain subsets of patients (7,27–31). The types of SPC vary with the primary diagnosis, the type of therapy received, presence of genetic predisposition, and the time from initial treatment.

Primary Diagnosis

Hereditary retinoblastoma, Hodgkin's disease, and soft tissue sarcomas are overrepresented among patients who develop SPCs relative to their incidence in the general population (7,31).

This could result from an interaction between the genetic predisposition to develop cancer and the specific cancer therapies, as is clear in patients with hereditary retinoblastoma and familial soft tissue sarcoma (31,32). In people with other primary malignancies, such as Hodgkin's disease, it is not clear whether the primary diagnosis is an independent risk factor for the development of SPC or whether the specific therapy needed to treat the primary cancer is the major contributor to the development of the SPC. Some associations between first and second cancers are summarized in Table 20-1.

Host-Related Risk Factors

Age at Diagnosis and Treatment of Primary Cancer

Younger age at diagnosis of the primary cancer has been reported to be associated with a higher risk of SPC (7,28,33). This association is seen primarily among radiation-associated SPCs. Conversely for secondary myelodysplasia and acute myeloid leukemia, which are strongly linked with specific chemotherapeutic agents, the risk increases with age at diagnosis and treatment of primary cancer (34,35).

Sex

Female sex is associated with a higher risk of SPCs, relating primarily to secondary breast and thyroid cancers among female cancer survivors (36,37). Moreover, some studies indicate a greater susceptibility of women to known carcinogens such as cigarette smoke (38). Possible mechanisms that underlie this greater susceptibility include greater activity of cytochrome p-450 enzymes, enhanced formation of DNA adducts, and the effects of hormones such as estrogen on tumor promotion (38).

Therapy-Related Risk Factors

Radiation

Although ionizing radiation is capable of causing most types of cancer, organs vary in their susceptibility. The risk is highest when exposure occurs at a younger age and increases with in-

TABLE 20-1. *Second cancers and their relationship with primary cancers*

Second cancers	Primary cancers	Median latency	Risk factors
Breast cancer	Hodgkin's disease Bone tumors Soft tissue sarcomas Acute lymphoblastic leukemia Brain tumors Wilms' tumors Non-Hodgkin's lymphoma	15–20 yr	Radiation Female sex
Brain tumors	Acute lymphoblastic leukemia Brain tumors Hodgkin's disease	9–10 yr	Radiation Younger age
Myelodysplastic syndrome and acute myelocytic leukemia	Acute lymphoblastic leukemia Hodgkin's disease Bone tumors	3–5 yr	Topoisomerase II inhibitors Alkylating agents
Thyroid cancer	Acute lymphoblastic leukemia Hodgkin's disease Neuroblastoma Soft tissue sarcoma Bone tumors Non-Hodgkin's leukemia	13–15 yr	Radiation Younger age Female sex
Bone tumors	Retinoblastoma (heritable) Other bone tumors Ewing's sarcoma Soft tissue sarcomas Acute lymphoblastic leukemia	9–10 yr	Radiation Alkylating agents Splenectomy
Soft tissue sarcomas	Retinoblastoma (heritable) Soft tissue sarcoma Hodgkin's disease Wilms' tumor Bone tumors Acute lymphoblastic leukemia	10–11 yr	Radiation Younger age Anthracyclines

creasing dosages of radiation and with increasing follow-up from radiation (39). Radiation-associated SPCs have a long latency period and typically develop in or at the edge of the radiation field. Some well-established radiation-associated SPCs include breast cancer (after Hodgkin's disease), thyroid cancer (after Hodgkin's disease and ALL), lung cancer (after Hodgkin's disease), brain tumors (after other brain tumors and ALL), osteosarcoma (after retinoblastoma, Ewing's sarcoma, and other soft tissue sarcomas), and nonmelanoma skin cancers (Table 20-1).

Several principles characterize radiation-induced cancer (40–42):

• A variety of histologic types of neoplasms can be induced by irradiation. These cancers are indistinguishable morphologically from naturally occurring cancers. The identification of a "radiation signature" in tumors would be important in evaluating SPC. There is evidence that radiation produces a different spectrum of mutations than other genotoxic agents. If these mutations could be discerned and characterized, then one could clearly identify radiation-induced tumors and understand, more completely, the radiation dose–response relationship for induced tumors. In this manner, molecular forensics may affect our understanding of attributable risk (43).

• Low–linear energy transfer (low-LET) radiation (gamma ray, x-ray) is generally less efficient in inducing tumors than high-LET radiation. In a murine hepatocarcinogenesis model, for example, neutron irradiation produced a greater incidence of hepatomas than did gamma irradiation (44). Low-LET radiation appears to become less effective at carcinogenesis per centigray as the dosage falls, whereas high-LET radiation (neutrons, alpha particles) does not (45). With low-LET irradiation there is less tumor induction when the dosage is fractionated or administered at low dose rates, implying that repair of carcinogenic damage is occurring. With high-LET irradiation, the radiobiological effect is higher at low dosages. The carcinogenic effectiveness of high-LET radiation is not diminished and may be increased by dosage fractionation or protraction (46).

- Comparison of the frequency of SPCs in different centers suggests that orthovoltage therapy is more likely to be carcinogenic than megavoltage therapy (42,47,48). This may be dose related: By delivering a higher dosage to bone, orthovoltage irradiation may increase the risk of an SPC of bone. The higher risk may also be related to the long follow-up available for orthovoltage patients.

- Although every tissue in the body is at risk for radiation cancer induction, sensitivity varies according to the tissue. For example, the thyroid gland and breast are sensitive to cancer induction after low radiation dosages; lymphoid tissue, lung, and liver are susceptible at moderate dosages, and bone at higher dosages. The relationship between dosage and response may vary according to the induced tumor. Cancer risk from radiation may be given per unit dosage (Gy or cGy) or per unit dosage equivalent (Sievert, Sv) where a "quality factor" *(Q)* is used to take account of the varying biological effectiveness of different radiation (e.g., for a gamma ray $Q = 1$, and for a neutron $Q = 20$). Therefore, dosage in Sv = dosage in Gy $\times$ Q. Detailed literature reviews indicate that the cancer mortality risk for the general population after whole body exposure is 1×10^{-4} to 4×10^{-4} per person-cGy. Pooled results of various partial body exposures give an estimated risk of 1×10^{-4} to 4×10^{-4} per person-cGy (4×10^{2} Sv^{1}). The risk based on incidence is about twice that for mortality (45,49). Leukemia data can be fit by a curvilinear dose–response model, whereas skin cancer appears to have a threshold dose–response function, and breast data fit a linear no-threshold model.

- The relationship of irradiation dosage to carcinogenesis is not clearly known. Data are available only for high dosages. Evaluation of risks for low dosages is of practical concern.

In the absence of measurement, extrapolation is used to predict the risk at low dosages (46).

- SPCs may also be induced by agents other than radiation (chemotherapy, environmental exposures, hereditary disposition). The low-dose radiation dose–response curve could be influenced by these confounding factors to produce a result that is the sum of two independent rates or may be greater than simple addition would indicate. A variety of chemotherapeutic agents (to be discussed), especially alkylators, are known to be carcinogenic, and they may be additive or synergistic with radiation. Immunosuppressive agents clearly influence the propensity for tumor induction, as is seen in the setting of organ transplantation (50).

- A large number of irradiated patients is necessary to calculate a radiation carcinogenesis risk with reasonable accuracy.

- Latent periods vary according to the induced tumor. At least two patterns of latent periods for radiation-induced cancer have been described. The first, exemplified by the risk of leukemia in atomic bomb survivors, consists of an early wavelike pulse of increased risk followed by a gradual decline to baseline levels. The second, more typical of solid tumors, is an increase in relative risk of SPCs over many years, which remains constant over time thereafter. The latter pattern suggests that a multi-event pattern of carcinogenesis is involved where the initiating initial event (radiation) is followed by promoting events (i.e., smoking, alcohol, environmental exposures) over many years (51). Long latent periods complicate the study of radiation-induced cancer because the presence of other carcinogens or disease processes may not be well documented.

- The duration of follow-up for any study population influences the frequency of tumors seen.

- It is unclear whether the risk of tumor development after exposure is simply an absolute increase that is proportional to the radiation dosage or a relative increase that builds on an underlying spontaneous risk (greater for some patients) of developing a malignancy.

- Age is a critical factor in determining radiation risk. In children, the most common SPCs occur in tissues undergoing rapid proliferation such as bone and thyroid. An actively proliferating tissue may be more susceptible to malignant transformation in any single cell because of the greater number of cell divisions. This might explain the higher frequency of secondary bone tumors in children than in adults (52,53). Childhood cancer survivors are likely to develop leukemias or sarcomas, whereas secondarily induced embryonal tumors are rare. Some cancers tend to aggregate in families, with specific constellations of tumor types observed (e.g., adenocarcinomas or sarcomas) (32,54). Some inherited syndromes clearly predispose patients to the development of second tumors (55). Patients with the nevoid basal cell carcinoma syndrome who are irradiated for medulloblastoma develop skin cancers in the irradiated fields 6 months to 3 years later (see Chapter 18). Children with ataxia–telangiectasia may be more prone to irradiation-induced malignancies.

Specific Examples of Radiation-Associated SPCs

Radiation-associated bone tumors and sarcomas exhibit a clear relationship with radiation dosage. The secondary bone tumors develop in the radiation field, typically after a latency period of 10 years. Both bone tumors and sarcomas may be aggressive and respond poorly to therapy (30,56,57).

Breast cancer has been increasingly reported among patients receiving radiation for Hodgkin's disease. The latency is typically 15–20 years from primary diagnosis, although it can occur earlier, and the risk is highest among patients diagnosed at a younger age, with the risk decreasing to that of the general population for patients receiving radiation for their primary cancer after the age of 30 years. Again, the risk appears to increase with radiation dosage, and the tumors typically develop in or at the edge of the radiation field (7,28,58–61).

Patients receiving radiation to the neck region are at a higher risk of developing thyroid cancers. Radiation therapy at a young age and female sex have been identified as risk factors for

the development of secondary thyroid cancers. Thyroid cancer has also been reported among patients receiving radiation to the craniospinal axis for ALL (62–64).

Brain tumors have been reported after cranial radiation for histologically distinct brain tumors or for prophylaxis or treatment of central nervous system disease among patients with ALL. Patients identified to be at greatest risk were those receiving radiation at age less than 6 years (7,33,65–69).

Chemotherapeutic Agents

Alkylating agents and topoisomerase II inhibitors have been shown to increase the risk of secondary myelodysplasia and acute myeloid leukemia (28,70,71). Alkylating agents have also been linked with bone tumors (56,57) and bladder cancer (72). The incidence of therapy-related myelodysplasia and acute myeloid leukemia typically peaks 4–6 years from diagnosis of the primary cancer and reaches a plateau after 15 years. The clinical observation that the risk of therapy-related leukemia does not extend beyond 15 years, despite an increasing risk of second neoplasms at other sites, indicates that the at-risk population of cells is no longer present (41). It may be that this period of time allows early pluripotential hematopoietic progenitors to undergo clonal extinction and be replaced from the compartment of resting stem cells by clonal succession. It is expected that stem cells in the resting phase of the cell cycle would be protected from the genotoxic effects of chemotherapy and radiation and that the excess risk of therapy-related leukemia would cease as undamaged cells were recruited into active hematopoiesis. Therapy-related leukemia is associated with a very poor outcome, with an estimated 12-month survival of 10% (73,74).

Alkylating Agent Associated Acute Myeloid Leukemia and Myelodysplasia

Table 20-2 summarizes the incidence, risk factors, and outcomes among patients with therapy-related leukemia after alkylating agent exposure

TABLE 20-2. Characteristics of therapy-related myelodysplasia or acute myeloid leukemia after treatment with alkylating agents and topoisomerase II inhibitors

Reference	Primary cancer	Cohort size	Cases of MDS and AML	Latency (yr)	Cumulative probability (%) (yr)	Risk factors	Percentage alive
Associated with alkylating agents							
10	HD	1,380	24	48 (10–168)	2.8 (14)	Alkylating agents Older age	0
42	HD	694	8	51.6 (16–148)	1.5 (20)	Chemotherapy Relapse	0
43	HD	1,641	7	NA	0.8 (30)	NA	NA
44	HD	667	5	49 (31–125)	1.1 (15)	Alkylating agents Increasing age	0
45	Childhood cancer	9,170	19	NA	0.8 (20)	HD, Ewing's Alkylating agents Doxorubicin	NA
Associated with topoisomerase II inhibitors							
38	Pediatric malignancies	16,422	10	NA	0.5 (5)	Etoposide Alkylating agents Radiation	NA
46	ALL	734	21	39.5 (15–100)	3.8 (6)	Etoposide: weekly or twice weekly	14
47	ALL	205	10	32	5.9 (4)	Etoposide	50
48	NHL	38	5	21	18.4 (4)	Etoposide, twice weekly	60

ALL, acute lymphoblastic leukemia; AML, acute myeloid leukemia; HD, Hodgkin's disease; MDS, myelodysplasia; NA, not applicable; NHL, non-Hodgkin's lymphoma.

(28,70,75–82). Increasing dosage of alkylating agent and older age at exposure have been identified as risk factors. The incidence typically is less than 5%, and patients with therapy-related myelodysplasia and acute myeloid leukemia after alkylating agent exposure have characteristic clinical and morphologic features (Table 20-3) (28,33–35,70,83,84). Cytogenetic abnormalities in patients who develop myeloid malignancies after therapy with alkylating agents characteristically involve losses or deletions of chromosomes 5 and 7 (37). The 5q31–33 region of the long arm of chromosome 5 contains at least nine genes involved in hematopoiesis. Defects in any of these genes could disrupt the balance between cell growth and differentiation and play a role in initiation and progression of leukemia. Complete or partial deletions of the long arm of chromosome 7 (7q- and –7) are nonrandom abnormalities observed in therapy-related leukemia.

Topoisomerase II Inhibitor–Associated Acute Myeloid Leukemia

Dosing schedule has been associated with epipodophyllotoxin-related secondary leukemia (80). Within the subgroups of patients who received epipodophyllotoxins (etoposide or teniposide) twice weekly or weekly, the cumulative risks were 12.3% and 12.4%, respectively. Of the remaining subgroups that included patients who received epipodophyllotoxins every 2 weeks, did not receive epipodophyllotoxins, or received them only during remission induction, the cumulative risk was 1.6%. After adjustment for the frequency of treatment, there was no apparent independent effect of the total dosage of epipodophyllotoxins in this study (80). Another large study from the Cancer Therapy Evaluation Program of the National Cancer Institute described the cumulative risks at

6 years for the development of secondary leukemia to be 3.3%, 0.7%, and 2.2% at the low (less than 1.5 g/m^2), moderate (1.5–3.0 g/m^2), and high (more than 3.0 g/m^2) dosages of etoposide, respectively, again suggesting a lack of dose–response relationship. A recent study using a case controlled design explored the dose–response relationship between epipodophyllotoxins and anthracyclines, and the risk of developing secondary leukemia. This study concluded that patients who received 1.2–6.0 g/m^2 of epipodophyllotoxins or more than 170 mg/m^2 of anthracyclines have a risk seven times higher than that of patients who received lower dosages or none of these drugs (85). Acute myeloid leukemia associated with exposure to topoisomerase II inhibitors is characterized by short latency (median, 24–36 months), predominance of monocytic phenotypes (M4 and M5), and an acute onset, often with a high blast count, rather than an initial myelodysplastic presentation (Table 20-3).

Topoisomerase II inhibitors induce chromosomal fragmentation, sister chromatid exchange, DNA deletions, and DNA rearrangements. Most of the translocations characteristic of leukemia disrupt a breakpoint cluster region between exons 5 and 11 of the *MLL* gene at chromosome band 11q23 and fuse *MLL* with a partner gene (86).

Genetic Predisposition

Members of families with Li–Fraumeni syndrome have been reported to be at higher risk of multiple subsequent cancers than the general population (29). The risk was highest among survivors of childhood cancer, and the excess risk was mainly for cancers characteristic of Li–Fraumeni syndrome, such as brain tumors and sarcomas. Patients with soft tissue sarcomas

TABLE 20-3. *Features of chemotherapy-induced hematopoietic malignancies*

Property	Alkylating agents	Epipodophyllotoxins	References
Median latency	4–6 yr (range, 1–20 yr)	1–3 yr (range 0.5–4.5 yr)	10, 15, 17, 37, 49
Presentation	Myelodysplasia	Abrupt, no preleukemia	37, 49, 50
Cytogenetic abnormalities	Loss of genetic material, often from chromosomes 5 and 7	Balanced translocations (often include 11q23)	37, 50
Age	Typically older patients	Younger patients	37, 50

who develop a second cancer are more likely to have a family history of cancer than those without a second cancer (32). The tumor types occurring in excess in family members are similar to those observed as second cancers, such as cancers of the breast, bone, joint, or soft tissue, thus indicating that the risk of second cancers is associated with a familial predisposition. Genetic predisposition also plays a significant role in increasing the risk of second cancers among patients receiving radiation therapy for hereditary retinoblastoma, with the risk increasing with increasing dosages of radiation (13). These studies suggest that germ line mutations in tumor suppressor genes might interact with therapeutic exposures to increase the risk of SPCs.

There is emerging evidence that polymorphisms in a drug-metabolizing enzyme thiopurine S-methyltransferase (*TPMT*) genotype might influence the risk of second cancers, including brain tumors (53) and acute myeloid leukemia (87). *TPMT* catalyzes the S-methylation of thiopurines, including 6-mercaptopurine and 6-thioguanine. *TPMT* activity exhibits genetic polymorphism, with about 1 in 300 people inheriting *TPMT* deficiency as an autosomal recessive trait. Several other genetic polymorphisms of enzymes capable of metabolic activation or detoxification of anticancer drugs, such as NAD(P)H:quinone oxireductase (NQO1), glutathione S-transferase (GST)-M1 -T1 and -P1, and CYP3A4, have been examined for their role in the development of therapy-related leukemia and myelodysplasia (88–91). There is evidence that an NQO1 polymorphism may be associated with a higher risk of therapy-related myelodysplasia (88). People with CYP3A4-W genotype may be at a higher risk of treatment-related leukemia through increased production of reactive intermediates that might damage DNA (89). Recently, Allan et al. (90) reported data suggesting that inheritance of at least one Val allele at GST-P1 codon 105 increases the risk of therapy-related leukemia.

Environmental and Lifestyle Factors

Environmental exposures and lifestyle factors such as tobacco, alcohol, diet, and hormonal factors and their association with second can-cers have been most commonly studied in survivors of adult-onset cancers. Smoking has been linked with lung cancer occurring as an SPC among survivors of Hodgkin's disease, with the risk increasing with increasing radiation dosages, suggesting a positive interaction on a multiplicative scale (92). Moreover, the increase in risk of lung cancer with increasing radiation dosage was much greater among the patients who smoked after the diagnosis of Hodgkin's disease than among those who refrained from smoking ($p = 0.04$) (92). Alcohol consumption has been shown to be a risk factor for oral, esophageal, and liver cancers occurring as SPCs (93–95). There are several anatomic sites, such as colon, breast, ovary, uterus, and prostate, where nutritional and hormonal factors play a role in carcinogenesis. Bidirectional associations across several hypothesized nutrition- and hormone-related cancers have been demonstrated across many registries. However, these studies are generally lacking in specific exposure information, and the support for a given etiologic hypothesis usually is indirect because the correlations between cancers hypothesized to share a common risk factor are examined without direct measurement of the putative common risk factors or potential confounders. Moreover, because the environmental exposures and lifestyle factors seem to be associated primarily with adult-onset cancers, a sufficiently large cohort of childhood cancer survivors must be followed until they reach the age at which they would be at risk for developing such cancers.

The next section focuses on certain primary cancers that are associated with a significantly greater risk of SPCs (e.g., retinoblastoma and Hodgkin's disease). It also focuses on primary cancers, with large, well-characterized cohorts of patients followed for sufficiently long periods of time to develop SPCs (e.g., acute lymphoblastic leukemia and Wilms' tumor).

Retinoblastoma

Children with hereditary retinoblastoma are at exceptionally high risk of developing multiple primary cancers, especially osteosarcoma and soft tissue sarcomas (relative risk [RR] = 30,

95% confidence interval [CI] 26–47) (31,96). On the other hand, patients with nonhereditary retinoblastoma appear not to be at greater risk for second cancers. The cumulative incidence of a second cancer at 50 years after diagnosis was reported to be 51% (±6.2%) for hereditary retinoblastoma and 5% (±3%) for nonhereditary retinoblastoma. The high risk of multiple primary cancers in patients with hereditary retinoblastoma is attributable primarily to germ line mutations in the retinoblastoma tumor suppressor gene, *RB1*. For second primary soft tissue sarcomas, the relative risks showed stepwise increase for all dosage categories of radiation therapy and were statistically significant at 10–29.9 Gy and 30–59.9 Gy. Third and additional nonocular tumors (soft tissue sarcomas, bone tumors, and skin cancers) have been reported among patients with retinoblastoma who had developed a radiation-related second tumor (97), with the 5- and 10-year incidence rates reported to be 11% and 22%, respectively. The cumulative probability of death from an SPC has been reported to be 26% at 40 years after bilateral retinoblastoma diagnosis (98). Radiotherapy for retinoblastoma further increased the risk of mortality from second cancers in this report.

These studies indicate that genetic predisposition has a substantial impact on risk of subsequent cancers in patients with retinoblastoma, which is further increased by radiation therapy. Moreover, patients with retinoblastoma are at a higher risk for developing third and fourth tumors, although the location and other risk factors are similar to those described for SPCs.

Hodgkin's Disease

Reports from large, well-characterized cohorts of patients reveal that in survivors of Hodgkin's disease the risk of developing SPCs is 7 to 18 times higher than in the general population (Table 20-4) (7,28,36,76,77,99,100).

Metayer et al. (60) reported their analyses of 5,925 patients with Hodgkin's disease diagnosed before 21 years of age and reported to 16 population-based cancer registries in North America and Europe between 1935 and 1994. A total of 157 solid (RR = 7.0, 95% CI 5.9–8.2) and 26 acute leukemias (RR = 27.4, 95% CI 17.9–40.2) were reported. The risk of solid tumors remained elevated among 20-year survivors (RR = 6.6) and persisted for 25 years (RR = 4.6). Temporal trends for cancers of thyroid, female breast, bone and connective tissue, stomach, and esophagus were consistent with the late effects of radiotherapy.

The risk of SPCs in a cohort of 1,641 patients diagnosed before the age of 20 years in the five Nordic countries was described to be 7.7 times that of the general population (77). The overall cumulative risk of subsequent neoplasms was 1.9% at 10 years, 6.9% at 20 years, and 18% at 30 years. High risks were observed for breast cancer (RR = 17, 95% CI 9.9–28), thyroid cancer (RR = 33, 95% CI 15–62), secondary leukemia

TABLE 20-4. *Second cancers after childhood Hodgkin's disease*

Reference	Cohort size	Time period studied	Number of second cancers	Cumulative incidence (%) (yr)	Standardized incidence ratio
10	1,380	1955–1986	135	31.2% (30 yr)	17.9
18	499	1962–1993	25	7.7% (15 yr)	—[a]
19	191	1969–1988	15	12% (15 yr)	Males: 18.0
					Females: 57
26	5,925	1935–1994	195	Solid tumors: 11.7% (25 yr)	7.7
42	694	1960–1995	59	Males: 9.7% (20 yr)	
				Females: 16.8% (20 yr)	Males: 10.6
					Females: 15.4
43	1,641	1940s to 1991	62	18% (30 yr)	7.7
69	182	1960–1989	28	26.7% (30 yr)	9.4

[a]Information not available.

(RR = 17, 95% CI 6.9–35), and non-Hodgkin's lymphoma (RR = 15, 95% CI 4.9–35).

A cohort of 694 children and adolescents followed for a median of 13 years for the development of SPCs revealed the relative risk of developing an SPC to be 15.4 (95% CI 10.6–21.5) for female and 10.6 (95% CI 6.6–16.0) for male patients (76). Breast cancer (n = 16) and soft tissue sarcomas (n = 13) were the most common solid tumors. The actuarial risk of SPC at 20 years of follow-up was 9.7% for men, 16.8% for women, and 9.2% for breast cancer.

The Late Effects Study Group followed a cohort of 1,380 children with Hodgkin's disease diagnosed at a median age of 11 years (range: 0.3–16) in North America and Europe between 1955 and 1986 to determine the incidence of second malignant neoplasms and associated risk factors (28). The cohort was recently updated to extend the median length of follow-up from 11 years to 15.1 years (101). The median age at last follow-up was 27.8 years (3.5–52.7), and the median length of follow-up was 17.0 years (0.1–45). An additional 103 subsequent neoplasms were ascertained (total n = 212). The cohort's risk of developing subsequent neoplasms was 18.5 times higher than that of the general population (Standardized Incidence Ratio [SIR] = 18.5, 95% CI 15.6–21.7). The cumulative incidence of any second malignancy was 10.6% (95% CI 8.6–12.7) at 20 years, increasing to 26.3% at 30 years; and of the cumulative incidence of solid malignancies was 7.3% (95% CI 5.5–9.1) at 20 years, increasing to 23.5% at 30 years. Breast cancer was the most common solid malignancy (SIR = 56.7, 95% CI 40.5–77.3). Other commonly occurring solid malignancies included thyroid (SIR = 36.4), bone (SIR = 37.1), colorectal (SIR = 36.4), lung (SIR = 27.3), and gastric (SIR = 63.9) cancers. Risk factors for solid tumors included young age at Hodgkin's disease and radiation-based therapy. Thirty-two patients developed third neoplasms, with the cumulative incidence approaching 21% at 10 years from diagnosis of second malignancy.

Follow-up of these large cohorts of survivors of childhood Hodgkin's disease for extended periods of time documents the increasing occurrence of radiation-associated solid tumors, especially breast and thyroid cancers and the emergence of other cancers common in the adult population, such as colon and lung cancer, at a younger age than expected in the general population.

Acute Lymphoblastic Leukemia

For survivors of childhood ALL, the estimated actuarial risk of developing an SPC has been reported to be 2.5–5% at 15 years from diagnosis (Table 20-5) (7,33,65–69). Among the second neoplasms observed after treatment of ALL, central nervous system tumors in patients treated with cranial irradiation, acute myeloid leukemia, and thyroid cancer are most commonly reported. Children under 6 years of age at the time of radiation to the central nervous system are at a higher risk of developing second primary brain tumors (7,33).

The incidence and type of SPCs after Berlin–Frankfurt–Munster treatment in 5,006 children with ALL diagnosed between 1979 and 1995 and followed for a median of 5.7

TABLE 20-5. *Second cancers after childhood acute lymphoblastic leukemia*

Reference	Cohort size	Time period studied	Number of patients with second cancers	Cumulative incidence (%) (yr)	Standardized incidence ratio
15	9,720	1972–1988	43	2.5% (15 yr)	7.0
32	1,597	1972–1995	13	2.7% (18 yr)	—[a]
33	981	1958–1985	8	2.9% (20 yr)	5.9
34	1,815	1962–1988	20	5.0% (15 yr)	—[a]
35	5,006	1979–1995	52	3.3% (15 yr)	—[a]
36	8,831	1983–1995	70	1.3% (10 yr)	7.0

[a]Information not available.

years were reported (68). This cohort's risk of developing an SPC was 14 times higher than that of the general population, and their risk of developing a brain tumor was 19 times higher. The cumulative risk of SPC was 3.5% at 15 years among patients treated with cranial irradiation but only 1.2% among nonirradiated patients.

A cohort of 8,831 children diagnosed with ALL and enrolled on Children's Cancer Group therapeutic protocols between 1983 and 1995 revealed the cumulative incidence ($\pm SE$) of any second neoplasm to be $1.3 \pm 0.2\%$ (at 10 years), representing a risk 7.9 times higher than in the general population. The risk was significantly higher for acute myeloid leukemia (RR = 52.3), non-Hodgkin's lymphoma (RR = 20.8), parotid gland tumors (RR = 33.4), thyroid cancer (RR = 13.3), brain tumors (RR = 10.1), and soft tissue sarcoma (RR = 9.1). Multivariate analysis revealed relapse of primary disease (RR = 3.5, 95% CI 2.1–5.8), female sex (RR = 1.8, 95% CI 1.1–2.8), and radiation to the craniospinal axis (RR = 1.6, 95% CI 1.0–2.6) to be independently associated with a higher risk of second neoplasms. Actuarial survival at 10 years from diagnosis of second neoplasms was 39%.

Follow-up of these large cohorts of children treated with contemporary risk-based therapy documents that the incidence of second neoplasms remains low after diagnosis of childhood ALL.

Wilms' Tumors

Between 1969 and 1991, 5,278 patients were enrolled in the National Wilms Tumor Study (NWTS) and by the end of 1993 had contributed 39,461 person-years of follow-up. Forty-three second neoplasms were observed, whereas only 5.1 were expected (RR = 8.4, 95% CI 6.1–11.4) (71). The cumulative incidence of an SPC after Wilms' tumor was 1.6% after 15 years from diagnosis of Wilms' tumor. Abdominal irradiation received as part of initial therapy was associated with a higher risk of a second cancer (RR = 1.4 per 10 Gy, 95% CI 1.1–1.8). Doxorubicin potentiated the radiation effect. Treatment for relapse further increased the risk for second

cancers. Seven of the 43 patients with second cancers were identified to have acute myeloid leukemia at a median of 3 years from diagnosis of Wilms' tumor (102). All 7 patients had received chemotherapy regimens that included doxorubicin or etoposide, and 6 of the 7 patients had received infradiaphragmatic irradiation. These results demonstrate the importance of current efforts to limit the use of intensive chemotherapy and radiation therapy to patients with aggressive disease.

The next section is devoted to the more commonly reported SPCs, such as breast, bone, and thyroid cancers, focusing on the incidence and risk factors associated with the development of these second cancers.

Bone Tumors

The estimated risk of subsequent bone tumors among 9,170 2-year survivors of childhood cancer was reported to be 133 times that of the general population (95% CI 98–176), with an estimated 20-year cumulative risk of $2.8 \pm 0.7\%$ (57). As compared with matched controls who had survived cancer in childhood but not developed bone cancer later, the risk (95% CI 1–7.7) of developing a bone tumor was 2.7 times higher in patients who received radiation therapy, with a sharp dose–response gradient, reaching 40 times higher after dosages to the bone of more than 60 Gy. After adjustment for radiation therapy, treatment with alkylating agents was also linked to bone cancer (RR = 4.7, 95% CI 1.0–22.3), with the risk increasing with cumulative drug exposure.

A report from the population-based National Registry of Childhood Tumours in Britain of a cohort of 13,175 3-year survivors of childhood cancer diagnosed between 1940 and 1983 revealed the cumulative probability to be 0.9% at 20 years, except after hereditary retinoblastoma (7.2%), Ewing's sarcoma (5.4%), and other malignant bone tumors (2.4%) (56). The risk of bone cancer increased substantially with the cumulative dosage of radiation to the bone ($p < 0.001$, linear trend). At the highest level of exposure, the risk appeared to decline ($p = 0.065$, nonlinearity). The risk of bone cancer increased linearly ($p = 0.04$, one-tailed test) with the cumulative dosage of alkylating agents.

A cohort study of 4,400 3-year survivors of a first solid cancer during childhood diagnosed in France and the United Kingdom between 1942 and 1986 revealed the risk of osteosarcoma to be a linear function of the local radiation dosage (30). Bilateral retinoblastoma, Ewing's sarcoma, and soft tissue sarcoma were found to be associated with a higher risk of subsequent osteosarcoma.

These three studies demonstrate that the risk of second primary bone tumors among survivors of childhood cancer is not very high, except among certain specific tumor types, and that the risk is associated with the use of radiation therapy and alkylating agents. These studies therefore provide a rational basis for targeted surveillance and modification of therapeutic protocols in certain high-risk groups.

Breast Cancer

Women with Hodgkin's disease who receive mantle irradiation are at a higher risk of breast cancer. Results from several registries show that 10 or more years after radiation, the overall breast cancer risk is approximately 4 times higher (7,59,60,103–110), and can be 55 to 75 times higher, in girls exposed to radiation at puberty than in the general population (28,101). The risk of developing breast cancer remains elevated for many years (Table 20-6) (28,101).

Follow-up of a cohort of female Hodgkin's disease survivors diagnosed and treated before 16 years of age showed that the actuarial estimated cumulative probability of developing breast cancer approached 28% at 30 years from diagnosis (101). The median age at diagnosis of Hodgkin's disease was 14 years, and the median age at diagnosis of breast cancer was 32 years. The median latency between the diagnosis of Hodgkin's disease and diagnosis of second primary breast cancer was 18 years (range 4–28 years). Twenty-seven of the 29 cancers developed in the radiation field. Ten of the 29 patients with breast cancer subsequently developed cancer in the contralateral breast. The estimated cumulative probability of developing breast cancer among women receiving irradiation approached 25% by 40 years of age.

The Childhood Cancer Survivor Study Cohort has evaluated the risk of breast cancer among 13,581 5-year survivors of childhood cancer (7). Breast cancer was the most common SPC ($n = 60$), and the cohort had a risk of developing a second primary breast cancer 16.2 times higher than that of the general population. The majority of second primary breast cancers occurred among survivors of childhood Hodgkin's disease. The median time to development of breast cancer was 15.7 years. The risk of developing a breast cancer appeared to remain elevated throughout the follow-up period (RR = 10.1 at 5–9 years of follow-up and 10.1 at 20–30 years of follow-up).

TABLE 20-6. *Risk of breast cancer in Hodgkin's disease survivors by age and latency*

Reference	Size of cohort	Length of follow-up	No. of BCs	Median age at diagnosis of HD/BC	Median latency	Relative risk	Risk factors	Outcome (% alive)
7	13,851	15.4 yr	60	—[a]	—[a]	16	Radiation therapy	—[a]
10	483	11 yr	17	11/32 yr	19 yr	75	10–16 yr Radiation therapy	82%
25	885	10 yr	26	28/40 yr	15 yr	13 (<15 yr at diagnosis)	Age <30 yr Radiation therapy	73%
26	5,925	10.5 yr	52	—[a]	—[a]	14	Radiation therapy	—[a]
27	257	10 yr	6	14/28 yr	14 yr	20	Radiation therapy	—[a]
28	3,869	—[a]	55	All ages	>10 yr	61	Age <16 yr at diagnosis of HD	—[a]

BC, breast cancer; HD, Hodgkin's disease.
[a]Information not available.

In a recent report, van Leeuwen et al. (92) evaluated the factors responsible for the higher risk of breast cancer among female survivors of Hodgkin's disease. They concluded that breast cancer risk increases with increasing radiation dosage up to at least 40 Gy. They explained the substantial risk reduction observed in their study associated with chemotherapy as possibly reflecting its effect on menopausal age, suggesting that ovarian hormones promote tumorigenesis after radiation has produced an initiating event. These findings are similar to those of Travis et al. (111), who found that hormonal stimulation appears important for the development of radiation-induced breast cancer, as evidenced by the reduced risk associated with ovarian damage from alkylating agents or radiation. The high radiation-related risk, which does not diminish at the highest dosages or the longest follow-up, suggests the need for lifelong surveillance.

To determine whether genetic factors predispose patients with Hodgkin's disease to develop breast cancer, Gaffney et al. (112) evaluated breast cancer specimens for loss of heterozygosity (LOH) at regions where BRCA1 and BRCA2, two breast cancer tumor suppressor genes, are located. They were unable to find statistical evidence of LOH at BRCA1 and BRCA2 in breast cancers from patients previously irradiated for Hodgkin's disease.

For women treated after age 30, however, no excess breast cancers have occurred (59). The high risk of breast cancer in women exposed to radiation for the treatment of Hodgkin's disease at younger ages raises important issues about cooperative efforts among institutions to mount prospective screening programs including breast physical examination, sonography, mammography, or quantitative magnetic resonance imaging for these patients. Moreover, most of the current combined-modality treatment approaches for children with Hodgkin's disease use lower radiation dosages and seek to exclude breast tissue from radiation fields.

Thyroid Cancers

The risk of thyroid cancer has been described after radiation therapy for several primary cancers, including Hodgkin's disease, ALL, and brain tumors, and after total body irradiation for bone marrow transplantation (7,28,33,62–64,69, 101,113). The long-term risk of developing a thyroid tumor in 4,096 3-year survivors of childhood cancer treated between 1942 and 1985 in France and Britain was reported to increase with increasing dosage of radiation: A dosage of 0.5 Gy was associated with a risk of developing a thyroid cancer 35 times higher than in the general population, and the risk increased to 73 times when the exposure increased to 3.6 Gy (63). Radiation therapy at a young age has been identified as a risk factor for the development of secondary thyroid cancers (62). The risk of thyroid cancer was reported to be 18 times that of the general population among 1,791 5-year survivors of Hodgkin's disease followed as part of the Childhood Cancer Survivor Study Cohort (64). Thyroid cancer has also been reported among patients receiving radiation to the craniospinal axis for ALL (7,33,101).

Future Directions

The absolute risk of SPC is small, with fewer than two excess second cancers occurring per 1,000 patient-years of follow-up (7). The ongoing efforts to improve survival after childhood cancer must not be overshadowed by the risk of SPC. However, of all possible late sequelae, SPC can be the most devastating. It is therefore imperative that patients and health care providers are aware of risk factors for SPC and the populations at greater risk for developing second cancers so that surveillance is focused and early prevention strategies can be implemented.

Examples of potential primary prevention strategies include use of gender-specific therapy for patients with Hodgkin's disease to reduce the risk of radiation-associated breast cancer among female survivors. Another example of a primary prevention strategy is tailoring therapy based on the identification of patients heterozygous for drug-metabolizing enzymes before therapy is initiated for the primary cancer.

Secondary prevention measures currently under consideration include programs to educate clinicians and survivors about the risk of SPC and about ways to decrease the risk of developing SPC by adopting healthful lifestyles. For example, both patients and health care providers need to be educated about the higher risk of breast cancer among the female survivors of childhood cancer. Patients must appreciate the importance of properly conducted self-examination as the foundation of breast cancer screening. In addition, clinical and mammographic screening should be instituted at a younger age and performed more frequently than recommended for the general population (114). Other measures include intervention programs for smoking cessation, screening for breast, lung, and cervical cancers, chemoprevention for specific cancers, and avoidance of unnecessary exposure to sunlight.

Finally, SPCs provide us with a unique opportunity to understand the pathogenesis of various cancers. The exact timing and magnitude of the primary exposure (i.e., cancer therapy) are known, and following the patients closely may lead to a better understanding of the progression of events and perhaps the identification of biomarkers that would identify patients who ultimately develop SPCs (70). Several such studies that involve prospective, longitudinal follow-up of patients are being undertaken to elucidate the sequence of events that ultimately lead to the development of SPC.

REFERENCES

Articles particularly recommended for further reading are indicated by an asterisk.

1. Reis L, Eisner M, Kosary C, et al. *SEER Cancer Statistics Review, 1973–1998.* Bethesda, MD: National Cancer Institute, 2001.
2. Sklar C. An overview of the effects of cancer therapies: the nature, scale, and breadth of the problem. *Acta Paediatr Scand* 1999;433[Suppl]:1–4.
3. Sankila R, Pukkala E, Teppo L. Risk of subsequent malignant neoplasms among 470,000 cancer patients in Finland, 1953–1991. *Int J Cancer* 1995;60:464–470.
4. Dong C, Hemminki K. Second primary neoplasms in 633,964 cancer patients in Sweden, 1958–1996. *Int J Cancer* 2001;93:155–161.
5. Curtis R, Boice J Jr, Kleinerman R, et al. Summary: multiple primary cancers in Connecticut, 1935–82. *Natl Cancer Inst Monogr* 1985;68:219–242.
6. Olsen J, Garwicz S, Hertz H, et al. Second malignant neoplasms after cancer in childhood or adolescence. *BMJ* 1993;307:1030–1036.
7. Neglia J, Friedman D, Yutaka Y, et al. Second malignant neoplasms in five-year survivors of childhood cancer: Childhood Cancer Survivors Study. *J Natl Cancer Inst* 2001;93:618–629.
8. Gurney J, Davis S, Severson R, et al. The influence of subsequent neoplasms on incidence trends in childhood cancer. *Cancer Epidemiol Biomarkers Prev* 1994;3:349–351.
9. Farber R. Cancer development and its natural history: a cancer prevention perspective. *Cancer* 1988;62:1676–1679.
10. Boice JD. Cancer following medical irradiation. *Cancer* 1981;47:1081–1090.
11. Marshall C. Tumor suppressor genes. *Cell* 1991;64:313–326.
*12. Cavenee W, White R. The genetic basis of cancer. *Sci Am* 1998;March:72–79.
13. Constine L, Marcus R, Halperin E. Molecular biology and the future of therapy for childhood rhabdomyosarcoma. *Int J Radiat Oncol Biol Phys* 1995;32:1245–1249.
14. Levine A. The genetic origins of neoplasia. *JAMA* 1995;273:592.
*15. Levine A. Tumor suppressor genes. *Sci Am* 1995;Jan–Feb:28–37.
16. Hartwell L, Kastan M. Cell cycle control and cancer. *Science* 1994;266:1821–1828.
17. Kai M, Luebeck E, Moolgavkar S. Analysis of the incidence of solid cancer among atomic bomb survivors using a two-stage model of carcinogenesis. *Radiat Res* 1997;148:348–358.
18. Hall E. *Radiobiology for the radiologist,* 4th ed. Philadelphia: JB Lippincott, 1994:323–350.
*19. Hall E. What will molecular biology contribute to our understanding of radiation-induced cell killing and carcinogenesis? *Int J Radiat Biol* 1997;71:667–674.
20. Riches A, Herceg Z, Wang H, et al. Radiation-induced carcinogenesis: studies using human epithelial cell lines. *Radiat Oncol Invest* 1997;5:139–143.
21. Trott KR. Radiation and cancer. *Eur J Cancer Prev* 1996;5:377–378.
22. Gibbs W. Roots of cancer. *Sci Am* 2003;289:57–65.
23. Duesberg P, Li R, Rasnick D, et al. Aneuploidy precedes and segregates with chemical carcinogenesis. *Cancer Genet Cytogenet* 2000;119:83–93.
24. Jallepalli P, Lengauer C. Chromosome segregation and cancer: curing through the mystery. *Nat Rev Cancer* 2001;1:109–117.
25. Hahn W, Weinberg R. Rules for making human tumor cells. *N Engl J Med* 2002;347:1593–1503.
26. Loeb L, Loeb K, Anderson J. Multiple mutations and cancer. *Proc Natl Acad Sci USA* 2003;100(3):776–781.
27. Robison L. Second primary cancers after childhood cancer. *BMJ* 1996;12:861–862.
28. Bhatia S, Robison L, Oberlin O, et al. Breast cancer and other second neoplasms after childhood Hodgkin's disease. *N Engl J Med* 1996;334:745–751.
29. Hisada M, Garber J, Fung C, et al. Multiple primary cancers in families with Li–Fraumeni syndrome. *J Natl Cancer Inst* 1998;90:606–611.
30. Le Vu B, de Vathaire F, Shamsaldin A, et al. Radiation dose, chemotherapy and risk of osteosarcoma af-

ter solid tumours during childhood. *Int J Cancer* 1998;77:370–377.

*31. Wong F, Boice J, Abramson D, et al. Cancer incidence after retinoblastoma: radiation dose and sarcoma risk. *JAMA* 1997;278:1262–1267.

32. Strong L, Stine M, Norsted T. Cancer in survivors of childhood soft tissue sarcoma and their relatives. *J Natl Cancer Inst* 1987;79:1213–1220.

33. Neglia J, Meadows A, Robison L, et al. Second malignant neoplasms after acute lymphoblastic leukemia in childhood. *N Engl J Med* 1991;325:1330–1336.

34. Bhatia S, Ramsay N, Steinbuch M, et al. Malignant neoplasms following bone marrow transplantation. *Blood* 1996;87:3633.

35. Darrington D, Vose J, Anderson J, et al. Incidence and characterization of secondary myelodysplastic syndrome and acute myelogenous leukemia following high-dose chemoradiotherapy and autologous stem cell transplantation for lymphoid malignancies. *J Clin Oncol* 1994;13:2527–2534.

36. Beaty O, Hudson M, Greenwald C, et al. Subsequent malignancies in children and adolescents after treatment for Hodgkin's disease. *J Clin Oncol* 1995;13:603–609.

*37. Tarbell N, Gelber R, Weinstein H, et al. Sex differences in risk of second malignant tumours after Hodgkin's disease in childhood. *Lancet* 1993;341:1428–1432.

38. Zang E, Wynder E. Differences in lung cancer risk between men and women: examination of the evidence. *J Natl Cancer Inst* 1996;88:183.

39. Garwicz S, Anderson H, Olsen J, et al. Second malignant neoplasms after cancer in childhood and adolescences: a population-based case control study in the 5 Nordic countries. *Int J Cancer* 2000;88:672–678.

40. Arseneau J, Sponzo R, Levin D, et al. Nonlymphomatous malignant tumors complicating Hodgkin's disease. Possible association with intensive therapy. *N Engl J Med* 1972;307:965–971.

41. Blayney D, Longo D, Young R, et al. Decreasing risk of leukemia with prolonged follow up after chemotherapy and radiotherapy for Hodgkin's disease. *N Engl J Med* 1987;316:710–717.

42. Haselow R, Nesbit M, Dehner L, et al. Second neoplasms following megavoltage radiation in a pediatric population. *Cancer* 1978;42:1185–1191.

43. Report on a workshop to examine methods to arrive at risk estimates for radiation-induced cancer in the human based on laboratory data. *Radiat Res* 1993;135:434–437.

44. Wiley A Jr, Vogel H Jr, Clifton K. The effect of variations in LET and cell cycle on radiation hepatocarcinogenesis. *Radiat Res* 1973;54:284–293.

45. Kohn H, Fry R. Radiation carcinogenesis. *N Engl J Med* 1984;310:504–511.

46. Okey A, Harper P, Grant D, et al. Chemical and radiation carcinogenesis. In: Tannock I, Hill R, eds. *The basic science of oncology,* 3rd ed. New York: McGraw-Hill, 1998:166–196.

47. Potish R, Dehner L, Haselow R, et al. The incidence of second neoplasms following megavoltage radiation for pediatric tumors. *Cancer* 1985;56:1534–1537.

48. Li F, Cassady J, Jaffe N. Risk of second tumors in survivors of childhood cancer. *Cancer* 1975;35:1230–1235.

49. Richardson R. Past and revised estimates for cancer induced by irradiation and their influence on dose limits. *Br J Radiol* 1990;63:235–245.

50. Matas A, Hertel B, Rosai J. Post transplant malignant lymphoma, distinctive morphologic features. *Am J Med* 1976;61:716–720.

51. Land C. Temporal distributions of risk for radiation-induced cancers. *J Chron Dis* 1987;40[Suppl 2]:45S–57S.

52. Meadows A, D'Angio G, Mike V, et al. Patterns of second malignant neoplasms in children. *Cancer* 1977;40:1903–1911.

*53. Tucker M, Coleman C, Cox R, et al. Risk of second cancers after treatment for Hodgkin's disease. *N Engl J Med* 1988;318:76–81.

54. Fraumeni J. Clinical patterns of familial cancer. In: Mulvihill J, Miller R, Fraumeni J, eds. *Progress in cancer research and therapy,* Vol 3: *Genetics of human cancer.* New York: Raven Press, 1977:223–234.

55. Hawkins M. Second primary tumors following radiotherapy for childhood cancer. *Int J Radiat Oncol Biol Phys* 1990;19:1297–1301.

56. Hawkins M, Wilson L, Burton H, et al. Radiotherapy, alkylating agents and risk of bone cancer after childhood cancer. *J Natl Cancer Inst* 1996;88:270–278.

*57. Tucker M, D'Angio G, Boice J. Bone sarcomas linked to radiotherapy and chemotherapy in children. *N Engl J Med* 1987;317:588–593.

58. Boice J. Radiation and breast carcinogenesis. *Med Pediatr Oncol* 2001;36:508–513.

59. Hancock M, Tucker M, Hoppe R. Breast cancer after treatment of Hodgkin's disease. *J Natl Cancer Inst* 1993;85:25–31.

60. Metayer C, Lynch C, Clarke E, et al. Second cancers among long-term survivors of Hodgkin's disease diagnosed in childhood and adolescence. *J Clin Oncol* 2000;18:2435–2443.

61. Travis L, Curtis R, Boice J. Late effects of treatment for childhood Hodgkin's disease [Letter]. *N Engl J Med* 1996;334:745–751.

62. Tucker M, Jones P, Boice J, et al. Therapeutic radiation at a young age is linked to secondary thyroid cancer. *Cancer Res* 1991;51:2885–2888.

63. de Vathaire F, Hardiman C, Shamsaldin A, et al. Thyroid carcinomas after irradiation for a first cancer during childhood. *Arch Intern Med* 1999;159:2713–2719.

64. Sklar C, Whitton J, Mertens A, et al. Abnormalities of the thyroid in survivors of Hodgkin's disease: data from the Childhood Cancer Survivor Study. *J Clin Endocrinol* 2000;85:3227–3232.

65. Kimball Dalton V, Gelber R, Li F, et al. Second malignancies in patients treated for childhood acute lymphoblastic leukemia. *J Clin Oncol* 1998;16:2848–2853.

66. Nygaard R, Garwicz S, Haldorsen T, et al. Second malignant neoplasms in patents treated for childhood leukemia. *Acta Paediatr Scand* 1991;80:1220–1228.

67. Pratt C, George S, Hannock M, et al. Second malignant neoplasms in survivors in childhood acute lymphocytic leukemia. *Pediatr Res* 1988;23[Suppl]:345a.

68. Loning L, Zimmerman L, Reiter A, et al. Secondary neoplasms subsequent to Berlin–Frankfurt–Munster

therapy of acute lymphoblastic leukemia in childhood: significantly lower risk without cranial radiotherapy. *Blood* 2000;95:2770–2775.

69. Bhatia S, Sather H, Pabustan O, et al. Low incidence
of second neoplasms among children diagnosed with
acute lymphoblastic leukemia. *Blood* 2002;99:4257–
4264.

70. Smith M, McCaffrey R, Karp J. The secondary leukemias: challenges and research directions. *J Natl Cancer Inst* 1996;88:407–418.

71. Hawkins M, Wilson L, Stovall M, et al. Epipodophyllotoxins, alkylating agents, and radiation and risk of
secondary leukaemia after childhood cancer. *BMJ*
1992;304:951–958.

72. Pedersen-Bjergaard J, Erbsoll J, Hansen V, et al. Carcinoma of the urinary bladder after treatment with cyclophosphamide for non-Hodgkin's lymphoma. *N
Engl J Med* 1988;318:1028–1032.

73. Neugut A, Robinson E, Nieves J, et al. Poor survival
of treatment-related acute non-lymphocytic leukemia. *JAMA* 1990;264:1006–1008.

74. Smith S, Le Beau M, Huo D, et al. Clinical–cytogenetic associations in 306 patients with therapy-
related myelodysplasia and myeloid leukemia: the
University of Chicago series. *Blood* 2003;102:43–52.

75. Smith M, Rubinstein L, Anderson J, et al. Secondary
leukemia or myelodysplastic syndrome after treatment with epipodophyllotoxins. *J Clin Oncol* 1999;
17:569–577.

76. Wolden S, Lamborn K, Cleary S, et al. Second cancers following pediatric Hodgkin's disease. *J Clin
Oncol* 1998;16:536–544.

77. Sankila R, Garwicz S, Olsen J, et al. Hodgkin's disease patients diagnosed in childhood and adolescence: a population-based cohort study in the five
Nordic countries. *J Clin Oncol* 1996;14:1442–1446.

78. Schellong G, Riepenhausen M, Creutzig U, et al.
Low risk of secondary leukemias after chemotherapy
without mechlorethamine in childhood Hodgkin's
disease. *J Clin Oncol* 1997;15:2247–2253.

79. Tucker M, Meadows A, Boice J, et al. Leukemia after
therapy with alkylating agents for childhood cancer. *J
Natl Cancer Inst* 1987;78:459–464.

80. Pui C, Ribeiro R, Hancock M, et al. Acute myeloid
leukemia in children treated with epipodophyllotoxins for acute lymphoblastic leukemias. *N Engl J Med*
1991;325:1682–1687.

81. Winick N, Mckenna R, Shuster J, et al. Secondary
acute myeloid leukemia in children with acute lymphoblastic leukemia treated with etoposide. *J Clin
Oncol* 1993;11:209–217.

82. Sugita K, Furukawa T, Tsuchida M, et al. High frequency of etoposide (VP-16)-related secondary leukemia in children with non-Hodgkin's lymphoma.
Am J Pediatr Hematol Oncol 1993;15:99–104.

83. Krishnan A, Bhatia S, Slovak M, et al. Predictors of
therapy-related leukemia and myelodysplasia following autologous transplantation for lymphoma: an assessment of risk factors. *Blood* 2000;95:1588–1593.

84. Bhatia S, Davis S, Robison L. Leukemia. In: Neugut
AL, Meadows AT, Robinson E, eds. *Multiple primary
cancers.* Philadelphia: Lippincott Williams & Wilkins,
1999.

85. Le Deley MC, Leblanc T, Shamsaldin A, et al. Risk
of secondary leukemia after solid tumor in childhood

according to the dose of epipodophyllotoxins and anthracyclines: a case-control study by the Société
Française d'Oncologie Pediatrique. *J Clin Oncol*
2003;21:1074–1081.

86. Felix C. Secondary leukemias induced by topoisomerase targeted drugs. *Biochim Biophys Acta* 1998;
1400:233–235.

87. Relling M, Yanishevsky Y, Nemec J, et al. Etoposide
and antimetabolite pharmacology in patients who develop secondary acute myeloid leukemia. *Leukemia*
1998;12:346–352.

88. Naoe T, Takeyama K, Yokozawa T, et al. Analysis of
genetic polymorphism in NQ01, GST-M1, GST-T1,
and CYP3A4 in 469 Japanese patients with therapy-
related leukemia/myelodysplastic syndrome and de
novo acute myeloid leukemia. *Clin Cancer Res*
2000;6:4091–4095.

89. Felix C, Walker A, Lange B, et al. Association of
CYP3A4 genotype with treatment-related leukemia.
Proc Natl Acad Sci USA 1998;95:13,176–13,181.

90. Allan J, Wild C, Rollinson S, et al. Polymorphism in
glutathione S-transferase P1 is associated with susceptibility to chemotherapy-induced leukemia. *Proc
Natl Acad Sci USA* 2001;98:11592–11597.

91. Woo M, Shuster J, Chen C, et al. Glutathione S-
transferase genotypes in children who develop treatment-related acute myeloid malignancies. *Leukemia*
2000;14:232–237.

92. van Leeuwen F, Klokman W, Stovall M, et al. Roles
of radiotherapy and smoking in lung cancer following Hodgkin's disease. *J Natl Cancer Inst* 1995;87:
1530–1537.

93. Rothman K, Keller A. The effect of joint exposure to
alcohol and tobacco on risk of cancers of the mouth
and pharynx. *J Chron Dis* 1972;25:711–716.

94. Flanders W, Rothman K. Interaction of alcohol and
tobacco on laryngeal cancer. *Am J Epidemiol* 1982;
115:371–379.

95. LaVecchia C, Negri E. The role of alcohol in
esophageal cancer in nonsmokers, and the role of tobacco in nondrinkers. *Int J Cancer* 1989;43:784–785.

96. Moll A, Imhof S, Schouten-Van Meeteren A, et al.
Second primary tumors in hereditary retinoblastoma:
is there an age effect on radiation-related risk? *Ophthalmology* 2001;108:1109–1114.

97. Abramson D, Ellsworth R, Kitchin F, et al. Second
nonocular tumors in retinoblastoma survivors. *Ophthalmology* 1984;91:1351–1355.

98. Eng D, Li F, Abramson D, et al. Mortality from second tumors among long-term survivors of retinoblastoma. *J Natl Cancer Inst* 1993;85:1121–1128.

99. Tucker M. Solid second cancers following Hodgkin's
disease. *Hematol Oncol Clin North Am* 1993;7:
389–400.

*100. Green D, Hyland A, Barcos M, et al. Second malig-
nant neoplasms after treatment for Hodgkin's disease
in childhood and adolescence. *J Clin Oncol* 2000;
18:1492–1499.

101. Bhatia S, Robison L, Meadows A. High risk of subsequent neoplasms continues with extended follow-up
of childhood Hodgkin's disease cohort: report from
the Late Effects Study Group. *J Clin Oncol* 2003;21:
4386–4394.

102. Breslow N, Takashima J, Whittam J, et al. Second
malignant neoplasms following treatment for Wilms'

tumor: a report from the Wilms' Tumor Study Group. *J Clin Oncol* 1995;13:1851–1859.

103. Janjan N, Zellmer D. Calculated risk of breast cancer following mantle irradiation determined by measured dose. *Cancer Detect Prev* 1992;16:273–282.
104. Chung C, Bogart J, Adams J, et al. Increased risk of breast cancer in splenectomized patients undergoing radiation therapy for Hodgkin's disease. *Int J Radiat Biol Phys* 1997;37:405–409.
105. Tinger A, Wasserman T, Klein E, et al. The incidence of breast cancer following mantle field radiation therapy as a function of dose and technique. *Int J Radiat Biol Phys* 1997;37:865–870.
106. Aisenberg A, Finkelstein D, Doppke K, et al. High risk of breast carcinoma after irradiation of young women with Hodgkin's disease. *Cancer* 1997;79:1203–1210.
107. Prior P, Pope D. Hodgkin's disease: subsequent primary cancers in relation to treatment. *Br J Cancer* 1988;58:512–517.
108. Carey R, Lingood R, Wood W, et al. Breast cancer developing in four women cured of Hodgkin's disease. *Cancer* 1984;54:2234–2236.
109. Cook K, Adler D, Lichter A, et al. Breast carcinoma in young women previously treated for Hodgkin's disease. *AJR* 1990;155:39–42.
110. Yahalom J, Petrek J, Biddinger P, et al. Breast cancer in patients irradiated for Hodgkin's disease: a clinical and pathologic analysis of 45 events in 37 patients. *J Clin Oncol* 1992;10:1674–1681.
111. Travis L, Hill D, Dores G, et al. Breast cancer following radiotherapy and chemotherapy among young women with Hodgkin disease. *JAMA* 2003;290:465–475.
112. Gaffney D, Hemmersmeier J, Holden J, et al. Breast cancer after mantle irradiation for Hodgkin's disease: correlation of clinical pathologic and molecular features including loss of heterozygosity at BRCA1 and BRCA2. *Int J Radiat Biol Phys* 2001;49:539–546.
113. Acharya S, Sarafoglou K, LaQuaglia M, et al. Thyroid neoplasms after therapeutic radiation for malignancies during childhood or adolescence. *Cancer* 2003;97:2397–2403.
114. Kaste S, Hudson M, Jones D, et al. Breast masses in women treated for childhood cancer: incidence and screening guidelines. *Cancer* 1998;82:784–792.

21

Anesthesia for External Beam Radiotherapy

Scott R. Schulman, M.D., and Edward C. Halperin, M.D.

Considering the awesome aspect of the therapy machines together with the fact that no one may be with the patient during the period of irradiation, it is surprising that the great majority submit to the complete course of therapy with little or no restraint and no sedation. . . . In a small number of patients in the infant-to-toddler age group of 1 1/2 to 5 years of age, patient co-operation may be impossible to obtain. . . . Complete immobility of the patient is absolutely essential for the accuracy and success of treatment. . . . Sedation of the patient becomes virtually a sine qua non.

Harrison and Bennet (1) made these observations more than 30 years ago. Their classic article, "Radiotherapy Without Tears," was the first published report describing anesthesia for radiotherapy in children. The problem of inadequate sedation prompted the authors to develop

the following simple method of anesthesia for radiotherapy of infants. . . . The method is applicable when the anesthetist must remain outside the treatment room, and consists of the insufflation of nitrous oxide, oxygen and halothane through the side-arm of the oropharyngeal airway (1).

Forty years of progress in anesthesiology have validated not only Harrison and Bennet's observation but also their solution to the problem of providing anesthesia for radiotherapy. This chapter will review issues in the sedation of children with an emphasis on monitoring the anesthetized child in the radiotherapy suite, develop a model of the ideal anesthetic for pediatric radiotherapy, explore anesthetic options for radiotherapy, and discuss the implications of the child's underlying disease that influence the anesthetic choice.

BEHAVIORAL TECHNIQUES TO AVOID ANESTHESIA

In some cases, a behavioral program to teach children how to cooperate with radiation treatment without sedation and anesthesia may be successful. Behavioral therapy techniques, called desensitization or exposure therapy, were originally developed for treating severe anxiety, fears, and phobias. The procedure involves inducing a relaxed state using music, cartoons, stories, or videos. Subsequently, one introduces the staff, equipment, and routines needed for radiation treatment.

A behavioral technique called differential positive reinforcement is used to strengthen cooperation and coping. Incentives such as praise, stickers, toys, and prizes are provided when the child attempts to cooperate. These are used to shape the child's ability to inhibit movement when instructed to do so. Shaping is a behavioral psychology technique whereby the criteria for reinforcement are gradually altered as the child improves performance. At the beginning, an approximation of the desired behavior is acceptable. After a while, more challenging and rigid criteria are set for reinforcement.

Videotaped cartoons and movies may be used to provide relaxation, distractions, and ongoing positive reinforcement in training young children to cooperate with radiation therapy. A small television monitor can be suspended near the linear accelerator couch and connected to a VCR so that movies or cartoons may be played during radiotherapy while the child is in the treatment position. Slifer et al. (2–4) demonstrated the efficacy of this technique in children between the ages of 2 1/2 and 7 years. Nine of 11 children were able to successfully undergo all of their radiation planning and treatment sessions without sedation.

TABLE 21-1. *Need for anesthesia in children as a function of age at initiation of irradiation*

Age (yr)	Total number of patients receiving external beam radiation therapy under anesthesia	Total Number of patients receiving external beam radiation therapy	Percentage of patients needing anesthesia
0–<1	25	26	96%
1–<2	24	27	89%
2–<3	30	35	86%
3–<4	20	41	49%
4–<5	16	44	36%
5–<6	4	38	11%
6–<7	2	28	7%
7–16	2	273	0.7%
Total	123	512	

From Fortney JT, Halperin EC, Hertz CM, et al. Anesthesia for pediatric external beam radiation therapy. *Int J Radiat Oncol Phys* 1999;44:587–591.

FREQUENCY OF ANESTHESIA FOR PEDIATRIC RADIOTHERAPY

When possible, children should be irradiated without anesthesia. Confidence-building measures and play therapy should be used to achieve patient stability and reproducible treatment. When these techniques fail, however, anesthesia must be used.

The frequency of anesthesia use as a function of patient age at the initiation of external beam radiation therapy in the Duke University Medical Center pediatric radiotherapy population is shown in Table 21-1. For very young children (3 years or younger) anesthesia is almost always needed. After approximately 5 years of age, however, anesthesia is rarely needed.

GOALS OF ANESTHESIA FOR RADIOTHERAPY

To accomplish the twin goals of irradiating the treatment volume while sparing healthy tissue, control of patient movement must be precise and absolute. How are these goals achieved in children? The approach varies depending on the institutional resources. Conscious or deep sedation is used in some centers, whereas general anesthesia is used in others. Regardless of the institutional practice, there is no substitute for vigilant monitoring and prompt intervention by people skilled in detecting and managing complications associated with the administration of sedative drugs to infants and children.

Anesthesiologists are increasingly asked to provide care outside the traditional operating room setting, such as in the radiotherapy suite (2). This is appropriate because the specialty has unique expertise in patient evaluation, selection, and monitoring and the ability to respond immediately to any complication of therapy. Expertise in drug selection and a comprehensive approach to the care of the child, which includes preanesthetic evaluation, postanesthetic care, and the provision of up-to-date feeding guidelines, are hallmarks of the anesthesiologist.

A prolonged fast before the induction of general anesthesia is no longer necessary. Infants, children, and adolescents can safely drink clear liquids (e.g., apple juice, water, popsicles) or (if applicable) breast milk until 3 hours before induction. Milk and solid food should be withheld for 4–6 hours for infants less than 6 months of age, for 6 hours for toddlers 6 months to 3 years of age, and for 8 hours for children older than 3 years of age.

The goals of anesthesia for pediatric radiotherapy are listed in Table 21-2. There are several options that, to varying degrees, accomplish the listed goals. There are no prospective, randomized studies in the setting of pediatric radiotherapy that demonstrate the superiority of one technique of general anesthesia over another.

Several routes of drug administration are available for sedation of children. Each drug and drug combination has its own set of side effects and contraindications. Several general guidelines

TABLE 21-2. *Goals for ideal anesthesia for outpatient pediatric radiation therapy*

Patient immobility
Rapid and smooth onset of effect with sedation, hypnosis, amnesia, and analgesia adequate for nonpainful radiation therapy procedures, along with a sufficient degree of muscle relaxation
Brief duration of action
Painless administration
Prompt recovery without postprocedure side effects but with residual analgesia and antiemetic effects during recovery
Minimal interference with eating, drinking, and playing
Safety for repeated administration
Low risk of tolerance to the anesthetic agents (tachyphylaxis)
Maintenance of a patent airway in a variety of body positions
Absence of side effects such as cardiovascular instability, respiratory depression, spontaneous movements, and excitatory activity
Cost-effectiveness

Modified from references 9 and 40, with permission.

TABLE 21-3. *Inhalation anesthetic agents commonly used in pediatric radiation therapy*

Sevoflurane (CFH_2-O-$CH(CF_3)_2$)
Nitrous oxide (N_2O)
Isoflurane (CF_2H-O-$CClH$-CF_3)
Enflurane (CF_2H-O-$CFCl$-CF_2H)
Halothane (CF_3-$CClBrH$)
Desflurane (CF_3H-O-CFH-CF_3)

may be considered. First, the route of administration of the drug should be the least traumatic for the particular child. Oral or rectal administration, avoiding intramuscular or intravenous administration, should be considered. Second, it should be kept in mind that some children will develop a tolerance to certain drugs used for sedation. Over time, the amount of drug and the amount of time needed to achieve sedation may both increase.

INHALED ANESTHETICS

Several general anesthetic options exist for radiotherapy. The anesthesiologist individualizes therapy based on data obtained from the patient's history, physical and laboratory examination, and discussions with the child, parents, and radiation oncologist. The physical limitations of the radiotherapy suite (such as the presence of an air exhaust system so that volatile anesthetic agents can be used) are also important in devising the anesthetic plan.

General anesthesia is accomplished with either inhaled agents (Table 21-3) or intravenous agents (e.g., barbiturates, ketamine, propofol). The first report of anesthesia for pediatric radiotherapy used halothane. Halothane is a halogenated hydrocarbon volatile anesthetic first in-

troduced for clinical use in 1956. Halothane has a long history of safe, effective use in pediatric patients. It has superior induction characteristics compared with isoflurane and enflurane, rapidly producing an anesthetic state when inhaled, with minimal airway complications such as coughing and laryngospasm. It is delivered by mask to the child and is painless to administer. Halothane has been demonstrated to be superior to isoflurane and enflurane for diagnostic and therapeutic procedures in children with malignancies (3). For anesthesia outside the operating room, Wolfe and Rao (6), "after considerable experimentation with various IV, intramuscular, and inhalation anesthetics, with and without intubation," recommended inhalation induction with halothane and nitrous oxide and oxygen and maintenance of anesthesia with halothane and oxygen without intubation. Halothane depresses respiration and cardiovascular function in a dose-dependent fashion. At dosages used for radiotherapy, these effects are negligible. Spontaneous respiration is typical with halothane anesthesia.

Sevoflurane is a disubstituted methyl ethyl ether inhalation anesthetic that surpasses halothane as the anesthetic of choice for infants and children (7). Sevoflurane has minimal pungency compared with halothane and may be more readily tolerated by children. Its lower solubility permits a more precise control over the delivery of anesthesia and a more rapid induction of and recovery from anesthesia. Sevoflurane also seems to have a lower respiratory irritant capacity than halothane and produces less coughing and breath holding than some other inhaled agents (8–11).

Inhalation anesthesia often is complicated by upper airway obstruction. Airway obstruction often is exacerbated in radiation therapy by the position of the patient. Positioning often entails immobilization of the child's head in a stabilization device, which can impede airway patency when an insufflation technique is used. This obstruction is relieved with an oropharyngeal or nasopharyngeal airway or a laryngeal mask airway. Although endotracheal intubation may be necessary in a small proportion of patients presenting for radiotherapy, it is preferable to avoid this technique because repeated laryngoscopy and intubation carry the risk of airway edema and trauma to the laryngeal structures.

An adjunct for airway management during pediatric radiotherapy is the laryngeal mask airway (LMA). The LMA (Fig. 21-1) is a silicone tube, the distal end of which has an elliptical-shaped cuff that, when correctly inserted and inflated, forms a low-pressure seal around the larynx and allows spontaneous ventilation in a variety of body positions without the need for

endotracheal intubation. Therefore, the LMA provides all the advantages of endotracheal intubation: a guaranteed patent airway without the disadvantages of repeated laryngoscopy and intubation. The LMA has been used for radiotherapy in children as young as 3 weeks of age. Grebenik et al. (12) reported the use of the LMA for pediatric radiotherapy in 25 children who received more than 300 anesthetics. They observed no complications directly related to the use of the LMA. Morris and Marjot (13) reported one case of posterior pharyngeal wall edema that corresponded to the area of contact between the posterior surface of the LMA and the oropharynx in a child repeatedly anesthetized with an LMA for radiotherapy. Moylan and Luce (14) reported more than 2,500 anesthetics given to 145 children with an LMA over

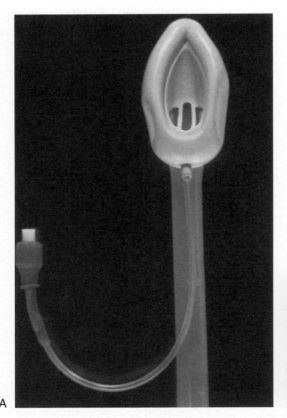
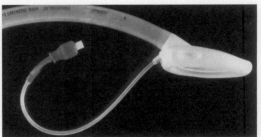

A   B

FIG. 21-1. The laryngeal mask airway is a silicon tube. The distal end of the tube has an elliptical-shaped cuff that, when correctly inserted and inflated, forms a low-pressure seal around the larynx and allows spontaneous ventilation without the need for endotracheal intubation. (Photographed by permission of Gensia, Inc. San Diego, CA.)

a 4-year period for radiotherapy. They raised the concern that a prone position for radiotherapy with the neck partially flexed can produce kinking of the LMA, with the possibility of airway obstruction. A new reinforced LMA may help alleviate this problem (15).

In summary, general inhalation anesthesia has many features that make it an attractive technique for pediatric radiotherapy. Onset is rapid, depth is easily controllable, it is not unpleasant to administer, recovery is rapid, the incidence of nausea and vomiting is low, and the airway is well preserved. This time-honored technique is widely used.

INTRAVENOUS ANESTHETICS

Intravenous anesthesia is also a popular and effective technique for pediatric radiotherapy. Intravenous anesthesia relies on either intermittent or continuous infusion of anesthetic agent into a peripheral or central vein in order to maintain a therapeutic concentration (16). Although it is not a new concept (sodium thiopental was administered by continuous drip as early as 1944), the advent of newer, short-acting anesthetic drugs, better equipment for infusing these drugs, and an improved understanding of pharmacokinetics in pediatric patients have led to a resurgence of interest in this technique. Postulated advantages of intravenous anesthesia include fewer peaks and troughs in serum concentration of drug, providing a steady-state serum concentration. Proponents of intravenous anesthesia contend that this steady-state concentration results in a more rapid induction of and emergence from anesthesia when compared with inhaled anesthetics.

There is an extensive body of experience with ketamine in the radiotherapy suite (17–19). Since its release in the early 1970s, this dissociative anesthetic has been widely used for radiation therapy in children. Ketamine produces excellent analgesia and amnesia of short duration. Ketamine is easy to administer (it can be given intramuscularly if there is no intravenous access), and an anesthesia machine is not needed when ketamine is used. Ketamine is felt to preserve respiration and airway patency more effectively than inhaled anesthetics. One series

described a child with a pharyngeal tumor who experienced airway obstruction with halothane anesthesia. When ketamine was substituted for halothane, the patient had an uneventful anesthetic treatment, which resulted in satisfactory conditions for radiotherapy (20).

Ketamine and midazolam can be used to produce repetitive intravenous anesthesia for a child undergoing radiation therapy. Ketamine is a phencyclidine derivative that produces dissociative anesthesia, characterized by electroencephalographic evidence of dissociation between the thalamus and the limbic system. The drug has a rapid onset of action, a short duration, and high lipid solubility. It does not produce significant depression of ventilation. There is an increase in systemic and pulmonary arterial blood pressure, cardiac output, cardiac work, and myocardial oxygen needs. The drug is metabolized extensively by hepatic microsomal enzymes. There have been case reports of tolerance developing with repeat administration of ketamine (21).

Ketamine is not a panacea. There are several caveats to its use. Ketamine has ocular effects that have implications for radiotherapy. The onset of ketamine anesthesia often is accompanied by nystagmus (more commonly horizontal than vertical). Nystagmus with ketamine usually is transient; however, if it persists, it may be impossible to use a hanging lens block in an anterior field for the treatment of retinoblastoma. Ketamine can also produce involuntary movement of other muscle groups (jerking), which is undesirable in pediatric radiotherapy. Ketamine raises blood pressure and heart rate. Its use in the setting of elevated intracranial pressure (ICP) is contraindicated because it causes ICP to increase. Although ketamine generally preserves respiratory drive and airway patency, apnea can occur after an intravenous bolus. In addition, it is a potent sialogogue, and copious secretions often accompany its use. Secretions can cause airway obstruction. Ketamine also sensitizes the airway to irritable stimuli, and reflex laryngeal closure (laryngospasm) often occurs. A drying agent such as atropine or glycopyrrolate should be given in conjunction with ketamine.

Finally, emergence from ketamine anesthesia often is characterized by hallucinations and nightmares. The incidence of emergence reactions ranges from 10% to 30% in adult patients. Emergence reactions are much less common in children. The reason for this difference is not known. Whatever the mechanism, the occurrence of these emergence reactions can be reduced if a benzodiazepine such as diazepam or midazolam is used.

Benzodiazepines such as diazepam and midazolam are rarely used as the sole agents for radiotherapy in children. Valium is painful to administer when given intravenously, and its duration of action exceeds the duration of most radiotherapy sessions. Versed is short acting and not painful when given intravenously, but when used by itself it does not produce satisfactory sedation for radiotherapy. A plateau in sedative effect often accompanies its use, so additional dosing does not produce the desired clinical effect. The release of flumazenil, a benzodiazepine antagonist, may improve the margin of safety for benzodiazepines. In the event that a patient receives an overdose or demonstrates an exaggerated clinical effect, the drug can be displaced from its receptor by flumazenil and the untoward effects can be reversed.

Midazolam is a water-soluble benzodiazepine with an imidole ring in its structure. This accounts for its stability in aqueous solution in rapid metabolism. It is two to three times as potent as diazepam. The short duration of anesthesia with midazolam is the result of its lipid solubility, which leads to rapid redistribution from the brain to an active tissue and to rapid hepatic clearance. It is almost totally metabolized by hepatic microsomal enzymes, and very little is excreted unchanged from the kidneys (21).

Barbiturates are sedative–hypnotic drugs that depress the activity of the central nervous system (CNS). These drugs produce sleep within seconds of intravenous administration. Awakening is rapid and occurs by redistribution of the drug from the CNS. Barbiturates are given as an intravenous bolus or as a bolus followed by a continuous infusion. The short-acting barbiturates thiopental and methohexital have been used in pediatric radiotherapy (18,19). Side effects include apnea, hiccoughs, laryngospasm, and paradoxical CNS excitation. Some radiotherapists use droperidol, a butyrophenone derivative with pharmacologic actions similar to those of haloperidol and phenothiazines, generally followed by pentobarbital for intravenous anesthesia.

Narcotic analgesics produce sedation as a side effect. Other side effects of opiates include respiratory depression, nausea, vomiting, and tolerance with repeated administration. These side effects of narcotics make opiate anesthesia undesirable for radiotherapy. Radiotherapy is not a painful procedure; narcotics should not be necessary.

Opiate use in pediatric radiotherapy is additionally limited by the pharmacokinetic profile of many drugs in this class. Opiates such as meperidine and morphine have long half-lives, which make them unsuitable for short procedures such as radiation therapy.

Potent synthetic opioids such as fentanyl, sufentanil, alfentanil, and remifentanil may have a role, but that role is limited by their ability to depress respiration, cause chest wall rigidity, and produce tolerance. Mixed opiate agonist–antagonists such as nalbuphine and butorphanol are touted as producing sedation and analgesia with less respiratory depression (plateau effect). These agonist–antagonists may be useful adjuncts in anesthesia for radiotherapy.

Propofol is an intravenous anesthetic that has hypnotic–sedative properties. Propofol is an alkyl phenol derivative that is insoluble in water. The active ingredient, 2,6-diisopropylphenol, is formulated in an emulsion of soybean oil, glycerol, and egg lecithin. This formulation gives it a milky-white appearance. It is a highly lipid-soluble compound and therefore has a rapid distribution into the CNS and a rapid elimination. This rapid elimination has made it a popular anesthetic agent for day surgery and short procedures. It can be given via a central venous line or a peripheral intravenous catheter (22,23). When it is given peripherally, pain on injection is common. This pain can be reduced by administering the drug with lidocaine. Propofol has been used by anesthesiologists in pediatric radiotherapy. It is given as an intermittent bolus or as a bolus followed by continuous infusion. Awakening is rapid, and the incidence of side effects is low. When it is administered as a rapid intravenous bolus, apnea and hypotension are common. However, when the dosage is fractionated and administered slowly, spontaneous respiration and blood pressure are preserved. Propofol appears to possess antiemetic properties, which add to its appeal.

Rapid and safe induction of anesthesia with propofol in children usually entails a loading dose of 2.5 mg/kg administered intravenously. The dosage is higher in non-premedicated children. Maintenance of anesthesia is achieved by continuous infusion of 2.5 mg/kg per hour if it is supplemented by analgesics and nitrous oxide. Tachyphylaxis with propofol is rare. Fast awakening after the propofol infusion is stopped results from its short elimination half-life and the lack of substantial accumulation during administration over a long period. The elimination half-life after a single injection is even shorter in children than in adults. Respiratory depression during injection of propofol anesthesia can occur primarily through an overly rapid injection. Controlled administration of the induction dose, using an automatic pump, guarantees a slow and steady injection. Clinically significant respiratory depression during the maintenance phase of sedation can be avoided by stabilizing the infusion rate using an automatic pump (26).

Scheiber et al. (24), from the University Hospital of Essen in Germany, reported 155 propofol anesthetic sessions performed on consecutive pediatric radiation therapy patients with a mean age of 30 months. The mean duration of anesthesia was 18 minutes. There were no clinically important complications involving respiration, circulation, or neurologic functions except for one transient episode of desaturation managed by suctioning and change in head position. children awakened spontaneously an average of 4 minutes after the propofol infusion was discontinued. No tachyphylaxis or unpleasant side effects were observed.

A lipid-based anesthetic agent such as propofol can support rapid microbial growth at room temperature. Bennett et al. (22) documented the association of propofol with postoperative in-

fections. This appears to be associated with a lapse in aseptic techniques. A significant anesthesia-associated complication of external beam radiation therapy in children is sepsis associated with the central venous access line. Eleven of 74 children receiving radiotherapy at Duke University Medical Center who had a central venous line developed proven sepsis (15%) with fever and a positive blood culture drawn through the central line. Of these 11 children, 8 had received prior chemotherapy (73%). Six of the 11 had been anesthetized with propofol (55%), 4 with a short-acting barbiturate induction plus inhalation anesthetic (36%), and one with inhalation anesthesia alone (9%). The pathogens cultivated from these 11 children included *Staphylococcus, Bacillus, Streptococcus, Enterobacter,* and *Candida* (23).

There are four potential sources of central venous access colonization producing sepsis: the skin insertion site, the catheter hub, hematogenous seeding of the catheter, and infusate contamination such as might be caused by propofol (25). In the setting of anesthesia for pediatric external beam radiotherapy, one is concerned about the possible contamination of the catheter through repeated use by the anesthesiologist. It is well known that there is a high incidence of central venous line sepsis in a variety of high-risk settings including patients receiving chemotherapy or total parenteral nutrition, burn unit patients, and those in the intensive care unit (23,25). The risk of sepsis with repeated catheter use in such settings ranges from 5% to 29%. Therefore, one should not be surprised by the occasional case of sepsis in the child whose central venous line is accessed repeatedly for anesthesia for radiotherapy.

SEDATION OR ANESTHESIA?

Conscious sedation as a medically controlled state of depressed consciousness allows protective reflexes to be maintained, retains the patient's ability to maintain a patent airway independently and continually, and permits appropriate response by the patient to physical stimulation or verbal commands (e.g., "open your eyes"). General anesthesia is a medical state of unconsciousness, usually accompanied by a loss of protective reflexes, including the inability to maintain a patent airway independently and to respond to physical stimulation or verbal commands.

The drugs commonly used for sedating young children in radiation therapy include chloral hydrate, which is administered by an oral or rectal route; phenobarbital, which may be administered orally, rectally, or intravenously; fentanyl, which is available for administration orally, intramuscularly, or intravenously; midazolam, for intramuscular or intravenous use; meperidine, which may be administered orally, rectally, or intramuscularly; promethazine, which is a sedative agent administered orally or intramuscularly; chlorpromazine, which may be administered orally or intramuscularly; or droperidol, which may be administered intramuscularly or intravenously. Chloral hydrate has principally a sedative effect. Pentobarbital has both sedative and hypnotic effects. Fentanyl has analgesic and amnesic effects. Meperidine is primarily an analgesic. Promethazine and chlorpromazine have principally sedative effects, whereas droperidol has both tranquilizing and sedative effects.

Some institutions first attempt to sedate a child for radiation before using general anesthesia. For physicians who first use chloral hydrate, the dosage is 75–100 mg orally or rectally. If adequate sedation is not achieved in 20 minutes, a second dose of 25 mg/kg can be given if the lesser dose of 75 mg/kg was used initially. The maximum dosage should not exceed 2,000 mg. An alternative is midazolam 0.05–0.2 mg/kg given by slow intravenous push over 3–5 minutes and titrated to effect. It is generally recommended to give oxygen by mask during the procedure. Some physicians prefer meperidine 0.5–1 mg/kg, with a maximum of 20 mg, to be given by slow intravenous push over 3–5 minutes. If sedation fails, general anesthesia is administered by an anesthetist. The criteria for consulting an anesthesiologist include the need for a regular boosting of chloral hydrate, unsatisfactory sedation, or unsatisfactory radiation therapy caused by patient motion.

A retrospective review of the clinical experience with sedation and anesthesia for pediatric radiation therapy has recently been published by investigators from the King Faisal Specialist Hospital and Research Center of Riyadh, Saudi Arabia (28). They attempted to sedate children and, if that failed, then moved to general anesthesia. In a series of 1,033 consecutive treatments, 86% included general anesthesia, and 14% were performed with conscious sedation. With the use of general anesthesia, satisfactory control of motion for radiotherapy was achieved in 97% of cases. Conscious sedation gave a satisfactory result in only 68% of cases ($p = 0.0001$). There was a high rate of unsatisfactory sedations, including complications with chloral hydrate. Meperidine was also unsatisfactory. The highest success rate was achieved with propofol anesthesia in 837 procedures. Only 7% of these procedures had at least one complication, and satisfactory treatment was achieved in 98% of cases.

Although the authors of this study argue that, except for retinoblastoma cases, physicians should use conscious sedation with midazolam before moving to general anesthesia, the data may not support this view. Conscious sedation often does not achieve a sufficiently stable child for precision radiation therapy, the uncertain duration of times to achieve anesthesia may make it difficult to operate a radiation therapy department on schedule, and the significant incidence of complications all may argue for a policy of moving directly to anesthesia under the direction of an anesthetist rather than conscious sedation administered by a radiation oncologist in an attempt to avoid anesthesia. Because anesthesia is almost always needed anyway, the attempt to use conscious sedation may create unnecessary delays (26).

It is crucial to have adequate monitoring capabilities when sedating children for radiation therapy. A daily evaluation process should include checking presedation vital signs and evaluating any contraindications such as presence of an upper respiratory tract infection, acute pulmonary problems, allergy, or other problems that may alter the appropriate drug dosage. The child is monitored during therapy with a closed-circuit television monitor that is clearly visible outside the radiation therapy room. A display of the pulse oximeter should be visible. Emergency equipment including a pediatric emergency cart, suction machine, Ambu bag, face mask, defibrillator, oral airway, and emergency drug box should be readily available. After each daily sedation, the child should be kept in the radiation therapy department until it is evident that the effects of sedation have worn off and the child is able to take fluids and has stable vital signs. Meticulous chart documentation is essential (27–29).

ANESTHESIA MONITORING

Unrecognized hypoventilation is the primary cause of morbidity and mortality in pediatric anesthesia (29,30). The respiratory depressant effects of many anesthetic agents combined with the propensity for airway obstruction as a consequence of positioning for radiotherapy make anesthesia for pediatric radiotherapy a risky proposition. The need to be physically removed from the patient during radiation delivery adds to the challenge of adequate monitoring.

What constitutes appropriate monitoring for children receiving sedatives and general anesthetics? The American Academy of Pediatrics Section on Anesthesiology and the American Society of Anesthesiologists have published guidelines (30,31). The standards for basic intraoperative monitoring of the American Society of Anesthesiologists state,

> During all anesthetics, the patient's oxygenation, ventilation, circulation and temperature shall be continually evaluated. Qualified anesthesia personnel shall be present in the room throughout the conduct of all general anesthetics, regional anesthetics and monitored anesthesia care. In the event there is a direct known hazard, e.g., radiation, to the anesthesia personnel which might require intermittent remote observation of the patient, some provision for monitoring the patient must be made.

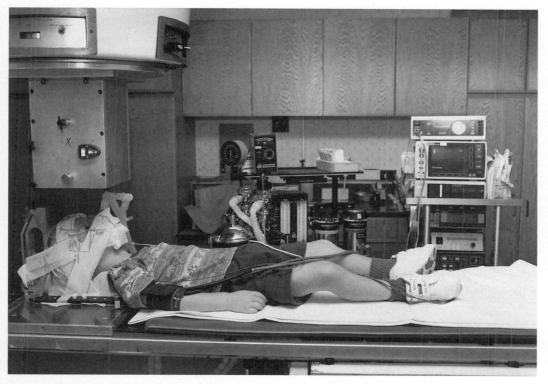

FIG. 21-2. The anesthetized child is monitored, in the accelerator vault, with electrocardiogram, pulse oximetry, and capnometry. Notice that the gas delivery mask is well integrated into the radiotherapy head stabilization device.

Provisions made for monitoring in radiotherapy suites include closed-circuit television screens on which are displayed the patient and the oxygenation, ventilation, circulation, and temperature monitors and leaded glass windows through which the patient and monitors can be viewed while the radiation treatment is delivered (Fig. 21-2).

Early reports of anesthesia for radiotherapy relied on visual inspection of patient color as a monitor of adequacy of oxygenation. However, the unreliability of direct observation for detecting cyanosis is known (32). Pulse oximetry is an accurate, noninvasive, continuous measure of arterial oxygen saturation. A pulse oximeter is an optical sensor that measures the concentration of oxyhemoglobin. Oximeters work according to the Beer–Lambert law, which states that when a parallel beam of light falls on a semitransparent homogeneous sub-

stance, the intensity of the transmitted light decreases exponentially as distance through the substance increases, and if a parallel beam of light is transmitted a known distance through a clear solution with a dissolved solute, the intensity of the transmitted light decreases exponentially as the concentration of solute increases. In clinical practice, pulse oximeters measure red and infrared light transmitted through tissue beds such as a finger, earlobe, or nose. The utility of pulse oximetry in detecting cyanosis in children has been demonstrated in large randomized controlled clinical trials (33). Pulse oximeters are used to closely monitor cardiorespiratory changes resulting from anesthetic agents. The reusable, clip-on Durasentor (Nellcor, Incorporate, Hayward, CA) is not generally recommended for patients weighing less than 40 kg. However, the Oxisensor (Nellcor, Incorpo-

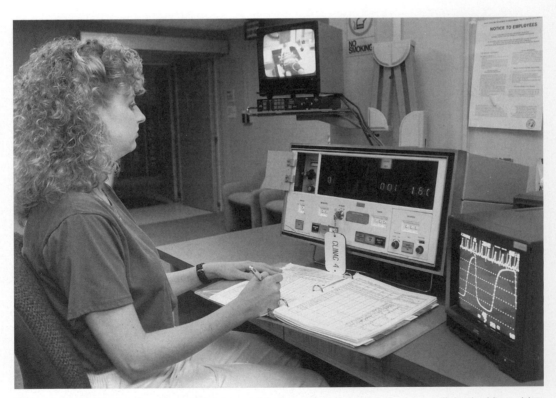

FIG. 21-3. Monitoring from immediately outside the treatment room is accomplished with a video screen displaying the child, an intercom system for audio, and a monitor displaying the electrocardiogram, respiratory wave, and fraction of inspired oxygen.

rated), a disposable pediatric digit oxygen transducer, can be used for these children. It is an expensive device, but with proper handling it can be reused from day to day (28).

How is ventilation best monitored? The first report of anesthesia for radiotherapy used continual visual observation of the thorax and abdomen combined with a wisp of cotton placed over the mouth. The cotton fibers moved in and out with inspiration and expiration, respectively, amplifying air movement. Amplifiers are used because the anesthesiologist cannot be physically present while radiation therapy is being delivered. Several amplifiers of ventilation have been described for use in radiotherapy. Visual amplifier methods include attaching a cotton-tipped applicator to the thorax and observing via a closed-circuit television monitor the excursions of the cotton tip with inspiration and expiration and placing a light box on the patient's abdomen or chest and observing on the televi-

sion monitor the movement of the lightbulb with each respiratory cycle. Aural amplifiers allow the anesthesiologist to hear the patient's breath sounds from outside the treatment area. An esophageal or precordial stethoscope can be connected to an audio amplifier, and the output can be heard on a speaker or earphone.

Observation of the movements of the reservoir breathing bag by the anesthesiologist is an excellent monitor of gas exchange. This technique is applicable to patients anesthetized with inhalational agents whose tracheas are intubated, those who have an LMA in place, or those who have a simple face mask applied over the nose and mouth. If the breathing bag cannot easily be seen on the closed-circuit monitor or through the leaded glass window, its movements can be amplified by a stick made of tongue blades. One end of the stick is attached to the neck of the breathing bag with a piece of tape, and a flag of white paper is placed at the

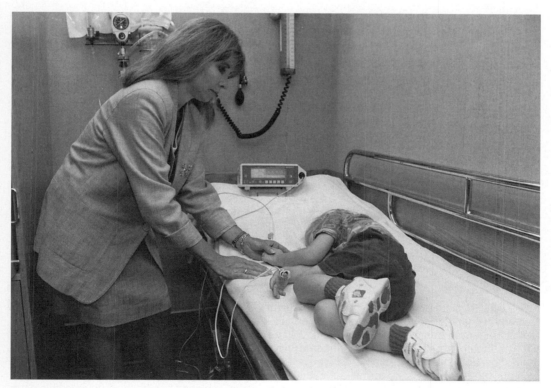

FIG. 21-4. The anesthesiologist is at the bedside in the recovery area in the radiotherapy department. Oxygen, suction, and pulse oximetry monitoring are immediately available.

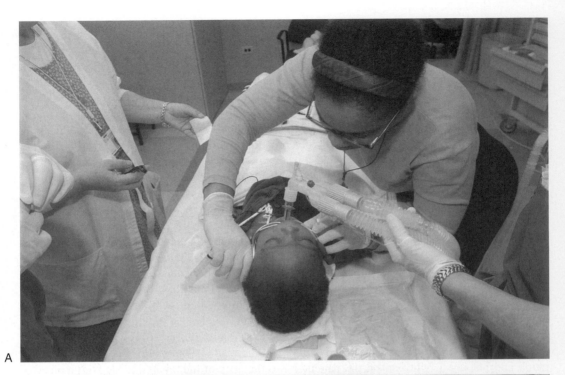

A

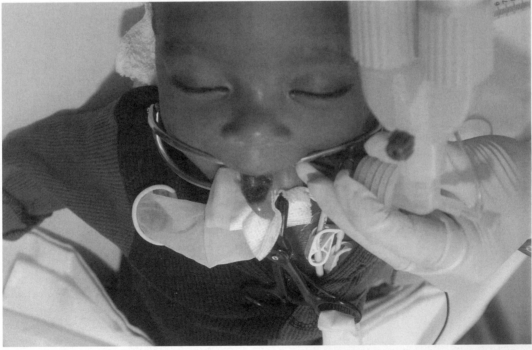

B

FIG. 21-5. To minimize the effects of external beam irradiation on the mandible and neck of this child with embryonal rhabdomyosarcoma of the tongue, resected with positive margins, daily fractionated radiotherapy was administered via an orthovoltage intraoral cone while the child was anesthetized. **(A)** The mouth is held open with a standard surgical mouth gag used commonly in the operating room. The anesthesiologist stabilizes the gas tubes attached to the airway. **(B)** The tumor bed is painted with methylene blue to make it easy to identify. The tongue is pulled forward with a plastic towel clip over gauze. A lead shield, inside a surgical glove, is placed behind the tongue to shield the floor of the mouth. **(C)** The intraoral cone is docked. The tongue is held in place by the towel clip, which is pulled taut by a strap seen in the far right of the picture. The child is alive and well, with satisfactory speech development, eight months after radiotherapy.

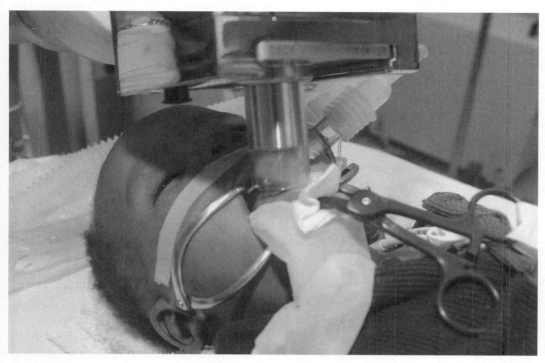

C

FIG. 21-5. *Continued*

opposite end of the stick. This long lever arm greatly accentuates the movements of the breathing bag and serves as an amplifier of ventilation.

The gold standard for assessing ventilation is capnometry. Capnometry is the quantitative measurement of the partial pressure of CO_2 produced by the patient during the ventilatory cycle. Capnography is the continuous graphic display of CO_2 concentration as a function of time. End-tidal CO_2 analysis is a means of assessing alveolar ventilation, airway patency, and the functioning of the breathing circuit and ventilator. End-tidal CO_2 monitoring has been shown to be an effective monitor in pediatric anesthesia, capable of the early detection of many potentially life-threatening events such as apnea, bronchospasm, and disconnections in the breathing circuit (34).

The adequacy of circulatory function during the administration of anesthesia is assessed by continuous display of the electrocardiogram (ECG) and by measurement of blood pressure. Noninvasive, automated oscillometric blood pressure determination (DINAMAP, Criti Kom,

Inc., Tampa, FL) is readily available and uniquely suited for remote monitoring of blood pressure. The ECG and DINAMAP displays are viewed indirectly on the closed-circuit monitor or directly through a leaded glass window if the radiotherapy suite is so equipped (Figs. 21-3 and 21-4).

In the Duke series of anesthesia for pediatric radiation therapy, the most frequently used monitoring techniques were ECG (95%), pulse oximetry (93%), monitoring of blood pressure via manual aneroid sphygmomanometer (71%), monitoring of the fraction inspired oxygen via polarigraphic electrode placed in the inspired gas limb in the anesthesia circuit (57%), pulse oximetry (93%), capnometry (55%), and blood pressure monitoring via an automated, noninvasive oscillometric device (DINAMAP) (15%). In most patients, multiple monitoring techniques were used (23).

In summary, standards for monitoring anesthetized children have been published. These standards and guidelines are intended to promote high-quality care. No matter how rigorous the adherence to these recommendations, it is impossible to guarantee specific patient outcomes. The provision of anesthesia for radiotherapy carries with it the additional challenge of remote monitoring of patients whose airways may be compromised not only by their underlying disease but also by the constraints of positioning for the procedure (Fig. 21-5).

ANESTHETIC IMPLICATIONS OF UNDERLYING DISEASE

Radiotherapy is used to treat several different pediatric malignancies. In the Duke series, the diagnoses leading to treatment with external beam radiotherapy under anesthesia were primary CNS tumor (28%), retinoblastoma (26%), neuroblastoma (18%), acute leukemia (9%), rhabdomyosarcoma (7%), Wilms' tumor (5%), Langerhans cell histiocytosis (4%), and other (3%). It is not surprising that the diagnoses leading to radiotherapy under anesthesia differ somewhat from the most common diagnoses of cancer in childhood. Leukemia is an uncommon indication for radiotherapy under anesthesia because it is, in general, a malignancy of older children, and the role of radiation therapy is limited. Diseases associated with younger children in which radiotherapy is more frequently used dominate the list (23). Many of these malignancies have implications for the pediatric anesthesiologist. Children with supratentorial brain tumors can have elevated ICP. Management of anesthesia for patients with elevated ICP includes the avoidance of drugs that can raise ICP, such as ketamine. Anesthetic techniques that result in elevations in arterial CO_2 tension can produce intracranial hypertension by increasing cerebral blood flow.

Some neuroblastomas secrete catecholamines and cause systemic hypertension. Blood pressure elevations are associated with abdominal palpation. This problem is rare in pediatric radiotherapy because the tumor is not manipulated.

Wilms' tumors often are massive and can impair ventilation by increasing intra-abdominal pressure. An occasional child with a Wilms' tumor will undergo endotracheal intubation for respiratory failure before presenting to the radiation oncologist for radiotherapy. These tumors can also extend into the inferior vena cava and

renal vein, producing renovascular distortion and systemic hypertension.

Children with Hodgkin's disease, non-Hodgkin's lymphomas, and T-cell acute lymphoblastic leukemia can present with anterior mediastinal masses. These masses can produce tracheal compression and impair ventilation. They can also produce superior vena cava syndrome by compressing the great veins. Some patients with anterior mediastinal masses are referred to the pediatric radiation oncologist for external beam therapy before tissue biopsy. Radiation therapy before tissue biopsy is recommended in some of these patients because the induction of anesthesia in some patients with anterior mediastinal masses can be fatal. Death on induction of general anesthesia in these patients is caused by either the inability to ventilate because of airway compression or the inability of the heart to circulate blood because of tumor encroachment on the right heart or pulmonary circulation (7). Prospective identification of children with anterior mediastinal masses who are at risk for cardiorespiratory collapse on induction of general anesthesia involves a thorough history and physical examination aimed at eliciting signs and symptoms of airway and cardiovascular impairment. Laboratory studies useful in assessing preanesthetic risk include a chest radiograph, computed tomography scan, and upright and supine flow-volume loops. The pediatric radiotherapist may treat patients with anterior mediastinal masses for whom the risks of general anesthesia are felt to outweigh the benefits of obtaining tissue before the institution of therapy. These patients should not receive anesthesia or sedation.

In addition to these considerations, the pediatric anesthesiologist must consider the associated implications of treating malignancy in children. These implications include the cardiac, hematologic, pulmonary, immunologic, and neurologic impairments caused by chemotherapy (34).

Anemia is one of the most common problems in children with cancer. Anemia decreases oxygen delivery to the tissues. Oxygen delivery is the product of the arterial oxygen content and the cardiac index. If oxygen delivery to the tissues is inadequate, organ system failure occurs. The minimum acceptable hemoglobin value in anesthetized children is unknown. Hemoglobin values as low as 7 g/dL may be adequate if the patient has normal cardiovascular compensatory mechanisms. However, many patients cannot compensate for low levels of hemoglobin because they have chemotherapy-induced myocardial dysfunction.

Cardiac toxicity is most notably caused by the anthracycline antibiotic chemotherapeutic agents doxorubicin and daunorubicin. These drugs have both an acute and a chronic effect. Acute toxicity manifests as rhythm and conduction disturbances such as supraventricular tachycardia, ventricular ectopic beats, and heart block. Chronic toxicity manifests as a cardiomyopathy, which can progress to left ventricular failure in 2–10% of patients. Factors that increase the risk of anthracycline cardiotoxicity include dosages greater than 550 mg/m^2, age younger than 1 year, concurrent use of other chemotherapeutic agents such as cyclophosphamide and cisplatin, and a history of mediastinal irradiation.

Pulmonary toxicity occurs in 5–10% of patients treated with the antibiotic chemotherapeutic agent bleomycin. Bleomycin produces interstitial pulmonary fibrosis, which results in restrictive lung disease. The damage is thought to be produced by oxygen free radical formation. The role of exogenous oxygen in promoting the pulmonary toxicity of bleomycin is controversial. However, it is prudent to avoid inspired oxygen concentrations greater than 28% when anesthetizing patients who have been treated with bleomycin, provided that they maintain satisfactory levels of arterial oxygen tension.

On rare occasions, the child undergoing anesthesia for radiotherapy has received a prior course of irradiation to the head and neck or lungs. The anesthesiologist should be aware that these children may be at higher risk for laryngeal edema after instrumentation of the airway and for difficulty in maintaining oxygenation (35–38).

REFERENCES

References particularly recommended for further reading are indicated by an asterisk.

*1. Harrison GG, Bennet MB. Radiotherapy without tears. Br J Anaesth 1963;35:720–721.

2. Slifer KJ, Cataldo MF, Cataldo MD, et al. Behavior analysis of motion control for pediatric neuroimaging. J Appl Behav Anal 1993;26:469–470.

*3. Slifer KG, Buckholtz JD, Cataldo MD. Behavioral training of motion controlling young children undergoing radiation treatment without sedation. J Pediatr Oncol Nurs 1994;11:55–63.

4. Slifer KJ. A video system to help children cooperative with motion control for radiation therapy without sedation. J Pediatr Oncol Nurs 1996;13:91–97.

5. Fisher DM, Robinson S, Brett CM, et al. Comparison of enflurane, halothane, and isoflurane for diagnostic and therapeutic procedures in children with malignancies. Anesthesiology 1985;63:647–650.

6. Wolfe TM, Rao CC. Anesthesia outside the operating room. Semin Pediatr Surg 1992;1:81–87.

7. Keon TP. Death on induction of anesthesia for cervical node biopsy. Anesthesiology 1981;55:471–472.

8. Eger EI II. New inhaled anesthetics. Anesthesiology 1994;80:906–922.

9. Eger EI II. New inhaled anesthetics. Int Anesthesiol Clin 1995;33:61–80.

10. Lerman J. Sevoflurane in pediatric anesthesia. Anesth Analg 1995;81:S4–10.

11. Smith I, Nathanson MH, White PF. The role of sevoflurane in outpatient anesthesia. Anesth Analg 1995;81: S67.

12. Grebenik CR, Ferguson C, White A. The laryngeal mask airway in pediatric radiotherapy. Anesthesiology 1990;72:474–477.

13. Morris GN, Marjot R. Laryngeal mask airway performance: effect of cuff deflation during anaesthesia. Br J Anaesth 1996;76(3):456–458.

14. Moylan SL, Luce MA. The reinforced laryngeal mask airway in paediatric radiotherapy. Br J Anaesth 1993; 71:172.

15. Wilson IG. The laryngeal mask airway in paediatric practice. Br J Anaesth 1993;70:124–125.

16. Jacobs JR, Reves JG, Glass PSA. Rationale and technique for continuous infusions in anesthesia. Int Anesth Clin 1991;29:23–38.

17. Amberg HL, Gordon G. Low-dose intramuscular ketamine for pediatric radiotherapy: a case report. Anesth Analg 1976;55:92–94.

18. Bennett JA, Bullimore JA. The use of ketamine hydrochloride anesthesia for radiotherapy in young children. Br J Anaesth 1973;45:197–201.

19. Edge WG, Morgan M. Ketamine and paediatric radiotherapy. Anaesth Intensive Care 1977;5:153–156.

20. Cronin MM, Bousfield JD, Hewett EB, et al. Ketamine anaesthesia for radiotherapy in small children. Anaesthesia 1972;27:135–142.

21. Worell JB, McCune WJ. A case report: the use of ketamine and midazolam in intravenous sedation for a child undergoing radiation therapy. J Am Assoc Nurse Anesthetists 1993;61:99–102.

22. Bennett SN, McNeil MM, Bland LA, et al. Postoperative infections traced to contamination of an intravenous anesthetic propofol. N Engl J Med 1996;333: 147–154.

*23. Fortney JT, Halperin EC, Hertz CM, et al. Anesthesia for pediatric external beam radiation therapy. Int J Radiat Oncol Bio Phys 1999;44(3):587–591.

24. Scheiber G, Ribeira FC, Khafaga Y, et al. Evaluation of the safety and efficacy of repeated sedations for the radiation therapy of young children with cancer. A

prospective study of 1033 consecutive sedations. *Int J Radiat Oncol Biol Phys* 2001;49:771–783.

25. Daghistani DH, Horn M, Rodriguez Z, et al. Prevention of indwelling central venous catheter sepsis. *Med Pediatr Oncol* 1996;26:405–408.

*26. Seiler G, DeVole Khafaga Y, Gregory B, et al. Evaluation of the safety and efficacy of repeated sedations for the radiation therapy of young children with cancer. A prospective study of 1033 consecutive sedations. *Int J Radiat Oncol Biol Phys* 2001;49:771–783.

27. Bucholtz JD. Cost savings in pediatric monitoring during sedation for radiation therapy. *Oncol Nurs Forum* 1991;18:1246.

28. Bucholtz JD. Issues concerning the sedation of children for radiation therapy. *Oncol Nurs Forum* 1992; 19:649–655.

29. Committee of Drugs of the American Academy of Pediatrics. Guidelines for the monitoring and management of pediatric patients during and after sedation for diagnostic and therapeutic procedures. *Pediatrics* 1992;89:1110–1115.

30. Committee on Drugs. Guidelines for monitoring and management of pediatric patients during and after sedation for diagnostic and therapeutic procedures. *Pediatrics* 1992;89:1110–1115.

31. American Society of Anesthesiologists. Standards for basic intraoperative monitoring. *Directory of Members* 1993;58:709–710.

32. Comroe JH Jr, Botelho S. The reliability of cyanosis in the recognition of arterial hypoxemia. *Am J Med Sci* 1947;214:1–6.

33. Cote CJ, Goldstein EA, Cote MA, et al. A single blind study of pulse oximetry in children. *Anesthesiology* 1988;68:184–188.

34. Tobias JD. Special considerations for the pediatric oncology patient. In: Berry FA, Steward DJ, eds. *Pediatrics for the anesthesiologist.* New York: Churchill Livingstone, 1993:287–303.

35. Ginsberg RJ. Surgical considerations after preoperative treatment. *Lung Cancer* 1994;10[Suppl 1]:S213–217.

36. Mark RJ, Bailet JW, Poen J, et al. Postirradiation sarcoma of the head and neck. *Cancer* 1993;72:887–893.

37. Mendel P, Anaes FC, Bristow A. New methods of dealing with the complications of panendoscopy. *J Laryngol Otol* 1992;106:903–904.

38. Glauber DT, Audenaert SM. Anesthesia for children undergoing craniospinal radiotherapy. *Anesthesiology* 1987;67:701–803.

22

Stabilization and Immobilization Devices

Edward C. Halperin, M.D., and Kim Light, C.M.D.

The pediatric radiation oncologist must strike a balance: Administer a sufficient radiation dose to achieve the desired goal of tumor control while not giving a dose that is so high as to engender an unacceptable risk of complications. For many tumors the clinically relevant dose–response curve is sigmoidal and steep. A small variation in dose can significantly influence the chance of tumor control and the risk of complications. Errors in dosage prescription can be the result of physician error. To eliminate physician error, proper training, education, and peer review must be conducted regularly. Another source of error is in treatment planning and administration. We can determine the location of the target volume with computed tomography, magnetic resonance imaging, positron emission tomography, and plain radiography. Computer technology allows three-dimensional tumor volume reconstruction and beam planning. Most patients undergo treatment planning and beam confirmation with virtual or conventional simulation. The linear accelerators used in clinical practice provide beams with sharply defined edges. Online portal imaging is becoming increasingly popular. A skilled dosimetrist can generate treatment plans using combinations of photons and electrons, wedges, beam weighting, intensity modulation, and compensators. However, all of this effort and skill can be for naught if the patient is not holding still or is not put in a reproducible and comfortable position at each treatment session. The need for reproducibility has become more widely recognized because smaller margins are used with conformal treatment techniques. For the anxious child, positioning and stabilization often is the weakest link in the chain of treat-

ment planning and implementation (1,2). Quality radiotherapy demands that a daily setup accuracy of a few millimeters be ensured (3–5). For the youngest patients, anesthesia is needed, a topic we reviewed in Chapter 21. In this chapter we will consider psychological, educational, and mechanical aids for patient immobilization.

PSYCHOLOGICAL PREPARATION AND PATIENT AND FAMILY EDUCATION

Before beginning radiotherapy, many children have undergone multiple venipunctures, lumbar punctures, bone marrow biopsies, surgery, and chemotherapy. Therefore, they may fear any attempt to be immobilized. It is unlikely that the physician can create such a strong relationship with the child as to ensure cooperation with treatment. The key to the child's cooperation is the parent's or caregiver's calm confidence. The child will pick up on the parent's positive or negative attitude. This is not to say that the physician should not try to develop a good relationship with the child. However, if the child's parents or guardians feel comfortable with the treatment plan and express confidence in the presence of the child, then more than half of the battle is won.

The therapy team should give the parents a tour of the radiotherapy department, a chance to see and touch the equipment, adequate time to meet the personnel involved in their child's case, and an unhurried time to ask questions and have them answered. It is often advisable to conduct this initial visit without the patient present so that conversation is not inhibited. The parents can also communicate ideas to the staff that will make the child more comfortable. The child must also be given a tour of the department and meet everyone involved in his or her case. The radiation therapist should be willing to demonstrate simulation and treatment on a favorite doll or stuffed animal toy (6). An unhurried atmosphere, pleasant background music, patience, and positive reinforcement are important to ensure the child's cooperation.

Many pediatric inpatient services benefit from the expertise of trained play (or recreation) therapists. These people should be made familiar with the routines of pediatric radiotherapy. They are often valuable allies in making a child more at ease in the therapy area. Special toy radiotherapy machines, art activities, and acting through the planned treatment are techniques play therapists use to prepare a child for treatment. Behavioral techniques to improve patient cooperation with radiotherapy are discussed in Chapter 21. Many children and parents are accustomed to receiving information from television. To meet this need, the physician may turn to specially prepared and commercially available videotapes describing external beam radiotherapy. Some of these videotapes are professionally made, use animation and professional actors, and are specifically targeted at a pediatric audience.

They can convey a significant amount of information in a short time and can be watched numerous times by the child and family if necessary. Some departments make it a routine to show instructional videotapes to most children and families. In addition, printed patient education materials are available. These include special coloring books about radiotherapy, pamphlets with drawings describing treatment, and more mature material for teenagers and parents. Some departments use desktop printing, photographs, and looseleaf binders to construct their own patient education materials.

The widespread availability of computers has created a new world of opportunity for patients to educate themselves about cancer treatment. It is not unusual for a family to have surfed the World Wide Web for information about a particular tumor or to have discussed their medical problems in an online chat room or bulletin board. Many pediatric oncology centers, comprehensive cancer centers, and radiation oncology departments have Web sites that go into detail about personnel and available protocols. Families may also learn about cancer treatment via the toll-free telephone numbers of the National Cancer Institute and patient advocacy groups.

ERRORS IN FIELD PLACEMENT

A field misalignment can result in a miss of some part of the tumor volume. With the use of conformal fields, a setup error may result in a significant decrease in tumor control probability because of steep dose–response curve models. Furthermore, poor patient immobilization necessitates greater tumor margins. Improper immobilization will result in treatment setup errors and increase the risk of normal tissue complications and compromised target coverage. To improve tumor control probability and reduce normal tissue complications, it is important to reduce setup error. This can be facilitated by proper use of immobilization devices.

Geometric misalignment of the patient relative to the incident beam can result from setup errors. These may persist throughout the course of treatment (systematic errors) or may vary unpredictably around a mean value (random errors). A systematic error probably is of greater clinical significance than treatment-to-treatment variability or random error. The implicit conclusion is that errors in treatment delivery, including unsatisfactory immobilization, may be a significant cause of marginal recurrence of tumor after treatment (7).

No matter what precautions are taken, there are uncertainties in the planning and delivery of external beam radiation therapy. Gunilla Bentel (1936–2000), the well-known author and dosimetrist, characterized these, and we are indebted to her for the following discussion (8–10).

In broad terms, uncertainties are of two general types. The first are uncertainties related to the delivery of radiation. These include inhomogeneities in the beam, problems related to dosage calculations, variables in the output of linear accelerators, instability of the beam-monitoring technique, and problems related to beam flatness. The second type of uncertainties in the delivery of radiation therapy can be divided into those related to mechanical inaccuracies in the equipment and those related to the patient. Mechanical uncertainties include errors in field size settings, rotational settings, errors in the crosshair alignment, deviations in the position of the isocenter, incongruency of the light beam with the actual beam, problems with the alignment system, couchtop difficulties, and errors in constructing the beam-shaping blocks. Patient-related uncertainties include uncertainty in target delineation, organ motion, movement of skin marks, day-to-day problems in repositioning, and patient motion.

Although the magnitude of uncertainties in radiation therapy treatment vary, some uncertainties may be additive, whereas others may cancel each other out. Thus, the net effect on any given day can be variable.

Mechanical immobilization of the awake radiotherapy patient is an adjunct to patient education and psychological preparation of the patient. Although there is no substitute for education and psychological preparation, mechanical aids can greatly facilitate accurate treatment. In adult radiotherapy, several studies show that field displacement can be minimized by stabilization. In studies in adults by Bentel et al. (8–10) on Hodgkin's disease, head and neck cancer, and lung cancer, it was found that stabilization devices decrease the number of field position adjustments per number of times tested. In general, more elaborate and firmer stabilization devices such as whole torso cradle stabilization and customized masks produce superior results. A randomized trial of 96 adults with prostate or bladder cancer used external beam radiotherapy with or without a pelvic immobilization device. The average simulation-to-treatment deviation of the isocenter was 8.5 mm in the non-immobilized group and 6.2 mm in the immobilization group ($p < 0.001$). In the non-immobilized arm, 31% of the port films had isocenter deviations more than 10 mm and 11% had isocenter deviations in the immobilized arm ($p = 0.001$) (10).

To the author's knowledge, there are no large-scale mathematical evaluations of the value of immobilization in pediatric radiation oncology. This is not surprising because with the small number of pediatric cases and the wide variety of sites treated, it would be difficult to generate a large series. Fortunately, there are many reports in the adult literature of the value of immobilization and comparisons of various types of immobilization. We will consider some of these.

In the treatment of adult pelvic malignancies such as colorectal cancer and gynecologic malignancies and, in particular, in the treatment of prostate cancer, studies have compared short and long Alpha Cradles (immobilizing only the legs or immobilizing the torso and legs), Hipfix devices, foam leg cushions, and no immobilization. In general, these studies consistently show that more extensive Alpha Cradle immobilization is superior to less extensive immobilization, that the Hipfix device is slightly superior to the Alpha Cradle, that both are superior to leg foam cushions, and all are vastly superior to no immobilization. Similarly, limb immobilization for the treatment of extremity soft tissue sarcomas appears to improve reproducibility of daily radiotherapy (7,12–14). It would be reasonable to conclude that in the treatment of childhood cancer, immobilization would show a similar improvement in treatment localization.

Even in the setting of anesthesia for radiotherapy, immobilization is worthwhile. One cannot be assured that the anesthetized child is placed in the same position every day or that the pulling, tugging, and adjusting necessary for the anesthesiologist to go about his or her work will not result in malpositioning. A customized immobilization device, adapted to the needs of the anesthesiologist, can minimize these problems.

THE IDEAL MECHANICAL AID

Mechanical immobilization of the pediatric radiotherapy patient is an adjunct to patient education and psychological preparation, not a substitute for it. The ideal mechanical aid to patient positioning will meet the following goals:

- The child must feel comfortable and secure; there must be no danger of falling.

- The device must satisfy the radiotherapy treatment plan regarding patient position for correct geographic irradiation.
- The setup should be quick and easy for the therapist.
- The body part treated should be rendered immobile.
- The position of the body part should be reproducible for daily treatment.
- Construction of the device should be reasonably quick. It should not be difficult to train therapists, dosimetrists, and physicians in the procedure.
- The stabilization device should not adversely affect beam buildup and backscatter characteristics.
- The system should be economical.
- If anesthesia is being used, the device must not interfere with the establishment of a secure airway, intravenous access, and the use of monitoring equipment (2,15–20).

Several immobilization systems meet these criteria to varying degrees. However, there is no perfect system. Techniques vary widely between institutions. The skilled radiation oncologist should know several techniques so he or she can use them as the situation demands.

STANDARD ACCESSORY DEVICES

There are a large number of commercially available radiotherapy accessories for patient stabilization. These devices have the advantage of being inexpensive and reusable. They have the disadvantage of not being customized to the individual patient and providing poor immobilization (21–23). The plastic head sponge provides stability for the head when the patient is supine. A device called a "doggie dish" because of its resemblance to a pet's feeding bowl is available in several sizes for head support also (Figs. 22-1, 22-2, and 22-3). Many linear accelerator couches are narrow and do not provide a comfortable resting place for a child's arms or legs. Plexiglas, plastic, or wooden sheets or boards may be used to widen the couch. These may be anchored by placing them, in part, under the child's body (21).

Every pediatric radiotherapy unit should be equipped with an assortment of canvas or other fabric straps to attach to the treatment couch and small sandbags. These cannot be used to restrain an uncooperative child or, by themselves, ensure a reproducible treatment setup. However, they can be used as an extra measure of safety against rolling or falling.

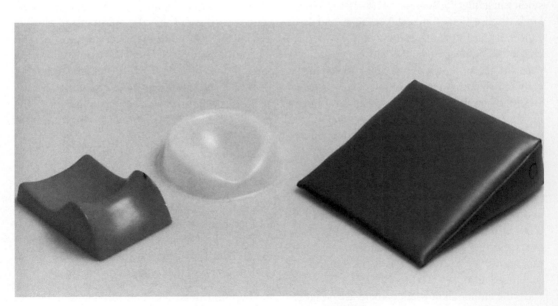

FIG. 22-1. Supine head supports.

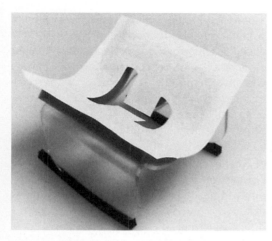

FIG. 22-2. A prone headrest.

THE BITE BLOCK

Bite blocks are used in head and neck radiotherapy to stabilize the child's jaw so that the same mouth position is reproduced at each treatment session, to deflect or depress the tongue away from the hard palate during irradiation of the nasopharyngeal or hard palate areas, to keep the mouth open during treatment, thus reducing the volume of oral mucosa, and to fill the natural airspace of the mouth (22).

They are also commonly used for head stabilization for highly conformal irradiation, intensity-modulated radiation therapy, and radiosurgery of intracranial tumors. A bite impression can be made in the radiation oncology department with rapidly setting dental material on a plastic bite plate of the sort used in dentistry. It is the custom in some depart-

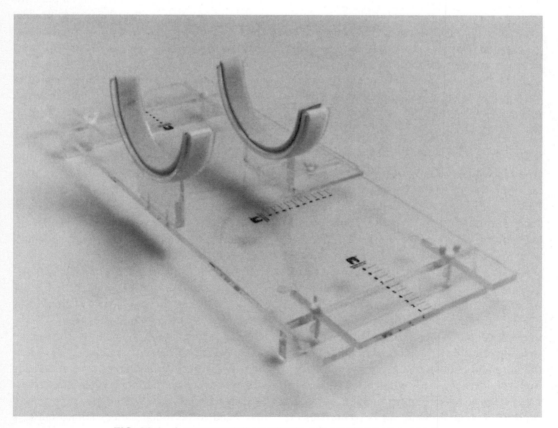

FIG. 22-3. A commercially available adjustable head support.

ments to place the barrel of a hypodermic syringe in the middle of the dental impression to provide an additional airway for the patient. Other departments embed tongue depressors in the modeling compound to provide extra pressure on the back of the tongue.

Some pediatric dentists have training in sophisticated techniques for making full and partial mouth impressions. These impressions can be adopted to create snugly fitting and elegant bite blocks. If the bite block is used as the sole patient-positioning device, the block is fixed to a calibrated arm that is, in turn, fixed to the treatment couch. Three-dimensional treatment planning, simulation, and treatment are done with the arm in the same position each day. Stability depends on the child's willingness to accept the dental impression in his or her mouth and bite down firmly. It is also very important that the staff and the child understand the purpose of the bite block because it can be used for various purposes. If the bite block is to be used in conjunction with a thermal plastic head stabilization device, then it is important to prepare the thermal plastic with the bite block already in place. Only in this way can one ensure that the plastic mask will fit snugly around the facial contour as it is distorted by the bite block.

THERMAL PLASTICS

A custom-made contoured thermal plastic device often is useful for immobilization. Thermal plastics are used by orthopedic surgeons for splints and casts and are commercially available from several suppliers (5,23–26). The plastic comes in perforated sheets that soften and become malleable when heated to 160–180°F (70–80°C) in a hot water bath. The material's stickiness and elasticity hold it in place during molding. The softened sheet is draped over the patient's face from the hairline to below the chin. It is molded to the bridge of the nose and chin to ensure a reproducible fit. Some children are more comfortable if a gauze pad is placed over bony prominences of the skull to alleviate pressure. In 7–10 minutes the plastic is cool and retains the desired shape.

The new cast may be clamped or screwed to a wooden or plastic board on the treatment couch. The perforations in the plastic allow air circulation and a partial view of patient anatomy. Setup marks may be drawn directly on the cast, or the cast may be cut away for treatment (Figs. 22-4, 22-5, 22-6, and 22-7). Stretched thermoplastic causes a slight increase in the radiation surface dosage from 6- or 18-MV photons (27). The thermal plastic device can be used with standard or customized head supports. A customized support usually is more comfortable and reproducible than standard head supports.

The Orfit Cast System, also called the Hipfix System, consists of a thermoplastic sheet that, when heated in a water bath, becomes malleable. It is then stretched and molded to the patient's body but may also be used with children. In adult radiotherapy, it is most commonly used to cover the pelvis and the upper part of the legs. It is then fixed on a fiber carbon plate inserted in a mattress on the treatment table. The sheet is locked into place on a rigid pelvic board (13,14).

Uvex casts are a transparent, lightweight, rigid form of immobilization. They are commonly used to contour the head and neck and the pelvis. An impression is obtained with plaster bandages. The Uvex cast is formed from the plaster.

Steroid use, weight loss or gain, or edema during a course of radiation can render a thermoplastic stabilization device ill fitting. Sections of the head holder can be cut away to make the device more comfortable as long as immobilization is not compromised; often a new head holder must be made (28).

If the child is to be irradiated under anesthesia, the thermal plastic head holder can be fabricated with the gas mask or CO_2 monitor as integral parts of the immobilizer. The anesthesiologist and radiation oncologist must agree on the head position and degree of neck extension to facilitate radiotherapy and anesthesia airway management. It is very important to establish a proper airway initially, or planning may need to be redone after another mask is made.

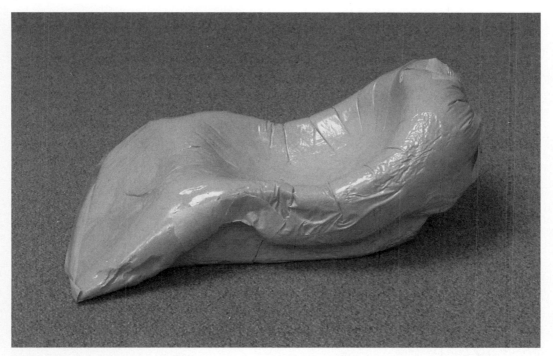

FIG. 22-4. A polyurethane foam mold of the head and neck in supine position provides stability and reproducible head position. This is combined with a thermoplastic head holder to create a tight fit and a stable patient.

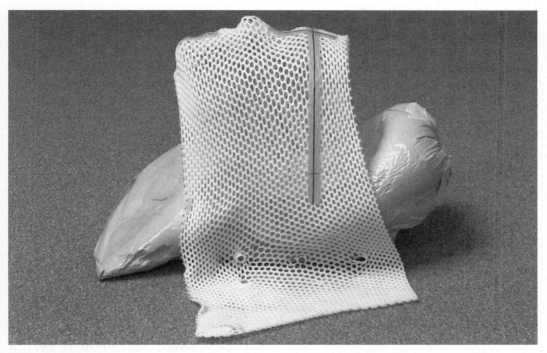

FIG. 22-5. A thermoplastic head holder made of a single sheet, combined with a polyurethane foam mold of the head and neck, provides the stability needed for three-dimensional conformal therapy of a brain tumor.

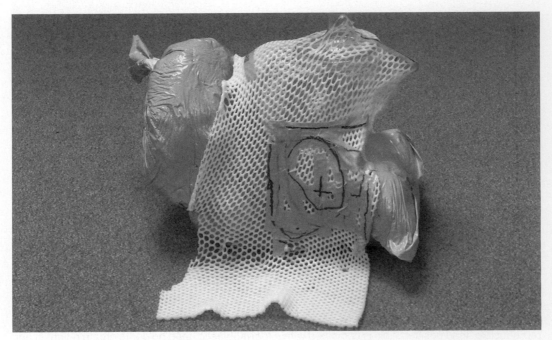

FIG. 22-6. This thermoplastic head holder and polyurethane foam mold of the back of the head and neck were created for treatment of child with posterior fossa ependymoma. The child needed anesthesia for daily treatment. Notice how the anesthesiologist's gas mask was built into the head holder for daily use. The markings on the mask, for laser alignment and port marks, may be drawn on tape placed on the mask.

PLASTER OF PARIS

Plaster of Paris is a fine white gypsum powder. In the past, plaster bandages were often used for radiotherapy purposes. They are now less popular because alternatives have become available such as thermoplastics, polyurethane foams, and vacuum bags. The plaster bandage consists of a mesh impregnated with plaster powder. The bandage is immersed in water, the excess water is squeezed out, and the material is ready for molding (16,21). An exothermic reaction occurs as the material solidifies. Heat is produced, and one must take care not to burn the child.

In order to make a cast, the body part to be immobilized is covered with stockinette or other soft lining for protection. Alternatively, one may coat the area with petroleum jelly. The plaster strips are applied in sufficient number to provide structural stability. The cast may be removed when partially dry and then allowed to harden. Casts may be reinforced, cut out, or drawn on as needed.

Plaster casts were used at one time for craniospinal irradiation, whole body casting for immobilization of young children, and head immobilization (29,30). They may be used in conjunction with vacuum-molded thermoplastics (27). Plaster casts can achieve excellent immobilization, but their production is time consuming (31). They have been supplanted, for the most part, by other techniques. At least one department uses a product that consists of sheets of plaster-soaked bandage sandwiched between cotton flannel and polyurethane foam. The flannel adds to the cast's structural strength when soaked with the plaster. The foam is in contact with the patient (1). The material becomes pliable when wet and is used in the same manner as the plaster bandage strips described previously.

VACUUM-MOLDED THERMOPLASTICS

Several types of clear plastics are available in flat sheets that may be used to construct clear,

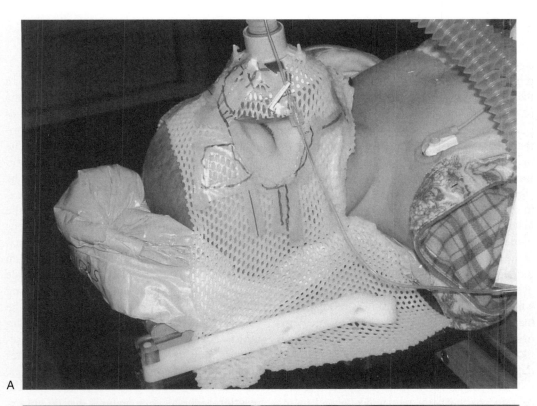

A

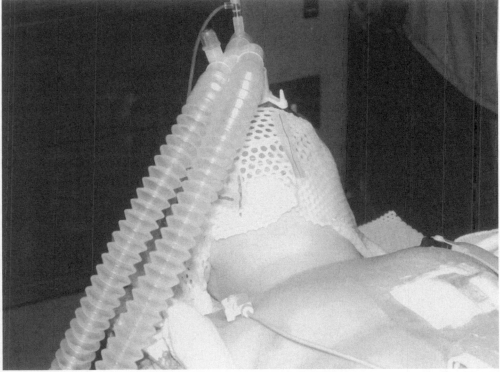

B

FIG. 22-7. A thermoplastic head holder is used to stabilize a child receiving external beam radiotherapy for retinoblastoma. **(A)** A custom-made foam headrest cradles the head and neck. Notice how the anesthesia mask is built into the thermoplastic head holder. **(B)** The head holder comes over the jaw to stabilize the neck in the desired degree of extension for airway management.

rigid immobilization devices (10,16,28,32). The initial step in the construction of these devices is the preparation of a plaster mold. The body part of interest is molded with plaster bandages. The plaster impression is allowed to dry, and then the ends are closed off to form a container for plaster casting. Plaster powder is mixed with water to a creamy consistency, and the impression is filled. After the casting has been allowed to dry, the impression bandages are peeled off, leaving a model of the body part. The plaster model is then placed in a vacuum molding machine that heats the clear plastic sheet and, with the aid of a vacuum, draws the plastic tightly over the cast (32,33). The plastic becomes hard when cool. Some technical skill is needed in using the vacuum-molding machine to avoid wasting the plastic material, tearing the plastic as it molds, or wrapping the plastic too far around the model, locking the plastic on the plaster.

When the plastic mold is completed, it may be fitted to the body part and attached to the treatment couch. Visibility is excellent, and one may draw directly on the plastic.

POLYURETHANE FOAMS

A commercially available system for creating a polyurethane mold, Alpha Cradle and Alpha Cradle Mold Maker (Smithers Medical Products, Inc., Akron, OH), is a popular way to immobilize for pediatric radiotherapy (6,25). The body part to be immobilized is placed on a polystyrene bag that is filled with chemicals. The chemical reaction that occurs generates an expanding polyurethane foam. The foam fills the bag and molds around the body part. Various frames may be used with this system for thorax, abdominal, or limb immobilization. Styrofoam sheets, 0.75–1 inch thick, may be placed inside the bag to be incorporated into the expanding foam and add strength to the device. After the chemical reaction is initiated, one has 4–5 minutes to position the patient. The child must remain motionless for approximately 15 minutes as the immobilizer hardens and cools (Figs. 22-4, 22-6, and 22-8). The exothermic chemical reaction generates temperatures that do not exceed 105.7°F. This degree of heat may be uncomfortable for some children. A sheet of paper

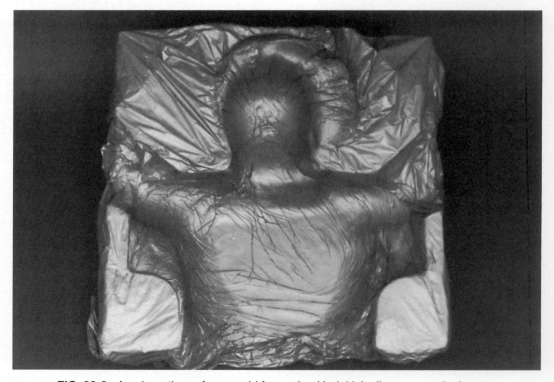

FIG. 22-8. A polyurethane foam mold for supine Hodgkin's disease mantle therapy.

or pillowcase on the bag usually allows enough heat displacement for comfort without interfering with molding. After the mold hardens, marks can be made directly on the cradle for setup purposes.

In the treatment of abdominal and pelvic malignancies, such as neuroblastoma, Wilms' tumor, retroperitoneal sarcoma, and lymphoma, it is generally desirable to avoid bowel irradiation. A variety of techniques have been used to exclude bowel from the treatment field. A prone position, the use of a full bladder to displace bowel, and compression devices all have proponents. A polyurethane mold and reinforcing Styrofoam sheets can be used to construct a "belly board" to exclude bowel from the treatment field. The child is simulated prone, with small bowel contrast. The polyurethane mold is made so that the hips are slightly elevated to allow gravity to pull the mobile bowel out of the pelvis. A hole is cut in the center of the board so that the abdomen falls slightly into the opening. By this means, a lateral field can be constructed that may exclude bowel. If the simulation is conducted with small bowel contrast, the degree of bowel protection can be documented (21,34).

The Alpha Cradle has a density of 0.03 g/cm^3 (32). For ^{60}Co, 6-MV, and 18-MV photon beams, the presence of an Alpha Cradle increases the surface dosage. The magnitude of the increase is a function of the thickness of the transited cradle and the energy of the beam (27,35). The authors of this book have occasionally noticed an increase in skin reactions in skin irradiated through an Alpha Cradle. The Alpha Cradle should be kept as thin as possible without compromising patient positioning.

Polyurethane casts are expensive. Mixing and pouring the chemicals takes speed and dexterity. Gases are produced during foam production, and dust is generated if the cast is cut for modi-

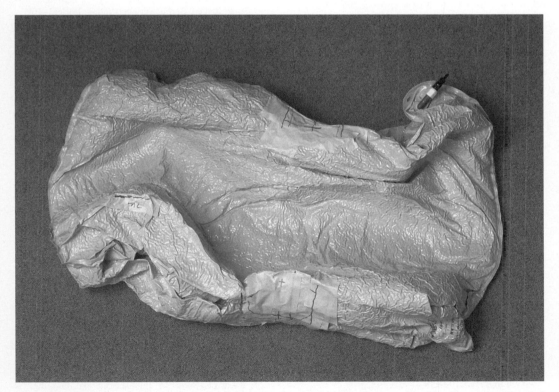

FIG. 22-9. This vacuum bag was created for the treatment of a 5-year-old girl with retroperitoneal embryonal rhabdomyosarcoma. The child was positioned in a right lateral decubitus position to allow small bowel to fall away from the treatment area. The mold held her in a stable and reproducible position each day. Treatment setup marks are drawn on tape on the device.

fication. Measures should be taken for fume exhaustion and chemical and dust containment (31). Although there are drawbacks, reproducible positioning is easily achieved with these cradles (11,36).

VACUUM BAGS

Many institutions use vacuum bags or pillows (e.g., VacFix, S&S Par Scientific, Inc., Brooklyn, NY). These systems consist of a bag filled with Styrofoam or plastic beads. The patient lies on the bag in the treatment position. Air is evacuated from the bag through a valve. This conforms the bag to the body. The shape is retained throughout the course of treatment.

A vacuum bag immobilizer can be created in a few minutes, it can be adjusted after forming, and it can be reused for several patients (Fig. 22-9). The surface dosage is higher for a beam passing through the bag. This could increase the skin reaction to radiation (35). Reproducibility of setup with the system is quite good (31).

REFERENCES

References particularly recommended for further reading are indicated by an asterisk.

1. Goldson AL, Young J Jr, Espinoza MC, et al. Simple but sophisticated immobilization casts. *Int J Radiat Oncol Biol Phys* 1978;4:1105–1106.
2. Williamson TJ. Improving the reproducibility of lateral portal placement. *Int J Radiat Oncol Biol Phys* 1979;5:407–409.
3. Hendrickson FR. Precision in radiation oncology. *Int J Radiat Oncol Biol Phys* 1982;8:311–312.
4. Van Arsdale ED, Greenlaw RH. Formalized immobilization and localization in radiotherapy. *Radiology* 1971;99:697–698.
5. Verhey LJ, Goitein M, McNulty P, et al. Precise positioning of patients for radiation therapy. *Int J Radiat Oncol Biol Phys* 1982;8:289–294.
6. Donaldson SS, Shastak CA, Samuels SI. Technical and practical considerations in the radiotherapy of children. *Front Radiat Ther Oncol* 1987;21:256–269.
7. Light KL. Immobilization and treatment of patients receiving radiation therapy for extremity soft-tissue sarcoma. *Med Dosim* 1992;17:135–139.
8. Bentel GC, Marks LB, Krishnamurthy R, et al. Comparison of two repositioning devices used during radiation therapy for Hodgkin's disease. *Int J Radiat Oncol Biol Phys* 1997;38(4):791–795.
*9. Bentel GC, Marks LB, Hendren K, et al. Comparison of two head and neck immobilization systems. *Int J Radiat Oncol Biol Phys* 1997;38(4):867–783.
10. Bentel GC, Marks LB, Krishnamurthy R. Impact of cradle immobilization on setup reproducibility during external beam radiation therapy for lung cancer. *Int J Radiat Oncol Biol Phys* 1997;38(3):527–531.
11. Kneebone A, Ggebski V, Hagendoorn N, et al. A randomized trial evaluating rigid immobilization for pelvic irradiation. *Int J Radiat Oncol Biol Phys* 2003;56:1105–1111.
12. Fiorino C, Reni M, Bolognesi A, et al. Set up error in supine position patients immobilized with two different modalities during conformal radiotherapy of prostate cancer. *Radiother Oncol* 1998;49:133–141.
13. Mitane C, Hoornaert MT, Dutreix A, et al. Radiotherapy of pelvic malignancies: impact of two types of rigid immobilization devices on localization errors. *Radiother Oncol* 1999;52:19–27.
14. Malone S, Szanto J, Perry G, et al. A prospective comparison of three systems of patient immobilization for prostate radiotherapy. *Int J Radiat Oncol Biol Phys* 2000;48:657–665.
15. Doppke KP. Treatment simulation organization. In: Write AE, Boyer AL, eds. *Advances in radiation therapy treatment planning.* New York: American Institute of Physics, 1983:131–137.
16. Watkins DMB. Patient positioning. In: *Radiation therapy mold technology: principles and design.* Toronto: Pergamon Press, 1981:7–18.
17. Pointon RCS, Studd D. Mould room practice. In: Pointon RCS, ed. *The radiotherapy of malignant disease,* 2nd ed. Berlin: Springer-Verlag, 1991:81–109.
18. Watkins DMB. The preparation of a larynx shell. In: *Radiation therapy mold technology: principles and design.* Toronto: Pergamon Press, 1981:19–32.
19. Watkins DMB. Appendix I: Technical considerations of some of the more commonly used impression, casting and molding materials. In: *Radiation therapy mold technology: principles and design.* Toronto: Pergamon Press, 1981:127–131.
20. Watkins DMB. Appendix II: photographs and constructional details of accessory equipment and positioning devices. In: *Radiation therapy mold technology: principles and design.* Toronto: Pergamon Press, 1981:132–137.
*21. Bentel GC. The treatment preparation process—I: target localization, treatment uncertainties, and patient immobilization. In: *Radiation therapy planning,* 2nd ed. New York: McGraw-Hill, 1996:162–218.
22. van der Geijn J, Harrington FS, Lichter AS, et al. Simplified bite block immobilization of the head. *Radiology* 1983;149:851.
23. Barish RJ, Lerch IA. Patient immobilization with a low-temperature splint/brace material. *Radiology* 1978;127:548.
24. Gerber RL, Marks JE, Purdy JA. The use of thermal plastics for immobilization of patients during radiotherapy. *Int J Radiat Oncol Biol Phys* 1982;8:1461–1462.
25. *Thermoplastic splinting material: Product information.* Chapel Hill, NC: M&N Consultants, Inc.
26. Product information. Wycoff, NJ: WFR/Aquaplast Co.
27. Klein EE, Purdy JA. Entrance and exit dose, regions for a Clinac-2100C. *Int J Radiat Oncol Biol Phys* 1993;27:429–435.
28. Sorensen NE, Sell A. Immobilization, compensation

and field shaping in megavolt therapy. *Acta Radiol Ther Phys Biol* 1972;11:129–134.

29. Mallion WE, White DR. Immobilization of the head in radiotherapy. *Br J Radiol* 1968;41:236.

30. Paterson R. *The treatment of malignant disease by radiotherapy.* London: Edward Arnold, 1963:150–166.

31. Jakosben A, Iversen P, Gadeberg C, et al. A new system for patient fixation in radiotherapy. *Radiother Oncol* 1987;8:145–151.

32. Devereux C, Grundy G, Littman P. Plastic molds for patient immobilization. *Int J Radiat Oncol Biol Phys* 1976;1:553–557.

33. Dickens CW. A machine for moulding thermoplastics. *Br J Radiol* 1960;33:64–65.

34. Shanahan TG, Menta MP, Bergelrud KL, et al. Minimization of small bowel volume within treatment fields utilizing customized "belly boards." *Int J Radiat Oncol Biol Phys* 1990;19:469–476.

35. Johnson MW, Griggs MA, Sharma SC. A comparison of surface doses for two immobilizing systems. *Med Dosim* 1995;20:191–194.

36. Gosselin M, Benk V, Charron F, et al. Postoperative radiotherapy for chondrosarcoma of the L1 vertebral body: a case report. *Med Dosim* 1994;19:217–222.

Index